MEDICAL PRACTICE AND THE COMMON MAN AND WOMAN: A HISTORY

A LIST OF COMMON PEOPLE

Jeanne d'Arc – daughter of a farmer
Astor – son of a butcher
Austin – daughter of a rector
Bach – son of a court musician
Beethoven – son of a singer for nobility
Bodin – son of a tailor
Boerhaave – son of a pastor
Botticelli – son of a tanner
Brahms – son of jobbing musician and a
    seamstress
Bunyan – son of a tinker
Cabot – son of spice merchant
Calvin – son of a notary and innkeeper's
    daughter
Cardano – son of a lawyer; illegitimate
Cervantes – son of a barber-surgeon
Columbus – son of a wool weaver
Comenius – impoverished
Copernicus – son of prosperous merchant
Da Vinci – son of notary and peasant
    woman, illegitimate
Dante – son of relatively low-standing
Davy – son of a woodcarver
Dee – son of a mercer
Diderot – son of a cutler
Donne – son of warden of ironmongers'
    Guild
Douglass – born in slavery
Drake – son of a farmer
Durer – son of a goldsmith
Einstein – son of partner in a featherbed
    company
Erasmus – son of a priest and his
    housekeeper, illegitimate
Faraday – son of a blacksmith's apprentice
Ferguson – son of a preacher
Fox – son of a weaver
Fulton – son of a farmer
Galileo – son of lute-player
Gauss – poor, working class
Gessner – son of a poor furrier
Goethe – son of prosperous parents
Goldsmith – son of assistant to parish priest
Gould – son of a farmer
Halley – son of a soap-maker
Harvey – son of a notary

Haydn – son of a wheelwright and a cook
Hegel – son of a secretary
Hobbes – son of uneducated village vicar
Hooke – son of a church curate
Jonson - son a bricklayer
Kant – son of a harness maker
Kepler – son of a mercenary
Kircher – little is known
Klaproth – son of a tailor
Knox – son of a merchant
Laud – son of a clothier
Linnaeus – son of a village curate
Locke – son of a legal clerk
Luther – mother "trading-class stock"
Marlowe – son of a shoemaker
Mendel – son of poor farmer
Mercator – son of a shoemaker
Mersenne – son of peasants
Michelangelo – son of a town administrator
Milton – son of a scrivener
Monteverdi – son of an apothecary
Mozart – son of violinist for nobility
Newton – son of a farmer
Ohm – son of a locksmith
Paine – son of tenant farmer
Petrarch – son of a notary
Pope – son of linen merchant
Priestley – son of a finisher of cloth
Pufendorf – son of a pastor
Rabelais – son of a lawyer
Rembrandt – son of a miller
Rousseau – son of a watchmaker
Scheele – son of a brewer
Servetus – son of a notary
Shakespeare – son of a glove-maker
Spenser – son of a journeyman clothmaker
Tesla – son of a priest
Truth – born in slavery
Van der Weyden – son of a knife
    manufacturer
Van Eyck - unknown
Van Leeuwenhoek – son of a basket-maker
Vanderbilt – son of a ferry boat owner
Villon – born in poverty
Voltaire – son of minor treasury official
Wollstonecraft – daughter of a drunk

This is a snippet from a list of common people, as estimated from the circumstances surrounding their birth and formative years. Primarily to extraneous factors is owed their renown, factors that permitted their aptitudes to surface. And it is the thesis of this book that comparable aptitudes are present in every person, but authoritarian social forces have, since the first societies, obstructed or perverted their appearance. Thus, the progress of mankind has been thwarted for thousands of years.

To Diana

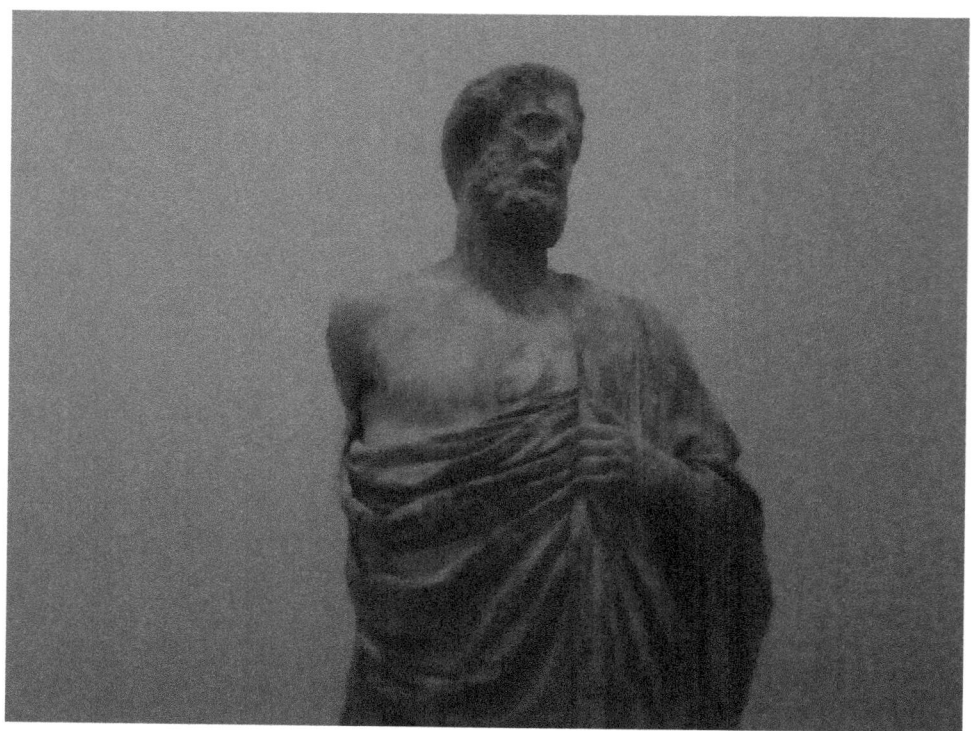

Ἱπποκράτης
Founder of the Medical Koinon

Hippocrates of Cos (460-380 BC), father of the medical koinon, the basis for the natural state of medical practice. This greater than life-size 4th C BC marble statue, thought to be Hippocrates as a representative Aesclepiad physician, was found in the Roman Odeon on Cos, purported island home of Hippocrates, and is now located in the Cos historical museum.

MEDICAL PRACTICE AND THE COMMON MAN AND WOMAN: A HISTORY

(Being an abridgment of *THE NATURAL STATE OF MEDICAL PRACTICE*)

ζήτειν αὐτῆς μὲν τὴν γένεσεν, ἢν δὲ δύνωμαι,
ἀποδιδοναι δὲ ἄνθρωπῳ τέχνην τὴν ἰατρικήν.

"To seek its origin and, if I can,
return the art of medicine to man."

Anonymous Fragment

by

William H. Adams, MD

XULON PRESS

Xulon Press
2301 Lucien Way #415
Maitland, FL 32751
407.339.4217
www.xulonpress.com

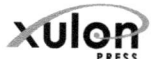

Paperback ISBN-13: 978-1-6312-9615-4
Hard Cover ISBN-13: 978-1-6312-9616-1
Ebook ISBN-13: 978-1-6312-9617-8

ARGUMENT

Doch uns ist gegeben
Auf keiner Statte zu ruh'n;
Es Schwinden, es fallen
Die leidenden Menschen
Blindlings von einer
Stunde zur andern,
Wie Wasser von Klippe
Zu Klippe geworfen
Jahrlang in's Ungewisse hinab.

[But man may not linger,
And nowhere finds he repose;
We stay not, but wander,
We grief-laden mortals,
Blindly, from one sad hour to another,
Like water from cliff unto cliff
Ever dropping, blindly
At last do we pass away.][1]

The Uncommon Man

Even the great Chesterton had it wrong, writing in an essay the following: "Progress has been merely the persecution of the Common Man."[2] As medical practice emerged from mankind's plebeian population and is used throughout this work as a marker of progress within a civilization, we must take exception with Chesterton's broad brush. Throughout his essay he considers the "uncommon" man, the victorious General, the famed scientist, the esteemed intellectual, the great political leader, and on and on, to be not the sources of beneficence to mankind, instead being partner to persecution of the Common Man. Amid many unassailably ingenious, truthful and thoughtful observations his deeper message unexpectedly falls flat on its face. The reason? An incorrect definition of the common man. Not that Chesterton defines him. Instead, he characterizes him: not well educated, not inclined to write a book, no particular interest in social movements, prone to spontaneous and genuine expression in song and speech sometimes accompanied by unappealing and embarrassing metaphors, not always admirable but always forgivable because all this is normal and because the Common Man loves his family more than notoriety.

Dictionaries tend to agree with Chesterton. Here are some of their definitions. Merriam-Webster: "the undistinguished commoner lacking class or rank distinction or special attributes." Thesaurus.com: "lowest common denominator," "average Joe."

---

[1] Final verse from the *Schicksalslied* (Song of Destiny), a poem by Friedrich Holderlin (1770-1843) set to music by Johannes Brahms (1833-1897). Translation of Rev. J. Troutbeck, D. D.

[2] Chesterton, G. K., *Persecuting the Common Man,* in *The American Mercury,* January 1936, pp. 67-71.

Cambridge Advanced Learner's Dictionary & Thesaurus: "the hoi polloi," "the man/woman in the street." The eminent historian, Hendrik Willem van Loon, went further and identified two classes of humans: *Homo agitans*, "those that do," and *Homo classificans*, "those who classify what the others have done." He estimated the latter to outnumber the former by a million to one![3]

Practitioners of medicine have always emerged from the common pool of humanity. In Part I of this work the evolution of medical practice is analyzed primarily in Western civilization. In Part II, however, while medical practice will remain prominent, generalized implications of conclusions from Part I are used as a guide to explore early attempts at human progress. It is an underlying principle of this book that every man and every woman is "uncommon," that unique skills, interests, aptitudes, and other qualities guarantee a species heterogeneity that is unique to *Homo sapiens*, a heterogeneity that exists for a reason. That reason will not be discussed herein, but its correctness has found comfortable lodging in medical practice from ancient Hippocratic physicians to physicians of the present day: every patient is unique and is to be treated as such. From this perspective, the common man becomes more like the literary "everyman," a person with his own story to tell but who is required to remain silent in the background. This volume is an inquiry into why he or she is, or has been, so required, an inquiry into what has led to the diminutive definitions of the Common Man and into what Chesterton identified as "the familiar routine of oppressing him [the Common Man] in practice and adoring him in theory."[4] The "uncommon" men that are the real object of Chesterton's disdain are, sadly, not uncommon enough, for he is referring to those persons who have, for whatever reason and through whatever means, willfully obtained power over the larger part of humanity, particularly that part which includes those unable to protect themselves from an authoritarian's gambit, a population that has had little or no access to education, little hope of improvement in their lot, and often not even a conception of what such improvement can mean, a population that can be so shielded from knowledge and influence that its personal interactions are limited to the narrow generational passage of unique and therefore sometimes distorted behavior, good and bad, in a way that makes them unable to see the difference, a population whose cognitive world has been so rationed that the idea of escaping it is inconceivable, a population of victims that has always been ripe for the rhetorician and politician.

Even if Chesterton's implied "uncommon man" were the superman as recognized by George Bernard Shaw in Cromwell, Napoleon, Julius Caesar, and Martin Luther, human society would still continue in its befuddled way unless the entire

---

[3] Van Loon, W. H., *Ancient and Medieval Civilizations*, in *Whither Mankind*, New York, 1930, Charles A. Beard, editor, p. 42.

[4] On this note reference is made to Aaron Copland's *Fanfare for the Common Man*, composed in support of Henry Wallace's 1942 "century of the common man" response to Henry Luce's "American Century." Wallace's eloquent cry was that of the internationalist with a plan to enforce equality upon the world. His rhetoric of freedom, therefore, was not a force for freedom of choice but freedom from want, for a face-off between his view of the common man who demanded his share of the wealth from the wealthy and powerful of any country, and a coercive redistribution of wealth if dialogue failed. Luce, in contrast, had based his American Century on the spread of individual liberty and resistance to authoritarian governments around the globe, whether totalitarian or communistic, with the goal of permitting the common man everywhere to include himself in the quest for opportunity rather than merely being someone else's means to it. The philosophical conflict between these opposing views runs throughout this book.

civilization were populated by similarly thinking superpersons.[5] In Shaw's view, therefore, the future was dismal indeed. But the "uncommon man" in this book should be, in contrast, the hope of the future. He is not only "everyone else" but he is also the potential source of beneficence in life for everyone. Rather than composed of millions of Cromwells and Napoleons who were to be in perfect agreement for their superman's dream to be fulfilled, heroes of the present work are the millions who disagree on almost everything but who have since the 18th C given Western civilization such a splendid start at making the future bright, and had they been permitted to materialize sooner many generations of our species would have been their beneficiaries.

Although authoritarianism, egalitarianism, natural law, spontaneous order and other charged terms will receive attention as the following chapters unfold, underneath it all is understood to be the story of "everyman," a chronicle of the effect of his suppression from the earliest times, sometimes by others, sometimes by himself. It may not be considered a very interesting chronicle in that it is more an accounting for what did not happen rather than what did happen, but the effects have been profound and are unceasing. And it is as a warning that this process may continue unabated forever that prompted the verse from the *Schicksalslied* that opened this narrative.

---

[5] See: Shaw, G. B., *Man and Superman*, first performed in 1905.

CONTENTS

LIST OF ILLUSTRATIONS

EXCURSI

DEFINITIONS

To avoid complex but nonetheless secondary sociological issues while describing the various civilizations to be deliberated in this work, the following basic definitions will be used. Some are simpler or more focused than dictionary or encyclopedia definitions, for scholarly articles offer a variety of definitions, sometimes conflicting, sometimes overlapping, for many of these terms. This listing reduces scholarly inferences considered irrelevant in present context.

1. Authoritarianism: Unconditional coercive social control at the expense of personal freedom.
2. City: A defined urban population held together by common enterprises.[6]
3. City-state: An autonomous or self-sufficient state consisting of a central city and its surrounding interdependent smaller settlements.
4. Civilization: An autonomous and self-sufficient urban and rural population sufficiently large to produce a surplus of food for trade that contributes to wealth and permits specialization of crafts and vocations.[7]
5. Corporatism: Central control of construction and production by special interest groups.
6. Culture: Learned social behavior.
7. Egalitarian: Archeologically defined, in whole or in part, as a society with no differential wealth in burials, dwellings, districts, or architecture, and no monumental structures, militarization or a distinct long-lived population.
8. Egalitarianism (social or coercive): A doctrine that would forcibly interfere with voluntary choice by imposing social or economic equality on a society.
9. Egalitarian kinship: A consanguineal and affinal group in which assigned status assists in implementation of opinions and traditions regarding redistribution of effort.
10. Empirical: "Originating in or based on observation or experience," and verifiable by observation (Merriam-Webster.com, not dated, Web. 27 May 2017).
11. Group: "A number of individuals having some unifying relationship."
12. Heterarchy: A multifocal system of management in a social system in which there is no permanent head.
13. Hierarchy: A fixed chain of command structure of constituents within a social system.
14. Individualism: Advocating or tolerating political and economic independence of the individual.

---

[6] By "defined" is meant a delineated space for a quantifiable population.

[7] This definition assumes that storage contributes to accumulation of wealth. It is a minimalist definition because the object of this volume is an analysis of the earliest stages of urbanization rather than urbanization in full flower. It differs from the definition used in the unabridged volume 1 of *The Natural State of Medical Practice: An Isagorial Theory of Human Progress* because a tiered governing hierarchy not specifically identified, but it is implied in the "settlement hierarchy" mentioned in later chapters. It is also somewhat at variance with that of Dr. B. G. Trigger (*Understanding Early Civilizations*, Cambridge, 2003, p. 46) who defined early civilizations as the "earliest and simplest form of *class-based* society." Social classes may have been a consequence of commercial success but not their cause or goal.

15. Kinship: A universal form of social organization based on real or alleged culturally defined family ties and rules of behavior.[8]
16. Koinon: An autonomous voluntary and democratic group sharing a common self-interest that meets in common council to freely exchange information and experience pertinent to all its members.
17. Network: Autonomous individuals or organizations that work together for a common goal.
18. Plebeian: A commoner.
19. Polity: An organized society not subject to the jurisdiction of a higher power.[9]
20. Profession: A livelihood that is a way of life and not bracketed by specified hours of employment.
21. Progress (noun): (1) For the group: a social concept based on the awareness of improvability of the human condition. (2) For the individual: a path toward a goal.
22. Rational: "Based on or in accordance with reason or logic," meaning that chance, coercion, rote, or mysticism play no role in a decision or judgment (Oxford English Dictionary).
23. Settlement hierarchy: The mechanism proposed as the natural way intergroup adjustments take place as an enlarging population center that has had no prior experience with a leadership hierarchy becomes more complex and must deal with new goods and services needed by the evolving society.
24. Socialism: "Any of various economic and political theories advocating collective or governmental ownership and administration of the means of production and distribution of goods." (Merriam-Webster.com. Merriam-Webster, not dated. Web. 19 Dec. 2018.)
25. Sodality: A non-kin social organization united around a specific purpose.
26. Society: "An enduring and cooperating social group whose members have developed organized patterns of relationships through interaction with one another."
27. Urban: Concerning a delimited populous area in relation to a non-populous rural area.

---

[8] The great value of the kinship is that it functions as a glue that holds somewhat disparate subgroups together. The structure of a kinship by itself may exert little authority if most authority resides within its constituent groups such as bands, clans, or tribes, for kinship is most prominently displayed in relations with non-kin. But what it does do is provide stability and credibility for the egalitarian groups under its umbrella, thus enhancing their powers of enforcement. The tighter the grip of kinship is on its members, the stronger is the hold on social norms.

[9] From: Piscitelli, M., *Pathway to Social Complexity in Norte Chico Region of Peru*, in *Feast, Famine or Fighting?: Multiple Pathways to Social Complexity*, https://doi,org/10.1007/978-3-319-48402-0_14, 2017, pp. 393-415.

PROLOGUE

ἔλεγχός εἰμ᾽ ἐγώ,
ὁ φίλος ᾽Αλεθείᾳ τε καὶ Παρρασίᾳ
Ἐλευθερίᾳ τε (συγγενέστατος) θεός,
μόνοισιν ἐχθρὸς τῶν βροτῶν τοῖς τὴν ἐμὴν
γλῶτταν δεδιόσι, πάντα τ᾽ εἰδὼς καὶ σαφῶς
διεξιὼν ὁπόσα σύνοιδ᾽ ὑμῖν (κακά,)
τὰ σῦκα σῦκα, τὴν σκάφην σκάφην λέγων.

"Confutation is my name, the friend of Truth and Frankness, and a deity close akin to Freedom, an enemy to those mortals only who fear my tongue, and one who both knows all things and makes clear all details, whatsoever evil of yours I know of. I call a fig a fig; a spade a spade."

Menander (342-290 BC)
Unidentified minor fragment 545K[10]

The primary objective of this book is to reveal the role of the common man and woman in the evolution of both the profession and progress of medicine and, by analogy and with supporting evidence, human progress in general. This was not its original intent, which was to identify features of earlier medical practices that might be useful in correcting the many deficiencies of modern medical practice.[11] It soon became apparent, however, that the overriding issues were social rather than medical. The present abridgement reflects that divergence of focus, beginning as it does with social influences affecting the maturation and progress of scientific medicine and only later analyzing those that prevent its initiation. But in this process the critical role of the common man and woman as the sole influence directing the progress of mankind was starkly revealed. Rather than invoking a "great man theory" with its heroic leaders, emperors, conquerers and exploiters of others as our source of beneficence, it is argued that it is to the mass of humankind, our plebeian ancestors, that such beneficence can be traced. For once released from under the authoritarian thumb the broadly distributed genius that resides in the variation of our species will promptly be made available as the times require. The constitutional freedoms of the West, by unleashing the natural and manifold genius of the common man and woman, are the source of our present unprecedented global healthful prosperity, its tardy appearance in human history the consequence of authoritarianism in its various guises.

Using medicine as a valid and objective gauge of human betterment, a point that will be justified later, we begin the analysis with a search for the natural state of medical practice, defined as effective medical knowledge effectively applied free from institutional influences. Hippocrates wrote that medicine comprises the patient, the

---

[10] *Menander: The Principal Fragments*, London, 1921, p. 489, translation of F. B. Allinson.
[11] This is explained in the unabridged three-volume work, *The Natural State of Medical Practice*, as released by Liberty Hill Publishing in July 2019, the individual titles being:
Vol. 1 - *The Natural State of Medical Practice: An Isagorial Theory of Human Progress*
Vol. 2 - *The Natural State of Medical Practice: Hippocratic Evidence*
Vol. 3 - *The Natural State of Medical Practice: Escape from Egalitarianism*

practitioner, and the disease, a reduction that bears no trifling.[12] A medical practice, on the other hand, comprises the patient, the practitioner,[13] and the practice environment, physical and social, and it is the latter that has played havoc with our profession over the ages.[14] Medical practices in some form have existed since mankind's first societies. Any inquiry, then, into the natural state of medical practice might seem impossible, for varieties of medical practice will be as boundless as man's societies, each having its own succession of unique interactions between the sick and those who they consult to get well. It would seem as reasonable and as useful to attempt to identify the archetypal medical practice from the lot as to fabricate one from fragments of them all, the latter being an eminently bureaucratic approach but hardly a sensible one.

But what is intended here is a historical search not just for an archetypal medical practice but for one that approaches the natural state. It is a state that implies that there is a sufficient quality, quantity and complexity of medical knowledge that a specialist is required for its proper use. It does not imply a practice free from social influences to which both physician and patient are equally exposed and susceptible. There is today much medical knowledge effectively applied. Why probe more primitive practices even if they be pristine? Is there something singular about the "natural" state that would justify the effort, something of value now or in the future? The answer is, the search for an ideal state, whether by a Plato or St. Augustine or Rousseau or Marx, is at the heart of some of mankind's most contentious thoughts in any age.[15] The "ideal state" is derived from someone's theoretical consideration of what should be best. But the "natural state" is one that works, however imperfectly, and conflict, sometimes violent, between idealism and realism is as menacing today as it has ever been. In the profession of medicine a practical question is whether some ideal state or the natural state should be its operational` goal. A better understanding of the natural state of medical practice is the second goal of this book, and it is implicit that the professional medical practitioner, rather than the dispenser of nostrums, is its focus.

A third aspect to the inquiry concerns classical education. Socrates argued, in Plato's *Gorgias* (sections 463-465), that rhetoric was ignoble (αἰσχρον), an irrational practice (ἄλογον πρᾶγμα), a bogus form of justice, and merely a variant of flattery (κολακείαν). Isocrates (436-338 BC), a rhetorician himself, is said to have commented that "Rhetoric is the art of making small things great and great things small."[16] Ignoring its noble critics, however, rhetoric has retained its full force, becoming far more potent,

---

[12] "The profession has three components: the disease, the patient, and the physician." ἡ τέχνη διὰ τριῶν, τό νόσημα καὶ ὁ νοσέων καὶ ὁ ἰατρός. (Translation by the author, as are all other Greek translations unless stated otherwise.) From *Epidemics* I, the Second Constitution, section 12, as found in volume 1 of the *Loeb Classical Library* series on *Hippocrates*.

[13] A practitioner according to Webster's 4th Collegiate Dictionary is a worker, "someone who does something." Here, of course, is meant a specified worker to whom the sick have recourse.

[14] Throughout this book the occasional use of the 1st person is justified insofar as the author has translated some of the citations from Greek, Latin, and German and holds an active professional license as a physician.

[15] W.H.S. Jones, in his Introduction to *Ancient Medicine* (*Loeb Classical Series, Hippocrates*, vol. 1) dramatically states the attraction for Plato: "The philosophical fervor which longed with passionate desire for unchangeable reality, that felt a lofty contempt for the material world with its ever-shifting phenomena, that aspired to rise to a heavenly region where changeless Ideas might be apprehended by pure intelligence purged from every bodily taint ...."

[16] ῥητορική τὰ μὲν μικρὰ μεγάλα τὰ δὲ μεγάλα μικρὰ ποιεῖν. Cited by Plutarch in his *Life of Isocrates* from his (Plutarch's) famous work, *Parallel Lives*.

if less proficient, with modern communications technology.[17] The public of today is faced with competing rhetoric containing so much information that it is easy to be caught up in the trivial or irrelevant or deceptive, whether literary or scientific. It would be wise to protect the younger generation from this assault by rhetoric until a basic classical education, including instruction on rhetoric itself, has been completed, thereby permitting intelligent selection of items for subsequent pursuit. Information is no substitute for knowledge, or, as Heracleitus (6th-5th C BC) said, and said better:

> πολυμαθίη νόον ἔχειν οὐ διδάσκει·
> "Much learning does not teach [good] sense; ..."
>   Heracleitus, *On the Universe*, XVI[18]

This is an essential task because new informational technologies can promote with increasing efficiency a distorted picture of man and his agencies, one being the practice of medicine. This book, therefore, is liberally provided with quotations from the past to demonstrate how ancient Western thinkers were at least the intellectual equal of their remote descendants, and that the great social issue of today is, in fact, well-worn, unchanged except in scale after thousands of years.[19]

---

[17] It may be at times the bane of democracy, but without rhetoric to galvanize an informed people there is a risk that neutral and unimpassioned logic will do worse and permit "evil" rhetoric, *i.e.*, rhetoric targeting the uninformed, to displace it. Thus was such great value placed on rhetorical skills in ancient forums. See R. Weaver's *The Ethics of Rhetoric*, Chicago, 1968, chapter one, and περὶ ὕψους (*On the Divine*) by Pseudo-Longinus (see p. 340 of the present work for information on Pseudo-Longinus). Plato decried rhetoric because, preferring the expert, he denied the wisdom of any appeal to the people. Aristotle on the other hand stated, "Those speaking the truth and doing so justly have an obligation to be persuasive." (*Rhetoric*, 1355 a21*ff.*)

[18] Taken from the *Loeb Classical Library*, *Hippocrates*, vol. 4, p. 476, translation of W. H. S. Jones. Heracleitus was ridiculing the sophism of Hesiod, Pythagoras, Xenophanes, and Hecataeus.

[19] Many of the citations herein are presented both in their original language and in translation, for naivete regarding the arbitrary nature of translation is a threat to attempts at an objective understanding of the historical past. It is important that the original text be readily at hand for those who wish to determine if another person's interpretation is sound. For example, biblical linguistics thrives, and healthily, because so many readers are determined not to be misled by the translator with a point of view. Finally, it should be useful to have, in one place, a broad spectrum of ancient thought in its original language that bears on the topic of the moment, for to locate a selection of learned statements secreted away in books of every description, even from a single library, is a daunting task that should not have to be shouldered anew by every interested party. Nevertheless, for the sake of brevity in this abridgement the longer citations have been deleted, but they are available in the unabridged volumes. For a succinct statement on the importance of exposure to classical texts see: Lord Hewart of Bury, *The Classics*, Manchester, 1926. Lord Hewart was Lord Chief Justice of England. In conclusion: (1) references in the footnotes are numerous, extensive, and usually include page numbers of the citations, for the author intends that the reader understand that his opinions and interpretations in this work are not the consequence of an overactive imagination, but have been contemplated by many prominent thinkers in the distant and recent past. The duplication of some references is for the convenience of the reader, for the number of the issues discussed may lead to selective reading of subjects by chapter, and a reference used in several chapters should not require a series of searches for the initial citation. (2) Many items referenced herein are from old editions of works rather than modern versions. One value of early editions of the classics is that, by seeing in ancient printings a subject of current importance being discussed by intellectuals from that distant age without modern glosses, a better comprehension of the

The final point of this work, and one that will be unequivocally established in the pages to follow, is a rebuttal of the following sentiment, as expressed by the eminent physiologist, Sir Michael Foster (1836-1907):

> "For indeed it is one of the lessons of the history
> of science that each age steps on the shoulders of
> the ages which have gone before. The value of
> each age is not its own, but is in part, in large part,
> a debt to its forerunners."

With regard to the field of medicine such humility will be shown to have been misplaced.

---

historicity of issues may be apparent. Since the inception of this book the Internet has become a practical source of early editions of printed works.

PART I – HISTORICAL ANALYSIS

INTRODUCTION

A. The Problem

In Western medicine the critical reaction in that cascade of events that flows from the hint of illness to, hopefully, recovery of health has traditionally involved two persons only, the physician and patient. Their interaction is an eminently human one, an inevitably emotional groping for a rational solution to an existential threat. To plot the clinical course amid a struggle for objectivity is the physician's daily task. And it is in the physician's office, amid the modern pressures of unrealistic promises and hopes of storybook endings, that perverse or deviant events in the practice of medicine will first declare themselves. And so they have, for the authoritarian is on the move and an evolutionary yet venerable medical tradition is being breached. That is the problem.

But the continual turmoil of human events, with its unpredictable dispersion of advantages and disadvantages, provides little opportunity for baseline measurements by which we may gauge our progress and identify the causes of success or failure. This opportunity is diminished further by a finite earthly existence during which cumulative experience is seen through a myopic lens: each generation feels justified, even compelled, to reinvent the wheel and considers itself especially favored by new ideas to forego the old ones.

To see whether the medical profession in its mission is now following some unnatural course or merely an alternative pathway, it is necessary to explore the practice of medicine in the days before technology, religious institutions, and government sank their talons of commercial, philosophical, and bureaucratic disinterest into that fragile pair. After all, we would not wish our descendants to view the consequences of the present structure and function of medicine with the pathetic eye with which we must view most of the profession's history. In the pages to follow it will be shown that many of the advances in medicine now enjoyed, and which have blossomed so in the last one hundred fifty years, were arbitrarily denied to mankind for many centuries, indeed millennia. It is time to restrain our pride in modern medical achievements. We are, after all, neither wiser nor kinder than our predecessors, nor should those in medicine presume that matters are now well in hand or that we have closed Pandora's box. Let us instead inquire as to why it took so long to get where we are today. In history books are found few reminders of that delay, which is facilely attributed to ignorance of the time. Ignorance it may have been, but not ignorance by chance. Someone or something is to blame.

B. The Participants

In Western society the generic term "doctor," in Latin a "teacher,"[20] is applied to those who have attained a high level of educational achievement in any of a broad range of endeavors. It is also applied to some with technical expertise but little relevant intellectual certification. Thus, physicians and many nonphysicians share a sobriquet of little specificity. The present enquiry concerns physicians only, and thus they will be called.[21]

---

[20] "Docere," to teach; "doctor, doctorus," *m.*, teacher.

[21] This includes dentists, if they will have it so, for all aspects of a practicing dentist's work find

But further delimiters are needed, and the essential one is that the physician be a clinician directly involved in patient care. Just as a young man becomes a fireman to save, through personal skill and bravery, people from fires, the primary desire for entry into medicine should be to help and, if possible, to heal, through personal contact, the sick. Career practices of non-clinical physicians are not addressed here. They include:

1) Research physicians: Clinical research should comprise all clinicians inasmuch as it is a professional responsibility to make useful clinical observations available to present and future colleagues so that better ways of doing things can benefit patients. Present purposes, however, are not relevant to the physician researcher whose personal career goal is one of research rather than clinical care or who considers the time commitment to clinical care subordinate to that research, although this in no way minimizes the value of basic research to benefit the sick.

2) Administrative physicians: Administrative medicine of all kinds, whether it be government or corporate, hospital- or clinic-based, is not included in this discussion. Institutional concerns are in no way analogous to health concerns of the individual. At the end of a working day the cares brought home by a clinician are of a different kind and magnitude from those of the administrator.

3) Wellness physicians: (a) Nutritional advice, including recommendations for a healthful diet, can be provided by non-clinicians. Plato has Socrates declare that the prescribing of medicines is a serious matter to be entrusted only to a true physician; nonphysicians, however, were the appropriate purveyors of advice on life-style.[22] (b) The allaying, in the healthy, of concerns over ill-health, the promotion of healthful living, and the avoidance of threats to good health can do without a clinician's involvement, in part because many such practices change from year to year and reflect regional social as well as medical trends. (c) Likewise, many health maintenance procedures do not require a clinician, for these are much regulated, or channeled, by regulatory institutions and greatly susceptible to social, economic, or sectarian pressures.[23] (d) Then there are practices, such as cosmetic surgery, that are clinical but which sometimes cater to certain patients who may not be ill but who seek advice or correction concerning an undesirable peculiarity that is not a

---

their equivalents among traditional physician attributes. There is even a court opinion that confirms this interpretation (see *Dental Brief*, Vol. 4, #10, Oct., 1899), ruling that dentistry is a specialized branch of the profession of the physician, a decision that does not diminish the profession of dentistry but rather enhances the profession of medicine. To which everyone must heartily agree, if for no other reason two of three practitioners vying for the honor of inventing practical gaseous anesthesia, Dr. William Morton and Dr. Horace Wells, were dentists.

[22] "..And while an inferior doctor is adequate for people who are willing to follow a regimen [a prescribed lifestyle] and don't need drugs, when drugs are needed, we know that a bolder doctor is required." Plato, *The Republic*, 459, c, translation of G. M. A. Grube, in *Plato, Complete Works*, J. M. Cooper, editor, Indianapolis, 1997.

[23] A standard feature of regulative institutional medicine is to force, however subtly, contemporary virtuous lifestyle changes, often with an eye to economy or promotion of a product or point of view. Yet a basic tenet taught for many years to the young physician is to not be judgmental about a patient's lifestyle, although specific items known to be harmful such as cigarette smoking are routinely discussed in the doctor's office. H. L. Mencken felt that those offering advice on healthful living debased their theories of the healthful life when they implied it would also be virtuous, for "The aim of medicine is surely not to make men virtuous; it is to safeguard and rescue them from the consequences of their vices. The true physician does not preach repentance; he offers absolution." (Mencken, H. L., *Types of Men*, [5] The Physician, in *Selected Prejudices*, London, 1926, p. 123.)

disease. Modern medicine has provided the techniques and modern economics the wealth for people to avail themselves of medical luxuries. Encompassing a risk-benefit in which the anticipated benefit is not derived from improved health places the physician and patient in a nontraditional relationship that will not benefit from this analysis. (e) Some patients seek to improve on health and request a physician's assistance to exaggerate, heighten, or prolong normal physiologic processes or sensations. Practices catering to such desires are not the domain of this book, for, while the science of medicine inevitably encompasses the healthy, the art of medicine exists only for the sick. Focus is henceforth on the clinician.

With so many physicians and their practices being considered irrelevant to this inquiry one may ask whether the inquiry itself has been made irrelevant. It will be maintained further on that it is in part the diversion of many in the medical profession away from care for the sick that has to a great extent diluted its effectiveness, brought down upon its membership much dissatisfaction from the community, and stifled its practice by inviting much regulation by society. There is instruction to be gained from the limitations imposed by Aristotle's uncomplicated definition of therapeutics: "the end of the science of medicine is health."[24] For society now sees physicians accommodating practices and expounding on matters outside their traditional arena of curing or palliating illness, often on matters in which nonphysicians may personally consider themselves expert.[25] Disillusion with the physician's effort is assured, and he who might have been considered the good doctor can no longer be distinguished from the bad one or the merely nice one.

Extension of the physician's influence outside of medicine is not a new phenomenon. The great Rudolph Virchow (1821-1902), the father of the field of cellular pathology, wrote, in 1849:

> "In reality, if medicine is the science of the healthy as well as of the ill human being (which is what it ought to be), what other science is better suited to propose laws as the basis of the social structure, in order to make effective those which are inherent in man himself. Once medicine is established as anthropology, and once the interests of the privileged no longer determine the course of public events, the physiologist and the practitioner will be counted among the elder statesmen who support the social structure. Medicine is a social science in its very bone and marrow,... ."[26]

Every man would be king![27] The hubris of those who would interpose the physician as

---

[24] a: ἰατρικῆς μὲν γὰρ ὑγίεια; I, i, 3; this is the H. Rackham translation to be found in the *Loeb Classical Library* series on Aristotle, vol. 19, *Nicomachean Ethics.*)

[25] The problem of "spilling over" of medical authority beyond its clinical boundaries is discussed by Paul Starr in *The Social Transformation of American Medicine*, New York, 1982. He views the profession's excessive privileges to be a consequence of economic and political, rather than professional, motivation. See also: Kass, L. R., *Towards a More Natural Science*, New York, 1985, p. 177, in which is discussed "a clear need to articulate and delimit the physician's domain and responsibilities," although in contrast to the present work Kass seems to feel the implications for implementation imply governmental rather than intrinsic professional policies.

[26] Virchow, R., *Scientific Method and Therapeutic Standpoints*, as translated by L. J. Rather in *Disease, Life, and Man*, Collier, New York, 1962, p. 80.

[27] Virchow expressed exuberant naivety and an exalted view of personal merit. But even the eminent Dr. Iago Galdston (1895-1989), psychiatrist and educator, echoed him in 1940: "The physician is conscious of his altered role. Till some thirty years ago it was the physician's job to cure and prevent disease. Now his job includes the production of health, mental as well as physical. He has become

legislator, adjudicator, or executor of government business just because he is a physician evokes Plato's philosopher king in Book 6 of *The Republic*, absurd, or perhaps whimsical, in formulation and treacherous in implementation. That is hubris in the extreme, and it is to the credit of the physicians in the United States that they have always been identified with the common man, rather than as nobility, church, or state functionaries.

The definition of "patient" is far simpler than that of "physician," namely, "a person receiving care or treatment, especially from a doctor."[28] The creation of a "patient" is instantaneous upon his meeting a physician, and the patient's potential spectrum of sickness extends from no sickness at all to imminent death.

The physician has a role even after death, for many of medicine's most basic truths derive from the work of Pathologists, those physicians, usually unseen by the public, who can expect no gratitude from patients or patients' families but to whom we all are so indebted.[29] It was the famous Morgagni (1682-1771), whose clinicopathological correlations were the basis for modern understanding of mechanisms of disease, who is credited with the motto found in many autopsy rooms around the world:[30]

> *Hic locus est ubi more vitae gaudet succurrere.*
> "This is the place where death delights to help the living."

C. The Solution ·

In approaching the solution one must understand the sequence of events that has made a solution necessary. Two pertinent questions can be raised. The first is, how did we get as far as we have? The second is, why did we not reach this point much sooner? The answer to the first is explained in Part I of this volume by exploring the natural state of medical practice. The answer to the second question is confronted in Part II.

---

social architect of the future, one who will have to co-operate with, and at times instruct or oppose the nursemaid, the schoolteacher, the business man and industrial expert, the journalist and the publisher, the film producer, the architect, the politician, and the parson, not to mention the raw materials - the people in their homes." (Galdston, I., *Progress in Medicine*, New York, 1940, p. 346.) Early in the 20th C the Chinese philosopher, K'ang Yu-Wei, stated, in his description of the utopian One-World he so desired, "Supreme at this time is the science of medicine... The power of the medical people being so great, it is necessary that we be watchful for the rise of some medical Napoleon, who might gather together a great following, and become a world ruler." At least this other-worldly philosopher, the darling of Mao Tse-Tung, recognized the dangers to the State of a medical man out of his element. See: Thompson, L. G., *Ta T'ung Shu, The One-World Philosophy of K'ang Yu-Wei*, London, 1958, p. 41, but note other eccentricities of K'ang Yu-Wei in the excursus on p. 281 of the present work.

[28] Webster's 4th Collegiate Dictionary.

[29] Many fields have opened for the Pathologist, whose subspecialties now include surgical pathology, autopsy pathology, forensic pathology, hematopathology, immunopathology, histopathology, and clinical pathology.

[30] Giovanni Battista Morgagni (1682-1771) at the age of eighty published his *De Sedibus et Causis Morborum per Anatomen Indagatus* (Venice, 1761), a classic in medical literature that correlated, in individual cases, careful autopsy findings with clinical signs and symptoms. A professor at the medical school in Padua for sixty years during which he collected voluminous data for his book, his comprehensive methodology and inductive conclusions formed the basis for all subsequent studies of anatomic pathology.

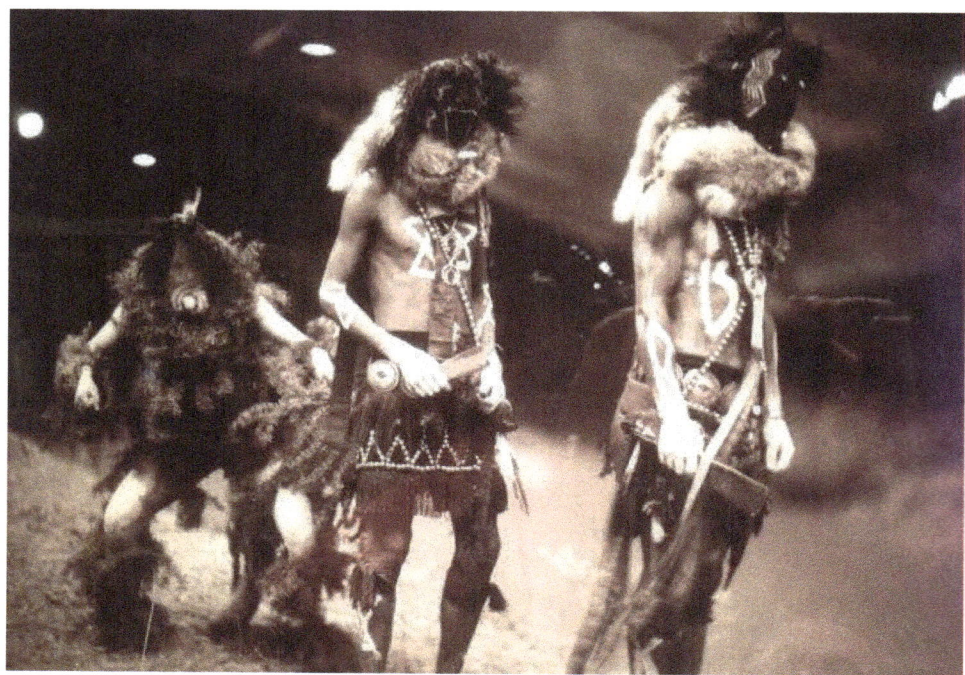

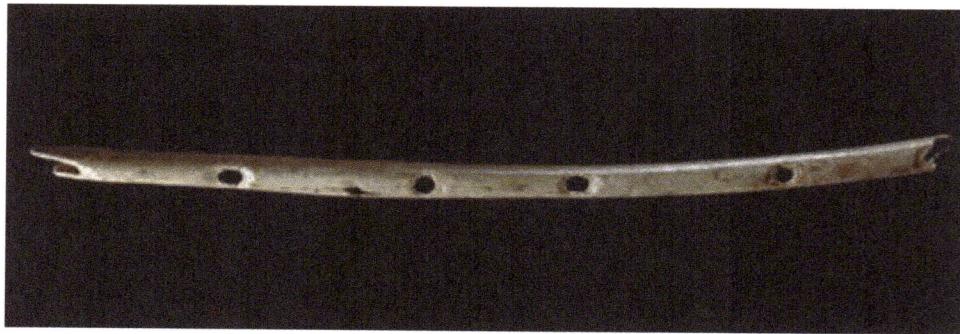

Fig. 1: Top - Photograph of Navajo Yeibichai dancers taken in 1900 by Edward S. Curtis, from the collection of the Wellcome Museum, London. Three "medicine-men" offered chants over several days to help a sick tribal member who initially is placed on a heated surface to induce sweating, and on the ninth and final day the Yeibichae dance, a curative ceremony for this very spiritual people, is performed. From the archives of the Wellcome Museum, London, as photographed by the author. Bottom - Carved bone flute from *ca.* 42,000 BC. The instrument may have been designed to play a pentatonic scale, which implies it was used for both group and solo performance. Lying near this flute was a female figurine and material used in cave painting. A fragment of a carved ivory flute of similar age was found in the same region in 2004: *Archaeologisches Korrespondenzblatt*, 34:447-462, 2004. A total of eight flutes have been found to date, suggesting music was a facet of normal human activity at that time. Photo credit: H. Jensen, Univ. of Tubingen, license of Wikimedia Creative Commons.

CHAPTER ONE

UNSTRUCTURED AND EARLY STRUCTURED SOCIETIES

"Recognition of facts and honest deductions are not natural to the human mind. The primitive instincts are for emotion and loose imaginings."

Howard W. Haggard, MD[1] (1891-1959)

The primitive forebear of the modern physician is thought by some to be the medicine-man or shaman. This is incorrect. The method of the medicine-man was devoted to controlling others, not disease. The medicine-man is the forebear of the psychic and the huckster. Empirical medicine finds its roots, instead, in the anxious observations of practical individuals in family units or tribes who sought, without official sanction, remedies for pain and disease for themselves and their families and neighbors.

A. Introduction: A Search for the Natural State of Medical Practice

In what time or place can an unglossed picture of the natural state of medical practice be obtained? There are three great forces that have influenced the course and practice of medicine: commercial, numinous, and political. The first has become particularly important as a consequence of technological advances of the last century. It follows that the age of a natural state of medical practice, implicitly pristine at its origin, may be old, perhaps ancient, for it must predate, or else have been isolated from, technologically advanced societies. As for the second, influence manifested through great religious institutions can so thoroughly permeate the mores and customs of societies that, assisted by appeal to the mystical, they can achieve the credence of legal authority. Independence from the latter is necessary. Lastly, the political nature of the society must be one that sought not to restrict, or was unable to restrict, individual initiative, thereby leaving both physicians and patients the freedom to search out each other's opinions and tolerances and to interact on a mutually agreed upon level. There are precious few lacunae in the story of mankind where these conditions have been met, even in part. The search begins in the most remote ages or places among primitive peoples.

B. Unstructured Societies

By "unstructured society" is meant a society that has not developed categories of workers or a premeditated social organization. It is a society that is organizationally paleolithic. Individual members carry out similar tasks, those being whatever is necessary for survival and daily living. The unstructured society is a most primitive one, whether Stone Age or contemporary, isolated from progress by time or geography. Dr. C. M. Bowra, in comparing several primitive societies, notes they are all

---

[1] Haggard, H. W., *Devils, Drugs, and Doctors: The Story of the Science of Healing from Medicine Men to Doctor*, London, 1913, p. 395.

hunter-gatherers whose fundamental social unit is the family.[2] They are, in general, nomadic, and, except for the dog, have no domesticated animals. They have little time for nonessential activities. In every society there is a natural receptiveness for discovery of the empirically useful. But the ability to initiate designs of the intellect in unstructured society is severely constrained by environmental necessity.

Constrained though the human intellect may be in primitive society, it is not absent. And there has yet to be presented any sustainable evidence to support the notion of inferior intellectual potential in primitive humans, just as there is no evidence of intellectual superiority of any particular racial or ethnic group. In the most telling of intellectual abilities, language, many primitive societies will have vocabularies numbering in the tens of thousands of words.[3] In one society there may be twenty different words describing maturational states of the coconut, whereas in another there may be twenty words describing developmental stages of the deer or other object of great local importance.[4] Dr. Samuel Kramer has stated that the ancient Sumerians (*ca.* 3000 BC) had some two hundred terms for "types and varieties" of sheep.[5] Among North American Indians the anthropologist Peter Farb cites several tribes with languages comprising approximately 25,000 words, a count that he thinks probably is an underestimate. The Roman's dictionary had no more than that number, although the ancient Greeks had two or three times as many. Furthermore, in all societies grammatical complexities seem commensurate with verbal.[6] There is, in addition, the discovery of inspired musical instruments and art forms produced by prehistoric people, such as a recently described flute carved from bone 42,000 years ago (Fig. 1) and an associated ivory "Venus" figurine. The flute, with five holes, is said to play a pentatonic scale, and if this were a purposeful design some suggest that the flute was used for group, rather than just solo, performance. All this is by way of stating that there is no reason, from

---

[2] Bowra, C.M., *Primitive Song*, Cleveland, 1962, chapter 1.

[3] Farb, Peter, *Man's Rise To Civilization*, New York, 1968, p. 231.

[4] Using this beautiful malleability of language, for example, Alexander `Scriabin selected from a repertoire of more than forty-five adjectives just to characterize the stylistic touch needed for playing his piano music, for example, and in translation, "crystalline," "limpid," "pearled."

[5] Kramer, S. N., *The Sumerians*, Chicago, 1963, p. 110.

[6] Estimating the number of words in a particular language is not simply a matter of counting dictionary entries, even if there happens to be a dictionary, which is often not the case. Significant variations in meaning of word roots come from prefixes, suffixes, inflections, and word admixtures that make up the great majority of words, a complexity common to all languages. Furthermore, since language exists because it is a social tool, growth in size and complexity of a language is profoundly influenced by its society's size and longevity, and its mechanism of growth from a basic vocabulary of 500 words has been analyzed by Robin Allott, a prominent scholar on the origin of languages. R. Goulden, P. Nation, and J. Read (*How Large Can A Receptive Dictionary Be?* in *Applied Linguistics*, 11:341-363, 1990) analyzed the vocabulary of Webster's *Third International Dictionary* (1961), the largest non-historical dictionary of English at the time it was published. Excluding compound or archaic words, abbreviations, proper names, alternative spellings and dialect forms, and when words were grouped according to word family consisting of a base word and derivative forms, this dictionary was found to have a vocabulary of around 58,000 word families (base words). Words and word families, of course, do not address the role of sentence structure, including length, as a determinant of complexity. The Chinese language in recent years has 50,000 or more characters and several times that number of words (made up for the most part of one to three characters), but the grammar, as spoken, includes no gender, number, tense, or voice and has few articles, and syntax clarifies meaning. In contrast, the early oracle script of the Shang Dynasty, *ca.* 1200 BC, had perhaps 5000.

available information, to assume innate intellectual superiority of individuals in any one society over another, whether separated by time or space, whether primitive or complex.[7]

The unstructured society is of interest because the absence of a ruling hierarchy would seem to offer a level of fairness and individual freedom that members of structured societies might envy. But, while individual freedom might exist in modern minds as a precious commodity applicable to all mankind, in practice the primitives have little time to take advantage of it, for their daily adversary is circumstance as well as the bully.[8] Therefore, in unstructured societies, where medical care is the province of the individual or perhaps a specified family member, there is no opportunity for a natural state of medical practice, the patient and practitioner often being one and the same. But such a simple arrangement was to be replaced as communities were established, for, as Dr. Bowra concluded, primitive societies universally believe in a supreme deity, and man's manipulation of this fact of life complicated much that followed.

C. Structured Societies: Tribal

The social organization that supercedes in complexity the immediate family or band is the tribe.[9] It is a grouping of bands, but one in which there exists extensions of family or kinships. This association creates social and political bonds among member families. In a tribal association law in the form of customs is dispensed by tribal leaders. Individuals have multiple responsibilities, some to themselves, some to the tribe. Latitude for individual expression is now limited not only by exigencies of nature but also by custom and custom's interpreters. As needed, specialists come forward to provide assistance in decision-making. These specialists render an elite service in that some are judged to have unique knowledge which they alone can use to interact with mystical forces emanating from objects or deities, thereby harnessing them for their own purposes. Since all primitive societies believe in some form of deity, in most of these societies can be found the sorcerer, who Sir James Frazer thinks is the natural progenitor of the medicine-man. And yet, while he may sometimes deal with illness in an empirical way, the medicine-man is, in fact, but a sorcerer. Often he is thought able to appear in different animal forms. In Borneo he conjures souls into a coconut for safe keeping, in Brazil he blesses the maize, in Africa he is the rain-maker, in North America Catlin described him as conducting religious ceremonies and acting as an oracle, and in Canada he bottles up souls in hollow bones. Abundant examples collected by Frazer bedeck antiquity and equate the two functions: ". . . magicians or medicine-men appear to constitute the oldest artificial or professional class in the evolution of society. For sorcerers are found in every

---

[7] The Sapir-Whorf hypothesis of the mid-twentieth century addresses the relation between language and thought. If proven to be true, it may modify this statement somewhat, for it states that language reflects, and affects, a people's worldview. Concepts in one language may not be comprehensible in another, and thereby reasoning and judgment may differ. In this sense one language might, in certain settings, provide a survival advantage over another. But the hypothesis does not imply intellectual inequality, and, of course, it is but a hypothesis.

[8] This simplistic statement receives much attention in Part II of this work.

[9] For an anthropologist's detailed view of social organization, incuding band and tribe, see, for example, E. R. Service, *Primitive Social Organization, an Evolutionary Perspective*, New York, 1962.

savage tribe known to us: [*sic*]."[10] Thus, the sorcerer and medicine-man have a common origin and serve a common purpose through common means. If there is any difference between them it is that the latter tends to be identified with larger societies having the luxury of greater specialization. See Fig. 1 (top) for medicine-men in action.

Medicine-men deal with or appear to induce life-or-death situations, often by trying to direct the progress of the soul. Both Sir James Frazer and Joseph Campbell have filled volumes with anecdotes of this sort of activity collected from around the globe. [11] Some are amusing but most are grotesque and pathetic, a continual reminder of what the human mind is capable of believing, a fact not to be lost sight of in the modern age. But the essential point is that there is not the faintest professional connection between the product of a tribe's medicine-man, a puffed-up sorcerer, and whatever empirical medicine was being pursued simultaneously by individual tribal members. If a medicine-man were called in to see a very ill person, his value lay not in empirical surgical or medical treatments. Instead, his role was to face and manipulate demons. For example, here is the definition of a medicine-man, as gathered from an array of scholarly studies of 19th C Native American tribes: [12]

> "Among American Indians the professions of medicine and religion are inseparable. The doctor is always a priest and the priest is always a doctor. Hence, to the whites in the Indian country the Indian priest-doctor has come to be known as the 'medicine man' and anything sacred, mysterious, or of wonderful power or efficacy in Indian life or belief is designated as 'medicine,' this term being the nearest equivalent of the aboriginal expression in the various languages. To 'make medicine' is to perform some sacred ceremony, from the curing of a sick child to the consecration of the sun-dance lodge. Among the prairie tribes the great annual tribal ceremony was commonly known as the 'medicine dance,' and the special guardian deity of every warrior was spoken of as his 'medicine.'"

Even if medicine-men, as specialists, were to be considered medical professionals, what would have been the nature of their medical practice? If the practitioners of this form of medicine can, for illustrative purposes, be designated "doctors," then the critical element of their medical practice would have been the doctor-totem relationship or doctor-spirit relationship. Any doctor-patient interaction was solely cajolatory in nature and subordinate in importance. It had this aspect as well: that the primitive practitioner,

---

[10]Frazer, J. G., *The Golden Bough: A Study of Magic and Religion*, vol. 1 of the abridged edition, New York, 1951, p. 121. The reference concerning the evolution of the sorcerer to medicine-man is on p. 106 of that work.

[11]Sir James G. Frazer published, in 1890, his first volumes of *The Golden Bough, A Study in Magic and Religion*, ultimately a twelve-volume compendium of primitive "magic, customs, social practices and religion," the most influential element being "fear of the human dead." Joseph Campbell, in *The Masks of God*, explored the "unity of the human race" by studying its myths, publishing his findings in four volumes over ten years (1959-1968). Both authors have collected and analyzed the anecdotal record of man's experience with the subjective. To add to this frightening collection an even more wretched account of primal practices, see: Devereaux, G., *A Study of Abortion in Primitive Societies*, New York, 1955.

[12] This definition of a medicine-man was presented in the *Fourteenth Annual Report of the Bureau of Ethnology to the Secretary of the Smithsonian Institution*, 1892-93, Washington D.C., 1896, p. 980. The terms "shaman" and "medicine-man" are often used interchangeably, the scholar's distinctions being nuanced. See: Hultkrantz, A., *The Shaman and the Medicine-Man*, in *Soc. Sci. Med.*, 20:511-515, 1985.

assuming he was not overtly psychotic, which he sometimes was, almost certainly understood the charade in which he was an actor. A satisfactory clinical outcome in a particular case may have occasioned a sigh of relief, but it did not produce even the smallest advance in true knowledge, seeing that neither the cause nor the natural course of things were predictably altered for the better, although they were certainly alterable for the worse. Ordinary mortals almost always know when what they are doing is ineffectual, and, given repeated observations, suspicion approaches certainty. Nevertheless, there have been curious instances of one shaman consulting another for relief of illness. There will always be some who would be fooled all the time.

The role of medicine-man traditionally devolved upon some of a community's most bizarre members. Prof. Eric R. Dodds writes: "A shaman may be described as a psychically unstable person who has received a call to the religious life."[13] Peter Farb has discussed the Eskimo shaman, pointing out that in contrast to the other tribal specialists the shaman has no traits that distinguish him from the general society except for bizarre behavioral or neurological manifestations that serve the same purpose.[14] His limited abilities in other areas provided the psychological basis for the social meddling that formed his livelihood, and his collusion with those in authority over the tribe provided him his insurance, an enviable position that was perhaps due to his susceptibility to easy manipulation. Oddness, then, seems to be a worldwide requirement for a shaman, an example being the "basir" shamans of Borneo, who, selected by virtue of being hermaphrodites, unite the earth (feminine principle) with heaven (masculine principle).[15] Shamans are not the equivalent of a priesthood, explaining and presiding over formal religious ritual. They are, instead, deemed capable by themselves of directing mystical power. They are regarded as "medicine-men" because of their presumed capacity to invoke or dispel, rather than medicinally cure, illness.

The prominent medical historian, Henry Sigerist, MD, stated, in his paean to the medicine-man, that "Today nobody doubts that they [the medicine-men] are sincere and believe in what they are doing, … ."[16] But harsh as it may seem to attribute base motives to simple and ignorant primitive practitioners, such an attribution is reasonable. It may, in fact, be overly fair. There is reason to allocate a lesser degree of humaneness to medicine-men and other mystics than their fellow citizens. It can be argued that they would likely have abused their special status to the detriment of society for personal ends beyond that of merely keeping their job. Such was the case 3,000 years ago with the priest of Apollo in Homer's *Iliad*, who, during the Trojan War, successfully invoked a deadly plague on the Greeks because of personal injury, but who had earlier wished them well in putting Troy to the sword.[17] Apollo, of course, was a deity closely identified with the practice of medicine, and his priest clearly had no humanitarian attachment to either side

---

[13] Dodds, E. R.; *The Greeks and the Irrational*, Boston, 1957, p. 140.

[14] Farb, Peter, *Man's Rise To Civilization*, New York, 1968, p. 50. And Dr. George Devereux, an anthropologist and expert in ethnopsychiatry, has described the Mojave Indian medicine-man as inevitably "a psychotic in partial remission." See *Mohave Ethnopsychiatry*, Washington, D. C., 1969, p. 12.

[15] Transgender phenomena have been inspirational for many primitive societies. For a more extensive review and interesting perspective see Jones, P., *Androgyny: The Pagan Sexual Ideal*, in *J. Evang. Theol. Soc.*, Jan., 2000.

[16] Sigerist, H. E., *History of Medicine*, New York, 1951, vol. 1, p. 177.

[17] Homer, *Iliad*, Book I. The *Iliad* has been described as the story of the wrath of Achilles. It can, however, also be described as the revenge of an exasperated priest.

in the conflict if his private interests were jeopardized.

The medicine-man was but a shade above a trickster, and Dr. Carl Jung wrote that "the trickster is a collective shadow figure, an epitome of all the inferior traits of character in individuals."[18] The practice profile of the modern medicine-man remains fully identifiable, and his call finds eager answerers. G. I. Gurdjieff (1872-1949) was a Russian-born mystic who established in Paris in 1922 his *Institute for the Harmonious Development of Man*. This man, who commented, "All evil deeds, all crimes, all self-sacrificing actions, all heroic exploits, as well as all the actions of ordinary life, are controlled by the moon," is survived by more than thirty Gurdjieff Centers around the world. Such is the power of certitude over the indecisive.

As social structures evolved in enlarging primitive populations, the medicine-man assumed greater importance. With centralized authoritarian control now dominating society, he began to use his special knowledge to invest some of that authority in himself. Ancient practitioners of sorcery and those in recent primitive societies, being elite interpreters of the supernatural and to maintain their claims of effectiveness, required the following: 1) a restriction on access to their sacred knowledge, not so much to limit the proliferation of practitioners as to prevent the layman from discerning the veneer of their knowledge, thereby allowing them to maintain their privileged status, a practice historically first recorded in ancient Mesopotamia;[19] 2) a protector, an authoritarian figure who maintained control over the community or society, thereby assuring no competition from other practitioners using "alternative" deities that might threaten the *status quo*; and 3) a scapegoat for their failures, which would naturally be either the will of some spirit or the ill-will of the patient.

And surely medicine-men and others of their ilk were no less inclined to wealth, power, and status than are men of the present day; salesmanship, patent protection, and a good lawyer remain key elements of successful entrepreneurship. But the fabulous nature of their knowledge exhibited no similarity to an effective medical practice, and medical prediction, if any existed, bestowed no ability to modify for the better the course of disease. It is, furthermore, impossible to discern any humane component in their practice. Simply put, they had no product to sell, but sell it they did, and well. The shamans in the Chavin culture of Peru (900-200 BC) were an elite class with great authority and capable of directing the course of an entire society, perhaps aided by manipulation of society with hallucinogens. George Catlin describes shamans sitting on councils of war and, in some American Indian tribes, often feared more than the chiefs.[20] Frazer gives medicine-men too much credit. From them, he posited, arose the sacred kingships, concluding with this statement: "Logically it [the shaman/priesthood] rests on a mistaken deduction from the association of ideas. Men mistook the order of their ideas for the order of nature, and hence imagined that the control which they have, or seem to have, over their thoughts,

---

[18] Radin, P., *On the Psychology of the Trickster Figure*, with commentary by C. G. Jung and found in English translation in: *The Trickster: A Study in American Indian Mythology*, New York, 1956, pp. 197-99, 209. Jung placed the Trickster between the Shaman and the Fool.
[19] "May he who knows instruct him who knows. And may he who knows not, not read this." And, "he who does not keep the secret will not remain in health. – His days will be shortened." Quoted (uncited, but perhaps early Babylonian from the 2nd millennium BC) by Sigerist, H. E., in his *History of Medicine*, New York, 1951, vol. 1, p. 433.
[20] Catlin, G., *Illustrations of the Manners, Customs, and Conditions of North American Indians*, London, 1848, 7th edition.

permitted them to exercise a corresponding control over things."[21] To which it can be responded that this "insight" was not restricted to the development of those who would later become kings. Indeed, such "insights" are ubiquitous, not sacred, and with but a moment's recall the reader can name a budding shaman who was in his class in school, or, briefly viewing afternoon television offerings, identify very active contemporary shamans at work, all of whom would be kings if they could.

It has been proposed that prehistoric societies and today's primitive societies share points of view. As examples, an African tribal society has been described in which its "modern" diviner, although practicing "placebo" therapy, was virtually a high priest, and, along with the tribal chief, was that society's dominant power,[22] and the Todas of southern India[23] were described in 1906 to have different practitioners for medicine and sorcery, but this availed the patient little for they both employed the same magical formulae in their respective treatments. And so, even into the 20th C the primitive practitioner of medicine remained but a medical sorcerer. There is, however, an alternative view of contemporary primitive societies, that being that they represent atavistic or degenerate branches of the greater societies.[24] In this case it may be unfair to equate motives and practices of a practitioner in an atavistic society with those of a pristine and perhaps high-minded ancient medicine-man. But this seems rather far-fetched. Regardless of the source of motivation, it is to be remarked that Dr. Henry Sigerist[25] gave the following perspective on being a modern physician: "The medicine man holds in primitive society an infinitely more important position than the physician does in a modern community, ..." and, further, "It is an insult to the medicine man to call him the ancestor of the modern physician." [26] We will note, in agreement with Sigerist, that the medicine-man is surely no ancestor of ours, but for quite different reasons. Sigerist's statement should be reversed: "It is an insult to the modern physician to call him a descendant of the medicine-man."

It is not only an insult; it is an error. But many textbooks on the history of medicine begin with stories of the medicine-man as a sort of natural precursor of the physician. The medicine-man, however, was as great a fraud in ancient times as he is now. There is no equating the medicine-man with the modern physician in any way whatsoever. The medicine-man is no "ur-physician," although there are, unfortunately, occasional examples of physicians acting the medicine-man.

---

[21] Sir James G. Frazer, *The Golden Bough*, vol. 1 of the abridged edition, New York, 1951, p. 121.

[22] Jansen, G., *The Doctor-Patient Relationship in an African Tribal Society*, Assen, 1973.

[23] Rivers, W. H. R., *The Todas*, London, 1906, p. 271.

[24] Guthrie, D., *A History of Medicine*, 1946, p. 2, for a brief mention of this possibility. At the end of the 19th C the concept of social Darwinism incorporated atavism of individuals and of primitive societies into an explanation for variations and deviations in the evolutionary progress of humankind.

[25] Henry Sigerist's life as a medical historian at, among other places, the Johns Hopkins University, is reviewed by Fel and Brown (*Making Medical History: The Life and Times of Henry E. Sigerist*, Baltimore, 1997). Sigerist (1891-1957), a physician whose career was primarily that of a medical historian, wrote much on the interaction of the medical profession and society, and he was a great admirer of the Soviets and their medical system. His popularity declined after he left the United States and returned to his European roots. Recently, however, Fel and Brown feel his significance is on the rise, noting that there is even a Sigerist Society. The contempt with which physicians were held by the leadership of the proletariat in the later years of the Soviet empire was shared, however subtly expressed, by Sigerist.

[26] Sigerist, H. E., in his *History of Medicine*, New York, 1951, vol. 1, p. 161.

There is a severe sentence awaiting the medicine-man and other political magicians, once the myth of the "noble savage" has been properly interred. Not only have they been detrimental to medicine, to scientific thought, and to logical thought in general, but they are also guilty of hijacking religion. Prof. Allier, who argues that magic was not the "origin of religious feeling," is not alone in concluding that the primitive, and not so primitive, mystical authoritarian thwarted true religious development.[27] By exploiting exotic theories of causation cultists have been able to commandeer religious awe for the purpose of acquiring power. This manipulation of fear to the detriment of the wonder of life has guided men down a dark and dreary road, leading even great thinkers such as Thomas Hobbes to promote overweening centralized governance as a necessary evil to contain it. Mysticism, both bane and balm of the primitive, can, in the hands of the authoritarian, insinuate itself like the intestine parasite it is into all aspects of society and be used to influence its hosts for despotic ends.

Returning to the idea of who might be the "natural precursor" of the modern physician, it is often assumed that medical practice has a chronologically continuous prehistory and history because in all ages man has sought relief from the afflictions of disease and trauma, and things are surely better now than they used to be.[28] But it arguably has not been evolutionary until recent centuries. As shall be shown in the following pages, there was a flourishing of scientific medicine in ancient Greece, but, as with a bronze masterpiece of Greek sculpture, the Roman Empire chiseled a crude imitation of it, barbarian invaders hacked off its head and arms, and the Dark Ages covered it over with silt. With the Renaissance there was a sputtering rediscovery of scientific medicine, but only now can the profession of medicine be described as evolutionary. The medicine-man and his congeners represent no part of this evolutionary chain, and it is odd that they have yet to disappear from erudite discussion. This is particularly so in that, while medicine has demonstrably evolved, the medicine-man has remained frozen in time, his likeness identifiable to every generation. Dr. Gerald Weissmann has succinctly documented its modern menace, soberly quoting many examples, a particularly grotesque one being:

> "... what the National Socialists wanted to do was to introduce a popular medicine, [they] had little regard for scientific medicine, and they were all attracted by natural medicine. All sorts of popular drugs which were not approved by the medical profession allegedly because we did not understand them or were too conceited or were financially interested in the suppression of them were used experimentally in concentration camps.... The source of these experiments was Himmler's conception of medicine as pure mysticism."[29]

To conclude this section, it is of no value to inquire further into a prehistoric

---

[27] Allier, R., *Magie et Religion*, Paris, 1935. An earlier work by Allier, *Le Non-civilisé et Nous* (Paris, 1927), had propounded his theory on the stunting of human intellectual growth by magic. There is a recent scholarly discussion of these issues in English: Styers, R., *Making Magic*, Oxford, 2004, pp. 137-138.

[28] One scholarly chronology of developmental stages of medicine that has been proposed is: 1) Prehistoric; 2) Ancient; 3) Classical; 4) Medieval; 5) Pre-scientific or Transitional; 6) Scientific or Modern. See the preface in: McKenzie, D., *The Infancy of Medicine*, London, 1927.

[29] Weissmann, G.; *"Sucking with Vampires," The Medicine of Unreason*, in: *The Flight from Science and Reason, N. Y. Acad. Sci.*, 775: 179-187, 1995. The quotation is that of the chief physician to the SS (the greatly feared *Schutzstaffel*), as told at the Nuremberg Tribunals.

or primitive physician-patient relationship. No such thing existed. It is a waste of time to attempt to draw anything of professional relevance from primitive medicine-men. The nightmare and universality of primitive behavior was captured by Fontenelle: "All men are so much alike that there are no people whose follies should not make us tremble."[30] And therefore we must not forget Dr. H. W. Haggard's warning, "The danger comes from intelligent people who...have not been educated to think rationally; it comes from sentimental and idle people in whom the primitive instinct escapes...."[31]

---

[30] *Oeuvres de Fontenelle*, 1790, v, p. 372. This is cited in: Allier, R.; *The Mind of the Savage*, London, 1929, translated by F. Rothwell, a book debunking the myth of the "noble savage."
[31] Haggard, H. W., *Devils, Drugs, and Doctors: The Story of the Science of Healing from Medicine Men to Doctor*, London, 1913, p. 395.

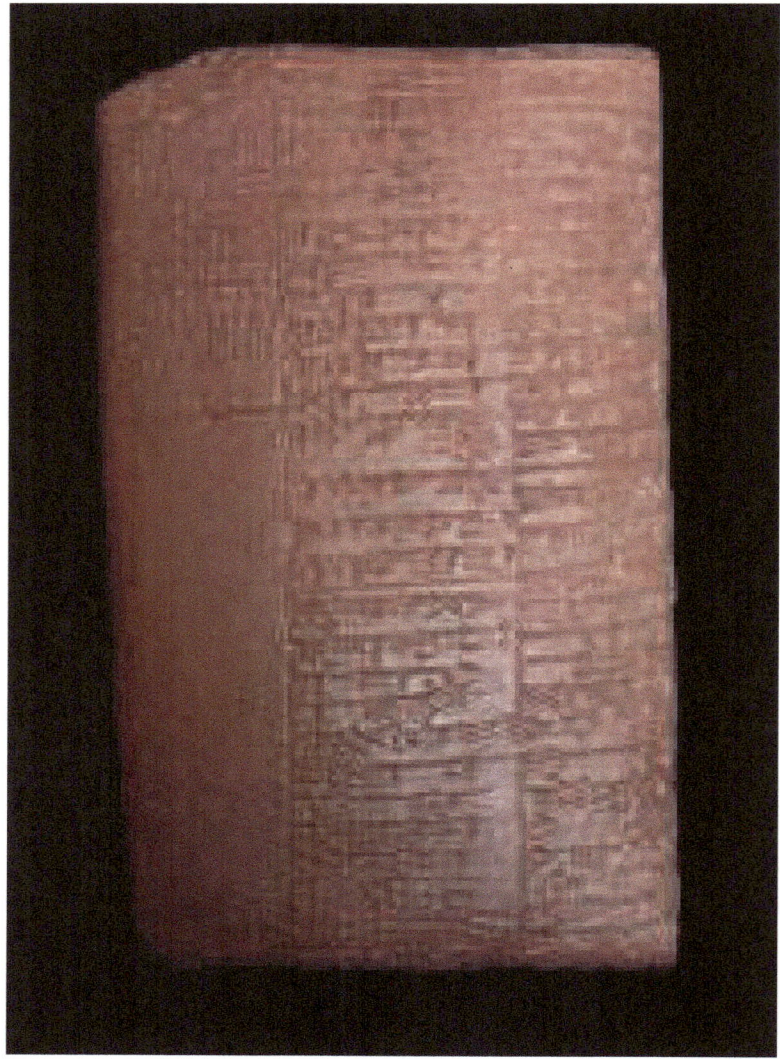

Fig. 2: Pharmacopoeia dated to between 2200 and 2100 BC, found at Nippur, an ancient city in what is modern-day Iraq. The original cuneiform tablet is presently at the University Museum, Philadelphia, Acc. #: B14221. It is among the earliest Sumerian documents relevant to medicine, describing fifteen rational prescriptions for poultices and infusions but including no charms or mystical references. Scientifically it is a most interesting document, for it appears that heat and alcoholic extractions of herbs were used to isolate active principles if water was not employed, something only scientific testing would have permitted. (See: Webb, J. L., *The Oldest Medical Document*, in *Bull. Med. Libr. Assoc.*, 45:1-4, 1957.) Photograph of this replica by the author.

CHAPTER TWO

LARGE STRUCTURED SOCIETIES, AUTHORITARIAN - MESOPOTAMIA

"In all ages the reason of the world has been at the mercy of brute force."

F. Marion Crawford[1]
(Cited by Dr. William Osler in his essay,
The Leaven of Science.)

Increasing regional populations resulted in larger societies and, ultimately, great civilizations. Chaos was prevented by authoritarian rule at the highest level and elitist interpretation of custom at lower levels. Mystical or theurgical beliefs accompanied the transformation of the medicine-man to priest. Early Mesopotamian society acquired an early form of rational medicine and a primordial physician, although the nature of that medicine and its practitioners is only now becoming appreciated. But consolidation of early city-states into kingdoms, followed by a succession of monarchical empires, was associated with domination of medicine by the exorcist-priest, the *asipu*. As the Common Era approached rational medicine in Mesopotamia had long since ceased to exist.

A. Introduction: The Universal Appeal of Authoritarianism

The penchant for authoritarian rule, whether pursued out of fear of chaos, fear of force, or anticipation of aggrandizement, has existed in all times and in all places, and seems to be a universal preference. Authoritarianism is the natural state of things, and there is never a lack of bold individuals who strive to lead those less so.[2] It follows the law of entropy by creating, from an irregularly charged and individualistic state, a monotonously structured, low energy society resistant to change. Authoritarian impulses are the rule in nature among vertebrates that live in societies, a fact that finds its proof in hierarchical displays of force, the exiled contender, and the docile herd. It could be argued that, among the various forms of governance, authoritarian rule represents Darwinian success, for in human society great civilizations have been the most profound construction

---

[1] Found in: *The Witch of Prague*, in *The English Illustrated Magazine*, London, 1890-91, p. 337.

[2] A description of an "authoritarian" was provided by Aristotle's successor, Theophrastus (371-287 BC), as listed as "Oligarchy" among his *Characters*: ("Authoritarianism would seem to be a desire for office that covets power and profit. The authoritarian is the sort who, when the people are debating which people to choose to assist the chief magistrate with the procession, takes the podium and says they need to have absolute power; if other speakers propose ten of them, he says "One is plenty – but he has to be a real man!" He remembers only one line of Homer – he doesn't know a single thing about the rest: "More than one leader is bad; let one alone be our ruler." (This translation of Theophrastus from the *Characters* is by Rusten and Cunningham in the 2002 edition of the *Loeb Classical Library* series.) Theophrastus is referring to a line from Homer's *Iliad,* 2.204: οὐκ ἀγαθὸν πολυκοιρανίη· εἷς κοίρανος ἔστω..., ("Rule by many is no good; there will be only one ruler here...") in which Odysseus ridicules the implication that any Achaean can be "king" and ignore the divine right of the one whom Zeus has honored, a statement that Aristotle repeats in his *Politics* (1292a13).

of authoritarianism.[3]   It is to be expected, therefore, that most information relevant to medical practice will be found in study of the great civilizations, inasmuch as almost all of humankind from the first man and woman up to 4 March 1789 knew nothing but authoritarian rule. [4]

Prof. Arnold Toynbee's *Study of History* enumerated twenty-three distinct civilizations in an analysis of societal progression and regression.[5]   In contrast, this chapter and the succeeding five provide a regional perspective on civilizations and medical practice, these being selected for global representation, with Greco-Roman civilization reserved for later chapters. In the context of a polity, the term "civilization" is applied here to those societies that have succeeded in developing a system of hierarchical administrative bureaucracies.[6] We begin with the Mesopotamian region, the "cradle of Western civilization" that centers on what is now Iraq but which also includes much of the modern Middle East.

B. Mesopotamia and Its Cuneiform Script

One justification for excluding primitive practitioners from any analysis of the natural state of medical practice is that practice profiles are better comprehended from written records and conclusions are less intuitive. The earliest civilization to develop a form of writing, presently considered by scholars to be Sumerian, was the forerunner of a series of authoritarian Mesopotamian civilizations geographically placed in the regions served by the Tigris and Euphrates rivers. Sir C. Leonard Woolley considered the Sumerian civilization to have been "old" prior to dynastic Egypt, and the earliest known forms of its writings date from *ca.* 3400 BC.[7] It was a complex and dispersed culture of city-states, unique among the great civilizations in that there is no clear record of a preexisting Paleolithic society in Mesopotamia, a consequence of the late formation of the delta at the north end of the Persian Gulf. A Bronze Age culture thus was introduced into pristine geography.

Clay inscriptions of commercial activity in early Sumer, *ca.* 3000 BC, are plentiful, but there is no mention of medical practices. Nor are there records of trade and craft guilds. Early documents refer instead to the equivalent of "state workshops," the palace often being the site of craft production. Even into the 3rd millennium craftsmen

---

[3] A religious argument against popular notions of Darwinism stresses its link to authoritarianism, pointing out that a Darwinian theory of evolution provides philosophical justification for violent social movements such as Nazism and Marxism, whereas individualism is a natural corollary of creationism.

[4] March 4, 1789 marked the opening of the first United States Congress under its new Constitution, although a quorum of attendees was not achieved for some days. But there was a predecessor that, although on a smaller scale, might be the world's first document to declare self-government: the *Fundamental Orders of Connecticut*, promulgated in January 1639, the product of the Puritan leader, Thomas Hooker, and his fellow citizens in what is now Hartford, Connecticut.

[5] Toynbee, A., *Study of History*, Oxford, 1934-1961, in twelve volumes.

[6] This definition is from *The Columbia Encyclopedia*, 6th editor, Columbia University Press, 2000.

[7] Just where the original Sumerians came from, and when, is debated, and some feel they arrived in Mesopotamia not much before 3000 BC. See: Woolley, C. L., in *The Sumerians*, New York, 1929, who gives inclusive dates as 4000 – 2600 BC. Modern scholarship considers 1950 BC as the time of their final political disappearance, although many aspects of their culture were assimilated by subsequent cultures.

lived in craft quarters. Much of the land in 4th and 3rd millennium Mesopotamia was under the control of religious temples as local rulers exchanged land governance for services. It has been pointed out that there are many similarities between the Sumerian "temples" and medieval monasteries in the West; they were the essential "business" activity for their cities, controlling irrigation waters, dispensing produce, land, prebends, and goods in return for services, offerings, and obedience.[8] By providing an administrative counterbalance to secular leadership they were a stabilizing influence on the economy and populace, in addition to being a mechanism for restraining activities of the king. Southern Mesopotamia, therefore, is thought to have been composed, to a great extent, of independent theocratic city-states in which most citizens were unable to own land. Woolley could only assume that medical practitioners maintained ties to temples, but this generally was not the case.[9]

Sumerian hegemony was replaced by a neighboring nomadic Semitic people, the Akkadians, who ruled from 2350-2150 BC. Then followed an intercalated period of re-emergent Sumerian dominance, a period noted for a "renaissance" in the arts and for extensive centralization of government. One of its kings, Ur-Nammu, provided a legal code for his minions. There followed, in approximate sequence, the Amorites (1900-1595 BC) to whom belonged Hammurabi (the Old Babylonian period), the Kassites (1595-1155 BC), the neo-Hittite kingdoms to the west (1150-700 BC), the Assyrians (1170-609 BC), the Neo-Babylonian empire (626-539 BC), and the Persian Empire.[10] Only two fragments of actual Sumerian medical texts have been recovered, and but few are from the subsequent Akkadian and Amorite periods. But archeologists have uncovered many descriptions of their medical practices from libraries of the Assyrian and Neo-Babylonian periods. This was enabled by cuneiform writing, invented by the Sumerians and subsequently modified to support the language of invaders and to remain the fundamental Mesopotamian script for over two thousand years. Most extant medical texts are late Assyrian (934-609 BC), and yet the cuneiform is Akkadian, a variant of the Sumerian script that served as a *lingua franca* for the region. So revered were the Sumerian and Akkadian writings that they would be repeatedly copied over the centuries, and so it is that many Assyrian tablets are now known to describe medical practices of Sumer some 1500 years earlier. There are even bilingual dictionaries for Sumerian technical terms that were composed by Babyonians as early as 1800 BC for the purpose of preserving a Sumerian intellectual tradition (Fig. 3), even though that spoken language (not the script) had long since been replaced in day-to-day use by the unrelated Akkadian.[11] It is thus indirectly that much of the nature of Sumerian medicine can be deduced.

---

[8] Fish, T.; *Catalogue of Sumerian Tablets in the John Rylands Library*, Manchester, 1932, Prefatory Note.

[9] Woolley, C. L., in *The Sumerians*, New York, 1929, p. 111.

[10] For the purposes of this synopsis these dates are all approximate, the list of empires incomplete, and the selected empires do not all reflect linear rule of Mesopotamia and contiguous regions. Modern scholarship on ancient Mesopotamia is voluminous, probing, and complex.

[11] Older bilingual dictionaries or word lists have also been recovered from excavations of Ebla, a prominent contemporary city-state located near the Mediterranean coast in present-day Syria. Prior to its destruction by the Akkadians *ca.* 2240 BC, Ebla scribes had adapted Sumerian cuneiform to serve a phonetic purpose for their own language. See L. Casson, *Libraries in the Ancient World*, New Haven, 2001, chapter one.

C. Early Mesopotamian Practitioners and Evidence for an Empirical-Rational Medical Practice

Noting that medical records contained many incantations and charms used as remedies for symptoms,[12] Sir E. A. Wallis Budge concluded that early Mesopotamian medicine had many similarities to the Egyptian. This might be expected, as writing may have developed at about the same time in the two empires, their principal centers of authority being separated by a mere nine hundred miles. And yet it was not necessarily so, for the Greco-Roman and Persian civilizations were face-to-face antagonists over a thousand years, and while there were purchased services never did one adopt characteristics of the other, and in this regard it may be relevant that in mathematics the Egyptians developed a decimal system whereas the Babylonians used a sexagesimal one.[13] Rather than representing interrelated practices, Egyptian and Mesopotamian medicine more likely were each unique, indigenous, and autonomous, any similarities merely reflecting the usual course of medicine in authoritarian societies, a thesis further developed below.

For some years scholars have reported that early Mesopotamians were cared for by at least two classes of medical practitioners: those of the "herb" (the *asu*), and the "word" (the *asipu*).[14] The latter is said to have been esteemed the more. The esteemed *asipu* traditionally has been viewed as a priest and exorcist, able to assist the gods in reversing a lunar eclipse and ridding a person of demons. Dr. Saggs states that the word *asipu* is related to the Greek word for "enchanter" (ἐπῳδός) as used in the *Book of Daniel*, 2:10, and that his medical role was to function as witchdoctor.[15]

The term *asu*, in contrast, has traditionally been interpreted as "physician." An earlier term for *asu* in Sumer was *azu.* Dr. L. A. Waddell, a physician, translated the latter as "diviner" or " physician" on Sumerian seals dated *ca.* 3000 BC, with the interpretation of "diviner" being one who practiced water divination, obviously not a clinical practitioner.[16] This suggests that the early *azu* was not solely an empirical medical

---

[12] Thompson, R. C., *Assyrian Medical Texts*, in *Proc. Roy. Soc. Med.*, Sect. Hist. Med., 1924, 17:1; 1926, 19:29. The two articles contain numerous examples of diseases of the eye, teeth, and mouth.

[13] Bengston, H., *The Greeks and the Persians*, London, 1969. Bengston notes that despite free communication between the two societies, Persia attached no value whatever to Greek achievements, and the Greeks, valuing the individual, viewed as barbarian the glorification of a monarch who rendered all his subjects faceless. There was no "spiritual contact" between the two.

[14] A third class of practitioner has been proposed, that of "the knife," *i.e.*, the surgeon, as alluded to by S. Bertman in *Handbook to Life in Ancient Mesopotamia*, Oxford, 2003, pp. 307-308, but his source of information on this class is merely the Hammurabi Law Code, in which the *asu* is the wielder of the "knife." Thus, the services of a surgeon are implied as subsumed by the *azu/asu*. This remains, however, an assumption that could benefit from closer scrutiny.

[15] Saggs, H. W. F., *The Greatness that was Babylon*, London, 1988, p. 297 (revised edition).

[16] See Dr. Waddell's discussion of Seals #5 and #15 in: *The Indo-Sumerian Seals Deciphered*, a 1980 reprint by Omni Publ. of a work first published in 1925. An opinion of the later *asu*, as expressed by C. Edwards in *The Hammurabi Code* (London, 1904), describes him as a "doctor" who, combining "exorcist, medicine man, physician, and surgeon," was to "pronounce a counter-spell" on a suspected wizard and whose victim was protected from unfair exorcism by the Hammurabi Code. In *A Sumer Aryan Dictionary* by L. A. Waddell (London, 1927) the *asu* in Sumerian was a "wise man, seer, priest, physician, conjurer, auger; literally, 'one who has deep knowledge'," whereas in Akkadian he was "a physician, wizard, diviner, soothsayer, conjurer." The Akkadian *asu's* antecedent was the Sumerian *azu*. It is later that the Akkadian *asipu* is mentioned.

practitioner. The *asu*, however, was responsible for carrying out empirical ministrations, including application of poultices, bandaging, and washing. He executed the many treatments for diseases described in clay tablets, which included "infusions" for fevers, diarrheas, and swellings, as well as application of liniments and treatments for worms.[17]

Edith Ritter defined more clearly the distinction between the *asu* and the *asipu*.[18] The former was a hands-on practitioner who prepared drugs, applied bandages, and gave enemas and massages. This person, who was poorly paid, was of lesser importance than the *asipu*, the academic practitioner who was an authority from the gods, a "man of rote and learning" who dealt with amulets, incantations, and other magical or religious procedures, who had expertise in prognosis, and whose aim was to exorcize the sick man of his disease rather than to treat it. Ritter, like Saggs, limited the *asipu's* function primarily to witchcraft. Medical judgments by the *asipu* were auguries, and even the walk to a patient's house could provide opportunities for prognostication: "If [the *asipu*] sees either a black dog or a black cat, that sick man will die."[19] Curiously, the function of the *asipu* was guided, in part, by examining the patient's physical condition, and perhaps he viewed an examination of the patient the same as he would the entrails of a sacrificial animal, more the stuff of omens than objective evidence of pathology.[20] The *asu* and the *asipu* were sometimes consulted individually for the same patient, and Dr. Saggs (see above citation, p. 415) thinks their functions overlapped. Ritter noted that certain stones, when pulverized, were used by the *asu* as a medicine, whereas the *asipu* used the same, but intact, stones as amulets.

Recent scholarship, however, has challenged the assessment of these medical roles and now assigns to the *asipu* the tasks of diagnosis and a search for causes of illness, whereas the *asu's* role has been restricted to the application of treatments. As a practitioner of "the herb," therefore, some scholars now identify the *asu* as akin to a pharmacist.[21] Essential to this thinking is the forty-tablet *Treatise on Medical Diagnosis and Prognosis*, written *ca.* 1600 BC and rewritten and edited *ca.* 1050 BC but recording information from many centuries earlier. It describes the role of the *asipu* in prognosis and causation. Some of its clinical descriptions seem objective and astute, inspiring Dr. Nils Heessel to call the *asipu* a "learned diagnostician."[22] For example, the frequent

---

[17] Bottero, J.; *Everyday Life in Ancient Mesopotamia*, translated by A. Nevill, Edinburgh, 2001, Chapter 10, *Magic and Medicine*. It contains clinical descriptions of external somatic pathology. There also is mention of the kidney from about 3000 BC and a votive offering of a model of the kidney has been dated to 1300 BC. See: Purkerson, M. L., *et al.*; *Depictions of the Kidney through the Ages*, in *Amer. J. Neph.* 17:340-346, 1997. A learned discussion of urinary tract disease as understood in ancient Mesopotamia, with some translations, is found in: Geller, M.J. and Cohen, S. L., *Kidney and Urinary Tract Disease in Ancient Babylonia, with Translations of the Cuneiform Sources*, in: *Kidney International*, 47:1811-1815, 1995.

[18] Ritter, E. K.; *Magical-expert (=ashipu) and physician (=asu): notes on two complementary professions in Babylonian medicine*, in *Assyriological Studies*, 16:299-321, 1965.

[19] Saggs, H. W. F., *The Greatness that was Babylon*, London, 1988, p. 417.

[20] Such is the essence of the *asipu*'s role as described by A. L. Oppenheim in his classic work, *Ancient Mesopotamia: Portrait of a Dead Civilization*, Chicago, 1977.

[21] Scurlock, J.; *Physician, Exorcist, Conjurer, Magician: A Tale of Two Healing Professionals*, in Abusch, T. and van ver Toorn, K.; *Mesopotamian Magic: Textual, Historical, and Interpretative Perspectives*, Groningen, 1999, p. 69-79.

[22] N. P. Heessel, in his *Diagnosis, Divination and Disease: Towards an Understanding of the Rationale behind the Babylonian Diagnostic Handbook*, found in: *Magic and Rationality in Ancient Near Eastern and Graeco-Roman Medicine*, H. Horstmanshoff and M. Stol, editors, Leiden, 2004,

references to ghostly visitations with which the *asipu* contended, while seemingly mystical, may actually have represented an attempt at describing and dealing with the organic brain syndrome or acute confusional state that encompasses the delirium and obtundation often seen in severe or terminal illness, states in which the patient may see and appear to discourse with phantoms, persons known or unknown. A previously missing chapter of the abovementioned *Treatise on Medical Diagnosis and Prognosis* makes quite clear that, despite references to demons, clinical acumen was in play, for prognosis was based on clinical observations and treatment was reasonable and not hurtful, if not particularly helpful.[23] An example is the knowledgeable translation and commentary of a section that suggests Bell's palsy:

> If a man has facial palsy, his (affected) eye deviates from the other and night and day remains open, so that he cannot lie down to sleep, he should not cease constantly to rub his face with honey and leban...so he will recover.[24]

Further impressive clarifications of a true clinical role for the *asipu* come from the insightful commentary by Dr. Paullisian, an anesthesiologist, about a variety of translations by different experts, and from translations by Dr. Scurlock and Dr. Andersen, the latter a specialist in internal medicine, of many cuneiform medical tablets, including the *Treatise on Medical Diagnosis and Prognosis* mentioned above.[25] Scurlock and Andersen devised a list of traditional modern medical specialties and then sought statements in the cuneiform tablets that seemed to be reasonably consistent with modern clinical knowledge in those specialties. The result is a far greater appreciation of the power of observation of the clinicians of Sumer. Dr. Paullisian, for example, cites a translation by Adamson describing an example that convincingly portrays a patient with Parkinsonian symptoms:

> "if his head, hands, and feet are trembling at the same time, when he walks, he falls forward, his words embarrass him in his mouth, his mouth forces itself into speech, in speaking saliva falls."

A resting tremor that can involve all extremities and head and neck, fenestrating gate, monotonal speech, and drooling are typical signs of advancing Parkinsonism, of which there are many causes, and the ancient observer has here identified not just some

---

pp. 97-116, has updated the nature of this *Treatise*, detailing its editing in the 11th BC by a prominent scholar named Esagil-kin-apli. The rational nature of the original clinical observations emerges with greater clarity, and at the same time the expressed mystical aspects of causation of disease do not interfere with diagnosis or treatment.

[23] Clinical distinctions between a Bell's palsy and hemiparesis were described, and various presentations of Todd's paralysis (a postictal paralysis) were recognized. See: Wilson, J. V. K. and Reynolds, E. H.; *Translation and Analysis of a Cuneiform Text Forming Part of a Babylonian Treatise on Epilepsy*, in *Med. History*, 34:185-198, 1990.

[24] Wilson, J. V. K. and Reynolds, E. H.; *On Stroke and Facial Palsy in Babylonian Texts*, in *Disease in Babylonia*, Leiden, 2006, I. L. Finkel and M. J. Geller, editors, Chapter 4, pp. 67-99.

[25] Paullisian, R.; *Medicine in Ancient Assyria and Babylonia*, in *J. Assyrian Academic Studies*, 5:3-51, 1991, and Scurlock, J., and Andersen, B.; *Diagnoses in Assyrian and Babylonian Medicine: Ancient Sources, Translations, and Modern Medical Analyses*, Urbana, 2005.

symptoms but a syndrome.[26]

From evidence interpreted in such disparate ways, what can be inferred about Mesopotamian practitioners, their origin and their functions? The original Sumerian *azu* had some role as a mystic healer. The etymology of his appellation is uncertain, but some

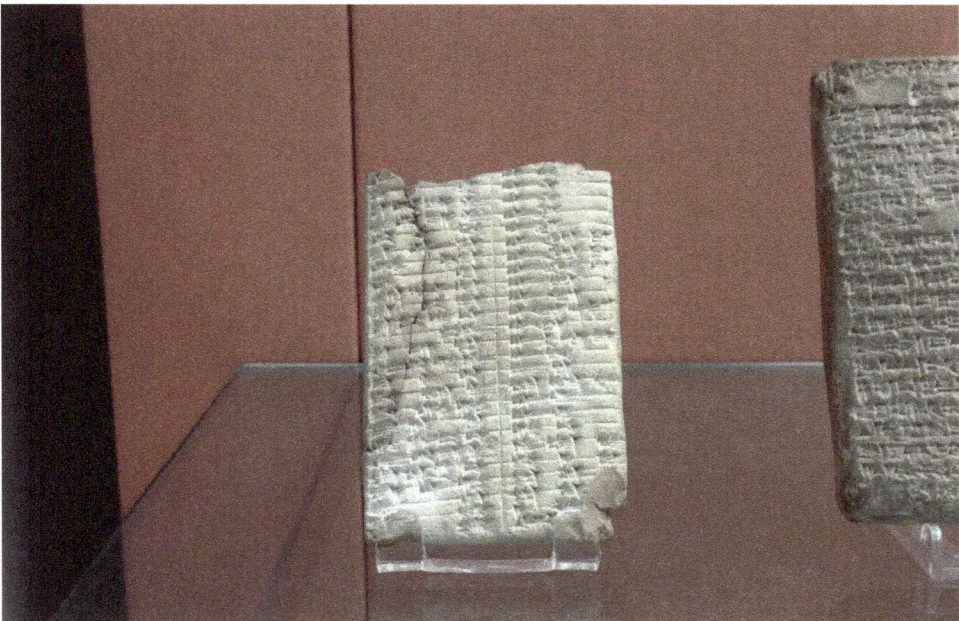

Fig. 3: Cuneiform tablet, Neo-Assyrian period, *ca.* 800 BC, with Sumerian words and phrases on the left and Akkadian equivalents on the right. Classified as a "scholarly" tablet, the Sumerian and Akkadian terms would originally have been in use *ca.* 2000 BC. Collection of the Metropolitan Museum of Art, New York. Photograph by the author.

consider it derived from "water diviner."[27] But he also was an empirical healer. There is little evidence for a temple affiliation. The 2200-year-old Sumerian pharmacopoeia shown in Fig. 2 contains no appeal to mysticism in its use of prescriptions, and the isolation of active principles by the processes of heating, alcoholic extraction, and precipitation by organic salts is implied.[28] This pharmacopoeia (or "therapeutic manual") was intended for use by the *azu*. Furthermore, in both the Laws of X (2050 BC) and the Code of Hammurabi (1754 BC) the *asu* is described in terms consistent with physician rather than as a mystic. It is proposed here that the azu was and would remain the only medical practitioner throughout early Mesopotamian history and into the Common Era.

With the advent of the Akkadians, however, there came a competitor, the *asipu*,

---

[26] The original article commented on by Dr. Paullisian is: Adamson, P. B.; *Some Anatomical and Pathological Terms in Akkadian*, in *Revue d'Assyriologie*, 84:27-32, 1990.

[27] As an aside, divining for water is an ancient and and still revered art in the eyes of some, and represents a psychic power instilled in a select few. See: Jones, C. E., *Water Finding*, London, 1907.

[28] Dr. G. Majno, in *The Healing Hand*, (Cambridge, 1975, p. 51) even describes what is reasonably interpreted to be an ingenious distillation apparatus in Sumer that might have been used to volatilize, then condense, active principles from resins or other fluids.

an exorcist, an employee of the temple or royal court. The *azu*, now termed an *asu* in Akkadian, became subordinate to the *asipu* as the Akkadians extended centralized control over the dispersed city-states. The *Treatise on Medical Diagnosis and Prognosis* (also termed the *Diagnostic and Prognostic Handbook*) now became the important medical text, and it was meant for use by the *asipu*. Thus, an exorcist was given an expanded role which included diagnostic and prognostic skills to guide the *asu's* hands-on therapy, and this division of labor recurs in the region until the Common Era. Furthermore, Sir G. E. R. Lloyd proposed that the *asipu* developed a concept of *prognosis* that could be considered a step forward in the progress of medicine. After reviewing a variety of medically related inscriptions, he concludes there was "a desire to anticipate the course sickness will take."[29]

But the desire to foretell the future is a common, if often ill-conceived, wish of mankind. By means of exsticipy, astrology, or other divining practices, any purported knowledge of the future can be used to gain ascendancy over others, a design to control, not to cure.[30] It would have been, in effect, the domain of the medicine-man. Barbara Bock has also stated that the *Treatise on Medical Diagnosis and Prognosis* is not written for purposes of treatment, but to determine prognosis and "supernatural cause" of the patient's symptoms.[31] It is relevant, therefore, that although evidence of an empirical-rational medical practice points to a Sumerian origin, it was the Akkadian *asipu* and his successors who would from then on be identified as the more important specialist in managing disease, with the consequences to the *asu* bearing heavily on the course of Mesopotamian medicine.

Dr. Scurlock suggests the extensive and scholarly *Treatise on Medical Diagnosis and Prognosis*, which was addressed to the *asipu* and edited in 1050 BC, to be the accumulated and therefore improved medical knowledge of more than a thousand years, a process that was to be continued in some circles for another thousand. If the hypothesis of Scurlock is correct, as the centuries passed the role of the *asipu* should have become progressively sophisticated in knowledge and procedures. But Dr. Oppenheim has stated that "all extant tablets of this type, whatever their date or provenience reflect only the medical practice and state of medical knowledge in the Old Babylonian period," *i.e.*, *ca.* 1800-1530 BC.[32] The idea that both the *Treatise on Medical Diagnosis and Prognosis* of 1050 BC and the Sumerian pharmacopoeia of 2200 BC each represent the full extent of medical knowledge in their respective eras separated by more than a millenium may be, therefore, an inaccurate generalization. Who can be confident that the totality of the knowledge in the *Treatise* did not also originate in early Sumer, its *editio princeps* waiting to be discovered?

During the subsequent Kassite era, *ca.* 1530-1170 BC, (1) the practice of the *asipu* as described in the nine-table *surpu* ritual was one of exorcism, (2) the *asu* is no longer mentioned in writings of that empire, (3) a profound increase in religious fervor appears, and (4) "wisdom becomes divine," *i.e.*, it was written and therefore available only to scribal elite, secretive and involving "knowledge of mysteries that had little to do

---

[29] Lloyd, G. E. R.; *The Ambitions of Curiosity*, Cambridge, 2002, p. 24. And: Contenau, G., in *Everyday Life in Babylon and Assyria* (New York, 1954, Chapter 4), cites a similar claim from a study published in 1907.

[30] Concepts underlying medical prognosis are discussed on p. 225*ff*.

[31] Bock, B., *The Healing Goddess Gula*, Leiden, 2013, chapter 3.

[32] Oppenheim, A. L.; *Ancient Mesopotamia: Portrait of a Dead Civilization*, Chicago, 1977, p. 291.

with the practical realities of life."[33]   In the ensuing Neo-Assyrian period, *ca*. 900-609 BC, there are letters from the *asipu* to royalty in which the advice of the *asipu* is via omens whereas the *asu*, once again mentioned in texts, is the caregiver for earaches and other infirmities.[34]   The *asipu* was still a formidable figure in the 4th C BC cuneiform and Aramaic writings and he was still retained by the temple, his role still the traditional "incantation" priest.   Thus, at all these chronological stages references to his function, even some Biblical references, are as an exorcist or conjuror.

Given the strong associations of the *asipu* with mysticism and exorcism, it is difficult to assign him a role equivalent to the modern internist who advises an "assistant" in patient care, whether pharmacist or nurse practitioner.   And yet the work of Scurlock and Andersen provides convincing evidence of careful medical inquiry at some point in Mesopotamian history.   Perhaps the *asipu* was a master at "inspection," the initial phase of the physical examination of any patient.   By merely observing a patient and obtaining an accurate medical history considerable clinical information becomes accessible.   The *asipu* could not inspect the entrails of a patient as a seer would inspect those of a sacrificial animal, but second best would be to look for external evidence, such as abnormal movements, abdominal distention, skin lesions, and neurological abnormalities.   With this information he might identify the demonic cause and the reason the disease manifestation assumed its particular manifestation, as well as the likely outcome.   Being observational rather than analytical, it required no real understanding of the disease process and would not lead to any such understanding, but for contemporary society it was completely credible, satisfactory, and consistent with traditional beliefs.   Such beliefs were made easy by the *asipu* when he imposed mysticism even when the mysticism itself was far-fetched. For example, here is Ritter's translation of a treatment for epistaxis (nosebleed):

> "let him hold a tampon of the seeds of … at the base of the nostril … they will then recite an incantation … and will put it into the nostril according to the text that I sent they should act …"[35]

This patient had a typical unilateral anterior epistaxis, a routine family encounter.   The exact bleeding site, Kiesselbach's triangle, is known to anyone interested in the problem for it is easily localized and its bleeding easily controlled by mild pressure on the side of the affected nostril.   What possibly could an incantation have added to management that could just as easily have been carried out by the patient's grandmother.   Probably at issue was recurrent epistaxis, but it must have seemed a farce to most of those involved, including the patient and his grandmother, for it was just that, except perhaps to the *asipu* whose daily bread depended on a faithful laiety.   But he could not have fooled everybody.

As a further contrast, the *asu* was a full-time clinician, whereas the *asipu* had a

---

[33] van der Toorn, K.; *Why Wisdom Became a Secret: On Wisdom as a Written Genre*, in *Wisdom Literture in Mesopotamia and Israel*, R. J. Clifford, editor, Atlanta, 2007. Prof. Van der Toorn argues that ideas that had earlier been discussed in open forum became, with the evolution of a scribal bureaucracy and writing, accessible only to "scribal elite." He gives the example of an "Old Babylonian" version, *ca*. 1600 BC, of the Gilgamesh epic as representing "human knowledge painstakingly acquired," whereas by *ca*. 1100 BC the "Standard Babylonian" edition described that wisdom as "divine."
[34] Parpola, S.; *Letters from Assyrian Scholars to the Kings Esarhaddon and Assurbanipal*, Winona Lake, 1970 (reprinted in 2007).
[35] Ritter, E. K.; *Magical-expert (=ashipu) and physician (=asu): notes on two complementary professions in Babylonian medicine*, in *Assyriological Studies*, 16:299-321, 1965.

variety of functions as part of his temple responsibilities. Another important point is that the *asu's* ancestor, the *azu*, had, at least as early as 2250 BC and prior to the advent of the *asipu*, the traditional doctor's equipment needed for examination and treatment.[36] Clinical medicine is a full-time occupation even when provided part-time, or so it is in modern medicine. It would have taken some time to examine and talk to a patient, not to mention the time necessary to walk to the patient's domicile, unpack one's necessary paraphernalia, clean up afterwards, hone one's clinical skills, and attend to all related minutiae. The *asipu's* other responsibilities, such as exorcism, attendance at rituals and consecrations, and combating witchcraft must have severely limited direct patient contact. He would, therefore, have had little opportunity to acquire new medical knowledge. Indeed, he had no need to acquire new knowledge, for his primary function was to reverse the ethereal causes of illness. The *asipu's* clinical handbook may have been but a handy guide based on the *asu's* work over the centuries or handed down from the earliest *asu(s)*, such as occurred with 5th C BC Hippocratic writings that found their way into the hands of medieval divines like the 6th C AD Bishop Isidore of Seville (see p. 332, footnote). In contrast to European integration of Hippocratic works, in ancient Mesopotamia the clinical handbook became a shortcut for determining the supernatural cause of the patient's problem, and it came into, and remained in, the *asipu's* hands because he was a temple adherent and able to read. But the true Mesopotamian practitioner was the *asu*. Over time his function was diminished, perhaps even to the point of being restricted to pharmacy, as suggested by Scurlock and Anderson. But the *asipu*, despite his sometime medical gloss, was from beginning to end little more than a state-sponsored exorcist.

D. Medicine and the Mesopotamian State

In early Sumer the city-state arrangement of society was notable for specialization of local trades and reverence for local deities. As for elements of governance, Prof. Herbert Muller makes the statement that initially there were popular assemblies, although a specific citation for this not provided.[37] That degree of liberty was not maintained, however, and it was King Urukagina of Lagash (perhaps a revolutionary, reigned *ca.* 2370 BC) who has been credited with reforming inequities and restoring liberties, with the implication that some concept of individual freedom was understood in early city-states.

Ancient Sumer was then conquered and integrated by its neighbors, the Akkadians, just as two thousand years later the Romans would subjugate the neighboring Greeks. It was Woolley who first recognized that many of the laws of Sumerian civilization, as well as many particulars of its art and religion, were retained by its more primitive conquerors, again resembling Roman assimilation of aspects of Greek culture. When Sumerian hegemony was temporarily restored (2125-2000 BC), the earliest extant written law code (Laws of Ur-Nammu) was promulgated *ca.* 2050 BC, of which fifty-seven laws have been identified so far. Four refer to the *azu*, translated below as

---

[36] This included bronze scalpels, needles, forceps, and even quartz magnifying lenses. See: Scurlock, J., and Andersen, B.; *Diagnoses in Assyrian and Babylonian Medicine: Ancient Sources, Translations, and Modern Medical Analyses*, Urbana, 2005, p. 6. Ebla, an ancient city about 500 miles from Sumerian Ur, was recently excavated and thousands of tablets written in Sumerian cuneiform were recovered. See footnote, p. 37.

[37] Muller, H. J., *Freedom in the Ancient World,* New York, 1961, p. 47.

"physician," all of which stipulate the fee required for "healing" some specified illness:

> "if [a man ...-s and] a physician [heals him, ...]
> "If a man [...-s and] a physician heals him, [he shall weigh and deliver] 5 shekels [of silver].
> "If [a man ...-s and] a physician heals him, [he shall weigh and deliver] 4 shekels [of silver].
> "If [a man ...s and] a physician heals him, [he shall weigh and deliver] one shekel [of silver]. [38]

It appears that fees were set by the State for performing a "cure," which might have been the draining of an abscess or extracting a tooth, such services as would have been provided by the *azu*. No laws stipulated fees for the *asipu* and there were no legislated penalties for poor outcomes, yet fees were specified for other trades such as innkeeping and weaving. It is unlikely that the laws stipulating fees were devised to enrich the *azu* or other tradesmen. The laws may be viewed as curbs on avarice or a black market, but fundamentally they indicate a State-regulated economy, if in fact the Code were meant to be enforced. The specified fees probably were for services purchased from medical practitioners within the community, the "private" *azu*, rather than those assigned to the palace.

Three centuries later Hammurabi, who rose from nomadic stock to be proclaimed the unifier of Mesopotamia, inscribed in stone what is called *The Code of Hammurabi* (1754 BC). The laws designated P215-P223 specify the fee for the (presumed private) practitioner, here again identified as the *azu* in cuneiform and translated as "physician," but for the most part and in contrast to the Code of Ur-Nammu they provide for punishment and decide malpractice claims based on outcome, and no exception is noted for those poor outcomes that inevitably accompany, in some cases, good judgment. Such laws would push any surgeon to treat only highly selected patients, specifically those likely to recover whether or not they would, in fact, respond to his bronze lancet. The *azu* at this time (1750 BC) must have been considered a lowly and readily expendible technician. Also note the continuum of worth of the free man, freed man, and slave, the Code's total literary contribution to the physician-patient relationship. Hammurabi's Code may have been wonderful protection for the poor and swift justice for the felon, but for the practitioner "of the knife" it was nothing to write home about. Whether the Code referred to a class of practitioner other than the *asu* who performed empirical minor surgery is unknown.[39] As in the Ur-Nammu code, the *Code of*

---

[38] Roth, M. T., *Law Collections from Mesopotamia and Asia Minor*, Scholars Press, GA, 1995, p. 37. This excerpt is listed by her under the *Law of X*, which may be a fragment of the *Code of Ur-Nammu*. Prof. Roth's valuable book contains many details, translations, and qualifying statements about the status of these and other ancient Mesopotamian writings. The "shekel" in this early period refers not to a coin but to a unit of weight of a substance, in this case silver.

[39] Some scholars, including E. A. M. Budge, have described three types of early Mesopotamian practioners, those of the word (*asipu*), the herb (*asu*), and the knife, this trio of skills being described by King Ashurbanipal. But there is apparently no separate appellation for a practitioner "of the knife." Parallels between the early barber-surgeon and Budge's lowly "practitioner of the *knife*" suggest themselves. Perhaps the practitioner of the knife was merely the early *azu* or *asu* who included minor surgery among his duties. Under the Babylonians it was the *asu*, not the *asipu*, who wielded "the knife" and is specifically referred to in the Code of Hammurabi, for that is the transliterative interpretation of the text. The nature of Mesopotamian surgery has benefited from

Hammurabi does not contain laws pertaining to the *asipu*, the exorcist/internist who represented an elite arm of a powerful temple or secular government. Sanctioned by authority and working under the ensign of a deity, perhaps the *asipu* was not susceptible to secular justice.

But consider the absurdity and self-defeating purpose of the penalties mentioned in the Hammurabi Code if the *asu* were indeed providing a valued medical service. It is small wonder that the *asu*, that brave individual who dared to flourish a scalpel, disappears from the cuneiform historical record near the end of the Old Babylonian period. The usefulness and practicality of surgical skills in managing life's daily traumas has always added to the prestige of the profession of medicine. Just why surgery has generally been less regarded than internal medicine over the ages is addressed elsewhere (p. 222*ff*), but it is appropriate to note the following: the *asipu* may have edged out the *asu* in the mid-second millennium just like the "learned" European medieval and renaissance physicians managed to overshadow the barber-surgeon to the point that only in 1800 were British surgeons able to claim their own Royal College, almost 300 years after the chartering of the Royal College of Physicians.[40] For the *asipu* there also may have been an institutional religious reticence toward surgery, similar to that which later emerged from medieval monasteries in response to ecclesiastical directives.

A further perspective on the control of medical practice in Hammurabi's time can be inferred from two of the Code's regulations on crafts and trades:

> P188 – If an artisan has undertaken to rear a child and teaches him his craft, he cannot be demanded back.
> P189 – If he has not taught him his craft this adopted son may return to his father's house.

---

the painstaking assemblage of information collected by archeologists and analyzed by Dr. Majno. (Majno, G., in *The Healing Hand*, Cambridge, 1975.) It fills in the shading, to a limited extent, on the type of empirical surgery that existed. Dr. Majno notes the scarcity of any Sumerian surgical literature, from which he infers that scribes wrote only about matters complex enough to require written, rather than memorized, guidance, for an apprenticeship in minor surgery would require observation and imitation rather than study. Alternatively, those performing surgical procedures may have been commoners beneath the dignity of imperial scribes, for surgery, as manual labor, probably included draining of abscesses, extracting teeth, removing foreign bodies, and managing trauma.

[40] So that the intrinsic importance of the *asu* in Mesopotamian society can be better appreciated, it is appropriate to recount here the origin of the Western barber-surgeon, a topic relevant to this work in later chapters. In early medieval times his original task was to shave the monks. By the 13th C there were two ranks of barber-surgeons, clerical and lay, and the latter had to be examined by the former. But, as the Church incrementally prohibited clergy from performing surgical procedures (see p. 324, the Council of Tours), the lay practice soon extended to phlebotomy, cupping, tooth extraction, enemas, treating wounds, and preparing and applying plasters. The practical value of the barber-surgeon in England led to the obtaining of a Charter in 1462 from Edward IV. It was from the humble status of barber-surgeon that the great French surgeon, Ambrose Pare (1510-1590), arose, and in 1660 a French royal decree by Louis XIV united barbers and the officious surgeons into a single guild. (See F. H. Garrison's *History of Medicine*, Phila., 1913, Chapters 7 and 9.) With the advent of the teaching of human anatomy in England a barber who passed an examination in anatomy was expected to become a surgeon. Although the College of Physicians of London was founded in 1518, it was only in 1745 that barbers and surgeons were separately incorporated, a flattering statement on the usefulness of barber-surgeons in English society as recently as the mid-18th C.

Assuming medical practice was included among the crafts and trades, as it was in other ancient societies, there are corollaries: (1) Empirical surgery, as a representative craft along with potters, tailors, and masons, must have been important to society for Hammurabi himself to address its activities and even its training. (2) There must have been sufficient benefits from association with a craft or trade to warrant State regulations for preventing abuse of craft or trade membership. (3) Crafts and trades were in effect state-controlled corporations assigned to provide specified services. For example, in his translations the scholar Chilperic Edwards renders a Babylonian term for "son of the people" to mean *artisan*, implying in Hammurabi's time State control of trades and crafts.[41] (4) Controlling entry into a craft or trade, as implied in sanctions should a father demand return of the fledgling craftsman from the master craftsman, must have been necessary to restrict competition that might have occurred if the newly trained craftsman decided to set up his own shop outside of royal purview. Thus, the new craftsman's principal obligation, once trained, was to the ruling authority and his new professional family, not his biological one. As the *asu* was ranked on the same level as the innkeeper and the baker, perhaps everyone was so regulated.

E. Shift from Empirical-Rational to Mystical Medicine

The Kassites, who ruled Mesopotamia between 1595-1155 BC, left no written records in their own language, although they used variant Sumerian and Akkadian cuneiform, which remained dominant well into the 1st millennium BC, analogous to the persistence of Latin as the language of the erudite nearly up to the present day.[42] Curiously, it was in the middle of the 2nd millennium that the professional scribe also disappeared, his duties likewise subsumed by the *asipu*.[43] And it was also during this hegemony of the Kassites that the whole of Babylonia was for the first time integrated into a single State. Prior to this the region had first been divided among numerous small theocratic city-states, and then, under Hammurabi, the fragmented region was integrated commercially. But, it was the centralization of authority by the Kassites that was contemporary with final empowerment of the *asipu* and disappearance of the practical practitioner, the *asu*, and the scribe. Prof. Tzvi Abusch ascribed the situation to the "expanding role of the male *asipu* as a result of increasing centralization and stratification of the state, temple, and economy."[44] Prof. Postgate has indicated that from *ca.* 2500 to 1500 BC there was a transfer of power from the temples to the palace.[45] The significance

---

[41] Edwards, C., *The Hammurabi Code*, London, 1904, p. 71.

[42] Following its inception (*ca.* 3100 BC) the Sumerian cuneiform evolved into a syllabic script, and thus civilizations subsequent to Sumer were able to represent their own languages using the same or similar cuneiform writing.

[43] Ritter, E. K.; *Magical-expert (=ashipu) and physician (=asu): notes on two complementary professions in Babylonian medicine*, in *Assyriological Studies*, 16:299-321, 1965, mentioned under (3), p. 303. Note as well that the absence of written records during the Kassite period preceded what is now called the Mesopotamian Dark Age, estimated to have started around 1200 BC, contemporaneous with the "dark age" that followed the decline of the Mycenaean empire and preceded the appearance of classical Greece.

[44] T. Abusch, *Mesopotamian Witchcraft*, Leiden, 2002, p. 28.

[45] J. N. Postgate, *Early Mesopotamia: Society and Economy at the Dawn of History*, London, 1992. He cites as an example King Shulgi (2095-2047 BC) who placed temples under secular supervision.

of this he contends is proof that "Mesopotamian religion is politics." What might be the reason for the apparent resurgent religiosity? Perhaps it represents an example of that universal mechanism for maintaining population control described by a prominent anthropologist: "Priesthood," wrote Dr. Carleton Coon, " is 'the most efficient and least expensive agency for law enforcement' in a homogeneous community."[46] And there was indeed a resurgence of religious activity during the Kassite dynasty, and many religious temples were restored in the sacred city of Nippur. With increasing piety being fostered within the population, greater political power was being claimed by the State, a tactic to be often repeated on a vast scale by other civilizations in centuries to come. Remarkably, as will be described in the next chapter, there was in contemporary Egypt a similar regression of empiric-rational medicine that also coincided with a dominant religious movement and empowerment of the priest caste.

As previously mentioned (p. 42), the *azu/asu*, with the end of the Amorite rule and subsequent social disruption, disappeared from view during the Kassite era. The *asipu* was now on his own and without competition. But his professional armamentarium, aside from garb and mantras, was archaic medical wisdom of which the "content, arrangement, and even wording is rather constant throughout the more than one millennium attestation." Who then carried on the minor surgery, pulled the teeth, drained the abscesses, and set the fractured bones, skills so valuable to daily life? Surely it was not the esteemed *asipu*. This person did, however, expropriate some of the knowledge of the *asu* and thereby invest himself with the aura of the *asu*, "akin to the relationship between chiropractors and the medical profession's physicians today."[47] The *asu* must have persisted in some guise but was now without official relevance or recognition.

The *asu* reemerges into the written record of the Assyrians in the 1st millennium and he is again mentioned alongside the *asipu*, their relative positions and functions unchanged from what they had been 1000 years earlier.[48] It is likely that this resulted from the Assyrian need for a military medical corps. Basically a military dictatorship with its strategic objective being military conquest, the Assyrians had a genius for organization and resurrected the lowly *asu* to provide medical care for a large and widely extended army. With few exceptions, however, his status was to remain lowly.

Doctors Scurlock and Andersen, as previously mentioned, consider Mesopotamian medical writing over two millennia, despite a series of profound societal changes, to represent a continuum of progressively improving medical knowledge. Such a claim requires careful validation. A textbook containing great clinical wisdom does not require centuries to create; one or two generations will suffice. In ancient times there was little or no technology involved, and many clinical features such as jaundice, abscess formation, and blood in the urine are obvious to the laiety and professionals alike. All

---

[46] Mentioned by Herbert J. Muller in his book *Freedom in the Ancient World*, New York, 1961, p. 27.

[47] Gabriel, R. A., *Man and Wound in the Ancient World*, Washington, D.C., 2012, p. 90.

[48] Finkel, I. L., *On Late Babylonian Medical Training*, in: *Wisdom, Gods, and Literature: Studies in Assyriology in Honour of W. G. Lambert*, A. R. George and I. L Finkel, editors, Indiana, 2000, pp. 137-223. Also note that the library of an as*ipu* has been uncovered and dated to the neo-Assyrian period in the city of Assur, 912-608 BC, and relative roles and appellations of *asu* ("pharmacist") and *asipu* (now translatable as "incantation priest") were retained even into Hellenistic times (Drawnel, H., *Between Akkadian "Tupsarrutu" and Aramaic* , in *Revue de Qumran* 24:373-403), a 2000-year-old terminology with little change in meaning even though the medical function of the *asipu* suffered degradation. A similar qualitative fluctuation over an even longer period would occur with the ancient Greek ἰατρός (iatros), often translated as "physician."

that is required is a small and efficient organization of clinicians and a written language that permits subsequent generations to judge the merits of written records and improve the statistical base. The idea that Mesopotamian "physicians" were able to hone their profession in some protected niche during centuries of destruction, carnage, and pestilence under a series of authoritarian masters and their contesting armies seems unlikely. It is more likely that with each subjugation the "profession" had to begin anew, with temple professionals being selected from the newcomers or sympathetic locals at the behest of the new claimants to the throne. A mitigating and confounding factor, however, was the cuneiform record available to the *asipu* associated within the temples or royal courts. This permitted continuity of medical thought over the centuries. The Kassite Empire relied heavily on assimilating Babylonian intellectual property and devotedly embraced its religious icons and written traditions. It has been proposed that the purpose for copying of already ancient texts was "tradition maintenance" and secret wisdom. Cuneiform libraries do not appear to have been available to the *asu* who some suggest may have been, in most instances, illiterate. In contrast, libraries were available to the *asipu*, either a personal library or one attached to a temple. By analogy, ancient Egyptian scriptoria attached to temples contained papyri that were restricted to use by temple priests (p. 70). Had a cuneiform medical legacy been widely available a true clinical corpus of medical texts might have evolved, one that might have equaled that of the later Greek Hippocratic physicians. Instead, the *asu*, who began as a private practitioner and equivalent to other professionals in ancient Sumer, was gradually reduced to a lowly, segregated, and menaced passive health care provider for most of subsequent Mesopotamian history, with no chance to organize and communicate with his colleagues in an association that might have logarithmically increased medical knowledge.[49] One can only speculate on how much of Esagil-kin-apli's scribal success can be attributed to transmission of the early Sumerian *azu's* cache of clinical wisdom.[50] For, should an empire manage to persist four hundred years, as did the Kassite, there was time enough to develop an advanced system of medical care that should have set a shining example for the ages, especially if a foundation for that process had been included, as it was, among the treasures of conquest. Why that did not happen then or now is, of course, the subject of this book.

Much information on the course of Mesopotamian medicine comes from the 30,000 clay tablets found in the Royal Library of the Assyrian monarch Ashurbanipal (685-627 BC). Of the more than six hundred that pertain to medicine, many are copies of earlier texts, which is indicated by cuneiform comments on the tablets, such as "like its old copy" and "like the ancient tablets of Sumer and Akkad." Dr. Oppenheim noted that

---

[49] This face of the *asu* was not without exception, for at least one *asu* was a prominent practitioner seconded to a neighboring dominion and some temples had a *rab-asu*, or "chief physician." But it is not surprising that the *asu's* role over 3000 years would not be categorically homogeneous.

[50] Esagil-kin-apli edited in 1050 BC the *Treatise on Medical Diagnosis and Prognosis* (see p. 483, footnote). It is notable in that the scholarly editing and canonization of the archaic *Treatise* was done at the behest of a Neo-Assyrian King Adad-apla-iddina (ruled 1068-1047 BC), similar to the compilations of archaic manuscripts on ancient Chinese medicine and botany/pharmacology periodically ordered by Chinese emperors. Such amalgamations, however lionized then and now, contained little that was new, reflecting primarily a codification of traditional thinking and a desire by the head of state to develop a unified medical canon that would reflect the eminence of central government and assist it ends. Perhaps further scholarship will determine if this applies to Esagil-kin-apli's work. He was, after all, not a medical person, had no credentials to judge medical merit, and would not have been selected by a medical community to represent its views.

Old Babylonian *medical, legal, and mathematical* texts originally composed prior to 2000 BC, including the pharmacopoeia in Fig. 2, were transcribed in Sumerian cuneiform, or at least had technical terminology that was Sumerian, and the use of Sumerian technical terminology was still extant in 1st millennium Akkadian medical tablets.[51] In contrast, Old Babylonian texts on divination were never written in Sumerian.[52] These striking analyses further support the notion that practitioners of empirical and probably rational medicine existed in early Sumer. The reason more evidence of empirical or rational procedures have not been uncovered may be that, other than clay tablets, perishable writing materials were used.[53] It is unfortunate that many tablets from the Royal Library of Ashurbanipal hinting at rational medicine and describing surgical procedures, including, perhaps, the draining of an empyema of the chest, are fragmented and illegible. But in any event they are a powerful reminder of the appeal to authority, for more than ten centuries elapsed between Hammurabi and the Assyrian ruler, Ashurbanipal, and of medical progress was there none, the witnesses being these clay tablets that represented a millennium of recycling of what was even then already ancient knowledge.[54] And it is remarkable that the later Assyrians, while perhaps unaware of their own deficiencies in medical practice, seemed in the 7th C BC to credit a superiority to early knowledge, assuming that in general the older the wisdom the better it was,[55] a pattern of thinking to be repeatedly encountered in pages to follow.

The contribution to medicine by the Assyrians, therefore, particularly in the New Assyrian period (911-621 BC), rests primarily in the copying of the earlier texts of Sumer/Akkad. Even their herbal remedies, while they did include some new discoveries, were thought to function by divine fiat rather than through innate pharmacological properties. Although the designations of both *asipu* and *asu* demonstrated their durability by retaining their meanings for almost 2000 years, magic and astrology were the *modus operandi* of Assyrian practitioners. Even King Ashurbanipal himself became a scholar in reading ancient cuneiform tablets, relying on incantations for his health and for guiding his kingdom. Indeed, that was the primary reason for the vastness of his library in the first place: "I deposited them within my palace for reference and for my repeated reciting

---

[51] Oppenheim, A. L.; *Ancient Mesopotamia: Portrait of a Dead Civilization*, Chicago, 1977, chapter 6; Kramer, S. N. *The Sumerians*, Chicago, 1963. As will be discussed later, the remarkable durability of ancient medical authority is not unusual, as attested by Egyptian medical papyri and Hippocratic writings.

[52] Furthermore, Dr. Irving Finkel noted that clay tablets on Late Babylonian medical training had items referring to the *asu* written with a vertical orientation, whereas those for the *asipu's* mysticism were horizontal (Finkel, I. L., *On Late Babylonian Medical Training*, in: *Wisdom, Gods, and Literature: Studies in Assyriology in Honour of W. G. Lambert*, A. R. George and I. L Finkel, editors, Indiana, 2000, p. 146), the stylistic distinction implying significant qualitative differences in content between the two.

[53] Waddell, L. A., *The Indo-Sumerian Seals Deciphered*, a reprint by Omni Publ., California, 1980, of the 1925 publication. On p. 23 he describes the earliest Sumerian writing as being more cursive and adapted to the equivalent of pen and paper rather than the more rigid format later used for incising clay tablets.

[54] It may be relevant as well to note that there was a Sumerian "renaissance" under Ur-Nammu (reigned 2112-2095 BC) that was associated with extensive government reforms intended to ease the authoritarian abuses of the Akkadian monarchs. This "renaissance" may have provided the opportunity for a renewal of rational medical practices, and perhaps the two early tablets, the Pharmacopoeia (Fig. 2) and the *Diagnostic and Prognostic Handbook*, were evidence of that.

[55] Fincke, J. C., *The Babylonian Texts of Nineveh*, in *Arch. fur Orientforschung*, 50:111-149, 2003.

of them."[56]

By the end of Assyrian rule (612 BC) most Sumerian empirical-rational medicine had long been forgotten, except to those few practitioners attached to State or religious institutions who could read the ancient tablets. This does not imply that those practitioners were the intellectual recipients of an ever-increasing hoard of medical knowledge which they then used for the betterment of their countrymen. Instead, they were the ignorant recipients of the dregs of a barrel of medical knowledge compiled many centuries earlier and with which they knew naught what to do.

F. The Legacy of Mesopotamian Medicine

Mesopotamian civilization, over two thousand years and under a series of masters, evolved at an early stage a strict temple or state-regulated system of quasi-medical practitioners. The earliest medicine, that of Sumer, had been empirical-rational. It developed at a time when Mesopotamian society comprised autonomous city-states. It is tempting to think that significant personal liberty existed, at least for some segments of society. Its medicine was then copied by the Akkadians, nobbled by the Amorites, co-opted by the Kassites and their priests, and become barely recognizable after the fall of the Assyrians.[57] Its original practitioner, the *azu* (and subsequently *asu*) had been diminished in opportunity and significance (see Table 1). There had been a relentless regression rather than progression in medicine over 2000 years. As documentation, in mid-5th C BC Herodotus made no mention of a medical practice whatsoever during his visit to the region, as the often-quoted lines from his *History* describe the medical scene:[58]

> I come now to the next wisest of their customs: having no use for physicians, they carry the sick into the market-place; then those who have been afflicted themselves by the same ill as the sick man's, or seen others in like case, come near and advise him about his disease and comfort him, telling him by what means they have themselves recovered of it or seen others so recover.

Thus, by the time of Herodotus (484-425 BC) there were no medical professionals at all. What he had observed was the expression, perhaps in a medical free market, of the practical value of personal experience, however limited, over the mystical mind.

It should be noted that much of the regression described above occurred in the second millennium, a period of ruralization and declining population in Mesopotamia. The climatic, political, and pestilential events leading to this and how they affected the

---

[56] Saggs, H. W. F., *The Might That Was Assyria*, New York, 1990, especially Chapter 14 which is devoted to medicine. The entire library of Ashurbanipal was reserved only for himself, not the general public, and its contents were primarily devoted to mystical and religious methods that permitted his continued domination of the empire, information he had no desire to share. For bibliographical material on Ashurbanipal's library. See: Casson, L., *Libraries in the Ancient World*, New Haven, 2001, pp. 9-15.

[57] This period, however, may not have been totally devoid of empirical observations in medicine, and it has been noted that there is more frequent mention of quantitation of components of written prescriptions in the late Babylonian era than in the earlier "late Assyrian" era, although the time separating the two was not great.

[58] Herodotus, I, 197. The English translation was by A. D. Godley for the *Loeb Classical Library* series of *Herodotus*.

medical profession are unknown. But even when large areas of the Middle East were again united under the Persian monarch, Cyrus the Great (ruled *ca.* 559-529 BC), and the empire entered a period of relative stability and great prosperity, medicine as a profession did not prosper.[59] Why? So immense and bureaucratically well-run was the Great King's dominion that it has been lamented that the defeat of the Persians by the Greeks at Marathon, in preventing world hegemony by that prince and loosing democracy on the world, was the greatest calamity ever to befall humanity! Great projects were undertaken by the Persian kings, even a medical school being established at the temple of Sais (Tais) in Egypt during the reign of Darius (521-485 BC) which Breasted claimed to be "the earliest known scientific foundation of any kind". But the chief "physician" of the "medical school" at Sais was not a physician. Characterized as a "priestly aristocrat," he may even have been a naval commander whom some have considered an enemy collaborator and one who was sent by the Persian monarch as a high priest to restore the dignity of the temple after an earlier desecration.[60] The idea of a true medical school at Sais seems fanciful.

Because there are so few documents from the Old Persian period (600 BC to 300 BC, during which the pre-Islamic Persian language was in use), the principal commentary on Persian medicine is in the *Avesta*, sacred writings of the Zoroastrians wherein is described the origin of medicine and the means through which the field of medicine is useful to humanity.[61] But the *Avesta* contains nothing relevant to clinical practice or medical science. In the verses of the *Yashts* are named some "spiritual beings" that oversee health-related functions. [62] In a subsequent set of ancient texts (*ca.* 1st C BC), the *Pahlavi*, medicine is divided into surgery, herbal therapy, and prayer, the last being the most important. The superior physician was the "prayer-physician" and "the one who cures in each man the soul of its sins and the body of its sickness." Despite some clinical statements in several chapters of the Pahlavi text known as the *Dinkard*, incantations, exorcisms, and confessionals were prominent in therapies to the point that, in the 3rd C

---

[59] The adulatory history of Cyrus the Great (Κυρου Παιδειας) compiled by Xenophon (430-355 BC), makes five references to medicine. One relates to the use of poison, one metaphorically to the necessity of the physician knowing both instruments and medicines, one expressing gratitude to physicians of his friends that survived injuries, and two involved caring for wounded soldiers or prisoners in which he himself worked alongside "physicians," which would suggest they were similar to medics in a modern army. This does not, therefore, describe medicine as a profession. There is also an equivalent situation during Xenophon's incursion into Persia, as described in his ἀναβασις (*Anabasis*) when his army, which numbered perhaps ten thousand, "elected" eight "physicians" from the soldiery to attend to battlefield injuries prior to a battle. Their conception of a "physician" was obviously not ours, even though this was the time of Hippocratic physicians in the Greek homeland.

[60] This was the famous Udjahorresne (active *ca.* 525 BC), whose statue in the Vatican Museum contains a long inscription of his services, of which those services that might be expected of a "chief physician" go unmentioned. See: *Ancient Egyptian Literature*, vol. 3: *The Late Period*, Berkeley, 1980, M. Lichtheim, editor, pp. 36-40.

[61] Zoroaster was a Persian prophet. His dates are unknown, and although his birth is traditionally given as *ca.* 600 BC some scholars now place it many centuries earlier. The religion he founded, which embraced a form of monotheism, became the central religion for Persia, and Artaxerxes I established a Zoroastrian calendar in 441 BC. Following the conquests of Alexander the Great the popularity of Zoroastrianism decreased, but it still has its followers around the world. Astrology has been prominent in its writings, just as it was during the age of Persian Empire.

[62] The *Avesta*, by oral tradition, is assigned a date of *ca.* 1000 BC, but the earliest extant writings date from *ca.* 300 AD, *The Book of Arda Viraf*.

AD, the entrance of Manicheanism into Persia popularized the idea of foreswearing the ingestion of medicines entirely.[63] Such was the persuasive power of what has been called "the religious sciences."[64] Finally, even though the vastness of the Persian Empire should have provided a convenient opportunity for intellectual contact with the Indian subcontinent, Africa, and Europe, incorporation of aspects of foreign medicine did not occur. The absence of any evidence of imported medical practices from regions abutting Persia does not reflect on Persian intelligence or intransigence. It indicates, instead, that a similar state of ignorance afflicted them all.[65]

As Mesopotamia proceeded through the first millenium of the Common Era, the spread of an extensive and relatively coherent Islamic empire incorporated many aspects of preexisting cultures, including medicine. But it was the realization of the significance of earlier Greek works that became the spur for medical inquiry in the Middle East in the 9th and 10th centuries, its first prominent physicians coming from Persia. The importance of this is discussed in a later chapter, but it is perhaps a droll observation that the famed *Thousand Nights and a Night* ("The Arabian Nights"), supposedly compiled about 1000 AD, barely mentions medicine, and in one of its tales a king beheads forty physicians and crucifies forty astrologers when they failed to cure his daughter's illness, which does not speak too highly for either profession as being indispensable, and suggests that one of the principle roles of physicians at this time was to rid a person of evil Jinns, or "genies."

What an auspicious beginning was squandered. With so much that can be learned by simple clinical observation, the absence of advancing knowledge following initial inroads by the Sumerians indicates severely restricted intellectual boundaries within which subsequent Mesopotamian practitioners were permitted to work. Dr. Oppenheim has decried the loss of practical medicine in ancient Mesopotamia as a curse of written tradition: "The history of medicine all over the world demonstrates this phenomenon."[66] But it is more than a curse of "written tradition." The problem is not in the writing; it is instead the victory of impressed orthodoxy over the individual as written tradition is commandeered by despotic institutions for their own ends. As the story unfolds, the full import of this culprit will be exposed.

And so it happened that in 1871 Heinrich Schliemann was excavating for the remains of Troy near the western coast of Turkey. Because he happened to have some quinine and tincture of arnica (a medically useless counterirritant rubbed on sprains and bruises), he attracted considerable local attention as a healer. "Without possessing the slightest knowledge of medicine . . ." he did what he could to help a population that often traveled many miles for his medical assistance, for priests were the parish doctors throughout the district and they disliked washing, had no medicines, and depended on bleeding as a mainstay of treatment.[67] Although Troy is geographically slightly removed

---

[63] For those who can read the Pahlavi text see the Madan edition of Dinkard III, p. 160, II. 4-7,

[64] J. K. C., *Illnesses and Other Crises*, in: *Religions of the Ancient World*, Cambridge, 2004, S. I. Johnston, editor, p. 464.

[65] E. A. W. Budge described Mesopotamian medical practice of this age as primarily *herbalism based on magic*. Most remedies in his translation of the *Syriac Book of Medicines* (London, 1913) appear strange to moderns, and there is a large astrological component. This work, however, was probably copied in the 5th C AD from various sources, including traditional writings of Mesopotamian practitioners and Greco-Roman manuscripts, and probably does not reflect the content of early Mesopotamian pharmacopoeias. Whatever pearls of empirical knowledge existed in the writings even at this late date are lost in recitations of magical formulae.

[66] Oppenheim, A. L.; *Ancient Mesopotamia: Portrait of a Dead Civilization*, Chicago, 1977, p. 298.

[67] Schliemann, H.; *Troy and Its Remains*, London, 1875, pp. 141-2.

from the Tigris-Euphrates (Mesopotamian) river system, clinical practice in the Middle East at the end of the 19th C was decribed by Dr. Allbutt thus: "In modern Islam...Medicine is now almost wholly in the hands of the barbers; the actual cautery is in much request; and cutting for stone, and operation for cataract are in the hands of specialists as they were from time immemorial in the West."[68] After a span of 4,300 years behold the apotheosis of Sumerian medicine.

Table 1: Chronological sequence of medical practices in Mesopotamian history

Culture	Type of Practice	Nature of Governance	Practitioner
Sumerian	Empirical-rational	Autonomous city-states, theocratic	*Azu* – empirical-rational
Akkadian	Empirical-rational (copied from Sumer) and magic	Militarily linked empire	*Asipu* – mystical *Asu*–subordinate, empirical-rational
Amorite	Empirical-rational and magic	Commercially linked empire	*Asipu*– mystical *Asu* - subordinate empirical-rational (copied from Sumer with rigid control}
Kassite	Magic	Bureaucratically linked empire	*Asipu*– mystical* *Asu* disappears
Assyrian	Magic, Astrology	Monarchical Empire	*Asipu* – mystical* *Asu* reappears as military medic and herbalist
Persian	Mysticism	Monarchical Empire	*Asipu* – mystical* (vanishes)

*There is evidence that at times some of those "mystical" duties included recognition of specific disease states, a function that might be considered clinical. But within that function diseases were caused by displeasure of the gods, were associated with particular gods, and the required treatment had to be appropriate for and agreeable to the involved god. For this reason the overall function of the *asipu* is listed as "mystical."

[68] Allbutt, T. C., *The Historical Relations of Medicine and Surgery to the End of the Sixteenth Century*, London, 1905, p. 21.

CHAPTER THREE

LARGE STRUCTURED SOCIETIES, AUTHORITARIAN – NORTH AFRICA

"If thou abasest thyself in obeying a superior, thy conduct is entirely good before god. Knowing who ought to obey and who ought to command, do not lift up thy heart against him."

The Precepts of Ptah-Hotep, X, (*ca.* 2200 BC)
(Translation of Phillipe Virey, in *Records of the
Past*, Second Series, vol. III, 1890)[1]

Ancient Egyptian medicine is renowned, athough enthusiasm is not unanimous. It is the writings of the earliest dynasties, *ca.* 3000 BC, as revealed in the famous 1550 BC copies known as Papyrus Ebers and the Edwin Smith papyrus that provide insight into empirical and perhaps rational medical practices. But, appropriated by the priest caste of the State, empirical-rational medicine became manipulated canon. A mere twelve papyri grace the medicine of a 3000-year-old empire, a component of many of the twelve being but repetitions of clinical cases or sections from the Papyrus Ebers, which thereby might be considered the high point of Egyptian medicine. Despite a promising beginning, medicine in North Africa, just as in Mesopotamia, came to nothing long before the Common Era.

A. Introduction: The Reputation of Ancient Egyptian Medicine

Although there were several notable ancient civilizations in North Africa, including Ethiopian, Aksumite, Kush, Berber, and Carthaginian, the extensive and remarkably enduring Egyptian civilization is the focus of this section. The fame of ancient Egyptian medicine is great, and, while there are those who would rather describe it as pervasive, many scholars proclaim it the foundation of modern medicine.[2, 3] For example, the founding of the Kingdom, the first dynasty dating from 2925 BC, was soon followed by the earliest named physician, Imhotep (*fl.* 2667-2648 BC), a master architect and later a magician-vizir who was posthumously declared a demigod. It was he who advised Pharaoh Zoser of Dynasty III to sacrifice to the god, Khnum, in order to stop a seven-year drought and famine from "a low Nile," apparently with a good result.[4] By

---

[1] This translation is similar to that by Charles Horne in *The Precepts of Ptah-Hotep*, found in vol. 2 of *The Sacred Books and Early Literature of the East*, New York, 1917.

[2] See: *Black Athena Revisited*, Chapel Hill, 1996, Lefkowitz, M. R., and Rogers, G. M., editors, the chapter by Robert Palter, pp. 209-266, for a review of relevant references.

[3] Ghalioungui, P., *Magic and Medical Science in Egypt*, London, 1963; Bernal, M., *Black Athena Writes Back*, Durham, 2001, the latest book in a scholarly melee on the geographic origin of modern medicine; Ebbell, B., *The Papyrus Ebers*, Copenhagen, 1937.

[4] This is recorded on a Ptolemaic-era stone, the sacrifice being the ceding of some eighty miles of the Nile and adjacent land in lower Nubia. The historical accuracy is, therefore, debated. Interestingly, there are some who think that Imhotep, perhaps a foreigner in Egypt, was none other than the biblical Joseph, whose interpretation of Pharaoh's dream is described in *Genesis* 41. Also, see: Drower, M. S., *Water-Supply, Irrigation, and Agriculture*, in: Singer, C. J., *et al.*, *The History of Technology*, Oxford, 1954, vol. 1, p. 537. And as a final comment, there are also those who

1600 BC he had become the patron of scribes.[5] His importance in the history of medicine, however, appears to have been acquired long after his death, for he was deified only in the Egyptian Late Period (664-332 BC) when "physician" was added to his attributes, as described by the 3rd C BC Egyptian historian, Manetho. The rise of a supernatural being from the dust of a legendary individual is not unique; it can take centuries to achieve sainthood in the Catholic Church. But the historical record does not identify any specific medical works of Imhotep the physician.[6] A reasonable justification for his persistent glorification in the medical realm must remain obscure.

External testimony by the ancient Greeks is said to acknowledge the superiority of Egyptian medicine. One source of this opinion, the writings of the Greek poet, Homer, was composed in the 8th C BC as Greece was emerging from the presumed chaos of its Dark Ages. The Trojan War, which had been fought during the time of the Mycenaean Empire (*ca.* 1500-1200 BC), was described in part in Homer's *Iliad*. It contains vivid and accurate descriptions of battlefield trauma. Except for superficial aspects of wound care, however, there are references only to theurgical cures. The "physicians" of the *Iliad* provided no relief from Apollo's plague with which that epic poem commences, nor do they ease other diseases, a feature first commented on by Celsus, the Roman medical writer of the 1st C AD.[7] Homer's descriptions of trauma management probably reflected Hellenic methods in use at the time of his writing. One might expect, therefore, that the simple Hellenic practices would pale beside those of a 2000-year-old empire such as Egypt. Such is what Homer implied in the *Odyssey*, where there is the following statement: "Egyptian physicians, most skilled of all countries."[8] But the medicine practiced in Egypt at the time of Homer, which would have been during the 25th, or Nubian (Ethiopian), dynasty (760-656 BC), was also of a magical or religious nature. It is likely, therefore, that Homeric-age medicine was everywhere poor medicine indeed, and that Homer's opinion of Egyptian medicine represents not laudatory testimonial but poetic license, one based not on an observed superiority of Egyptian medicine in which "every man is a healer" but on wonder at the extensive canonical organization of its bureaucracy, a concept alien to the Greeks. Another testimonial, vague and indirect, is found in the *Book of Jeremiah*, where Egypt is implied as prominent for its medicines, but it speaks volumes that the Hebrews took no Egyptian medicines or medical practices with them as they left captivity (*ca.* 1400 BC).[9]

---

postulate that the Biblical Joseph, whose grandfather Abraham is thought to have lived in Mesopotamia (Ur), was an *asipu* (see preceding chapter), also a debated topic.

[5] *The Oxford Encyclopedia of Ancient Egypt*, Oxford, 1954, chapter 19.

[6] Hurry, Jamieson, *Imhotep: The Vizier and Physician of King Zoser and afterwards the Egyptian God of Medicine*, Oxford, 1926.

[7] "quos tamen Homerus non in pestilentia, neque in variis generibus morborum aliquid attulisse auxilii, sed tantumodo ferro et medicamentis mederi solitos esse proposuit." (...whom, however, Homer has stated, as not having brought any relief in plague, nor in the various kinds of diseases, but were accustomed to heal wounds only by the knife, and medicine.) Celsus, *De Medicina*, Book I, Preface, translation of J. Steggall in: *The First Four Books of Aur. Corn. Celsi De Re Medica*, London, 1837, p. 2, meaning there was treatment only of war wounds.

[8] *Odyssey*, Bk. 4.219-232, translation of A. Murray, from the *Loeb Classical Library*.

[9] Wootton, A.C., *Chronicles of Pharmacy*, London, 1910, available in a reprint by USV Pharmaceutical Corp., Tuckahoe, NY, 1972, p. 48. Wootton points out that there is no Biblical evidence that any "medical lore" was taken by the Israelites after leaving Egypt, even though the Ebers papyrus and other medical papyri were copied/written at approximately the time of Moses. He also makes the point that there is no definite Biblical evidence that the Israelites used any

B. Documentary History of Ancient Egyptian Medicine

But information about Egyptian medicine need not be sought only from foreigners. Splinting of bone fractures has been documented in the 5th Dynasty (2450 BC), and Breasted comments that there were medical texts then in use, although they have not survived the sands of time.[10] Breasted, in his famous translation of the Edwin Smith surgical papyrus (from *ca.* 1550 BC), included a photograph of a skull from 2500-3000 BC showing two perforations bored into the mandible, presumably to drain a complicated dental abscess.[11] There is also a written record of Egyptian medicine in subsequent centuries, both on stone and in medical papyri, although the Smith surgical papyrus, notable for its sensible approach to traumatic injury, is the only one exclusively anchored in empiricism. And yet Dr. Majno, a surgeon himself, has commented on the nature of Egyptian wound care, noting that nowhere is there mention of surgical incision, only surgical dressing.[12] He states also that there appears to have been no subdivision of the physician class given solely to performing surgical procedures.

There is in the Smith papyrus, however, an indication of a physician-patient relationship above and beyond the naming of a complaint and the giving of a prescription. Physical contact between physician and patient, the intimate nature of mere touching, has often been stressed as a powerful mechanism for bonding the two as together they deal with the same illness. And Dr. Majno has underscored the significance of this in his analysis of Case 47 of the Smith surgical papyrus:

> "If thou examinest a man having a gaping wound in his shoulder,...thou shouldst palpate his wound."
>
> Case 47, 1st examination. Translation of J. H. Breasted
> (Dr. Majno's wording is, "Thou shouldst lay thy hand on it.")

The injunction to the physician to "lay the hands on" is repeatedly found in other papyri, and thus Dr. Majno's interpretation seems appropriate. Even if the purpose of the contact is merely estimating the physical extent of a wound, such palpation cannot be impersonal. It is far simpler to ignore than to become involved in another's tragedy, especially if risk is involved. Humaneness is implied in Case 47, and it is also a feature of the other cases cited in the papyrus, including Case 2.[13] And so it is from Egypt that an essential virtue

---

medications other than topical ones. "Go up to Galaad, and take a balm for the virgin daughter of Egypt; in vain hast thou multiplied thy medicines; there is no help in thee." *Jeremiah* 46:11, in the Septuagint. Gilead, of course, was in Palestine, and it is the "multiplied thy medicines" (ἐπλήθυνας ἰάματα σου) reference that implies an Egyptian connection. See *The Natural State of Medical Practice: An Isagorial Theory of Human Progress*, Maitland (FL), 2019, p. 117, for more details of Hebrew medicine after the exodus.

[10] See: Breasted, J. H., *Reign of Neferkerere*, in: *Ancient Records of Egypt*, Chicago, 1906, vol. 1, pp. 111-113.

[11] Breasted, J. H. (1865-1935), *The Edwin Smith Surgical Papyrus*, Chicago, 1930, two vols. The recto of the papyrus describes 48 surgical cases, diagnosis and treatment. The verso includes a magical incantation that Breasted concluded was unrelated to the empirical surgical text.

[12] Majno, G., *The Healing Hand*, Cambridge (MA), 1975, chapter 3.

[13] An interesting point about the instruction to palpate is that it represents a standard directive to the intended reader to personally and physically involve himself in care of the sick one, rather than to manage the case indirectly or at a distance through an intermediary or incantation. The reader is therefore assumed to be a "real doctor," *i.e.*, a fellow professional and clinician.

of medical practice can first be historically identified. This is not a simple issue, however, and concern for friends and family has always found expression. Despite the absence of a directive for their use, the Sumerian *azu* with his bronze scalpels obviously had physical patient contact, suggesting the motive of humaneness. Evidence of concern may even exist among nonhuman primates such as the chimpanzees described in the opening chapter of Dr. Majno's remarkable book,[14] although it has been argued that the motive for that aid tended to be pleasure rather than empathy, and gorillas appear to display grief.

In a similar vein, Breasted gives credit to the ancient Egyptians for deriving a basis for moral principles outside of medicine, for such was expressed as part of the worship of Ptah, the Sun-god. This probably preceded the First Dynasty, *ca.* 3000 BC, but can only be verified from later historical evidence. Breasted concluded that the Nile Valley was "a unique arena," a place of "human brotherhood and friendliness" to which man had arisen from the "bestial savagery of physical man." He gives no medical implications of his opinion.[15] But it is an unreasonable assumption that friendship and concern for others could have been derived from only one place and one point in time. Human virtues, not assigned to nucleotide sequences in DNA, have surely been around since the origin of humanity itself, and their expression in the First Dynasty merely reflects a technical innovation, writing, that could for the first time transmit evidence of their existence. As Samuel Johnson viewed virtue and the human condition, "Prudence and justice are virtues and excellencies of all time, and all places. We are perpetually moralists, but we are geometricians only by chance." We are humane by design, bestial by circumstance.[16]

With but two other exceptions, all medical papyri so far discovered contain magical incantations. One of those exceptions is the Kahun papyrus, a series of thirty-four clinical scenarios and treatments relevant, in part, to gynecology that are resistant to knowledgeable modern interpretation.[17] The other is the *Papyrus Ebers*.[18] Like the Smith papyrus, it was transcribed about 1550 BC, the original manuscript perhaps dating to *ca.* 3000 BC. In it the ancient Egyptian term for physician, *swnw*, was given to those who practiced conventional medicine, in contrast to the priests and magicians, although modern opinions support the notion that differences among physician, priest, and magician may have been more quantitative than qualitative. Dr. Jamieson Hurry noted that, while there were twelve "spells" mentioned in the Ebers papyrus, even in these it can be inferred that their purpose was intended for psychological assistance. He appreciated the apparent ancient Egyptian use of magical rituals for psychological needs of the patient, particularly if there was not a cure for a particular affliction, in which case the person casting the "spells" should have understood that humaneness rather than cure was their

---

[14] Majno, G., *The Healing Hand*, Cambridge (MA), 1975, pp. 10-14.

[15] Breasted, J. H., *The Dawn of Conscience*, New York, 1933, chapter on Nature and Friendliness.

[16] The relevance of this and "natural law" is explored in depth in Part II of this book.

[17] The *Kahun* papyrus, dating from 1825 BC and dealing with gynecology, contraception, and pregnancy testing, contains procedures such as vaginal fumigation and the infamous instilling of crocodile excrement for contraception. Still, only one incantation is present.

[18] Translation of the Ebers papyrus has posed problems. Although a replica was published by Ebers, it was translated from the original hieratic into German by Joachim in 1890, from which it was then translated into English by C. P. Bryan, an effort considered to be unsatisfactory. Then Wreszinski transcribed the hieratic into hieroglyphic in 1913, and it was from the latter that B. Ebbell made his 1937 English translation. Publication of a more knowledgable translation is awaited, an undistributed one by Ghalioungui being mentioned by John Nunn in his *Ancient Egyptian Medicine*, London, 1996, found in the Red River Books edition, 2002, on p. 31.

intent.[19] A list of other medical papyri is provided below.[20]

Traditional thinking concludes that Papyrus Ebers was written for the equivalent of the specialist in internal medicine, the modern-day "internist," whereas the Smith papyrus was for those dealing with surgical illness. And Dr. Chauncey Leake pointed out that in the Ebers papyrus eighty percent of the oral therapies are quantitated, whereas only thirty percent of topical therapies are so treated.[21] This implies a rational attempt to avoid iatrogenic toxicities. The ancient Egyptian use of honey and copper salts, both having antibacterial qualities, was intentional pharmacotherapy, not mysticism, that helped wound healing.[22] It has been calculated that the average number of ingredients in the recipes of the Papyrus Ebers was 4.2, and that many of its prescriptions contained at least one component, primarily herbal, that would be expected to produce a physiological or pharmacological effect.[23] Lest it be concluded, however, that a scientific Egyptian pharmacopoeia existed, it is appropriate to consider the basis of herbal medicine. It takes no effort at all to seek out a biologically active botanical. The first to come to hand will be such, for there is no such thing as a biologically inactive living entity.[24] This provides

---

[19] Hurry, Jamieson, *Imhotep: The Vizier and Physician of King Zoser and afterwards the Egyptian God of Medicine*, Oxford, 1926.

[20] The *Hearst* papyrus from about 1450 BC contains much that is similar to or the same as Papyrus Ebers, along with incantations. The *Chester Beatty* papyri of the 13th C BC include many magical and religious incantations and a section on diseases of the anus, the function of which was so central to Egyptian medical theory at that time. The *Berlin* papyrus, also 13th C BC, contains much material found in Papyrus Ebers plus sections on vaguely defined breast diseases and on fertility tests. The *London* papyrus is primarily magical, although it has parallels to Papyrus Ebers. Papyrus *Carlsberg VIII* may be from the 13th C BC and involves sex of the fetus, ability to conceive, and items mentioned in the Kahun papyrus. The *Ramesseum* papyri include three that deal with medicine. Mostly magical, there are sections on diseases of children and women, the earliest of the three apparently being more empirical in its advice. See: Nunn, J. F., *Ancient Egyptian Medicine*, London, 1996, p. 34*ff*. Also see the slightly longer listing of papyri in *Medicine in the Days of the Pharoahs*, B. Halioua and B. Ziskind, Cambridge, 2005, endmatter, p. 189, translated by M. B. DeBevoise. A similar list of the important medical papyri and relevant discussion are found in: Nunn, J. F. and Tapp, E., *Tropical Diseases in Ancient Egypt*, in *Trans. Royal Soc. Trop. Med. and Hygiene*, 94:147-153, 2000. There is also a 2nd C AD papyrus from Egypt, the *Anonymous Londinensis*, that was brought to the British Museum in 1891. It is a recounting of earlier Greek medical writings, mentions Hippocrates, is written in Greek, and is valuable for the light it sheds on Greek rather than on Egyptian medicine.

[21] Leake, C., *An Historical Account of Pharmacology to the Twentieth Century*, Illinois, 1975, p. 51.

[22] Honey as an effective anti-infective agent will be mentioned several times in this work, so it should be made clear at the onset that honey can harbor dormant spores of some bacteria and molds, the significance of which is under investigation. At present it is not to be given to infants.

[23] See the review of Parkins, M. D., *Pharmacological Practices of Ancient Egypt*, in: *Proceedings of the 10th Annual History of Medicine Days*, W. A. Whitelaw, editor, Calgary, 2001, p. 5-11. For an older but insightful discussion of the Egyptian pharmacopoeia as extracted from papyri see: Leake, C., *The Old Egyptian Medical Papyri*, Lawrence (KA), 1952, a Logan Clendening Lecture on the History and Philosophy of Medicine, second series.

[24] The ancients were well aware of this. After seven years apprenticeship Jivaka (later to be named one of India's great physicians and personal physician to the Buddha) was given the following test by his Master: "Bring me all local plants that are not medicinal!" When Jivaka reported back that he had not come across any plant that had no medicinal qualities, his Master informed him he had passed the test. (Cited by Mookerji, R. K., *Ancient Indian Education*, London, 1947, Chapter 11.) Mankind has carried on a perpetual search for active botanicals. Some think the use of cinchona

enormous confidence to those who deal with botanicals and who claim that biologically significant activity can rightfully be attributed to their particular botanical product of interest, for they know that somewhere will be proclaimed, if not today, then tomorrow, a biochemical basis for that claim, whether real or not. The primitive empiricist could take leaves or roots from any plant and be assured that something would happen if he ingested enough of it. Indeed, the most critical step in the empirical search for botanicals as food and medicine is not the identification of efficacy but the avoidance of toxicity.[25] This is still with us today in "health foods" and in the daily expositions by the news media, for their *avant-garde* recommendations, while advertised as promoting healthful foods, often can be more correctly viewed as advising experimental dietary alternatives. The purpose of this sermon is to point out that every botanical, indeed every living thing, contains an enormous range of biologically active molecules in order to be a living thing, and most of those molecules are found in every other living thing, plant or animal, although their proportions and activities vary.

Expert opinion holds that the Ebers and Smith papyri of *ca.* 1550 BC are actually copies of medical treatises composed many centuries earlier. For the Ebers papyrus that date may have been as early as the 1st dynasty (*ca.* 3000 BC), and for the Smith papyrus it may have during the Old Kingdom (3rd through the 6th Dynasties, *ca.* 2686-2134 BC).[26]

---

bark for fevers, from which was derived quinine for malaria, was a Western hemisphere discovery of the remote past, although there is no supporting documentation that the Incas knew anything of its medicinal value, just as it is unproven that malaria existed in pre-Columbian America. Others, therefore, date its discovery to the Jesuits working in Peru in the early 17th C, for wherever the Jesuits went one of their activities was to acquire knowledge of local flora and fauna, which included a search for substances of medicinal value. The bitter taste of the cinchona tree bark may have prompted them to assess its therapeutic potential. See: Taylor, N., *Cinchona in Java; The Story of Quinine*, New York, 1945, chapter 3. Corporations and individuals today continue a worldwide search for therapeutic botanicals.

[25] Hippocratic works frequently mention "strong" foods (τὰ ἰσχυρότατα μάλιστα, "those especially strong [or virulent, harsh, dangerous]," *Ancient Medicine* VI, 16). "Strong" thus used implies toxicity, not physical state or taste, as such foods "treat with indignity both the healthy and the sick" (λυμαίνεσθαι τὸν ἄνθρωπον καὶ τὸν ὑγιᾶ ἐόντα καὶ τὸν κάμνοντα. *Ancient Medicine* VI, 17-18. Translation by the author.)

[26] Edwin Smith (1822-1906) was an American expatriate who profited from buying and selling ancient Egyptian artifacts. He was a competent amateur in reading hieratic script. In 1862 he bought several papyri from some grave robbers for £12. One, containing forty-eight surgical settings, is famously known as the Edwin Smith Surgical Papyrus. Another he sold to Prof. Georg Ebers (1837-1898) . It contained, in 877 numbered paragraphs, a potpourri of texts and recipes relevant to internal medicine. It is the now famous Papyrus Ebers. The reason the two papyri are thought to be copies of much more ancient works is that antiquated hieroglyphic terms are used that prompted explanatory glosses at a later date. This is fascinating, especially for the Smith papyrus, now thought to have been copied from an Old Kingdom original, for the 6th Dynasty is thought to represent a transition period into the First Intermediate Period of Egyptian history. The latter period was a divisive time, with local leaders replacing the Pharaoh of a no longer unified Egypt. The lower classes began to acquire tastes previously restricted to the aristocracy. Art of the period, while less refined, reflected the now unfettered efforts of those formerly unable to acquire it. This easing of constraints on individual effort may have coincided with the original compositions from which the Smith papyrus would later be copied. It is also remarkable that this coincides with the Papyrus *Prisse* in which the virtuous life is described for the first time, *ca.* 2200 BC. For this bit of history and a translation of "*The Instruction of Ptahhotep*" from Papyrus *Prisse* see: Lichtheim, M., *Ancient Egyptian Literature, vol. 1, The Old and Middle Kingdoms*, California, 1973, p. 5*ff* and p. 61*ff*.

It is possible, therefore, that in the formative years of ancient Egypt empirical medicine was practiced in predynastic communities, a point made in Part II of this work. Support for this hypothesis was recently strengthened by the finding of amphorae from 3150 BC that contained traces of herbal wines.[27] If confirmed it would suggest that alcohol extraction of medicinal herbs was known to practitioners at this early date, a procedure also known to the early Sumerian *azu*. The Ebers papyrus implies this type of medicine was useful, and thus that papyrus from 1550 BC was apparently restating what had been known 1500 years earlier. This would be objective evidence that other items in the Ebers papyrus could have been from that earlier date. What was Egyptian society like 5000 years ago and who were its medical practitioners?

With an increasing population in the region of the Nile the necessity for irrigation to support farming led, in predynastic Egypt, to group cooperation and development of small communities with local leaders.[28] Subsequently, during the Naqada II period, 3500-3300 BC, there was a coalescence of populations into towns and small cities, the rise of specialists in many fields including metalworking, new artistic endeavors, and inequality of wealth. There were sufficient regional differences to support the notion of an Upper and a Lower Egypt, the latter distributed about the Nile delta and being more agricultural and thereby more diffuse and egalitarian in social structure. That area was also especially exposed to trade with the Levant and elsewhere. Upper Egypt, in contrast, developed more rapidly, the population collected into fewer and larger settlements, hierarchical leadership was more pronounced, and a considerable differential in wealth was evident in house size and burial arrangements. Ultimately Upper Egypt came to dominate the Lower to form dynastic Egypt. Of interest are indications about this time (Naqada I-II periods) of Mesopotamian influence in architecture and design.[29] And it is this social background that may have promoted the accumulation of empirical medical knowledge by local practitioners.[30]

The nature of predynastic medical practice can only be inferred from later writings and peripheral sources, and there are precious few of these. There is no candidate available for the presumptive prehistoric practitioner, nor is there information on his clinical procedures and medicines. Dr. Richard Sullivan has reviewed the evidence for early surgical efforts ("proto-surgery") during this era, and he concludes (1) that as there is no evidence for opiate use for analgesia/anesthesia down to at least 2000 BC, even though they were in use in surrounding regions, and if anything at all was used it probably was alcohol intoxication, although in the Ebers and Smith papyri no suggestion of

---

[27] McGovern, P. E., *et al.*, *Ancient Egyptian Herbal Wines*, in *Proc. Nat. Acad. Sci.*, 106:7361-7366, 2009.

[28] For a review of this period see: David, A. R., *The Ancient Egyptians: Beliefs and Practices*, Portland, OR, 1998, 2nd edition.

[29] For evidence of considerable Mesopotamian influence in early (primarily predynastic) Egypt see: Rice, M., *Egypt's Making: The Origins of Ancient Egypt 5000-2000 BC*, London, 2003, 2nd edition, chapter 2. As for a mechanism for transmitting that influence Rice states: "It is significant that all the principal archeological evidence which indicates contact with Mesopotamia and western Asia is found in the predynastic and Early Dynastic sites which are concentrated along this stretch of the Nile." That region is the Wadi Hammamat, a natural course leading from the Red Sea to the Nile in the vicinity of Naqada.

[30] Despite the statement in the preceding chapter on Mesopotamian medicine that there was no reason to consider it in any way subordinate to Egyptian medicine, one cannot but wonder about the converse, and that the anonymous predynastic source of clinical material that found its way into the Smith and Ebers papyri was, in fact, the *azu*.

sedation is mentioned, (2) no evidence of a therapeutic incision or surgical scar had been found in examinations of 90,000 mummies as noted in Dr. Rowling's 1986 report, nor have knives or other medical instrumentation ever been recovered, suggesting that true surgical procedures must have been uncommon and perhaps forbidden,[31] (3) there is no evidence of trephining, despite its use in nearby Jericho and in contemporary Europe and England, and (4) antisepsis was probably used based on the contents of salves and ointments as listed in later writings.[32] This is consistent with the Smith papyrus, which, as noted by Dr. Majno, mentions no "invasive" procedures, only wound dressings.[33] Thus the limited information on medical practices that predate dynastic medicine does not support the notion of professional surgeons as presently understood unless, as postulated by Dr. Sullivan, they practiced in secret to avoid temple or palace imperatives. But there must have been some type of medical practitioner, for there not to have been would seem an inexplicable anomaly in any large society.

From this postulated nebulous beginning must have come the medical knowledge that found its way into the Ebers and Smith papyri. That is to say Papyrus Ebers contains in its eight hundred prescriptions and incantations the accumulated wisdom of Egyptian empirical internal medicine of at least 5000 years ago.[34] It can be considered the equivalent of a "Harrison's" textbook of Egyptian medical practice for 2500 years, and, also like "Harrison's," it is considered a collection of writings by different authors.[35] But the origin of the ancient but insightful Ebers papyrus is unknown. Perhaps it represents the thoughts of predynastic practitioners during an age yet unencumbered by pharaonic or priestly directives. One might even suspect a Mesopotamian origin for the work, so patent is the dearth of medical information from other Egyptian sources. The more important point, however, is that papyrus Ebers conclusively documents, like Ashurbanipal's library of clay tablet copies of 1500-year-old Sumerian medicine in Mesopotamia, no advance in Egyptian medicine over the same period.[36] In fact, as shall now be shown, there is good evidence that a monumental decline

---

[31] Rowling, J. T., *Some Speculations on the Rise and Decline of Surgery in Dynastic Egypt*, in *Science in Egyptology*, A. R. David, editor, Manchester, 1986, p. 399-412.

[32] Sullivan, R., *Proto-Surgery in Ancient Egypt*, in *Acta Medica*, 41:109-117, 1998.

[33] Majno, G., *The Healing Hand*, Cambridge (MA), 1975, p. 86.

[34] Dr. John Nunn, in his *Ancient Egyptian Medicine* (London, 1996), states that paragraph 856a of Papyrus Ebers provides a reference from about 3000 BC. Papyrus Ebers is thought to have been derived from several medical texts and is not coherently organized. In contrast to the Smith papyrus there is no attempt at prognosis. Near the end of the papyrus are several indications for surgery other than trauma.

[35]Harrison's *Principles of Internal Medicine*, first published in 1950 by Dr. Tinsely R. Harrison (1900-1978) while Chief of the Department of Medicine, Univ. of Alabama, is now in its 16th edition and describes 4,700 diseases and disorders in 2,607 pages. It weighs 9.5 pounds and is the most widely used medical textbook in the world. New editions are released about every three years, whereas the Ebers papyrus text has had only one edition in 5000 years, some abridgements excepted. The multiple authorship of the Ebers papyrus represents a composite of unrelated medical statements rather than a planned and focused scholarly treatise such as the modern Harrison's textbook of medicine and the ancient Edwin Smith papyrus. The ancient Chinese medical classic, the *Huang Ti Nei Ching Su Wen*, is also a composite, but, as will be discussed at length in the next chapter, it may represent a reassembly of fragments of a lost ancient original.

[36] Indeed, most of the tablets in Ashurbanipal's library are now known to have been looted from Babylon or confiscated by Ashurbanipal from other sources, and their use was for the him alone, a "library" in name only, not reflecting of a period of enlightenment but instead being an "omen

in the quality of medicine actually took place. That decline has received little attention, however, for the emphasis on the good sense found in the Smith and Ebers papyri has been overwhelmingly portrayed as representing Egyptian medicine as a whole, which it surely does not.[37]

C. The Disappearance of Empirical-Rational Egyptian Medicine

To understand the failure of Egyptian medicine to progress beyond its primitive empirical-rational beginnings, the chronological sequence for medical discovery as perceived by the modern mind must first be reviewed. (1) In its earliest stage, medical discovery is expected to be "empirical," which is to say, based on pragmatic trial-and-error. (2) In the second stage, as discovered knowledge accumulates beyond what each person can experience or manage, specialists are defined in society, and their job is to bring together the successes and failures of the trial and error approach. This advance is also pragmatic, but, because reason and practical choice among alternative substances are involved, it can now be called "rational." (3) The most advanced stage is the "scientific," and, although varied procedures assist to this end and at times extend the original knowledge to include a new area, it is basically through confirmation that exactitude in technique and certitude in result are more closely approximated, the exactness and certainty providing a solid basis, in modern research, for a working hypothesis that may lead to a theory and ultimately to a fundamental principle.[38] The spectrum covered by the three stages is one of degree of a process, that process being improvement in the quality of knowledge. In this scheme, experimentation is by no means restricted to "scientific," for empirical medicine is nothing if not experimental. Furthermore, confirmation of an experiment is but another experiment. The terms "empirical," "rational," and "scientific," therefore, at least in the context of clinical medicine, represent a continuum of improvement in the quality, not quantity, of knowledge. The types of medicine they represent, as well as modern definitions of the terms themselves, overlap to an extent, but the three terms as defined will be frequently used in the pages to follow.

Returning to the subject of Egyptian medicine, empirical medicine may have evolved to the rational stage in the predynastic period and the early dynasties, if modern scholarship is correct about the source of the information found in the Ebers and Smith papyri.[39] This is similar to evidence of rational Sumerian medicine that is inferred from

---

reference library" for management of the empire (L. Casson, *Libraries in the Ancient World*, New Haven, 2001, p. 15).

[37] Not only is literary support for an advanced ancient Egyptian medical practice based on fragile evidence, but Breasted commented in his introductory notes (Breasted, J. H., *The Edwin Smith Surgical Papyrus*, Chicago, 1930, two vols., p. 10) that the Smith papyrus may well have been known earlier as *The Secret Book of the Physician*, an indication that what little medical knowledge was available was closeted for the use of an elite few. But there are contrary views regarding a regressive Egyptian medicine, and an interesting and well-stated but still unconvincing review can be consulted: see Ritner, R. K., *Innovations and Adaptations in Ancient Egyptian Medicine*, in *J. Near Eastern Studies*, 59:107-117, 2000.

[38] This sequence is nicely discussed by J. W. Powell in *Darwin's Contributions to Philosophy*, included in C. F. Holder's book *Charles Darwin, His Life and Work*, New York, 1899, p. 214.

[39] There is apparently a more recent opinion that the Smith papyrus is a copy of a text only a few centuries older than the extant manuscript (which belongs to the New York Academy of Medicine), being composed shortly *after* the end of the Old Kingdom.

the few medical tablets of the late 3rd millennium and the copied tablets in the library of Ashurbanipal in 7th C BC Nineveh. Such wisdom accumulated in the early Egyptian dynasties should not have disappeared overnight, and it did not. But it was permitted no healthy longevity, for one of the consequences of the stabilization of the great Egyptian empire was the intertwining of medicine with government agencies, in this case the priesthood.[40] That unhealthy mix led to a usurpation of a nascent medical profession by the pharaonic families and priests, and thence forward all "physicians" would be priests. As a consequence there was a transformation of medicine not from rational to the scientific, but from rational to irrational, or magical, medicine. From approximately 2500 BC to the time of its subjugation by the Persians 2000 years later Dr. Nunn concluded there was no change in content of Egyptian medical practice, an optimistic assessment.[41] There is an artistic parallel, as suggested in Fig. 4 where the figures on the Narmer Pallette (3100 BC, predynastic) can be compared to those of the Pyramidion of Wedjahor (630 BC, Late Kingdom, perhaps the 26th dynasty). Little stylistic change is apparent over a period of 2500 years, although craftmanship has clearly deteriorated.

In the early dynasties, Egyptian "physicians," identified as *swnw*, were divided into many classes, including the simple physicians, physician inspectors, chief physicians, palace physicians, inspectors of palace physicians, and chief palace physicians, and as centuries passed many subspecialties were identified, including eye doctors, belly doctors, and anus doctors. There was also a hierarchy of administrative physicians and royal physicians, including the "chief of doctors to the queen." Nunn has estimated that half of the named physicians in the Old Kingdom had some association with the royal house. At various times a *swnw* inspected the butchers, examined sacrificial animals, provided scribal services, was in charge of "liquids" (perhaps referring to urine examinations), provided dental care, veterinary services, and undertook priestly duties. It seems the *swnw* provided a range of services so broad that even "health care provider" inadequately comprehends them. The term "physician," therefore, is misleading in this context for it lends the prestige of a modern physician to an Egyptian medical profession, if indeed such a profession existed, that it does not deserve. There was a class of priest physicians superior to the *swnw* but their function was religious rather than clinical, so the appellation of "physician" to them also is problematical. At least superficially there

---

[40] Pharaohs from the very beginning of dynastic Egypt were considered representatives of god, a justification for their monumental pyramids. Thus, they held both secular and divine dominance over the population, one of their titles being "High priest of every temple" in the land. The next layer of priesthood, selected by the Pharaohs, often had both religious and bureaucratic responsibilities within the government. From these a chief priest was assigned to individual temples. Some appointments became hereditary. Peter Clayton (*Chronicle of the Pharaohs*, London, 2006) states that in 1080 BC the Amun priesthood owned two-thirds of all temple land and ninety percent of the ships plus "many other resources," at times being more powerful than the pharaohs. The idea that Egyptian priests were both devout practitioners of a hallowed religion and pious ascetics who served the spiritual needs of their congregations is incorrect. Priests were an essential component of government that comprised both legislative and judicial components, for the Pharaoh was considered both the "upholder of Ma'at," goddess of law and order, and the chief administrator of government, and priests were his minions. It has been estimated that at one point approximately twenty percent of the population was involved in maintaining the religious institutions of ancient Egypt, a remarkable category for such a bevy of civil servants. The present number of government employees (federal, state, local) in the United States is approximately eight percent of the total population.

[41] Nunn, J. F., *Ancient Egyptian Medicine*, London, 1996, p. 206.

is a resemblance between the priest physician and the *swnw* in Egypt and the *asipu* and the *asu* in Mesopotamian medicine. But lacking from the historical record is information about the practitioner outside the palace or temple environment who cared for the commoners. Could the early *swnw* prior to the centralization of power in the hands of early pharaohs have had a role similar to the early Mesopotamian community *azu* prior to the arrival of the *asipu*?

In vain does one look for meaningful descriptions of medical practice originating during the Middle Kingdom, the 2nd Intermediate Period, the New Kingdom, and the 3rd Intermediate Period, spanning the years 2080-664 BC. The deficiency is notable as well in dentistry, for, despite the presumed drainage of a mandibular abscess in 3000 BC mentioned by Breasted in his publication of the Smith papyrus, a survey of dental specimens from 6000 individuals interred in Nubian cemeteries and spanning approximately 3000 years of Egyptian history revealed not a single instance of dental manipulation.[42]

On the other hand, mysticism, always evident in Egyptian medicine where it is likely that all "physicians" were priests, became increasingly prominent as the centuries passed.[43] The appearance of particularly pious theocratic governments of the New Kingdom (1570-1085 BC) set the stage for a fully developed medical priesthood, and the Ramesside collections of papyri, dating from approximately 1300 BC, contain only magical therapies. At this point recall that the Sumerian/Akkadian "physician," *i.e., asu*, disappeared from Babylonian cuneiform writings at about this same time during a similar period of religious revival (p. 42*f*).

With the Late Dynastic Period (664-332 BC) the prominence of the priest physician and magicians persisted, along with an increase in animal worship and tomb decoration. The *swnw* now included embalming among his chores. At this time there was a resurgence of Egyptian prosperity. Foreign commerce was permitted and Greek mercenaries were employed to put down rebellions. Despite the prosperity it is notable that no medical manuscripts whatever are available from the Late Period, although it must be acknowledged that there was a disruption of society upon entry of the Persians beginning in 525 BC.[44] Research has revealed that there was actually a relative decline in the number of named physicians.[45] And so, after 2500 years, ample time for development, Egyptian medicine had come to nothing. Despite the considerable attention Egyptians focused on their *swnw* and personal hygiene, Warren Dawson wrote that the ancient Egyptians were "incapable of abstract thought," and the value of their medical

---

[42] This study (*The Archaeological Survey of Nubia 1907-1908, ii; Report on the Human Remains*, G. E. Smith and F. W. Jones, 1910) is cited and augmented by A. Ruffer. See: *Study of Abnormalities and Pathology of Ancient Egyptian Teeth*, in *Amer. J. Phys. Anthrop.*, 3:335-382, 1920.

[43] Much of the information in this paragraph comes from Chapter 6 of a superb book: Nunn, J. F., *Ancient Egyptian Medicine*, Norman (OK), 2002.

[44] This is surprising because there are stones at Abu Simbel that were inscribed by Greek mercenaries from Kolophon, Teos, and Ialysus in 590 BC. Furthermore, these Greek cities were not considered wealthy and therefore less likely have a well-educated populace, for it was the poorer cities that were the source of mercenaries. See: Dunham, A. G., *The History of Miletus*, London, 1915. It appears that Egyptian literacy was, at that time, far behind that of Greece.

[45] P. Ghalioungui, in *Magic and Medical Science in Egypt*, London, 1963, states the numbers to be: Old Kingdom – 52, Middle Kingdom – 20, New Kingdom – 40, Late Period – 15. Hippocrates (460-380 BC) would have lived during the later 26th and into the 27th dynasties of the Late Period.

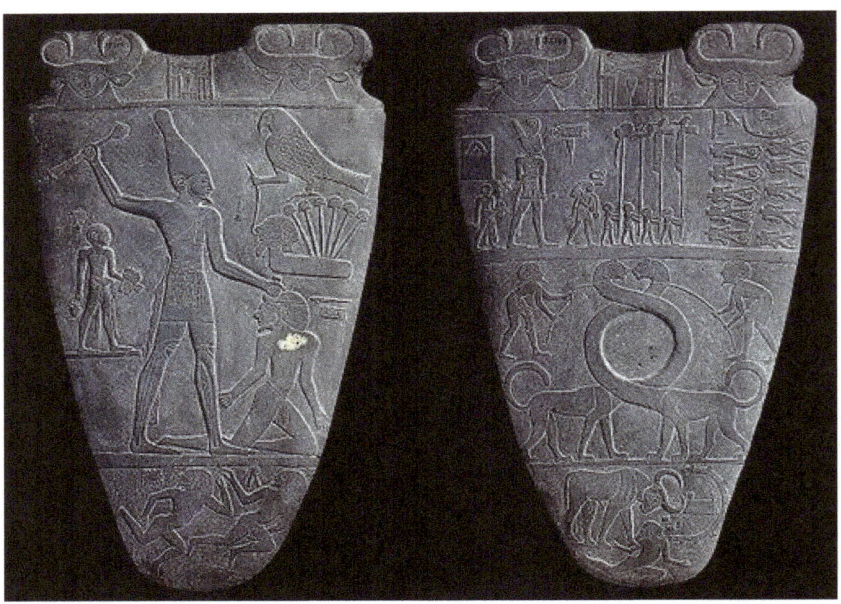

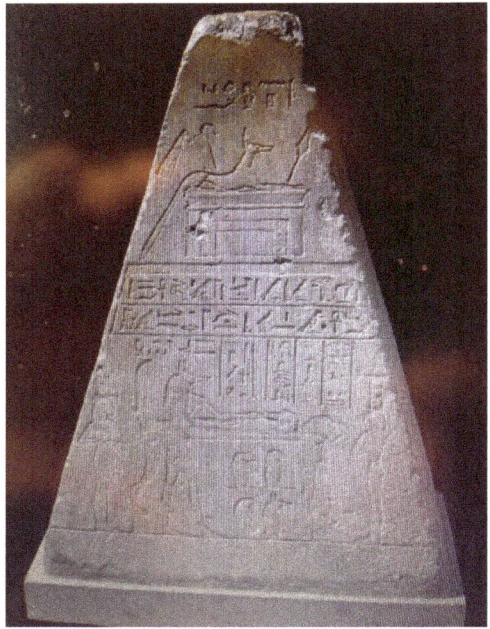

Fig. 4: Top - Photograph of the Narmer Pallette, approximately two feet tall and dated to about 3100 BC, which some think documents the joining of Upper and Lower Egypt under a predynastic or early dynastic king. It was found in Hierakonpolis on the Nile, 100 miles from the ancient Red Sea port along the trading route known as Wadi Hammamat. Bottom – Photograph pyramidion Wedjahol, also two feet tall, the topmost stone of a pyramid, the 7th C BC burial site of a wealthy New Kingdom individual. Compare its style and artistry with the Narmer Palette, 2500 years older. Photo credits: Top: public domain, Wikimedia Creative Commons; Bottom: British Museum, license of Creative Commons.

texts he deemed to be historical rather than medical.[46]

The subject, however, was not entirely forgotten. Midway in the Late Period (*ca.* 440 BC), Herodotus wrote on the subject of Egyptian medicine:

> The art of medicine among them is distributed thus: - each physician is a physician of one disease and of no more; and the whole country is full of physicians, for some profess themselves to be physicians of the eyes, others of the head, others of the teeth, others of the affections of the stomach, and others of the more obscure ailments.[47]

Herodotus was not describing a plethora of subspecialists of rational medicine in a population so well served it should have lived forever. It was, instead, a plethora of civil servants invoking archaic medical and mystical canon, a national health service in which all practitioners were under direction of the State.[48]

After the death of Alexander the Great in 323 BC Egypt was under the hegemony of the Greek Ptolemys (323-30 BC). By means of taxation they supported native practitioners in the royal medical service and those carrying out sanitary duties such as burials. But the practice of Greek (Hippocratic) medicine served only the Greek population of Alexandria, not the native population.[49] And so Prof. Rostovtzeff writes, "As regards the "laoi" [the common people in the East and in Egypt, who were, in effect, the king's tenants], I am afraid that it was left to the gods and the priests to help them die in peace."[50]

To advance the timeline further, in the 1st C BC Diodorus Siculus noted that Egyptian physicians were required to follow historical therapies, at least if they were to receive public funds, and infractions were punishable by death, a testament to fully deployed authoritarian coercion applied even to benevolent effort. Egypt had been under Greek (Ptolemaic) rule for almost three centuries, during which time the Greek colony of Alexandria became known as a center for medical research and perhaps training. But political administration under the Ptolemies had been structured according to language, with bureaucratic dominance being accorded the Greek-speaking population. As Nunn points out, the first Ptolemy to speak Egyptian was Cleopatra VII (69-30 BC). Thus, traditional Egyptian medicine, rather than Greek (Hippocratic) medicine, continued to be practiced among the general population. Diodorus states:

---

[46] Stated in an essay by Dawson, W.R., in *Science, Medicine and History*, London, 1953, E. A. Underwood, editor. Prof. Halliday came to a similar conclusion. He praised the Egyptian pyramids as masterpieces of empiricism, "but they were, at the least, repetitive in their construction," and the two civilizations of Sumer and Egypt "hardly ventured beyond patient empiricism." Halliday, W. R., *The Growth of the City-State*, Boston, 1923, p. 17.

[47] Herodotus, *Histories*, II.84. Translation of G. C. Macauley in *The Histories of Herodotus*, London, 1890.

[48] Jonckheere, F., *Les Medicins de l'Egypte Pharaonique*, Brussels, 1958, pp, 95-137, as referenced by von Staden, H., *Herophilus: The Art of Medicine in Early Alexandria*, Cambridge, 1989, p. 23 (footnote).

[49] The Egyptians found this quite satisfactory, as Herodotus stated: Ελληνικοῖσι δὲ νομαιοισι φεύγουσε χρᾶσθαι, τὸ δὲ σύμπαν εἰπεῖν, μηδ᾽ ἄλλων μηδαμὰ μηδανῶν ἀνθρώπων νομαίοισι. ("The Egyptians shun the use of Greek customs, and (to speak generally) the customs of any other men whatever." Herodotus, *The Histories*, II, 91, translation of A. D. Godley, *Loeb Classical Library*.)

[50] Rostoftzeff, M., *The Social and Economic History of the Hellenistic World*, Oxford, 1953, vol. 2, p. 1094.

"On their military campaigns and their journeys in the country they all receive treatment without the payment of any private fee; for the physicians draw their support from public funds and administer their treatments in accordance with a written law which was composed in ancient times by many famous physicians. If they follow the rules of this law as they read them in the sacred book and yet are unable to save their patient, they are absolved from any charge and go unpunished; but if they go contrary to the law's prescriptions in any respect, they must submit to a trial with death as the penalty, the lawgiver holding that but few physicians would ever show themselves wiser than the mode of treatment which had been closely followed for a long period and had been originally prescribed by the ablest practitioners."[51]

At a later date, while priests were not always physicians, physicians were always priests, and low-level ones at that, based on statements by Clement of Alexandria (2nd C AD).[52] Treatments remained, as they had for 3000 years, symptom-oriented rather than disease-oriented, although elements of Greek medicine, especially botanicals and metals, finally found a place in Egyptian medical canon in the *Crocodilopolis Medical Manual*, a composite of elements of Egyptian and Greek medicine dated *ca.* 170 AD.

It is extravagant to conclude that the Crocodilopolis manuscript represented contemporary practice, for how much significance can be inferred from a single manuscript, one that probably is in part a copy of a deteriorating 6th C BC one and from which some of its text can be traced to the 16th dynasty, the time of the copying of the Ebers and Smith papyri. In striking contrast, there is a myriad of well-preserved papyrus manuscripts on all sorts of other matters from Roman Egypt, an indication of the rarity and insignificance of Egyptian medical writing at that time.[53] In summary, the Crocodilopolis manuscript provides a colophon to ancient Egyptian medicine, for it is said to contain not only features of several of the earlier medical manuscripts, especially the Ebers papyrus, but for the first time included elements of Greek medical knowledge. As a final comment on the decline of ancient Egyptian medicine, that decline took place in a single kingdom (albeit with several masters) over 3000 years, whereas Mesopotamian medicine met a similar fate over a similar period but under a series of distinctly different authoritarian regimes. The relative coherence and stability of Egyptian civilization provided no protection against its medicine's demise.[54]

---

[51] *Diodorus Siculus*, Bk. I, 82, 3, the *Loeb Classical Library* translation of C. H. Oldfather. A notable feature of this passage is absence of the concept of progress, for it indicates that perfection in medicine was considered to have been reached 2,500 years earlier, and to attempt any improvement was perilous, a comment not on the medicine but on ancient Egyptian governance.

[52] A function of medical care has been ascribed to the *pastophori*, processional idol-bearers classed below that of priests. There is variance in opinion as to their medical role, and Clement of Alexandria classified physicians as low-level priests, but R. E. Witt, in *Isis in the Ancient World*, Baltimore, 1977, p. 190, identifies them as interpreters of traditional medical and magical works at the 3rd C BC Serapeum in Alexandria, a large temple dedicated to the god Serapis, protector of Alexandria.

[53] *From the Contents of the Libraries of the Suchos Temples in the Fayyum. Part I. A Medical Book from Crocodilopolis. P. Vindob. D. 6257*, Vienna, 1976, E. A. E. Reymond, editor.

[54] Although there were intruders who did impose changes from time to time, essential institutions were retained.

D. Overview of Ancient Egyptian Medical Practice

Summarizing the written record of ancient Eqyptian medicine, there are twelve known medical papyri that represent 3000 years of medical tradition. Of these, only the earliest, the Smith, Ebers, and Kahun papyri, are relatively free of magic. Of the three the Ebers papyrus represents the most ancient medicine, and it provides many of the cases mentioned in most of the remaining nine papyri, to which spells, incantations, and amulets were added. And so by about 200 AD the last medical papyrus available, the Crocodilopolis, contains clinical cases that include eye disease, fevers, and bites, but its therapies are almost all magical.[55] In light of the preceding it is remarkable that even in 363 AD the Roman Emperor Julian stated: "…in place of every testimony it is enough to commend his [the physician's] knowledge of the art, if he has said that he was trained at Alexandria."[56] But here the reference is to Alexandrian medicine, about which there will be much mention in later chapters, and Greek medicine as practiced in Alexandria must not be confused with Egyptian medicine.

The prominent Greek historian, Diodorus Siculus (*fl.*, 60-30 BC), provided interesting but limited insight into Egyptian medicine, and perhaps the punitive penalties against medical practitioners that he cited were, in part, to prevent abuse of patients from those who would experiment on them, an unlikely event but nevertheless a laudable position. But it also indicates (1) little faith in contemporary Egyptian practitioners, (2) inordinate faith in Egyptian physicians of more than 2,000 years earlier, and (3) a powerful deterrent to medical innovation. And so it is instructive to compare the observations of Egyptian physicians by Diodorus with contemporary comments on Greek physicians in Rome made by the Roman orator, Cicero (106-43 BC), in letters to his friends. In them Cicero (1) laments the loss of "so skillful a physician," (2) reassures a sick friend he will seek assistance from his own physician, (3) notes, concerning a friend's physician, "What a delightful physician he, . . .," while to another friend he expresses dissatisfaction with the friend's choice of physician, (4) writes that physicians favor recovery, whereas trainers favor appearance, and (5) he volunteers to quicken a physician's interest in a friend's illness by contributing to payment of the physician's fee.[57] Cicero's attitude was a practical and somewhat favorable view of the profession, but more importantly it indicates the Greek physician was very much an interactive participant in a patient's illness and able to pursue, even in Rome, an independent course of action, the antithesis of the Egyptian practitioner.

Ancient manuscripts do not identify the clinicians responsible for the wisdom found in the Ebers papyrus. It can be postulated that the equivalent of the Sumerian *azu* briefly existed in Egypt's formative years. Although their history is murky and implied, great credit must be given to those early clinicians. Nevertheless, that historical Egyptian therapies that survived down to the Christian era were the remnants of medicine 3000 years old is less a comment on their quality than on their master, less an expression of durability than inflexibility. It comes as no surprise that ancient Egyptians had, with the

---

[55] There is also the "magical" London-Leiden papyrus from the 3rd C AD that contains some medically relevant material, including a few botanicals and a recommendation for gout, namely: writing on a slip of precious metal that is then wrapped in deerskin and tied to the leg that is the location of the problem. Most of that manuscript's contents are invocations.

[56] *Julianus*, XXII, 16, 18, translation of W. C. Wright, *Loeb Classical Library*.

[57] These comments are extracted from: *Cicero's Letters to Atticus, Cambridge*, 1965-1970, 7 vols., D. R. Shackleton Bailey, editor.

exception of some restricted temple scriptoria, no libraries.[58] Some have suggested that the knowledge in the Egyptian papyri, especially the notably objective Edwin Smith papyrus, represents the acme of cumulative medical wisdom up to that point in time. This is not likely to be correct. The papyri more likely embody the embers of a flickering flame of superior knowledge acquired in predynastic Egypt, a flame that would be smothered by the confines of empire. The Egyptian empire survived far longer than Sumer, a fact most likely explained by the natural protections afforded the former by a bordering vast desert and a sea. Nevertheless, as in Mesopotamia, North African medicine deteriorated under Pharoanic management as early empirical-rational medical practices succumbed to a petrifying social system, providing but another brick to reinforce the wall of class distinction. Here was no natural state of medical practice.

---

[58] This has been explained in part by poor preservation of Egyptian writings; see: Casson, L., *Libraries in the Ancient World*, New Haven, 2001, p. 16. Papyri from as early as 2500 BC (4th Egyptian dynasty) have been recovered, however, and thus any deterioration of written documents as an explanation for the absence of libraries requires more certain documention.

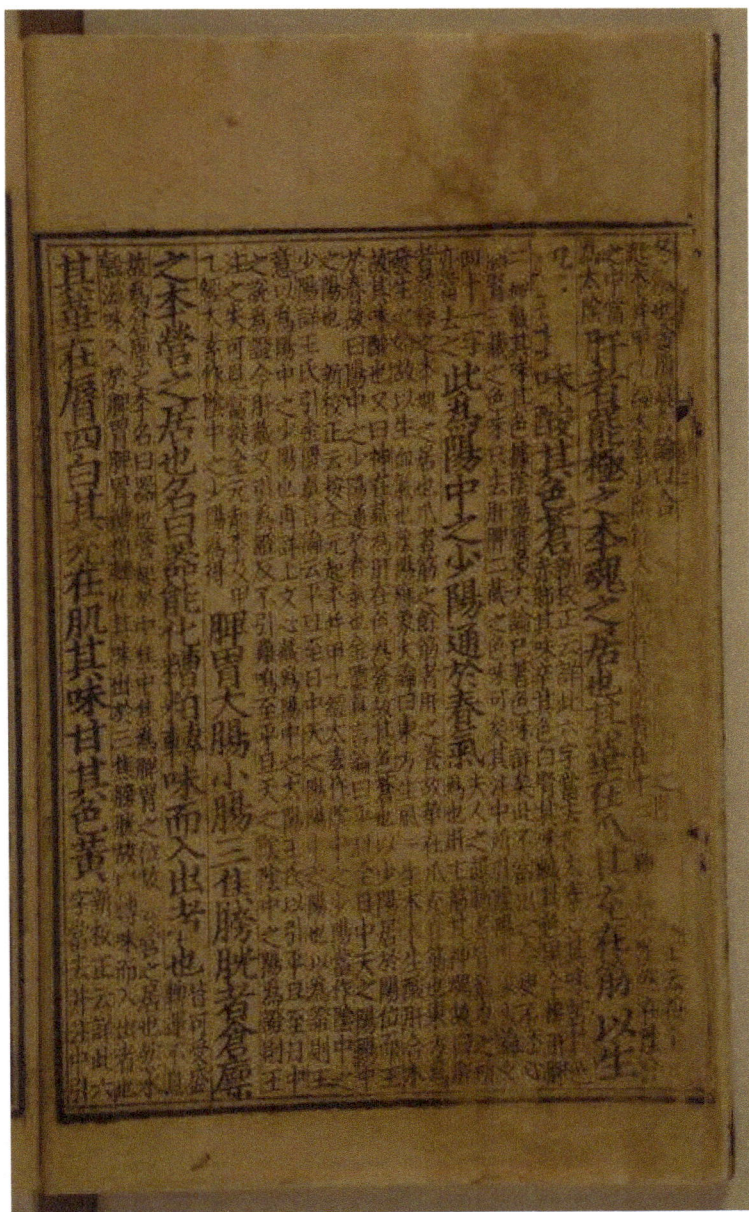

Fig. 5: A page, from the Jin Dynasty (1110-1234 AD), of the *Huang Ti Nei Ching Su Wen*, one-half of the masterpiece of traditional Chinese medicine, the other half being the *Nei Ching Ling Shu*. This is thought to be the earliest printed edition of the work, although its content was essentially established by Wang Bing in 762 AD during the T'ang dynasty (see p. 78). Photo credit: courtesy of the World Digital Library of the Library of Congress with support of the United Nations Educational, Cultural and Scientific Organization (UNESCO).

CHAPTER FOUR

LARGE STRUCTURED SOCIETIES, AUTHORITARIAN – THE FAR EAST

*"The relation between superiors (*chun-tzu*) and inferiors is like that between the wind and the grass. The grass must bend when the wind blows it."*

The Analects of Confucius, XII.19

There is a tenuous historical record for early Asian medicine, but the *Huang Ti Nei Ching Su Wen*, assembled in the 1st C BC, is said to encapsulate ancient Chinese medical thought. This may be called into question, but there are undoubtedly valid clinical diagnostics in that document, and it acknowledges the uniqueness of the individual patient. Nevertheless, its theories and treatments reveal a codified system of disease and physiology with no basis in fact, more a fabrication than a misunderstanding. It is remarkable that a civilization known for its many manifestations of brilliance would validate such a basis for medical practice, but the fault can be traced to a restrictive system of education by a central authority and to a society willing to tolerate, or unwilling or unable to challenge, that authority. There were, unquestionably, significant empirical medical discoveries, particularly in herbal therapies, but they were made by local, often itinerant, practitioners who will remain forever unknown, their ideas and medical practices for the most part unrecorded, of only local value and relegated to folklore. Instead, authoritative medical canon such as the *Huang Ti Nei Ching Su Wen* assumed dominance concurrently with the rise of imperial China, and it persisted up to, and was revived during, the twentieth century, and, to the dismay of many, has widely proliferated today.

A. Introduction: Ancient Medicine without Ancient Documentation in Early Unification

In contrast to Sumer and Egypt, the oldest Chinese medical texts date only from the early 2nd C BC, as established by recent scholarship. It has been concluded, for example, that there is no historical evidence of acupuncture being used as a medical treatment prior to the 1st C BC. With this relatively new information, the prehistory of Chinese medical practice, traditionally dated to *ca.* 2500 BC, has become even further removed from reasoned assessment than it previously was. This does not mean that a system of medicine did not exist in earliest times, for most writing was done on perishable materials, usually wood surfaces or more durable bone. Had Chinese population centers been in arid regions, survival of those materials may have mirrored the survival of clay tablets and papyrus in Sumer and Egypt, and historical evidence of an ancient medical practice at the time of mythical Emperors might proudly stand beside the Sumerian *asu* and the postulated predynastic Egypt practitioner. But that is not the case. Indeed, the discovery of silk manuscripts from a burial site in Hunan Province in 1973 has produced evidence suggesting none of the classics of Chinese medicine, including their theoretical foundations to be discussed below, predate *ca.* 100 BC.

Nevertheless, it has been said that the earliest form of Chinese medicine, practiced *ca.* 3000-2000 BC as deducible from a few ancient non-medical writings, was of a type known as ancestral healing. This period in Chinese prehistory has been termed the Longshan era. It was a period that saw a developing cultural homogeneity of the future China. There was a myriad of small communities in the region surrounding the Yellow River, perhaps the equivalent of the city-states of Sumer and predynastic Egypt. It is thought that communal adhesion was based on kinship, whereas Sumerian city-states were often theocracies. There is no information available concerning medical practices of the Longshan era, and an early form of character-writing would not appear for another five hundred years, although several pieces of Longshan pottery with scratched symbols suggest an earlier attempt. But it was during this era that the first legendary "sages" are said to have lived, including Huang Ti, the Yellow Emperor, of whom more later. As time passed there developed the concept of demonological medicine, in which, for example, local inflammation or swelling was thought to identify the presence and specific location of a demon. Therapies, including needling, were said to be guided by this. A description of day-by-day clinical practice of that age does not exist, but there are references to medicines, exercises, spells, and minor surgery.[1] Although it would be expected that shamanism would have been a prominent force, it was not until the evolution of dynastic China in the subsequent millenium that such a practice is discerned.

A formal Chinese medical system is known to have existed contemporaneously with the Greek physician, Hippocrates (460-380 BC), for the ancient Chou dynasty (1050-256 BC) developed an official ranking of court professionals, including medical practitioners, based on written examinations.[2] Notably, medical practitioners were distinct from priests.

But a change in society occurred during China's march to unification when the Chou dynasty attempted to bring under control the turmoil of the Warring States period (481-221 BC). Heavy-handedness characterized its approach to the social upheaval that was under way. With the subsequent monarchical Qin Dynasty (221 – 206 BC) and Han Dynasty (206 BC – 220 AD), an imperial China was created and possession became an issue for the State rather than the local war-lord. Assimilation of city-states occurred. The examination system for civil service promotion, a centralized mint, and the standardization of weights and measures were manifestations of national bureaucratic centralization. The conservative and tolerant philosophies of Lao Tzu (5th C BC), who praised simple living, honesty, and avoidance of hostility, and Confucius (551-459 BC),

---

[1] See: *Cambridge Encyclopedia of China*, Cambridge, 1991, 2nd edition, for an overview.

[2] The *Chou Li* ("Ritual of Chou") is discussed by Majno, G., in *The Healing Hand*, (Cambridge [MA], 1975), p. 293, who concluded a rigid state-sponsored system of medical care existed. The *Chou (Zhou) Li* served the early Han Dynasty as a Confucian classic that was an all-inclusive guide to officials of government. It specified in great detail the proper way to fulfill the administration of State affairs, including city planning, architecture, protocol, and etiquette, and was important in fostering stability of the early Chinese State. Its examination system, used to identify appropriately qualified applicants for schooling and college, targeted the young, an apparatus that promoted desireable characteristics in its graduates, from whom the royalty would then select those who were to enter public service. It is, however, difficult to imagine such a system, essentially one that was run by the palace, representing in totality the vast regions of China. The Eastern Chou dynasty encompassed many city-states, but most were between the Yellow and the Yangtze rivers. The examination system, for which China is justifiably famous, actually began in earnest in the Song dynasty (960-1279 AD) when its benefits were extended beyond the aristocracy. Prior to that the examination system was devised to maintain monarchical control over the ruler's favorites and a necessary bureaucracy. (See: Dien, A. E., *State and Society in Early Medieval China*, Stanford, 1990.) It is naive to think that the purpose of the earlier examination system was to guarantee a supply of high-quality medical practitioners.

who described the merits of being a humane, dutiful, and educated gentleman, were, in general, welcomed by the Han government. Certain Taoistic and Confucian beliefs, however, represented opposing political perspectives and led to factions. Thus, late in the Former Han Dynasty (206 BC - 9 AD) the Confucians prevailed, and thereafter Confucian writings provided philosophical guidance and justification for governmental policies. To ensure this convenient philosophy was imbued into those seeking a position in government bureaucracy, a National University, or "Imperial Academy," was begun in 124 BC, and a nationwide system of education was put in place in 3 AD. A policy of formal examination as the basis for civil service preferment that had been instituted *ca.* 165 BC was now based primarily on an understanding of Confucian texts, a mechanism for educating a cadre of Confucian practitioners philosophically sympathetic with, and professionally invested in, the dynastic government. This course of government policy, including its subsequent versions of the Imperial Academy, was considered necessary for social uniformity among the elite classes and was pursued into the 20th C.[3]

B. The *Huang Ti Nei Ching Su Wen*, Medical Classic and Guide for Traditional Chinese Medicine, and the Hunan Medical Treatises

The preceding comments on political centralization of early China have been required for a discussion of the famed *Huang Ti Nei Ching Su Wen* ("The Yellow Emperor's Classic of Internal Medicine.") "The *Nei Ching* undoubtedly contains the fundamental principles of traditional Chinese medicine." Thus wrote the famous western scholar of Chinese literature, Dr. Joseph Needham, and Lu Gwei-djen.[4] The first mention of this classic textbook of ancient Chinese medicine is found in the *Annals of the Former Han Dynasty* (206 BC-9 AD). Nevertheless, popular and traditional views hold the *Huang Ti Nei Ching Su Wen* origin to have been about 2500 BC during the purported reign of the legendary third Chinese emperor, Huang Ti. If there is any truth in the traditional view, the original *Huang Ti Nei Ching Su Wen* would have been contemporary with the earliest medical compositions of Sumer and Egypt. There are aspects of the *Huang Ti Nei Ching Su Wen* reminiscent of medical practice in other ancient civilizations. For instance, there is a similarity between the Yellow Emperor of the *Huang Ti Nei Ching Su Wen* and the first named Egyptian physician, Imhotep. Both are either mythical or legendary figures, both are purported to have lived about 2500 BC, and both have been credited with ingenious inventions outside the field of medicine, Imhotep in architecture, and Huang Ti as the inventor of the wheel and other useful items. Both were subsequently elevated to the rank of a deity.

But it now appears certain that the *Huang Ti Nei Ching Su Wen* was not composed, nor its theories developed, prior to the 1st C BC. What might have transpired during that century to produce such a change? The Han Dynasty (206 BC – 220 AD) is considered by many as one of the most glorious eras of Chinese history, during which

---

[3] The Quozijian, in literal translation "School for the Sons of the State" but known in Western translation as the Imperial Academy, officially closed in 1905, although its educational functions had been incorporated into the Imperial University of Peking in 1898. See: Yuan, Z., *Local Government Schools in Sung China: A Reassessment*, in *History of Education Quarterly*, 34:193-213, 1994.

[4] Needham, J. and Gwei-djen, L., *Hygiene and Preventive Medicine in Ancient China*, in *J. Hist. Med.* XVII, Oct. 1962, #4, pp.429-470.

China's borders were enlarged, approaching those of the modern nation. And it was midway during the Former Han Dynasty (206 BC – 9 AD) that centralization of power was pursued by a ruling faction that found Confucianism more consistent with its aims than other philosophies, including Taoism. The latter embraced at that time the concept of "action by inaction," a philosophical system guided by introspection and noninterference with fate, which in part meant a *laissez-faire* approach to many matters. There was an expectation that difficult situations would, on their own, often find a natural path of resolution and that the superior course of action was the "natural" one. This approach was sometimes applied to mercantile interests and outlying territories. It opposed an excessively centralized bureaucracy, preferring, for example, to permit large city-states on its borders to exist under local warlords who were to keep barbarian tribes in check. The *Yan tie lun*, written in the late 2nd C BC, contained opposing arguments drawn from a formal discussion of the merits of ways to remedy a State exhausted by war and to bolster imperial strength.[5] The opposing ideas have been described as "greater freedom of action" *vs.* "greater measure of control," the former meaning a relaxation of onerous burdens on the population, the latter meaning a tighter monarchical control on means of production. Neither implied a diminishing of government involvement, however, a course that would seem to have been more consistent with Taoism, but even Taoism designated those characteristics of a ruler that would lead to a happy people rather than limitations on that ruler.[6] This was a critical time in formation of the governing philosophy of the Chinese State, and it was at this time that standardization of medical theory resulting in treatises like the *Huang Ti Nei Ching Su Wen* were compiled, perhaps a peripheral manifestation of the trend towards centralized power and system of government. The Imperial Academy, founded to instill Confucian principles in candidates for government office, was the likely mechanism for its implementation.

But whatever the reason, concurrent with the formation of an Imperial China, Chinese medicine would develop in two totally distinct ways, one being the scholarly practice as portrayed in the *Huang Ti Nei Ching Su Wen* that was available to the bureaucracy, and the other an unregulated system comprising a myriad of autonomous individual practitioners that provided care to the vast majority of the population and of which virtually nothing is known. The bipolar nature of ancient Chinese medicine was the consequence of the profound effects of that nation's authoritarian governance: at one end of the spectrum were elite practitioners who assumed a protected but dependent status within a political framework; at the other end was the common practitioner, parochial, untutored, and unprotected, but with the ability to observe and innovate, by exclusion accepting the burden of providing care for China's vast number of commoners.

---

[5] *Yan tie lun*, usually translated as "Discourses on Salt and Iron," centered around a debate by a panel of invited experts concerning fiscal policies of the central government in 81 BC, during which its monopoly on mining and production of salt and iron was attacked by a faction claiming it caused great hardship on the people. This open debate, evoking the "liberal vs. conservative" dispute of modern politics, offers great insight into serious intellectual social thought of the early Han dynasty, although similarities to the present are limited.

[6] Major, J., *et al.*, *The Essential Huainanzi*, New York, 2012, a fascinating document of which several sections are devoted to describing ideal management of a kingom. Democratic process goes unmentioned.

C. Characteristics of the *Huang Ti Nei Ching Su Wen*

The *Huang Ti Nei Ching* has been the focus of extensive commentary for 2000 years. In its present embodiment there are two main components, the *Su Wen* and the *Lin Shu*. Each comprises eighty-one chapters, and the format is a dialogue between Huang Ti, the Yellow Emperor, and one of several ministers. The *Su Wen*, the primary focus of this chapter, addresses questions considered basic to medicine, whereas the *Lin Shu* primarily addresses acupuncture. The true nature of the composition of the *Huang Ti Nei Ching Su Wen* has yet to be agreed upon, for it is considered to be a compilation of extracts from an estimated twenty earlier works that in themselves include items from as many as three hundred authors from unknown periods in early Chinese history. Even the name of the compiler(s) is unknown. The various treatises were acquired by individuals who emended and perhaps amended them, transmiting them via the teacher-pupil tradition over many generations.[7] From the variable content of the many early versions of the composition it seems that there is no *editio princeps* from which all other versions derive. Apropos the present discussion the *Huang Ti Nei Ching Su Wen* contains material relevant to internal medicine.

In reviewing the *Huang Ti Nei Ching Su Wen* it is obvious that some clinical observations of an empirical and perhaps rational nature were indeed made. As described by Dr. Ilsa Veith in *The Yellow Emperor's Classic of Internal Medicine*, (Berkeley, 2002, a paperback reprint of Dr. Veith's 1949 work), the pulse of the pregnant woman was noted to be especially full,[8] and different fever patterns were recognized. Cyanosis was properly related to respiratory failure, and if a patient had six pulse beats to one respiration there was probable heart trouble.[9] Such observations as these are described in Book 4 of Dr. Veith's translation and, if accurately translated, suggest valid attempts at associations. Also in Book 4 is a probable description of debridement of a septic wound.[10] At the beginning of Book 9 there is a description of what could conceivably be typhoid fever.

---

[7] The scholarly work of D. J. Keegan has removed much of the mystery surrounding the origin of the *Huang Ti Nei Ching Su Wen*. See his *The Huang-ti nei-ching: The structure of the compilation; The significance of the structure*, Ph.D. thesis, Univ. of Calif., Berkeley, 1988. Works that might be confused with the *Huang Ti Nei Ching Su Wen* are the *Nan-Ching* (Manual of Difficult Issues), which is especially relevant to acupuncture, and the *I Ching* (Manual of Change), an interpretation of "universal laws" that is oracular and is meant to permit control of the future. The latter's only mention of illness (Hexagram 45 in *I Ching*, translated by K. and R. Huang, New York, 1987) is to assert that it builds character, although some commentators attribute considerable clinical usefulness to the *I Ching*. See: Shima, M., *The Medical I Ching*, Boulder (CO), 1992. The *Nan-Ching* is undergoing a revival, and a new translation has revealed material of a clinical nature that places its value at least to that of the *Huang Ti Nei Ching Su Wen*.

[8] The pulse in pregnancy is indeed "full," a consequence of the maternal increase in blood volume and cardiac output that accommodates the fetus.

[9] Curiously, and assuming the examiner's respiratory rate at rest was fourteen per minute (a bit more rapid than today's "normal" of twelve), "heart failure" would have been indicated when the actual pulse rate was only 84 per minute (6 X 14). This suggests a transcription error, for six pulse beats per respiration *of the patient*, if the patient's breathing were labored at a rate of twenty per minute, the resulting pulse rate of 120 per minute would have been more consistent with heart failure. Factors other than pulse and respiratory rate were probably involved in reaching a final diagnosis.

[10] This particular entry is interesting in that the cause of the wound, or ulcer, is deemed to have been the entry of "minute particles" through the skin, a suggestion consistent with a theory of microorganisms.

This description is awash in theoretical consideration of Yin and Yang, but it has this great merit: demons or divinities were not identified as the cause of illness. And there is a final but equally important point: ancient Chinese medicine recognized the complexity of illness and the great variability of its manifestations in individual patients.

Diagnosis as proffered by the *Huang Ti Nei Ching Su Wen* was performed by observing two features, the countenance, including complexion, and the pulse. The examination of the latter had to be performed in a specified setting at a specified time, usually early in the morning before it was disturbed by activities of daily living, and the procedure could take half an hour. Apparently timing of the pulse was standardized against the respiratory rate of the examiner and was usually four to one.[11] In Book II, Treatise V, Dr. Veith has rendered a section thus: "Nothing surpasses the examination of the pulse, for with it errors cannot be committed." Clinical descriptions sound inviting: "the feeling of the pulse should be done according to method: for when it is slow and quiet it acts as protector and guardian. In days of Spring the pulse is superficial, like wood floating on water or like a fish that glides through the waves."[12] With use of this "sphygmology" further physical examination was thought to be unnecessary, a claim of remarkable hyperbole. Yet even the English physician, Caleb Parry (1755-1822), could note that, in spite of daily evidence of its shortcomings, ". . . we ought to wonder at the confidence with which physicians look to the condition of the pulse in the radial arteries as the general evidence of the state of disease, and the chief rule of the administration of remedies."[13] Inspecting the patient from a distance and assessing the pulse are powerful diagnostic tools even today. Preoccupation of the ancients with the pulse may, therefore, seem understandable, if not fully justifiable, but one cannot help but suspect that the practitioner who does not examine the rest of the patient has, purposefully or not, little time, little knowledge, or little interest concerning his work.

Had the early enthusiasm for the pulse and inspection of the countenance been extended to other aspects of medical biology and pathology great progress might have ensued. This did not happen. Instead, the *Huang Ti Nei Ching Su Wen* offered frequent admonitions about the necessity of strict adherence to rules of diagnosis and specifics of therapy, a tactic by which imperfect adherence was virtually guaranteed, thereby providing a perfect scapegoat for a bad outcome. Often the value of prognosis was used not to determine therapy but to identify those who would or would not die. In addition, it was the nature of the users of the work to present its knowledge in a nonnegotiable

---

[11] Bedford, D. E., *The Ancient Art of Feeling the Pulse*, in *Heart*, 13:423-437, 1951.

[12] From Book 5 of the *Huang Ti Nei Ching Su Wen*, found in: Veith I., *The Yellow Emperor's Classic of Internal Medicine*, Berkeley, 2002, p. 124. (This is a paperback reprint of Dr. Veith's 1949 work.) It must be acknowledged that simile has great value in the absence of a technical vocabulary, and it may at times be its equivalent. Today's medical students are taught, for example, the "water-hammer" pulse of aortic valve insufficiency and the "machinery" murmur of a patent ductus arteriosus.

[13] Parry, C. H., *Elements of Pathology and Therapeutics*, London, 1825, p. 50. Dr. Parry was a careful observer, and he described the first patient with what would be called Graves' disease in 1786, long before the description by Graves (1835). In that description of hyperthyroidism he associated the rapid and forceful pulse with thyroid enlargement. Overweaning concern about the pulse in the 18th C is not unexpected. A work by Theophilus, *De Pulsibus* (Concerning the Pulse), written in the 7th C AD and based on the writings of Galen, was one of several treatises comprising the *Articella*, a famous collection of works used for medieval medical education in the West well into the 16th C that thereby conditioned generations of practitioners to accept the overarching importance of the pulse in diagnosis until it was finally displaced by new ideas.

posture regarding medical practice; its practitioners expected patients to be malleable and compliant. Indeed, one might consider the most notable feature of the *Huang Ti Nei Ching Su Wen* to be the ingenious way in which a medical tract that repeatedly stresses curability was able to maintain its good reputation for centuries in the face of what had to be repeated evidence of its uselessness. There were many attempts at clarifying archaic Chinese characters of the *Huang Ti Nei Ching Su Wen*, but their purpose was always to restore the accuracy of the original text, not to improve or update it. The resistance of subsequent medical writers to improve on its archaic contents is a striking characteristic of ancient Chinese medicine. Thus, it is unfair to be critical of the original *Huang Ti Nei Ching Su Wen*, just as it is unfair to berate the work of Galen just because no one came forward to challenge it for many centuries. If there were fault to be laid, it should be with those who venerated rather than questioned archaic writings (for reasons for this see the Excursus on Appeal to Authority, p. 230).

The *Huang Ti Nei Ching Su Wen* did not reach its approximate final form until 762 AD, when it was edited by Wang Bing. Although Wang Bing was apparently given some kind of instruction in medicine by a teacher it is not known whether he was a "physician." Prof. Paul Unschuld states that it is primarily through his writings that he is known, as his personal history is unavailable.[14] He apparently held a position within the government bureaucracy, and Dr. Veith's translation mentions that he was "one of the highest ministers."[15] His motives for editing the *Huang Ti Nei Ching Su Wen* are also unknown, but it took twelve years for him to meet with many scholars and to peruse some forty-eight major texts for information relevant to his work, obviously a great personal effort and commitment. His alterations, additions, and commentary were extensive and have remained the essential text of the work to this day, similar to the version of the Mesopotamian *Treatise on Diagnosis and Prognosis* of ca. 1800 BC as edited in 1150 BC by the Assyrian scribe, Esagil-kin-apli (see footnote, p. 50). There were many changes in the text over the centuries, and it is notable that most are said to have been additions to the corpus, not replacements for knowledge that might have become obsolete.[16] Indeed, the older the knowledge the less "obsolete" it was viewed, because reverence for earlier writings has been a persistent feature of Chinese medicine just as it has been in many other cultures.

Such was the nature of the *Huang Ti Nei Ching Su Wen*, fashioned for the medical intellectuals. What a contrast it posed to the illiterate common practitioner, the itinerant doctor.

D. The Itinerant Doctors

Like Egyptian medicine, the true face of ancient Chinese medicine has been hidden behind a handful of treatises. These treatises began to be compiled concurrently with the inauguration of an imperial China. They were then brought forward by a handful

---

[14] Unschuld, P., *Huang Di Nei Jing Su Wen*, Berkeley, 2003, p. 39.

[15] Veith I., *The Yellow Emperor's Classic of Internal Medicine*, Berkeley, 2002, Appendix III. This is a paperback reprint of Dr. Veith's 1949 work.

[16] Needham, J., Gwei-Djen, L., in *Science and Civilization in China*, Vol. 6, Part VI (Medicine), Cambridge, 2000, Sivin, N., editor. The *textus receptus* of the *Huang Ti Nei Ching Su Wen* is the product of emendations and compilations, the work of many writers, much as the papyrus Ebers and the *Hippocratic Corpus* are considered multi-authored collections of treatises.

of elite scholars or encyclopedists who edited and codified their contents over many centuries.[17] But what was the true face of Chinese medicine?

Consider the observation of Prof. Nathan Sivin: "The classics are documents of the scholarly traditions that developed on the edges of the small, literate, officeholding elite, and which treated few of those outside it (and few of its women)."[18] Even more relevant is his observation that: "We know practically nothing about the practitioners who could not be called physicians… who actually were the peasant majority's only source of therapy."[19] The peasant's practitioner was usually a travelling medical craftsman now called an "itinerant doctor," although another term was a "bell doctor," which referred to the practitioner's bell that was rung as he announced his entrance into a village or street. It is unfortunate that no itinerant doctor wrote a book or, if written, one that survived, for a truer depiction of medical practice would then have emerged, one far more complimentary to Chinese ingenuity than the cryptic theoretical tracts of a few sophisticates writing for the most part under imperial dictate (see Table 2, p. 83).

There is a superficial resemblance of the itinerant doctor of early China with the peripatetic doctor of early Greece: both were entrepreneurs and both were apparently valued insufficiently to warrant government attention. As with all other early societies in the absence of shamanism, medical practitioners posed neither a threat to the State nor a venue for sufficient profit or influence to bother regulating. They were socially insignificant and their only judges were their patients. Although the quality of itinerant doctors must have ranged from the charlatan to the clever, caring, and observant, these were the people who carried the physician's burden even though they had no physician's training. The State favored homogeneity of theory rather than augmentation of knowledge, but theories were of little value to the itinerant practitioner, whose interest was more likely to have been herbal therapies suggested by local folklore or by other practitioners. To some extent the latter was a successful strategy. One indication that itinerant doctors were appreciated among the general population was their mention in ancient Chinese novels.[20] Another was the regional canvassing of practitioners by Imperial command so that comprehensive catalogues of therapeutic herbs and other agents could be developed, implying an appreciation of the itinerant practitioner's empirical knowledge. If a specific therapy cured a prominent person that itinerant doctor might be well rewarded and remembered in folklore or even admitted into the bureaucracy. But beyond that the itinerants sadly constitute a faceless profession. It is unfortunate that one must attempt to infer from the *Huang Ti Nei Ching Su Wen* or other classics what passed for instructions on curing. Instead, one wishes for the notebooks of

---

[17] Whether Chinese medicine was scientific in ancient times depends on definitions: Dr. Needham and Lu Gwei-Djen note that translation of the modern Chinese word for "science" is "classification knowledge," which suggests science is viewed as a field of study rather than a method of study or a means of acquiring new knowledge.

[18] See the review by Nathan Sivin in: *Social History of Medicine,* 19:334-336, 2006, p. 336.

[19] Sivin, N., his Introduction to volume 6, part VI, of the classic series *Science and Civilization in China,* by Needham, J., and Gwei-Djen, L., Cambridge, 2004, p. 195, footnote.

[20] A flattering review by an acupuncturist of the itinerant doctors attributes to them some of the Chinese medical classics, stating, for example, that Wang Shuhe, compiler of the famous 3rd C work on the pulse (the *Mai Jing*) was itinerant. See: Yuxia Que, *Itinerant Doctors in Chinese History*, in *J. Chin. Med.*, 86:28-31, 2008. Elsewhere, however, he is described as of noble origin who studied with a prior master of medicine, not at all an "itinerant." In a reference the author cannot relocate it is stated that Wang Shuhe obtained some of his information on the pulse from itinerant practitioners, but the point is moot because the essence of the *Mai Jing* is pure fantasy.

the itinerant doctors. Periodically there would be all-inclusive surveys of herbal remedies, and such surveys were then "published" by the State and are now referred to as "classics" of *materia medica*, some of which are listed in Table 2. But the practitioners who originally discovered the relatively few entries that were clinically useful, based on painfully extracted personal experience, will never receive recognition. Those few but admirable discoveries raise a critical point: there is no reason to think that there was any difference between the ancient Chinese and Greek travelling practitioners in their ability to identify signs and symptoms of disease and to observe the results of their therapies. What prevented the itinerant doctors of China from developing and propagating their discoveries among their colleagues in a fashion similar to their ancient Greek colleagues?

Several explanations suggest themselves:

1) Any attempt to insert new findings by an itinerant doctor into classical texts would have been resisted by the bureaucracy unless the finding was consistent with contemporary theories found in the *Huang Ti Nei Ching Su Wen*.

2) The secretive nature of the knowledge held by individual practitioners would have been inaccessible to scientific scrutiny. An example of secrecy in ancient Chinese medicine is discussed by Dr. Sivin in his recounting of the life of Ch'un-yu I (2nd C BC).[21] Several "books" on aspects of medicine existed at that time, and the elderly teacher of this young nobleman made them known to him because: "My family is well provided for. I love you, and intend to teach you all my secret formularies." Ch'un-yu later notes that, although his teacher was skilled, he had been "unwilling to treat the illnesses of others [*i.e.*, other than family and friends]. It must be due to this that he was not renowned. He also told me 'Take care that you do not let my sons and grandsons know you have studied my formulas.'" Medical knowledge as secretive as this must have been remained profoundly provincial, rarely extending beyond the individual practitioner's domain, much less to another city.

3) This region of the world was no ancient Greece composed of relatively isolated small city-states. Instead, the estimated population of China at the end of the Han Dynasty has been set at 60,000,000. To control even the relatively homogeneous population such as existed in an agrarian China of that era required (a) a large and dedicated elite bureaucracy, and (b) no organized opposition. These two goals were sought by purposefully maintaining an agrarian economy and by making membership in the bureaucracy the goal of those families and individuals who sought its tangible benefits, which included exemption from taxation. The results were brilliantly successful, but as a consequence individual enterprise was restrained and innovation discouraged.

4) There was little possibility that itinerant doctors would join together as a force for improving medical care when they knew that there was an elite cadre learned in the medical treatises that had been declared by bureaucratic sages as "classics" that had behind it the force of the monarchy.[22]

In any event, the itinerant doctor pursued a path quite different from his elite counterpart, his profession being ignored and his limited knowledge periodically raided

---

[21] Sivin, N., *Text and Experience in Classical Chinese Medicine*, in Bates, D. G., *Knowledge and the Scholarly Medical Tradition*, Cambridge, 1995, pp. 177-201; Harper, D. J., *Early Chinese Medical Literature: The Mawangeui Medical Manuscripts*, London, 1998, pp. 55-67.

[22] Some "guilds" of itinerant doctors apparently were formed during more recent dynasties, but Yuxia Qiu (*J. Chinese Med.*, 86:28-31, 2008) states these guilds were for itinerant craftsmen that included sellers of combs and sweetmeats, and medical practitioners were managed by these guild representatives just as were the other craftsmen. Early guilds are not described..

by the State for its encyclopedic productions. Their failure to progress was imposed by the authoritarian society within which they worked.

E. Chinese Medicine and Society

In reading the Veith translation of the *Huang Ti Nei Ching Su Wen* it seems unfathomable why such a treatise would become the structure upon which the medical practice of an immense empire would be based for two thousand years. Its bizarre descriptions of causes and effects of biological phenomena would seem to have precluded any serious consideration by even a medically naive but educated population, or by the village butcher with his observations of animal anatomy. The problems with translations of the *Huang Ti Nei Ching Su Wen* are discussed by Dr. Veith in the excursus to her work. To explain the lionization of the *Huang Ti Nei Ching Su Wen* either her translation must grossly error or the population for which the *Nei Ching* was composed was poorly educated. The former is not a likely explanation. Dr. Veith, who received a doctorate in the History of Medicine, spent four years translating the classic while working at The Johns Hopkins University with the famous medical historian, Dr. Henry Sigerist (see footnote, p. 31). Furthermore, other modern translations may read better, but they have improved little on the technical insight of Dr. Veith. Dr. Majno, who consulted Chinese experts in the field, cites the remarkably disparate range of meanings that can be applied to *Huang Ti Nei Ching Su Wen* medical terminology,[23] and the medical historian, Dr. Nathan Sivin, wrote in 1998 that "no available translation is reliable."[24]

On the other hand, ancient Chinese intellectuals can hardly be considered to have been uneducated. Education in Confucian China was assigned the highest priority. But to be poorly educated does not mean one must be uneducated. There can exist a qualitative deficiency in education, a systematic error in its application. The ancient examination system as devised for medicine probably played a role in perpetuating medical myths, the examinees knowing that their professional success lay in the hands of a political class that rigidly relied on canonical standards as a guide for assessing excellence or, more to the point, compliance. A parthenogeneic government perpetuated its interests by reiterating its theories through bureaucratic functionaries. Thus, early errors remained in force, no corrective measures could be applied, and a basically useless medical manifesto like the *Huang Ti Nei Ching Su Wen* was revered for millennia in a civilization known throughout the ages for its otherwise many manifestations of brilliance. Indeed, by this same mechanism the State even guided medical research. As shown in Table 2, many, if not all, of the important medical treatises known to us today were compiled under imperial directives. In this sense the Emperors functioned as a National Institute of Health. Being the Chief Bureaucrat rather than a Physician Scientist, the most an Emperor could do as a "research scientist" was to command subordinates to glean his provinces for contemporary information on promising herbs and to have the ancient canons rewritten in the vernacular of his day. Being ignorant of the significance of clinical signs and symptoms that might suggest new avenues of investigation of human pathology he was, by the nature of his commands for updated texts, able only to ensure that his minions' ignorance of clinical medicine was shared by all those under him,

[23] Majno, G., in *The Healing Hand*, Cambridge, 1975, p. 241.
[24] Sivin, N., *Science and Medicine in Imperial China*, in *J. Asian Studies*, 47:41-90, 1988.

including those whom history has blithely termed "physicians."

A factor contributing to defective medical education is that Chinese medicine reflected cultural preferences of its elite classes. In one area the appeal of the *Huang Ti Nei Ching Su Wen* can be readily appreciated, and that is its attitude toward hygiene and preventive medicine. This attitude, if not its application, has been favorably compared by Dr. Needham and Lu Gwei-djen with that of ancient Greece and Rome.[25] It is consistent with the philosophical orientation of intellectuals in ancient China, that being the welfare of the State rather than the state of the individual. Chinese medicine has always been part of a larger concept, one that includes religious belief and philosophy. Thus, the wisdom of its texts is considered to lie in preventive methodology. Its medical sages "do not wait until sickness is present to cure the sickness, they cure it before it takes place … .[26] Ruiping Ruii in the same reference expands on this by noting that in Confucian bioethics the human body is "part of the onto-cosmological body that comprises the totality of Heaven, Earth, and myriad things." Sun Szu Miao, a 6th C AD Confucian doctor, is quoted as stating "a superior doctor takes care of the state, a mediocre doctor takes care of the person, an inferior doctor takes care of the disease." This statement will stand as a classic of political rhetoric, a brilliant medical *non sequitor* that has and will continue to inspire shallow intellects forever.[27] The "superior doctor" is reminiscent of Dr. Sigerist's extraordinary view of the medicine-man (p. 31*f*).

In summary, the Hunan discoveries and knowledge of contemporary political realities point to a defective system of medical erudition that need not be assigned to clotured knowledge, lack of curiosity, or lack of patronage. It is more likely to have been the offspring of an intellectual contrivance, a response to contemporary political demands as Confucianism was implemented as State doctrine. For Chinese medical canon was based on an epistemological maze devised by one or a few individuals, a maze unfounded on biological reality and designed to fit a theoretical body of knowledge with its roots in Confucian philosophy. And from this bureaucratic trap of authoritative theory, a fine example of the eternal search for the profound generalization, the siren's call of the *panacea*, ancient Chinese medicine never escaped.

---

[25] Needham, J. and Gwei-djen, L., *Hygiene and Preventive Medicine in Ancient China*, in *J. Hist. Med.* XVII, Oct. 1962, #4.

[26] Peimin Ni, *Confucian Virtues and Personal Health*, in *Confucian Bioethics*, (Philosophy and Medicine, Bk. 61), 1999, Ruiping Fan, editor, p. 31. And, of course, the ideal patient would benefit from going to see the physician *before* he became ill, for there would be little reason to go once he had become ill as little could be done. This was also important in acupuncture. As it was the stimulation of selected points on the body surface that was postulated to reverse an illness, the earlier that stimulation occurred the more likely therapy would be effective.

[27] The statement may be of much earlier origin, being reported in the *Kuo Yu* ("State Discourses") complied by Tso Chiu-Ming, 4th C BC, and is also translated as:

   The top physician heals a nation,
   The middle physician heals patients,
   The mediocre physician heals diseases.

Table 2: Some Chinese medical treatises compiled under Imperial command*

600 AD *Zhu Bing Yuan Hou Lun* (Treatise on the Causes and Symptoms of Diseases) 50 vols. The Sui Dynasty Emperor's physician ("tai yi"), Chao Yuang Fang, authored this important work as ordered by the Royal Court, perhaps Emperor Yang.

652 AD *Qui An Jin Fang* (Prescriptions Worth a Thousand Gold) 30 vols. Authored by the famed physician, Sun Si Miao, the authority requesting the work is uncertain. Perhaps it was solely an individual effort, but it is generally acknowledged that Sun Si Miao spent most of his adult years in a hermit-like existence, living in a cave. How he would have acquired the knowledge for his writings is a matter for debate, for his patients must have sought him out in the mountains. Many must also have remained in his presence for extended periods for him to know the true consequence of his therapies. Perhaps more relevant to his famous writings are his travels with Emperor Gao Zong. Thus, while he is often praised as declining to work for three emperors, in fact he may have had some significant intercourse with them, and his writings may have reflected their indulgence. Sun Si Miao has been called the Chinese "Hippocrates." He was born in 581 AD, roughly a thousand years after the Greek physician.

657 AD *Xinxiu Bencao* (Newly Revised Herbal of Tang) 54 vols. Emperor Xianqing of the Tang Dynasty mandated this compilation, which was carried out by Su Jing and twenty other scholars.
659 AD *Ying Gong Tang Bencao* (Duke Ying's Tang Pharmacopoeia); then edited to become the *Tang Bencao* (New Tang Pharmacy) 53 vols. This work was sponsored by Emperor Gao-Zong, who set Li Ji, Minister of Works, to the task, which was later improved with the help of twenty-two scholars.

973 AD *Kai-Bao Bencao* (Pharmacopoeia of the Kaibao Reign) 21 vols. Emperor Song Tai-Zu commissioned the Imperial Pharmacist, Liu Han, and a Taoist monk to compile this work. Some say Liu Han was a physician.

992 AD *Tai Ping Sheng Hui Fang* (Tai Ping Benevolent Prescriptions) 100 vols. Emperor Zhou Jiong ordered a national collection of medical information by his Department of Medicine. It was an encyclopedic work covering all aspects of medicine.

1111-1117 AD *Sheng Ji Zong Lu* (General Collection for Holy Relief) 200 vols. Emperor Song Hui Zong commanded his Royal Physicians to compile the work, which is a pharmacopoeia but one that also includes theory, specialties, diagnostics, and other aspects of medicine.

1556 AD *Gui jin Yitong Daquan* (Complete Medical Book, Ancient and Modern) 100 vols. Written by Xu Chunfu, this was an encyclopedic work. Xu Chunfu was in the "Institute of Imperial Physicians."

1742 AD *Yi Zong Jin Jian* (Golden Mirror of Medicine) 90 vols. The Qian Long Emperor commissioned this encyclopedic work covering all aspects of medicine, which was carried out by Wu Qian, of whom little is known, and eighty others of the palace bureaucracy.

*Several Chinese classics of medicine are of unknown authorship, including the *Huang Ti Nei Ching Su Wen* (it was the work of many authors), *Shen Nong Bencao Jing* (the first *materia medica*, containing 365 prescriptions), the *Shang Han Lun* (the classic on cold injury), and *Jin Gui Yao Lue* (Essential therapies from the Golden Cabinet). These works were often edited and altered under the aegis of the State, though the stimulus for their original composition is unknown.

Seeking a Grand Unified Theory has prompted the most brilliant of men to err.[28] And thus it happened in China. Any valid clinical observations within the classical texts, however well described and astute, represent a parallel event to the theoretical constructions of the *Huang Ti Nei Ching Su Wen* and related works rather than a consequence of their logic. Important medical advances might have occurred had there been surgical practitioners, for the practical and beneficial nature of surgery has helped the medical profession survive repeated displays of its profound ignorance. But that specialty's progress was hindered by the Confucian concept of sacredness of the body. Knowledge of anatomy was considered unnecessary, for knowledge of the theories of internal medicine was felt to have made surgery unnecessary. Such is the tight embrace and far-reaching consequence of a Grand Unified Theory taken too seriously.

Opportunities for escaping the maze did present themselves. Concurrent with the eastward spread of Buddhism from India, dated to 67 AD by Mookerji, were aspects of Indian medicine, including some interchange of pharmacopoeias and medical theory.[29] Then, beginning in the 2nd C AD, there was the invention of paper, permitting a far wider dispersion of knowledge, along with its usefulness in standardizing aspects of culture.[30] In the 7th C AD a Chinese account of medicine in India concluded, after a discussion of the value of diets and fasting in therapy, that they were ". . . an effective cure – by which each man is himself the king of physicians. . . ." Even when the medical knowledge of Islam and of Nestorian Christianity, the latter a sect associated with the famed medical center in Persia that preserved much ancient Greek learning (in Gondeshapour, see p. 317), entered the Chinese empire during the Tang Dynasty (617-907 AD), there was no change in Chinese medical theory.

A proper medical school might have remedied medical ignorance, and there is historical mention of what some have termed a "medical school" within the National University. Its formation was commanded by the Emperor and it included a specified faculty for acupuncture and massage. Significantly, however, although the Imperial Academy became a large institution, students enrolled in the various medical divisions at one point numbered as few as twenty individuals, and the duration of study was as long as seven years.[31] Thus, medical practitioners, or even medical instructors, for the empire could scarely have been a serious role of the "medical school" at this time. This is consistent with the opinion that the National University was, in fact, more a Directorate

---

[28] Albert Einstein (1879-1955), on reviewing Hubble's work indicating an expanding universe, declared his "cosmological term," which he had invoked for convenience to put his theory into accord with what he thought was a stable universe, to be "the worst mistake of my life." That that term now may be scientifically acceptable makes his "worst mistake" statement but another mistake. The modern use of the phrase *Grand Unified Theory* refers to a unifying theory of particle physics, its acronym being GUT.

[29] Mookerji, R. K., *Ancient Indian Education*, London, 1947, chapter 11.

[30] It is one of the mysteries of Chinese inventions, however, that rarely did one succeed in becoming socially beneficial. Dr. Joseph Needham (his Introduction to *The Genius of China*, edited by R. K. G. Temple, Rochester [VT], 2007) identified some 271 inventions that followed this pattern. For the reasons, see: Lowrey, Y. and Baumol, W. J., *Rapid Invention, Slow Industrialization, and the Absent Innovative Entrepreneur in Medieval China*, a paper read at a meeting of the American Economic Association, Atlanta, Jan. 3-5, 2010. As for printing, Chinese characters, which number in the tens of thousands, pose a significant difficulty for moveable type, and this probably made it impractical for extensive medical texts to be printed until recent times.

[31] Tao, L., *Achievements of Chinese Medicine in the Sui (589-617 AD) and T'ang (618-907 AD) Dynasties*, in *Chinese Med. J.*, 71:301-320, 1953, especially the Table, p. 316.

of Education under the patronage of the Emperor, that its role was primarily oriented to printing Confucian classics and to providing medical practitioners for the Royal family and its bureaucracy, and that the "medical school" component actually began about 1000 AD and was short-lived.[32]

F. Conclusion and Legacy

The classic medical texts of ancient China provide little information regarding the actual practice of medicine. It is uncertain whether there even was a discrete occupational group identifiable as physicians, which Dr. Sivin answered in the negative.[33] And perhaps relevant is recent scholarship that suggests that "the most important interlocutor of the Yellow Thearch," *i.e.*, the Yellow Emperor in the *Huang Ti Nei Ching Su Wen*, was none other than Hippocrates himself (460-380 BC), whose message may have reached China about 200 BC. Thus, some of those nuggets of rational medical thought found in the *Huang Ti Nei Ching Su Wen* may have been imported.

There is one final consideration. In contrast to ancient Sumer and Egypt, the medical practice of ancient China can be pursued up to the present day in a search for the natural state of medical practice, for, of the three civilizations discussed so far, only the Chinese version has functionally survived. Modernization of China's medical profession was attempted in the 1920s by the Ministry of Health of the Kuomintang, even to the point of abolishing what is now termed "traditional Chinese medicine."[34] But traditional Chinese medicine was given new life with the victory of the communist People's Republic in 1949, when the economics of providing health care necessary for popularizing the government led to legitimization and official promotion of this cheap alternative to scientific medicine.[35] A translation of the term used to describe today's Chinese medicine is "confluence of medicine," the consequence of drawing on two medical traditions since the repopularization of Western medicine in recent years. All practitioners of traditional medicine have since been encouraged to learn modern Western medicine. Both types have government recognition.[36] There was a setback during the Cultural Revolution of

---

[32] See: Chapter 7, C. Clinical Medicine of the *Huang Ti Nei Ching Su Wen* and the "National University" in Huff, T. E., *The Rise of Early Modern Science*, Cambridge, 2003, 2nd edition, p. 284. Medical writings at this time mimicked those of medieval Europe and the Middle East, most being commentaries on ancient writings, just as medieval European writings were commentaries on Galen rather than on new discoveries.

[33] Referring to Chinese medical professionals, "At no point in the past can we speak of a single autonomous occupational group." See: Sivin, N., Introduction to volume 6, part VI, of the classic series *Science and Civilization in China*, by Needham, J., and Gwei-Djen, L., Cambridge, 2004.

[34] Founders of the Kuomintang, or Chinese Nationalist Party, included Dr. Sun Yat-sen, a physician trained in Western medicine who became China's first President.

[35] For information on the extraordinary changes in 20th C Chinese medicine see: Unschuld, *Chinese Medicine*, Brookline, MA, 1998; the original was in German. Also see the Foreword by Ken Rose in a recent reprinting of Veith's work, *The Yellow Emperor's Classic of Internal Medicine*, Berkeley, 2002.

[36] Cai Jing-Feng, in Jan Van Alphen, Anthony Aris, editors, *Traditional Medicine in China Today*, Boston, 1996. Care should be taken to not equate *traditional* and *scientific* Chinese medicine, and to unify them in an attempt to justify retention of ancient and venerable ways for political or economic aims will not be useful. For example, *artemisinin* is an effective antimalarial, a compound extracted from one of many hundreds of herbs used for many centuries to treat fever in China. This

1965, requiring the government to popularize the "barefoot doctor." This "doctor" was, in fact, the layman himself, who was provided in 1970 with a "do it yourself" booklet by the State.[37] It contained advice on management of trauma, childbirth, and disease in terms understood by those untrained in medicine, plus information on preventive medicine, sanitation and public health issues. Thus, during this recent extreme manifestation of authoritarian governance in China there was an extreme, albeit temporary, regression of health care to the point that there were not even "itinerant doctors" to help the sick.

To what can the disparate paths that medicine took in the great civilization of China and in the West, as first represented by ancient Greece, be attributed? Prof. G. Lloyd, formerly chairman of the East Asian History of Science Trust, has written extensively on the subject, and a summary is presented in the following table:[38]

Table 3: Ethos and success, East and West

Ethos	China	Greece
1. Fundamental concepts	refining of abstract theory	objective observation
2. Livelihood	patronage	reliance on manual skills
3. Cosmology	State is part of the Whole	analogies only
4. Pluralism/deviance	a negative virtue	a positive virtue
5. Public/private spheres	public interest	private interest
6. Consensus/disagreement	emphasis on orthodoxy	emphasis on disputation
7. Persuasion	avoided	a tool for advancement

Overall, conforming to authority was the path to advancement that permeated ancient Chinese thinking, whereas in the West, beginning with ancient Greece, success from individual prowess favored survival and/or prosperity.

In large and varied countries such as China there will always be the sporadic but important medical advance that results from singular empirical discovery or insight. And surely the *Huang Ti Nei Ching Su Wen* does not represent the gold standard of medical practice in a country of mountains, jungles, and deserts now encompassing 3,800,000 square miles and 1.4 billion people. Take, as an example, the Chinese therapy

sounds like a triumph of traditional Chinese medicine. This is not so. The true recognition of its effectiveness was the result, forty years ago, of scientific investigation by a Chinese pharmacist with a background in Western medicine, Ti YouYou, who finally received the Lasker Prize for clinical medical research in 2011. Otherwise, in the hands of traditional Chinese medicine practitioners the artemisinin-producing herb would have remained virtually unknown, undistinguished, and sporadically employed. Any "triumph" for artemisinin must be credited solely to Tu YouYou and her scientific screening of hundreds of botanicals, not to the ancient philosopher, part-time government official, medical layman, and prolific social critic of his age, Ge Hong, and not to the government that, out of military necessity and in secrecy, commanded a malaria cure, funded the search, then lost interest in the project once it was able to copy modern drugs already developed elsewhere. There is a perennial search for botanicals in all cultures useful for fevers. The 1814 edition of Culpeper's Herbal lists ten botanicals out of four hundred that were effective for "agues," most being "tertian" and "quartan." The question is not whether one or another was thought to be effective; the question is which were proven to be effective.

[37] It is available in English translation, one being an edition issued by the U. S. Dept. of Health, Education, and Welfare: *A Barefoot Doctor's Manual*, Bethesda, 1977.

[38] Adapted from G. Lloyd and N. Sivin, *The Way and the Word*, New Haven, 2002, p. 239*ff*.

of goiter in the 7th C AD using thyroid glands obtained from domestic animals, sometimes with added seaweed, a source of iodine.[39] It was a clever invention, and in various forms it has been included in traditional Chinese therapies. Writings from as early as 700 AD may have recognized forms of beriberi and associated them with a change in preparation of rice, although this information lay dormant for centuries, awaiting 20th C elucidation and exploitation.[40] But it is not enough to have an isolated empirical discovery. There must be action taken that betters the lot of individuals within society. It has been repeatedly noted that despite the numerous discoveries and inventions in China over many centuries none became the stimulus for commercial exploitation that might have been a basis for prosperity and societal improvement.[41] And so it was that Marco Polo would describe the 13th C medicine of southern China and "throughout Cathay," *i.e.*, northern China, in these terms: In Kara-jang, Vochan, and Yachi provinces, "there are no physicians. When someone falls ill, he sends for magicians,"[42] and, "the same practice is observed throughout Cathay and Manzi and by almost all idolaters owing to their lack of physicians." In conclusion, the great discoveries in China that placed that civilization so in advance of medieval Europe were paralleled neither in the practice nor the profession of medicine.

---

[39] The thyroid gland, high in iodine, was recommended for goiter by Sun Si Miao, a 7th C physician. Desiccated pig thyroid for medicinal use is still available but rarely used, and then only by prescription. It does indeed have biological activity.

[40] Huang, H. T., *Science and Civilization in China*, Cambridge, 2000, Vol. 6, Part V, Chapter 7, Needham, J., Yates, R., *et al.*, eds.

[41] This problem is discussed and referenced in: Lowrey, Y., and Baumol, W. J., *Rapid Invention, Slow Industrialization, and the Absent Innovative Entrepreneur in Medieval China*, in *Proc. Amer. Philosophical Soc.*, 157:1-21, 2013, in which the commitment of medieval Chinese government was to agrarian stability, one consequence being a stunting of entrepreneurship. See also: Needham, J., in his Introduction to *The Genius of China: 3,000 Years of Science, Discovery, and Inventions*, Rochester, VT, 2007, R. K. G. Temple, editor.

[42] This statement is then followed by two pages of description of the ceremony of magic. See: Latham, R. E., *The Travels of Marco Polo*, London, 1958, p. 182.

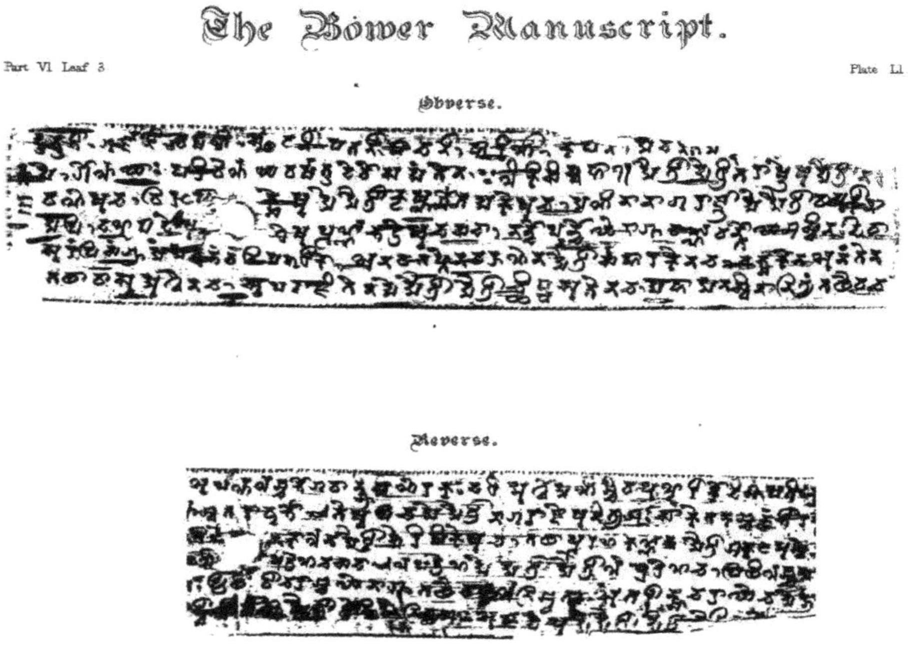

The Bower Manuscript.

Part VI Leaf 3

Plate LI

Obverse.

Reverse.

Fig. 6: The Bower manuscript, a 6th C AD Indian Buddhist work written on birch-bark, is the earliest extant writing on Ayurvedic medicine. Comprising seven chapters written on fifty-one leaves, five contain comments about pharmaceutical agents, eye diseases, hair dyes and washes, aphrodisiacs, a long section on the uses of garlic, and many other items. The remaining chapters are on divination. (See: Hoernle, A. F. R., *The Bower Manuscript; facsimili leaves, Nagari transcript, romanised transliteration and English translation with notes*, Calcutta,1908-1912.) Photo credit: Wujastyk, 26.06.2011, license of Creative Commons. The photograph is of one of the Plates in Hoernle's book.

CHAPTER FIVE

LARGE STRUCTURED SOCIETIES, AUTHORITARIAN – THE ASIAN SUBCONTINENT

"Make all the men on every side, Parna, obedient to my will."

> *Hymns of the Arthavaveda*, Book III, 5, vi, vii; "A King's
> address to an amulet which is to strengthen his authority."
> The amulet (of wood) was considered a gift from Indra, Leader of the
> Gods, to a king. Translation of R. T. H. Griffith, 1895. The *Hymns* date
> to *ca.* 1000 BC.

"Artisans, musicians, physicians, buffoons, cooks, and other workmen, serving of their own accord, shall obtain such wages as similar persons employed elsewhere usually get or as much as experts (kusalah) shall fix.".

> From Kautilya's *Arthashastra*, thought to be the work of the
> Prime Minister of the great Mauryan emperor, Chandragupta (340-298
> BC), who unified virtually the entire Indian subcontinent. Book III,
> describing laws of the kingdom. (The 1915 translation by R.
> Shamasastry, reprinted, Mysore, 1960)

The earliest historical record of Indian medicine, which has much of empirical worth, can be dated only to *ca.* 100 BC. Nevertheless, traditional Indian medicine, Ayurveda, is far more ancient. With the advent of the caste system, it came under the hegemony of the Brahmin, or priest, caste, even medical training being their purview. Equally important to development of Indian medicine was centralization of medical authority within medical guilds that were integrated into regional monarchical governments. Despite the insertion of elements of Hippocratic medicine as a consequence of Alexandrian and Islamic intrusions into the subcontinent, traditional Indian medicine would have changed little up to the present time were it not for assimilation of elements of modern Western medicine since the 18th century. The popularity of Ayurveda in part rests on its being a less expensive alternative to scientific medicine.

A. Introduction: Indian Medicine's Early History

Indian medicine has a long and continuous history, making itself known about 1000 BC in the first drug prescriptions of Ayurvedic practitioners and continuing to this day. Ayurvedic medical practice has been described as the Hindu medical science of longevity, and the prescriptions have been those of herbalists. Some consider it the oldest system of medicine in the world.[1] Holy books of the Hindus, the derivative of an oral

---

[1] The National Center for Complementary and Alternative Medicine (NCCAM), a component of the National Institutes of Health, U. S. Department of Health and Human Services, states "Ayurvedic medicine (also called Ayurveda) is one of the world's oldest medical systems. It originated in India and has evolved there over thousands of years." (Extracted from NCCAM website, 2014.)

tradition supposedly traceable to perhaps 2000-3000 BC, are thought to be the source of the theory of humours, from which elements came to be found in the writings of Hippocrates in ancient Greece.

An early historical account of the medicine of ancient India comes from Herodotus in the 5th C BC, who wrote of one group, "And whenever any of them falls into sickness, he goes to the desert country and lies there, and none of them pay any attention either to one who is dead or to one who is sick."[2] But in his statement the level of fantasy or misinformation, or even the true identity as Indians, as he calls them, is uncertain. His comments cannot be taken to represent the status of Indian medicine. A Greek physician who accompanied the forces of Alexander the Great, Megasthenes (*ca.* 350-290 BC), wrote τὰ ᾽Ινδικά (ta Indika, "the Indians"), a work in four books of which little remains. Dr. J. H. Baas, the prominent historian of medicine, cites him as stating that the Indians used few drugs, although other sources show the Indian pharmacopeia to have been most extensive, a point with which Dr. Baas agreed.[3] Megasthenes wrote:

> "... the second in estimation are the Physicians [ἰατρίκη or ἰατρός, "iatros"],[4] philosophers, who are conversant with men, simple in their habits, but not exposing themselves to a life abroad, living upon rice and grain, which every one to whom they apply freely gives them and receives them into his house: they are able by the use of medicines to render women fruitful and productive either of males or females: but they perform cures rather by attention to diet than the use of medicines. Of medicines they approve more commonly of unguents and plaster, for all others they consider not free from deleterious effects. These, and others of this sect, so exercise their patience in labours and trials, as to have attained the capability of standing in one position unmoved for a whole day."[5]

Now there has never been a drug that could guarantee the sex of a fetus. Had there been one, the race that developed it surely would have long since ceased to exist. It is better

---

[2] ὃς δ᾽ ἂν ἐς νοῦσον αὐτῶν πέσῃ, ἐλθὼν ἐς τὴν ἔρημον κέεται· φροντίζει δὲ οὐδὶς οὔτε ἀποθανόντος ουτε κάμνοντος. (*The Histories of Herodotus*, Bk. III, 100, translation of G. C. Macaulay, London, 1890.)

[3] Baas, J. H., *Outlines of the History of Medicine and the Medical Profession*, New York, 1889, H. E. Handerson, translator, p. 48.

[4] The Greek word for "physician" is ἰατρός (iatros). But, as discussed later, the classification of a medical professional trained in medicine according to recognized standards as a "physician" probably did not exist in ancient Hellas. Thus, the phrase "healthcare provider," today's catch-all phrase for a variety of medical practitioners with a great range of skills, is probably closer to the ancient meaning of the Greek word. The criticism directed against incompetent "physicians" mentioned in Hippocratic writings does not, therefore, indict "physicians" as a class, and certainly not Hippocratic physicians, but refers only to those medical practitioners viewed as inferior in training and skills as compared to the Hippocratic practitioners themselves and unworthy to be listed among their ranks. Despite these very important semantic limitations, the traditional translation of ἰατρός as "physician" will be used in this book.

[5] Megasthenes was a diplomat sent to a Mauryan king. He gives the earliest Greek account of India. Describing castes, he discusses first the Brahmin caste. Then, under the Germanes sect he cites the Hylobii as the most honorable, living "in the woods upon leaves and wild fruits" and wearing clothes of tree bark. The Greek text for the cited quation can be found in: Cory, I. P., *Ancient Fragments*, a Wizard edition reprint, Minneapolis, 1975, p. 239-240, translation of E. Richmond Hodges. This tract is not readily available and it is therefore quoted in the original Greek, which is from Strabo, Bk. 15.

to rely on internal rather than external sources for a history of Indian medical practice.

B. The Three Stages and the Three Ages of Indian Medicine

Indian medicine of today has three divisions, the consequence of its chronological stages: the Ayurvedic, the Unani or Greco-Arabian system, and the Modern, which some consider Greek in origin but with Western post-Renaissance changes. The first is ancient and traditional; the second, practiced more by the non-Hindu population, is a derivative of Greek-Hippocratic medicine introduced with the Alexandrian conquests of the 4th C BC and the Muslim incursions of about 1000 AD; and the third is a consequence of intrusions in the 17th C by European colonial powers.[6,7]

Prof. Kenneth Zysk has divided Indian medicine into three ages. The first is the *Vedic age*, 1200-800 BC. The ancient Vedic works contain poetically enshrined concepts transmitted orally from generation to generation for thousands of years. The essence of the Vedas was the "right moral order" on which were based the four goals of life: prosperity (*artha*), satisfaction of desires (*kama*), moral duty (*dharma*), and spiritual perfection (*moksa*, or liberation from finite existence). But, as noted by a 19th C German historian of Indian medicine, Prof. Julius Jolly, there are no specific Vedic tracts on medicine.[8] The *Atharva Veda*, 1.22, for example, includes a short tract used to counteract jaundice, but it does so by charms, not empirical therapy:

> Unto the sun let them both go up - your heartburn and your yellowness;
> with the color of the red bull do we envelop you.
> with red colors do we envelop you for the sake of long life;
> so that this person may be free from harm and may become non-yellow.
> Those cows/herbs that have Rohini [the Red One] as presiding divinity, as also cows which are red –
> their every form and every power - with them do we envelop you.
> Into the parrots do we put your yellowness and into the yellow-green *ropanaka*-birds.
> Similarly into the turmeric [or yellow wagtail?] do we deposit your yellowness.[9]

Thus, medical peculiarities are mentioned in the Atharvaveda, or "science of incantations," that represent signs of disease, including ascites, fever, and dementia.[10]

---

[6]Bhatia, S. L., *Greek Medicine in Asia and Other Essays*, Bangalore, 1970. The author of this well-written small volume makes the suggestion that contributions from Indian medicine were introduced to Greece via Alexander the Great (356-323 BC). He also argues that Hippocrates "introduced ethical principles into the practice of medicine, which are much the same as those laid down by Charaka and Sushruta, who preceded Hippocrates by centuries," an argument made less tenable by recent studies on the age of ancient Indian texts.

[7] European medicine in India focused initially on hospitals for Europeans. It was only in the 19th C that Indians enrolled in medical colleges.

[8] Kashikar, C. G., *Indian Medicine*, New Delhi, 1977, a reprint of Julius Jolly's 1901 well-regarded history of Indian medicine (*Medicin*, a volume of a larger work), having been translated into English from the original German.

[9] This example is quoted in: *Sources of Indian Tradition*, W. T. de Bary, editor, New York, 1958, vol. 1, p. 18. The practice of putting a string of yellow flowers around the neck of a jaundiced person is still common on the subcontinent.

[10] Zysk, K. G., *Does Ancient Indian Medicine Have a Theory of Contagion?*, in *Contagion*, L. Conrad., editor, Aldershot, 2000, chapter 5. The chants and anatomical terms of the Vedic age are

They are mentioned, however, as evidence of demonic visitations on man because of sinfulness, not as something to be understood and treated by mortal means. "Hindu classic medicine stems from priestly magic; unlike pioneers of modern thought who became famous through their persecution by the Church for contradicting traditional ideas, Hindu medical men never were at variance with the authority of Brahmin priestcraft and revealed sacred lore."[11]

The second stage identified by Dr. Zysk is the *classical*, extending from 800 BC to the time of Muslim invasions in about 1000 AD. At the beginning of this stage some postulate that Hinduism came firmly under the control of an elite Aryan class, from which the Brahmins would soon claim the highest position in the caste system. It is also the age of Ayurveda. Medical practice now became a fact of history, for a series of great writings emerged. The theory of humors, of balance of forces, became formalized. Strong religious and mystical ties remained part of medical canon, however, even though it has been stressed that Ayurvedic medicine is not a branch of Hinduism. There is, furthermore, evidence that Ayurveda is an indigenous production and that there was no Aryan "invasion" that introduced the Vedas into the subcontinent. A parallel development at this time was the rise of a guild system in many professions and crafts.

The third stage Dr. Zysk calls the *syncretic*, in which features of Unani, Muslim, and Western practices became integrated. This stage, dating from about 1000 AD, has persisted up to the present time. As stated by Prof. Pareti, *et al.*, the "theory of Ayurvedic medicine was handed down through generations of physicians (vaidya), and is still widely followed in India today."[12] But today's Ayurvedic medicine has been modified by adopting some Western concepts and pharmacopeia and has come to be a low-cost alternative to Western medicine, encompassing standardized medicines made by Ayurvedic pharmaceutical companies. In a similar fashion, Unani medicine continues to this day with its own medical schools and bureaucracies. It also has appropriated much Western medicine, including diagnostic tools. Being relatively inexpensive, it, too, is undergoing something of a revival. Analogies with the evolution of osteopathy in the United States, apart from its longevity, seem appropriate.[13]

---

also discussed in a series of articles in the *J. Royal Asiatic Soc.*, 1906-1909, such as one by Hoernle, *Studies in Ancient Indian Medicine, II*, in *J. Royal Asiatic Soc.*, 39:1-18, 1907.

[11] Zimmer, H. R., *Hindu Medicine*, Baltimore, 1948. Zimmer contrasts, favorably, the status of Indian medicine with that of contemporary Western Dark Ages, perhaps correctly. But that status reflects defects of the latter rather than strengths of the former, as will be described later in this work.

[12] Pareti, Luigi; *History of Mankind: Cultural and Scientific Development*, Vol. 2, *The Ancient World*, London, 1965, p. 750.

[13] Andrew Still (1828-1917), son of a Virginia preacher and "physician," developed his osteopathic system of therapeutics after being unable to save the lives of family members and fellow Civil War soldiers with the medical knowledge he acquired from some medical reading and from an apprenticeship with his father. Inventing osteopathy in 1874, he opened the first School of Osteopathy in 1892 in Kirksville, Missouri. His unconventional approach to medicine minimized the use of drugs and stressed physical contact and reassertion of proper anatomical relations. This was not popular, even in an age of unconventional approaches. But with the opening of his school of Osteopathy it became enthusiastically accepted, thus demonstrating the importance of disciples nd institutional credentials in fashioning public opinion. Over the years osteopathy has progressively accommodated diagnostic and therapeutic procedures of allopathic medicine, to the point that osteopathic and allopathic physicians now have equal standing and closely similar procedures.

C. Indian Medical Classics

The most venerable and oldest book on Indian medical practice is the *Charaka Samhita*, the "medical compendium of Dr. Charaka." Like China's *Huang Ti Nei Ching Su Wen*, it has been amended and emended many times, but it presumably represents medical thought of a much earlier age as preserved by oral tradition. Both Drs. Baas and Bhatia state that the *Charaka Samhita* and the *Susruta Samhita* (to be discussed below) preceded Hippocratic writings by centuries.[14] Dr. Gerrit Meulenbeld, who recorded all the great Ayurvedic writings, begins his monumental work with the *Charaka Samhita* and the *Susruta Samhita*.[15] He agrees that they are the earliest of the writings, the *Charaka* preceding the *Susruta*. Both were written in Sanskrit when finally committed to history, as are all other medical writings of the classical period. There is a great range of estimates concerning the age of the *Charaka Samhita*, but on the basis of style, language, and content, it has been dated by some as not later than 200 AD and not earlier than 100 BC, the *Susruta Samhita* not later than the 5th C AD. And yet, despite the preceding, the oldest extant Indian medical manuscript is the one acquired by Hamilton Bower in 1890 and which has been dated to the late 6th C AD. The "Bower" manuscript, found in Chinese Turkestan (now the Chinese autonomous region of Xinjiang), is a composite of manuscripts and is said to mention Susruta and to include elements of the *Susruta Samhita* (Fig. 6). In contrast, the *Charaka Samhita* is represented by no extant ancient manuscript, although contemporary versions have been traced back to a famous version made in the 9th C AD by Drdhabala, a scholar who is said to have edited a modified version, adding an extensive component of his own work that he considered to represent some of the missing sections of the *Charaka Samhita*.

The *Charaka Samhita*, probably composed in northwest India, is long, complex, and esoteric. Dr. Avinash Chandra Kaviratna, a noted translator of the *Charaka Samhita*, states: "No summary, however skillfully framed, can afford an adequate idea of the real contents of Charaka's compilation," surely an intimidating introduction for any student of Indian medicine.[16] Dr. Meulenbeld includes the following analysis in his work: ". . . it consists of a mosaic of elements derived from diverse schools of thought, often modified in the service of medicine, and mixed with concepts not found elsewhere." The *Charaka Samhita*, like the *Susruta Samhita* to follow, comprises one-hundred-and-twenty chapters written in verse and prose. The author is unknown, for there were several prominent Charakas in early Indian history. Charaka has been described as a "half-mythical" figure, and the term "charaka" was also applied to itinerant teachers, perhaps analogous to the Greek use of the term "sophist" in the 5th C BC. The *Charaka Samhita* also has a section suggesting input from Hippocratic sources, and Hippocratic features, both ethical and professional, are present in its Oath.[17] Beyond the cultural appendages peculiar to the

---

[14] Baas, J. H., *Outlines of the History of Medicine and the Medical Profession*, New York, 1889, H. E. Handerson, translator, p. 40, and Bhatia, S. L., *Greek Medicine in Asia and Other Essays*, Bangalore, 1970.

[15] Meulenbeld, G. J., *A History of Indian Medical Literature*, Groningen, 1999, in five volumes. Meulenbeld's review of the classical medical literature of India is a remarkable accomplishment that unfortunately has no equal among the civilizations reviewed thus far in this work.

[16] A. C. Kaviratna's quotation is found in the "Notice" of his translation of the first part of *The Charaka-Samhita*, Calcutta, dated 1896.

[17] See translation of *The Medical Student's Oath of Ancient India* by A. Menon and H. F. Haberman, in *Med. Hist.*, 14:295-299, 1970; also see Veatch, R. M., *Cross Cultural Perspectives in Medical*

time and place of its composition, similarities of many lines with the Hippocratic Oath are obvious, although the Greeks did not include the requirement of celibacy nor did they attempt to coerce moral perfection of the practitioner, preferring, instead, to merely specify his professional obligations.[18] Obedience to authority and witholding of treatment from unattended women or haters of the king are but two of the many differences. Both oaths imply an intimate association of teacher and student, but the Oath of Initiation suggests a degree of commitment on the part of the novice that surpasses that of the Hippocratic Oath.

A medical school was not specified as integral to training. In the early centuries of the Common Era there was an intellectual center located in Taxila, in today's Punjab, that suggests an analogy with the academic center in Gondeshapour in contemporary Persia. But despite the statement that a famous physician, Jivaka, took seven years to complete his medical studies there, identification of an ancient medical school in the region of Taxila is lacking. Three kinds of physicians are described by Charaka: the "hypocrites," or quacks, who look like physicians, the physicians "by report," who not only look but act like physicians but have no medical knowledge, and the true physicians, who know, among other things, drugs and the medical scriptures.

There is no testimony regarding the physician-patient interaction, although instruction is given to both. Advice to the physician includes the following: "A thorough mastery of the scriptures (bearing on the science of life), large experience (of actual results), cleverness, and purity (of both mind and body) are regarded as the four (principal) qualifications of a physician."[19] As to the patient, "Memory, obedience to the directions (given by the physician), fearlessness, and communicativeness are the qualifications of the patient."

Topics of the early chapters of the *Charaka Samhita* include matters relating to divine descent and medical theory, drugs for emesis and purgation, preparations for external purification, evacuative preparations, daily regimen (clothing, diet, massage), and seasonal changes in physiology. Clinical observations in the compendium are often astute and extensive. Twenty varieties of "worms" and twenty varieties of diseases of the sexual organs of women are described, as are other categories of disease, often containing twenty varieties. Just what the "worms" might have been is a mystery, for visual, *i.e.*, macroscopic, inspection of stool and skin lesions today from around the world would identify only *nine* worms infesting humans: ascarides, strongyloides, schistosomes, tapeworm, whipworm, hookworm, guinea worm, onchocerca, and pinworm. Without a microscope one wonders what were the other eleven types of "worms."[20] Drug treatment and therapeutic diets are given in some detail.

The embellishments on theories such as the Tridosha[21] of Ayurvedic medicine, which some feel was the predecessor of early Western humoral theories, reveal

Ethics: Readings, Boston, 1989. It is obvious that there are more points of difference between the Hippocratic Oath and The Oath of Initiation than there are similarities.

[18] See: Adams, W. H., *The Natural State of Medical Practice: Hippocratic Evidence*, Maitland (FL), 2019, p. 512*ff*, for the Hippocratic Oath and its translations.

[19] Lesson IX of the *Charaka-Samhita*, Calcutta, 1896, Part I, p. 102*ff*, translator: A. C. Kaviratna.

[20] To be fair, there are six types of tapeworm that can infect humans.

[21] The Tridosha comprises three biological components: metabolism, movement (including visceral), and structure (including stability and fertility).

similarities to those ascribed to the Hippocratics.[22] But treatment has a tendency to be directed toward a specific symptom at a specific point in time, rather than at an identifiable symptom complex of a definable disease process evolving over time. The Hippocratic admonition not to treat an incurable disease is maintained by Charaka, although the motives might be questioned:

> The course of treatment which a physician, conversant with the distinction between curable and incurable diseases, commences at the proper time with the aid of intelligence, verily succeeds (in accomplishing its object).
> That physician who takes up the treatment of a disease that is incurable incurs loss of wealth, loss of knowledge, loss of fame, censure of the world, and incapacity for practice.[23]

The other prominent Ayurvedic writing is that by Susruta, although there have been some who think the writings of Susruta are but later Arabian transcriptions of some of the Hippocratic works.[24] Dr. Bhagavat Sinh Jee has written on Aryan medical science. He includes in his work more than a hundred drawings of surgical implements, such as forceps, bougies, and tongs. But the source of his detailed engravings is not stated, being attributed to "old writers" who are not specified in his bibliography.[25] Others have commented that no genuinely ancient or medieval surgical instruments from India have survived, and that Susruta's work does not develop surgical ideas but describes, primarily in Book II, only empirical management. The types of surgery listed in the *Charaka Samhita* comprise excision, incision, rupturing, scraping, scarification, suturing, probing, caustics, and leeches, but there are no other early sources of information regarding Indian surgery, perhaps because of caste taboos. Dr. Bhagavat Sinh Jee affirms this in noting

---

[22] There may have been early contacts between Greek and Indian medicine given their similarities in theory and in practice as expressed by Dr. Charaka. It has been stated that the theory of disease described in some works of Plato and in the earlier chapters of περὶ φύσιος ἀνθρώπου (*Concerning the Nature of Man*) of Hippocrates may have come from Indian sources. Although the classic Sanskrit medical texts of India first appear in manuscript perhaps four hundred years after Plato (427-347 BC), it is claimed that their body of knowledge actually preceded Plato by many centuries. (Pareti, L., *History of Mankind: Cultural and Scientific Development*, vol. 2, *The Ancient World*, London, 1965, p.750.) There is the conjecture that philosophical concepts such as "the one and the many," reincarnation, and cosmic cycle came to ancient Greece from India, reaching across borders during the period when Persia had "united" Greece and India. Greeks at this time, including the physician Democedes (5th C BC), may have had the opportunity to travel in Persia, learn from Indian medicine, and return that knowledge to medical centers in Sicily, Italy, and Greece. Later, during the Hellenistic period, the offspring of this exchange would return to India. (McEvilley, T., *The Shape of Ancient Thought: Comparative Studies in Greek and Indian Philosophies*, New York, 2000.) Another opinion is that Greek medicine came from Egypt, where it had been received from India. (Bhagvat Sinh Jee, *A Short History of Aryan Medical Science*, London, 1896, p. 192f.) Whatever the sequence, it is notable that there are no attributions to Greek medicine in the Sanskrit writings, whereas some credit is given to Greeks for discoveries in astronomy (Hunter, W. W., *The Indian Empire; Its People, History and Products*, London, 1886, chapter 6). This suggests little Greek influence in Indian medicine before the Common Era. Ayurveda is a uniquely Indian system of healing.

[23] Lesson X, the *Charaka-Samhita*, Calcutta, 1896, p. 109.

[24] This is attributed to E. Haas in J. H. Baas' *Outlines of the History of Medicine*, New York, 1889, transl. H. Handerson, MD, p. 44, footnote, and the reasoning is surely circuitous. (See: Raju, V. K., *Susruta of Ancient India*, in *Indian J. Ophthalmol.*, 51:119-122, 2003.)

[25] Bhagvat Sinh Jee, *A Short History of Aryan Medical Science*, London, 1896, chapters 2 and 10.

that surgery declined in India because of an aversion to physical contact with not only the patient, but also "blood, pus, and other matter" necessary for the study of anatomy and practice of surgery, this because the Brahmin caste maintained full control over medical teaching.[26] The Brahmins appealed to the Vedas as justification for declaring that "healers were corrupt as a result of the defilement they incurred from contact with unclean people" and were to be avoided.[27] Thus, a change occured about 750 AD as the Brahmin caste removed itself from studies that required physical contact with patients or products of the diseased body, leaving that responsibility to the lower Vaidya caste, which in time followed a similar course.[28] This same opinion has been expressed by Chari, who concludes there is little evidence that any of the surgical practices mentioned in the *Susruta Samhita* were ever performed from the time of its writing up to the 19th C.[29]

As a consequence of early Brahmin policies, village medicine was left to pursue its own course. Thus, the daily surgical and medical practices of the average ancient Indian practitioner remain unknown, despite modern emphasis on some technically unique ophthalmological procedures, plastic surgery that included rhinoplasty, and *Susruta*'s mention of sweet-tasting urine now attributed to diabetes. Again, the fascinating work of Dr. Guido Majno reviews not only these techniques, but also their significance.[30]

D. Brahminization and the Social Context of Indian Medicine

Prof. Zysk proposes an explanation for the appearance of empirical medical practices in the classic era Ayurvedic works of Charaka and Susruta. He argues that the evolution of the dominant Brahmin priesthood, or caste, by distancing itself from medical practice in the Vedic age, relegated that occupation to practitioners who were peripatetic and sometimes ascetic. Being viewed as of little importance, however, such practitioners were open to new ideas because of their "intellectual freedom." Over time there was a merging of their practical labors and discoveries with those of mendicant Buddhists who considered Buddha a healer and who had also acquired a catalog of therapies. At the same time, the traditional songs and incantations of the Vedas used for illnesses fashioned a "Brahmanization" of this empirical merger of empirical knowledge by an insertion of its origins into Hindu mythology in such a way as to make the final product appear to be an inherently Hindu art. This is implied, Dr. Zysk continues, in the opening statements of the *Charaka* and *Susruta* Samhitas. Thus, those two works, the epitome of classical era medical ayurvedic treatises, obtained the imprimatur of Hindu philosophy that would serve as a basis for Hindu science despite their disparate origins.[31]

But there may now be evolving a more interesting history of the *Charaka*

---

[26] Ibid., 1896, p. 186.

[27] Zysk, K. G., *Mythology and Brahmanization of Indian Medicine: Transforming Heterodoxy into Orthodoxy*, in *Categorisation and Interpretation*, J. Folke, ed, Goteburg, 1999, pp. 125-145.

[28] Hunter, W. W., *The Indian Empire; Its People, History and Products*, London, 1886, p. 104.

[29] Chari, P. S., *Susruta and Our Heritage*, in *Indian J. Plastic Surg.*, 36:4-13, 2003. This brief but excellent review of Indian medicine by a practicing Plastic Surgeon acknowledges a documentary limitation on Indian medical history.

[30] Majno, G., *The Healing Hand*, Cambridge (MA), 1975, chapter 7.

[31] Zysk, K. G., *Mythology and Brahmanization of Indian Medicine: Transforming Heterodoxy into Orthodoxy*, in *Categorisation and Interpretation*, J. Folke, ed., Goteburg, 1999, pp. 125-145.

compendium. The complicated story is presented by Dr. Debiprasad Chattopadhyaya.[32] He noted that the 9th C AD editing of the *Charaka Samhita* by Drdhabala was termed a "reconstruction" by the editor himself, indicating the likelihood of extensive changes, and one-third of the compendium was solely Drdhabala's own work, a factor that Chattopadhyaya thinks is due in part to the editor's religious affiliation and which can explain the "jumble of science and superstition" now found in a venerable writing that traditionally is claimed to be based on objectivity. But in exploring more ancient origins for the *Charaka* compilation that Drdhabala modified, it may be that Charaka himself was also a compiler and editor of but an earlier version of the work and of a much earlier era. The name Atreya has been attached to the individuals who might have been the source of the initial version. Atreya are considered to have descended from one of Hinduism's sages, Atre, and a disciple, Agnivesa, is credited with formulating, according to Atre's instructions, the Ayurvedic method of medical practice that has been handed down to the present day, after its modification by Charaka as the *Charaka Samhita*. If this is so, the ancient work would from its inception have been a Brahmin effort.

But other scholars suggest that it was the Hindu sage, Bharadvaja (*ca.* 1500 BC) who first formulated the Ayurvedic principles upon which the various schools, or areas, of medicine would be founded.[33] Those principles were: (1) belief in causality, (2) acknowledgement of a disease as an entity rather than a status, and (3) acceptance that curability (of curable diseases) can reside in the actions of a physician. As pointed out by Dr. Chattopadhyaya, each of these principles strongly implies objectivity and the acknowledgement of natural laws that can be understood by man. A basis for medical science is thus provided by Bharadvaja, and the continued existence of Ayurveda can be attributed to that factual clinical base that can still be found in some chapters of the *Charaka Samhita* despite much that is medically irrelevant or spiritual. Although Bharadvaja has been proposed, therefore, as the source of Ayurveda, how could one person have acquired the massive amount of knowledge that has endured in the *Charaka* and *Susruta* Samhitas?

Again, Dr. Chattopadhyaya has proposed the answer: the medical knowledge was the accumulated wisdom and experience of many practitioners. Thus, a pattern emerges, one that is similar to that discussed in the preceding chapters on Mesopotamian and Egyptian medical practice although not so apparent in Chinese medicine. In the earliest days individual practitioners, relatively unfettered by tradition, regulation, or intimidation, were able to develop an archaic and empirical but objective medical practice that was sufficiently useful that their practices became a guide to others who might wish to join them in what might now be called the profession of medicine. But as time went by the knowledge and the process of acquiring that knowledge became enmeshed in extrinsic social developments that diminished the scientific component but added a new dimension consistent with orthodox religion. This would have begun during the age of the Atreyas and subsequently maintained, compiled, and supplemented by Charaka and later by Drdhabala, and perhaps by other unknown hands. Although the time scale over which this sequence occurred is vague and the factual nature of the parties involved is

---

[32] Chattopadhyaya, D., *Science and Society in Ancient India*, Amsterdam, 1977, especially the interesting Introduction.

[33] As a Hindu sage in early Vedic times Bharadvaja's hymns are considered to have been prominent *ca.* 1500 BC in northwest India among a semi-nomadic people, thus approximately coeval with the Mycenaean Empire in ancient Greece, although the first appearance of the earliest hymns is thought to have occurred centuries earlier.

debatable, the significance of such a transfiguration will become obvious below.

It is in its social context, more than its medical teaching as expressed by the two practitioners, Charaka and Susruta, that Indian medicine distinctly diverges from that of the contemporary West. One area of divergence was the Indian medical profession's inflexible social integration. Prior to 400-500 BC, in the later Vedic age, there were many highly structured societies within India, and "each part of society [was] busy in a particular duty prescribed to it." This was the caste system of Hinduism.[34] It was codified in the *Laws of Manu* which date from about 500 BC (the date being very uncertain), and initially its hierarchy of castes was based on occupations.[35] Many medical practitioners on the Indian subcontinent have the name of Vaidya or its equivalent. This name is derived from the trade or craft caste-name and often indicates a practitioner of Ayurvedic medicine. During the Vedic period medical practitioners were held in poor repute, at least by the upper classes. Their pay from the Mauryan State (321-185 BC) was the same as that of water-carriers and horse-grooms, and in the ranking within the existing social system "they were considered no better than whores, hunters and followers of other despicable professions," a consequence of "pollution" the medical practitioners acquired in direct patient contact.[36] Later their status improved, and Brahmin, Kshatrya, and Vaidya castes would provide physicians. Within the caste system Brahmins could teach all three castes, the Kshatrys could teach Kshatrys and Vaidyas, and the Vaidyas could teach other Vaidyas and any lower castes.[37]

But the social response to the caste system as it was integrated into Hinduism was the introduction of two great egalitarian religions (Buddhism and Jainism) that bred

---

[34] Beena Jain, *Guild Organization in Northern India*, Delhi, 1990. The origins of the caste system is obscure. Some consider it the consequence, over many centuries, of ethnic (some say "color") struggles as Aryan migrations came to dominate native Indian populations in the 1st millennium BC, something reminiscent of the invading Dorian Spartans as they subdued the native Laconians. The subdued populations provided manual labor for production of food and services, thus necessitating a martial arm of governance to maintain order. Class distinctions comprised, therefore, the Brahmins, Kshatrya, and Vaishya; priests, military, and laborers.

[35] There is a translation of the *Laws of Manu* by G. Buhler, found in: *Sacred Books of the East*, M. Muller, editor, vol. 25, and the caste system is defined in Book 10 (of 12) in that volume (Oxford, 1886). The earliest extant copy of the work has been dated to *ca.* 200 AD. The original castes included the Brahmins, the Kshatriya (warrior class), the Vaidya (Vaishya) (farmer and commercial class), and the Sudra (the once-born). Over centuries the caste subdivisions have come to number into the thousands.

[36] Chari, P. S., *Susruta and Our Heritage*, in *Indian J. Plastic Surg.*, 36:4-13, 2003.

[37] The success of the caste system has been profound, and while the defects of such a system have been frequently and vigorously discussed and denounced, the reason for its resounding success in crowd control over two thousand years has been neglected, and it may explain the existence today of caste systems in many parts of the world. In authoritarian states underclasses are essential to the stability of social stratification because those "less low" than others will view themselves as fortunate not to be as low as others and at the same time feel superior to them. As a consequence, they tend to resist a risk in change of social status. The greater the number of strata, or castes, the greater the stability of the whole, for in this way those of the lowest strata become relatively fewer (even though from the higher strata's viewpoints those lower than they are remain numerically unchanged) and thereby less likely to destabilize society. The logic at work in the survival of the caste system demonstrates, in the simplest way, a corrective for the inherent instability of undemocratic government (with few in the highest stratum). Other correctives include having a military or warrior caste (such as the Kshatriya caste in Hinduism) given the status of a high stratum or implementing regulations via a large civil service.

dissatisfaction in the lower castes, the result being a rapidly growing influence of the new philosophies.[38] This was, in turn, a signal for greater independence for the caste-related trades, and it was also at this time that the number and size of towns were increasing. With a greater social mobility that attended the religious changes, crafts and arts became organized. Guilds developed and became powerful. The influence and vested interest in these trade and craft guilds became so great that, over the centuries, some even organized to function as banks.

Because of the growing power of guilds, they came under governmental control about 400 BC. In contrast to the castes, which were social institutions, the guilds were economic ones that, like the later medieval Western guilds, served their members in matters of common welfare and protection, especially from competitive infringements. Although guild activity had improved social mobility, independent action by individual guild members was not an option. Rigid management, emanating from either the executive of a guild itself or from the royal court, required conformity. When revolts within the guilds arose, the local monarch would pass judgment, including punishment. Concurrence by the guild was assured because the local ruler could subsidize guild funds. These early guilds have been described as "semi-states within a state." Strict authoritarian containment of trades and crafts within rigid caste and economic systems thus marked the social environment in which early Indian medicine existed.[39]

Another divergence was the early appearance, in 4th C BC India, of the hospital. There is a legendary attribution to Gautama Buddha of hospitals for man and for animals. The nature of the hospitals is unclear, for there is no contemporary documentation of their existence. Of the "hospitals" subsequently established by King Ashoka in the 3rd C BC the available inscriptions suggest they functioned as "religious retreats, asylums or resting places, refectories or free hotels, medical-supply stations or storehouses" primarily for the use of Buddhist pilgrims. But Buddhist influence in the subcontinent was increasingly prominent from 200-750 AD, and Sir William Hunter stated that Buddhist princes established hospitals in all the important cities, often with associated medical schools.[40] After some centuries, however, any nascent Indian hospital system disappeared as traditional Hinduism reclaimed religious dominance and hospitals were abolished, to the detriment of subsequent progress in Indian medicine. It was not until 4th C AD that the public hospital appeared in the West, and even then it was often a former pagan temple used as a way-house for those without hope rather than a center for medical expertise.

In summary, the *Charaka* and *Susruta* compendia may not represent the true substance of the earliest Indian practice of medicine. Intriguing anecdotes invite explanation, such as the ancient Hindu observation that black ants are attracted to sweet urine, inspiring the physiologist, Homer Smith, to propose this as the world's oldest

---

[38] For a discussion of the *Laws of Manu* and other seminal ancient works, see their analyses in *Eight Decisive Books of Antiquity* by F. R. Hoare, London, 1952.

[39] A comprehensive review of the guild system is: Thaplyal, K. K., *Guilds in Ancient India*, Delhi, 1996. It covers the period from 600 BC to 600 AD. Importantly, medicine is not listed among the guilds studied, but the author acknowledges that there likely was a variety of guilds that developed in reponse to local exigencies and whose history is unknown.

[40] Hunter, W. W., *The Indian Empire; Its People, History and Products*, London, 1886, p. 108. Also see: Garrison, F. H., *Newer Sidelights on the Antiquity and Provenance of Indian Medicine*, in *Bull. N. Y. Acad. Med.*, 6:523-535, 1930, p. 529. He cites inscriptions from the time of the great Buddhist King, Ashoka (304-232 BC), as translated by R. Muller.

diagnostic test, one that would detect diabetes mellitus.[41] The Indian subcontinent has always been the home of grand and diverse cultures, and it seems unreasonable to apply the general interpretation expressed in these paragraphs to such a vast region. Is it realistic to extrapolate from the manuscripts of Drs. Charaka and Susruta a coherent method of contemporary medical practice being followed by physicians serving a hundred million people distributed over a geography that ranged from the high Himalayas to tropical jungle within an area of 1,250,000 square miles? It is not likely. Perhaps it was limited only to Charaka and Susruta themselves or to a relatively few medical practitioners in some large cities. How many of the mendicant medical practitioners travelling among the villages could even read? Classical Sanskrit first appears about 300 BC, and Megasthenes (p. 90) denied the presence of a written language in the regions visited by him but a few decades earlier. By the time of the writing of the *Charaka Samhita* alphabetic literacy may not have been widespread among even the elite classes. In any case, such organizational structures and empirical procedures of the medical profession as existed during the classical age (800 BC-1000 AD) were lost when released from religious management, reverting to empiricism and magic. This was, in part, due to disruptions by Muslim invaders, internal dissention, and the further introduction of Unani medical practices. Thus Marco Polo (1254-1324) related the following during his travels: in the kingdom of Coilum (in Malabar, southern India) "They have very good astrologers and physicians. Man and woman, they are all black, and go naked, all save a fine cloth worn about the middle."[42] This sounds more like the description of Megasthenes in the 4th C BC, a return to the age of mendicant practitioners rather than the professional practice of a descendant of Dr. Charaka.

Indian medical professionals in ancient times had little hope of improving on Ayurveda. Ayurvedic wisdom was thereby guaranteed to remain "ancient." There probably were clinicians superior to Drs. Charaka and Susruta living in many villages throughout the subcontinent and throughout India's history, but they will remain unknown. Had they written down their findings, and had they been able to form groups whose purpose was to foster a better product or service rather than to erect exclusionary barriers that they thought were necessary to retain what little they had, their efforts might have succeeded. Most likely, however, they would have been regulated out of existence if their knowledge were interpreted as inconsistent with contemporary religious dogma. Perhaps somewhere will be found personal documents that will clarify this issue.

---

[41] Smith, H. W. S., *De Urina*, in *J. Am. Med. Assoc.*, 155:899-902, 1954. Reinhold Muller, however, could not confirm this discovery (*Die Harnruhr der Alt-Inder*, in *Arch. Ges. Med.*, 25:1, 1932.) And see paper of Folke Henschen, *On the Term Diabetes in the Works of Aretaeus and Galen*, in *Med. Hist.* 13:190-192, 1969.

[42] Yule, H., *The Book of Ser Marco Polo*, London, 1903, ii, 376.

CHAPTER SIX

LARGE STRUCTURED SOCIETIES, AUTHORITARIAN – THE WESTERN HEMISPHERE

"No prince was ever more feared by his subjects, both in his presence and his absence."

> Hernando Cortes describing Moctezuma II, King of the Aztecs, in Letter 2 to Charles V, published in 1522[1]

"And since the Incas had no other aim in their method of government than to place their vassals daily in a state of greater subjection and servitude, to please them each of their governors and caciques, both high and low, applied himself to the attainment of their objective, which was to exhaust the strength of the Indians until they were unable to raise their heads."

> Bernabe Cobo, *Historia del Nuevo Mundo*, III, published in 1653, but reflecting his experiences in Cuzco (1609-1613) and subsequent researches into Inca civilization[2]

With virtually no written medical literature, the practice of medicine is barely definable in the ancient Americas. Some idea of the medical environment can be derived from figurines and herbal lore, but, with no evidence of communication between professionals, the conclusion is that virtually all practitioners were local medical empiricists or shamans. In many pre-Columbian societies the shamans were positioned to influence social direction. No medical organization, professional or otherwise, has been identified. There is no evidence of medical inquiry in pre-Columbian art or other archeological finds.

A. Introduction: The *Badianus Manuscript*

There is no equivalent of the Eber's papyrus or the *Code of Hammurabi* by which a glimpse of ancient medicine in the Americas can be obtained. The most secure source for pre-Columbian medical practices is the *Badianus manuscript* (Fig. 7).[3] It is an herbal written in 1552, thirty years after the conquest of Mexico. It is thought to represent Aztec medicine as it was practiced prior to contact with European culture. Composed by an Aztec medical practitioner who wrote using native glyphs and then assisted in translating the text into Latin, the manuscript contains no incantations. There may have been, however, a disinclination after the conquest to display non-Christian practices to a Spanish audience.

---

[1] Found in second letter of Cortes to Charles V, as translated in: *The Dispatches of Hernando Cortes, the Conqueror of Mexico*, New York, 1843, translated by G. Folsom. See *Early Americas Digital Archive*, a resource of the University of Maryland Libraries' e-Publishing Initiative.

[2] *History of the Inca Empire*, by Father Bernabe Cobo, as translated and edited by Roland Hamilton, Austin, 1979.

[3] Emmart, E. W., *The Badianus Manuscript*, a facsimile of the original, published by the Johns Hopkins University Press, Baltimore, 1940. The original, since 1991, has resided in Mexico City.

The *Badianus manuscript* clearly indicates, nevertheless, that medical diseases were inflicted by divinities, and some treatments, such as placing a tooth from a corpse on a sufferer's head to treat fever and treating certain eye problems by tying the eye of a fox to the patient's arm, indicate their use was for their mystical rather than pharmacological properties. Both priestly and empirical Aztec healers could be called in consultation for an illness, at least into the 16th C. Practitioners used herbs and steam baths, cleaned wounds and drained abscesses, and applied drug treatments that included astringents, antihelminthics, narcotics, laxatives, and emetics. Prominent in treatment was that cosmopolitan medicament, honey, and egg yolk.[4] The treatment of eye disease

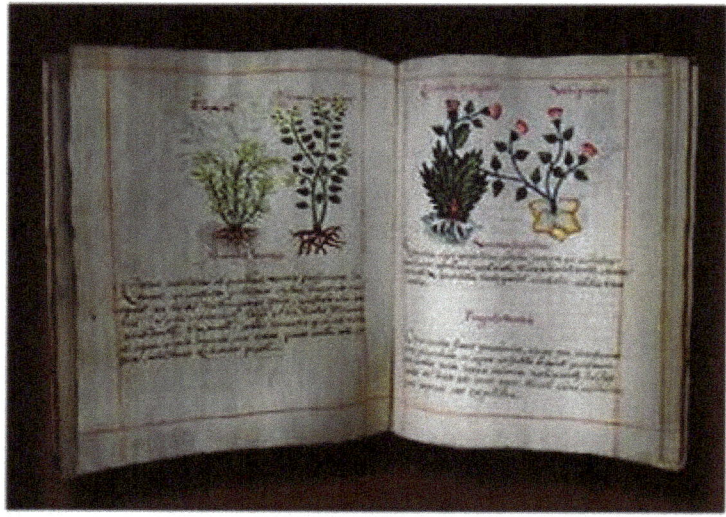

Fig. 7: Pages from the Codex Barberini, Latin 241 (Badianus Manuscript) of 1552. Photograph licensed under Wikimedia Creastive Commons Attribution 4.0 International.

was, as in Egypt, a particularly prominent branch of therapeutics, and, like the Egyptians, sometimes required the dust of a corpse (cited in Emily Emmart's translation of *Badianus manuscript* on p. 44). Although not mentioned in the manuscript, cataract removal may have been practiced. Contemporary Andean medicine included phlebotomy, therapeutic enemas, and an extensive pharmacopeia.

There are several older manuscripts that survived the targeted destruction of pagan writings during the Spanish conquest, the earliest being the Mayan *Codex Dresdensis*, composed about 1200 AD. None of these older manuscripts, however, are of a medical nature. Interestingly, they were written on *amatyl*, a writing surface made from processed tree bark that is thought to have been invented as early as 500 BC. Perhaps an early medical treatise remains to be discovered in the Yucutan or elsewhere in Mesoamerica.

---

[4] Honey remains the subject of active investigation for wound care, and the U. S. Food and Drug Administration in 2007 gave approval for marketing by prescription of a particular form of honey for chronic wound care. Also see: Israili, Z. H., *Antimicrobial Properties of Honey*, in *Am. J. Ther.*, 21:304-323, 2014, a discussion of the value of topical honey. Egg yolk has some antimicrobial activity, and it can contain specific antibodies to pathogens given to hens.

B. The Earliest Medical Practice

But there is a much older record from the western hemisphere. The major ancient civilizations of the Americas can be geographically grouped thus: (1) the Olmec, dating from 1500 to 100 BC, predecessors of the Aztec, and possibly in contact with the early Maya; (2) the Chavin, Paracas, Nazca, and Moche dating from roughly 900 BC and predecessors of the Inca; and (3) the Maya, whose identity some date back to perhaps 2000 BC. All the foremost early American civilizations were completely authoritarian. The Olmec civilization had both a ruling class and prominent shamans. Centuries later Prescott described the Aztec government as an elective monarchy, but a familial monarchy nonetheless. The Moche people, initially comprising many small agricultural communities that were apparently autonomous, subsequently coalesced into a single authoritarian state under "supernatural authority," and it is thought that the importance of their shamans was so great that they ultimately functioned as its rulers. As the Moche had no system of writing, however, their medical practices are unknown to us. Domination by shamans has also been proposed for the Chavin people. The early Paracas society, 700-400 BC, is thought to have been theocratic, with powerful shamans guiding secular leaders, and its replacement, the Inca, was ruled by a king who was considered divine, all land being owned by the State. The ancient Mayan cities were ruled by monarchs who were perceived as demigods, theocracies of absolute authority and a pattern that endured for millennia. Recent excavations concerning the Caral Supe culture in Coastal Peru have permitted carbon dating of a 200-acre city of pyramidal temples and even an amphitheater to almost 3000 BC.[5] The nature of the governance of Caral Supe is explored further on p. 548. The Ecuadorian coastal Valdivian culture is of equivalent antiquity, although it is speculated that the latter was controlled by powerful shamans aided by hallucinogens.[6]

While the relevance of the *Badianus manuscript* to earlier pre-Columbian medical practice must remain speculative, the earlier Americans left remarkable ceramics and scuptures of diseased persons. Specific anatomical diagnoses can be made from many of their artful figurines, which figures therefore represent inspection of the infirm and provide visual rather than written testimony, in a sense a more intimate description of that infirmity. Their figurines may not have been used by medical practitioners, but their accurate portrayal of external evidence of disease was surely the equivalent of ancient Egyptian or Chinese descriptions of signs of disease such as "jaundice," "fever," and "edema."[7] The Hippocratic facies was noted by the Aztecs, who first came to

---

[5] Caral was discovered in 1948, but it is the research of Dr. Ruth Shady that has revealed the size and significance of the city and culture of Caral Supe. Its population is estimated to have been about 3000, although with all related "suburban" sites it might have been as high as 20,000. Its area was some 160 acres (65 hectares). C. McEvedy, in *The Penguin Atlas of Ancient History* (New York, 1967), p. 26-27, estimated Mesopotamian city-state size in 2250 BC to be in the range of 10,000-15,000. An estimate of population density for these urban areas is 250 persons per hectare. For Caral, however, 3000 persons/65 hectares = 46 persons per hectare, a low figure, but just one of Caral's many pyramids, while only 60 feet high, took up an area of 25,000 sq. yds., the size of four football fields.

[6] Cocaine and some of its metabolites have been identified in the hair of Chilean mummies dated to 1000 BC. See: Verano, J. W., *Health and Medical Practices in the Pre-Columbian Americas*, in *Perspectives*, Vol. 4, WHO, 1999.

[7] The collection of medical figurines of A. J. Weisman (see: *Medicine before Columbus*, New York, 1979) contains convincing examples of yaws, cretinism, emaciation, orbital cellulitis (or some form

prominence about 1200 AD. But ceramic figurines were being made by the Valdiva culture, in what is modern-day Ecuador, in the 3rd millennium BC. Realism in facial expression from Xochipala ceramics of 1500 BC could rival sculpture from the Renaissance (Fig. 8). Tlatilco figurines from 1200 BC representing a rare congenital abnormality have been described as the "oldest scientific medical images in world history."[8] Olmec figurines of the 12th C BC show a man with a gibbous deformity of a tuberculous spine, striking terracottas of fetuses, and a remarkable portrayal of a human heart.[9] Olmec sculptures of fetuses are described by Tate and Bendersky.[10] A 2nd C BC Moche facial sculpture displays a prominent enophthalmos. Particularly interesting are Moche figurines lacking a foot. Skeletons have now been found that reveal evidence of amputations that healed, suggesting successful surgical technique of no mean skill, attended by procedures said to be similar to those of the 19th C surgeon, Dr. James Syme.[11] There were even wood prostheses. Facial palsies, accurate representations of stages of pregnancy that apparently include dystocia and its correction, cleft lips, and "hemifacial spasms" can also be identified. Etruscan art, so innovative, is mirrored in 4th C BC Colima art from Mexico. There are instruments that were used for trephination by the Moche of Peru. Trephination of the skull has been identified from Paracas specimens dating from 500 BC, although some think evidence supports an earlier date, perhaps by as much as 2000 years. Suturing of wounds was well established and splinting of fractures has been documented.[12]

Specific infectious diseases seen by pre-Columbian practitioners are being discovered. Tuberculosis may have been endemic in the region of modern-day Peru in 900 AD. It is likely that the bacterium, *Helicobacter pylori*, a causative agent for gastric

---

of exophthalmos), splinted fractures, scoliosus, ascites, a mother feeling the temperature of a child, a woman with stomach pains, various stages of pregnancies with accurate portrayal of abdominal muscles, dystocia, identical twins, thalidomide-type birth defects, priapism (?), and models of beds with openings for excretion (like the Philips cot for cholera patients). The specimens date from the Mochica (1st C AD), Nayarit (3rd C AD), and Colima (3rd C BC) cultures.

[8] The abnormality is "diprosopus," fully explained by G. Bendersky, in *Tlatileo Sculptures, Diprosopus, and the Emergence of Medical Illustration*, in *Persp. in Biol. and Med.*, 43:477-501, 2001. The condition is rare, but duplicated facial structures are so striking that supernatural causes have always been blamed for the lesion in the past, and thus producing an image of such an abnormality is not unexpected. The same investigator identified a terracotta figure of the human heart dated from about 1000 BC.

[9] Tate, C., Bendersky, G., *Olmec Sculptures of the Human Fetus*, in *Persp. in Biol. and Med.*, 1991, pp. 1-20. The importance of tuberculosis in pre-Columbian America is described by G. P. Lombardi and U. G. Caceres in their fascinating paper, *Multisystemic Tuberculosis in a Pre-Columbian Peruvian Mummy: four Diagnostic Levels, and a Paleoepidemiological Hypothesis* (*Chungara*, 32:55-60, 2000). They present evidence that tuberculosis, as caused by *Mycobacterium tuberculosis* rather than *M. bovis*, was endemic in southern Peru about 900 AD, citing the frequency of gibbous deformity. They further suggest that tuberculosis arrived in the Americas from Asia via migratory populations some 10,000 years earlier.

[10] Tate, C., and Bendersky, G., *Olmec Scultpures of the Human Fetus*, in *Perspectives in Biology and Medicine*, Spring, 1999, pp. 1-20.

[11] Verano, J. W., *et al.*, *Foot Amputation by the Moche of Ancient Peru: Osteological Evidence and Archaeological Context*, in *J. Osteoarchaeology*, 10:177-188, 2000.

[12] Marino, R. and Gonzales-Portillo, M., *Preconquest Peruvian Neurosurgeons: A Study of Inca and Pre-Columbian Trephination and the Art of Medicine in Ancient Peru*, in *Neurosurgery*, 47:940-950, 2000, an interesting, if exuberant, recounting of pre-Columbian neurosurgery, including numerous photos and a description of surgical instruments.

and duodenal ulcers, gastric cancer, gastritis, and even gastric lymphoma, existed in pre-Columbian America, having been found in gastric biopsies of mummies from 1350 AD, although it has been proposed that it was present in 1000 BC.[13] Newer DNA techniques using the polymerase chain reaction have recently permitted the diagnosis of Chaga's disease (7000 BC) and leprosy (7th C AD) in the Americas, although this provides no insight as to their epidemiology. Whether malaria and syphilis existed in the western hemisphere prior to Columbus or were subsequently released into the Old World remains under active investigation.

That there were empirical therapies and procedures in pre-Columbian medicine that were the equivalent of treatments and procedures used in other areas of the globe is not a debatable point. A statement of the eminent American historian, William Prescott, supported by documentation, is consistent with this:

> "I must not omit to notice here an institution the foundation of which in the Old World is ranked among the beneficent fruits of Christianity. Hospitals were established in the principal cities, for the cure of the sick and the permanent refuge of the disabled soldier; and surgeons were placed over them, "who were so far better than those in Europe," says an old chronicler, "that they did not protract the cure in order to increase the pay."[14]

Many aspects of ancient pre-Columbian culture paralleled a global trend. Both Cyprus and the New World had their first permanent settlements *ca.* 9th or 10th millennium, and, in a comparison of their population centers of the 2nd millennium, are, except for metallurgy, equally developed. By 3000 BC a written language was in use in Mesopotamia, whereas it is proposed that the Olmec had devised a system of writing by 900 BC. Herbal therapies by the Paracas *ca.* 600 BC included coca leaf anesthesia and alcoholic beverages for control of pain and infection, and hair from Chilean mummies from 1000 BC document cocaine use (see footnote, p. 103), whereas opiate use for pain is described about 1500 BC in Egypt and in Homeric times (*ca.* 800 BC) among the ancient Greeks, although poppies were cultivated for opium in Sumer about 2500 BC as a "joy plant," and its value in pain management must have been known.[15] The parallels continue up to recent times, as noted by Dr. Sigerist in the Foreward to Emily Emmart's book on the *Badianus Manuscript*: "At the time of the Renaissance mediaeval herbals were still popular in Europe and were printed and reprinted. In other words, in the sixteenth century patients were treated along the same lines on both continents." Given the unproven status of all theories of a cross-cultural exchange between the pre-Columbian American Indians and other civilizations, it is thought that cultural attributes of western hemisphere inhabitants arose *de novo*, except for those traits transported across

---

[13] *Helicobacter pylori* is the most frequent modern cause of duodenal and gastric inflamation and ulceration, as well as predisposing to gastric malignancies. See Castillo-Rojas, G, *et al.*, *Presence of Helicobacter pylori in a Mexican Pre-Columbian Mummy*, *BMC Microbiology*, 8:119, 2008, and Allison, M. J., *et al.*, *Further Studies on Fecal Parasites in Antiquity*, in *Amer. J. Clin. Pathol.*, 112:605-609, 1999.

[14] Prescott, W. H., *History of the Conquest of Mexico*, Bk. 1, Chapt. 2, first published in 1843. He cites the work of the historian, Friar Juan de Torquemada, the famous *Monarchia Indiana*, published in 1615 and based on observations during a productive lifetime spent in the New World.

[15] Brownstein, M. J., *A Brief History of Opiates, Opioid Peptides, and Opioid Receptors*, in *Proc. Natl. Acad. Sci. USA*, 90:5391-5393, 1993.

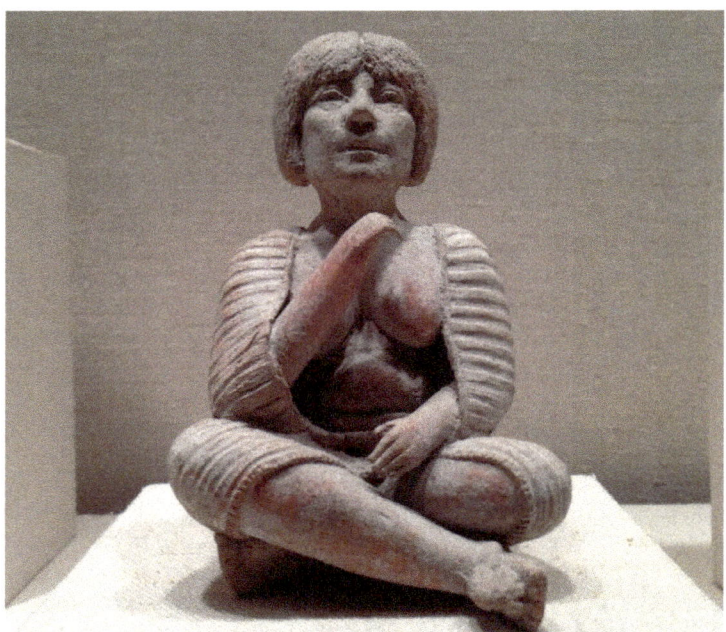

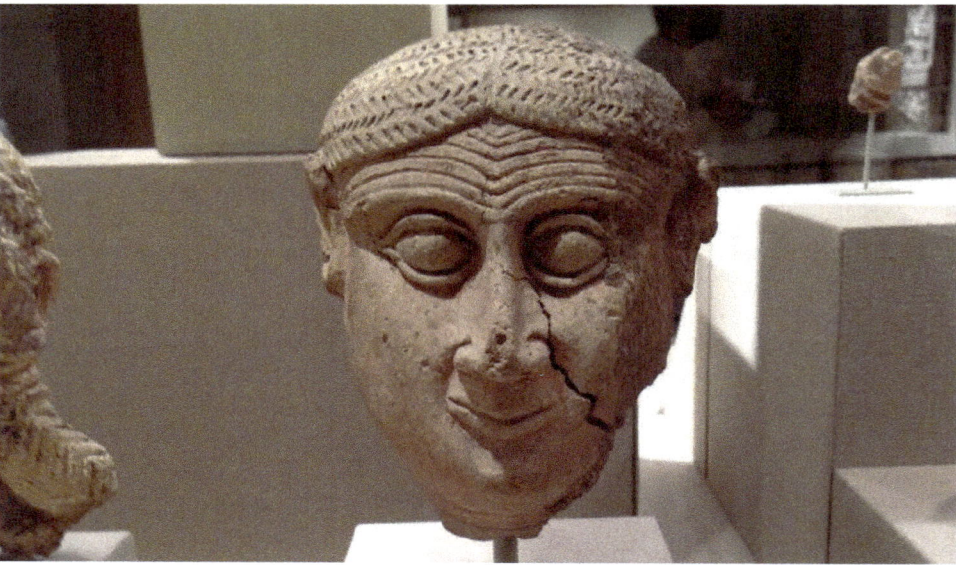

Fig. 8: Top - A Xochipala woman. This five-inch Mexican ceramic figurine, perhaps as ancient as 1500 BC, is from the collection of the New York Metropolitan Museum of Art.
Bottom - Ceramic head, perhaps as ancient as 1500 BC, southern Mesopotamia, collection of the New York Metropolitan Museum of Art. Compare facial features of the two ceramics. The sizes of the two heads greatly differ, the bottom one being about nine inches in height, whereas the top one is about one inch. Both photographs by the author.

the Bering Straits by the early arrivals.[16] The relevance of these observations will soon be made clear.

To conclude this chapter, a summary of ancient medicine of the Western Hemisphere is necessarily brief and unsatisfactory, for, without any early medical treatises like those described in the preceding four chapters, archeology alone provides the fundamentals for our understanding. Other civilizations have left their scraps of written history to assist us, as Derozio wrote:

> Then – let me dive into the depths of time
> And bring from out the ages that have rolled
> A few small fragments of those wrecks sublime.[17]

And yet, had the Nineveh library of Ashurbanipal in Mesopotamia and the Ebers and the Smith papyri in Egypt remained undiscovered, what different pictures would now be painted of medical practice in those regions. On those scraps of evidence a vast history of medicine has been erected. On those scraps, and in the absence of the printing press and the radio and in the presence of overwhelming ignorance, average life spans of thirty years, and unremitting conflict, legendary progressive and self-sacrificing medical professionals humbly and ably serving hundreds of millions of people have been inferred. But what this presumption has, in fact, erected is an artful but deceptive fiction of history, one that exalts, for purposes of tribal pride and politics, some institutional grandeur or power. Were a single 2500-year-old document on empirical medical therapy to be found in the jungles of the Yucatan, how quickly would the alarming and manipulative shamanistic medicine described above be transformed into a picture extolling the professional triumphs of a superior New World race. Or, were the Nineveh library and the Ebers and Smith papyri waiting to be discovered, would not the ghoulishness and mysticism of the medicine of Mesopotamia and North Africa, when compared to early pre-Columbian medicine in the Western hemisphere, seem little more than differences in kind? Embellishments of ancient cultures epitomize a global vogue, the desire to be identified as a member of one of those powerful institutions, especially those receiving the initial credits and thereby implicitly intellectually superior. And so now the distinction between ancient Chinese and Greek cultural ethic noted on p. 86 can be viewed in a broader perspective: all the regional civilizations discussed so far share the same consequences of varied, but always authoritarian, command structures. But a break with this system was beginning, as the next chapter will describe.

---

[16] For a recent overview of the migration and early dissemination of humans throughout the Americas, see: Dillehay, T., *The Settlement of the Americas*, New York, 2000.

[17] Henry L. V. Derozio (1809-1831), in his poem *To India - My Native Land*.

CHAPTER SEVEN

LARGE STRUCTURED SOCIETIES, LIMITED AUTHORITARIAN – THE LEVANT

ἡ γὰρ ψυχὴ πάσης σαρκὸς αἷμα αὐτοῦ ἐστι·
"For blood is the life of all flesh; ..."

Leviticus 17:11[1]

In the contested lands between Mesopotamia and Egypt have arisen epochal creeds and ideas. But historical assessment of their nomadic tribes is limited because of disruptions among their societies and the disappearance of perishable textual materials. The Bible is the principal source of their histories, in part supported by archeological finds, in part at odds with them. Amid the flux of cultures and migratory tribes just to the east of the Mediterranean it is ancient Hebrew medicine that is best documented, and that can be credited to religious writings which began to accumulate in the 8th C BC. Notable features of Hebrew medicine were (1) intolerance of magical devices and (2) a distinction between medical practitioners and priests. Although the nature of medical practice is uncertain, it probably had rational as well as empirical components. An unsettled tribal existence could explain why a formal, and ultimately scientific, medical organization did not develop. Roman domination provided the colophon to indigenous medical practices. A profound inhibitory effect on medical progress has often been attributed to religions, and it is with this in mind that the Levant has been chosen to conclude this brief review of primitive and ancient authoritarian societies and their effects on medical practice, for it was Hebrew prophets who first began to neutralize earthly authoritarianism using the morality of the individual as judged by an almighty God, thus opening a path to social equality.

A. Introduction: Ancient Levantine Cultures

The Levant, as employed here, includes the area now occupied by Lebanon, Syria, Jordan, Israel, and the Palestine territories. It is a region notable for the historical introduction of the common man as a compelling force on the grand stage of human events, a first rift in the armor of earthly authoritarianism. "The prophets of the Old Testament were the first to preach social justice."[2]

---

[1] The Greek text is from the diglot Septuagint version as published by S. Bagster and Sons, Ltd., London, *ca.* 1884. New Testament translations are from the King James version, the original of 1611 as edited in 1769. This particular statement of Moses about 1400 BC was chosen because of its medical implication. In context it refers to ancient dietary restrictions as commanded by God. It is not stating that blood represents (or "is" or "carries") the "breath of life" (soul) of an individual, without which there is no life. Had that been the intent, terms for "body," "man," or "soul" would have been used rather than σάρξ, which specifically means "muscle" or "tissue" and which would not have been a substitute for the aforementioned three terms. Thus, the intent of the Commandment, if correctly translated into Greek, is stating that blood is required for sustaining life of bodily tissues (here identified as "flesh.") All societies know that loss of blood can be associated with loss of life, but this statement acclaims blood as biologically, rather than spiritually, necessary for life. Some may disagree with this interpretation by the author.

[2] Wallace, H. A., *Democracy Reborn*, New York, 1944, p. 190. Amos and Micah, 8th C BC Hebrew prophets, were, in addition, common men themselves. This entry into history of the common man

Incessant conflicts among tribes and creeds in the western arc of the Fertile Crescent and trading centers of the Levant prevented development there of a powerful, coherent civilization, although there could hardly have been another great civilization squeezed between the Nile and the Euphrates. Indeed, the area now under consideration acted as a buffer between the Mesopotamian and Egyptian civilizations, and by averting a face-to-face confrontation may have contributed to their longevities. Nevertheless, the region was developed at an early age, for Jericho, in the Jordan Valley, was a walled city by 7000 BC, and Ugarit, on the eastern coast of the Mediterranean, by 6000 BC. While not supporting a monolithic long-lived empire, the Levant is a large region now being better characterized through archeological finds than through documents, with the exception of the Bible and a few, but important, inscriptions. Although the Assyrians and Persians temporarily extended their control into the region from a distance, the early dominant groups were the Canaanites and Hebrews, and the history of the region is to a great extent a history of their disputes with each other and with surrounding cultures, Egyptian to the southwest, Mesopotamian and Persian to the east, Crete/Minoan to the west, and Assyrian/Hittite to the north.

The Canaanite culture had notable city states such as Ugarit, although it was otherwise poorly structured and tended to be nomadic.[3] There were many named kings but no unitary and cohesive kingdom, although it later became an important power as its culture evolved into what would be called Phoenician. Early Canaanite society probably served as an important commercial link between Egypt and Mesopotamia, although Egypt's suzerainty in mid-2nd millennium BC impoverished it. Its coastal cities may have hosted medical practitioners from Egypt, for it is known from extant Egyptian letters that medical assistance was on occasion requested by Canaanite kings. A Canaanite anthropomorphic jar exhibiting the characteristic leontine facies of lepromatous leprosy was found at ancient (*ca.* 1300 BC) Beth-Shan in present-day Jordan, but there is apparently no Canaanite or Phoenician medical literature. The Canaanite practice of ritual sacrifice of children is mentioned in *Deuteronomy*, 12:31. Although there was already a form of Canaanite writing, one that would be adopted and modified by other cultures, there is now little written record of the Canaanites except for that on ancient Egyptian monuments and papyri and in much later Hebrew scrolls. Papyrus was more perishable in the Fertile Crescent's rainfall than in Nile-watered Egypt. Thus, no information is available at present from which Canaanitic medical practices might be surmised.

Hebrew origins were tribal, nomadic, and patriarchal. There are those who consider Canaanites and Hebrews as representatives, from some earlier age, of a common ancestral Western Semitic culture, and it is in Canaan that the patriarch Abraham promulgated his peoples' covenant with God. Centuries later, following the exodus from

---

also represented a dramatic shift away from social morality, in which morality was solely vested in maintaining society as a whole and in which the individual was a nonentity. "Morality and commonweal were identical ideas." (See: Moses, A., *The Religion of Moses*, Louisville, 1894, p. 109.) Instead, it was to be individual morality ("moral emancipation" in the cited reference) that guided a man's interaction with other men, as indicated by "Thou shall not..."

[3] Ugarit was a prominent trading center for Egypt, Cyprus, and Mycenae, reaching its apogee about 1300 BC. A cuneiform listing of items from that period is thought to represent items belonging in a physician's office. The list included strainers, cups, bowls, a whetstone, forceps with sheath, a chest, scales, two scalpels, two lancets, a tine, and a bed and coverlet. See: Stieglitz, R. R., *A Physician's Equipment List from Ugarit*, in: *Journal of Cuneiform Studies*, 33:52-55, 1981. Others have considered them to be "commercial goods."

Egypt under Moses during the 15th C BC, Hebrews were governed by "judges" during times of peril. These judges, selected without regard to their social status, were empowered for a defined period and were reputed to have served their tribes well for several centuries. But the expedient appeal of authoritarianism during crises prompted the people to call for a king, and from about 1050 BC onward Hebrew kings led armies and attempted a national unification that had been urged forward by military necessity. The first three kings were the famous Saul, David, and Solomon. But with subsequent north/south schism of the Hebrews, followed by deportation, captivity, and assimilation of the majority, the earliest known date of their internal historical documents is the 8th C BC.

B. Hebrew Medicine

Earlier it was noted that some scholars feel Mosaic law, specifically the Covenant Code,[4] and the Code of Hammurabi have a common origin. The former has been placed in the 13th C BC, some four or five centuries after Hammurabi.[5] Prior to the exodus the Hebrews lived as vassals in Egypt for several centuries, and perhaps aspects of an earlier Akkadian tradition persisted in Hebrew folklore up to the time of Moses. Indeed, Abraham is thought by many to originally come from Ur, a Chaldean city in Mesopotamia. The Dartmouth Bible leaves the resemblance unresolved, although equating the two is inconsistent with a Divine attribution, and religiosity is not expressed in the Code of Hammurabi, a civil code. Relevant to present discussion, in contrast to the Hammurabi Code the Hebrew Covenant has no regulations pertaining to physicians.

The difficulties in determining ancient Israelite medical practices was highlighted by Dr. Harry Friedenwald who stated in 1935 that medical writing in the Talmud, which was completed by the 5th C AD, "is 'popular medicine'; most, if not all, having been translated by laymen."[6] But Biblical writings are now being more accurately dated. For example, the Book of Job is probably contemporary with the Greek tragedy, *Prometheus Bound*, which is ascribed to Aeschylus (525-456 BC). In biblical texts there is almost no mention of anything pertaining to physician practices, even though it has been suggested that Job himself was a physician. Overall there is the assumed fact of supernatural interventions in the form of disease or cure thereof, the basis of it being derived from the concept of retribution for sins against commandments of an Almighty God: "And Asa was diseased in his feet in the thirty-ninth year of his reign, until he was very ill; but in his disease he sought not to the Lord, but to the physicians."[7] Asa died the next year. And it is thought that the Chonicler frowned on pre-exile physicians, probably because they used spells and incantations along with medicines. On the other hand,

---

[4]Covenant Code: *Exodus,* 20:23 – 23:33.

[5] In fact, C. Leonard Woolley (1880-1960), the noted archeologist who led the British Museum excavations at Ur, thought the Code of Hammurabi "embodied regulations much older than his time." See *The Sumerians*, New York, 1965, p. 111.

[6] For this statement and a dated but scholarly and convenient review and bibliography on the topic of Hebrew medicine see: Friedenwald, H., *The Bibliography of Ancient Hebrew Medicine*, in *Bull. Med. Libr. Assoc.*, 23:124-157, 1935.

[7] II Chr., 16:12. The translations of all Old Testament passages are from the diglot Septuagint version as published by S. Bagster and Sons, Ltd., London, *ca.* 1884. New Testament translations are from the King James version, the original of 1611 as edited in 1769.

Hezekiah, very ill, was to die, or so he was told by the prophet Isaiah. In despair Hezekiah turned his face to the wall and prayed. His prayers were heard by God, and he was healed.[8]

Respect for a supernatural power as an influence over man's health is universal, and there is a parallel between divine retribution in the form of plagues described in Hebrew sacred texts and that of its contemporary polytheistic counterparts. In Samuel I, 5:6, after removing the Ark of the Covenant, the Philistines are visited by a plague, highly lethal, associated with mice and "emerods."[9] The plague that opens Homer's *Iliad* was caused by Apollo, and one of Apollo's names, Σμινθεῦ (Smintheus), or "mouse god," may have been based, like the Philistine plague, on recognition of some sort of association between rodents and certain epidemic diseases of humans.

In contrast to other societies, however, there was an "antipathy toward idolatry" that expelled mysticism from Hebrew medical practice, as expressed in Deut. 18:10-12:

> "There shall not be found in thee one who purges his son or his daughter with fire, one who uses divination, who deals with omens, and augury, a sorcerer employing incantation, one who has in him a divining spirit, an observer of signs, questioning the dead. For every one that does these things is an abomination to the Lord thy God; for because of these abominations the Lord will destroy them from before thy face."[10]

This admonition in various forms was echoed by the Prophets throughout early Hebrew history, for mysticism is a perennial attractant requiring perpetual vigilance. It has been pointed out that the Sumerian terms, *asipu* and *asu* (p. 38*ff*), share a root with phonetically similar Hebrew words for "sorcerer," "witch," and "enchanter," the latter term in Hebrew being *'assaph*, the equivalent of the *asipu* of Sumer/Akkad and of *assia* in Aramaic, "the principal priest of Mesopotamian incantation rituals."[11] Although prophets might occasionally heal, this represented Divine intervention. Hebrews always distinguished between the physician and the priest.

It is noteworthy that seven of the most important medical papyri discovered in ancient Egypt are dated not long after the Hebrew exodus, and yet, with the exception of circumcision, no Egyptian medical legacy is found in Hebrew medical practices.[12] Even embalming, so important in ancient Egypt, was for the most part forbidden by the

---

[8] II Kings, 20:1.

[9] I Samuel, 5:6 ("And the hand of the Lord was heavy upon Azotus, and he brought evil upon them, and it burst out upon them into the ships, and mice sprang up in the midst of their country, and there was a great and indiscriminate mortality in the city." (From the diglot Septuagint version as published by S. Bagster and Sons, Ltd., London, *ca.* 1884. New Testament translations are from the King James version, the original of 1611 as edited in 1769.) From the popular translations of "emerod" it appears that there is no consensus as to what medical lesion is being described, "buboes" (large lymph nodes) and hemorrhoids consequent to dysentery being two of the suggestions (see Shrewsbury, J. F. D., *The Plague of the Philistines*, London, 1964, chapter 1).

[10] Deut. 18:10-14

[11] Nash, T., *Devils, Demons, and Disease: Folklore in Ancient Near Eastern Rites of Atonement*, in *The Bible in Light of Cuneiform Literature: Scripture in Context III* (pp. 59-60), Lewiston, NY, 1990, W. W. Hallo, *et al.*, eds.

[12] The work of J. Preuss, *Biblish-Talmudische Medizin*, (Berlin, 1911), makes it clear that the principal preventive and therapeutic options of the Egyptians were not used by the Hebrews. And recall that at least two of the seven papyri, those of Ebers and of Smith, were 16th C BC copies of much earlier works and would have had centuries for their knowledge to be dispersed and become well-known. As for circumcision, this is a practice found in many parts of the ancient world, including aboriginal Australia, equatorial Africa, and pre-Columbian America.

Pentateuch (Torah). Finally, the remarkable and salutary sanitation practices of the Hebrews do not find their origins in the medicine of their Egyptian overlords, being derived, instead, from Moses as expressed in the Pentateuch and as construed later by rabbis in the Talmud, although this is not to deny the extravagance of some elements of personal cleanliness described among the Egyptians. The primary purpose of the Hebrew practices has been interpreted as promotion of health, although Talmudic injunctions regarding public and personal hygiene also were seen as religious obligations.[13]

Health and disease were viewed by the Hebrews as emanating from the same source, and, in Exodus 15:26, they were told that ". . . no disease which I have brought upon the Egyptians will I bring upon thee, for I am the Lord thy God that heals thee." And it was in this sense that physicians, executing the will of God, were to be considered messengers of God. In the 2nd C BC there is the famous statement about honoring the physician, but the context is as follows: First pray, [next] leave off sin, [next] cleanse the heart, "then give place to the physician...."[14] Listed last, it was nevertheless an important feature of society, unshared by some great ancient civilizations, that enforced an essential separation of powers, for the ancient Hebrews there is no instance of a priest performing the functions of the physician, although a priest might foretell death or survival. In *Isaiah* 38:21 the prophet Isaiah told Hezekiah, "Take a cake of figs, and mash them, and apply them as a plaister, and thou shalt be well." Here the prophet is acting as a practitioner, and perhaps he was considered one, but it is likely that he was merely administering a generally understood empirical remedy of a local nature. Dr. Fielding Garrison comments that priests were "medicine's police," but this was in reference to the sanitary laws that functioned as public health policies, not to the practicing physician.[15] A different medical role of the priest is found in Leviticus XIII, where a cutaneous manifestation of disease named λεπρά (lepra) is, after a complex differential diagnosis, declared by the priest to be a reason for isolation of the afflicted person from the rest of the community.[16] As Dr. Max Weber points out, this was an instance in which the "ritualistically impure" were subject to priestly management, and thus it was not an infringement on the physician's

---

[13] See Hart, M. D., *The Healthy Jew: The Symbiosis of Judaism and Modern Medicine*, Cambridge, 2007. Herodotus noted in the 5th C BC that Egyptians had high standards of personal cleanliness. But it is uncertain whether earlier Egyptian practices such as embalming, use of wells for drinking water, circumcision, and prohibitions on using certain animals for food were, strictly speaking, public health measures, religious observances, or both.

[14] *The Wisdom of Ben Sira* (The Sirach, *Ecclesiasticus*) discusses the physician and sickness in 38:1-14. It begins: τίμα ἰατρὸν πρὸς τὰς χρείας τιμαῖς αὐτοῦ, καὶ γὰρ αὐτὸν ἔκτισε Κύριος. ("Honour a physician with the honour due unto him for the uses which you may have of him: for the Lord has created him.") *Ecclesiasticus* is thought to have been written near the beginning of the 2nd C BC. Sira states that God gave to man the intelligence to manage his own ills through the use of earthly means, whether healing herbs or the technical knowledge of the physician. He implies that this is how God administers man's health, rather than through direct intervention or through select devout intermediaries, meaning priests.

[15] Garrison, F. H., *History of Medicine*, Phila., 1913, p. 47; also: *Leviticus*, chapters X-XV, from the diglot Septuagint version as published by S. Bagster and Sons, Ltd., London, *ca.* 1884. New Testament translations are from the King James version, the original of 1611 as edited in 1769.

[16] Leviticus, chapter XIII. The differential diagnosis in this instance is laid out by Divine authority to Moses, and so it is arguable that the clinical acumen therein expressed is not attributable to either priests or physicians and therefore not an issue whereby priests were usurping physicians' prerogatives. The careful description thus given to a people with no knowledge of pathophysiology sufficed to both protect the public and those with skin lesions that were not "lepra."

role by priests.[17] Another possibly useful practice, and one related to the foregoing, was the incineration of material that might contain a contagious agent.[18]

Surgical procedures were limited, as in all ancient societies. The only ones listed in the Bible are circumcision, castration, and the closing of wounds. Circumcision receives extensive commentary, and, as first mentioned in Genesis, it was even performed by mothers themselves, including the wife of Moses on her new son (*ca.* 1500 BC).[19] But this practice has been identified in ancient Egyptian inscriptions as early as 2374 BC. The early popularity of circumcision, which the ancient Hebrews considered ordained by God, may have been due to concerns about the development of pathological phimosis and its complications later in life, although in Egypt Herodotus clearly states that it was meant for the purpose of cleanliness.[20]

Licensing of Hebrew physicians has been diffidently inferred from biblical terms suggesting the "proven" and "expert" physician, and every settlement was to have at least one physician. In contrast to the superabundance of specialists in Egypt, Hebrew practitioners were not so portrayed and probably were more like general practitioners. Some biblical interpreters think the profession of medicine passed from father to son, perhaps a familial guild, and a vague idea of guilds has been inferred from *Genesis* 4:20-22 as suggesting the ancient nature of such associations.[21] The collection of fees by physicians was sanctioned, at least in the Talmudic period: "A physician who heals for nothing is worth nothing."[22] Physicians were accompanied by apprentices when visiting the sick.

The advent of Christianity introduced the New Testament. Dr. Cyril Elgood has commented that the freedom from magic, including exorcism, in the Old Testament (or Tanach) does not extend to the New Testament,[23] and even St. Augustine granted that magical powers could be ascribed to non-Christians.[24] It is notable, therefore, that the Babylonian Talmud displays commentary with its basis in both "Akkadian" medical practices and magic. It is proposed that contemporary scholars in the Talmudic period (70 BC – 500 AD) still had some early cuneiform tablets available to them, and this information was melded with elements of Hippocratic medicine in an exposition of the

---

[17] Weber, M., *Ancient Judaism*, Glencoe, 1952, p. 174.

[18] See, for example, *Lev.* 13:52 and 11:33.

[19] καὶ λαβοῦσα Σεπφώρα ψῆφον, περιέτεμε τὴν ἀκροβυστίαν τοῦ′ υἱοῦ αὐτῆς· ("And Sepphora, taking a small stone ["flint knife"], excised the foreskin of her son;...." *Exodus* 4:25.)

[20] This, of course, was written almost 1000 years after Moses: τά τε αἰδοῖα περιτάμνονται καθαρειότητος εἵνεκεν, ... "They practice circumcision for cleanliness' sake;...." Herodotus, *The Histories*, II, 37, translation of A. D. Godley, *Loeb Classical Library*.

[21] "And Ada bore Jobel; he was the father of those that dwell in tents, feeding cattle. And the name of his brother was Jubal; he it was who invented the psaltery and the harp. And Sella also bore Thobel; he was a smith, a manufacturer both of brass and iron;...." (The translations of all Old Testament passages are from the diglot Septuagint version as published by S. Bagster and Sons, Ltd., London, *ca.* 1884. New Testament translations are from the King James version, the original of 1611 as edited in 1769.) This vaguely suggests the original assigning of familial trades. See: Gordon, Cyrus H.; *The Common Background of Greek and Hebrew Civilizations*, Scranton, 1965.

[22] Babylonian Talmud, *Bava Kamma*, 85a.

[23] Elgood, C., *A Medical History of Persia and the Eastern Caliphate*, Cambridge, 1951, a discussion in chapter 2.

[24] St. Augustine: *Confessions*, Book X, see chapters 35 and 42.

practices of physicians in Hebrew society.[25] The complexity of Rabbinical analyses over those centuries cannot be easily summarized, but one would hope that the opinion of some experts, as expressed in Kiddushin 82a, did not reflect the general opinion of Hebrew society, for it states "the best of doctors is destined for hell." The simply stated reason is that being a physician was a privileged position that unduly subjected its practitioners to temptation and was therefore not an appropriate profession for a godly person. Perhaps the point to be construed here is that the devastating events that ushered in the Talmudic period led to a codification of ritual and laws that drew on a variety of local resources in an attempt to supplant a vanishing oral tradition. Thus, the nature of Hebraic medicine and its place in society may have fundamentally changed from what had traditionally been practiced.

C. Conclusion

Knowledge of the physician-patient relationship in early Levant society is extremely limited. As Prof. Max Weber states, "The state of medical arts in ancient Israel [in pre-Hellenistic times] is quite unknown."[26] Nevertheless, based upon limited writings the following apply to Hebraic medicine: 1) there was generally a clear distinction between physician and priest, 2) the value of the physician to the community at large was acknowledged, 3) magic was forbidden to the medical profession, 4) the merit of a physician earning a fee was accepted, and 5) there is no mention of any attempt to regulate physicians. If the final intellectual destination of biblical pre-Christian medicine in the Levant were to be assigned, it most likely would belong to empiricism. Perhaps it extended beyond empirical, for there was no obvious institutional obstruction to improvement, but it was not scientific for it had no organization for scientific pursuit. But biblical era medicine, of all those mentioned heretofore, was the only one that remained solely the purview of individual practitioners. One might argue that Hebraic medicine avoided mysticism because it avoided being caught up in any great authoritarian civilization or institution, being instead a feature of a culture that, but for three centuries, shunned authoritarian governance. That culture surely had laws, but they came from the Highest Authority. Biblical chapters abound in infractions of those laws, but an important part of the Bible is the recounting of the consequences of those infractions. Almost all chastisements emanated from that Highest Authority, not a secular leader. To protect the people from error the Hebrew leaders cajoled, warned, and wept. But theirs was not the authority to govern with impunity, and their guidance was surely not arbitrary. Hebrew practitioners, therefore, protected from earthly authoritarianism, remained autonomous except for local social pressures to which all were subject. Had ancient Hebrew medicine existed in a stable environment with the opportunity to grow in public esteem it might have acquired the attention necessary for progression to a science. Lower level empirical practitioners with no professional organization, but protected by their religion's interpreters who, steadfastly defending it from usurpers, made possible their autonomous existence. The interpreters of their religion also provided another reason Hebrew medicine avoided a slide into priest medicine or its equivalent.

---

[25] Geller, M. J., *Akkadian Healing Therapies in the Babylonian Talmud*, Issue 259 of Preprint, Max Planck Institute, Berlin, 2004.
[26] Weber, M., *Ancient Judaism*, Glencoe, 1952, p. 175.

At the opening of this chapter there is mentioned the common man and "social justice," and the propagation of the idea of social justice throughout society was the work of early Hebrew prophets. Although social justice, *per se*, is irrelevant to medical practice, the essence of social justice in Hebrew society was equality, and the effectiveness of the appeal for social justice suggests the prophets' words fell on ears attuned to the idea. In the first place, there was equality of all persons before God. Secondly, it has been pointed out that in having common ancestors, Adam and Eve, the first man and woman, there is logic to a system of justice that rates no man above another. Third, although democracy was in no way a feature of biblical life, there is repeated in many places in the Book of Judges and of Samuel, a span covering centuries, the following statement:

> "And in those days there was no king in Israel; every man did that which was right in his own sight."[27]
>
> Judges, XXI, 25

Fourth, the "judges" who guided Israel during turbulent times were often of humble origin. Fifth, the prophet Samuel listed the dangerous consequences of foregoing "judges" for a monarchy (I Samuel, VIII, 11-18). Even when the ancient Hebrews begged for a king, the one chosen by God, namely Saul, while large in stature, was from the weakest clan of the smallest of the tribes of Israel.[28] Thus, resistance to authoritarianism pervades this period of Hebrew history, although it was not sufficient to prevent a subsequent voluntary descent into monarchical governance, the source of many ensuing woes. After this it is likely that social disruption caused by wars, plagues, and captivities prevented establishment of a professionally organized medical practice.

The title of this chapter is in a sense misleading, for there is the implication that theocratic authoritarianism inevitably frustrates medical progress, and it is true that theocracy has been blamed for many ills of society. But ancient Hebrew society, while theocratic, does not deserve such censure. The Authoritarian at the head of their society was God, and the commands of God were not to be subject to modification by earthly politicians and were equally apportioned to every member of society, a pact of equality before the ultimate Law their leaders took pains to obey. This was a Divine covenant with an independent nomadic people, and so their medicine was not co-opted by an authoritarian institution in those days.

---

[27] ἐν δὲ τὰς ἡμέραις ἐκείναις οὐκ ην βασιλεὺς ἐν Ἰσραήλ· ἀνὴρ τὸ εὐθὲς ἐνώπιον αὐτοῦ ἐποίει. From the diglot Septuagint version as published by S. Bagster and Sons, Ltd., London, *ca.* 1884. New Testament translations are from the King James version, the original of 1611 as edited in 1769.

[28] Also see: Everdell, W. R. *The End of Kings: A History of Republics and Republicans*, Chapter 2, Chicago, 1983. Parallels with ancient Greece are presented that are striking, especially that between Samuel and Solon. Samuel, who preceded Solon by approximately 300 years, continually inveighed against monarchy and its faults.

CHAPTER EIGHT

ANCIENT AUTHORITARIAN SOCIETIES AND MEDICAL PRACTICE - CONCLUSION

> *"Except the blind forces of Nature, nothing moves in this world which is not Greek in its origin."*
>
> Sir Henry Maine (1822-1888)[1]

A review of selected ancient societies suggests that several had evidence of a transient period in their earliest histories consistent with a rational medical practice. But within authoritarian society medicine did not benefit from the social advantages of a metropolis or the efficiency of centralized services, inevitably becoming, with the limited exception of Hebrew medicine, manipulated canon. None of the regions cited can claim precedence in originating a natural state of medical practice or of progress toward scientific medicine for none reached a steady state beyond that of the empirical. But the unheralded arrival of a new political system was soon to challenge, then surpass in greatness, all that had gone before.

A. Early Medicine and Its Final Common Pathway

Some predominant ancient civilizations have now been surveyed in a search for the natural state of medical practice and they have been found wanting. But surely these were not periods of medical vacuum. Empirical knowledge was available, if not cumulative. In the opening chapter it was argued that the medicine-man was irrelevant as a practitioner of primordial medicine. Who, then, was relevant at that early stage? Some prefer the explanation put forth in 1894, in which women were described as the ". . . chief discoverers of medical herbs and the first empirical physicians who learned to brew and prepare different remedies."[2] This was also the opinion of Alan Wootton, who described the earliest medical practitioners as herbalists and "women in many cases."[3] This may well be close to the truth, for surely each family looked after its own, perhaps sharing its own medical discoveries and disappointments with other families.

But, whatever medicine's origin, man's curiosity and his ability to innovate in the face of necessity did result in the acquisition of medical knowledge. Innumerable observations were made of pharmacological effects of all kinds of substances in a virtually infinite number of clinical trials, carried out, of course, without informed consent. Most produced inconsequential, and many produced disastrous, results. The information gained, along with the identification of clinical signs of health and disease and the

---

[1] Maine, the great philosophical jurist and historical scholar, made this statement in his famous work, *Village-Communities in the East and West*, London, 1871, p. 238.

[2] *Womens' Share in Primitive Culture*, Otis Tufton Mason, 1894, p. 17.

[3] Wootton, A.C., *Chronicles of Pharmacy*, London, 1910, available in a reprint by USV Pharmaceutical Corp., Tuckahoe, NY, 1972, p. 1. Wootton interpreted the art of pharmacy as beginning when early herb seekers began "to prepare their remedies so as to make them easier to take or apply." He uncharitably ascribes the beginnings of the medical profession, however, to the day when these discoveries were kept as secrets by certain persons or families, mystical theories being added to increase the exclusivity of their knowledge.

formulation of some idea of the course, if not the cause, of illness, was collected hither and yon but promulgated through limited time and space. The same limitations were also found in other aspects of culture. In Upper Paleolithic Period, from approximately 40,000 to 12,000 years ago, implements of stone and bone, similar in structure and function and with no local evidence of a gradient of improvement over time, are observed in widely separate parts of the world. There was a basal level of discovery and invention, but one consistent with bare subsistence, and it was held in common by man wherever he wandered. It was the wandering, in fact, that seemed to assure only bare subsistence. With the formation of tribal societies there was increased efficiency in propagation of knowledge, but the quality of knowledge remained unchanged. It is in this way that empirical medical knowledge, however overshadowed by illusion or delusion, has existed since the dawn of mankind: it was circumscribed, superficial, unsystematic, and circumstantially insusceptible to improvement, knowledge found along byways that began everywhere but led nowhere.

B. The Prologue Concludes

With the arrival of the Neolithic, however, there came large permanent settlements, complex societies, and domestication of plants and animals. This transition was not easy, for risks abound in highly populated settlements as well as in sparsely populated nomadic societies, but it was successful, at least in the sense that it might be analogous to a school of fish whereby a mechanism for survival of the species allows for the sacrifice to a predator of many within the school. In any event, in settled societies around the globe inventions and discoveries could now take root. Ideas were no longer necessarily fleeting; they could be acted upon and built upon. Inventions and discoveries differed from place to place, but over millennia there has been a global similarity in their emergence. As an example, for ten thousand years the Western hemisphere was isolated from the rest of the global population. It is in a sense a laboratory for comparative observations on societal evolution uninfluenced by Old World cultures. Despite the presumed disadvantage of isolation, the advent of farming in approximately 6000 BC, squash cultivation in 8000 BC in northern Peru (squash did not grow wild there), and domesticated llamas and alpacas about 5000 BC,[4] astronomical inscriptions and constructions about 6000 BC, mummification in 5000 BC, irrigation in 4000 BC,[5] Peruvian step pyramids in 2500 BC, glyph writing perhaps as early as 1500 BC, and many other discoveries are surprisingly similar to those elsewhere in the world, even though their impact was of a more restricted nature. One estimate is that the "colonialization" of the entire Americas by new arrivals from across the Bering Strait required no more than a thousand years. Thus, a powerful argument favoring a similar course in development of all the world's large civilizations as they traversed the Neolithic and

---

[4] This estimate is based on genetic linkage studies with llama and alpaca ancestors: Kadwell, M., *et al.*, *Genetic Analysis Reveals the Wild Ancestors of the Llama and the Alpaca*, in *Proc. Royal Soc.*, London, B, 268:2575-2584, 2001.

[5] For a recent review see: *From Foraging to Farming in the Andes*, Cambridge, 2001, T. Dillehay, editor, especially his Introduction.

Bronze ages is demonstrated in pre-Columbian America.[6] It is true that the earliest copper implements have been found in Mesopotamia. This invention quickly spread regionally, soon followed by the invention of bronze. Such a useful invention has led to the idea of dominance of certain civilizations, whereas it is, in a sense, but a local response to a local commodity, copper being one of the few metals that can be found naturally unalloyed or uncompounded. Metal tools, after all, merely happen to be a more useful invention, not necessarily a cleverer one, than a myriad of other early discoveries and inventions, and thus their exploitation represents to a significant degree geological rather than intellectual peculiarities. Moreover, recent information has revealed smelting of copper by western Great Lakes Indians at the Old Copper Complex as early as 4000 BC.[7] In contrast, rubber, obtained from sap of certain vines, was a discovery by the Olmec of Mesoamerica, perhaps by 1500 BC. The point is, with permanent settlements new cultural options were everywhere opened.

New cultural options, however, would not include any options for medicine. Empirical medical knowledge, as handed down by nomadic societies, did not constitute a medical practice, the essence of which has been described as "a consultation of a sick person with a compassionate medical scholar."[8] There could have been no such consultation prior to the accumulation of sufficient medical knowledge that the average person had neither time nor ability to comprehend, an amount sufficient to require a "scholar." Now the great civilizations had the luxury of acquiring scholars to manage what became, in medicine, a burden worthy of a scholar. Manuscripts of several of those civilizations reveal vestiges of antecedent medical practices that, although transient, might be classified as rational. But social evolution resulted in centralized authoritarian governance and bureaucracies, with the apparent exception of Hebraic medicine. Those bureaucracies, whether political or theocratic, came to incorporate or control "medical scholars" who were employed to the benefit of the bureaucracies. Thus, medical decisions by State-appropriated practitioners were based on authoritarian necessities rather than ethical principles, the former being defined by the bureaucracy, whereas the latter would, in modern Western medicine, be defined by the patient and his society.[9] Medical organization sought monopolistic power and economic certainty in collaboration with government, whether temporal or spiritual. Such an organization often extended the authority of the State, thereby replicating the role of the medicine-man in primitive society. Working under the restrictions imposed by such a goal, early regional medicine up to the time of its demise, or, in the traditional medicine of China and India, up to the present day, continued on much as it had for thousands of years.

For those of the view that mankind had its origins "scuttling across the floors of silent seas" there may seem to be an inevitable Darwinian logic at work in the gradual progress of human knowledge since the days of the caveman, and that ancient Egyptian, Mesopotamian, and Asian knowledge represented an improvement, perhaps vast, over the knowledge of even more ancient societies. But that is a conjecture or, at least in medicine,

---

[6] "As one of the last continents occupied by humans but one of the first sites of preindustrial civilization, America offers an important study in rapid culture change." Dillehay, T., *The Settlement of the Americas*, New York, 2000.
[7] For a recent overview of this subject see: Fregni, G., *A Study of the Manufacture of Copper Spearheads in the Old Copper Complex*, in *The Minnesota Archeologist*, 68:121-130, 2009.
[8] This elegant phrase the author owes to a former clinical colleague, Dr. Frederick Newsome.
[9] The present-day trend to replace virtue-based ethics with "rule-based ethics" is a throw-back to this authoritarian vision and is discussed in detail on p. 224*ff.*

a presumption. The artistic artifacts of 10,000 years ago, long preceding the great civilizations, do not suggest an intellectually inferior species of humanity. The 42,000 year-old flute of ivory found in Germany (Fig. 1), the magnificent twenty-foot-long Panel of Horses drawn on the walls of a cave near Chauvet in southern France 35,000 years ago, the 26,000-year-old Altamira cave paintings in Spain, the 28,000-year-old picture of a rhinoceros in South Africa, the 21,000-year-old carved ivories from the Angara River in Siberia, and the 12,000-year-old picture of a kangaroo from Australia must astonish. And so each man must question the significance of the civilization of his own ancient forebears, a civilization to whose inhabitants he can more distinctly relate his origins, and to which he is inclined to offer so much obeisance, for that civilization merely represented the steady state of human things on earth, continually recycling since the dawn of mankind. Thus, with allowances for variations in flora and fauna, the level of medical care prevailing in the developing civilizations of ancient Egypt, Mesopotamia, Asia, and the Western hemisphere was similar, each representing a spontaneously devised primeval form of medicine that has existed at all times and in all places in the absence of organized scientific thought. The possibility for medical progress that had been raised by human settlement had not been realized despite the passage of time and the concentration of talent. Now what would happen?

C. The Curtain Rises

Consider the following scenario. With regression of the last glacial period, perhaps 12,000 years ago, there was an abrupt flourishing of human activity that occurred earliest in those warming geographical locales that would prove especially conducive to human survival. It was as if a flower garden, dormant during the cold season and then subjected to sun and warm rain, suddenly blossomed forth. This seems to have been the case with *Homo sapiens*, for the birth of culture appears to have been a spontaneous, simultaneous, and unambiguously global event, one unlikely to have required an international communication network to set it going. If the plow were not invented *de novo* in both the Middle East and China, then it took 3600 years (from 4000 BC to 400 BC) for good news of that Mesopotamian invention to reach China, surely no argument for an ancient World Wide Web.[10] Thus mankind proceeded as if endowed, given the right environment, with equivalent abilities to undergo, in all places and at the same time, a series of events that would lead to societies and cultures, all being, with allowances for local peculiarities of geography, of a similar nature. It is as if the human intellectual thermostat had been preset, or by some unknowable agency instilled, with the consequences now appearing as if predetermined by mankind's DNA. The great barrier to social development of humans had been extrinsic and climatic. It was now overcome.

Then, within the new social frameworks that developed, patterns are once again seen, this time in social evolution. These patterns are notable, again making allowances for local geographical and biological variations, more for their similarities than for their differences. For example, coca and ipecac were New World discoveries, opium and senna discoveries of the eastern Mediterranean and Near East, ephedra and camphor discoveries of Asia, and eucalyptus a discovery of ancient Australians. They are distinctly different

---

[10] McNeill, W., *The Rise of the West*, Chicago, 1963, p. 27. A technologically advanced plow was in use in China during the Han Dynasty, its forerunners unknown.

medicinal herbs, but the event of their ancient discovery was the same. Simultaneously, families merged into tribes, and tribes into realms. Then, given man's indomitable proclivity to obtain the products of another man's labor by force or fraud, the great civilizations appeared. Unique cultures developed. Nevertheless, the sequence of stable communities, farming, pottery production, irrigation, artistry, and metallurgy seemed to flow from each as if triggered by the action of the same permissive genes.

Focus now on medicine and the usefulness of certain herbs, the antiseptic actions of honey and resins, the invention of trepanation, circumcision, suturing and setting of fractures. Evidence for all this is found throughout the ancient world, including the Americas. The *Solanaceae* botanical family is found worldwide, and primitive man everywhere discovered the psychogenic effects of some of its species, including mandrake from Europe through Asia, henbane in China, *Datura* species in South America, pituri (*Duboisia hopwoodii*) in Australia, *Datura metel* (*e.g.*, "apikan") in Africa, and *Datura stramonium* (or related species) in Greco-Roman times. The bark of many trees, containing tannins, has been used globally for management of diarrheas, and *nux vomica* was used as an emetic in Australia, India, and China. The universality of the search for herbal medicines fostered, in all civilizations presented in these chapters, medicinal therapies of a similar nature.[11] It is as if there were a certain basic level of empirical medical knowledge and expertise to which man could naturally aspire but could not surpass. Now the nature of these empirical achievements was such that each was capable of being the product of one person's efforts. None required the combined intellects of a group for either discovery or application. This is not inconsistent with John Stuart Mill's assessment: "The initiation of all wise or noble things comes and must come from individuals; generally at first from some one individual." But then he goes on to write, "The honor and glory of the average man is that he is capable of following that initiative...."[12] While Mill's reason for assigning inferior status to the average man and his "honor and glory" is in no way apparent, at least to the author, the authoritarian state is a profound obstruction to individual "initiative." Consequently, ancient civilizations were able to erect only a limited base for objectively observing and, in medicine, to sustain only a primitive level of practical knowledge. The potential for development, for progress, was minimal; the quality of medicine could even regress.

And yet, if one looks at cultural progress, what a vast improvement the great civilizations seemed to represent over the preexisting state of affairs. Should anyone wish to experience vicariously the nature of man in his pristine state he should consult not the Book of *Genesis*, which is disquieting enough, but the twelve volumes of Dr. Frazer's *The Golden Bough*. And Montaigne gave us a description of man's wide-ranging barbarity: ". . . there is nothing barbarous or savage, ...save to the extent that everyone

---

[11] A similar global pattern is also apparent for non-medical discovery. One example might be the use of a lodestone for determining direction. In China there is evidence for such use in the 4th C BC and recently studies suggest the same for the Olmec civilization in Mexico (1500 BC – 100 BC). See: Klokocnik, J., *Pyramids and Ceremonial Centers in Mesoamerica and China: Were They Oriented Using a Magnetic Compass?*, in *Stud. Geophys. Geod., 51:515-533, 2007.* To carry this concept a giant step further, there are those who consider purposeful self-medication for relief of symptoms a behavioral feature of the Great Apes and perhaps other animals. See: Huffman, M. A., *Self-medicative Behavior in the African Great Apes: An Evolutionary Perspective into the Origins of Human Traditional Medicine*, in *Bioscience*, 51:651-661, 2001.

[12] John Stuart Mill (1806-1873), *On Liberty of Individuality*, in *On Liberty*, London, 1869. His monograph was discussing "... the nature and limits of the power that can be legitimately exercised by society over the individual."

regards as barbarous the things to which he is not accustomed."[13]

Dr. Fielding Garrison, the medical historian, commented that the long-lived civilizations were "the cold storage plants of knowledge acquired in the past," by which he meant that a rigid system of social control of authoritarian governance, brought about by an entrenched elite consumed with a need for self-preservation, evolved state- and self-serving priesthoods or brotherhoods of medical mystics.[14] There was a "virtual enslavement of the individual unit." The scope of Garrison's criticism encompassed Egypt, Babylonia, China, and Byzantium. And the celebrated Dr. Charles Singer, went a step further.[15] He declined to even discuss any of those same systems of medicine, for they were unworthy of his attention, instead focusing solely on scientific medicine.

It is time to dispense with the traditional notion of the evolution of medicine and replace it with something more consistent with objective observations of mankind's past. That traditional notion has, for many years, pitted group against group, nation against nation, and even continent against continent, in vying for the laurel as to whom goes the credit for inventing the profession of medicine. As it turns out, no one person, group, or even civilization can be credited with such a discovery. The laurel goes, instead, to a *process*, a new political system. That new political system would permit the release of the natural ingenuity of man, an ingenuity that had existed, dormant, in all societies and civilizations. Just where the people came from who developed that political system is still debated. Therefore, no individual or society can step forward to accept the award. But at long last came that age when the combined intellects of men could be applied to their problems. In the areas of philosophy, politics, art, law, science, and medicine, society was no longer to rely on an individual's discovery, as interpreted, abandoned or exploited by another individual, a characteristic of authoritarian society. Instead, an age now appeared in which mankind's collective intellect would be empowered to solve problems that authoritarian societies had barely been able to name. The impediment to social development had been extrinsic and climatic, but the impediment to intellectual development was intrinsic and political. And so, 2500 years ago mankind's steady state was turned on its head, for its equilibrium was punctuated in ancient Hellas where for the first time free men were able to break through the opaque ceiling of authoritarianism that had contained them from their earliest days.[16]

---

[13] *The Essays of Michael Seigneur de Montaigne*, London, 1776, Book I, chapter 30, as translated by Peter Coste: Writing on *Cannibals*, "I do not find by what I am told, that there is any thing wild or barbarous ..... excepting, that every one gives the denomination of Barbarism to what is not the custom of his country."

[14] Garrison, F., *Medicine as an Agency in the Advancement of Science, Art and Civiliation*, in *Bull. N. Y. Acad. Med.* V, p. 305-327, 1929.

[15] Singer, C., *Medicine*, in *Legacy of Greece*, Cambridge, 1921, G. Murray, editor, pp. 201-248.

[16] "Hellas" (ἑλλάς) is a name that has been applied to ancient Greek culture at a time when there was a cultural but no national identity and the word "Greek" had yet to be devised. Aristotle is often cited as the source of the word "Greek" when he wrote, in *Meteorologica*, I, xiv, that γραιχος (graikhos) was the equivalent of "Hellene" as a name for certain Hellenic people. There is occasionally some resistance to use of "Greek" in describing this ancient culture, and in the Archeological Museum in Izmir, Turkey, (the ancient Smyrna), the word "Greek" is not to be found on any displayed items, such terms such as "Ionic" and "Achaean," or their equivalents being used instead to describe the inhabitants of the famed ancient cities of the west coast of Turkey and nearby Greek islands. For the purposes of this work, however, the popularly understood phrase "ancient Greece," whenever used, will refer to any Hellenic or proto-Hellenic people, although occasionally Hellas will be used in the context of the more ancient Greek societies.

CHAPTER NINE

LARGE STRUCTURED SOCIETIES, DEMOCRATIC - HELLENIC

"ἐλευθέρους ἔθηκα."
"I set them free."

Solon (638-558 BC), fragment 36.15
(Translation of John Lewis, from his book,
Solon the Thinker, London, 2006)[1]

The societal strata, or coordinates, of reasoning are: μονολογιζομένος (monologizomenos, or *that which is being reasoned by a solitary individual*), ἀνισολογιζομένος (anisologizomenos, or *that which is being reasoned by unequals*), and κοινολογιζομένος (koinologizomenos, or *that which is being reasoned in common council*). The first describes empiricism of the individual in primitive society, the second introduces the ruler or patron that characterizes authoritarian relationships, and the third describes a consequence of the democratic trend that first developed in ancient Hellas. Mycenaean Greece, the Greek Dark Ages, and the Archaic Period provide little evidence for rational Greek medicine. But by the 6th-5th C BC matters had changed. Many Greek city-states demonstrated broad acceptance of democratic governance. This preference demonstrated the principle of κοινονία (the "koinon," or *common council*), and it was applied not just to government by the people, but also to political, trade, and craft coalitions. Simultaneously there emerged the availability of, and a public preference for, community practitioners of rational medicine, as corroborated by Thucydides' description of the plague of Athens.

A. Introduction: Characteristics of Democratic and of Authoritarian Governance and Their Implications for Medical Organization

It was the focus of the opening chapters that modern medicine owes nothing to the medicine-man or to authoritarian governance, ubiquitous agents pernicious to progress. Now approaches a phase of societal development that is traditionally associated with scientific medicine.

When society at large is directed by all its members, this delegation of power to the people is termed democracy. The Greek etymology is: δεμός (demos) = the people of a locality, and κράτειν (kratain) = to rule. The word δεμοκρατία, or "democracy," was first used by Herodotus in his *Histories*, begun in approximately 455 BC, although an early stage of democracy had been outlined by Solon in 596 BC and a fully developed form of democracy was institutionalized in Athens in 507 BC. The power of the people in 5th C Athens was restricted to adult male freeborn citizens, but it is ironic that the possibility of the average citizen obtaining political office was far greater then than now. For, recognizing the undue influence of rhetoric in the hands of the powerful and the power-seekers, "It is scarcely too much to say that the whole administration of the state

---

[1] This book by Dr. John David Lewis is a judicious and authoritative review of Solon's political philosophy and role in the early evolution of Athenian democracy.

was in the hands of men appointed by *lot*: (italics added)."[2] There may, in fact, have been no important elected positions in Athens at all. This was done to protect the polity from the influence of an elite clique, just as was the introduction of the *ostracism*, by which a person perceived to exercise undue influence over the community could, by popular vote, be banished for a specified period to avert unwarranted concentration of power and influence in any one man. Undue reverence of and deference to prominent or popular persons was recognized by ancient Greeks as the source of many problems.

Why do societies proceed as they do, some failing, some thriving, some appearing as bright meteors in history, others as great ocean vessels, bearing for millennia a momentum capable of repelling all shocks to survival? Historians will provide a long list of contributory factors, but, while seldom mentioned, among them should be the following:

1. The power of the leader: The more powerful the leader, the more powerful he tends to become, just as the speed of a falling object increases with the distance traveled per unit time per unit time ($s=d/t^2$). A force may be small at onset, as in a single man, but as other men hang on his coattails, reflecting the natural desire of most subjugated men to perceive themselves as strong, they identify and ally themselves with strength, and the consequence has been exponential expansion of influence and threatened world domination by clerks and corporals [Stalin, Hitler], kings and caliphs [Alexander, Umar]. In a world conditioned to servitude, all passions cower before force, and those most effective in wielding force are acclaimed by their cultists as the most virtuous. John Locke commented that virtue and vice always go together, that what constitutes virtue varies from society to society, but that ". . . nothing else but that which has the allowance of public esteem is called virtue."[3] Facility in the use of force, sometimes a vice, can now be redefined as a virtue, for history has shown that no virtue surpasses that of being victorious.[4]

2. The power of dogma: The more demanding a dogma, the more passion it provokes. As Prof. Froude noted, "Once possess people with a belief, and never fear that they will find facts enough to confirm it."[5] But beyond this, undemanding principles are viewed as frivolous, whereas those requiring an investment of effort, sacrifice, and discomfort over time invent their own

---

[2] Headlam, J. W., *Election by Lot at Athens*, Cambridge, 1891, p. 2. And Prof. Headlam makes this interesting observation: judicial actions of the Athenians were based on simple and clearly defined laws, unlike the complex mass of *Lex Romana* that would follow, because reliance on the *lot* precluded a privileged class of lawyers and bureaucrats. Even judges of the annual contests of tragedies and comedies were selected by lot, so steeped in democracy and confident in its citizenry were the Athenians. Aristotle was of the opinion that in poetry superior judgment lay with average citizens, not a few experts.

[3] Locke, J., *Concerning Human Understanding*, Bk. II, Chapter 28, 11.

[4] Furthermore, in authoritarian societies the losers, should they be permitted to survive, seldom have the means of expressing the merits of their opposition, no one to whom they can disclaim the new virtue. The next generation, therefore, begotten by the winners, will know no better.

[5] Froude, J. A., *Short Studies on Great Subjects*, New York, 1872, chapter entitled "Scientific Method Applied to History," p. 454.

significance, the original nature of the dogma even becoming irrelevant to action.[6]

And so the usual course of human society has been, for the mass of humanity, to acknowledge the preeminence of force and the demands of dogma, political or religious. Dogma and the threat of force are antithetical to the expression of genius. How does this bear on medicine?

Historically, much effort has been spent on unproductive speculation as to the origin of medicine in ancient primitive or authoritarian societies described in preceding chapters. Whether the pulse was first discerned by this or that person is of no importance. It cannot be doubted that the pulse has been discovered repeatedly, and by countless individuals, over the millennia. Any mother bathing or clothing an infant, especially a febrile one, would do so. The critical question, however, is what permitted the accumulation of observations of the pulse in various clinical settings that replaced a simple observation within a complex association, such as that between the pulse and fever, or the increased warmth of the body in the presence of a focus of inflammation or a skin rash, and ultimately a description of the course a child's illness was likely to take over time. Complex associations of this sort can be accurately assembled only from experience or shared experience with similarly sick children.

For certain clinical signs are apparent to all. It takes no skill to diagnose advanced jaundice, and minimal skill to spot mild jaundice.[7] The first diagnosis of jaundice was probably made about the time early man realized that a well-aimed rock could down small prey. Far subtler signs have been recorded by nonphysicians: Gentile da Fabriano (1378-1427) perfectly portrayed the plantar reflex of an infant Jesus in his famous 1423 painting *Adoration of the Magi*, but it would not be until 1896 that Dr. Joseph Babinski published a paper on the clinical significance of the plantar reflex, or what is now called the "Babinski reflex," a physician's assessment of which is part of every neurological examination. The person with abundant ascites or with a generalized exanthem or with a hemiparesis is often identified by a lay person, usually by the patient himself; a physician is not needed for the obvious. But jaundice, ascites, skin rash, and hemiparesis are not diseases; they are *signs* of disease. Simple descriptions such as these are commonplace observations, not profound medical discoveries; observation in no way implies comprehension. They are mentioned in writings or portrayed in figurines from all ancient civilizations.

A more complex step than simple *observation* is the linking of one observation or symptom to another.[8] This is the concept of *association*. Like simple observations,

---

[6] Dogma: "2. A principle, belief, idea, or opinion, especially one authoritatively considered to be absolute truth: tenet." (Webster's II New Riverside Dictionary, 1984). Notably, a dogma is not required to be true, or, as Froude pointed out, its confirmation can be added later. Dogma of the Catholic Church, however, is Divine revelation and is binding, the subornation of which is heresy.

[7] This was obvious to the Hippocratics, as stated in *Prorrhetic* II (Προρρητικων Β): πρῶτον μὲν γὰρ τοὺς ὑφύδρους τε καὶ φθινώδεας τίς ἂν οὐ γνοίη·, ("In the first place, who *wouldn't* recognize patients with dropsy or consumption?") II, 18-19, *Loeb Classical Library*, *Hippocrates*, vol. VIII (italics added, translation of Potter).

[8] A *sign*, in medicine, is physical evidence relevant to an illness found by the examiner in the course of physically examining a patient, for example, tenderness on palpation of the abdomen. A *symptom* is an observation concerning that illness as expressed by the patient himself, for example, "I have pain in my chest" or "I have developed a lump on my chest."

associations are easily made. They can be quite complex, even fanciful, and are routinely made by everyone throughout the day, every day.

But it is the next step, *causation*, that poses problems, for by that step men attribute to an observation or association a particular cause, and in that attribution humans are almost invariably wrong: he has a cold because of a change in weather; I have a headache, so my blood pressure must be high; she has arthritis because of radiation exposure from Three Mile Island; you are sick because you have sinned. Elaborate theories of causation have dogged medicine since its earliest days, and even Samuel Johnson could claim with confidence in the mid-18th C that, "It is incident to physicians, I am afraid, beyond all other men, to mistake subsequence for consequence, to use the fallacious inference *post hoc, ergo propter hoc*."[9] The compulsion to ascribe causation remains very much with us today. The consequence of that compulsion is undisciplined action, which caused John Locke to state, regarding his own medical practice, ". . . it being better in my opinion to doe no thing, than to doe amiss."[10]

A vital feature of clinical practice is knowledge upon which action might be taken to improve chances for a favorable outcome of an illness, and to do this the usual outcome of that illness needs to be clearly defined. This can only be achieved by experience. The variability in disease presentation is infinite, no two patients being identical. To determine the usual course of an illness observation of many patients is necessary. Modern medical journals indicate on a daily basis the profession's keen awareness of this need. The week this paragraph was written the *Annals of Internal Medicine* reported a case control study of the risk factors associated with kidney infections in healthy women. The study identified, after interviewing 1,334 women, two factors associated with an increase in risk of kidney infection: (1) history of a previous urinary infection, and (2) sexual behavior. Specifically, these two factors predispose to kidney infection in healthy, non-pregnant, community-dwelling women, "profound" results that assuredly will come as no surprise to most people. This study was reported by six co-authors, supported by federal funds, carried out not by examination of sick patients but by computerized telephone interviews, and had its conclusions based on likelihood as determined by a complex analysis that acknowledged statistical limitations of the study. In the same journal another article profoundly concluded from a study of 38,156 male health professionals that "light and moderate average alcohol use was generally not associated with an increased risk for ischemic stroke, although drinking pattern and beverage type modified this relation." The considerable effort required to complete these two studies, the conclusions from which required so many qualifiers that one must wonder why anyone bothered to publish them, was funded by grants from the National Institutes of Health of the US Department of Health and Human Services. But the point to be made is that these are everyday examples of the type of effort exercised by modern researchers to even vaguely anticipate the consequences of illness-related behavior for two very common medical events.[11] Such efforts require input from many observers, indeed, an organization.

---

[9] Cited by Samuel Johnson in *Literary Magazine*, 1756, for a review of "*Essay on Water*" by Dr. Lucas. The Hippocratics agreed, but there is no reason to select out physicians more than any other group for an obsession with *causation*; see p. 238, footnote on Francis Bacon.

[10] John Locke (1632-1704), the English philosopher, was also a physician (p. 363, footnote). The quotation is recorded by John Brown, MD, in his *Locke and Sydenham*, Edinburgh, 1858.

[11] The two articles are: Scholes, D., *et al.*, *Risk Factors Associated with Acute Pyelonephritis in Healthy Women*, p. 20-27, and Mukamal, K. M., *et al.*, *Alcohol and the Risk for Ischemic Stroke in*

The critical factor in achieving effective organization is the social setting, for medicine, as a profession, has been trying to be born since the first communities. But ancient attempts had their miscarriages, some early in gestation, as when alert mothers spotted a disease association in their families suggesting communicability of an illness but had no opportunity to pass their thoughts on to others. And some occurred near term, perhaps in Sumer, Old Kingdom Egypt, and possibly even ancient China and India, where rationally organized collections of empirical medical observations may have existed prior to the time medical practitioners or their knowledge were purloined and integrated into a bureaucracy.

To read, therefore, of the identification, by ancient practitioners of any land, of jaundice, wheezing, or edema implies nothing whatever about the medical knowledge or medical practice of the time. Moderns may declare that an ancient description of wheezing is synonymous with asthma, and thereby credit the ancients with a modern diagnosis. Crediting them with knowledge of the etiology and comprehension of pathophysiology of asthma, *i.e.*, causation, however, is presumptuous. In modern Western medicine the physician, by his training, is able to state either the true proximate cause of the patient's signs or symptoms, or, equally important, that the cause of the problem is as yet unknown, both responses being enormous improvements over previous ages. This is because organized data collection is the multiplier of personal experience. Organized data collection and analysis, not dogma, now guide Western medicine, and there is now at least some intellectual control over concepts of causation. How came this to medicine? It came about because of medical organization. And the history of medical organization is the key to any true history of medicine. The initial question in this Section (third paragraph) of how dogma and threat of force bear on medicine can now be answered. They do so by affecting its organization.

B. Coordinates of Reasoning

There is a grid upon which intellectual potential within a society becomes manifest. At its most basic the grid comprises three strata, or coordinates,[12] the names of which can be conveniently expressed in words derived from the Greek root λογός (logos), or "reason":

1. μονολογιζομένος (monologizomenos), "that which is being reasoned by one person"

Through cave paintings, ivory flutes, figurines and other works of intellect the reason and ingenuity of man's distant ancestors speak to their descendants. Allied against a threatening world but disunited by nature, early man maintained himself in small groups. The energy-intensive effort of hunting and a nomadic life can explain the dispersed and tiny social groupings of early Stone Age man that were his social heritage since creation. But it has been the ability to reason, then as now, that has been mankind's intellectual

Men: The Role of Drinking Patterns and Beverage, p. 11-19, in: *Annals of Internal Medicine*, Jan. 4, 2005, vol. 142, No. 1.

[12]A coordinate can be defined as one of a set of variables used in specifying the state of something.

heritage, and a Stone Age infant bred within a family of today might well become class valedictorian.

But the constraints of nature and the limitations imposed by low population density, social groupings, and brief life spans did not permit the propagation of ideas.[13] Therefore, a man's novel thought, no matter what its potential, went no further than the geophysical limits of the immediate family or tribe. Writing had not yet been invented. Therefore, the reasonings of the individual remained isolated and, ultimately, given the arduous world in which he lived, died out when that individual died. And this is the pattern that has existed for most of man's time on earth. Minimum dates can be assigned to the pattern during which it was the exclusive form of intellectual propagation: from approximately 40,000 BC to 10,000 BC. But it should be obvious that this pattern remains very much in force today. Most of our potentially constructive thoughts each day are known to no one outside ourselves. They are "things being reasoned by one person." Should all else fail, this most fundamental pattern of reasoning will permit the survival of some *Homo sapiens*, although we should hope that day never arrives.

2. ἀνισολογιζομένος (anisologizomenos) or, "that which is being reasoned by unequals"[14]

Beginning about 10,000 BC with the retreat of the glaciation period, a new human association came into existence, the settled community. Now there was a social pattern in which one person could easily communicate his idea to another, but with this improvement over μονολογιζομένος: because of the larger social groupings, the concentrated energies of many people could be applied to a single individual's idea. No longer was honey in a poultice a family remedy for a wound. From the larger society there was the possibility that honey as a treatment for wounds would become widely used, perhaps even an official recommendation by the society's leadership, thereby extending its therapeutic usefulness to many who previously had been ignorant of its value. This benefit could be provided because societal leadership was centralized and authoritarian, the better to control chaos and greed among the many, limiting it instead to the benefit of one or a few. Similarly, what had been a small cairn placed over the body of a deceased could now become, in the larger society, the Great Pyramid; a man who earlier, through his superior strength, might have been the domineering ruler of his family, might now become a tyrant who, with an army, could rule millions.

Yet honey remained but honey, a tyrant but a man, and a pyramid but a pile of rocks. For in this social pattern an idea, in the vise of authoritarianism, could be either stifled or chiseled into stone, depending on the whim and threat of force of one man or a few. This pervasive pattern has always hindered the progress of mankind, just as it does today, although it is less evident now because innovations of free societies have been purchased, stolen, or copied by authoritarian ones, thereby camouflaging the profound distinction between the two.

Nevertheless, authoritarianism did have one great advantage: now there was a way to harness the efforts of many men. In authoritarian societies where there were cities

---

[13] These and other factors will be analyzed in detail in volume 3 of this work.

[14] The sense of "aniso..." is "unequal," as found in: anisocoria – pupils of unequal size; anisocytosis – cells of different sizes; anisoploid – "a chromosomal number that is an odd multiple of the basic number ...." (Merriam-Webster's Unabridged Dictionary, 1986).

many people's efforts could be applied to the common task or the uncommon event, sometimes with great efficiency. But such efforts were directed at implementation of the patron's decision, usually with an eye to maintaining his hegemony. Whether an idea, be it good or bad, originated from a peasant or a pharaoh, it remained unadorned, limited by the intellect or goals of an authoritarian figure who made life or death decisions regarding not only his subjects but also their intellectual property. Thus, mankind's progress was stalled at a certain level of achievement, one that is recognized in all the large societies of the past and most of those of the present day. But the time was approaching when a new social pattern would emerge. This time the pile of rocks would become the Parthenon, the tyrant would be replaced by the voice of the people, and the profession and practice of medicine would be invented.

3. κοινολογιζομένος (koinologizomenos), or, "that which is being reasoned in common council"

City-states have existed since the founding of the earliest cities. And if any institution is commonly identified today with ancient Greece, it is the πόλις (polis) or city-state. Other societies had evolved city-states, but the Greek version was different. Aristotle noted its uniqueness and he called the Greek city-state a κοινον (koinon), an association of men engaged in "common council," noting that each Greek city-state was autonomous, regulated from within and reflecting the moral character of its members.[15] These associations sought out mutually acceptable ways of living together. The outcome of this happy effort was democracy, and its ornament classical Athens. The same principle of a koinon, or "common council," could be applied to small groups such as craft and trade associations within the city-state, and with remarkable results. Demosthenes said that a man's greatest blessing was good fortune, but equally important was good counsel.[16] Surely one of the greatest blessings for any society is the good counsel that emerges from the "common council," the koinon.

---

[15] αὕτη δ᾽ ἐστὶν ἡ καλουμένη πόλις καὶ ἡ κοινωνία ἡ πολιτική. ("And it is this that is being called the city-state or the common council [koinon] or political association.") Aristotle, *Politics*, I,1,7, translation of the author. And it is in a political sense of "partnership" that the term is most used, some considering it the equivalent of a federated state. It superseded the ἔθνος (ethnos), which was a loose tribal or clan organization. See: Scholten, J. B., *The Politics of Plunder*, Berkeley, 2000. He discusses koinons in the process of detailing the history of the Aitolian koinon of the 4th and 3rd C BC. The koinon was based on urban settlements and later was applied to a federation of such settlements, each city being an autonomous voting member of the organization. There were, at one time, as many as a thousand Greek city-states, large and small. There were exceptions to equitable city-state associations; centralized political and military authority marked certain leagues. (For a discussion of various confederacies see: Ehrenberg, V., *The Greek State*, New York, 1960.) In this regard it is interesting to reflect on the Mycenaean age, for evidence from archeological finds, as well as that from the *Iliad* of Homer in his "Catalogue of Ships," indicates that Agamemnon's military assemblage was not summoned to Troy by the monarch of some mighty empire. It was more a confederation where each constituent community or city-state determined whether or not to join and sought to advance its own interest within the confederation by argument and inveigling.

[16] "Demosthenes expresses the view, with regard to human life in general, that good fortune is the greatest of blessings, while good counsel, which occupies the second place, is hardly inferior in importance...," cited by Pseudo-Longinus in *On the Sublime*, translation of W. R. Roberts, London, 1899.)

Excursus on the Koinon

Definition of "koinon:" A voluntary autonomous and democratic group allied in self-interest and acting in common council.

1. An abridged definition of the classical era Greek word "koinon," taken from the Liddell and Scott Greek-English Lexicon (Boston, 1875):

Verb: κοινόω - I make common, communicate, impart; to make a sharer in.

Noun: κοινωνία, ἡ - communion, fellowship, intercourse.
κοινῶν, ὁ – a companion, comrade, counsellor
Adjective: κοινός, ά, όν - common, shared in common.

2. A definition of "koine," taken from Merriam-Webster's Collegiate Dictionary, 10th edition:
Noun: 2: a dialect or language of a region that has become the common or standard language of a larger area.

"Koine" is the term applied to the common dialect of Greece that, arising from the armies of Alexander, superseded classical Attic Greek, the conversion occurring mainly in the 3rd C BC.[17]

3. "Koinon" in its various forms was frequently used by the ancient Greeks, and, as an incentive for moderns to reintroduce the concept of "common council" in preference to the "gifted" or "natural-born" leader, "koinon" will be frequently used in the pages to follow. Another reason for its employment herein is efficiency, as there is no equivalent term in English.[18]

4. Scholarly use has concentrated on the koinon's larger political ramifications that suggest a "federation," or union of self-governing states, but its functional application in this book will primarily refer to small groups. As such, the koinon was a group of individuals engaged in common council, and here a preliminary comment on the aptitude of the individual is required.

While at a certain level of creation all men may be considered equal, this neat egalitarian expression is, in human experience, blatantly quantitatively and qualitatively errant. The modifier "equal in opportunity" in this context is moot. Some are simply stronger, some smarter, some more thoughtful, bigger, smaller, quicker, and on and on. In any single

---

[17] Koinon was a respectable, even honorable, term initially, and Philo (20 BC – 50 AD), in his ethical theory, considered κοινωνία, by which he meant "fellowship," a virtue. But it came to mean over several centuries something that was ordinary, common, or mediocre and representative of the public at large, ultimately even something profane.
[18] In modern American English "koinon" is preferred as more euphonic than "koinonia," although the latter would be technically the more correct usage for a group.

category of ability a graphic population distribution of that ability may or may not be Gaussian, but there will always be wide-ranging inequality.[19] But were the entire list of man's abilities to be lumped together and regraphed according to the usefulness of any individual quality at the appropriate moment in time, a sharp peak would be apparent because every person's unique ability at something would be viewed as equal to that of any other person's ability at something else should the occasion arise that would put each ability to the test when the time is right. The person who was an outlier in one category, for example "strength," might be the perfect example of success in another category such as "endurance" or "composure." With the addition of more and more categories, fewer and fewer of the total population would be perpetual outliers, for each individual possesses some unique and useful capabilities. Everyone has an aptitude for something.[20] Faith in the ability of the individual is the unwritten creed of democracy, and so it is also for the koinon. The thermostat of the individual that determines his choices in life will, like the polyglot of qualities that creates the impression of inequality, vary from individual to individual, each ideally capable of being activated at the appropriate moment, no one quality being superior to any other from the vantage point of society until the moment of testing arrives.[21] The koinon permits that individual merit to surface. Note that this has

---

[19] Sir Francis Galton (1822-1911) described what might be considered a Gaussian distribution of intellectual ability in his *Hereditary Genius* (London, 1892) in which he divided men into classes based on the degree of separation from an "average." He believed men are far from being equal, that genetic factors are extremely important in determining this, and he made the extraordinary statement that the smartest dog is far brighter than the most stupid human. In retrospect his interpretations of the data were based on a ludicrously simple understanding of biology. He also had an extremely restricted and elitist definition of "abilities," even as he acquired data on matters such as the mathematically symmetrical variation in chest sizes among men. It did not occur to him in his value system that at times, and perhaps most of the time, physical ability is more important to individual or group survival than intellectual ability. In a pleasant contrast there is the opinion of the Irish educator, Edmond Holmes, Chief Inspector of Elementary Schools, whose experience indicated "that under favorable conditions the average child can become the rare exception..." (Holmes, E., *What Is and What Might Be*, London, 1928, p. 303).

[20] This is an ancient conjecture. In the *Huainanzi*, the 2nd C BC book of Chinese Masters, is the following: "Uncut jade can never be thick enough; jade inlay can never be thin enough; lacquer can never be black enough; rice powder can never be white enough. These four are opposites, yet when [urgently] needed, they are equal, their usefulness is the same." (From *The Huainanzi*, J. S. Major, S. A. Queen, A. S. Meyer, and H. D. Roth, translators and editors, New York, 2010, p. 401.) Dr. E. G. Browne of Cambridge, at the outset of his FitzPatrick Lectures, implied almost as much when he repeated an Arabic proverb: "I have not stored thee up, O my tear, save for the time of my distress," meaning, he wrote, "the time comes when the services of a person or thing provided for a particular contingency are at last actually required." (See *Arabic Medicine*, Cambridge, 1921, Lecture I.) The koinon, from its entire membership, has a gamut of services available for contingencies, rather than merely those of a single leader. It is thus that Aristotle could develop the theory of what has been termed as "the wisdom of the many" (See: *Politics*, Bk. 3, 1281, b.) He thought that virtue and reason were universal characteristics of mankind, and given the necessarily broadened spectrum of perception a group (obviously of free people) was superior to the reason of a single yet superior man. This has been put into a fascinating modern perspective by Josiah Ober (*Democracy's Wisdom: An Aristotelian Middle Way for Collective Judgment*, in *Amer. Polit. Sci. Rev.*, 107: 104-122, 2013) and his cited reference of Aristotle's *Politics*, III, 1281a42-b10. Also see p. 201 for another Aristotelian relevancy.

[21] And none can say who that man is and when is that moment. Alfred Zimmern (*The Greek Commonwealth*, New York [Modern Library printing of 1931 5th ed.], Part II, chapter 6) cites an ancient Greek proverb, ἀρχὴ ἄνδρα δείξει ("Office will bring out the man.") Hidden quality can

nothing to do with "fairness" or "morality" or "popularity." What it does is provide an arsenal of abilities that can assist a society to survive its challenges, whereas the exclusion of variety in a society's abilities will limit its ability to survive the variety of challenges it will confront. Finally, Socrates, in Plato's *Theaetetus* (149a *ff*), makes a related point: He, Socrates, does not disagree with those who claim he is not wise, that his wisdom is sterile, and that he has produced no new invention. Wisdom and invention were to be found, instead, in those youths from whom, with his assistance as a metaphorical "midwife," he had "delivered" their nascent ability to think clearly and logically. In other words, he had permitted their merit to surface.

5. The professional koinon was not a function of the Greek city-state. Except for the silver mines and a few other critical ventures, the sources of Greek wealth were not state operations. Koinons were not taxed. In a sense, a modern-day koinon might be the Chamber of Commerce in a community, a local collection of individual interests seeking to improve, through periodic meetings, their image and commercial advantage through discipline in maintaining quality and pursuing an integrated approach to marketing.[22] The koinon is not the equivalent of a guild or a Roman collegium, organizations that Haywood has described as where an individual "would combine his own puny individual forces with the resources of his neighbours and friends that what he alone could not do he might do through cooperation. Through pooling their money, their knowledge, their influence, and their good will the dim multitudes of common people learned to hold their own in a great hard world."[23] The koinon might pool its knowledge and ideas, but this was done not "to hold their own," but to permit each member to promote his own interests, although in so doing benefits for the others often would follow.

6. The "magic" of the koinon is to be found in the application of several minds to a common problem. For all the rhetoric about the individual being the best judge of his own interests, a quick look around one's neighorhood will prove that this is often not the case. The other fellow may be right after all. On the Bowery there are many individualists who, by themselves, have proved unequal to the daily task. And in this is found the value of the koinon. It is superior to individual application, although only if each member has free rein to venture his opinion. But it is precisely this feature that has so greatly effected a delay in development of the koinon, indeed, has led to its being ignored. Even the great Descartes stated than an edifice or organization conceived by a single mind is patently superior to one that has been conceived and assembled by several. His political inference was that admirable Sparta could trace its superiority to the fact that its laws represented the genius of a single man, Lycurgus, and this because there was no rift or fragmentation in pursuing a singular goal. Descartes would have been no advocate of the koinon.[24] How

---

emerge from unexpected quarters, which is one reason character carries inordinant weight in electing officials: democracies, and thus the koinons, know that the "unexpected" is not the same as "rare." John Stuart Mill expresses and extends this thinking in another way: "All errors which [a person] is likely to commit against advice and warning are far outweighed by the evil of allowing others to constrain him to what they deem his good." (*On Liberty*, chapter 4.)

[22] Chambers of Commerce, first organized in 1599, are of two types, public and private. The latter is voluntary; the former, European, is compulsory. A koinon would, of course, represent the private type.

[23] Haywood, H. L., *Freemasonry and the Roman Collegia*, in *The Builder*, June 1923.

[24] Descartes, R., *Discourse on the Method*, 1637, Part Two.

grateful the West should be for his English contemporary, John Locke! For the koinon requires freedom for each individual to pursue self interest within the group rather than for the group or for someone else's interest. Thus, many minds in the group can be freely applied to what may be a singular issue or a general goal. As an example of the former, a member may invent a useful tool, in which case the magic of the koinon lies in vetting and promoting the new device, for it may prove useful to the koinon's individual members. Although the community and the koinon will benefit from the invention, rewards or distinction will accrue to the individual who invented it. On the other hand, if the koinon members have a goal in common for improving their business prospects through, for example, advertising or setting standards, all members are rewarded if their combined efforts meet with success.

Related benefits include: (1) Just as democracy displaces other less desirable forms of government, a koinon substitutes freely organized group knowledge for a single individual's "all-knowing" intelligence that inherently finds its basis in self-preservation and tends naturally to preclude competition,[25] and (2) individual members will have less incentive to turn to special interest groups for promoting self-interest, for a koinon, in contrast to a guild or a union, will pose no obstacles to self-interest to which all members aspire. There would be little reason to avoid, subvert, or bypass procedures of the koinon that are intended to facilitate rather than exploit the membership or any part thereof.

7. The koinon would not likely administer a corporation or a government, for members of a koinon should know the whole range of issues on a particular problem. It fits best, therefore, with a profession or trade. Its validity in the Greek city-states probably rested to considerable extent on their relatively small populations of citizens and on the specificity of political goals.

8. Membership in a koinon is selective, for members must have a common purpose, differences being for the most part in the area of implementation. Democratic government, on the other hand, must resolve what may be wildly disparate purposes. The koinon should be a relatively small group, and the mechanics of a small group apply to its functioning.[26] Procedures of a koinon do not come naturally for there is no obligatory

---

[25] The general idea expressed here, and some of the terms used, can be traced to Friedrich Hayek's 1945 essay *The Uses of Knowledge in Society*.

[26] A group can have as few as two people. The term, therefore, is applicable to the physician-patient relationship, and "group dynamics" have been scientifically studied, both in its psychology and its decision-making processes. See: Bion, W. R., *Experiences in Groups and Other Papers*, New York, 1961. But modern interest in small groups focuses on a small group's status within the larger group, *i.e.*, attempts by the former to improve its position within the latter, and its relations with other groups. This is more akin to medieval guilds, with focus primarily on trade unions and mercantile interests, protectionism, and monopoly. Individuals in the group receive a benefit when the group advances. But the consequence of the small Greek koinon was to advance the status of individual members within the group, any advancement of the group as an organization being but a secondary effect. A modern formal definition of a group is broad and fits both purposes: "associations exist to fulfill purposes which a group of men have in common." (Laski, H., *A Grammar of Politics*, London, 1939, p. 67.) It is relevant that the Aristotelian concept of the city-state koinon, as a democracy, was applied to relatively small populations such as composed the Greek polis. Interestingly, the Greek Classicist, H. D. F. Kitto, viewed the small size of the polis as part of an inherently unstable social assemblage because, by urging that every citizen be part of its

hierarchy, no preferred rules of order, no coercion. For persons unaccustomed to freedom of thought and action the koinon would be chaos. To ancient Egyptians, Mesopotamians, Asiatics and pre-Columbian Americans a koinon would have been inconceivable.

9. In one sense, however, the koinon can be likened to a government. A nation is but one of a family of nations. Those nations may be large or small, rich or poor, but they have this in common: they are in unspoken but implacable competition for survival, and the nation that disavows its leadership and or subverts cohesion will fall under domination of another, a perpetual truth disregarded at great peril. Similarly, a koinon is but one group among many groups vying for survival. Edith Hamilton commented that "The Romans were wonderful organizers, and an organization is not a place where people are encouraged to seek or to be free."[27] Roman organizations undoubtedly were not koinons. Nevertheless, the craft or trade koinon, like a nation, is not a communal variant of Speaker's Corner at Hyde Park. It requires decision and cohesion. Despite frequent and even necessary differences of opinion, its members must assume both decision and cohesion are necessary and ideally should either voluntarily adhere to the conclusions of their deliberations or renounce membership in the koinon. Otherwise there will be other groups, whether koinons or not, that will eliminate it. Unanimity of thought or action is not required, but weaknesses are displayed if fragmentation is excessive.

10. Implicitly, the koinon is an arena where there can be compromise, and an important feature is that a member need not compromise his principles in a koinon. When concerted action is required, its aggregate decision represents the sum, within established procedure, of many strongly held opinions. It is, in fact, the koinon itself that permits survival of the uncompromising principle, for a principle, even if voted down, continues to exist in the face of defeat; it is part of the record, an argument archived until again of potential value. This is in no way a compromise of one's principles. Defeat is merely one strikeout in a nine-inning game. The holder of that uncompromising principle is not excommunicated, jailed, or executed. There yet may come his day of victory. The ability of the koinon to preserve rather than bury contrary opinion is a source of its strength, for potential validation of any opinion, however personally uncompromising its author, is ever in the wings.

11. Of extreme importance, the existence of a koinon depends not only on its members, but on the δῆμος (demos, "all the people of a place") as well. For without free choice, the koinon presents no advantage. The deck is easily stacked against it. Its existence relies on a public that has the freedom of choice. Therefore, the koinon was not only inconceivable in ancient civilizations, it was utterly impractical, for its success lay not with the "demos." It would have been manipulated by the central authority, either by carrot or by stick, and the koinon would not have remained a koinon for long. For successful functioning a koinon requires a public (1) possessing choices, and (2) capable of choosing. It requires an intelligent public supportive of differences, supportive of competition, and able to offer rewards. It requires, in a word, freedom. But here is a note of caution. The concept of koinon assumes the fortunate society that permits its

---

management, it was run by "amateurs" rather than professionals and thereby unable to properly manage its propensity for "progress." See: Kitto, H. D. F., *The Greeks*, Harmondsworth, 1963, chapter 9. (First edition was in 1951.)

[27] E. Hamilton, *The Echo of Greece*, New York, 1957, p. 216.

unrestricted functioning is a society that is not hindered by those who are slothful, purposefully ignorant, psychologically unfit for personal survival, or lead a parasitic existence within the greater society, i.e., their number is insufficient to affect social direction.

12. The term "koinon" has not disappeared. In the southeastern United States there is a utopian community founded in 1942 named "Koinonia Farm." Its website is www.koinoniapartners.org. This noteworthy community has interpreted "koinon" to mean "loving fellowship," a phrase in no way implied by the ancients.[28]

13. The fundamental benefit of a koinon to society is in the realm of ideas. Marketing, self-interest, the summation of "puny forces," and integrated approaches to managing a problem are benefits a koinon brings to individual members. But its value to society is in its validation and dissemination of ideas, and it is in the realm of ideas that the spectrum of individual merit will be most on display. In the "chicken or the egg" debate, the koinon is the mother hen.[29]

14. "Koinon" is not in modern English or American dictionaries. There is no contemporary equivalent of the word, the essence of which is found in the phrase "common council." But given modern embellishments to the American dictionary such as "mouse potato," soul patch," and "big-box," it should be no imposition to add "koinon."[30] In lexical development of the term for modern dictionaries the following might be considered. Prof. Donald Morrison has stressed a distinction between two

---

[28] *Interracialism and Christian Community in the Postwar South; The Story of Koinonia Farm*, Virginia, 1997. More recently, in 1984, was the founding of the Koinonia Academy, a Catholic private school. The term is thus most used in the context of a religious brotherhood. See also: De Mare, P. and Piper, R., *Koinonia: From Hate through Dialogue to Culture in the Larger Group*, London, 1991, where koinonia refers more to an impersonal fellowship.

[29] There also may be societal benefit on a larger scale. R. Nisbet, in *History of the Idea of Progress* (New York, 1980), discussing society as a whole but focusing on the great value of smaller social units and the importance of their remaining autonomous, provides an interesting parallel to the koinon as a force for progress. In the present work the medical koinon is an essential component required for progress in the profession of medicine. On a grander scale, however, Nisbet assessed features necessary for societal progress as a whole. Importantly, he regards smaller social groupings (churches, unions, local legislatures) as the mechanism for progress of a society. An all-embracing government, by usurping individual freedom and impressing lesser minds, limits the options for free expression and will inhibit the generation of both the passion, variety and quality of ideas that can emanate from smaller groups. Authoritarian options rarely include room for novelty or originality. The mind of the authoritarian is, for whatever reason, molded to obtain and retain control of the present, whereas the collective mind of a free society is free to break that mold and to consider a better tomorrow, implicitly including its progeny. It would be appropriate to add "koinon" to Nisbet's list of smaller societal groups. Axiomatically, as Nesbit was speaking of social groupings in general, one can infer that a threat to the koinon is an example of the threat that authoritarianism presents not only to an individual group but to society at large. For a difference between Nisbet's concept and the one espoused in this book see the Excursus on Religion and Medicine, p. 347, of the present volume.

[30] "Mouse potato" – a person who spends an inordinate amount of time using a computer; "soul patch" – a small patch of hair allowed to grow between the lower lip and the chin; "big-box" – a "physically large chain store" or its company. These three terms are among new entries to the 2006 *Merriam-Webster's Collegiate Dictionary*, 13th edition.

expressions of koinon as used by Aristotle[31]: κοινον ἀγαθον, meaning, literally and emblematically, "common good," and κοινει συμφερον, meaning, literally, "a benefit of the commonality [shared aims]," and idiomatically, "mutual advantage." The use of "koinon" in this excursus and book is more consistent with the latter. The momentous importance of the koinon to medical practice is developed in the following chapters.[32]

End of excursus

At this point a broad overview of concepts expressed thus far will be useful. The coordinates of reasoning relate generally to social framework thus:

μονολογιζομένος (that being reasoned by one person) = unstructured society
ἀνισολογιζομένος (that being reasoned by unequals) = authoritarian society
κοινολογιζομένος (that being reasoned in common council) = free society

These societies can in turn be related to the evolution of an authentic medical profession and of the medicine-man (Table 4, p. 136).

C. The Earliest Hellenic Medicine

A *precis* of one of the greatest inventions of the early Greeks requires a perspective of early Greek history. It appears that between, roughly, 3000 and 1600 BC a formative Hellenic civilization existed.[33] For the next 500 years, from 1600 BC to the time of its disintegration in about 1100 BC, mainland Greece and the Peloponnese were under the hegemony of the Mycenaean empire, a truly Greek civilization with a written syllabic, recognizably Greek, language.[34]

Mycenaean civilization became extensive, even dominating the first defined European civilization, the Crete/Minoan, in about 1500 BC. Despite its significance in history, virtually nothing medical has been identified from the Mycenaean period, though

---

[31] Morrison, D., *The Common Good*, chapter 7 in *The Cambridge Companion to Aristotle's Politics*, Deslauriers, M., and Destree, P., Cambridge, 2013.

[32] That small koinons have sporadically emerged in many societies, including hunter-gatherer groups, is not debated. For example, "What should we do now?" is asked in any threatened small society in its attempt to get the best ideas from any of its desperate members. But it was the ancient Greeks who implemented and sustained the concept with the force of law and to the exclusion of alternative governance on what might almost be called a national scale.

[33] In Grecian prehistory the onset of the Neolithic is taken as 6000 B.C. The Bronze Age, which runs from 3000 to the end of the Mycenaean period, 1100, is also termed "Helladic."

[34] This is the famous Linear B. See: Ventris, M., Chadwick, J., *Documents in Mycenaean Greek*, Cambridge, 1956. Linear A, considered to be older (18th-15th C BC), may have been an early form of Greek and the precursor of Linear B, but it remains undeciphered. See: Duhoux, Y., *Linear A* (translated by Lillie, W. J.) in "*A History of Ancient Greek*," A.-F. Christidis, editor, Cambridge, 2007, chapter 10, p. 229.

Table 4: Relation of Social Structure to Type of Medical Practice

Type of Governance	Professional Medicine (Objective therapy)	Numinous Medicine (Subjective or "placebo" therapy)[35]
Unstructured (primitive)	Empirical medicine	Shamanism
Authoritarian*	Rational medicine	Canonic medicine
Free society	Scientific medicine	Huckster

*Note that (1) while rational medicine should logically fit within large authoritarian civilizations and is so here portrayed, this intercalation has only rarely, and even then transiently, been permitted, and (2) canonic medicine includes both priest medicine of a theocracy and State-sponsored medicine, terms that are functionally synonymous.

votive terracotta anatomical figurines from Crete that date from about 1800 BC are to be seen in the Archeological Museum in Heracleion, Crete. A term suggesting "physician" has been found to be phonetically similar to the later Greek word for physician, ἰάτρος (iatros).[36] It was inscribed on clay tablets preserved at Mycenae on the Peloponnesian peninsula, but nothing indicates a physician's duties and methods, nor describes continuity of the profession from an earlier age or into later times.

The collapse of the Mycenaean civilization around 1100 BC has been variously attributed to a society weakened by an extended war against an eastern kingdom centered at Troy and to a Dorian "invasion," although the nature of the invaders and whether there was an actual invasion is debated. But for the next three centuries Greece suffered through its "Dark Ages," reemerging fragmented into city-states on the one hand but more homogeneous in culture on the other.[37] It was then that Homer recited his poetry, at the onset of what is called the Archaic period of Greek history, dating from 750 BC. Although the two Homeric epics, the *Iliad* and the *Odyssey*, were composed at this time, they related

---

[35] Placebo: "a medication prescribed more for the mental relief of the patient than for its actual effect on a disorder," *Merriam-Webster'sCollegiate Dictionary*, 10th ed.; "any dummy medical treatment," *Dorlands' Medical Dictionary*, 27th edition, 1988; "a psychological treatment, in contrast to a pharmacological treatment," *A Dictionary of Psychology*, Oxford, 2001. None of these definitions grasp fully the intent of this heading, for early practitioners would not have known what therapy was inert, or "dummy," nor would they have been able to reliably distinguish a psychological benefit from a pharmacological one, a problem even today. Perhaps "an agent not shown to have, however infrequently, a predictably favorable effect," would be more accurate in this context.

[36] A syllabary of Linear B, the written language of the Mycenaens, has been established, and the term for physician is phonetically "i-ja-te" and in ancient Greek "ἰατήρ," just as pater (father) is phonetically "pa-te" and in classical Greek "πατήρ," and pharmakon (medicine) is phonetically "pa-ma-ko" and in classical Greek "φαρμακον." For a brief account of the discovery of Linear B see: Chadwick, J., *The Decipherment of Linear B*, Cambridge, 1958.

[37] See: Morris, I., *The Eighth-century Revolution*, the fourth chapter in *A Companion to Archaic Greece. Blackwell Companians to the Ancient World*, Malden, MA, 2009, Raaflaub, K. A. and van Wees, H., editors, for a modern perspective on the emergence of Greek culture and related topics from its Dark Ages.

events surrounding the Trojan War some four centuries earlier. Their descriptions of battlefield first aid performed by talented nonphysicians have been scrutinized, some experts concluding that all events of a medical nature in Homeric writings were associated in some way with divine intervention. But what is germane is that they suggest only an empirical approach to trauma management, surely not unexpected in a warrior society.[38] They are a synopsis, perhaps, of medical practice in the 8th C BC, for who would suggest that any medical progress had occurred in Greece between the 12th C and the 8th C. In the poetry of Hesiod of a slightly later 8th C date no reference to medicine as a profession is found, although Hesiod was a poet of a different stamp, writing of things commonplace, a dramatic change from Homer, who wrote of war and aristocratic grandeur. It appears from these sources, however, that down to 750 BC Hellenic medicine had neither organization nor noteworthy resources. Its practices, as described by Homer, were mystical and empiric, of a kind identified with primitive or early structured society.

The Archaic Period (750-500 BC) ushered in by Homer and Hesiod was the time of Thales the natural philosopher, Sappho the esteemed poetess, and many other great thinkers and artists. It saw the development of the Greek alphabet, the flourishing of trade, the founding of Syracuse and other Greek colonies, and development, in Asia Minor, of the first coinage. The Greek traditions in art, science, and letters were established. Most importantly, the Archaic period saw the sunset of the monarchies and the dawning of democracy.

Still, there was virtually no mention of the practice of medicine.[39] Dr. Sigerist, in his unique way, speculated that the "late" appearance in Greek history of medical writings was due to physicians being illiterate tradespeople rather than priests.[40] But the reason was unlikely to be illiteracy. Hellenic society by the 6th C promoted literacy, surpassing other societies in literacy among the common people, as documented by inscriptions of all kinds on tombs, monuments, and edifices. "Graffiti" written by common Greek soldiers can be found as far away as Nubia in southern Egypt, where they campaigned as mercenaries of Psammatichos II from 594-589 BC.[41] Herodotus described a sizeable school on the island of Chios that held 120 boys *ca.* 500 BC, not far from the island of Cos, home of Hippocrates, and Aristophanes, later in the 5th C, addresses a

---

[38] The first use of the Greek term for "physician," ἰήτηρ, is applied to Machaon in *The Iliad*, Bk. IV, 190, when he is called to remove an arrow and apply a dressing: ἕλκος δ' ἰητὴρ ἐπιμάσσεται ἠδ' ἐπιθήσει φάρμαχ', ἅ κεν παύσησι μελαινάων ὀδυνάων. ("and the physician will probe the wound, and apply a medicine that can stop the severe pain." Translation by the author.) When Machaon himself was wounded in the battle, the famed statement that "the physician is worth many men" (ἰητρὸς γὰρ ἀνὴρ πολλῶν ἀντάξιος ἄλλων) was made by Idomeneus (Bk. XI, 514). Even though Achilles was also trained in medicine by the centaur, Cheiron, only the "sons of Asclepius," Machaon and Podaleireus, are termed ἰάτροι.

[39] The topic of 6th C BC Greek medicine is typically mentioned in the context of the natural philosophers of that period, the assumption being that natural philosophy was the prelude to Greek medical progress. This may be unwarranted (see next page), but the point here is that there is no description of any aspect of clinical practice available from 6th C Greece.

[40] Sigerist, H. E., *History of Medicine*, Oxford, 1961, vol. 2, p. 84. The striking feature of Sigerist's statement is not that it may be false, for who really knows, but rather that among the myriad of explanations from which to choose he chose this one.

[41] They were "scratched on the left leg of a colossal statue of Rameses II" in Nubia: Tod, M. N., *A Selection of Greek Historical Inscriptions*, Oxford, 1933, p. 6.

literate audience in his classic, *Frogs*.[42] [43]

During the Archaic period the cause of democratic government was set on a winning course by Solon (638-560 BC) with the Constitution of Athens in 596 BC. This eminent lawgiver was cognizant of and considerate of the medical profession, although he does not imply existence of any medical organization. He does not equate the physician with the seer in the realm of prognosis. Also in the 6th C there appeared many great thinkers in Greece, some to be included among the civic leaders described as the Seven Sages, others as the natural philosophers of Ionia. Dr. Sullivan considered the roots of rational medicine to be detectable in works of Thales, Anaximander, Anaximenes, Pythagoras, Heraclitus, Alcmaeon, Anaxagoras, and Empedocles, the first three being representatives of the Miletos school.[44] Spanning the years 639-544 BC the latter thinkers formulated a basis for "rational medical logic" by stating, in an astonishing burst of reason, that natural phenomena, including biological ones, were analyzable and therefore understandable in their own right, objectively rather than supernaturally. Perhaps the Miletos School and those philosophers who followed can be credited with formulating concepts that would support a scientific discipline, but it does not prove that what will be called Hippocratic medicine found its inspiration in their works. With the doubtful exception of Alcmaeon and an even more unlikely Empedocles, none of the philosophers listed by Dr. Sullivan were clinical physicians. As for their providing the "roots of rational medicine," there is no *a priori* reason why the inspiration for the natural philosophers of Miletos, the Ionian philosophers, and the soon to appear Hippocratic medicine could not have been one and the same, events that were parallel rather than in series. It has been stated that "The early Milesians were, in fact, men of science rather than philosophers in the strict sense,"[45] and thus were akin to medical science. Still, the practice of medicine in Hellas late in the Archaic period, *i.e.*, 550 BC, may not have been much different from that at its beginning, nor significantly different from the medicine of any of the contemporary great civilizations described in the preceding chapters.

D. Pre-Hippocratic Medicine

It is undeniable that great works have been attributed to contemporary authoritarian leaders, including the Hanging Gardens of Babylon, the circumnavigation of Africa, and the subterranean tunnels of Jerusalem, all wonderful examples of monarchical power and efficiency. But an educated king is no match for an educated public, as ancient Greece in the subsequent two centuries would show.

Now approaches the age of particular interest to medicine, Classical Greece (500-338 BC). At its outset overwhelming Persian armies and navies had been memorably repelled by small, Athenian-led forces at Marathon and Salamis, and by a

---

[42] The occasion in Chios was the collapse of the schoolhouse while the boys were at their studies, from which only one child survived (Herodotus *Histories*, 6.27.2). Chios is an island off the west coast of Asia Minor (Fig. 9).

[43] Woodbury, L., *Aristophanes' Frogs and the Athenian Literacy*, in *Trans. and Proc. Amer. Philol. Assoc.*, 106, 349-357, 1976, especially footnote 13.

[44] Sullivan, R., *Thales to Galen*, Part I, in *Proc. R. Coll. Physic.*, Edinburgh, 26:135-42, 309-15. 1996

[45] See the chapter by J. Burnet, *Philosophy*, in *The Legacy of Greece*, R. W. Livingstone, editor, Oxford, 1921.

Spartan-Athenian effort at Plataea. As a consequence, Athenian power and authority rapidly grew. Despite recurring wars that ultimately led to its ruin, Athens became, and for centuries remained, the intellectual center of Greece and beyond. During its meteoric career, Athens witnessed the appearance of democracy in unbridled form, the construction of the Parthenon, the birth of political thought, the composition of the world's greatest tragic plays, and artistic expression, likes of which the world had never seen. It was the home at one time or another of Solon, Themistocles, and Pericles; Socrates, Plato and Aristotle;[46] Aeschylus, Sophocles, and Euripides; Antiphanes, Simonides of Ceos, and Cleophon; Herodotus,[47] Thucydides, and Xenophon; Phidias, Praxiteles, and Demosthenes. It was also the age of Hippocrates.

Having reviewed the Mycenaean age, the Greek Dark Ages, and the Archaic period there is no historical evidence of a sophisticated medical practice prior to the time of a legendary physician named Hippocrates (460-380 BC). He is thought to have come from the eastern Greek island of Cos. The feats of an earlier Greek physician, Democedes, recounted by Herodotus,[48] have invited much comment and speculation, but what generalizations should be derived from the secondhand account of one man's adventures? And so, in the writings attributed to Hippocrates and with little evidence of precedent, there is the abrupt appearance of a full-fledged medical profession in Greece during the age of Pericles (495-429 BC). Was this an outgrowth of "temple" (sacredotal) medicine? Leonard Whibley gives reasons why this was unlikely to have been the progenitor of rational medicine, pointing out the health resort nature of temples, including the important one at Epidaurus.[49] Some say, and with well-marshaled argument, that Hippocratic medicine did not suddenly appear, that a form of "natural" medicine already existed and, far from being novel, had been widely accepted in early Hellas even though little discussed.[50] And with this there is no disagreement, for such was revealed by the

---

[46] Aristotle was born in Stagira, a city in Macedonia settled by Ionians from the island of Andros in the Cyclades. Prof. J. Burnet (University of St. Andrews), in *Legacy of Greece* (Oxford, 1921, R. W. Livingstone, pp. 57-96), therefore, considered him Ionian and thereby susceptible to Ionian scientific reasoning. Aristotle moved to Athens when he was 18 years of age.

[47] Herodotus was born in Hallicarnasus, but he applied for Athenian citizenship, received an award from the Athenian assembly, and may have died there.

[48] In Bk. 3 of Herodotus' *History* Democedes is described as the most skillful physician of his time and the principal reason for the good name of the "medical school" of Croton. Called from a prison sometime about the year of 520 BC to attend an injured Darius, the Persian monarch, Democedes was richly rewarded. Democedes' story has been often recounted by historians of ancient Greece and ancient medicine, including works by Garrison, Baas, Durant, Grote, Sigerist, and Prioreschi, usually citing his salary as an example of the wealth of physicians in general, or at least a significant proportion of them. Democedes, the son of an Asclepian priest, was a "social lion," not a common man. For the usual pay of physicians see: Zimmern, A. E. *The Greek Commonwealth*, Oxford, 1915, Part III, chapter 7, p. 271.

[49] Whibley, L., *A Companion to Greek Studies*, Cambridge, 1931, p. 665*ff.* For example, Whibley references the 3rd C poet, Herondas, who in Mime IV describes a scene at the Temple of Asclepius on the island of Cos. Two women sacrifice a cock in thanksgiving for recovery from illness, but their thanks go to a broad range of deities, not to a physician or other secular healer, implying the latter are unconnected in any way with the temple.

[50] Wickkiser, B. L., *The Appeal of Asklepios and the Politics of Healing in the Greco-Roman World*, U. of Mich., 2003, doctoral dissertation. See also: Longrigg, J., *Greek Rational Medicine*, London, 1993, and the chapter entitled *Death and Epidemic Disease in Classical Athens*, in *Death and Disease in the Ancient City*, eds. V. M. Hope and E. Marshall, London, 2000. Prof. James Longrigg comments on the unlikely possibility that Hippocratic medicine arose from temple medicine,

Athenian response to the plague of Athens, although Hippocratic medicine will be shown later to be far more than empiric, or "natural." [51]

Excursus on Physicians and the Plague of Athens

οὔτε γὰρ ἰατροὶ ἤρκουν τὸ πρῶτον θεραπεύοντες ἀγνοίᾳ, ἀλλ᾽ αὐτοὶ
neither for the physicians being adequate at first treating in ignorance, instead they
μάλιστα ἔθνησκον ὅσῳ καὶ μάλιστα προσῆσαν, οὔτε ἄλλη ἀνθρωπειά τέχνη
especially died much the more in that especially they were at hand, nor other human art
οὐδεμία· ὅσα τε πρὸς ἱεροῖς ἱκέτευσαν ἢ μαντείαις καὶ τοῖς τοιούτοις
not one; likewise and before altars they supplicated or to priests or to those like them
ἐχρήσαντο, πάντα ἀνωφελῆ ἦν, τελευτῶντές τε αὐτῶν ἀπέστησαν ὑπὸ τοῦ
they employed, everything useless was, by the dying and of them they gave up by the
κακοῦ νικώμενοι.
evil being defeated

"For in the first place neither the physicians, treating in ignorance, prevailed, as they themselves died the most frequently in proportion as they above all were in the forefront, nor [in the second place] any other human art; and likewise [in the third place] the people made supplications in the temples or to the priests and employed those of this sort, [but] all were of no use, and finally resigning themselves they were defeated by the evil."

Thucydides' *History*, Bk. II, 47, interlinear and vernacular translation by the author,[52] bracketed words added for clarity

Thus begins the description by Thucydides (471-400 BC) of the Athenian plague of 428 BC, during the second year of the Peloponnesian War between Athens and Sparta. The horror of this calamity is given in vivid and wrenching detail by the great historian, who was himself a victim of that plague but fortunate to survive it. It is this epidemic that, according to Galen (130-200 AD), was ended by Hippocrates, who had been called in specifically for that purpose.[53]

---

particularly that of the Asclepeion, and on the significance of the Athenians' preference for rational practitioners at the onset of the plague.

[51] The Hippocratic physicians would have agreed. In *Regimen in Acute Diseases*, V, an early work traditionally attributed to Hippocrates himself, this statement is made: "The severe diseases are those the Ancients classified as being associated with (1) pleuritic chest pain, (2) lung disease, (3) delirium, or (4) kausos fevers and diseases that, like kausos fever, have a "continuous," or unremitting, fever pattern." Here Hippocrates not only recognizes a preexisting body of clinical knowledge, but agrees with its astuteness. (Translation by the author.)

[52] Here for comparison is a more fluid translation of this section by the composer of *The Leviathon*, Thomas Hobbes (1588-1679): "For at first, neither were the Physicians able to cure it, through ignorance of what it was, but died fastest themselves, as being the men that most approached the sick, nor any other Art of man availed whatsoever. All supplications to the Gods, and enquiries of Oracles, and whatsoever other means they used of the kind, proved all unprofitable, insomuch as subdued with the greatness of the evil, they gave them all over." See *The Natural State of Medical Practice: Hippocratic Evidence*, p. 519*ff*, for the author's full translation of Thucydides' description.

[53] Galen, *De Theriaca ad Pisonem*, 16. But the meticulous Thucydides mentions no Hippocrates, nor do any other authors up to the time to Galen, six hundred years after the event. Furthermore, it

The account by Thucydides is important in the way it throws light on the status of the medical profession in Athens at that time. (1) Of the three venues for attempts at stopping the plague, *viz.* physicians, the other arts, and sacrificial offerings or appeals to seers, that of the physicians is listed first and is given the greatest commentary. (2) The opening statement about the physicians' efforts describes them as το πρῶτον ("in front, before, precedent") which implies priority over the others, whether it be precedence in time or in deemed importance.[54] (3) Among the three venues only the physicians are described as voluntarily facing the full force of the plague, and they do so in a professional manner that is presented by Thucydides in such a way as more to be expected than exceptional, for he does not praise them. In a sense, the latter may represent the epitome of praiseworthiness. To praise them was an unnecessary and redundant battlefield promotion and demeaned their ineffectual but heroic efforts. (4) Finally, Thucydides describes the response of "the physicians," not that of a single physician or a few, or a named physician. Many community physicians stepped forth to do their job, and no exceptions were noted.[55]

The historian Victor Ehrenberg wrote that "Thucydides had accepted the main principle of the Hippocratic school of medicine that observation and experience, not philosophical theories or general hypotheses, lead to the discovery of truth." Yet Thucydides was ten years older than Hippocrates, who would have been 32 years of age at the time of the plague, and therefore perhaps Thucydides' rational impartiality reflected a "main principle" of practitioners preceding Hippocrates.[56] Is it realistic to conclude that an exalted reputation, method, and linguistic heritage of young Hippocrates of Cos had become a feature of the Athenian medical landscape by 428 BC? This seems unlikely.

End of Excursus

---

seems highly unlikely that any man, by the age of 32 years, would have been so precocious as to have accumulated the knowledge, experience, and reputation to do what Hippocrates is said to have been invited to do for the Athenian plague. Finally, the same plague recurred among Athenians elsewhere within a few years, as, described by Thucydides in Book III, 87, and no mention is made of Hippocrates nor the use of any Hippocratic contrivance or intervention that might have halted the plague the first time in Athens, a testimonial in denial of any effective remedy in the first place.
[54] Prof. Longrigg came to the same conclusion based on his own translation of the plague as described by Thucydides. See *Death and Epidemic Disease in Athens* in: *Death and Disease in the Ancient City*, London, 2000, V. M. Hope and E. Marshall, editors, p. 59.
[55] The population of Athens in 430 BC, shortly before the plague, has been estimated at 172,000, to which must be added an estimated 115,000 slaves, a total of 287,000. Over a quarter of a million people provide a sizeable statistical sample from which to extrapolate the significance of public opinion of physicians implied by Thucydides. (Data from A. W. Gomme, *The Population of Ancient Athens*, Oxford, 1933.)
[56] Ehrenberg, V., *From Solon to Socrates*, London, 1973, p. 365. Ehrenberg's opinion was shared by John Finley, Jr., who wrote that Thucydides must have been very familiar with Hippocratic writings, noting a similarity between his description of the plague and the *Epidemics* of Hippocrates (*Thucydides*, Cambridge MA, 1942, in the Introduction, p. xii.) He based this on Thucydides' rejection of speculation on origins of the Peloponnesian War, similar to Hippocratic rejection of medical theories as a basis for action.

For Athenians to have developed by 428 BC a preference for rational medicine over temple medicine and magic there must have been a preceding period of rational medical practice by physicians, not to mention time needed for adjustments within society to the practitioners of this, perhaps, unique approach to medicine. For example, Herodotus (484 - 425 BC), who began his famous *History* when Hippocrates would have been a child, writes with the assumption that at least some diseases did not have a supernatural origin, and four Hippocratic treatises have been dated by some scholars as prior to the writings of Herodotus.[57] And for Athenian practitioners to have been properly established in such a practice would have required at least one and probably two generations of physicians. If there were some thirty physicians of the usual age distribution practicing in a given city and if medical careers spanned thirty years, at least a generation would be necessary to see all the old-style practitioners replaced by new ones. That rational medicine was being taught to medicine's professionals prior to Hippocrates' birth in 460 BC is, therefore, a reasonable conclusion. External evidence for this is limited, but Aeschylus (525-455 BC), Sophocles (496-406 BC), and others were able to rely on the physician rather than the mystic.[58]

It is difficult, therefore, to credit a physician of Hippocrates' day with freeing up the medical profession from the thralls of religion and magic. It was already so.[59] How could a widespread and popular medical practice evolve so quickly and influence so profoundly the distant population of Athens by 428 BC? Hippocrates can be discounted as the sole, or even an important part of, the explanation.

---

[57] In *The Histories* of Herodotus the mental derangement of Cambyses II, perhaps associated with epilepsy, was attributed to either the god, Apis, or "from some other cause, as many ills are wont to seize upon men; for it is said moreover that Cambyses had from his birth a certain grievous malady, that which is called by some the "sacred disease":..." (translation of G. C. Macauley, Bk. III, 33). The four Hippocratic works are: Diseases II (450 BC), Airs, Waters, Places (pre-Herodotus), Places in Man (early 5th C BC), and gynecological texts (480 BC.)

[58] Aeschylus: "and to whom one must attempt to turn back the suffering of disease with healing medicines, cautery, or judicious surgery." *Agamemnon*: 848-850, translation of the author, first performed in 458 BC: "This first and foremost: if ever man fell ill, there was no defence – no healing food, no ointment, nor any draught – but for lack of medicine they wasted away, until I showed them how to mix soothing remedies wherewith they now ward off all their disorders." *Prometheus:* 478-483, translation of H. W. Smyth in the *Loeb Classical Library* edition of Aeschylus, perhaps performed in about 460 BC, with this section describing the medical practices Prometheus taught to mankind. Sophocles (496-406 BC): οὐ πρὸς ἰατροῦ σοφοῦ θρηνεῖν ἐπῳδὰς πρὸς τομῶντι πήματι. ("[It is] not for a wise physician to chant magical incantations in the presence of a surgical disorder.") *Ajax*: 581, first performed in 441 BC, and: πολλὰ τὰ δεινὰ κοὐδὲν ἀνθρώπου δεινότερον πέλει·.....νοσων, δ᾽ ἀμηχάνων φύγας ξυμπέπρασται. ("... man has contrived refuge from illnesses once beyond all cure.") *Antigone*: 361, also performed in 441 BC, when Sophocles was fifty-four years old. In addition, fables ascribed to Aesop (?d. 564 BC) are critical of physicians with only book-learning and what are best described as "quack" physicians (see Fable #133), thus suggesting there were true physicians as well.

[59] And this was not a characteristic of medicine alone. In Pericles' funeral oration in 430 BC shortly after the start of the Peloponnesian War and shortly before the plague, he renders not a single tribute to the gods. On the other hand, Aelian, in his *Historical Miscellanies*, states that Athenians were always very superstitious, and even in the days of the playwright, Aeschylus (525-455 BC), stoning was approved for impiety. But there is no equivalence between superstition and piety.

It is far more likely that rational medicine characterized medical practice simultaneously in mainland Greece and/or Ionia. This is consistent with the theory advanced by Dr. Wickkiser.[60]

While the puzzle is not solved, an Age of Reason seems to have descended on 5th C BC Hellas just as two thousand years later it was to descend on a renascent Europe and engender the Enlightenment. The application of reason to all endeavors seems to have been endemic, being reflected in its great natural philosophers rather than being produced by them. Sir Alfred Zimmern wrote, "He is a Greek who thinks for himself, ... "[61] And, to paraphrase James Froude, "There are epidemics of brilliance as well as epidemics of disease."[62] The epidemic of brilliance in Hellas was well under way by the 5th C BC, and had become a fact of everyday life contemporary with the development of democracy. Peter Farb described the circumstances in this way:

> "No claim for the superiority in intelligence of one race over another has ever withstood scientific scrutiny. Nor does a greater number of biological mutations occur in some races or cultures than in others. Actually, biological mutations produce humans with the potential to grow into geniuses at a steady rate at all times and among all peoples. That virtually no geniuses are recorded for a thousand years in ancient Athens does not mean that they were not produced. Nor does the astonishing cluster of geniuses that appeared in the fifth and fourth centuries B.C. in Athens mean that biological mutations were produced in greater number at that time. The rate of mutation remained the same; what changed was the culture, which allowed great men to flourish."[63]

In the culture of emerging democratic popular governments in Greek city-states practitioners of medicine were able to act using their common sense by engaging in common council. Common sense was not cloistered in an Ionic city such as Miletos or on a Doric island such as Cos. Rational medical thought had both a spontaneous and multifocal origin in Hellenic society. That that origin coincided with the arrival of democracy shall now be shown.

---

[60] Wickkiser, B. L., *The Appeal of Asklepios and the Politics of Healing in the Greco-Roman World*, U. of Mich., 2003, doctoral dissertation, especially chapter 3.

[61] Zimmern, A., *The Greek Commonwealth*, Oxford, 1924, p. 95.

[62] Froude made his comment in regard to Calvinism: "There are epidemics of nobleness as well as epidemics of disease;...."; *Short Stories on Great Subjects*, London, 1877.

[63] Farb, P., *Man's Rise to Civilization*, 1968, pp. 20-21.

CHAPTER TEN

ANCIENT GREECE AND THE CONCEPTS OF PROGRESS AND DEMOCRACY

κρείττων ἡ πρόνοια τῆς μεταμελαίας.
"Forethought is better than repentance."

Dionysius of Halicarnassus (60 BC – *ca.* 10 AD)

Progress is possible when there can be purposeful improvement over a preexisting state. Earlier chapters provided examples exposing authoritarian management of medicine as a guarantor of its survival but not its progress. Progression through monarchy, aristocracy, tyranny, and thence to democracy reflected political progress that led to the triumph of democratic Athens and many other Hellenic city-states. In contrast, Sparta, which purposely chose to retain firm authoritarian governance, remained silent in medicine as in other things despite its proximity to Athens. It was at this time that the medical profession, defining its path for progress, opened its ranks to those outside the traditional medical families, and persons having a special interest in medicine and biology could enter the field and provide a base for scientific inquiry. But it was the democratization of medical practice itself, the interaction of physician and patient rather than the admission of outsiders, that led to: (1) the recognition of the uniqueness of each patient, (2) the recognition of the complexity of diseases, and (3) acknowledgement of the patient's role in directing his own medical care. This democratization of Hellenic medicine, often attributed to Hippocrates, represented the beginning of the true physician-patient relationship, the *natural state of medical practice*. In this κοινόν (koinon) of two it was not the physician's role that had changed; it was the patient's role, a revolutionary transformation. Engaged in common council against illness, the patient and physician could contribute equally to decision-making, the physician being the advocate for his patient and for no one else.

A. Introduction: The Concept of Progress

Aeschylus (513-455 BC) wrote perhaps ninety plays, of which seven survive complete. Aeschylus' life spanned the waning years of the 6th C Greek tyrants and the maturation of Athenian democracy. *Prometheus Bound*, a play thought by many scholars to have been written by him, is an allegory of rebellion against tyranny, a confrontation between the mind and brute force. The name, Prometheus, or Προμηθεύς (πρό [pro] = beforehand; μητιάω [metiaw] = I deliberate), means "forethought." In the play this Hellenic god is chained to a high peak by Zeus as punishment for bestowing fire, hope, inventions, and crafts on primitive man. Prometheus described the objects of his pity as he had found them:

ἔφυρον εἰκῆ πάντα.
"Being without comprehension, they made a mess of everything."

Aeschylus, *Prometheus Bound*, line 450

Prometheus boasted that he gave to man comprehension and the tools necessary to plan for the future, including a written language to assist memory, astronomy to foretell the seasons, and divination to predict coming events; in other words, the tools the playwright considered necessary for improving man's existence, a means to escape the bonds of tyranny and ignorance, a means to progress. In *Prometheus Bound*, Aeschylus has presented man in "a position of full authority for his actions and for the judgment of his actions, thus emancipating him" from the arbitrary power of the universe, a cognomen of Zeus.[1]

"The reasonable man adapts himself to the world; the unreasonable one persists in trying to adapt the world to himself. Therefore, all progress depends on the unreasonable man." So wrote G. B. Shaw in his pamphlet *Maxims for Revolutionists* that was attached to his philosophical play, *Man and Superman*, in 1903. The inference is that progress did not occur prior to the appearance of the unreasonable man. As Western civilization can be viewed as the cradle of progress, progress both as a concept and as a fact of daily life, the West has the dubious honor of being the fountainhead of unreasonableness. But what is implied in the term "world" is "established authority," a risky, even unreasonable, target for the faint of heart. And, therefore, matters are exactly the opposite. Since the West owes to the concept of progress its technical and cultural dominance, what Shaw calls a "reasonable" man might better be defined as one who is intimidated, his "unreasonable" the indomitable man of reason.[2]

The birth of Shaw's unreasonable man as a force in history occurred in ancient Greece, and its first spokesmen were the natural philosophers of Ionia: "It seemed to them that, if only they (the pioneers of philosophy) could strip off all the modifications which art and chance and fate had introduced, they would get at the ultimate real."[3] Prior to this virtually all mankind survived by bowing to authority. But in Hellas societies developed in which, at least among freeborn male citizens, action would be based on objective self-interest as legitimized by the many, not the one or a few. The ancient Greek citizen's perspective, or "point of view" as summarized by Hutton, included the following attributes: the Greek was oriented toward individualism rather than collectivism, his interest was centered on the intellectual rather than on force, and he was "humanitarian" only "so far as compatible with scientific self-interest."[4] Hutton did not include the concept of "progress." But Aeschylus, writing in the early days of Athenian democracy, did. The Hippocratics did as well:

> "In medicine everything [necessary] has hitherto been put at its disposal, both a foundation and path having been found, by which many admirable discoveries have already been made. And all the rest will be discovered provided that the researcher proceeds competently, being aware of previous discoveries and using them as his point of departure."

Ancient Medicine, 2, 1-4[5]

---

[1] See the insightful essay on the philosophical position of Zeus in the Greek pantheon by Leon Golden, *"Zeus, whoever he is...,"* in *Transactions and Proceedings of the American Philological Association*, 92:156-167, 1961, p. 166.

[2] Maxim #124, in *Maxims for Revolutionists*, attached to his play, *Man and Superman,* and found in *Man and Superman; A Comedy and a Philosophy*, Westminster, 1903, p. 238. Shaw, a committed socialist, might have been at some variance with this interpretation of his maxim.

[3] Burnet, J., *Early Greek Philosophy*, London, 1892, p. 11.

[4] Hutton, Maurice, *The Greek Point of View*, London, n.d. [1931].

[5] ἰητρικῇ δὲ πάντα πάλαι ὑπάρχει, καὶ ἀρχὴ καὶ ὁδὸς εὑρημένη, καθ᾽ ἣ καὶ τὰ εὑρημένα πολλά τε καὶ καλῶς ἔχοντα εὕρηται ἐν πολλῷ χρόνῳ, καὶ τὰ λοιπὰ εὑρεθήσεται, ἤν τις ἱκανός τε ἐὼν καὶ τὰ εὑρημένα εἰδὼς ἐκ τούτων ὁρμώμενος ζητῇ.

Excursus on Progress

Progress (n.) – 2: a forward or onward movement (as to an objective   or to a goal)
Merriam-Webster's Collegiate Dictionary, 10th edition

Progress can mean the physical act of forward motion, but it must be directed at or for something, not random, although the goal itself may not be specifically defined. But progress can also result from an active search for an improved state of something rather than forward motion. This type of progress builds on what is already known. Proof of the latter type of progress requires an existing state to have changed, as far as can be determined, for the better. It can be categorized as an abstraction or a tangible.

In his *The Idea of Progress*, Prof. John Bury notes that "general Progress of humanity belongs to the same order of ideas as Providence or personal immortality. ... Belief in it is an act of faith." As such it is an idea that requires one to "conceive that it is destined to advance indefinitely in the future," and that "it is based on an interpretation of history which regards men as slowly advancing in a definite and desirable direction." But this is an abstract presumption, a relatively recent intellectual innovation, and is inappropriate for scientific conclusions.[6]

The tangible is the better telltale of progress, but it can be complex. As an example, some might consider simple discovery to represent progress. A stream discovered to be dammed up by beavers could provide insight to a man whereby he might similarly raise the water level in a stream to irrigate a field or unleash the kinetic energy of stored-up water. The application of his discovery might be considered progress, bringing benefit to him and to his society. Others think progress implies newness. Elizabeth Cady Stanton (1815-1902) wrote "Progress is the victory of a new thought over an old superstition." Progress as a process has also been viewed since the 19th C as an equivalent to biological evolution in which societies and their members exhibit characteristics of organisms under competitive pressures, the result being that the various societies have taken similar courses in their escape from savagery.

But "progress" as development rather than motion is not characterized by a single unadorned discovery, by an adjective, or by genetic variation. The *modus operandi* of this form of progress is a purposeful mechanism that leads toward a goal. A singular or fortuitous discovery does not necessarily represent movement toward a goal, particularly a goal of society, even though that discovery may prove useful.

Progress, therefore, is more a product of searching than discovering, of inventing rather than mimicking. A discovery may seem a panacea when first encountered, only to be later found to induce harm in greater proportion than good. But, if an existing state is improved upon by invention, the consequences will tend to be good rather than bad, for

---

The Greek text is provided because it so clearly defines "progress" as understood by the Hippocratics.

[6] Bury, J. B., *The Idea of Progress*, London, 1921, Introduction. He concluded that this abstract idea of progress was not elucidated until the 16th C.

the unintended bad will be more likely to have been anticipated in the process of inventing and the problem avoided. Discovery and invention, each critical to man's survival, often act in concert.

First hinted at by Ionian natural philosophers such as Xenophanes (570-480 BC),[7] and then described in allegory by Aeschylus, the actual implementation of a mechanism for realizing progress occurred first in early Hellas in the Hippocratic writings. For this reason, Dr. J. H. Baas, in his classic *Outlines of the History of Medicine* assigns all but one of the ancient great civilizations to a short introductory section of 66 pages entitled:

> "*The Medical Culture of Those Nations Whose Development in Medicine is either Already Closed or is Stationary (or not Independent). The history of the most ancient medicine and the medicine of primitive peoples.*"

But the bulky remainder (1,020 pages) of Baas' volume is an insightful history of Greek medicine and its consequences in the West, entitled:

> "*The Medical Culture of Those Nations Whose Development in Medicine has been or is **Progressive** [emphasis added].*"[8]

An authoritarian society is not devoid of discovery and invention, and once a discovery has come to the fore the authoritarian society can efficiently propagate it, for better or for worse. The outcome is determined by the patron of the man who made the discovery, the patron being either an individual in a position of power or his committee. And should some enlightened totalitarian leader desire an improved water supply for his people, the necessary reasoning and true progress may follow, an example being the famous tunnel dug through a mountain at the direction of Polycrates, the tyrant of Samos.[9] **Therefore: in the realm of implementation the distinction between the authoritarian and the free society can be blurred, leading to a serious underestimation of the threat posed by authoritarian governance. Indeed, there is no other statement in this book that is at the same time more important and less obvious in its implications. For both history and experience have shown that most ideas for improvement in authoritarian states will have been stolen from, copied from, or purchased from, a freer society.[10] It is allotted only to a free society to provide a sustained intellectual environment whereby ideas can be systematically improved, can, in a word, progress.[11]**

---

[7] Xenophanes was from Colophon, an Ionian city near Ephesus in Asia Minor.

[8] Baas, J. H., *Outlines of the History of Medicine and the Medical Profession*, (translated by H. E. Handerson), New York, 1889, p. 81.

[9] The tunnel was constructed during the reign of Polycrates (ruled: 538-522 BC) by initiating its excavation from both sides of the mountain, which required the excavators from both ends to meet midway under the mountain. In a clever engineering *tour-de-force*, they did.

[10] Or a relatively free subunit within that authoritarian society. As for Polycrates of Samos, he, like many ancient tyrants, relied upon popular support to maintain his authority. His famous tunnel, therefore, probably represented the wishes of some of his citizens, whom a tyrant must appease and which serves to mitigate his authoritarian tendencies. See p. 151*ff re*: tyrannies.

[11] In this sense the Renaissance did not represent progress, and, indeed, may have been the opposite. Many of the great names of the Renaissance considered their age as rescued from decadence by the rediscovery of ancient writings. As for medicine: "In that year [1514] a collection of Galen's works,

The concept of inevitability of progress as the natural course of things is expressed in Plato's "little by little" advancement of mankind to a better world, and similar to the flow of time. This is a huge generalization and a concept that sadly is tenable only by those who consider their particular perspective as representing the spearhead of "progress." Prof. Robert Nesbit, in contrast, would define the concept of progress as applicable to all mankind from its very beginning to the present day, as manifested in the change from the primitive to the modern, but he considered it a phenomenon of Western society, an "amalgamation" of ancient Greek and Judeo-Christian millenianism from which all mankind would benefit. In so doing, he viewed it as an idea that has been embedded in Western society for 3000 years.[12] The eminent historian, Prof. Leopold von Ranke, was one of many who considered, and consider, the unfolding of history to be directional, the direction being determined by Divine will, although Prof. Ranke qualified his position: "But historical development does not rest on the tendency towards civilization alone."[13] The Greeks, however, identified both the role of the individual in bringing about progress and the authoritarian will to stop it. Xenophanes (6th C BC) stated mankind's position:

> ". . . the gods have not revealed to mortals things from the beginning but [mortals], by long seeking, discover what is better. "

> Stob. *Ecl.* I, 8.2, Flor. 29, 41, Fragment 18
> Translation of Kathleen Freeman, *Ancilla to the Presocratics*, Oxford, 1966

This is an expression of faith in man's abilities rather than acquiescence to man's fate. In conclusion, it seems at first glance folly to consider the discovery of a beaver dam that prompts a man to devise a method of irrigation as not representing progress. But if progress is movement toward a better state, what role did progress play in this discovery? It played little or no role, as the discovery was fortuitous. But if food supply was tenuous and a dam had been planned to assure food sufficiency, then it was indeed true progress. Throughout most of man's prehistory and history discoveries have represented only sporadic, however temporarily useful, phenomena akin to "punctuated equilibrium."[14] The concept of progress of a society, however, is not one whereby society improves and regresses by dribs and drabs directed by chance or opportunity. Instead, progress requires

---

translated directly from the Greek into Latin by Nicolo Leoniceno (1428-1524), was published in Paris and seized upon with enthusiasm. .... Physicians, seeing for the first time the works of Galen and Hippocrates stripped of their dross [*i.e.*, freed from centuries of errors and emendations accumulated through translations from Greek to Syriac to Arabic and thence to Latin], believed that now they had captured the essence and spirit of the great classical authors and were at last about to enter a new Golden Age." (From: Saunders, J., O'Malley, C., *The Illustrations from the Works of Andreas Vesalius*, Cleveland, 1950, p. 13.) A return to thinking already two thousand years old does not suggest progress, but at least it represents profound dissatisfaction with the status of medical knowledge in the early 16th C.

[12] Nesbit, R. A., *History of the Idea of Progress*, London, 1980, p. 18. Dr. Nesbit notes that his opinion coincides with that of the Greek poet Hesiod, who had a "vision of a progressive, rather than a degenerative, mankind."

[13] Von Ranke, L., *Universal History*, New York, 1885, p. xii.

[14] This term is borrowed from: Eldredge, N., and Gould, S.J., *Punctuated equilibria: An alternative to phyletic gradualism*, in *Models in Paleobiology*, San Francisco, 1972, T. J. M. Schopf, edition, pp. 82-115, although William Bateson, in his *Materials for the Study of Variation* (London, 1894), presented a much earlier theory for the discontinuity of variation.

a perpetual search for the successful expedient. It must be a process permeating society, one in which the most recent evidence of progress will disappear when improved upon. To develop such a sense a society must first become aware of its improvability. The earliest proponents of such a society were the natural philosophers of Ionia, who described worldviews that did not rely on arbitrary forces of a divine nature, noting, instead, that there was a natural order of things that was predictable and therefore subject in many instances to control by man. Societies contemporaneous with the Ionian thinkers such as the several states of China, the Mauryan age of India, the Late Period of Egyptian pharaohs, the reigns of the Persian monarchs, and the Olmec civilization of Central America, reveal nothing comparable and therefore nothing that could be a basis for progress. Things might get bigger but not better.

End of Excursus

There is a tendency to conflate, to bring together into a whole, disparate ideas touching on a single topic, to find relevance of one idea to another even though no relation may exist. Thus, when we speak of "religion," under this rubric some equate Buddhism, Christianity, Hinduism, Confucianism, and Zoroastrianism, although each is utterly different from the others and the relevance of each to religion (see *Excursus on Religion and the West*, p. 347, for definitions) is a matter of semantics. Some speak of "medicine" the same way, viewing the medicine-man, the barber-surgeon, the herb-seller, the colon-cleanser, and the modern physician as part of a unified panorama of "healers," when in fact each represents a distinct phenomenon. The ancient Greeks did not clarify the matter, for they often applied ἰατρός (iatros) to any practitioner who dealt with matters pertaining to health. A similar inclination to conflate events unrelated in both origin and purpose is seen with the term "progress." Here it is the perspective of social benefit that provides the glue combining disparate, even incongruent, discoveries and inventions into a latticework upon which humans appear to mount to an ever-higher state. Such false analogies and wishful thinking have helped obscure the true basis of religion, medicine, and progress. Remarkably, the *Ethics Manual* of the American College of Physicians, 5th edition, 2005, implies a superiority of Aesculapian (temple) magical medicine over Hippocratic medicine in that the latter tolerated different standards of care for the rich and the poor. This equates the Hippocratic physician with contemporary slave practitioners, which is patently a falsehood, for the latter were not physicians, and the two went their separate ways. Had there been enough Hippocratic physicians to go around, who is to say that everyone would not have preferred access to them? Those who *would* say it hopefully will read this book.

B. Ionia, Mainland Greece, and Political Progress

A sequence of the Greek dramatic arts has been proposed in which mythology assumes different purposes according to the political status of the age:[15] (1) The Greek

---

[15] O'Neil, James L., *The Origins and Development of Ancient Greek Democracy*, Rowman and Littlefield, Lanham, MD, 1995.

heroic age was the age of epics, on which were based the Homeric poems. Mythological creations helped control and sustain monarchical establishments among men. (2) Monarchies were superseded by aristocratic governments. It was then that the Greek theatrical chorus was invented, and in ancient performances questions were first raised by the chorus regarding choices of actions.[16] Links to mythological characters were maintained in family lineages, but the association of mythology with leadership of society was now an indirect one as vested interests vied for power. (3) The aristocracies then gave way to the tyrant, who rose to power by means of his appeal to the many. At this time the earliest tragedies were being staged.[17] (4) With the approach of democracy, there was the advent of comedy, and now there were only the faintest allusions to mythology. Members of society could laugh at themselves and at one another. Examples of political leaders from each of these four stages would include, respectively, Agamemnon in Mycenae, Lycurgus in Sparta, the Peisastrati in Attica, and Pericles in Athens. The political changes actually observed in each of the four ages are as follows:

1. Monarchy

Agamemnon was a king over other kings and one of the chiefs that, for four centuries, managed the affairs of the centralized monarchical bureaucracy of the Mycenaean kingdom. His authority was sanctioned by Zeus, as Nestor says: ". . . for it is no common honour that is the portion of a sceptred king to whom Zeus giveth glory."[18] Thus the divine right of kings has a long history in the West. The Mycenaeans built grand palaces and were in contact with other civilizations. This is attested by its art, poetry, and commerce. It was Agamemnon's leadership of the West in the Trojan War that contributed so to his notoriety, his actions and motives being immortalized by the Greek tragedians. Some attribute the beginning of the end of the Mycenaean civilization to the war against Troy, even though the Mycenaeans, early Greeks, were victors.

2. Aristocracy

There then followed a period of destruction and presumed political chaos of which little is known, the Greek Dark Age. Society at this time was fragmented, each social grouping evolving its own division of labor and a pyramidal system of power. This power structure laid the basis for a hereditary and elitist leadership. Still, the overarching control of large kingships of the Mycenaean age was now gone and the

---

[16] Arion of Methymna (late 7th C BC), according to Herodotus (*The Histories*, Bk. I), was a harpist and singer who is credited with formal development of the Greek chorus. None of his works have survived.

[17] Thespis of Icaria (6th C BC) is credited by Aristotle as the first actor to perform opposite a chorus. His works, none of which survive, were first termed *tragedies*, a word derived from τραγῳδία (tragoidia), meaning a song relevant, for example, to sacrifice of an animal such as a goat, for "male goat" is the English translation of τράγος (tragos). Aeschylus increased the number of actors to two (each of whom could play multiple roles), and his earliest play, presented in 472 BC, was *The Persians*.

[18] ἐπεὶ οὔ ποθ' ὁμοίης ἔμμορε τιμῆς σκηπτοῦχος βασιλεύς, ᾧ τε Ζεὺς κῦδος ἔδωκεν. Homer, *The Iliad*, Bk.I, 278-9. The translation is by A. T. Murray for the *Loeb Classical Library* series of Homer, vol. 1.

early Archaic period was now underway (750 BC). There were at that time few powerful monarchies remaining in Archaic Greece. In Attica, the office of πολέμαρχος (polemarch), a military commander set apart from the king, had been instituted by election and proved to be the first Hellenic limitation on kingly power. Later, archonships were established, and annual elections of archons began around 700 BC.[19] There was also a change from somewhat nomadic life of the Dark Age to a settled life that included personal land ownership, especially in the colonies.[20] Private ownership ultimately received the sanction of legislation.[21] A new basis for social groupings was devised, the φρατρίαι (phratries), which were extended kinships that also incorporated unrelated families who provided ancillary services. The affairs of the local society then came to be managed by a royal council, or βουλή (bouleh). Overall, however, leadership remained hereditary for it lay in the hands of wealthy private estate owners who intended to retain it. Lycurgus, who is credited with providing the city-state of Sparta with its rigid law code, was an advocate for the aristocracy in that his Council of Elders and the Assembly fixed the leadership and control of the military in the hands of a few elite. Even in Athens the laws of Solon in 594 BC, while representing an early stage in development of democracy, permitted continuation of aristocratic control.

3.   Tyranny

Aristocracies then suffered a powerful challenge: the increasing wealth of other segments of society. This was the consequence of overseas trade, which led to an expanding upper class. Colonization was brought forth by both overpopulation of established mainland Greek cities and, more importantly, by aristocratic intolerance of dissent. Early colonies were often like family businesses, a form of private enterprise, although they maintained close ties with their mother cities. Even merchants founded cities. The resulting wealth led to an unintended consequence: social mobility began to weaken established nobility. It has been pointed out that wealth which had accumulated in some aristocratic families was diluted whenever one or two generations of several male heirs divided that wealth proportionately, whereas a non-aristocratic family that became wealthy but had only one heir would continue to amass wealth. Class distinction became less clear. Concurrently, Greek commerce expanded and Greek trade prompted the development of an industrial base. By 650 BC it has been stated that "wealth is competing with descent as a political test...."[22] An elected judicial system incorporated some representation of

---

[19] The Archons were chief magistrates or governors. In contrast to a monarch, or "single" leader, Athenian Archons had divided responsibilities and ultimately would be chosen by lot rather than by election.

[20] Discussed by Bury, J. B., in *A History of Greece to the Death of Alexander the Great*, London, 1900, p. 99. Over the next fifty years, colonization produced a change in which the "aristocracy of birth gave way to an aristocracy of wealth."

[21] This system of land ownership and its management were first described by the poet, Hesiod, who noted "Work is no disgrace." (ἔργον δ᾽ οὐδὲν ὄνειδος, in *Works and Days*, line 310, translation by H. G. Evelyn-White, *Loeb Classical Library* edition of Hesiod, vol. 1.)

[22] Bury, J. B., *A History of Greece to the Death of Alexander the Great*, London, 1900, p. 177. Also, Plutarch notes that trade was not a socially inferior activity, Plato sold oil to pay for travel expenses, and Thales in the preceding century had engaged in trade.

the lower classes. Κοινονίαι (koinons, or brotherhoods and guilds), previously restricted to nobility, now included commercial enterprises. Another key change occurred around 600 BC with the development of the privately armed soldier, or *hoplite*, and organization of the *phalanx*. Even some farmers could now afford military armament necessary to be a hoplite. Prof. McNeill concluded it was in part to prevent the decay of the phalanx that led Sparta and Athens to take on major political reforms.[23] Growing realization that safety resided in interdependence of all levels of society further diluted aristocratic influence.[24]

With more numerous powerful families, inevitable leadership struggles led to the seeking of society-wide popular support for *selective aristocratic control*, the *tyranny*. Thus was born the Age of the Tyrants, a phrase some scholars have applied to 6th C Hellas, although there were many tyrants in the 7th C BC, including some on the Peloponnese. It was a time when the voice of the people was first heard *en masse*. Colonial expansion and discontent with the nobility led to local revolutions and to transient tyrannies. These some consider to have been a necessary precursor of democracy, in that aristocracy as an institution was held in check by the tyrant and yet existing civil law was retained so as to satisfy the tyrant's constituency. Indeed, Profs. Winspear and Silverberg go so far as to state: "Throughout the sixth and fifth century in Greece, wherever we meet the word tyrant, we should usually understand "leader of the democratic movement."[25] The tyranny of the Peisistratus family in Athens, which lasted from 546 to 510 BC, was attended by good judgment in foreign policy, numerous good works for city improvement, and generous donations to friends and constituents. It is an example of the salutary face that on occasion can grace the authoritarian figure. Dr. Breasted even equated the Age of the Tyrants, when the Greeks pulled ahead of the rest of the world, with the Industrial Revolution.[26] It therefore happened that the tyranny was a "positive concept" in the 6th C BC, and Dr. Muller could equate tyrants with "the first professional politicians."[27] As Sir William Halliday has nicely stated,[28] "a contented proletariat is a condition of the tyrant's tenure of power," a restatement of Euripides (*Antigone*, frag. 14; "The tyrant must the many strive to please."). Tyrants remain popular today, although the modern tyrant has assumed, justifiably, a far more odious public image.

---

[23] McNeill, W., *The Rise of the West; A History of the Human Community*, Chicago, 1963, p. 199*ff*. The response of Athens was to turn to Solon for assistance. There had been a period when the agricultural population was repeatedly repressed, but the laws of Solon reformed the constitution, fostered the interests of the lower classes, and promoted democratic change. See: Bury, J. B., *A History of Greece to the Death of Alexander the Great*, London, 1900, p. 179*ff*. Solon also devoted himself to commerce. He fostered the trades because there was limited subsistence to be gained from the poor soil of Attica. He urged every man to have an occupation, and immigration of trained artisans was promoted.

[24] A critique of this "pre-Dorian" theory is presented by R. Sealey (*A History of the Greek City States ca. 700-338 B. C.*, Berkeley, 1976, p. 56*ff*) who questions the importance of hoplite and phalanx in promoting a greater role of the lower classes in city-state governance. He also concludes that a peasant hoplite caste would have been unlikely to enthusiastically embrace the uncertainties of a warrior state, prefering instead the stable lifestyles necessary for an agricultural society.

[25] Winspear, A. D., and Silverberg, T.: *Who Was Socrates?*, New York, 1939, p. 60, footnote.

[26] Breasted, J., *Ancient Times: A History of the Early World*, Boston, 1916, Chapter XII.

[27] Muller, H. J., *Freedom in the Ancient World*, New York, 1961, p. 165.

[28] Halliday, W. R., *The Growth of the City-State*, Boston, 1923, p. 64.

There is an additional nuance to this change from aristocracy to tyranny. No longer was the preponderance of the population entailed, in one form or another, to fulfill the needs of the aristocratic class. They could now begin to think about fulfilling their own needs. This natural desire had been expressed earlier in the works of Hesiod and Solon in their praise of work and of pride in its results. Hesiod (*ca.* 700 BC) had written, "In the race for wealth each man will strive his neighbor to excel and all the world's the better for the strife,"[29] and "Work is no disgrace; the disgrace is idleness." Solon (638-558 BC), although upper class by descent, was of limited means and traveled much while engaged in business activities. Pindar (522-433 BC) wrote that, "Success for men, if it comes ever, comes not unattended with difficulty [*i.e.,* work]." Sophocles (496-406 BC) has Electra say, "Success, remember, is the meed of toil." Euripides (480-406 BC) has Menelaus say, "With little labor how can man acquire great profit?"[30] Pericles (495-429 BC), in his famed funeral oration, stated:

> ". . . and with us it is not a shame for a man to acknowledge poverty, but the greater shame is for him not to do his best to avoid it."

> *The Histories* of Thucydides, Bk. II, 40, translation of C. F. Smith for the *Loeb Classical Library* series on Thucydides, vol. 1

Finally, Plutarch wrote that in this earlier age the Greeks did not associate work with "social inferiority." That this vigorous outlook was transient is apparent a century or so later in Aristotle's claim that:

> "…one should [live] neither a laborer's nor businessman's life (for such a life is ignoble and incompatible with virtue), nor, in the best State, are [citizens] even to be farmers, (for there is need of leisure for the development of both virtue and competent citizenship)."[31]

> Aristotle, *Politica*, Bk. 7, 1328b, 1329a
> W. D. Ross, editor, Oxford, 1957

The social approval of work consequent to the decline of aristocratic power and felt at all levels of society, including, as the above evidence proves, the upper classes, was to have relevance to medicine.[32]

---

[29] From Hesiod's *Works and Days*, 23, translation of T. B. Harbottle, *Dictionary of Quotations (Classical)*, London, 1902.

[30] Hesiod, *Works and Days*, 311. The Pindar quotation comes from *Pythian Ode* 12, 50: εἰ δέ τις ὄλβος ἐν ἀνθρώποισιν, ἄνευ καμάτου οὐ φαίνεται. The translation is by J. W. Donaldson. The quotation from *Electra* is: ὅρα, πόνου τοι χωρὶς οὐδὲν εὐτυχεῖ. Translation is by F. Storr, *Loeb Classical Library*, series of Sophocles. More literally it would be: "Look, nothing good happens in a place without toil." The quotation from Euripides' *Orestes* (lines 694-5) is: σμικροῖσι γὰρ τὰ μεγάλα πῶς ἕλοι τις ἂν πόνοισιν· Translation is by T. B. Harbottle, *Dictionary of Quotations (Classical)*, London, 1902.

[31] This opinion of Aristotle is commonly expressed in the unattributed quotation, "All paid jobs absorb and degrade the mind."

[32] The social disapproval of work over the next century was also to have consequences, for it was associated with an increase in the importance of slavery, to which Prof. Benjamin Farrington (*Greek*

4. Democracy

Democracy appeared first in Ionia, the west coast of modern-day Turkey, near which lay the island of Cos, later to be known for its production of superior physicians. But historical documentation of the stages in democracy's development is best found in Attica, where, in 594 BC, the Constitution of Athens was proclaimed.[33] The upper classes no longer had exclusive control over high office, and an assembly of citizens was now involved in decisions affecting society. Athenian democracy was then extended in city-state management by Cleisthenes in his reforms that began in 507 BC. He made δῆμοι (demes), or regions, rather than φράτραι (phratries), or extended tribal associations, the basis for citizenship. By this means the average citizen was no longer a tribal cipher. Then, in 487 BC, with the selection of Athenian leaders by lot, Athenian democracy was fully expanded throughout the age of Pericles, which encompassed the early years of Hippocrates. At this time it was the persuasive power of Themistocles (524-460 BC) that strengthened the demands of average citizens in managing city-state affairs when he brought about the formation of a large navy, for by this act, which required recruitment of large numbers of rowers on the military triremes, the importance of the average citizen in protecting Athens was undeniable.[34] A strong-willed democrat who saved Athens from the Persians by means of that large fleet, Themistocles also fostered an industrial base of "craftsmen of free birth." A generation later the importance of work remained paramount, and Pericles could state in 428 BC that Athenians had no bias against poverty unless no attempt was made to rise from it. Trade was also greatly bolstered by the increasingly efficient use of the Lydian invention of coinage. The introduction of money, Prof. Toutain writes, by apposing "landed wealth" with "moveable wealth," prompted the emergence of banking and capitalism. Imported foodstuffs were paid for by a profusion of processed articles of exchange.[35] Democracy and capitalism were proving their worth in fostering prosperity.[36, 37]

Science, Harmondsworth [UK], 1953, p. 34*ff*) attributes the loss of Greek "technical" proficiency as well as causing a greater disparity in wealth.

[33] Perhaps earlier indications of popular governance are an inscription indicating isonomia on Chios and the Dreros Law on Crete, both dated about 650-600 BC.

[34] Slaves were not used to power military vessels.

[35] Toutain, J., in: *The Economic Life of the Ancient World*, New York, 1930, p. 74.

[36] Plutarch, *Parallel Lives*, Solon, 2.

[37] "Capitalism" is a modern economic term, and the history of capitalism is modern as well. Merriam-Webster's Collegiate Dictionary, 10th edition, defines it as "an economic system characterized by private or corporate ownership of capital goods, by investments that are determined by private decision, and by prices, production, and distribution of goods that are determined mainly by competition in a free market." State capitalism is an incongruous variant of the term. But capitalism in its philosophical sense has been described as a social system based on the principle of individual rights. At this point some discussion of its place in ancient life may be helpful. Capitalism describes a rational economic system in which all means of production are privately owned and for profit, being controlled by a free market. It permits the accumulation of wealth exceeding need. Evidence of capitalistic practices existed in 6th C BC Greece, and the importance of a multiplier effect that followed on the invention of coinage and its subsequent use in commerce and market speculation has been described by Rostovzeff. Indeed, the Greek word

The political progression from monarchy to democracy was now accomplished, but to what end? It has been often stated that the progress of mankind has depended on the rare appearance of extraordinary minds, geniuses such as da Vinci, Newton, and Einstein. But good ideas are common; it is the social environment that is critical. The intellectual crop depends on societal weather. There have been many who have pondered the fall of an apple. Segments of Hellenic society had determined on democracy to resolve internal conflicts by words rather than force and to guide the city-state in its external relations. The result of their effort was resoundingly successful in producing a wealthy and powerful state. But it was more than this, for there is in democratic process the implicit assumption that the people themselves are capable of discussing options, resolving differences, seizing opportunity, and choosing wisely. It represented a profound faith in the ability of all men to reason. And yet this was not a matter of individual rights, for, as an example, Pericles praised the Athenian's toleration of his neighbor's individuality, not the promotion of it.[38] Also, unlike every other society before and after it up to 19th C Western morally-derived sanctions, some in Hellenic society found fault with the institution of slavery (see footnote, p. 371, its reference to Aristotle).

---

for the "interest" charged on a loan is τόκος (tokos), or "childbirth," for it represented both the birth of money from money and the birth of commercial enterprise from the borrowed money.

Normal expenses of Greek government were small. According to L. Whibley (*A Companion to Greek Studies*, 4th edition, Cambridge, 1931, p. 491*ff*), it was unusual to have a Ministry of Finance, and economic stores were not laid up. Much of State revenues came from customs and market "dues." There were few protective tariffs, and property taxes were uncommon. Although a progressive income tax was not used, the poor were exempt from taxes. Likewise "...the direct taxing of the soil, of trades and occupations, or even of the person, was considered in Greece, pressing emergencies excepted, as tyrannical." (Boeckh, A., *The Public Economy of the Athenians*, London, 1857, p. 407*ff*, translated by Anthony Lamb.) Additional income came from expected contributions from the wealthy. This minimized the need for taxation, for money was required for the military, fortifications, public service, festivals, policing of the slaves, poor relief, and engraving inscriptions. Sources of revenues included the royal mines, market dues, harbor toll, poll taxes on resident aliens, fines and confiscations, and tributes.

Most commercial activity in ancient Greece occurred in the ἄγορα (agora), or market place, the center of public life in Greek cities. The classes of commercial interests included the ἔμποροι (emporoi), or wholesale dealer in foreign goods, the κάπηλοι (kapaloi), or retailers of local goods, and the αὐτοπώλης (autopoleis), or sellers of products of their own manufacture. W. A. Becker, in his *Charicles or illustrations of the private life of the ancient Greeks* (translated by F. Metcalfe, London, 1845), states: "The legal restrictions were few. There were no trade-guilds, in the modern sense of the word, nor, properly speaking, any monopolies...." Also in the agora were found the τράπεζαι (trapezai), or money-changers, whose activities were carried out within sight but beyond earshot of the public, and which included extending loans and a number of other money-marketing services. Silver and copper coinage was for general use. Apparently there was an overseer of the agora, his purpose being to prevent fraud. It cannot be denied, therefore, that from these economic benefits that capitalism, long before it was given a name, was alive and well in freer societies. Even Solon (638-558 BC) traveled extensively because of his business interests. As for the means of production, Greeks employed slaves, had no large factories, and no large reservoir of workers who could bargain their product, labor. This consequence of capitalism would come much later.

[38] "...for we do not feel resentment at our neighbour if he does as he likes, nor yet do we put on sour looks which, though harmless, are painful to behold." *Thucydides,* Bk. II, XXXVII, translation of C. Forster Smith, *Loeb Classical Library.*

Greek democracy was revolutionary in that every adult male citizen contributed to the course of the Ship of State, although the nature of democratic process in the various city-states was diverse. But the purpose of ancient democracy was, to those who chose it, a way of best preserving the State rather than a means of ensuring individual freedom. It was a way to survive in an antagonistic world by enlisting shareholders of self-interest. It was based on the recognition (1) that objective self-interest expressed in unenjoined discourse can expose the superior idea – or amalgamation of ideas, and (2) that voluntary implementation of that superior idea was more effective than coercion as a basis for action.[39]

It was, therefore, an unintended consequence of faith in the average man's ability to reason that saw a relatively small population garner the blessings of an individual's opportunity to pursue self-interest. The result would be progress, a consequence of individual freedom, whereas other larger and richer but authoritarian populations remained stagnant except for an occasional change of master. Those happy conditions that would support progress, namely a sufficiency of population as the soil and intellectual freedom as the climate, were met in some 5th C Greek city-states. Sparta, however, was an example of a city-state that pursued a different course.

C. Sparta, an Exception

While Greek city-states with democratic institutions were prospering, industries were born only with reluctance in oligarchical states. An example of this was Sparta where labor was viewed as "civic degradation." For an anomalous event had occurred on the Peloponnesian peninsula. The early development of Sparta had been similar to that of the other Hellenic communities. Then in the 12th C BC the Mycenaean empire, centered on the Peloponnesian Peninsula, was replaced by Dorian Greeks, an ill-defined population migration from the mountainous northerly reaches of present-day Greece and Macedonia. Sparta became an important Dorian city. It had its own fledgling artistic and literary figures such as the famous poet, Tyrtaeus. But with the threat of internecine chaos, an 8th C lawmaker declared his views. Lycurgus,[40] passing his laws by obtaining agreement from prominent citizens of Sparta, turned Sparta away from democracy. It became, instead, an elective monarchy, secretive and warlike, subjugating nearby Hellenes. By displacing or dispersing the population of the Peloponnese, those Dorians inhabiting Sparta obtained, by the 7th C, control over much of the peninsula. Therefore, while the voluntary acceptance of the ancient laws of Lycurgus can be taken as a token democratic tendency early in Sparta's history, its subsequent political development was, by the nature of the laws it adopted, quite to the contrary. This course was the result of conscious action, for Sparta was never ruled by a tyrant, and it never had laws imposed on it from the outside. After 556 BC it was ruled by five Ephors, two hereditary kings, and the Gerousia, the latter being a council of elders over sixty years of age and officeholders for life. In fact, if not in theory, the Gerousia was aristocratic, its members

---

[39] A role for democracy *per se* in fostering a fragmentation of public opinion sufficient to hinder formation of undemocratic groups of sufficient size to carry forward disruptive or destructive policies cannot be discounted.

[40] Lycurgus is arguably a historical figure. He is credited with the rigid militaristic reforms that preserved the Spartan state, reforms that produced a legendary army and a much-admired code of personal conduct.

of noble family, and included in its numbers two prior kings. The Ephors, in contrast, were elected annually, and this gives the impression of democracy in government. But Xenophon equated them with tyrants, and others suggest that at times they were subordinate to the kings, their office being a mechanism for mollifying the public. The exclusion from the vote of those under thirty years of age and precluding the "undistinguished" from holding office belie any democratic quality to Spartan governance. [41] It must be acknowledged that in today's democracies the party system for nominating candidates for public office often shows utter disregard for opinions of the "undistinguished" public.

Given the rigid laws that the Ephors were to administer, there could be few displays of individualism at any level of Spartan society. From the 7th C Spartan youth lived in barracks from seven to twenty years of age, and not until the age of thirty were men permitted to live at home. The inconvenience of iron money was used to prevent diversion into luxury. Seventh and early 6th C Laconian bronzes, pottery, and ivories were similar to those of other city-states.[42] But, whereas the 6th C saw varying degrees of democratization occurring elsewhere in Greece, in Sparta the opposite took place. By the time democracy was fully established in Athens, about 500 BC, Sparta was a xenophobic, illiterate, and parasitic militaristic state.[43] Like the pyramids, Sparta survived, barely, even for a thousand years,[44] but its entire literary production from the early 4th C down to the 2nd C BC consisted of but three political pamphlets.[45] The city has been characterized as a "cosmos of silence," and even the power of the Ephors was to some extent based on "silent inspection" that body language often supplied in lieu of words as the Ephors strode the byways of ancient Sparta.[46]

Sparta was Greek and an autonomous city-state in the proximity of Athens, the two cities being separated by ninety-five miles. Yet rational medicine did not take hold there. Whereas Thucydides was to describe the Athenian physicians honorably attempting to stem the plague of 428 BC, Pausanias, a 5th C BC Spartan general, said, concerning the chronically ill, "The best physician is he who does not allow his patients to linger but buries them as quickly as possible."[47] This judgment on the quality of life

---

[41] O'Neil, J. L., *The Origins and Development of Ancient Greek Democracy*, Lanham, MD, 1995, chapter 1.

[42] Laconia refers to the region around Sparta, including the large valley that extends south to the Laconian Gulf.

[43] Powell, A., *Athens and Sparta*, Routledge, 1988. Thebes and Grecian (Dorian) Crete, like Sparta, were never democratic, and ancient Cretan communities, with their communal dinner tables, may have been the source of some Spartan laws. Prof. J-P. Vernant (*The Origins of Greek Thought*, Ithaca, 1982, p. 65) concurs with the early 6th C BC as the time of Sparta's "turning in on itself." He particularizes that change, unique among the Hellenic city-states, describing the process as one that both permitted Sparta to escape the monarchical world of the Mycenean kingdom and then avoid many of the defects that afflicted the other city-states. He then identifies the Spartan militarism as a major influence that would lead that society to use fear rather than persuasion to adhere to a balanced system of law and order.

[44] Cartledge, P., *Sparta and Laconia: A Regional History, 1300-362 BC*, Oxford, 2002, 2nd ed.

[45] Boring, T., *Literacy in Ancient Sparta*, Leiden, 1979, p. 54. During this time, however, Spartan influence was declining, subsequent to its defeat at the battle of Leuctra in 371 BC.

[46] Ephraim, D. *Sparta's Kosmos of Silence*, in: *Sparta, New Perspectives*, Duckworth, 1999, p. 117.

[47] κράτιστον δὲ ἔλεγε τοῦτον ἰατρον ειναι τόν μὴ κατασήποντα τοὺς ἀρρωστοῦντας, ἀλλὰ τάχιστα θάπτοντα. "He stated the best physician to be [that one who lets] those of the sickly not be subject to decomposition (further deterioration), but to be quickly buried." Plutarch,

of others is in perfect accord with authoritarian realities, whether fascist or communist. There is no other mention of physicians or of the profession of medicine in Sparta, although this may merely reflect the minimal contribution of Sparta to Greek letters.

Apart from the medical profession was the Asclepeion at Epidaurus, located on the Peloponnesian peninsula fifty-five miles from Sparta itself. The site of the Asclepeion had previously been associated with worship of Apollo, then being replaced in the 6th C BC to honor Asclepius. Whether the evolution of this famed Asclepeion and its mystical practices near Sparta was in any way associated with the xenophobic tendencies of 6th C Sparta is unknown, but two hundred years had to pass before the cult of Asclepius was introduced to Athens in the midst of the Peloponnesian War. Dr. Wickkiser concludes that the asclepeion as an institution was devised to address medical illness unresponsive to therapy by the physician and therefore deemed incurable, that there was no competition between physicians and Asclepios cult, and that Athens had political motivations for acquiring a relationship with Asclepios and the city of Epidaurus.[48] The cult of Asclepius is said to ultimately have exceeded in popularity that of Hippocratic physicians elsewhere in Greece and its colonies, although it is notable that Athenians acquired their association with the deity of Asclepius only under the duress of military expediency rather than by losing confidence in their Hippocratic clinicians. The serpent entwining the staff of Hippocrates that is medicine's icon is a reminder of the nature of that mysticism, for each Asclepeion had a labyrinth housing non-poisonous snakes that were able to roam the temple where patients came for relief of their ills. The curative value of the snakes required that they lick the patient's afflicted part such as a site of infection, although at times even dogs were applied to this office.[49]

Moralia, Cambridge, MA, 1931, translation by the author. In this translation it is understood that the traditional translation of κατασήποντα as "rotting" is not technically accurate, for the sickly were still alive. Thus, this is a figure of speech, and the meaning is closer to "further deterioration" of the already weakened patient. It seems that euthanasia is not the intended sense but that restriction to further medical care is implied. A similar, but "non-Spartan," opinion was ascribed to the sons of Asclepius in Plato's *Republic* (III, 408a,b): "But they thought that the life of a man constitutionally sickly and intemperate was of no use to himself or others, and that the art of medicine should not be for such nor should they be given treatment even if they were richer than Midas." (Translation of P. Shorey, in *The Collected Dialogues of Plato*, edited by E. Hamilton and H. Cairns, Princeton, 1961.)

[48] Wickkiser, B. L., *The Appeal of Asklepios and the Politics of Healing in the Greco-Roman World*, U. of Mich., 2003, doctoral dissertation. Wickkiser argues that the small city of Epidaurus was considered a potentially strategic location during the Peloponnesian war, and it was thus courted by Athens as an ally, one means being a close association with its most popular feature, the Asclepion and its claim to be the birthplace of Asclepius.

[49] It is thought that in its earlier decades the cult of Asclepius was entirely mystical or divinely inspired. Prof. Longrigg, however, has discussed the evidence that Asclepian temples were more influenced by Hippocratic medicine than the converse (Longrigg, J., *Greek Rational Medicine*, London, 1993, p. 25), and by the third century BC elements of empirical or rational medicine had been inserted into their operations. For a detailed description of the cult and the Asclepeium (*sic*) at Epidauros see: R. Caton, *The Temples and Ritual of Asklepios at Epidauros and Athens*, London, 1900. It is ironic to note that healing powers have recently` been ascribed to a non-poisonous snake saliva, the consequence of an endothelial cell growth factor (ECGF) that has been isolated from that substance. See the scientific but tongue-in-cheek article by R. Angeletti: *A Biomedical Roll for Sacred Serpents in Aesculapian Healing Rituals?*, in *Proc. IXth Eur. Mtg. Paleopathol. Assoc.*, Barcelona, 1995, p. 15.

Why focus so on Sparta? In a fascinating comparison, by controlling for the effects of 1) a common Hellenism, 2) a common social organization, the city-state, 3) a common language and a common knowledge and (limited) experience with democratic process, and 4) a free Athens only ninety-five miles distant, the Spartan experience greatly strengthens the negative correlation between authoritarianism and rational/scientific medicine, a correlation so consistent that it virtually assures a causal association.

D. Democracy and the Rise of the Individual and the Koinon

Insofar as it was a socialist military commune that Lycurgus introduced into the Spartan city-state, it is instructive to review de Tocqueville's comparison of democracy and socialism: "Democracy extends the sphere of individual freedom; socialism restricts it. Democracy attaches all possible value to each man; socialism makes each man a mere agent, a mere number. Democracy and socialism have nothing in common but one word, equality. But notice the difference: while democracy seeks equality in liberty, socialism seeks equality in restraint and servitude."[50]

There is fear in authoritarian societies of disruptive ideas that can result from education. This apparent threat in Sparta led to active promotion of illiteracy and conformity. How could any society purposefully permit such repulsive measures? It could, and did, and there are many who yet admire the regimentation of authoritarianism and the security to be found in an ignorant, monolithic, and well-controlled populace. Sparta was admired by many great thinkers, then and now.[51] Centuries after Sparta the Catholic Church would use this approach to a very limited degree when it forbade some Biblical translations viewed as threatening. Whereas the American educational system is primarily in the hands of the public, absolute state control of education exists in Cuba, Russia, China, and many other nations, a mechanism supported by state censorship in disingenuous attempts to mimic Spartan conformity. A literate society means nothing, however, if the State is the agency of education.

But democracy was controversial from its earliest days. Many feared that those with limited knowledge or experience in making decisions affecting the State would lead it to disaster.[52] Monarchs, including the Great King of Persia, feared it because if it

---

[50] A. de Tocqueville, *Discours pronounce a l'assemblee constituante le 12 Septembre 1848 sur la question du droit au travail*, in *Oeuvres completes*, vol. IX, p. 546, the translation cited in F. A. Hayek's *The Road to Serfdom*, Chicago, 1944. The famed writer and publisher Elbert Hubbard is said to have defined a prison as "An example of a Socialist's Paradise, where equality prevails, everything is supplied, and competition is eliminated." (*Roycroft Dictionary and Book of Epigrams*, East Aurora, 1923, p. 47.)

[51] These have included Plato, Rousseau, Thomas Arnold (1795-1842, British educator influential in public school reform), and Adolf Shicklgruber (Hitler). Even Aristotle commented that "…: living in accordance with government regulations ought not to be considered slavery, but a shield." Οὐ γὰρ δεῖ οἴεσθαι δουλείαν ειναι τὸ ζῆν πρός τὴν πολιτείαν, ἀλλὰ σωτηρίαν. *Politics*, V, 1310a, translation by the author. A less contentious, but in context somewhat less accurate, translation is that of Dr. Jowett: "…: men should not think it slavery to live according to the rule of the constitution; for it is their salvation."

[52] Early writings on constitutions were not complimentary to democracy, including a 420 BC work, *Athenaion Politeia* (author unknown), *Lakedaimoniwn Politeia* (Lakedaimonion Constitution) by Xenophon, and Xenophon's *Cyrou Paideia*.

succeeded their positions of power were threatened.[53]   Socrates had an aversion to selection of officials by lot, for why should not society want to be led by the most informed and capable leaders? As for a political philosophy, Plato likened a democracy to a beehive, a society run by drones (politicians) who survive by taking honey made by the "orderly" class (entrepreneurs) and distributing it to the largest class, the workers, after, of course, taking a goodly share of the honey for themselves. Ultimately the entrepreneurs tire of being "stung" by the drones and the drones mislead the masses to incite a reaction against the entrepreneurs, the result being a push by the former for an oligarchy and a push by the latter for a tyranny, the tyrant winning out.[54] Plato was no admirer of democracy.

Disgust with authoritarian governance, however, was the temperament of many citizens in autonomous Greek city-states. Herodotus described democracy's attributes that would be identified with city-states for many years.[55] A century after Herodotus Aristotle concluded that, while all forms of government had grievous faults, the great value of democracy was that it permitted emergence of the individual, and the opinions of a group of free individuals was likely to be superior to those of a few oligarchs, just as "a feast to which many contribute is better than a dinner provided out of a single purse."[56] And this freedom of the individual and its corollary, the freedom of individuals to organize to augment freedom's benefits, was the key to the success of Greek democracies.

But there is more. Consider again the playwright, Aeschylus. From time to time one man may be capable of surpassingly elegant epic drama that sees to the heart of a particular problem of his society. But all that insight and artistry cannot be considered a work of genius until the play is publicly performed and declared so. The immortality of the *Oresteia*, therefore, is explained by both the author and his audience.[57] Genius, with which mankind has been so frequently blessed, accounts for nothing unless the product of one's genius can be seized upon, discussed, and adjudged as genius by the community at large. There can be no genius in a strictly authoritarian society, for that man or woman will be either a factotum or a slave, the audience in either case being his or her master(s). For only in a free society will true genius be recognized and acclaimed, whereas those acclaimed as genius who emerge from under authoritarian rule are those few who render

---

[53] Herodotus, *Histories*, Book III, 82, the speech of the Persian monarch, Darius I.

[54] See a standard translation by Jowett, B.: *The Works of Plato*, vol. 2, *The Republic*, Bk. 8, "Tyranny naturally arises out of democracy." Οὐκ ἐξ ἄλλης πολιτείας τυραννὶς καθίσταται ἢ ἐκ δημοκρατίας.

[55] "But the virtue of a multitude's rule lies first in its excellent name, which signifies equality before the law; and secondly, in that it does none of the things that a monarch does. All offices are assigned by lot, and the holders are accountable for what they do therein; and the general assembly arbitrates on all counsels. Therefore I declare my opinion, that we make an end of monarchy and increase the power of the multitude, seeing that all good lies in the many." Speech of the Persian, Otanes, as imagined by Herodotus and as translated by A. D. Godley in the *Loeb Classical Library*, *Herodotus*, III, 80.

[56] *The Politics of Aristotle*, Bk. III, 11, translation of B. Jowett, Oxford, 1885.

[57] An analogous argument was made by Prof. Herbert Muller about cities as discussed in his book, *The Uses of the Past* (Oxford, 1954): "Without London and Boston Thoreau could have had no Walden, or no spiritual interests to take there." As a modern example, this thinking is mirrored in the association of great opera not just with Verdi, Puccini, and a few other gifted individuals, but with the Italian people as well. A further nuance to the topic is the "test of time," for an audience that establishes a work of genius may belong to a later generation.

service to the State and who are declared "genius" whether or not they are.[58] The more authoritarian the society the more true genius will remain anonymous unless recognized by outside agencies that learn of its existence. There is no profit to mankind in a lone man's brilliant insight if only one man is its judge and beneficiary. In a sense the society that will hear him out exhibits a collective genius; brilliant ideas are perennial, but a society open to contemplation of new thoughts has been rare indeed. For democracy to work, therefore, democratic thinking must extend throughout society; the magic of the koinon is not a function of a leadership.

Benefits of a free society, therefore, are 1) an expanded range of options about which an individual can think and thereby act, 2) the freedom of individuals to associate in groups to explore those options, and (3) the ability of a free society to pick and chose among options thus presented. The advancement, through organization, of individual goals can bring great benefits. For, in the competition of ideas, the more successful ones can be not only identified but improved on and widely adopted, and the benefit devolves as much on society as it does on the individual. In Greek governance it led to Periclean Athens, in the trades it led to wealth, and in medicine it led to the scientific method. No other civilization has a claim to such a remarkable invention as a free society because no other civilization had enough faith in the individual to put it to the test. The ancient Greeks did, and the honor is theirs alone.

Hellenic individualism, however, would have lasted but a short time without a parallel phenomen: its protection. Without that protection it likely would have followed the well-worn path to oblivion that all other civilizations have forced on their freethinkers. But in inventing democracy, the individual citizen and citizen groups were institutionally protected.[59] Laws for the first time applied equally to all citizens rather than arbitrarily serving the ends of a ruler or a ruling class. Democracy, unintended though it may have been, revolutionized society as well as government, for it secured equitable protections not only for the individual, but also the koinon, or common council, as practiced in the forums of government, the meetinghouse of the guild, and over the dinner table or in symposium at home.[60]

E. Democracy and the Natural State of Medical Practice

1. The cause of democratic enlightenment

---

[58] A perfect, albeit tragic, example is the Russian biologist, T. D. Lysenko (1898-1976), who was lionized by the dictatorship of the proletariat because his biological speculations on environmentally-induced genetic change, found conveniently adaptable as a condemnation of the bourgeoisie, thereby provided a justification for a disastrous experiment in social planning (p. 454*f*, footnote). On the other hand, a wonderful example of the occasional coincidence of genius with authority might be the *Brandenburg Concerti*, most of which were composed by Bach while living at the castle of his patron, Prince Leopold of Anhalt-Kothen. See also the Excursus on Patronage, p. 355.

[59] This point is made by Prof. Zimmern in his discussion of early Greek communities and Sparta (Zimmern, A., *The Greek Commonwealth*, Oxford, 1924, Part II, chapter 4).

[60] A Greek *symposium* was an evening banquet at someone's house, usually associated with drinking alcoholic beverages, hence the name (συμ – sum, "with"; πόω – poaw, "I drink"). It was a time for fellowship and often erudite discussion. "Symposium" is the name of a dialogue written by Plato that took place at such a banquet.

How did democracy settle on the ancient Greeks? (1) Consideration might first be given to personal characteristics of the Greeks themselves. But the success of the Renaissance and the later propagation of democracy and aspiration to individual freedom into the modern age belie any hypothesis of special genetic fitness of the ancient Greeks for the event. Consider also that the road from kingship to democracy was a rocky one, and that road had surely been attempted over and over again in other early societies. (2) Another possibility is that democratic evolution of Greek politics was a consequence of an ethnic trait of the Hellenes, a greater appreciation of man and his abilities, or, as Dr. John Lewis has stated in his lecture on *Political Thought in Ancient Greece*, a greater sense of self-worth.[61] But the proud name for China, *chung kuo*, meaning "the central country" in the sense that all other countries are, in effect, subsidiary, does not suggest the Chinese over the ages suffered from any deficiency in feelings of self-worth, at least for Han Chinese relative to the worth of non-Han. The same can be said of certain nationalistic notions of Aryan superiority early in the 20th C. (3) Perhaps a communal trait can be invoked. Sir Francis Galton provided the astonishing explanation that inadvertent eugenics over a single century produced in ancient Greece a superior breed of man.[62] (4) Prof. Zimmern concludes that much of the presumed antipathy that the ancient Greek citizen had against physical labor is actually a misinterpretation of their reticence to accept wages, that their work was their pleasure, and to acquire more wealth than was their due was considered an unworthy goal. How closely this idyllic picture reflects the actual day-to-day life of the ancient Greek craftsman can be debated, for the motives and the economics of it fly in the face of both human nature and historical evidence. (5) Then there is the Greek language itself. It is malleable, and the proposed role of language in affecting one's worldview is discussed on p. 27, the Sapir-Whorf hypothesis. Prof. Bruno Snel has highlighted the importance of the definite article, among the great civilizations a Greek invention, in unfettering human reason to cultivate philosophical and scientific thought.[63] And the doctoral thesis of Dr. Jessica Whisenant[64] discusses several scholarly perspectives on the role of literacy and oral tradition in the context of ancient Greece, the current "consensus" being: a) that there is great overlap between oral and literary chronicling, b) that only rarely did classical Athens use writing for collation, cataloging, and other forms of institutional memory, c) that artistic expression was equally served by oral and literary forms, and d) that even well into the 4th C BC complex writing was not an accomplishment of the common man. The conclusion to be derived from these arguments, as far as is relevant to present discussion, is that the role of literacy was relatively unimportant in determining the course of political Greece.[65] (6) It has recently

---

[61] This lecture by Dr. John Lewis is available throught the Ayn Rand Bookstore, operated by the Ayn Rand Institute.

[62] Galton F., *Hereditary Genius*, London, 1914, p. 329*f*.

[63] For example, ἡ ἀήρ ("the air"), now transformed into a noun, becomes susceptible to concepts concerning its being, in contrast to definitions of air, such as "something that we breath." From this linguistic development the Greeks, without any outside influence, had a basis on which to formulate scientific and philosophical concepts. See: Snell, B., *The Discovery of the Mind*, Cambridge, 1953, chapter 10, The Origin of Scientific Thought.

[64] Whisenant, J. N., *Writing, Literacy, and Textual Transmission: The Production of Literary Documents in Iron Age Judah and the Composition of the Hebrew Bible*, Univ. of Mich., 2008, chapter 2, pp. 19-47.

[65] It might even be postulated that it was the persistent dependence on oral tradition and oral discourse and the avoidance of written tradition and regulations by a privileged and literate few that helped democratic process to mature. But there are major exceptions to this conclusion. First,

been noted that mathematical processing, as studied by metabolic imaging of the brain, differs between those who speak Chinese and those speaking English even though both cultures use Indo-Arabic numerals.[66] The role of language in this regard must remain conjectural., but a broad-based literacy such as the Greeks had, could only be the consequence of practical phonetic writing, a Greek invention.[67] (7) Greek achievement may have become possible because of an increase in population density. A sufficient population is required for propagation of any idea, good or bad, just as it is necessary for epidemic disease. But here again the Hellenic city-states were not at all unusual, for many cities and regions elsewhere greatly exceeded them in population and population density. (8) Finally, the mountainous terrain of Greece posed strategic advantages in that, being physically demanding, it was a protective geography. Greece was also opportunistically mercantile in that it was at a crossroads of cultures that surrounded the eastern Mediterranean. But isolated city-states and cities astride trade routes were common and not restricted to the Greeks.

The key to the puzzle of Greek democratic enlightenment is found not in genetic fitness, economics, or geography, but in the rationality of the people themselves. Their new government, a democracy, granted citizens equal voice in good times and equal liability if things went awry, but it did not grant them individual freedom. Their invention of democracy was, instead, a manifestation of individual freedom, or appreciation thereof, already in existence. Their democracy did not produce a love of freedom; it was, instead, the result of it. Their new government was *them*. Did this respect for freedom flow from a virtuous acknowledgement that one's neighbor was one's equal and it was only fair that he be treated as an equal? No, for selfishness was a characteristic of all their actions. Furthermore, it took them a century and more to overcome resistance to democratic governance. Was it viewed as a moral good, as something intended by their religious pantheon? Hardly. Was it given to a neighbor because he needed it? No, unless that neighbor was a family member. Was it the need to cede prerogatives to one's neighbors so that those neighbors would in turn recognize one's own rights? Yes. For the answer to the puzzle is compromise. "Let us agree that if I let you alone you will let me alone."[68]

Sparta, perhaps alone among the city-states, remained illiterate and, perhaps as a consequence, endured as a militaristic commune. Second, the *Hippocratic Corpus*, insofar as it is a scientific document, is evidence that recorded clinical experience must have permitted some of its perspicacious clinical axioms to become convention.

[66] Tang, Y., *et al.*, *Arithmetic Processing in the Brain Shaped by Cultures*, in *Proc. Nat. Acad. Sci.*, 103:10775-10780, 2006.

[67] Goody, J. and Watt, I., *The Consequences of Literacy*, in *Comparative Studies in Society and History*, 5:304-345, 1963.

[68] It is but fair to cite the insightful and ingenious alternative explanation for Greek freedom expressed by the prominent cultural sociologist, Prof. Orlando Patterson. Pre-Classical Era wars took few male captives, for the losers were systematically killed. Thus, slaves were for the most part females. Beyond this, females could be ransomed from captivity, and their slavery was not considered demeaning. It was women, therefore, who lived in the fear of slavery, and it was women who first appreciated their personal freedoms and who could appreciate the misery of those who had none. It was Greek women also who sought to expand their freedoms, infringing on masculine prerogatives. Patterson also discusses two other pillars of Western freedom, "civic" freedom, which was basically comfortable survival within tyranny, and "sovereign" freedom, a consequence of uninhibited power of a dominant state. These he feels contributed to perpetuation of slavery, a point much debated. See his *Freedom in the Making of Western Culture*, New York, 1991, Part II, *The Greek Construction of Freedom*.

The ancient Greeks recognized that, absent authoritarian governance and its threat of force, compromise is the only way to avoid chaos if a society is to remain intact, for humanity will be unanimous in nothing. As Dr. Boris De Wiel has nicely described it, democracy is "an irresolvable contest [in a society] of priorities among common values,"[69] a contest manifested by the perpetual bickering in democratic assemblies. Compromise, a rational and noncombative process, is an indispensable component of democracy. A "compromise in the common interest" was the method by which freedom was permitted and retained, thereby becoming the basis for the freedoms of the Greek polis. As a consequence, Greek democracy was able to procure the good ideas of many men.[70]

2. The cause of medical enlightenment

Explanations for the march to Greek exceptionalism in medicine might include the following. (1) Social changes that began in the Archaic period, such as the growth of commercialism with its cosmopolitan cross-fertilization of ideas that follow on travel and distant trade, may have combined to foster medical creativity. However, cross-fertilization of ideas is moot, for there is little to suggest that Greek medicine was anything but indigenous (p. 179*ff*). (2) There also was a growth of wealth. This is likewise an unlikely explanation, for focal centers of opulence had occurred throughout late prehistory and history, and progress in medicine did not result. Furthermore, the general prosperity of Periclean Greece would have had little effect on the medical profession, for medicine was but a local occupation, required little financial outlay, and was not lucrative. To this can be added the extraordinary economy of simple clinical observation as medicine's principal scientific tool. (3) Similarly, there was the new wealth consequent to early forms of capitalism. But as important as capitalism was to the creation of a wealthy city-state, capitalistic practices were of little relevance to the course of Hippocratic medicine, for the reason previously stated. It is more likely that any temporal association between the two did not reflect cause and effect; rather, both could claim a common origin for their successes.

There was a more important phenomenon in play, and that was a work ethic that extended throughout much of a society during its reversal of authoritarian governance. In contrast to most authoritarian societies, evolving democratic city-states realized that physical labor was both necessary and thereby desirable for all its citizens. No longer could an aristocratic upper-class disdain physical or commercial enterprise. Personal and communal survival required everyone's participation in wealth creation. At the same time, the lower classes could now concentrate more on following their own dreams and creating their own wealth, rather than merely contributing to the goals and wealth of others. As described in Section B-3 of this chapter, there is testimony to the importance of work in the 6th and 5th C BC, just as there was in the early days of republican Rome. To be self-supporting was a matter of pride. This was to benefit Hippocratic medicine, for that profession required manual labor on the part of the practitioner. A man of a high socioeconomic class who in an earlier generation would have disparaged the hands-on clinical procedures of a physician might now overcome that prejudice and join whole-heartedly in their performance, although how often this occurred is unknown. As

---

[69] De Wiel, B., *Democracy: A History of Ideas*, Vancouver, 2000, p. 3.
[70] Muller, H. J., in *Freedom in the Ancient World*, New York, 1961, chapter 6, *The Uniqueness of Greece*.

prosperity grew and wealth accumulated, however, it again became admirable to delegate physical work, except for that associated with the military or overseeing estates. And so, by the 4th C BC physical work was again viewed negatively, for it interfered with intellectual pursuits and philosophical inquiry alleged to be necessary for optimum social leadership and social conditioning.

But Hippocratic medicine had evolved long before this, and it is likely that work ethic contributed to its success. The more educated classes were not disuaded from entering medicine, and this introduced into local practices physicians attracted by interest and self-interest rather than by obligation to tradition or to a familial guild. Thus, in the early democratic city-states, and perhaps beginning in the 6th C BC, the physician was left to his own devices. And the greatest good to come from noninterference was an opportunity to appreciate, for the first time, the uniqueness of the individual patient. The physician, not instructed or expected to give a predetermined response to a specific sign or symptom, could now inquire into the entire course of illness, making note of personal characteristics of the patient and how they might be affecting the course of illness. From these observations he could modify the usual therapy to respond to peculiarities of a particular case and do so without fear of sanctions like those meted out from the days of Hammurabi down through Roman Egypt. On the contrary, if he did a good job he was a likely recipient of greater remuneration, an inevitable spur for improvement. As the physician began to chronicle and share his findings with colleagues, patterns of disease were distinguished. The usual course of a disease could be anticipated, divergences from which he might attribute to identifiable factors previously unsuspected. Also important was the opportunity to judge the effectiveness of his treatments, for he had but to compare the effect of his treatment to the usual course of the disease without treatment or with some other treatment.

Management of each case was taken up in partnership with the patient who was also "free," assuming he was a citizen, rather than "partnering" in management with a superior. And this was the greatest advance, for medicine cannot be practiced by committee.[71] Patients helped tailor their own treatments, becoming partners in managing their own illnesses. And they were able to select from among practitioners whose abilities

---

[71] In practicing medicine by committee the committee members are in partnership with each other, not with the patient. The patient will have little input and may have little leeway to refuse a recommended committee option. Alternatively, the committee may invalidate other options. Another defect in the committee approach to practicing medicine is politicization. When several voices are involved in making a particular management decision for either a patient or a health policy, there will be a spectrum of opinion from which one might be particularly popular with the patient or with the general public. The committee member who most closely espouses that view will have a political advantage regardless of the wisdom of his choice. Indeed, public sentiment may influence some committee members to disregard the best choice of action for the patient in a conscious or subconscious attempt to court public opinion or to avoid being seen to advocate an unpopular recommendation. In either situation, personal interest can befog objectivity. Montaigne (1533-1592) noted the variety of opposing medical opinions regarding a patient's management. He wrote: "There is no great danger in mistaking the height of the sun, or in the fraction of some astronomical computation: but here, where our whole being is concerned, it is not wisdom to abandon ourselves to the mercy of the agitation of so many contrary winds." (*The Essays of Michael Seigneur de Montaigne*, London, 1776, vol. 2, p. 589, translated by P. Coste.) And there also is the "bystander effect" in which diffusion of responsibility can be used as a sometimes tragic justification for individual inaction (see: Stavert, R. R., and Lott, J. P., *The Bystander Effect in Medical Care*, in *N. Engl. J. Med.* 368:2013, 8-9, 2013).

must have been public knowledge. To do this entailed effort, but one in which there was to be another advantage: the patient had to be talked into agreeing to treatment. This meant, in some cases, cajoling, and in other cases, education. Finally, the patient was directly involved in risk assessment. He had to decide, on the basis of what the physician could tell him, what he was willing to undergo or risk in following some recommended treatment or lack thereof. The patient thus helped shape both the type of therapy and the goal of therapy. Every patient has his unique set of priorities, values, and tolerances. To impose those of the physician on the patient has, since the days of Hippocrates, been anathema in the West, its avoidance one of the glories. To impose those of the State on the patient has always been anathema in America, its avoidance a source of both pride and progress. The patient benefited as well from the focused attention of a physician who was not directed to see him, but who, by natural sentiment and training and self-interest, voluntarily and willingly accepted him as a patient. With this acceptance came a personal obligation to the patient. The motive for this obligation was to be found in personal honor, and its enforcement was through public opinion. It is often stated that the foundation of medical practice is trust. Disregard of this obligation, being dishonorable, was certain, in an open society, to be no secret. In contrast, the more authoritarian the system the less is the role of personal honor, the greater the role of impersonal legal commitment, and the greater the ease of concealment. But moral obligations are far better than laws. In the first place, laws may be wrong or bad. Second, laws are intimidating. Third, laws dampen enthusiasm, which is not surprising in that, except for revenge or to undo the effect of another law, the function of any law is to limit freedom of someone to do something. Fourth, laws inevitably lead to other laws and ultimately to bureaucracy, a system ridiculed throughout history as being expensive, unwieldy, and insensitive. Fifth, laws can bridle innovation and risk-taking. Sixth, and very important, laws can make thought superfluous. Seventh, and even more important, laws can render virtue unnecessary, sometimes impossible. The honorable physician with an obligation is far preferable to the legislated physician in an amoral State.[72] To add to this, the physician's obligation to the patient was not shared by any obligation to other persons or to government. The physician was the advocate for his patient, and for no one else.

What has just been described is not the currently popular phrase "patient-centered medicine," for focusing on the patient to some degree has always been part of any practitioner-patient interaction. It is, instead, the basis for the natural state of medical practice. Its defining feature is that the patient be a counterpoise to the practitioner, which the patient could not be with a medical functionary, whether shamanistic or bureaucratic. In this new system the status of the practitioner was not really changed, for practitioners of any sort, with their special knowledge, have always had privileged status when dealing

---

[72] Traditionally it has been the moral character of the Western physician that guided, and guarded, the profession. "Virtue ethics provided the conceptual foundation for professional ethics," but now virtue is being supplanted by principle- and rule-based ethics. See the important book: Pelligrino, E., and Thomasma, D., *The Virtues in Medical Practice*, New York, 1993. And the ethical issue was even touched on by the famed physician, Erasistratus (304-250 BC), who went further: "Most fortunate indeed wherever it happens that the physician is both, perfect in his art and most excellent in his moral conduct. But if one of the two should have to be missing, then it is better to be a good man devoid of learning than to be a perfect practitioner of bad moral conduct, and an untrustworthy man ..." See: V. Rose, *Anecdota Graeca et GraecoLatina*, Berlin, 1864, vol. II, section on Pseudo-Soranus, *Questiones Medicinales*, p. 244, 16-23. The Latin and its translation are found in: L. Edelstein, *Ancient Medicine*, Baltimore, 1987, a paperback reprint of the 1967 work, p. 334.

with the sick.[73] It was the status of the patient that changed. How important and yet unheeded this concept is. No longer were patients the passive object of disinterested authority. Now they had the authority to personally interact with, question, and judge their practitioner, just as the δῆμος (demos, the citizens of a place) of 5th C Athens could question, judge, and replace authority in their new democracy. Patients had a similar upper hand when it came to employment of the practitioner, for they could withhold payment or select a dream-interpreter or other seer, herbalist, or any of a variety of practitioners, all of whom extracted payment. Payment of the physician was not a new thing, for it has been described in other ancient civilizations. But now the payment was more likely to be for the practitioner and circumstances of the patient's choosing. The physician now had to listen closely to the patient in order to convince the patient that he was not only better qualified than his competitors, but also that he was better at looking out for that patient's welfare. The physician-patient relationship was now a matter of power-sharing, a democracy. What a revolution this was.

This new koinon of two, profoundly shaped by competition among a variety of practitioners, was to have scientific reverberations. For scientific medicine hinges on recognition of the complexity of disease, a complexity reflected in the unique expressions of illness in the individual patient. Abraham Flexner put it exactly right: "In a very real sense, indeed, every case is unique, so that there never comes a time when the watchful intelligence, observing and interpreting, absolutely necessary in investigation, becomes superfluous or irrelevant in practice."[74] What before might have been just another cough was now a recent cough or a chronic one, a dry cough or a productive one, one with fever, high or low, or without fever, and so on. Realization of the complexity of medicine led to more detailed study of diseases and to an appreciation of the broad spectrum of diseases, their patterns, and ultimately their causes. But the freedom of the individual physician to practice and to associate with colleagues, the opening of the profession to those with special interest in medicine and biology, the disconnecting of myth and superstition from disease causation, and the entrepreneurship of physicians' organizations would have advanced the profession but little had not the patient been equally free to offer a detailed personal history of his illness and his situation, as well as his opinion, advice, and, directly or indirectly, his economic threat, just as the audience of Aeschylus, while not the source of Aeschylus' inspiration, was the source of his success and with its hisses could have been the source of his failure. In a word, as with the Aeschylean audience, the patient could express judgment regarding the quality of his care, and if sufficient numbers of patients agreed, the practitioner could claim success based on his "audience."

Surely some of the Egyptian sick appreciated the attention of Pharoah's priest doctors or *swnw(s)*. The most grateful of all people are those having nothing to whom something is offered. And it is unfair to assume that all patients in other social systems had no right of refusal of treatment. But the ability to choose and work with one's personal physician is a mainstay of Western medicine. In free societies citizens can vote with their feet, an effective spur to competition, thereby opening the prospect of progress.

---

[73] In the USSR in the 1980s there was this difference: physicians had the upper hand over their patients not because of their knowledge, but because a powerful bureaucratic machine sanctioned, even required, the physician's hegemony in the physician's office. See also footnote, p. 440.

[74] Flexner, A., *Medical Education, A Comparative Study*, New York, 1925, p. 8. Flexner, who was pivotal in redirecting American medical education in the 20th C is further discussed on p. 198, footnote.

In summary, one characteristic of the Athenian democracy was toleration of the individual, from which emerged (1) freedom of individuals to organize to advance personal, rather than public or group interests, (2) an appreciation of the uniqueness of the individual, an appreciation that, in medicine, extended not only to the sick person but also to the expression of the disease in that individual, and (3) the ability to interact free from any outside interference, which, in medicine meant that both physician and patient were constrained only by social pressures to which both were equally subject. This, the closest approach to the natural state of medical practice, was not a purposeful societal undertaking, it did not represent organizational efficiency by leaders of the city-state, and it was not one man's bright idea. It was, instead, the effort of a small group of like-minded individuals who saw personal objectives best achieved by this invention, and they were able to achieve their objective because they were not prevented by others from doing so. There is no reason to think that the potential for action by similar small groups did not exist in other times and places. After all, some consider God to have provided all the earth and its manifold variety for man's preservation and enjoyment, and it is not far-fetched to argue that even mankind's great variety is but another manifestation of that plan.[75] The Greek invention was nothing more than an uncovering of potential that lay in wait, and the reason that it occurred in ancient Hellas was that those having a personal interest in medicine, both as a vocation and as a means of self-preferment, were enabled to come together freely in common council. In stark contrast, the medical practices of all other times and places of which we have written knowledge were not formed by the coming together of like-minded individuals for the purpose of rendering improved services to the sick, satisfying personal curiosity, and at the same time bettering themselves, but, reflecting the authoritarian nature of their times, to submit themselves, without exception, to a patron in order to obtain or retain some form of privileged largess.

As a backdrop for the natural state of medical practice, democratization did not so much foster freedom as it deterred those forms of government that would have it checked; it provided a defensive wall for both the individual and the koinon. And that is the great blessing of democracy. While people will argue and politick to obtain personal advantage, and while a semblance of chaos sometimes arises as they do so, as long as authoritarianism is kept in check they will advance and will resolve differences. Few, perhaps none, have declared democracy to be the ideal form of government, for human nature makes a democracy a haven for perpetual bickering and can sometimes give the craven an upper hand. But what it does that has been of such wonderful consequence is to displace alternative forms of governance. And this is all the difference. It explains why different forms of democracy, even its partial variants, are inevitably effective in improving the lot of society: authoritarianism has been diminished. It was only with the advent of a free citizenry that the full range of natural abilities could be exposed to public opinion. The key element in the flourishing of medicine lay not within the profession itself but in the structure of the society in which it existed. Man's progress in medicine, and in most other areas, has been due not to sudden flares of genius or to an ever-increasing intelligence or to brilliant institutional guidance, but to the removal of obstructions that prevent exploitation of his natural abilities. The culture that did this best

---

[75] On the author's daily bus ride to and from his hospital in recent years an elderly woman happened to board from time to time, and as she would slowly progress down the central aisle she would alway say, "Good evening, children," at which everyone in unison would respond, "Good evening." This was often followed by a brief homily: "For God planned that, like flowers, his children should be of different colors and varieties, that they were all beautiful and should love one another."

was to become the dominant culture. That culture arose around the Aegean because its political and social institutions played a permissive role for the display of reason and compromise. Rather than emancipating the profession of medicine, the Greeks, in emancipating man, invented it.

F. Postscript:

Evidence has been presented that supports the notion of a simultaneous, widespread, multifocal, autochthonous "epidemic" of rational activity in several spheres of human endeavor in ancient Hellas. No particular person, no particular political party, and no particular group jumps out at the modern scholar to assert priority in the invention of democracy, liberty of the individual, or a physician-patient relationship founded in trust. It is time, therefore, to recall the opening words of the Introduction to this work: "The essence of equitable human social existence is compromise." The Authoritarian thwarts compromise, for the Authoritarian has his favorites, whether it be in the Star Chamber, in a smoke-filled back room, or in a government office over expense account donuts and coffee. It was the recognition by the ancient Greeks of the practical merit of open dialogue and compromise that led, by stages and by stealth, to democracy and its blessings. True, their compromises were not always fair, and motives were often less than virtuous. After all, arising from the bleakness of tribalism, they did not begin their efforts with a *tabula rasa*. And the motivating force may often have been fear that, by not compromising, all might be lost. But compromise is, if nothing else, an exercise in rationality. As we, in our assemblies and board meetings, in the voting booth, in discussions over the backyard fence, in legislative deliberations, hash out our differences with words rather than with swords, we see the wisdom of the ancient Greeks still at work. While all other societies plagiarize what is convenient of that wisdom for their own purposes, beyond reach of such effrontery stand those Greeks, who first acknowledged, and in such an age, that the same rational intelligence they knew to be part of their own psyche must also abide in their neighbor, and it must be met on equal terms and acknowledged rather than subdued.

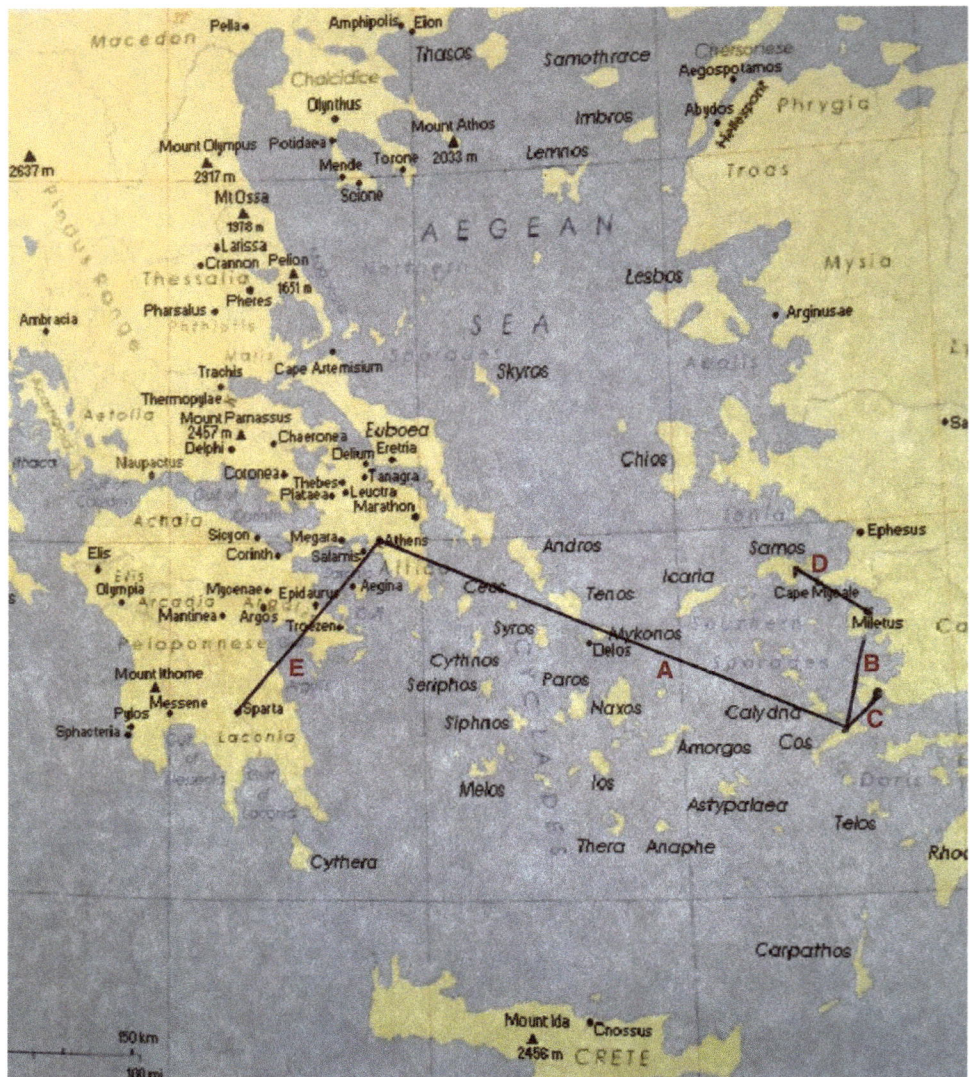

Fig. 9: The ancient Aegean Sea, with direct distances between selected ancient Greek cities for reasons discussed in the text.

A – The island of Cos, purported home of Hippocrates, to Athens: 260 miles.

B – The island of Cos to the preeminent Ionic city of Miletos: 50 miles.

C – The island of Cos to Halicarnassus, home of Herodotus, and Cnidos: 10 miles.

D – Miletos to the island of Samos, its commercial competitor: 30 miles.

E – Athens to Sparta: 95 miles.

CHAPTER ELEVEN

HIPPOCRATES AND THE PROVENANCE OF GREEK MEDICINE

πάλαι ποτ' ησαν ἄλκιμοι Μιλήσοποι.
"Once upon a time long ago the Milesians were brave."

Aristophanes, in *Plutus*, 1002

Hippocrates is the legendary icon for the modern physician. The association of Hippocratic medicine with the modest Doric settlement on the eastern Mediterranean island of Cos is unexpected, for neither geography nor demographics support the idea of a "medical school" on that small island. A more likely source for the origin of medical enlightenment was the ancient city of Miletos located on the coast of Ionia about fifty miles from Cos. Hippocratic medicine, the foundation of modern scientific medicine, was an indigenous Hellenic product, owing nothing to prior or contemporary societies.

A. Hippocrates the Great

Dr. Oswald Spengler wrote of the decline of the West.[1] Others, of a less pessimistic age and place and bolstered by subsequent history, have noted that the West has not declined, has in fact risen.[2] Furthermore, it has "risen" to the point that a future history of mankind will be, barring global calamity, an embellishment on the history of the West. And the history of the West is but the history of ancient Greece in all its manifestations.[3] There will be some debate over such a qualitative statement of Greek transcendence upon the subsequent course of world events, but in one discipline there has been, in the West, little controversy.[4] That discipline is Medicine, its disciple was

---

[1] Spengler, O., *Der Untergang des Abendlandes, Welthistorisches Perspektiven*, Munich, 2 vols., 1918, 1922. The Engish translation, *The Decline of the West*, was published in New York, 1926, 1928.

[2] McNeill, W., *The Rise of the West*, Chicago, 1963. McNeill judged diffusion of innovation from a sequence of superior cultures as promoting a general advancement of mankind, but the unprecedented rise in changes emanating from the West in recent centuries is now permanently installed. More recently McNeill has moderated the role of the West and has cited new scholarly investigations that have uncovered or increased in significance factors that will also likely modify his thesis. See: McNeill, W. H., *The Rise of the West after Twenty-Five Years*, in *J. World History*, 1:1-21, 1990.

[3] This is not just an opinion of the author. The eminent scholar, Bruno Snell, stated: "In Greece, and only in Greece, did theoretic thought emerge without outside influence, and nowhere else was there an autochthonous formation of scientific terms. All other languages are derivative; they have borrowed or translated or got their terms by some other devious route from the Greeks." See: *The Discovery of the Mind*, Cambridge, 1953, translated by T. G . Rosenmeyer, chapter 10, p. 227, The Origin of Scientific Thought.

[4] But see Prof. M. Bernal, *Black Athena Writes Back*, Durham, 2001, the latest in a series of scholarly exchanges regarding the role of Africa in the early development of Western civilization. The exchanges cite and briefly review much of the earlier work on the supposed controversy. Especially relevant are the sections on Greek science.

Hippocrates, and its embassy was located on the island of Cos off the western coast of Asia Minor, modern-day Turkey. While the actual existence of such a person as Hippocrates has been questioned,[5] both Plato[6] and Aristotle,[7] the former a contemporary of Hippocrates, affirm his existence and significance, and Aristophanes, in his comedy *Thesmophorizusai* of 411 BC, makes a seemingly unequivocal mention of the Hippocratic Oath.[8] Current scholarship, popularly presented by Prof. Jouanna, affirms the existence of Hippocrates the Physician.[9]

Some seventy treatises comprise the medical writings attributed at one time or another to Hippocrates. The individual works of the *Hippocratic Corpus*, as the collected writings are called, were composed between approximately 450 and 300 BC. Only a few of the works could have been written by Hippocrates, if indeed he wrote any of them, an opinion shared by Aristotle. They were composed, for the most part, by physicians for physicians, although a few may have been directed at, or even written by, nonphysicians. The earlier writings include the most important and objective treatises. As the 4th C progressed, deductive theory, acknowledgements of divine intervention, and perhaps elitism began to creep into the works.[10] The *Hippocratic Corpus* may have originally come from a library on Cos and then transferred to Alexandria in the 3rd C, but the truth is that its origin(s) is unknown.[11] That there could have been a library on Cos is supported

---

[5] The great student of the *Hippocratic Corpus*, Ludwig Edelstein, maintained lifelong that none of the works were by Hippocrates.

[6] "suppose you had your mind set on going to your namesake, Hippocrates of Cos, the famous physician, to pay him a fee for his services to you, ..."), *Protagoras* 311b. Translation of S. Lombardo and K. Bell, in *Plato, Complete Works*, J. M. Cooper, editor, Indianapolis, 1997. Note that from this quotation it can only be *inferred* that Hippocrates charged a fee for teaching. The second reference to Hippocrates is in Phaedrus, 270, c, d.

[7] "....in the same sense of the word great in which Hippocrates might be called greater, not as a man, but as a physician, ...," Aristotle, *Politeia*, 7.4.1326a15-17, translation of Benjamin Jowett, as included in *The Basic Works of Aristotle*, R. McKeon, editor, New York, 1941.

[8] See: *The Greek Classics: Aristophanes*, El Paso, 2006, translation of The Athenian Society, J. H. Ford, editor. *Thesmophoriazusai* (line 270). Comment: This is a controversial dialogue because some scholars conclude that the Hippocrates referred to in the play was an Athenian general, of whom there were several of this name, but the πάντας θεούς is suggestive of the first line of the Hippocratic Oath.

[9] Jouanna, J. *Hippocrates*, translated by M. B. DeBevoise, Baltimore, 1999. The original version, in French, was published in 1992.

[10] περὶ τεχνης (Concerning the Art) is considered by its translator, W. H. S. Jones, to be a lay composition, and he thinks περὶ φυσων (Breaths) was for public presentation. περὶ εὐσχημοσυνης (Decorum), νομός (Law), and παραγγελιαι (Precepts) he interprets as implying secretive medical knowledge and proceedings. See the *Loeb Classical Library Hippocrates*, volumes I-IV. Nevertheless, the very fact that the seventy or eighty Hippocratic tracts were written down does not suggest any intention of secrecy, a point made by L. Dean-Jones: *Literacy and the Charlatan in Ancient Greek Medicine,* chapter 5 in *Written Texts and the Rise of Literate Culture in Ancient Greece*, Cambridge, 2003, H. Yunis, editor, p. 119.

[11] Jouanna, J., *Hippocrates*, Baltimore, 1999, translated by M. B. DeBevoise. In chapter 4, "Writings in Search of an Author," Jouanna summarizes various opinions on the origin of the Hippocratic manuscripts. To further cloud the issue of authorship of the *Hippocratic Corpus*, Blum has described the dilemma facing modern scholars posed by the 2nd C AD papyrus, *Anonymous Londinensis*, in which its writer criticized those efforts that identified the medical works as Hippocratic based on a bibliographer's presumed knowledge of Hippocratic teachings rather than

by Dr. Elizabeth Craik who provides evidence of a library located on Rhodes, a nearby larger Dorian island, stating that most likely it was housed in the local gymnasium.[12] And there is an inscription listing donors to a Coan library dating from about 200 BC.[13] It is also unknown which, if any, Hippocratic writings were published and which were but collected observations intended for analysis, collation, personal use or proposed for publication.[14]

Dr. Baas, the prominent medical historian, begins his section on Hippocrates by noting the remarkable assemblage of great men in classical Greece, of whom Hippocrates was one: "That he appeared in such an age is an expression of that ever active law of national development, by virtue of which the great minds of any people appear together or in close succession to each other, and as a rule occupy but brief periods of time. In these periods too the nation itself passes through its golden age in a political, social and economical point of view, ere national vigor is corrupted and overwhelmed by the general prosperity." The conclusion of Dr. Baas regarding the decline of national greatness aches for debate, but his statement on the rise of great men rings true: "great men are far more the offspring than the creators of their epochs...."[15] Paraphrasing Oswald Spengler, this great Greek civilization, while fragmented in structure, was cohesive in culture. It has been suggested that its greatness and, ultimately, its destruction are traceable to lack of a central authoritarian figure so prominent in eastern cultures. Nevertheless, ancient Greece, with its "discrete beginning and ending and with no ties or obligations to the past," spanned an epoch that witnessed many great men.

Hippocrates was born on Cos in 460 BC, between the emergence of democratic governance in Athens (507 BC) and the classical Athens of Pericles (*ca.* 450 BC). Just how these two events affected political and intellectual development on the island of Cos is uncertain, for Cos was 260 miles across the eastern sea from Athens and quite the

---

on quotations directly attributable to Hippocrates. See: Blum, R., *Kallimachos, The Alexandrian Library and the Origins of Bibliography*, Madison (WI), 1991, translated by H. H. Wellisch, p. 45.

[12] Information relevant to this and other statements to follow is presented by Craik, E. M., in: *The Dorian Aegean*, London, 1980, the libraries being mentioned in chapter 5, p. 96*f.*

[13] οἶδε ἐπαγγείλαντο εις τὰν βιβλιοθήκαν ("announcing those who [gave] to the library" – BCH (*Bulletin de Correspondance Hellenique*), 59:421, 1935.)

[14] Just how a written work was published in eras dependent on manuscripts is, to a great extent, conjecture. The "publication" of the poems of Solon (early 6th C BC) is thought to indicate the time of their *formal public recitation* rather than a release of manuscripts for sale, and for centuries the masterpieces of Greek playwrights were dated according the date of their first public performance, not the date of written copies. Nevertheless, as time passed there were scriptoria where copyists worked, and in the marketplace, or agora, of Socrates' day there was an area where booksellers could be found, and in Plato's *Apologia*, 26e, it is stated that the books of Anaxagoras were readily available for young men to purchase. Copies of a work might be made at the request of a patron or in anticipation of sales, for copies were apparently available for purchase. Parameters of quality depended on veracity. There were no copyright laws, and no profit accrued to the author from these sales. Athens was a center for the book trade, and citizens in many cities probably had no such local industry and had to purchase books from Athens. If Hippocratic works were solely intended as reference works for use by Hippocratic physicians they may not have been "published" at all, for what general bookseller would take the risk of copying technical works useful to only a few specialists. See also: Croiset, A., Croiset, M., *An Abridged History of Greek Literature*, London, 1904, translated by G. F. Heffelbower, for a general review of the subject, although Hippocratic works are not specifically addressed.

[15] Baas, J. H., *Outlines of the History of Medicine and the Medical Profession*, New York, 1889, H. E. Handerson, translator, p. 99.

antithesis of the bustling city presided over by Pericles. The father of Hippocrates supposedly was a physician and his mother a midwife. His genealogy is said to have been one of a succession of healers to which the term Asclepiadae has been applied, a designation derived from Asclepius, a legendary individual assigned demigod attributes in post-Homeric times as a son of Apollo who was given healing powers by the centaur, Chiron. A wingless serpent entwining the staff of Asclepius is a popular symbol of medicine (p.158 *re*: snakes). The Drs. Edelstein[16] quote Cornutus (*fl.* 60 AD) who states "Asclepius was named from [the words] 'to be gently healed' and 'the withering occurring with [the approach of] death to be delayed.'"[17]   The family of Asclepiads was likened to "all great aristocratic families" by Prof. Jouanna.[18]

Wherever the truth may lie concerning the life of Hippocrates the physician, the Hellenic society that raised him as an icon deserves close attention. Thus, the term "Hippocratic medicine" will be used hereafter to refer to the medicine of Classical Greece (450-323 BC) as expressed in the *Hippocratic Corpus*, even though Hippocratic writings were not the work of one man and included additions well into the post-Classical period.

B. Miletos and the Island of Cos; Portraits in Contrast

Despite the association of Hippocrates with the island of Cos, the ancient centerpiece of Greek culture was not that small island and its Dorian inhabitants. It was, instead, the city-state of Miletos and its Ionians. Sir James Chadwick describes women from "Milatos" as being in the Mycenaean palace at Pylos, *ca.* 1300 BC,[19] suggesting Miletos was either a Mycenaean colony or within its sphere of influence at that early date. But Miletos is presently considered to have been founded about 1050 BC, with the people who settled there from the northern Peloponnese having replaced the preexisting Mycenaean community. At the onset of the Greek Dark Ages (*ca.* 1100 BC) they had fled to Attica, the site of Athens, and thence migrated to the western coast of Asia Minor, at that time already called Ionia. Modern scholars, therefore, consider Milesians as "Attic-Ionians," although it is likely that other refugee groups joined them. Miletos, a port city, early became a prosperous center of commerce by virtue of its shipping. Its neighbor to the east was the emerging powerful inland Lydian state, a factor that, by restricting inland trading, may have led to Miletos' reliance on maritime trade for wealth, one consequence being that it would maintain command of the sea. It was also known for its wool, furniture, and purple dye. Although not a military power, its inhabitants established more than fifty colonies, about one-fifth of all Greek colonies founded between 800-500 BC, and opened trading outposts in Egypt. Glotz reports that at one point it had ninety colonies around the Black Sea.[20]   Miletos was the first Greek city-state to use coinage, thus acquiring commercial advantage, and concurrently metallurgy became a prominent

---

[16] Edelstein, E. J. and Edelstein, L, *Asclepius, Collection and Interpretation of the Testimonies*, Baltimore, 1945.

[17] The probable derivation, found on p. 124 of the above citation, is: σκέλλω (skello) = "I dry up, wither," and ἠπίως (epios) = "gently."

[18] Jouanna, J., *Hippocrates*, translated by M. B. DeBevoise, Baltimore, 1999, Chapters 1 and 2, for a review of sources of the Hippocratic legend.

[19] Chadwick, J., *The Mycenaean World*, Cambridge, 1976, p. 80.

[20] Glotz, G., *Ancient Greece at Work*, New York, 1926, p. 121. Glotz also makes the statement that 6th C BC Milesian guilds contributed to democratic governance.

technology. Perhaps as a consequence of its prosperity and its convenient coastal location with exposure to many cultures, Miletos became the "intellectual center of the Greek world."[21] During the 6th C BC its population may have reached 65,000. Although archaic Greece left relatively little in the historical record, the great natural philosophers first made their appearance in Miletos, along with early historians, geographers, poets, and musicians. The first map, the first writings on navigation, and even suggestions of an evolutionary theory of life emerged at this time and in this place. Lest one think that Miletos was without its own serious problems, it was ruled by tyrants throughout much of the 6th C BC, and despite its flourishing commercial enterprises it is not considered a particularly artistic city for that time. Even its prominent thinkers have been attributed not to its freedoms but to a significant leisured class.[22]

The early governments of some Ionic city-states were more democratic than any on mainland Greece, and this may have been because colonizers lost some of their fealty to ancient customs and, if their number included proportionately fewer of the aristocratic class, were inclined to extend their liberties.[23] A column dated to about 600 BC has been found on the island of Chios that provides clear evidence of democratic participation in governance, and Dr. Tod quotes Dr. Ulrich von Wilamowitz that the column "makes us realize that 'the foundation for the organization of Greek society and the Greek state was laid in Ionia, exactly as for poetry and philosophy.' "[24] James O'Neil also concluded that the concept of democracy was understood in that region.[25] Prof. John Cook stated that among the Ionian cities was found "the first certain and unambiguous apparition of the organized Hellenic polis."[26] He concluded that Ionia led the Hellenic world in the 6th C BC, for it was relatively unsusceptible to "eastern" influences that operated elsewhere in Greece. Dr. Carl Roebuck has described the tribal changes in Ionia as Ionic city-states integrated newer arrivals and local Anatolians into a political system similar to one that, a century later, would be instituted by Cleisthenes in Athens.[27] Perhaps the opportunity for this political maturation was provided in part by protective shielding by the Latmos mountain range just to the east of coastal Ionia as it existed at the time. Contemporary Athens was but a landlocked small city derived from a coalescence of small towns. It had no colony, did not mint coinage until 510 BC, its culture adopting aspects of the more advanced Ionian cities, and in mid-6th C BC its acropolis was little more than a bald and

---

[21] Gorman, V.B., *Miletos, the Ornament of Ionia*, Ann Arbor, 2001, p. 72.

[22] See Dunham, A. G., *The History of Miletus down to the Anabasis of Alexander*, London, 1915, chapter 7, *The influence of commerce and politics upon Milesian literature and art*. And Gorman attributed them to its geography, cultural exposure, and affluence (see preceding citation).

[23] Heeren, A. H. L., *Reflections on the Politics of Ancient Greece*, Boston, 1824, chapter 5 discusses migration, loss of leading families, and a loosening of the "bonds of attachment to the soil and ancient customs...."

[24] Chios is a 325 sq. mi. Greek island three miles off the formerly Ionian coast and about eighty miles from Miletos (see map, Fig. 9.) For the inscription see: Tod, M. N., *A Selection of Greek Historical Inscriptions to the End of the Fifth Century B.C.*, Oxford, 1933, pp. 1-3. It is contained in the section entitled *The Constitution of Chios.*"

[25] O'Neil, James L., *The Origins and Development of Ancient Greek Democracy*, Lanham, MD, 1995, p. 21*ff*. He includes the Greek text on the column.

[26] Cook, J. M., in *Cambridge Ancient History*, Cambridge, 3, II (2), 804.

[27] Roebuck, C., *Tribal Organization in Ionia*, in *Transactions and Proceedings of the American Philological Association*, 93:495-507, 1961.

rocky hill.[28]

Unfortunately for the Greeks, Persia ultimately conquered the cities of the Ionian coast. Miletos had been an independent oligarchy until 560 BC when it was subjugated, along with the rest of Ionia, first by the kingdom of Lydia and then by the Persian monarch, Cyrus the Great. Mardonius, son-in-law of the Persian monarch, Darius, promoted democracy in several Ionian cities in the early 5th C, from which one might think that democracy was not a Greek invention. But Mardonius was merely reintroducing, as an expedient, what had previously functioned in those particular cities. Notwithstanding this expedient, many Ionians foresaw the ultimate consequences of Persia's expansion to the Aegean coast and therefore fled the region for the west.[29] The remainder attempted, unsuccessfully, to withstand the eastern intrusion by force of arms. Bengtson has concluded that the Ionian rebellion in 499 BC, centered at Miletos, had its origins, like the Stamp Act in America, in abridgments of freedom by the Persians rather than in economic or other factors.[30] Whatever the final incitement, Miletos was destroyed in 494 BC by the Persians, and, relevant to the origin of Greek scientific medicine, Persia maintained control over Ionia and nearby Dorian cities until defeated by the Greeks at Salamis and Plataea in 480/79, which was about twenty years before the birth of Hippocrates on the island of Cos, less than fifty miles from Miletos (Fig. 9).[31]

The island of Cos was the antithesis of Miletos. With an area of 109 square miles, it is located a few miles off the southwest coast of modern Turkey.[32] The residents of ancient Cos claimed descent from Sparta. As a center of medical learning its fame predated Hippocrates. Yet, this sleepy Dorian settlement had, until the 5th C BC, no written records of any kind, and furthermore it has been suggested that the absence of any Coan record concerning Hippocrates is consistent with the apparent absence of literature from Cos throughout the 5th C BC.[33] Dr. Susan Sherwin-White has commented on "…our almost complete ignorance of Coan institutions before the foundation of Kos [city] in 366…"[34] Its rugged coastline, especially the southern, and its single harbor permitted only a pastoral society known for its cabbage, and perhaps its modest means preserved it from destructive wars in that part of the Mediterranean. Cos had been included by Homer among the contributors of ships to the fleet of Agamemnon during the Trojan War, and even at that early date, ca. 1200 BC, may have been Dorian. When the Ionian Greek colonies along the coast revolted against the Persians, the Dorian segments of society were not prominent in their support of the Ionians, although, being Greek, their sympathies were not with the Persian. And when the revolt was put down in 546 BC Cos,

---

[28] For a brief description of 6th C Athens with a comparison to the cities of Ionia see: Linforth, I. M., *Solon the Athenian*, Berkeley, 1919, p. 30*ff.*

[29] For a comprehensive review of the dramatic events of 6th C Ionia see: Hurwit, J. M., *The Art and Culture of Early Greece*, 1100-480 BC, Ithaca, 1985, especially chapter 5.

[30] Bengtson, H., *The Greeks and the Persians*, London, 1969.

[31] The lack of evidence for a medical heritage attributable to early Miletos is profound. The subject is not mentioned in the histories of Miletos by Dunham, A. G. (*The History of Miletus*, London, 1915), Laale, H. W. (*Once They Were Brave the Men of Miletus*, Bloomington, 2007), or Gorman, V. B. (*Miletos, The Ornament of Ionia: A History of the City to 400 B.C.E.*, Ann Arbor, 2001).

[32] Cos is roughly thirty miles long and an average of two-three miles wide, with a rugged ridge extending along much of its southern coast. As for its size of 109 sq. mi., the area of ancient Attica, the location of Athens, was about 700 square miles.

[33] Paton, W. R. and Hicks, E. L. *Inscriptions of Cos*, Oxford, 1891, footnote p. xxvi.

[34] Sherwin-White, S. M., *Ancient Cos*, Gottingen, 1978, Chapter 4, *The Social Structure of the Community*, p. 153. She in fact generalizes this to include all the Dorian colonies (*ibid.*, xviii).

along with other Dorian islands, was under Persia's control and even contributed some ships to the Persian cause at the battle of Salamis. But with the defeat of the Persians in 480 BC Cos became a member of the Delian League of Greek city-states and remained an ally of Athens up to the time of the Peloponnesian War in 428 BC, although it had little political influence.[35]

Prior to the last half of the 4th C it was not a wealthy island, for its Athenian tribute in mid-5th C was modest compared to most other city-states, and it never did develop a commercial trading area on the coast of Asia Minor just a few miles opposite (Fig. 9).[36] Although a visitor to Cos city today will enjoy a small, charming, and thriving community on a small harbor and can explore excavations of a magnificent Asclepeion bordering its suburbs, this city was built in 366 BC. But the city of Hippocrates in the mid-5th C BC was located near Kephalos on the opposite (western) end of the island. Named Astypalaios and not to be confused with the nearby island of Astypalaia, it lay near a small cove that now harbors a modern but out-of-the-way resort. In contrast to the magnificent 4th C Asclepeion near Cos city on the eastern end of the island, only a few crude foundations are to be seen in the area of 5th C Astypalaios, with the exception of an early Christian church built within the ruins of an ancient temple. The coastal remnants of ancient Astypalaios for the most part remain to be discovered under modern hotels and eateries, but, surrounded by formidable hills, it is unlikely to have been a populous and wealthy city.[37]

There were other Dorian settlements nearby. To the east of the island of Cos was Halicarnassus. Being on the mainland, Halicarnassus was more open to Ionian culture and literature. Herodotus was born there when it was under Persian rule. Dr. Sherwin-White commented that Herodotus used a comprehensive approach to writing history, combining geography and ethnography with such factual or anecdotal history as he was able to obtain, similar to the approach of Hippocrates, who uniquely interweaved

---

[35] Nelson, E. D., *Coan Asylia: Small-State Diplomacy and the Hippocratic Legend*, in *Regionalism and Globalism in Antiquity*, F. DeAngelis, editor, Walpole, MA, 2013, pp. 247-266, which describes Coan attempts to heighten its reputation among among the greater powers in Hellenistic times. This most interesting study also casts the popular perception of Hippocrates in a new light, separating the legendary figure from the authentic one.

[36] Apparently fragmentary lists limit conclusions regarding tribute, but a tribute of three talents is given for 450 BC, increasing to five talents ten years later, significant sums, indicating Coan prosperity after it joined the Athenian confederation.

[37] Mention should also be made of the island of the Samos, 62 miles north of Cos. Artifacts and excavations indicate that in the 8th through the 6th C this island was far in advance of Attica. A walk around the cities of Pythagorion on Samos and Astypalaios on Cos quickly confirms the likely preeminence of the former. Herodotus, in his *Histories* (III, 139), delared Samos to be the greatest of all Greek cities. Also, Samos was the center for the greatest quantity of imported goods of all Hellenic regions. Despite this, there is only one mention of a medical item in the two present-day Samian archeological museums, and that one is a Roman-era scoop that could just as well have been used for cosmetics. There was not one reference to healing at a local Asclepeion nor a single Asclepian rod. Despite the earlier richness and extensive trade of Samos, medicine as a profession left no mark, suggesting that if scientific medicine did originate in the region it is more likely to have been in Miletos or other mainland city-state. Samos was often in conflict with Miletos, probably because of trading competition, whereas the nearby island of Chios was consistently sympathetic to Miletos. The ancient history of medicine in Chios is an unexplored subject.

medicine with environmental and social considerations.[38] Were the course of history nicely balanced the two would have been neighbors, or at least would have known each other. But Herodotus makes no mention of Hippocrates, his younger contemporary, and it is even more remarkable that he makes no mention of a medical school on Cos, merely ten miles distant.[39] He does, however, name Croton, about 900 miles distant in Italy, as the source of the foremost physicians in the late 6th C, second place going to Cyrene in North Africa, although even here he does not use any term that might, with certainty, be translated as "school."[40, 41]

William Paton concluded that in early 4th C Cos ("B.C. 394 onwards") the "political life of Cos was still very backward and undeveloped."[42] Subsequently, its influence and prosperity grew, Cos becoming prominent only after 350 BC, some time after the presumed date of the death of Hippcrates (380 BC). With the suzerainty of Ptolemaic Egypt Cos retained an autonomy that was enviable when compared to other islands and colonies in the region. Aristotle claims that Cos became famous for its silk. Furthermore, Cos was located on important trade routes connecting Egypt, Rhodes, Sicily, and the Dardanelles. With the founding and prominence of Alexandria, close communication with that center of learning was maintained. Physicians were attracted to Alexandria from Cos, which Dr. Sherwin-White has described as a "brain drain,"[43] and perhaps for this reason there have been few 4th C BC medically relevant inscriptions found on Cos. Nevertheless, its wealth and freedoms were retained through the 3rd C BC.

It is puzzling as to why Cos became the Hellenic center of medical excellence. Cos is not mentioned as the residence of a single patient in the Hippocratic works called Επιδημιων ("Of the Epidemics," or, more accurately, "House Calls"), of which there are seven Books that include approximately 380 case histories, whereas cities in Thessaly, Thrace, Scythia, Macedonia, the Peloponnese, Attica, and in some Aegean islands are mentioned.[44] Overall, the very few Coans identified in the entire *Hippocratic Corpus* do

---

[38] See the Introduction of: Paton, W. R., and Hicks, E. L., *Inscriptions of Cos*, Oxford, 1891, and also see: Sherwin-White, S. M., *Ancient Cos*, Gottingen, 1978, p. 39. These excellent books are well-researched histories of Cos in its early years.

[39] Herodotus (c. 484-420 BC) published his history not before 425 BC, as the latest information in it is from that year.

[40] ἐγένετο γὰρ ὢν τοῦτο ὅτε πρῶτοι μὲν Κροτωνιῆται ἰητροὶ ἐλέγοντο ἀνὰ τὴν Ἑλλάδα ειναι, δεύτεροι δὲ Κυρηναῖοι. "For it occurred thus that the Croton physicians were the foremost throughout Hellas, and the next [were] Cyrenes." Herodotus, *The Histories*, Bk.3, 131, 3, translation by the author.

[41] Galen himself refers to Cnidus, Cos, and the "schools" of medicine in Italy as χοροι, meaning "a band or troop of persons" and from which is derived the English "chorus," rather than a σχολή (skola; "school") or διδασκαλεῖον (didaskalion; "school") (Galen, X, 5 [Kuhn]). Galen, of course, lived six hundred years later.

[42] Paton, W. R., and Hicks, E. L., *The Inscriptions of Cos*, Oxford, 1891, p. xxvii.

[43] Sherwin-White, S., *Ancient Cos*, Gottingen, 1978, p. 256*ff.*

[44] The 380 patients are, for the most part, specified by name. Their descriptions vary in detail and a few are mentioned in more than one Book of the *Epidemics*. The number of 380 is, therefore, approximate. The reader may be interested in comparing a relatively modern version of the *Epidemics* by consulting Dr. R. C. Cabot's book, *Differential Diagnosis* (Phila., 1911), in which he gives case histories of 383 of his patients. Cabot, apart from his clinical prowess, initiated the field of medical social work, personally paid the salaries of its first employees that his hospital declined to support, and in 1923 introduced the venerable Case Records of the Massachusetts General Hospital into what would be renamed the *New England Journal of Medicine*.

not support a Coan source for a significant portion of its clinical material. An alternative explanation, therefore, is that medicine first flourished elsewhere in Hellenic lands, perhaps in Miletos, with Hippocrates and Cos being given more credit than is their due. After all, the Hippocratic works were written in Ionic Greek, the dialect of Miletos, rather than the Doric Greek of Cos.[45] And since the story about Hippocrates curing the famous Democritus is apocryphal, perhaps an Ionian in Miletos was the originator of what would be the *Hippocratic Corpus*. Furthermore, Apollo, by whom the Hippocratic Oath is sworn, was the traditional protector of Miletos.

Unfortunately, the medical establishment of Miletos will be forever unknown. While the Persian domination of Ionia from 540-479 BC was not initially severe, a succession of revolts occurred among Ionian Greek cities. "The Mede [Cyrus] was feared and hated, and his rule abhorred, and the great intellectual development which characterized Ionia ceased. One is tempted to draw an analogy between the dispersal of the Ionian philosophers by the Persians and the persecution of the Jews by modern Nazism."[46] As a consequence of the revolts, Darius, the son of Cyrus, destroyed Miletos in 494 BC as an example to the rest of Ionia. So devastated was the city that Gorman has stated ". . . there is not a single artifact that can be securely dated to the years between 494 and 479 ... ."[47] But Miletos came to employ secular leadership and accepted an Athenian-style constitution.[48] Conceivably this redeployed social environment was promoting scientific medicine about the time Hippocrates was born. But as there is no record of this, and given the turmoil surrounding the revolt, destruction, and reconstruction of Miletos and surrounding towns, there must have been a powerful check on the development of local medicine, perhaps erasing any earlier documentation of the type of medical practice subsequently termed "Hippocratic." Population estimates of Miletos in the 5th C are as low as 7,500, as reviewed by Gorman, down from the estimated 65,000 a century earlier. Had Persia been restrained and had not Miletos been razed, virtually, to the ground, there may have been the Milesian School of Medicine, the Milesian Corpus of medical writings, and the Classical Age of Miletos rather than of Athens. In support of this opinion, Prof. Craik, referring to the postulated medical school on the island of Cos, states: "The growth to prominence of the school of medicine in Kos owed much to the Milesian activity, ..."[49]

C. The Provenance of Greek Medicine

The early Greeks assumed the foundation for their medicine was ancient. In περὶ ἀρχαιης ἰητρικης ("Concerning Ancient Medicine"), a treatise of the *Hippocratic*

---

[45] Perhaps relevant is that Ionic prose writing also originated in the late 6th C BC in the hands of Milesians such as Hekataios, and as such was used by Herodotus in his histories. The earliest "Hippocratic" treatises, also prose works, may predate Herodotus. See Gorman, V.B., *Miletos, the Ornament of Ionia*, Ann Arbor, 2001, p. 81-82. Parenthetically, there is no known Hippocrates of Miletos, although a near contemporary and famed mathematicion named Hippocrates was from Chios, ninety miles distant. Interestingly, the name "Hippocrates"

[46] Gask, G. E., *Early Medical Schools*, in *Annals of Medical History*, Third Series, Vol. 1, 1939, pp. 128-157.

[47] Gorman, V.B., *Miletos, the Ornament of Ionia*, Ann Arbor, 2001, p. 212.

[48] Freeman, K. *Greek City-States*, London, 1950, p. 170.

[49] Craik, E. M., *The Dorian Aegean*, London, 1980, chapter 5, p. 90.

Corpus some consider the most likely to have come from Hippocrates himself, it is stated that "very long ago there already existed in medicine, both the first principles and the means having been discovered, ..."[50] There is little to support this claim. Citations expressing admiration for prehistoric medicine in ancient Hellas merely followed the same path as those citing the medical practices of ancient civilizations in China, Egypt, and India in that they attempted to make venerable a distant and unknowable past that tradition would not permit to be controverted. They also assumed that something could not have arisen from nothing, and logic demanded a precursor to the profession.

Sir John Mahaffy, on the other hand, thought Greek medicine found its origin in hygiene rather than in early attempts to ease illness.[51] He noted that, in Olympic competition, Greeks knew that "amulets and spells were of no use against better physical condition," and thus rational means were used to optimize the latter.[52] Clinical medicine, however, deals with the urgent practicalities of human suffering. There is no natural progression from the science of attaining the optimal fitness for already healthy athletes to the profession of medicine. The Hippocratics realized this:

> "Gymnastics and medicine are by nature opposites, for gymnastics is not intended to bring about any changes whereas medicine must, since the healthy person is not benefited by changes from his present state, but the ill one is."

> περὶ τοπων των κατὰ ανθρωπον (*On Places in Man*, 35, translation of P. Potter, *Loeb Classical Library*, *Hippocrates*, vol. VIII)

Greek medicine was not the outgrowth of an Olympic fetish.

And medical plagiarism did not assist in the birth of Greek medicine. In the first place, there is no evidence of foreign influence. The medical vocabulary of the *Hippocratic Corpus* was totally Greek. It was a makeshift vocabulary that used common everyday terms in a formulaic way, pressed into service for describing newly recognized physical phenomena. There are no medical terms that can be tied in any way to the medicine or language of any other prior or contemporary civilization.[53] Ancient Greek terminology as applied to medicine was indigenous, and the roots of individual medical terms are, as is the Greek language itself, solely of Indo-European origin. Prof. Longrigg states that nowhere do classical age Greeks attribute the origin of their medicine to any other culture, although he points out they were typically generous in acknowledging the

---

[50] "ἰητρικὴ δὲ πάλαι πάντα ὑπάρχει, καὶ ἀρχὴ καὶ ὁδὸς εὑρημένη...," *Ancient Medicine*, 2, 28-9, from vol. 1 of the *Loeb Classical Library* series on Hippocrates, translated by W. H. S. Jones.

[51] Mahaffy, J. P., *Social Life in Greece from Homer to Menander*, London, 1902, p. 291.

[52] Plato dates "modern" medicine from Herodicus, by "modern" meaning the age that actively combatting disease (playing "nursemaid" to disease) first entered mankind's experience. How did Herodicus torture himself? "By making his dying a lengthy process. Always tending his mortal illness, he was nonetheless, it seems, unable to cure it, so he lived out his life under medical treatment, with no leisure for anything else whatever. .....because his skill made dying difficult, he lived into old age." *Republic* III, 406,a,b. Translation of G. M. A. Grube in: *Plato Complete Works*, Indianapolis, 1997, J. M. Cooper, editor.

[53] Most entries of an American medical dictionary are partly or wholly derived from other languages. Were all the words with transparent affiliations with Greek or Latin removed from the modern American medical dictionary, it would be a slim volume indeed.

priority of others.[54]   But there are other arguments for an autochthonous Hellenic medicine.

1. It is illogical that a burgeoning and popular medical practice emerging in flourishing mid-5th C BC Greece should be derived from archaic remnants of a mystical medical system in a society that "had fallen into powerless decay"[55] and had squandered, over two millennia, its options for improvement. This argument is supported by the statement of Prof. von Staden, who felt that there was no progress in "pervasive magico-religious" Egyptian medicine between the Middle Kingdom (1986-1759 BC) and the 2nd C AD.[56]

2. Prof. Mark Geller cites some basic differences in Babylonian and Greek texts: (1) Babylonian texts were anonymous, whereas Greek physicians were able to identify with their works; (2) Babylonian texts, in contrast to Greek texts, do not refer to diet or to regimens for healthfulness; (3) differing opinions are absent from Babylonian texts, whereas alternative viewpoints are common in Greek texts; (4) case histories are found only in the Greek writings; (5) Greek treatments included dietary manipulation, whereas the Babylonian remained strictly herbal. Dr. Geller concludes that there is no certain evidence of any borrowing by the Greeks of Babylonian medical practices.[57]

3. Incantations, important therapies of organized medicine in many archaic societies, had no role whatever in Hippocratic medicine. This is not to say that expressions of religious piety and faith were not at times displayed.

4. Doctrinal similarities have suggested that some writers of the *Hippocratic Corpus* may have accepted and expanded the Ayurvedic concept of four humors, thus indicating influence emanating from the Indian subcontinent. It is proposed, however, that the initial Hippocratic reference in *Medicine I* to humors was in fact a description of the process of inflammation, not humoral imbalance.[58]

5. One example given by Saunders as indicating Egyptian influence on Greek medicine in this age was the latter's adoption of the Egyptian practice of temple incubation in which

---

[54] Longrigg, J., *Greek Rational Medicine*, 1993, p. 11.

[55] Hamilton, E., *The Echo of Greece*, New York, 1957, p. 16.

[56] Von Staden, H., in his Introduction to: *Herophilus; The Art of Medicine in Early Alexandria*, Cambridge, 1989. He gives extensive evidence against any Egyptian influence on Hellenic medicine as it evolved in Alexandria at the beginning of the 3rd C BC. Isocrates, in *Busiris* 21-23 (*Isocrates, Loeb Classical Library*, vol. I, translated by G. Norlin), attributes medical excellence in drugs to Egyptian priests, a consequence of the privileged status given to them by mythical King Busiris, the founder of Egypt, but Isocrates admits his opinion to be mere speculation. There was a cult of the Egyptian goddess Isis on the Greek island of Delos in the 3rd C BC, but it was initiated by an Egyptian priest, *i.e.*, it was an export of the Egyptians rather than an import by the Hellenes. (See: Bergman, J., *Ich bin Isis*, in *Acta Univ. Upsal*, Uppsala, 1968.)

[57] Geller, M. J., *West Meets East: Early Greek and Babylonian Diagnosis*, p. 11, and *Bloodletting in Babylonia*, p. 305, in: *Magic and Rationality in Ancient Near Eastern and Graeco-Roman Medicine*, H. Horstmanshoff and M. Stol, editors, volume 27 in *Studies in Ancient Medicine*, Leiden, 2004.

[58] See: Adams, W. H., *The Natural State of Medical Practice: Escape from Egalitarianism*, Maitland (FL), 2019, p. 321*ff.*

dreams were used to guide therapy.[59] This is said to have led to the cult of Asclepius becoming popular throughout Greece after appearing in Athens in 420 BC. But no matter wherever or in what form it was espoused, it had nothing whatever to do with the course of rational, then scientific, medicine of the Hippocratics, and the sooner the accounts of magical snake healing and the rest are forgotten the better. They are no longer amusing. And while dreams were given some clinical attention by the Hippocratics, it has been noted that dreams were considered by them to reflect the health status of the body, just as might mood or facies.[60] Temple healing should be recognized for what it was and no more: hope for the hopeless or the impatient.[61]

6. There appears to have been no transmission from Egypt to Greece of knowledge of the medicinal value of foodstuffs.

7. There is no evidence that regions to the east of India had intellectual contact with early Greek medicine. A multifocal origin for commonplace observations is to be expected.[62] And virtually all Egyptian items now displayed in Greek archeological museums were imported rather than of local manufacture, and their displays are impossible to confuse with Greek ones. Intermediate forms are not seen. But the *sine qua non* is that 7th C BC medicine was nothing to be proud about, no matter where it was found, and even if an element of some Egyptian medical practice did in fact find a place in Greek medicine it would remain but an irrelevant fact in the bigger picture.

8. The absence of any written record of medical achievement in Greece prior to the Classical Age was reviewed in the preceding chapter. Had Egyptian medicine been introduced in Greece's formative years, there should be evidence of this, for medical writing in Egypt had already existed for two thousand years. As an example, up to recent times in the West there was panache attached to a physician's prescription written in Latin.

---

[59] Saunders, J. B. de C. M., *The Transitions from Ancient Egyptian to Greek Medicine*, Kansas, 1963, pp. 11-12.

[60] Dreams were part of the practice of incubation healing in Asclepian temples, and it is proposed that sleep following a ritual act invited the gods to reveal some beneficial portent or cure via a dream. See: Harrisson, J., *The Classical Greek Practice of Incubation and Some Near Eastern Predecessors*, found at *www.academia.edu*, 2007. Also see: Holowchack, M. A., *Interpreting Dreams for Corrective Regimen: Diagnostic Dreams in Greco-Roman Medicine*, in *J. Hist. Med. and Allied Sci.* 56:382-399, 2001. And the distinction between interpreters of prophetic dreams and physicians is made clear in *Regimen* IV, 87 and 88, in vol. 4 of the *Loeb Classical Library* series on Hippocrates, p. 423*ff.*

[61] See especially chapters 2 and 3 of: Wickkiser, B. L., *The Appeal of Asklepios and the Politics of Healing in the Greco-Roman World*, U. of Mich., 2003, doctoral dissertation.

[62] But there is another most important factor affecting diffusion of knowledge, and that is the portability of that knowledge. Medical knowledge over the ages has been *parochial*. It was not a commodity for barter or trade, its practice useful only on a local scale. A written language, on the other hand, was a most useful implement for commerce, local and distant. Thus, the Phoenician alphabet of 1000 BC, once its value became clear, was rapidly integrated, with modifications, in many regions, from India to ancient Greece and its colonies. Its propagation was still "hand-to-hand," but those hands travelled far and wide that diffused that most practical invention. It is important to keep this distinction in mind as these chapters unfold, for the parochial nature of medical knowledge and medical practice prior to the modern age has influenced its history.

CHAPTER TWELVE

ANCIENT COAN MEDICAL ORGANIZATIONS

Greek democracy in the 5th C BC tolerated autonomous small groups, and as population increased so did trade and craft guilds. There existed on the island of Cos and nearby Cnidus medical families belonging to an ancient guild(s) of physicians, the Asclepiadae, an exclusive and protectionary hereditary organization. This guild disappeared in the 4th C BC at a time when guild membership was otherwise on the rise. It had been replaced with another type of medical organization, one presumably initiated by Hippocrates on the island of Cos. The type of organization that best fits with the course of Hippocratic medicine is a medical koinon, a small but democratically interactive group of autonomous practitioners. It was with the koinon that the science of medicine would be invented.

A. Introduction: The Source of Hippocratic Achievement

There have been many reasons advanced to explain the ascendancy of ancient Greeks, including those Prof. Gomperz:
1. "[a] conjunction of natural gifts and conditions"
2. "teeming wealth of constructive imagination"
3. "sleepless critical spirit which shrank from no test of audacity"
4. "...sharpest faculty for descrying and distinguishing"
5. "The religion of Hellas, which ... left the intelligence free"
6. "...rival centers of intellect, of a friction of forces"
7. "...order of state and society strict enough to curb the excesses"
But such generalizations present no competition for the simple message that fits best: the freedom of the common man and woman to pursue self-interest through common council. In this chapter the koinon is characterized as a common council for advancing parochial self-interest for professionals in general and medical professionals in particular.

Sir Alfred Zimmern flatly states, "City State life was, in fact, democratic."[1] But the benefits of democracy to the autonomous Greek city-states resided not just in democratic decision-making that guided city-state policy. They were also to be discerned in internal democratically-arrived-at decisions exploiting commercial opportunities within the city-state. With the advent of democracy protection was now pledged by laws which each citizen had a hand in devising, and tribal protections were no longer essential. The individual was now able to make his own selection of alliances. In the bigger picture freedom to pursue self-interest within a group through a membership with similar goals is of greater moment than individual action.

Arthur Koestler discusses the principles of organization as they relate to the individual: a system of feedback controls and external and internal sensors are the basis for the act of creation, the "domain of the individual."[2] But without implementation the "act" of creation is but an entertaining thought. The act of creation, when restricted to an individual, is a personal triumph, and genius and personal satisfaction can be found in the

---

[1] Zimmern, A., *The Greek Commonwealth*, Oxford, 1922, 3rd editor, p. 271.
[2] Koestler, A., *The Act of Creation*, New York, 1964.

domain of the slave, but who would ever know? A koinon, by announcing, improving, preserving, and amplifying a new idea, helps ensure it is not wasted, and society is the better for it. The famous medical organization of Cos that was associated with Hippocrates may have represented a successful implementation of this concept. Through a physicians' organization whose goal was to improve its members' service, public image, and, presumably, income, the intelligent efforts of many men could be applied to common problems. Frances Parkman (1823-1893) wrote of the opportunities of American democracy to the individual: "...men, lost elsewhere in a crowd, stand forth as agents of Destiny," referring to the benefits that freedoms offered by the New World gave to the minions of the Old.[3] This might be rephrased: "self-interest groups, suppressed elsewhere lest they confront and threaten established order," can do the same. What was the nature of the medical organization of Cos? This chapter poses the koinon to explain the ascendancy of Greek medicine.

B. Was There a Medical Guild of Cos?

Dr. Tod commented on the existence of voluntary Greek mercantile or craft associations as early as the 6th C BC, but he felt their significance to be limited, which he attributed to the fact that the many traditional Hellenic allegiances, such as those to *phratrie* or to *gens*, left little time or interest for guild development.[4] Later, in the 5th BC city-state, trade associations remained ill-defined and guilds were more common but small, usually with no more than ten or twenty members. Among them were the physicians of 5th C BC Cos and nearby Cnidus who are said to have traced a common professional and ancestral origin back to the demigod, Asclepius. How important the promotion of this ancestral religious affiliation was to medicine is uncertain, but it may have been essential to survival of their local medical monopoly, or medical guild. Declaration of a linear descent from a demigod likely prompted the laity to infer that members were not only imbued with communal values but also had privileged divine assistance in addition to technical skill, an advertising triumph.

When the traditional and political structure of Greek society underwent major disruption in the 4th and 3rd C BC, Greek guilds were common. They served primarily as niduses of religious and social activities for tradesmen and their families in a world of increasing social instability. Prof. Zimmern describes associations that provided opportunities for their membership to socialize and to "talk shop," although he terms them θίασοι (thiasoi).[5] Membership in a guild included all employees, both labor and management, who pursued a particular trade. The 4th C BC guild was not a political or

---

[3] Parkman, F., *Pioneers of France in the New World*, Boston, 1907, Revised edition, Introduction, p. 10.

[4] Tod, M., *Sidelights on Greek History*, Blackwell, 1932, esp. pp. 76-96.

[5] Zimmern, A., *The Greek Commonwealth*, Oxford, 1924, p. 269. But the *thiasoi* were a structural part of the tribal *phratries* and provided services to the ancient family lines (*gens*) to which they were attached by time and custom, and as such were not free-standing groups of like-minded individuals or familial trades as proposed for the Asclepiadae. Furthermore, W.H.S. Jones points out that *thiasoi* uniformly had some form of religious affiliation (*Loeb Classical Library, Hippocrates*, vol. II, p. 335). Recapitulating, tribes were composed of *phratries* (brotherhoods), which were in turn composed of *gens* (families) and their associates (*thiasoi*). The basic unit was the household, or οἶκός (oikos).

economic force, but it was a significant social presence. In medicine, however, what had been called the family "guild" of the Asclepiadae had ceased to be mentioned in the historical record by that time, although identification of certain physicians with the legendary family name of Asclepiadae (derived from the deified Asclepius of many generations earlier) was still being applied in the 1st C AD to, among others, the infamous physician, Xenophon. Also, Asclepiad has been suggested as the name for priest-healers attached to Asclepian temples, some of which remained popular well into the Roman era. Confusion, therefore, surrounds the meaning of "Asclepiad" as used over several centuries, and the Drs. Edelstein consider that it is the "hero" Asclepius, rather than his later status as a physician/healer assigned to him by Hesiod, from which physicians derive their icon.[6] But it can be inferred that the association(s) to which the term was applied must have been very loose to have escaped a more careful description by contemporary writers. It certainly was no labor union as generally understood today.

There also were individual Greek physicians employed under contract by cities and demes around the eastern Mediterranean. Termed δημόσιοι ἰατροί (demosioi iatroi, or "public physicians"), Prof. Louis Cohn-Haft noted that such physicians were retained under contract by cities in order that there would always be some fee-for-service medical care available to the community, in addition to contractural obligations relevant to the health of the community at large. Obtaining such a post was competitive. Some of these "public physicians" were identified with the island of Cos. Thus, rather than an agent of a guild, this connection of dispersed physicians with an attachment to a single location suggests a common feature of their profession. Perhaps it was a place of medical education, for Plato had declared it required payment of a fee, something like a medical school.

C. Was There a Medical School of Cos?

Greater focus is needed on ancient medical institutions rather than on a famous handful of sometimes notorious ancient medical personalities. Most textbooks of medical history do not do this. The earliest known "medical school" some say was founded at the Temple of Sais in the western Nile delta at the direction of the Persian monarch, Darius I (558-486 BC). Associated with that temple was Neith, usually described as a goddess of war, weapons, and wisdom, but apparently also a protectress during childbirth. The Temple of Neith at Sais, however, along with many other ancient Egyptian temples, contained an "archival" chamber, sometimes referred to as the *House of Life*. This chamber, or hall, included a scriptorium or library and other accessories of knowledge, and its use was restricted to priests of the temple. It was not a scientific institution and certainly was not a medical school. [7] About this time there also was a "medical school" at Croton in Magna Graecia, and Herodotus wrote that "the best physicians in Greek countries were those of Croton, and next to them those of Cyrene."[8] He does not, however, use any word that might be construed as indicating a "school." Furthermore, he states that the reputation of the Croton physicians was due primarily to the reputation of

---

[6] E. J. Edelstein and L. Edelstein, *Asclepius: Collection and Interpretation of the Testimonies*, Baltimore, a 1998 reprint of the 1945 original, pp. 53-64.

[7] Gardiner, A. H., *The House of Life*, in *J. Egypt. Archeol.*, 24:157-79, 1938; Galinghouli, P., *Early Specialization in Ancient Eqypt...*, in *Med. Hist.*, 13:383-386, 1969.

[8] Herodotus, *The Histories*, III, 131, translation of A. D. Godley, *Loeb Classical Library*.

but one man, the physician, Democedes. Despite this, it is often stated that the Croton "medical school" was started by a Milesian natural philosopher, Alcmaeon (*fl. ca.* 500 BC). Dr. Arcieri has described Alcmaeon as one "who initiated scientifical or experimental medicine," who used inductive reasoning, and who pursued dissection and vivisection of animals and "direct studies" of corpses to further the understanding of human biology and pathology.[9] Alcmaeon's fame, however, reflects his reputation as a Greek philosopher-scientist rather than as a clinician, a "real doctor." And yet, it is a "real doctor" who is given the responsibility of teaching clinical medicine, and it is as a "real doctor," rather than a sometime investigator in the health sciences, that Hippocrates of Cos has been accorded fame in perpetuity. Nevertheless, Arcieri claims ten of the greatest schools of medicine came from a common source, Alcmaeon's medical school at Croton, although he does not list them.

It is best to disregard the idea of a traditional medical school when considering ancient medical training, and even the advice of Dr. Jouanna regarding the probable nature of a school, or σχολή ("skoleh"), as the work of individual "masters" centrally located in population centers, while realistic, is hypothetical, at least for 5th C BC Greece.[10] Medical schools now have professors, classrooms, buildings, and the paraphernalia of organization. Nothing of the sort is identifiable of a Coan medical school, nor did any ancient writer provide a physical description of such a place.[11] Medical instruction was meted out not through books or classes. It was instilled through direct intercourse between a master and his apprentice, with mutual transmission of knowledge, questions, and clarifications. This form of medical apprenticeship was the norm in the West well into the 19th C. Just how a pattern of apprenticeships in medicine might have accommodated a "class" of medical students on the island of Cos is unknown, and indeed is difficult to imagine.

Prof. Vivian Nutton has also cautioned against exaggerating the importance of the so-called "schools" of ancient medicine (see preceding footnote). This is sound advice, for, small in size and population and with uninviting commercial prospects and a Spartan heritage, the island of Cos could have supported the aspirations of few medical students. Probably the concept of a formal "school" on Cos is misleading in all but one

---

[9] Arcieri, G. P., *Why Alcmaeon of Croton is the Father of Experimental or Scientific Medicine*, New York, 1970. Alcmaeon was a pupil of Pythagoras of Samos (580-489 BC) whose school, although perhaps it should be termed a "cult," was established at Croton about 550 BC. This religious sect instilled unique views of natural philosophy, not medicine, relying heavily on deductive reasoning. But Alcmaeon proceeded differently, using dissection and perhaps vivisection, both of which were proscribed by Pythagorean tenets, in his studies on physiology and anatomy. See also: Singer, C., *Evolution of Anatomy*, New York, 1925, for a brief unreferenced mention of Alcmaeon's work; Codellas, P. S., *Alcmaeon of Croton: His Life Work and Fragments*, in *Proc. Royal Soc. Med.* 1041-1046, 1932. Codellas provides translations and citations of "fragments" of Alcmaeon's work as presented by early authors.

[10] J. Jouanna, *The Birth of Western Medical Art*, in *Western Medical Thought from Antiquity to the Middle Ages*, Boston, 1999, edited by M. D. Grmek and translated by A. Shugaar, p. 29. Also see: Dales, R. C., *The Intellectual Life of Western Europe in the Middle Ages*, Washington, D.C., 1980, p. 210, for a discussion of the "medical school" of Salerno, where the following statement is made: "Still, throughout the entire period we have been describing, there is no evidence to indicate that there was any formal association of teachers and students at Salerno. Apparently teaching was private,..." Definitions of "medical school" down through the ages, as applied by modern writers, can be capricious.

[11] Nutton, V., *The Medical Meeting Place*, in *Clio Med.*, 27:3-25, 1995.

sense, that being the matriculation of its membership in return for a fee. It may be more reasonable, therefore, to consider these enrollees as not being novices but practitioners. Thus the "school" may have been an organization to which practicing physicians could apply for membership, and it was the offer of membership in a medical "Cooperative" for a fee that was the innovation of Hippocrates.

D. Η Κοινωνία Ιατρῶν Κώων (ΚΙΚ)
The Coan Physicians' Cooperative (CPC)

Dr. Sherwin-White concludes that there was a medical koinon on Cos, that it may have extended beyond the island to include Cnidus and Rhodes, and that a koinon was not a feature of tribal hierarchy.[12] Dr. Jouanna and others have also used the term "koinon" for the organization of kindred physicians who belonged to the Asclepiadae on Cos, even though it came to include physicians who had no family ties to the Asclepiadae.[13] These opinions buttress the argument that the physician network associated with the island of Cos was neither a guild nor a school of medicine, but rather a koinon, in the sense of a physicians' cooperative.

The professional koinon of ancient Cos would incorrectly be considered the equivalent of the modern guild, for "guild" and "koinon" are not in the least synonymous. Guilds as now understood will be discussed in greater detail later, for they evolved in medieval times to protect organizational interests. Thus the attribution of "guild" to the Asclepiadae, the familial organization of early Greek medicine, probably is not far from the mark, for the interests of members of the Asclepiadae were thought best served by maintaining exclusivity, protecting knowledge, and ensuring conformity of its members. Insofar as the community leadership had some say in the placement of physicians of the guild of the Asclepiadae, there is a resemblance to the medieval guilds in that the latter were controlled by municipalities. But Dr. Sherwin-White concludes that, while municipal leadership on Cos may have assisted in the placement of physicians, it did not interfere with the internal organization of the medical organization itself.[14] If this is true, that organization could set its own standards, educate its membership, watch over its finances, and organize its collective wisdom. It is postulated, therefore, that the educational organization that replaced the archaic guild-like Asclepiadae was not a school, but a koinon. This democratic institution would have served to advance individual interests by promoting professional excellence, doing so by promoting openness in the relations among physicians and between physicians and patients, improving the quantity and quality of professional knowledge, expanding its membership to qualified applicants, and maintaining a high standard of medical practice, as manifested in its famous Oath.

Among the many innovations attributed to Hippocrates the greatest may have been the inauguration of this new physician's professional organization for a fee to those outside the Asclepiad guild.[15] The democratic innovation of matriculating outsiders

---

[12] Sherwin-White, S., *Ancient Cos*, Gottingen, 1978, p. 257.

[13] Jouanna, J., *Hippocrates*, translated by M. B. DeBevoise, Baltimore, 1999.

[14] Sherwin-White, S. M., *Ancient Cos*, Gottingen, 1978, pp. 273-274. The author also provides evidence for internal organization of a physicians' organization.

[15] Plato reports this in *Protagoras*, 311, c: Socrates – "...suppose you had your mind set on going to your namesake, Hippocrates of Cos, the famous physician, to pay him a fee for services to you, and if someone asked you what this Hippocrates is that you were going to pay him, what would you

would have increased the number of physicians identified with Cos, improving the quality of their practice by pooling their observations, and efficiently communicating any improvements to member physicians, a further boost to reputation. There would have been superimposed a financial incentive for matriculating physicians to maintain high standards, for economic commitment or investment is a strongly motivating factor. The result was a furthering of the fame of Cos, which did surpass that of other named "medical schools," perhaps forcing them out of business.[16]

In this koinon, which might have been called something like the Coan Physicians' Cooperative, or CPC, there may even have been a network of physicians who rotated through specified cities on a prearranged schedule, perhaps like early judicial circuit riders in America. Membership in the koinon would have permitted access to the educational scrolls, lectures, and demonstrations, all of which would improve the practice and reputation of the affiliated practitioner, whose original training, obtained through the usual apprenticeship, could have been anywhere around the Aegean or beyond, but preferably with a Master who had a Coan affiliation. A Hippocratic treatise, therefore, was written for members of the koinon rather than being a memo for the physician writer himself. It also was not written to be passed on only to that physician writer's apprentice. The Hippocratic treatises were intended for a wider audience, one versed in their terminology, namely the physician writer's medical colleagues. Some works of the *Hippocratic Corpus* contain case histories that could be acceptable modern progress notes in patients' charts, notes to be read by the next physician who would visit that particular city. Prof. Craik reviews the prominent physicians associated with the name of Cos in the years after Hippocrates,[17] and a reasonable assumption is that their basic medical training was elsewhere and that they desired an affiliation with a Coan institution, not for a medical apprenticeship or guild membership, but for something like postgraduate education. A present-day analogy might be the short and intensive courses or reviews on medical topics and techniques frequently offered for a fee by prestigious medical institutions, whereby a small-town practitioner can obtain updated knowledge, and some cachet, by taking a two-week summer course at a Harvard University medical institution or The Johns Hopkins University, for example, courses that educate, a form of "continuing medical education" that usually does not involve or require hands-on clinical training.

A clue supporting the existence of a physicians' koinon is provided in that component of the *Hippocratic Corpus* known as the Επιδημιων (epidemion), or

---

say?" Hippocrates – "I would say a physician." Translation of S. Lombardo and K. Bell, in *Plato, Complete Works*, J. M. Cooper, editor, Indianapolis, 1997.

[16] Sherwin-White, S. M., *Ancient Cos*, Gottingen, 1978; see Cnidian school, p. 263; Rhodian school p. 259. The Rhodian school disappears from history with the advent of the "school" of Cos, and the nearby school of Cnidus became unidentifiable in the 4th C BC. Another feature of the Hippocratic koinon that may have contributed to its prominence and durability was that, as far as is known, it was the only "school" to write down (some might say "publish") its works. Admittedly, however, some "Hippocratic" works are thought to have been products of other "schools."

[17] Craik, E. M., in: *The Dorian Aegean*, London, 1980. Tellingly, on p. 115 of chapter 6 she distinguishes Hippocrates the Coan physician from Hippocrates, "the corporate Hippocratic writer,' one implication being that the writer(s) of the *Hippocratic Corpus* could have been a member of a physician association such as a koinon.

"Epidemics."[18] These seven collections of case histories are explained by W. H. S. Jones in the Introduction to his translations of Epidemics I and III found in the *Loeb Classical Library* series on Hippocrates. A medical information network whereby physicians funneled information to a central office that returned analyzed data to the field would have provided Hippocratic medical practices with both a scientific and an educational base (the scientific nature of Hippocratic medicine is discussed in the next chapter). It would have permitted individual physicians to report clinical observations from home. The central office would then scrutinize disease patterns, returning a synthesis of more accurate information to the same clinicians for improvement of their practices, a reporting system predating the modern medical journal by 2200 years. A noteworthy feature of these case histories is that many individuals are identified by name or address. For the most part this information adds little to an understanding of either the clinical problem encountered or its epidemiology. But it would have been information of great value to another physician in locating the same patient on a subsequent visit. This would have permitted follow-up of patients over a longer period, providing opportunity for gauging the effectiveness of treatment, for clarifying the natural history of the illness, and, perhaps, permitting some continuity of care that a single peripatetic physician could not provide. The case histories, therefore, functioned like today's hospital summaries or progress notes, something to be read by another physician, or perhaps the same one, prior to a visit to the same city or locale. This would explain why the grammatical structure of the histories is fundamentally spare and why they sometimes contain personal information of no medical value: they were never intended for "publication."[19]

Pliny reported that Hippocrates was responsible for removing the profession of medicine from the temple cults and establishing clinical medicine.[20] Thereafter, Hippocrates was acclaimed the great teacher of clinical medicine. But rather than a Greek Osler,[21] Hippocrates might better be likened to a Chief Executive Officer of the medical organization of Cos. Perhaps the medical profession should have another icon, the

---

[18] The author's preferred translation of "epidemics" as used in these Hippocratic works, *i.e.*, "House Calls," is justified in *The Natural State of Medical Practice: Hippocratic Evidence*, Maitland (FL), 2019.

[19] See, for example, *Epidemics* 2.2, 18b: "A woman carrying in the third or fourth month had eruptions on the lower left leg and on the right hand next to the thumb, eruption of the sort for which we give frankincense. I do not know what her baby was. I left her six months pregnant. She lived, I believe, in Archelaus' property near the cliff." (*Loeb Classical Library*, *Hippocrates*, VII, translation of W. D. Smith.) The last sentence is clinically irrelevant and was solely provided to assist in locating her on a future visit.

[20] Pliny's *Natural History*, book 29, chapter 2. He uses the Latin term, *clinice*, related to the Greek κλινώ (bed, couch), which indicates the Hippocratic physician visited his patients in their bed (*e.g.*, reclining). It is from this term that our "clinic" is derived. Interestingly, Pliny states that Hippocrates first shed his light on medical practice at the time of the Peloponnesian War (431-404 BC). Hippocrates would then have been at least thirty years of age.

[21] Sir William Osler (1849-1919), from western Ontario, was a famed physician and clinical teacher, the first professor of medicine at the new Johns Hopkins University Medical School in 1888, author of the enduring textbook, *The Principles and Practice of Medicine*, and advocate for establishing the *Quarterly Journal of Medicine*, a famous British medical journal. Of the clinical entities that have received his name, one is Osler-Vasquez disease, or polycythemia vera, a blood disorder usually requiring phlebotomy as mainstay of therapy. Having said this, he was but a man of his time, sparing in his approval of women as physicians and presumptious as were many of the Victorian elite, for which see G. Weissmann's essay, *Against Aequanimitas*, found in *The Woods Hole Cantata*, New York, 1985, p. 211.

medical cooperative at Cos, the KIK, ἡ κοινονία ἰατρων Κώων, (Coan Physicians' Cooperative, or "CPC"). Given the many cities served by Hippocratic physicians, including Crannon, Perinthus, Larissa, Abdera, and Thrasos, it would have been similar to today's physician employment services that provide temporary staffing for remote or specialized clinics or hospitals, a system of *locum tenens* (or "place holder," a temporary appointee). This would have been popular with the cities, who no longer had to rely on sporadic and unscheduled visits of solitary itinerant physicians. By collecting a fee the central organization on Cos would have been able to maintain administrative records, schedule physician visits with various municipalities, collate clinical observations useful for the physician network, and recruit more physicians. The reputation of the network required that it ensure that its physician members demonstrate comparable levels of knowledge and uniformity of comportment and ethical behavior, for, if its reputation in a particular municipality sustained a blemish, business would surely suffer. Thus, Hippocratic writings such as the *Oath*, *Precepts*, *Laws*, and *The Art* would have been directed not at medical practitioners everywhere but only to members of the koinon. Rather than being pretentious generalizations of idealists they were, instead, practical advice to fellow members for a successful medical career in the context of a koinon and, for the koinon, a practical way to pressure a member to behave as he should, a protection for the other members.

The extent to which a medical organization such as the Coan Physicians' Cooperative favored Coan prosperity and vice versa is unknown. But on epitaphs and honorific stele the appreciation of Coan physicians was frequently memorialized. Some Cos-affiliated physicians removed themselves to the new center of learning in Alexandria beginning late in the 4th C BC, where some attained fame for their medical studies.[22] Cos nevertheless remained a favorite of the Ptolemies, its arts and sciences were courted, and democratic institutions persisted, whereas elsewhere in the region the post-Alexander leadership of Egypt established traditional authoritarian control. Cos island remained a source of practicing physicians throughout the Hellenistic period and into the days of imperial Rome.

In summary, although it was demographically unfit for sustaining a sizeable clinical presence, the geographically, politically, and economically favored island of Cos may have provided a stable environment for a progressive medical institution. That institution almost certainly was not a guild or a medical school. Instead, it is likely that the business of medicine, at first under the watchful eye of the Asclepiadae of Cos, developed a regional physicians' network that transcended ethnic and political borders. Details of this organization remain inferential, and stories of its success seem something of a surprise. But of all the possibilities it is the one that best fits with the facts and the lack thereof. Furthermore, that organization, unlike a guild or a medical school, apparently eschewed a physical facility, declaring implicitly that its value resided not in its edifices, but in the intellects of its dispersed clinicians. The merit of those clinicians is the subject of the next chapter.

---

[22] Sherwin-White, S. M., *Ancient Cos: An Historical Study from the Dorian Settlement to the Imperial Period*, Gottingen, 1978. Chapter 7 provides documentation for many named physicians.

CHAPTER THIRTEEN

HIPPOCRATIC MEDICINE AS A PROFESSION AND AS A SCIENCE

δύο γάρ, ὧν τὸ μὲν ἐπίστασθαι ποιέει, τὸ δὲ μὴ ἐπίστασθαι, ἡ δὲ δόξα τὸ ἀγνοεῖν.

"For there are two [systems], of which one leads to understanding and one does not, and the one that does not is opinion [alternative translation: 'and thus opinion is ignorance']."

Law (from the *Hippocratic Corpus*),
Section 4

Many books can be written by a single author, but a lifetime in medicine affords limited opportunity for the tedious acquisition, by firsthand clinical experience, of new data or observations sufficient for publication. Thus, Hippocrates and Galen, as individuals, have received far too much credit for making medical discoveries. The lionization of these two early physicians is to a great extent attributable to the naivete or clinical incompetence of their medical successors and biographers. It is obvious that complex clinical analyses from assembled observations of Hippocratic physicians were used to transcend the limitations of individual clinical experience. Within the collective experience of the Hippocratic koinon the correctness of so many medical analyses proves that scientific revision, *i.e.*, confirmation of or improvement on preexisting knowledge, was made over time. The profession of medicine could now be defined as a science as well as an art and a profession.

A. Introduction: The Limits of Individual Clinical Experience

The assumption that the clinical writings of several prominent ancient physicians represented their extensive personal experience must be countered. Such vast first-hand knowledge as they sometimes describe would have been quite impossible to individually acquire. Consider Galen of Pergamon (130-200 AD), who started the study of medicine when seventeen years of age, which study spanned eleven years and four cities, one being Alexandria.[1] It was not until age twenty-eight years that he began his medical practice, which involved tending wounded gladiators. At age thirty-five he established a long-term residence in Rome. He no longer pursued surgery, instead devoting himself to (internal) medicine until the age of sixty-two, when he left Rome to spend his time in meditating and writing. Galen wrote at least 129 works on medicine, including topics such as anatomy, pathology, therapeutics, commentaries on Hippocratic works, hygiene, physiology, the pulse, medical philosophy, and related fields. He also wrote treatises on the soul, on logic, and on Plato's *Republic*. He compiled dictionaries, one in 48 books for the Attic language and one of medical terms in 5 books, and he was a book collector.[2] He

---

[1] Sarton, G., *Galen of Pergamon*, Kansas, 1954, and Garcia-Ballester, L., *Galen and Galenism*, Burlington (VT), 2002.

[2] Carolus Gottlob Kuhn published *Medicorum Graecorum opera quae extant*, Leipzig, 1821-1830. Being the collected works of Galen, they filled twenty-two volumes, the index required 676 pages,

was a favorite in the Roan Imperial court where he successively tended four Emperors, sometimes accompanying them on prolonged journeys, and he served as physician to the son of Marcus Aurelius, the infamous Commodus. He also provided public lectures and dissections. Such a career would have allowed, in the twenty-seven years he spent in Rome, little time for the painstaking and detailed personal accumulation of clinical data necessary to support his compendium of medicine, even with scribes taking dictation.

Hippocrates likewise is thought to have traveled much in acquiring a mass of clinical data and therapeutics now included in the *Hippocratic Corpus*. But consider how much time is spent assembling Resident staff, nurses, students, and others for morning rounds in the modern hospital, rounds that take place in one building, often on just one floor, rather than in houses scattered about town. And consider case V of *Epidemics* I in which the patient was observed in her home at least fifteen times over eighty days, the result being the observations of only one "case." With travel time between houses and between distant cities, meals, rest periods, conversations, protection from the elements, occasional civil strife, and the inevitable acute and chronic infirmities that would affect both the practitioner and his family as much as the patients he visited, surely the number of patients from whom detailed clinical observations were obtainable during the course of a physician's active professional career would not have been great, even with the assistance of apprentices, who of course would have to be conscientiously taught both the facts and the procedures needed for their future practices. Add to this that no two patients are alike, which the Greek physicians astutely recognized and which implies time-consuming questioning and examination of each patient, and that Hippocratics both practiced internal medicine and performed surgery, compounded their own medicine, and were called as witnesses in trials and performed other forms of civic duty, not to mention their family obligations, and it is indisputable that the clinical experience recorded in the *Hippocratic Corpus* must be the accumulated experience of many physicians.[3] Even today's health maintenance organization primary care practitioner, forced to provide just nine minutes, on average, for each patient in a streamlined setting, has, at the end of the day, only the occasional clinical observation which would, if it could, attract his pen. The point is a critical one. It cannot be gainsaid that the clinical experience embedded in the *Hippocratic Corpus*, its many truths being confirmed yet today, was the organized medical intelligence of many clinicians.

A final point directs attention to the population from which clinical experience was to be derived. Ancient Cos, the island home of Hippocrates, would have had far too small a population to provide the clinical experience required to train many physicians. Its population in 2005 was 28,000, and a century earlier it had been 10,000. It is unlikely to have been much greater 2,500 years ago.[4] Dr. Sherwin-White concludes Cos was

---

and, according to Prof. Sarton, the collection is incomplete. Nutton cites over 350 authentic works of Galen, ranging in size from 30-500 pages, and considers this will be substantially increased as new information is gained (Nutton, V., *Roman Medicine*, in *The Western Medical Tradition*. 800 BC to AD 1800, Cambridge, 1995, p. 60).

[3] See Aelian, *Var. hist*. iii, 7 and Plautus, *Amphitryon*, iv, I, 3 for doctors' offices as places of casual coffee-shop conversation.

[4] It has been estimated that the island of Samos, near to Cos and almost twice its size (190 vs. 109 sq. mi.,) may have had a population, inclusive of slaves, as high as 50,000 under the prosperous rule of Polycrates (ruled 546-522 BC). See: Shipley, G., *A History of Samos, 800-188 BC*, Oxford, 1987, p. 12*ff*. For whatever this analogy is worth, it suggests a Coan population as high as 30,000 in the age of Hippocrates might have been obtainable. Yet, the Hippocratic era population of Cos was probably concentrated near Kephalos, located on the west end of Cos island, and there are no

always "sparsely populated."[5] Cos island could have provided extensive experience to only a handful of physicians, and it would have required a lifetime of their service to acquire it.[6]

Now the profusion of information expressed by some of those early medical writers could have reflected that tendency to exaggerate one's personal experience, a commonplace even today. There is the risible testimony that seeing one case of a particular problem is sufficient for "in my experience," seeing two cases is "in my series," and seeing three cases is sufficient to attest that one has seen a particular problem "over and over and over again." Medicine is not immune to exaggeration. But the good sense and solid descriptions revealed in many of the writings of Hippocrates, Galen, and others support the inference that their conclusions were based on a much stronger statistical base than that obtainable through personal experience. Such a repository of data must have been collected, in an organized fashion, over time and from a wide area, by numerous practitioners and, at least for the Hippocratics, within the purview of their corporate headquarters.

B. Hippocratic Medicine as a Profession

Medical progress in ancient Greece paralleled political progress, although there are many that did not, and many still do not, view democracy as evidence of "progress." True progress must show purposeful improvement. But it has been claimed that the Hippocratics accomplished nothing except for observing the patient until he died.[7] Furthermore, Hippocrates never performed an experiment. Instead, he and his colleagues merely practiced medicine at the bedside. Is this sufficient to be called scientific? And just what is the art and science of medicine?

---

first-hand descriptions suggesting a city there that would in any way have rivaled the principal city of ancient Samos, where the modern city of Pythagorion is now located.

[5] Sherwin-White, S. M., *Ancient Cos*, Gottingen, 1978.

[6] Grenada, a Caribbean island of 130 sq. mi. with a population of 85,000 does indeed have a medical school, but at the time of this writing it offers only two years of training in preclinical courses, and its graduates must pursue their clinical studies requiring access to patients elsewhere.

[7] Aesclepiades (124-40 BC), the earliest Greek physician to establish a reputation in Rome, described Hippocratic treatment as "a meditation on death," a damning comment on the clinical expertise of Aesclepiades himself. The 19th C French physician, Houdart, passed a similar judgment (see: *Etudes Historiques et critiques sur la vie et la doctrine d'Hippocrate*, Paris, 1840). Old concepts die hard. Even if limited to just surgery, Greco-Roman era physicians performed more than 110 different surgical procedures according to Lawrence Bliquez (*Roman Surgical Instruments*, Mainz, 1994), hardly a "meditation on death," although even today surgical colleagues occasionally refer jokingly to a consultant internist's tendency to give a seemingly endless list of differential diagnoses and to his inexhaustible patience in waiting and observing. In the Hippocratic physician's eyes, however, the issue was not "meditating"; he was merely giving time for an "interior" problem to externalize, as seen, for example, in the tendency of many deep abscesses to burrough externally and then spontaneously drain. Once external evidence of the nature of the internal disease process was available to the Hippocratic physician, objective means to manage the problem would then be crafted.

Excursus on τεχνή (techne)

τεχνή, ἡ - art, skill, regular method of making a thing[8]

The Hellenes considered medicine a τεχνή (*techne*), traditionally translated as "art" in the famous first aphorism of Hippocrates:

ὁ βίος βραχύς, ἡ δὲ τέχνη μακρή, ὁ δὲ καιρὸς ὀξύς, ἡ δὲ πεῖρα σφαλερή, ἡ δὲ κρίσις χαλεπή.

"Life is short, the art long, opportunity fleeting, experiment treacherous, judgment difficult."

> Aphorisms, I, i (Translation by W. H. S. Jones, *Loeb Classical Library*, Hippocrates, vol. IV)

Hippocrates, in *Ancient Medicine*, II, praises empirical practices and their discoverers. But he agrees that practitioners of empirical medicine are not physicians, and empirical medicine was not, in his eyes, a *techne*: "That it [empirical medicine] is not commonly considered an art is not unnatural, for it is inappropriate to call anyone an artist in a craft in which none are laymen, but all possess knowledge through being compelled to use it."[9]

The popular modern phrase used to define *techne* as it applies to the field of medicine is "the art and science of medicine." The "science" of medicine refers to the quality of knowledge, not the nature of the knowledge sought.[10] It is objective, subject to confirmation, and is usually an extension of prior knowledge.[11] The "art" of medicine is the process of personal interaction, being the means by which the physician enlists a patient's assistance in diagnosing and optimally managing the patient's illness. Science involves learning, curiosity, and experimentation. Art, in medicine, concerns relationships, specifically the physician-patient relationship, and involves personality, humaneness, and aspects of physical presence. W. H. S. Jones, in his introduction to *Decorum*, assigns both art and science to be comprehended in the term "techne."[12] But neither of these terms reflects the Greek concept of medicine as a techne, and if medicine is viewed as only art and science, a critical element of a medical practice has been omitted. Dr. Iago Galdston almost made the point: "But here we must make sure that we understand

---

[8] *A Lexicon Abridged from Liddell & Scott's Greek-English Lexicon*, Boston, 1875, 14th ed.

[9] *Ancient Medicine*, IV, the translation of W. H. S. Jones, *Loeb Classical Library*, *Hippocrates*, vol. 1.

[10] The difference between science and religion "does not lie in their subject matter, but in the form of the interrogation and nature of their reply. Science begins where a conceptual problem takes the place of curiosity, as to sequences, and where, therefore, fancies and fables are replaced by the investigations of permanent relations." Windelband, W., *History of Ancient Philosophy,* translation by H. E. Cushman, New York, 1910.

[11] An exposition of τεχνή as a mechanism of scientific progress that builds on itself is given by H. W. Miller in *Techne and Discovery in On Ancient Medicine*, in *Transactions and Proceedings of the American Philological Association*, 86:57-62, 1955, Walton, F. R., ed.

[12] W. H. S. Jones, who translated *Decorum* (περὶ εὐσχημοσύνης) for the *Loeb Classical Library*, feels this work to be a late addition to the *Hippocratic Corpus*.

precisely what we intend by "medicine," for Medicine may mean the science and art of healing the sick and caring for the well, and it may also mean the practice of that science and art. In the one it is a body of knowledge. In the other it is the performance of a profession."[13] But he did not develop that thought. Abraham Flexner also understood: "An education in medicine involves both learning and learning how; the student cannot effectively know, unless he knows *how*" (italics added).[14] The Greeks identified "techne" as paramount. Had they wished to limit medicine to the art of relationships or to a field of knowledge they might, for example, have used terms that pertain to relationships, such as συγγίγνομαι ("I am with, associate or converse with"), or to scientific knowledge, such as ἐπιστήμη ("knowledge," "understanding"), rather than τεχνή. Relationships and scientific knowledge are important, but without competency in application their value is disputable. Preoccupation with only the science and the art of medicine can be unhealthful. A number of ancient commentators on medicine caution against both the haphazard practitioner who knows only what is in books and the counterfeit physician with his pleasing presentation.

An ancient Greek definition of techne can begin with Socrates, who considered it a "disciplined body of knowledge founded on a grasp of the truth about what is good and bad, right and wrong, in the matters of concern to it." [15] Plato provided a more specific definition, writing that a techne entailed knowledge based on understanding of the real nature of its object, not just its vocabulary. One might infer that the procedures of a techne would necessarily be explainable, objective, and subject to confirmation in order that real understanding be achieved in the first place, but the formation of a techne was not specifically addressed. Finally, it had to serve the good of its object, in medicine that being the patient. He explicitly pointed out that a techne was not a "knack acquired by experience."[16] From this it is clear that the term was not intended to mean just an "art" or scientifically acquired knowledge. For a treatment to be effective it had to be effectively employed. Aristotle agreed: "...just as to practice medicine and healing consists not in applying or not applying the knife, in using or not using medicines, but in doing so in a certain way."[17] He then extended the definition, noting that a techne required communication from one generation to another, thereby implying both ever increasing knowledge and collective utility,[18] also noting that the true physician, as a professional

---

[13] Galdston, I., *Progress in Medicine*, New York, 1940, p. 322.

[14] From Flexner, A., *Medical Education in the United States and Canada*, New York, 1910. And see footnote, p. 198 of this volume, for information on Flexner.

[15] *Plato, Complete Works*, Indianapolis, 1997, J. M. Cooper, editor. See footnote by translators, Grube, G. M. A. and Reeve, C. D. C., *Plato*, p. 977.

[16] Socrates, speaking of oratory, says to Gorgias: "And I say that it isn't a craft, but a knack, because it has no account of the nature of whatever things it applies by which it applies them, so that it's unable to state the cause of each thing. And I refuse to call anything that lacks such an account a craft." *Gorgias*, 465a, translation of D. J. Zeyl, in *Plato, Complete Works*, J. M. Cooper, editor, Indianapolis, 1997. The "it" refers to oratory as a *techne*; "knack" is ἐμπειρίαν. Jowett's translation begins thus: "An art I do not call it, but only an experience, ..."

[17] *Nicomachean Ethics*, V, ix, 15, 16, translation of Sir W. D. Ross, 1923.

[18] *Paideia*, vi, p. 1. Aristotle also understood the distinction between the basic and the applied sciences: ".... it is for the doctor to know the fact that circular wounds heal more slowly, but it is for the geometrician to know the reason for the fact." *Post. Anal.* 79, a, 15-17, translation of H. Tredennick, in the *Loeb Classical Library* series of Aristotle.

(τὰς τέχνας), does not treat contrary to principles despite the impulse of friendship.[19] The distinction of "profession" was also identified by Scribonius Largus, 1ˢᵗ C AD freedman physician to the Royal Court during the reign of Claudius, who defined it as being ethically compelled to be fully proficient in the merciful and humane application of medicine.[20] In all these senses, therefore, medicine seems to be a true techne. There is no current definition of "art" or "science" that provides equivalent illumination. With the definitions provided by Plato and Aristotle, a techne is, therefore, roughly equivalent to "profession" just as the word ἀτεχνίη is best translated as "unprofessional." [21] The Hippocratic quotation translated by Dr. Jones in the opening paragraph of this Excursus, its Greek cited in the footnote, can now read as follows:

> "And if it [empirical medicine] is not to be accepted as a profession, it is not unreasonable; for that in which none is a novice but all understand because of need or necessity, it is not fitting that this be called a profession."

Prof. Craik uses the word "profession" as a translation of "techne" in the Hippocratic Oath. It is the application of good judgment based on thorough understanding.[22] Von Staden views the term similarly in his discussion of Hippocrates in the *Dictionary of Ancient Greece*.[23] A summary of the elements of medicine may be useful:

Table 5: Three Elements of Medicine and Their Characteristics.

	Art	Science	Profession (τεχνή)
Function	Relationships	Knowledge	Application
Components	Personality Humaneness Presentation	Learning Curiosity Experimentation	Experience Judgment Expertise

End of Excursus on Techne

In conclusion, Hippocratic medicine was more than an art and a science. It was indeed a profession.

---

[19] Aristotle, *Politics* III, 16, 1287.

[20] See the first paragraph of the Introduction to the *Compositiones* by Scribonius Largus.

[21] A noncommittal definition of "profession" is "a calling requiring specialized knowledge and often long and intensive academic preparation" (*Webster's New Collegiate Dictionary*, 1979). For ἀτεχνίη used as "unprofessional" see the Hippocratic work, *The Art*, 1. Indeed, the better translation of the title for that work would be *The Profession*.

[22] Craik, E. M., in: *The Dorian Aegean*, London, 1980, chapter 6, p. 112. For another view of τέχνη as used in the Hippocratic work περὶ τέχνη in which a similar perspective is given although not identified with a "profession," see: Wickkiser, B. L., *The Appeal of Asklepios and the Politics of Healing in the Greco-Roman World*, Ph.D. thesis, 2003, chapter 1, III, B, available through UMI Dissertation Services.

[23] *Dictionary of Ancient Greece*, New York, 2006, Nigel Wilson, editor, entry "Hippocrates."

C. Hippocratic Medicine as a Science:

There are several arguments that support the scientific nature of Hippocratic medicine:

1) Disentangling objectivity and subjectivity

The Hippocratics dissociated medicine from pagan mysticism.[24] The hazards of theory unsupported by observation were obvious to them, and so they stated: 1) "Each of them [*i.e.*, each disease] has a nature of its own, and none arises without its natural cause."[25] 2) "Wherefore I have deemed that it [medicine] has no need of an empty postulate, as do insoluble mysteries, about which any exponent must use a postulate, for example, things in the sky or below the earth. ... For there is no test the application of which would give certainty."[26] 3) And in *On the Sacred Disease* is written: "This is about what is being called the "being possessed" [commonly translated as "sacred"] disease. It does not appear to me to be more divine nor more possessing than any other disease, but has a natural course and cause, ..."[27]

The distinctive natures of objective Hippocratic medicine and of subjective medicine are easily defined, their putative evolutionary paths shown in Table 6.

2) Application of inductive reasoning:

The principles of Hippocratic medicine were listed by Haggard: (a) there is no authority except facts, (b) facts are obtained by accurate observation, and (c) deductions are made only from facts.[28] Dr. Singer points out that this inductive reasoning, in which an observation is subject to confirmation, was rare among other intellectual efforts of the Greeks,[29] but Hippocratic writings quite clearly spell this out. Here is their method:

> "consequent to a foundation and resources and very many accounts and by small increments of knowledge, the collecting together and analyzing for a resemblance within a group, as well as the dissimilarities among them, and for resemblances among groups, so that from the differences there comes one similarity; thus [is] the path; thus verifying, by scrutiny, those having accuracy, and refuting those that do not."[30]

This was the method that would be rediscovered in the 17th C, the diminutive value of the alternative being stated by John Locke:

---

[24] Solon had much earlier declared the responsibility of man in determining his own fate: "If by your own actions you have suffered these most grievous calamities do not place the blame for your fate on the gods!" (Translation by John Lewis of Poem 11 as found on p. 110 of Lewis' book, *Solon the Thinker*, London, 2006.

[25] *Airs, Waters, Places*, XXII, translation of W. H. S. Jones in vol. 1 of the *Loeb Classical Library* series of *Hippocrates*.

[26] *Ancient Medicine*, I, 20-27, translation of W. H. S. Jones, *ibid*.

[27] *The Sacred Disease*, I, 1-4, in the *Loeb Classical Library* series on Hippocrates, vol. IV. Translation by the author.

[28] Haggard, H. W., *Devils, Drugs, and Doctors: The Story of the Science of Healing from Medicine Men to Doctor*, London, 1913, p. 387.

[29] Singer, C., *Medicine*, in *The Legacy of Greece*, Oxford, 1921, p. 212*f*.

[30] *Epidemics* 6.3.12, translation by the author.

"He that in Physick shall lay down fundamental maxims and from thence drawing consequence and raising dispute shall reduce it into the regular forme of a science has indeed done something *to enlarge the art of talking and perhaps laid a foundation for endless disputes*. But if he hopes to bring men by such a system to the knowledge of the infirmities of men's bodies he is mistaken" (italics added).[31]

Table 6: Historical Evolution of Medicine; Distinctions between Objective and Subjective Pathways

Objective Medicine	Effectors	Subjective Medicine	Effectors
Individual empiricism	Mothers	Magic	Medicine-man (to control others)
Collective empiricism (Rationalism)	Itinerant physicians	Mysticism	Seer (to control events)
Scientific analysis	Hippocratics	Faith	Priest (to control epistemology)
Investigative study	Alexandrians	Canon	Bureaucracy (to control preferment)
Modern expression	19th C Scientists	Salesmanship	Alternative Medicine

*If an alternative medicine procedure or drug is confirmed as useful by scientific analysis and investigative study, it has been thereby objectively evaluated and thenceforth should be incorporated into the objective path of the evolution of medicine. In this sense there is no ethical dilemma between allopathic and alternative medicine; if a medication is proven effective by objective and quantitative analysis, and if its toxicology is understood, both disciplines should, and would, welcome it.

Thomas Huxley narrowly defined science to be "classified knowledge," but one of today's definitions of science is "systematized knowledge, derived from observation, study, and experimentation, carried on in order to determine the nature or principles of what is being studied."[32] From this definition proceeds scientific inquiry and the scientific method. But Abraham Flexner (1866-1959), who has been credited with reorganizing medical education in the United States early in the 20th C, commented that clinical instinct was nothing more than rapid induction, the extrapolation of conclusions from observed data. Flexner, a nonphysician, made thoughtful observations regarding science and

---

[31] Antsey, P., and Burrows, J., *John Locke, Thomas Sydenham, and the Authorship of Two Medical Essays*, in *Electronic British Library Journal*, article 3, 42 p., 2009, a sophisticated and multidisciplinary study that establishes the authorship of both essays (*De Arte Medica* of 1689 and *Anatomie* of 1688) to have been solely the work of John Locke. The quotation comes from the former work.

[32] Webster's 4th Collegiate Dictionary.

medicine:[33] "Science resides in the intellect, not in the instrument." He applied the term "scientific" to the bedside work of the physician: "The clinic is scientific, ... to observe, explore, interpret, unravel," and this, he wrote, was "what scientific clinicians have always done."[34] It was understandable, therefore, that he viewed medicine not as an art, which he described as an "empirical venture," but as a science, one that clarified conceptions, extended and organized knowledge, and purified that knowledge by purging from it superstition and errors by confirmation based on repeated observation. This was also the thinking of Aristotle, who advised those who came after him to ignore what he had written if it conflicted with subsequent observations.[35] While the scientist is often envisioned as working at the laboratory bench, Flexner felt that the clinician was to be considered as much a scientist as his laboratory-based counterpart. It is this thinking that makes Hippocratic physicians scientists. For them, deductive reasoning would have to wait for a later age; there was no reason to waste time deducing from prearranged premises, for in the 5th C BC there were as yet no premises worthy of the effort, one unworthy example being the theory of the four humors.

3) Mechanisms for verification and refinement

The Hippocratics developed an organization that systematized medical knowledge by a process that incorporated self-correction and improvement. Formal logic can be applied to scientific method, but at its core it merely describes a process that

---

[33] Abraham Flexner (1866-1959) brought about a revolution in medical teaching in the United States. Arguing that medicine had no analogy with business, "Like the army, the police, or the social worker, the medical profession is supported for a benign, not a selfish, for a protective, not an exploiting, purpose," he wanted to eradicate the proprietary schools of medicine as "mercenary concerns that trade on ignorance and disease." He favored small classes, urged hands-on teaching so that medical students would both know and know how, and championed full-time faculty at medical schools. One unforeseen problem that emerged, however, although it was foreseen by Sir William Osler, was the prominence in medical school faculties of the full-time research physician to the exclusion of the clinician, a schism still felt today. But Flexner's opinion of the scientific clinician does not suggest that schism was of his doing. See: Flexner, A., *Medical Education: A Comparative Study*, NY, MacMillan, 1925, p. 7; also see: Ludmerer, K., *Learning to Heal: The Development of American Medical Education*, Baltimore, 1996; Bonner, T. N., *Iconoclast: Abraham Flexner and a Life in Learning*, Baltimore, 2002; and Altschule, M. D. (ed.), *Essays on the Rise and Decline of Bedside Medicine*, Lansing, 1989.

[34] As for science at the bedside, Claude Bernard, the eminent French physiologist, noted: "Observation is a passive science, experimentation an active science." (Found in his *An Introduction to the Study of Experimental Medicine,* 1865.) As any clinician will affirm, however, bedside medicine is anything but passive. The intellectual distinction between observation and experimentation implied by Bernard may be true, but eliciting a *pulsus paradoxus* or the murmur of mitral stenosis and locating the exact site of tenderness by palpation are but a few of innumerable examples of an active search that underlies clinical observation. And seeking new physical examination findings to explain an uncertain clinical condition is also not passive.

[35] Aristotle, *De Generatione Animalium*, Bk. III, 760b: "Such appears to be the truth about the generation of bees, judging from theory and from what are believed to be the facts about them; the facts, however, have not yet been sufficiently grasped; if ever they are, then credit must be given rather to observation than to theories, and to theories only if what they affirm agrees with the observed fact." Translation of Arthur Platt, found in *The Works of Aristotle*, Oxford, 1912, vol. 5, J. A. Smith and W. D. Ross, editors.)

is both objective and verifiable, one that moves further up the continuum of quality of knowledge:

> Empirical knowledge = experimental[36]
> Rational knowledge = practical
> Scientific knowledge = accurate

The clinical descriptions of many Hippocratic patients were not exercises in conciseness, nor were they literary efforts. Instead, they give all the details that could be obtained by a busy practitioner who was uncertain which of the details were the more important or relevant and might be found in another patient having a variant of the same disease. This represented, therefore, the casting of a broad net in order to isolate features of a disease process that might turn out to be peculiar to it or characteristic of it.[37]

4) Internal evidence:

Objective support favoring a Hippocratic scientific method can also be extracted from Hippocratic clinical writings themselves:[38]

a) *Prognostics* IX, describes the difference between *cyanosis* and *dry gangrene*:

And in the presence of the heaviness and should the fingernails and fingers seem cyanotic, anticipate an imminent death. But for the fingers or feet to be completely blackened is less deadly than if they are cyanotic. Thus, it is necessary to look for other signs, for should the patient appear to be bearing the illness well or should some other relevant signs appear in addition, expect the illness to progress to sloughing [of the digits] such that the blackened parts will autoamputate and the person will survive.

Comment: Cyanosis is the dusky hue seen in patients in whom blood flow is usually sufficient but oxygenation is deficient. Peripheral cyanosis of digits is here differentiated from the darkening that is a consequence of insufficient blood flow to digits leading to cell death, often the result of arterial occlusion. (1) The former is characterized not just by the color, but also the significance, of cyanosis, for it often indicates an imminent systemic threat from impaired oxygen delivery throughout the body and a mortal sign if not promptly reversed. In clinical terms it means there are at least five grams of unoxygenated hemoglobin per hundred milliliters of arterial blood, whereas normally

---

[36] Experimentation has become so exalted in modern conceptions of science that its elemental, trial-and-err, nature is often overlooked. One reason for this is the obfuscation often used by authors in modern journal articles when a theoretical justification is retrospectively given for a particular research approach that makes the outcome seem logical, which it seldom is.

[37] There are many examples of this in the Hippocratic works, a typical one presented in *Epidemics* VII, 85. The patient died after a brief illness, but the history included the distant past, interim symptoms, several new symptoms and signs, responses to several treatments, a varying mental status, and peculiar terminal behavior. There is no attempt by the practitioner to limit his history to a few points relevant to, or consistent with, a previously determined diagnosis. The diagnosis is uncertain. The medical history may, in fact, encompass two or more separate disease processes, acute and chronic. The author, in good scientific tradition, made no assumptions.

[38] The six sections of the *Prognostics* from which the following examples were taken are fully translated in interlinear and vernacular forms in: Adams, W. H., *The Natural State of Medical Practice: Hippocratic Evidence*, Maitland (FL), 2019, p. 105*ff*.

there would be virtually none. (2) The latter acknowledges the better prognosis of the patient with the blacker digit because the problem is more likely to be the result of local pathology rather than a systemic failure to adequately oxygenate the blood, and the digit may undergo autoamputation, or, as stated by the Greek physician in the last sentence of the paragraph, it may, if left alone, "fall off." This course is permitted to a limited extent even today for what is sometimes termed "dry gangrene" in which the afflicted digit or extremity, in the absence of infection or other complication and if left alone, shows a line of demarcation that is a guide to the extent of amputation that will be needed.

The distinction between the fingers in systemic cyanosis and fingers with locally impaired blood flow is easy, and an office-based physician in primary care is today likely to see both pathologies occasionally, perhaps every year or two. Thus, this passage from Prognostics is clinically astute, and conceivably it could represent the experience of a single experienced physician based on observations made over some years. But the course of events in both situations would have to have been observed over time, several times, for such a confident statement to be made that would stand the critical eye of other physicians. This sort of information could have been observed, analyzed, and passed on from father to son, from physician to apprentice. In terms of the division given on p. 200), this clinical description is closest to being "empirical," as it was basically personal observation.

b) *Prognostics* XIII describes *emesis*, and it is more complex than the preceding example:

XIII - Vomiting of a mixture of mucus and greenish [fluid] that is scanty and not of a thick consistency is the most favorable [type of emesis]. Worse are those that are homogeneously either mucus or bile. But if the vomitus is leek-green, burgundy-colored, or black it is important to know that any one of these is dangerous. And if all the colors are present in the same person's vomitus death is imminent; burgundy-colored emesis indicates the quickest death, if the smell is foul, although a putrid and foul smell is bad in any type of vomiting.

Comment: This Section first describes the usual appearance of benign vomitus with mucous and greenish secretions, the latter termed, correctly, bilious. But then the author describes vomitus that is leek-green, purplish, and black, stressing that they are more dangerous. To the clinician of a century ago, the leek-green color might have suggested typhoid fever, now rarely seen in the United States. Purplish emesis would indicate partially digested blood (a burgundy color), and black would be a more advanced auto-digestion of blood in gastric contents (colloquially called "coffee-ground" vomitus), both indicating, usually, upper gastrointestinal bleeding. The Hippocratic physician knew that the unfortunate patient displaying several colored components was in an especially bad way, and that the earliest death was most likely to occur in the patient with the purplish vomitus (it is an indication of brisk, perhaps massive, upper gastrointestinal bleeding), whereas he knew that "coffee-ground" (black) vomitus would often evolve more slowly, be less acutely threatening, and be in the long run usually, but not necessarily, less dangerous. He then added an additional variable, putrid smell. This is a consequence of bowel obstruction or advanced ileus, and its presence would be of great concern, especially in the days prior to abdominal surgery; if burgundy-colored blood was vomited by such patients, lethal bowel necrosis had occurred.

The short Section XIII, therefore, describes four colors of vomitus, two smells, putrid and not putrid, and seven possible clinical presentations, each presentation including the likely clinical course to follow. This knowledge the individual Hippocratic physician was unlikely to arrive at on his own; this had to be taught to him. The volume of information is not great, but the time over which seven dangerous and distinct sequellae of vomiting would have been not only observed but reliably distinguished from one another must have been years. This is an example not only of linearly accumulated knowledge, but knowledge that required analysis, something that a small professional group, a local koinon for example, could manage by sharing personal experiences, by "talking shop." In the scheme of the list in section C-3 of this chapter the knowledge expressed here is closest to "rational," practical judgment having been made after clinical discussion of repeated observations regarding prognosis.

c) *Prognostics* XIV-XVII – These Sections describe the possible consequences of the combination of *cough and chest pain*:

XIV - Sputum should be easily and promptly expectorated in all lung and chest wall problems, the yellow to seem as mixed thoroughly in the sputum. If late in the course of the illness one should bring up [sputum] that is yellow or tawny, or should develop a severe cough, or the yellow is not thoroughly mixed, matters will go badly. For sputum being a homogeneous yellow is dangerous, and that which is whitish and slippery and ropey is not helpful. But if the sputum is greenish-yellow or frothy it is very bad, and if it is homogeneously thus or appears dark it is to be even more to be feared. And it is grave should the lung produce or clear out nothing, instead being filled with bubbles in the throat [death rattle]. Nasal catarrh and sneezing are not good signs in any lung problem whether preceding or following upon the problem. But in other serious diseases sneezes are beneficial. A small amount of blood intermixed with yellow sputum is often associated with the onset of pulmonary disease, but being present for seven days or longer [the outcome] is less certain. All sputa are of concern whenever associated with unremitting aching; and worst is dark [sputum], as was discussed above. But the situation is improved once everything has been coughed up, thus terminating the discomfort.[39]

XV - When pains around the chest do not stop either in response to clearing of the sputum, emptying of the bowel, or by phlebotomy, medicines, and diet, it is important to realize that a collection of pus is developing. Of these collections it is very grave if the sputum being coughed up is still green, whether it is only partly or entirely so. Notably, should the purulent drainage of this type of sputum be led to decrease, the disease now having been present seven days, expect the sick person to die in forty days, unless something else favorable happens to him. Those favorable [signs] are: the patient is bearing the sickness well, has a good frame of mine, a lessening of the discomfort, the sputum is easily coughed up, body warmth being evenly distributed and moderate, absence of thirst, and urines, stools, sleep, and perspiration being "good" as discussed earlier. If all these signs develop the patient may well not die; if only some of them develop he may well survive longer than the forty days. In contrast, [if he does not develop any favorable signs] the contrary signs are: difficulty in bearing the illness, deep and rapid breathing, unremitting discomfort, difficult sputum production, extreme thirst, uneven distribution of body surface heat while febrile with the abdomen and chest wall being hot but the forehead and extremities cool, and urines, stools, sleep, and perspiration of the unfavorable type as described earlier. And should the person develop these he likely will expire before fourteen days have been reached, even by the ninth to the eleventh day. Thus, it is necessary for this information to be brought together and the very lethal nature of this kind of sputum and the evolution in fourteen days to be opposed. It is necessary, from all of these, to consider all the good developments and the bad, and from them predictions [are] to be made, as they should permit a

---

[39] This section is self-explanatory. The comment on sneezing being a bad sign can be correct in the sense that bacterial pneumonias are known to sometimes follow and complicate common viral respiratory infections, the latter often exhibiting sneezing.

correct foretelling. As for most of the other collections of pus, they rupture, arriving at this point in some twenty to sixty days.[40]

XVI - One should look close for the beginning of an empyema calculating from the day on which the patient first became febrile, had chills, or when heaviness [first] appears to be developing in place of tenderness in the region in which he had pain, for these indicate the onset of the empyema. Thus, from this time one can anticipate the discharge of pus according to the times predicted. And if there is an empyema on one side only, one ought to turn these [persons] over and consider carefully whether the patient has pain in the chest, or whether one side is hotter [to the touch] than the other, [and] asking, [while] he is lying on the healthy side of the chest, if something heavy seems to be hanging from the upper side. For if this is the case the empyema is on whichever side of the chest the heaviness occurs.

XVII - One ought to know all about an empyema from these signs: first, there is continuous fever, minimal during the day but higher at night and associated with heavy perspiration. Then there develops a desire to cough, although they expectorate nothing of what would be expected. The eyeballs become sunken, the cheeks flushed, the fingernails of the hands curved, and the fingertips hot.[41] In the feet there is fluctuating edema, blisters develop on the body, and they lose their desire to eat.

Therefore, whenever the patient has a delayed evolution of the empyema one must firmly trust in these signs. But whenever the evolution is more rapid as indicated by these signs or if they are present at the onset, the patient at the same time becomes more dyspneic. Thus, one should also be aware of signs indicating early or late rupture [of an empyema]: if there is incessant dyspnea, cough, sputum production, and general distress from the very beginning, expect [the empyema] to rupture within twenty days. On the other hand, if the distress and other symptoms occur as usual [for an empyema], expect it to rupture later. The symptoms of discomfort, breathlessness, and expectoration necessarily precede any breaking through of the empyema.

Those likely to recover after the draining of an empyema are those in whom fever clears the same day, and in whom there is prompt return of appetite, relief of thirst, the abdomen not distended. The pus, if it is white, smooth, homogeneous, should resolve, with phlegm cleared, cough relieved, and distress absent. Thus, they are relieved quickly and optimally, although, if not, relief will come soon. But if the fever does not quit the same day, but, seeming to quit, promptly resumes, and if there is thirst, anorexia, and watery stools, and if the pus is a dark green or a frothy mucus, such patients will expire, whereas if only some of these things occur and some do not, then some die and others recover after a long time. In all these cases and in others conclusions must be drawn from all the signs.[42]

---

[40] This is a fairly straight-forward and accurate account of the development of an empyema or lung abscess from a pneumonia. The sputum can be green from some kinds of pus, especially that produced in response to *Pseudomonas aeruginosa*, a particularly virulent bacterium. The time intervals are reasonable guesses, given the clinical status of the patients described.

[41] Increased warmth of the fingertips, only occasionally mentioned in modern texts (see: *Medical Management of Pulmonary Diseases*, Davis, G. S., editor, New York, 1999, p. 97). is a notable part of this Hippocratic description of clubbing, for classical clubbing of the nails is easily recognized as abnormal by anyone, whereas the increased warmth radiated by the fingertips, probably due to increased vascularity, is subtle and documents the Hippocratic scientific attention to detail.

[42] The varying time required for an empyema to form and then to rupture depends on several factors, including the infecting organism(s), host response, anatomic variability, and general health and nutritional status. It is not clear, in paragraph three, why there should be expectoration prior to rupture of the empyema, so perhaps the pain, breathlessness, and expectoration occur at the time of rupture, and, if the rupture is into a bronchus rather than externally through the chest wall, that surely would be the case. This interpretation depends on the translation of προ.

Comment: In these sections the author of *Prognostics* previously distinguished the combination of cough and chest pain from either cough alone or chest pain alone. He subsequently divides this combination of symptoms into those having a brief course and those of a chronic course. Of sputum production he describes that which is easily coughed up, that which is brought up with difficulty, that which is brought up early, and that which is brought up later in the course of the disease. Of the sputum composition he describes that which is visibly a mixture and that which is homogeneous. There is also the frothy. Then he describes possible sputum colors: yellow, red-yellow, white, pale green, black, and bloody. Under the cough and chest pain combination with a chronic course he describes those patients that develop an early-draining empyema and those that are late-draining. Finally, he describes the course of those experiencing an early easing of symptoms following drainage of the empyema and those that are incompletely eased. The theoretical number of distinct clinical scenarios based on these variables is 336. In addition, the author gives detailed descriptions of several good and bad signs and symptoms, both for the combination of cough and chest pain and for empyema. For the latter, bad signs included chronic remitting fever, sweats, sunken eyeballs, curved nails on hands with warm fingertips (now ascribed to pulmonary osteoarthropathy, commonly called "clubbing"), anorexia, swelling of the feet (perhaps the result of anorexia and protein depletion), and blisters (for unknown reasons). The author ends Section XVII with the following: "In these cases, as in all others, it is from the sum-total of the symptoms that an appreciation of the illness should be made."

A total of 336 combinations of signs, symptoms and clinical courses can be mathematically postulated for the descriptions of pneumonia and its complications from the above information.[43] But many of the combinations simply do not occur, many would be exceedingly rare, and the majority would have been impossible to differentiate from one another. Furthermore, the descriptions are based on a spectrum of pulmonary infection that is unknown to modern physicians. The role of tuberculosis, contemporary causes of simple pneumonia, the incidence of lung abscess and empyema, and prevailing factors such as malnutrition that might predispose to or complicate pulmonary infections are also unknown. But it is absolutely inescapable that the breadth of knowledge about pneumonia, its varieties, and its complications as expressed in these few sections of *Prognostics* is the result of the work of many clinicians over a long time. In addition, the correctness of many of the observations is a clear indication that the atypical, the aberrant, and the incorrect observations and conclusions that would inevitably occur in such an effort have been culled from the final version of the Hippocratic work. This would have required as great an intellectual effort as the initial collation, and it also includes additional observations of secondary findings. Furthermore, the medical data incorporated into it have undergone highly knowledgeable analysis and revision to arrive in its final and remarkably brief form.[44] It should make us pause in amazement.

---

[43] See: Adams, W. H., *The Natural State of Medical Practice: An Isagorial Theory of Human Progress*, Maitland (FL), 2019, p. 262, for the calculations and their basis.

[44] Take, for instance, the book by Sturges, O., and Coupland, S., *The Natural History and Relations of Pneumonia*, London, 1890. These authors review the difficulties in discerning causation and optimal treatment of pneumonia in the pre-antibiotic era, noting the following variables: age, sex, season, location, severity, stage at seeking treatment, various physical findings and symptoms. To this maze of presentations they reviewed reports of various therapies: phlebotomy (frequent or infrequent, large quantities or small, stage of disease at time of bleeding, etc.), antimony, gruels, tartar emetic, chloroform inhalation, digitalis, iron salts, copper salts, hydrotherapy, quinine, *etc.*

In the list given in section C-3 of this chapter, p. 200, this effort displayed by the Hippocratic physicians comes closest to "scientific." Intentional data collection and analysis on a broad scale were necessary to make such a clinical pronouncement. Consider modern-day statistics regarding pneumonia, the cause of most cases of empyema. The incidence of pneumonia in the United States might approximate one case per 300 persons per year.[45] Of patients treated for pneumonia, about one in twenty will develop empyema, or one case of empyema per 6,000 persons per year. [46] Assuming one generalist physician per 1,000 of a general population, on average a physician in an office practice might expect to see a *de novo* case of empyema every six years. In all of the United Kingdom there recently were approximately 4000 cases of empyema per year in a population of 60 million, or one case per 15,000 persons per year, and there are about 20,000 general practitioners available to them, meaning that, on average, the office-based physician would see a primary case of empyema every five years. Turning attention back to ancient Hellas, it would certainly take experience with hundreds of cases of empyema to develop the range of descriptions comprised by the *Prognostics*, and perhaps twenty times that number would have been the number of pneumonias examined at the onset of their illnesses; in other words, thousands of cases of what would now be termed "pneumonia." The number of physicians and the time require to do this was great. And it was an international effort, for in Prognostics XXV it is stated: "....about sure signs and about symptoms generally, that in every year and in every land bad signs indicate something bad, and good signs something favourable, since the symptoms described above prove to have the same significance in Libya, in Delos, and in Scythia. "[47]

If the Hippocratic physicians relied on the population of Cos for clinical experience they would have been hard pressed to acquire such statistics. Even today the population of the entire island is not much above 20,000, and if the American statistics

---

Importantly, they differentiated uncomplicated pneumonia from that which was associated with other disease processes, either separate diseases (*e.g.*, erysipelas, herpes, quinsy) or complications of the pneumonia itself (*e.g.*, meningitis, empyema, and other septic complications). They concluded that it slowly dawned on people that it was usual for pneumonia to resolve by itself, that it was rarely fatal under the age of fifteen years, and that, in those days, treatment results depended less on the method than on the source (*i.e.*, the institution, the physician, the location) of the treatment, one that helped the patient tolerate, or bear, the disease, now called "supportive care." Neither the authors nor the Hippocratics had radiographs to diagnose pneumonia, thus "lung problem" rather than "pneumonia" is used in translations herein.

[45] This would include all types of pneumonia, including viral, and many of this type of patient are not exceptionally sick, the diagnosis often being made on auscultatory grounds alone, indeed, sometimes even by standing in the hallway because of the patient's incessant nonproductive cough. On the other hand, patients with nonbacterial pneumonias may have quite severe coughs, and they often consult physicians. It is impossible to state what pneumonias the ancient physicians treated, although the variety of sputa they described might fit the modern picture of rust-colored for pneumococcal infection, currant-jelly for Klebsiella infection, viscous white for staphylococcal infection, and green for Pseudomonas infections, to use not entirely outdated terminology and descriptions.

[46] In the United States the actual rate of parapneumonic empyema in 2008 was six hospitalized patients (all ages) per 100,000 population. (Grijalva, C. G., *Emergence of Parapneumonic Empyema in the USA*, in *Thorax*, 66:663-668, 2011.) With the United Kingdom statistics given here the rate would be 6.7/100,000.

[47] *Prognostics* XXV, 11-16. Translation of W. H. S. Jones, *Loeb Classical Library Hippocrates*, vol. II. Libya comprised the region west of Egypt, Delos is one of the Greek Cyclades islands, and Scythia was an extensive region that included present-day Ukraine north of the Black Sea.

given above represented the prevalence of empyema in ancient Cos, there would have been no more than one or two cases per year. Although there is no way to determine whether the ancient prevalence was greater or less than at present, Hippocratic medicine must have relied heavily on a large and dispersed patient population, unless, of course, the source of its data was populous Miletos prior to destruction of that city. But more importantly, it required a physician organization.

d) *Epidemics* 6.7, paragraph 1, a clinical description of diphtheria:

It is usually stated that the first clinical description of diphtheria is found in the writings of Aretaeus (1st C AD).[48] Chadwick, however, cites the earlier *Hippocratic Corpus*, specifically *Prognostics*, 23, and *Coan Prenotions* 357.[49] But in none of these writings are there descriptions of neurologic symptoms that frequently are present, indeed, are a predominant symptom in many cases of diphtheria. Dr. Grmek has given an extensive scholarly dissertation on the "cough of Perinthus," as the disease described in *Epidemics* 6.7, paragraph 1, is called.[50] He concludes that that illness was indeed diphtheria, for neurologic abnormalities were prominent in the outbreak. Below is an interlinear translation by the author, followed by a smoothed-out version in the vernacular of modern medicine, that is in agreement with Dr. Grmek. It is cited in full because of its great importance in understanding ancient Greek medicine.

Epid. 6.7, 1 – The Cough of Perinthus[51]

βῆχες ἤρξαντο περὶ ἡλίου τροπὰς τὰς χειμερινὰς
coughs began around the winter solstice
ἢ πέμπτῃ καὶ δεκάτῃ ἢ εἰκοστῇ ἡμέρῃ ἐκ μεταβολῆς
either in a fifteen or twenty day from a change
πυκνῆς νοτίων ἢ βορείων καὶ χιονωδέων· ἐκ τούτων τὰ
frequent of southern or northern and snow; from these some
μὲν βραχύτερα, τὰ δὲ μακρότερα ἐγίνετο· καὶ περι-
shorter, and some longer it was developing; and lung
πλευμονικὰ συχνὰ μετὰ ταῦτα. πρὸ ἰσημερίης αυτις
disease frequently after these. before the equinox [March] again
ὑπέστρεφε τοὺς πλείστους, ὡς ἐπὶ τὸ πολύ, τεσσαρα-
it turned back for the most part, generally, forty
κοσταίους ἀπὸ τῆς ἀρχῆς· καὶ τοῖσι μὲν πάνυ βραχέα
[days] from the onset; and in these very brief
καὶ εὔκριτα ἐγένετο· τοῖσι δὲ φάρυγγες ἐφλέγμη-
and good resolution occurred; in some but throats were swollen and red,
ναν, τοῖσι δὲ κυνάγχαι· τοῖσι δὲ παραπληγικά· τοῖσι
and in [some of] these exudative pharyngitis ; and in [some of] these paralysis; and in

---

[48] Aretaeus: On Ulcerations About the Tonsils, chapter IX (περὶ των κατὰ τὰ παρισθμια ἑλκων, κεφ. Θ) of his work *On the Causes and Symptoms of Acute Diseases*, Book I.

[49] See: Adams, W. H., *The Natural State of Medical Practice: Hippocratic Evidence*, Maitland (FL), 2019, p. 138*ff*.

[50] Grmek, M. D., *Diseases in the Ancient Greek World*, Baltimore, 1991 (paperback edition, translated by M. Muellner and L. Muellner, chapter 12).

[51] Perinthus was an important city located some 70 miles to the west of present-day Istanbul, formerly in Thrace on the Propontis.

δὲ νυκτάλωπες,   μᾶλλον δὲ παιδίοισιν· περιπλευμονικά
[some of] these loss of visual accommodation, especially in children; lung disease

δὲ πάνυ βραχέα ἐγένετο.   νυκτάλωπες   μὲν ουν οὐδὲν
and very brief occurred. of loss of visual accommodation on the other hand then not one

βήξασι τὸ ὕστερον ἢ πάνυ βραχὺ ἀντὶ τῆς βηχὸς ἐγί-
in those coughing later or very briefly compared with of cough developed,

νοντο, φάρυγγες δὲ βραχέαι, μᾶλλον δὲ   νυκταλώπων.
but the [sore] throats brief, especially with the loss of accommodation.

κυνάγχαι δὲ   καὶ παραπληγικά, ἢ σκληρὰ καὶ ξηρά, ἢ
and exudative pharyngitis and paralysis, either encrusted and dry, or

σμικρὰ καὶ ὀλιγάκις ἀνάγουσι πέπονα, ἔστι δ' οἷσι
minimal and seldom they bring up purulence, and it is in them

καὶ κάρτα. οἱ μὲν ουν   ἢ φωνῇσι πλέον ταλαιπωρήσαν-
extreme. and those then either in the speech more being distressed,

τες, ἢ ῥιγώσαντες, ἐς κυνάγχας   μᾶλλον ἐτρέποντο.
or having chills, in the exudative pharyngitides especially they turned into.

οἱ δὲ τῇ χειρὶ πονήσαντες ἐς χεῖρας μοῦνον παραπλη-
and they by the hands working into arms only paralytics,

γικοί, οἱ δ' ἱππεύσαντες ἢ πλείω ὁδὸν πορευόμενοι ἢ
and they horsebackriding or more road being travelling or

ἄλλο τι τοῖσι σκέλεσι ταλαιπωρήσαντες τούτοισιν ἐς
other some by means of their legs being distressed in them into the

ὀσφῦν ἢ σκέλεα ἀκρασίαι παραπληγικαί, καὶ ἐς μηροὺς
low back or legs flaccid paralysis, and into the thigh

καὶ κνήμας κόπος καὶ πόνος· σκληρόταται δὲ καὶ
and lower leg fatigue and discomfort; most firm and

βιαιόταται αἱ   ἐς τὰ παραπληγικὰ ἄγουσαι. πάντα δὲ
most forceful [those muscles] into the paralysis to be induced. and all

ταῦτα ἐπὶ τῇσιν ὑποστροφῇσιν ἐγένετο, ἐν ἀρχῇσι δὲ
of these after the relapse developed, although at the beginning

οὐ μάλα. πολλοῖσι δὲ τούτων ἀνῆκαν μὲν αἱ βῆχες ἐν
not much. and in many of them eased then the coughs in the

τῷ μέσῳ,   ἐξέλιπον δὲ τελέως οὔ· ἀλλὰ ξυνῆσαν τῇ
middle [of the illness], remitted but completely not; but were with

ὑποστροπῇ. οἷσι φωναὶ ἀπερρήγνυντο   ἐς τὸ βηχῶδες,
in the relapse. in those voices having been broken into [something] like a cough,

τούτων οἱ πλεῖστοι οὐδὲ ἐπυρέτηνον, οἱ δέ τινες
of them most not being febrile, but some of them

βραχέα· ἀτὰρ   οὐδὲ περιπλευμονικὰ ἐγίνετο τούτων
briefly; nevertheless neither lung problems developed of them

οὐδενὶ οὐδὲ παραπληγικὰ οὐδὲ ἄλλο οὐδὲν ἐσημάνθη,
nor a single paralysis nor other any sign,

ἀλλ' ἐν τῇ φωνῇ ἐκρίνετο.   τὰ δὲ νυκταλωπικὰ   ἱδρύετο
but in the speech it was noteworthy. and the loss of visual accommodation was established

ὡς καὶ τὰ ἐξ ἄλλων προφασίων γινόμενα· ἐγίνετο δὲ
as if it from some other cause was occurring; and it happened

νυκταλωπικὰ τοῖσι παιδίοισι μάλιστα· ὀμμάτων δὲ τὰ
loss of accommodation in the children mostly; and of the eyes the

μέλανα ὑποποίκιλα, οσα τὰς μὲν κόρρας σμικρὰς ἔχει,
dark variegation, as large as [the iris] the small pupils it has,

τὸ δὲ ξύμπαν μέλαν ὡς ἐπὶ τὸ πολύ· μεγαλόφθαλμοι
and on the whole dark generally; large eyes

δὲ μᾶλλον, καὶ οὐ σμικρόφθαλμοι, καὶ ἰθύτριχες οἱ
more,   and not small eyes, and straight-haired
πλεῖστοι καὶ μελανότριχες.
and   black-haired.
γυναῖκες δὲ οὐχ ὁμοίως   ἐπόνησαν ὑπὸ τῆς βηχός,
and of woman not the same they suffered from the cough,
ἀλλ᾽ ὀλίγαι τε ἐπυρέτηναν, καὶ τούτων πάνυ ὀλίγαι ἐς
but   a few were febrile, and of the very few into
τὸ περιπλευμονικὸν ἦλθον, καὶ αὗται πρεσβύτεραι, καὶ
lung disease   came on, and the elderly,   and
πᾶσαι περιεγένοντο. ἠτιώμην καὶ τοῦτο καὶ τὸ μὴ
all   survived.   and this   and   not
ἐξιέναι ὁμοίως ἀνδράσι καὶ ὅτι   οὐδ᾽ ἄλλως ὁμοίως ἁλί-
to go out similiarly to men and because not otherwise similarly they are
σκονται ἀνδράσιν.   κυνάγχαι δὲ ἐγίνοντο μὲν καὶ
seized [by the disease] as men. but exudative pharyngitis developed and
ἐλευθέρησι δισσῆσι, καὶ αὗται τοῦ εὐηθεστάτου τρόπου,
in freewomen two,   and these of a well disposed nature,
περισσοτέρως δὲ δούλησιν,   ὅσησί τε   ἐγίνοντο βιαιότα-
but excessively in women slaves, in those in whom they developed the
ται καὶ ταχύτατα ἐπώλλυντο. ἀνδράσι δὲ πολλοῖσιν
most severe and rapidly they died.   but   in many men
ἐγίνοντο καὶ οἱ μὲν διέφυγον, οἱ δὲ ἀπώλλυντο. τὸ δὲ
they developed and some lived,   and some died. and
ξύμπαν οἱ μὲν μὴ δυνάμενοι   καταπίνειν   μοῦνον πάνυ
for the most part they not being able to swallow liquids only completely
εὐήθη καὶ εὔφορα, οἱ δὲ καὶ διαλεγόμενοι πρὸς τούτοι-
well disposed and borne well, but those distinguishing before in
σιν ἀσαφέως καὶ ὀχλωδέστερα καὶ χρονιώτερα· οἷσι δὲ
them indistinctly both more turbulent and prolonged; and in those
καὶ φλέβες αἱ περὶ κρόταφον καὶ αὐχένα ἐπήροντο
both the blood vessels near the temples and neck were distended
ὑποπόνηρα· οἷσι δὲ καὶ πνεῦμα ξυνεμετεωρίζετο κάκι-
somewhat suffered; but in those breaths   were raised
στον, οὗτοι γὰρ καὶ ἐπεχλιαίνοντο.
worst,   for these   grew very warm.

Translation: In December, coughs began two or three weeks after an abrupt onset of a cold spell [i.e., villagers probably spent more time indoors, perhaps with crowding]. Some [coughs] were brief, others long-lasting, and some developed subsequent pulmonary problems. In March they [the coughs] came back again, for the most part over a six week period, some being brief and with a good resolution, but others developing sore throats with swelling, some with exudative pharyngitis; in some of the latter there were paralyses and loss of visual accommodation, especially in children, and any associated pulmonary problems that occurred were very brief. No loss of visual accommodation followed in those with coughs or [if they did were] very brief along with a cough. But any loss of visual accommodation lasted longer [even when] the sore throats were brief. As for the paralytic exudative pharyngitides, whether or not they were encrusted and dry or mild with the patients bringing up slight purulence, in such patients [the illness] was severe. Those especially distressed in the voice and with chills more often turned into an exudative pharyngitis. And laborers using their hands might have paralysis only in the arms, those travelling by horse or walking (or otherwise using their legs) had flaccid paralysis in the lower back or legs in addition to fatigue and discomfort into the thighs and legs; the most firm and powerful [muscles] being caught up in the paralysis. And all of this developed after the recurrence [of the cough] [was over], although not much at first. The coughs in many eased during the course of the illness, but they never completely remitted, still being present when the relapse occurred. Those that had voices sounding something like a cough had no or little fever; neverthless none developed pulmonary problems, paralysis, or any other sign, but in the voice it was identifiable [*i.e.*, the characteristic abnormal speech pattern featured in the epidemic]. The loss of visual accommodation presented as if it were caused by something else [a separate disease]; it developed mostly in children, and the variegated iris that usually contains a small pupil became to a great extent black [the pupil was enlarged: "cycloplegia"]; [the loss of visual accommodation] was mostly in those with large eyes [pupils] rather than small ones, and with straight black hair.

But the women did not suffer in the same way from the cough, with few being febrile and with few [of these] developing lung problems, as was also seen in the elderly, and all survived. The reason for this was they did not go outside as the men did and because they were not as susceptible as men. Exudative pharyngitis also occurred in two freewomen of a well-disposed nature, but it especially developed in women slaves, and those who developed it most severely rapidly died. But in the men [slaves?] some lived, some died. And for the most part, even though unable to swallow liquids, they bore it well, although those distinguished by indistinct [speech?] had a more turbulent and prolonged [illness]; and those patients especially suffered if the blood vessels near the temples and in the neck were distended; but even worse were those with rapid respiration, for these grew very warm.

Comment: The preceding description is surely one of diphtheria. Here follows a succinct description of the neurological associations in diphtheria as given in a 1945 textbook, a modern description based on clinical testimony for the most part prior to development of antibiotics for widespread use and prior to widespread vaccination of children:[52]

> "Diphtheria as a cause [of neuritis] is very apt to be overlooked, especially as the diphtheria itself may have been slight and the neuritis may not develop for two or three weeks after the sore throat. .... The diphtheritic nature of the case may be suggested by a nasal alteration in the voice, or by inability to swallow liquids owing to their regurgitation through the nose – evidence of paralysis of the palate that is almost characteristic of diphtherial neuritis; the pupil reflexes are also apt to be affected, and the patient may be thought to have an error of refraction because paresis of the ciliary muscle renders accommodation difficult or impossible for the time being. The symptoms may stop at the palate and eye; but in bad cases – perhaps as the result of a toxin different from that which directly affects the palate – both paralysis and extreme atrophy of the limbs, without much sensory disorder, follow."

Several points can be made that confirm the diagnosis of diphtheria as the cause of the illness described in *Epidemics* 6.7, paragraph 1. The first is an understanding of the term νυκτάλωψ (nyctalopia) which some have interpreted incorrectly as "night blindness" and postulated as due to vitamin A deficiency. The neurotoxin of the bacterium *Corynebacterium diphtheriae* that causes diphtheria produces paralysis of the ciliary muscles with resulting loss of accommodation of the lens of the eye as part of the loss of the accommodation reflex, a complex response that involves constriction of the pupil when switching from distant to near vision. The Hippocratic physician noted the dilated pupils of some patients, and, recognizing that pupils normally dilate in the dark, termed

---

[52] French, H. F., Douthwaite, A. H., *An Index of Differential Diagnosis of Main Symptoms*, Baltimore, 1945, pp. 96-97. This publication was chosen for reference because it would present the best understood clinical features of diphtheria, as classical signs are now rarely observed by modern physicians working with a vaccinated population.

this finding, in effect, "pupils as they are at night" in the context of ambient light that was not normally associated with a large pupil. That this term for dilated pupils was meant for generic use by physicians is suggested in *Prorrhetic* II, paragraph 34, where the association of "nyctalopia" with headache is discussed as part of a non-diphtheritic illness: bilateral or unilateral pupillary dilatation is an important sign in many disorders that affect the central nervous system. The second point is that diphtheritic paralysis is more generalized as it becomes more severe, and it is in those muscles used most often that weakness and flaccid paralysis would be most apparent to the patient. But the third and most important point is use of the verb ὑποστρεφω (hypostrepho) and its derivatives, for it is certain that the physician was describing a recrudescence, return, or reestablishment of the same illness described at the outset, even though its manifestations were different, rather than a new or superimposed illness. They even state that it seemed as if it could have been due to some other cause. Finally, the concluding paragraph suggests the possibility of congestive heart failure with rapid respiration and distended neck veins, although the "very warm" seems unrelated to the congestion. In modern descriptions, diphtheritic myocarditis is clinically evident in more than ten percent of cases, and its prognosis is poor in over half of the afflicted patients. Earlier descriptions of disease indicate it became apparent after the acute diphtheritic symptoms had passed.[53] It is remarkable that the association of diphtheritic pharyngitis with the delayed development of various types of paralysis was not rediscovered, or at least not redescribed, until 1888, and even then the discovery was a laboratory observation rather than a clinical one.[54] Bretonneau mentions only palatal paralysis, the cause of regurgitation through the nostrils, and he had access to hundreds of cases of the disease and had performed autopsies on sixty.[55] But finally in 1898 a standard medical text stated, "Thus, paralysis is to diphtheria what dropsy is to scarlet fever – proof positive of the disease."[56] In interpreting all other ancient descriptions of "diphtheria," therefore, one must consider them all suspect because a neurological association was not mentioned, although surely some of the described cases were in fact diphtheria. The Hippocratic physician(s) describing the epidemic in Perinthus stated specifically that the paralysis followed pharyngitis, not pulmonary disease, although there is often some cough in diphtheria, and it is a measure of the clinical shortcomings of subsequent translations over the next two thousand years that this clear exposition of diphtheria was overlooked for that period. It is also a measure of the careful observations of the Hippocratics.

  To conclude this section, the scientific nature of Hippocratic medicine is

---

[53] For example, see: Von Pfaundler, M. and Schlossmann, A., *Diseases of Children*, Phila. 1908, translated by Shaw, H. L. K. and Linnaeus, F., vol. 3, p. 514.

[54] A reading of *Memoirs of Diphtheria* (which contains selected descriptions of diphtheria by the famed Bretonneau, Guersant, Trousseau, Bouchut, Daviot, and Empit, as translated by R. H. Semple, MD, London, 1859) finds no mention of paralysis, although the unusual voice and palatal insufficiency are mentioned. Pneumonia is the only late manifestation of the disease they describe. It was not until 1888 that Roux and Yersin reported that a sterile filtrate from a culture of *C. diphtheriae* produced a paralysis in those rabbits that did not die from the acute effects of the toxin. Earlier clinical descriptions of paralysis either cannot be ascribed definitely to diphtheria. Hamilton in 1826 postulated respiratory paralysis from "morbid secretions" in ulcerating "sore throat" (*Edin. J. Med. Sci.*, ii, p. 325), or they describe only nasal regurgitation of fluids. See: *Diphtheria*, by Andrewes, *et al.*, Medical Research Council, 1923, chapter I.

[55] Bretonneau, P., *Sur les moyens de prevenir le developement et les progres de la dipterie*, in *Arch. gen. de med.*, 5th series, 5:1-14, 6:257-279, 1855.

[56] Anders, J. M., *A Text-Book of the Practice of Medicine*, Philadelphia, 1898, p. 187.

incontrovertible. While Student t-tests and other statistical procedures were (apparently) not applied to the collected Hippocratic data, common sense prevailed.[57] And common sense is still needed today in the complex world of medical statistics. Even with the most sophisticated computerized analyses virtually every issue of a clinical journal will include articles whose authors declare that their statistics controvert the statistical analysis of some previous sophisticated publication on the same subject by others in the field. In this regard, one of the great 20th C research physicians, Dr. Eugene Cronkite, author of some five hundred peer-reviewed scientific publications, commented on the complexity of modern statistical mathematics by stating "If something looks statistically significant, it probably is statistically significant."[58] The mathematics of probability are but embellishments or refinements on common sense, not its replacement. Hippocratic physicians would have understood this perfectly.

---

[57] Another great 20th C physician, Dr. Maxwell Finland, stated with regard to statistics that when "unequivocal value...is not definitely apparent, the application of statistical analyses serves only to salve the conscience of the person who presents the data." (Quoted by D. M. Musher in his *N. Eng. J. Med.* review (355:2051, 2006) of S. H. Podolsky's book, "*Pneumonia before Antibiotics*," Baltimore, 2006), and a recent article in the *Annals of Internal Medicine* (Vol. 143:184-189, 2005) compared the probability of correct prognosis (termed "probability estimates") as made by clinicians to those made by clinicians aided by probability estimates based on the Bayes theorem, a procedure that permits mathematical quantification of sensitivity and specificity. The added statistical information did not result in improved accuracy in prognosis.

[58] Personal communication to the author.

CHAPTER FOURTEEN

ANCIENT GREEK MEDICAL PRACTICE

"Asclepiades very properly called all medical science which does not end in action, a meditation upon death."[1]

Early Greek clinicians, who, like the early sophists, were peripatetic, understood that diseases of civilization were not god-inflicted, a prerequisite for rational medicine. With population growth and enlarging cities whereby physicians could cease their itinerant existence, the profession became more responsive to societal pressures. Therapeutic options were limited and the pharmacopoeia was small, the latter reflecting a critical assessment of its components by Hippocratic physicians. Medicine was a profession requiring hard work to obtain a livelihood, and the Hippocratic practitioner engaged in both medical and surgical treatments. By the 4th C BC it was becoming an unattractive sinecure for the upper classes, although there was familiarity with its theories by intellectuals of the day. Diseases encountered by Hippocratic physicians are difficult to identify.

A. Introduction: The Origin of Disease

Standard textbooks of internal medicine contain about three thousand pages.[2] This size permits brief accounts, in small print, of most medical diseases and a thumbnail sketch of their pathophysiology. The *International Classification of Diseases (ICD-9-CM)* as of October 1, 2003, had in its "Tabular List of Diseases" some 7,734 coded disease categories, exclusive of those related to injury and poisoning.[3] Where do all these diseases come from?

For most of man's time on earth it has been presumed that gods or demons inflict disease as vengeance or punishment, a common attitude throughout the world today. But in ancient Greece, as in China, and surely in the minds of perceptive individuals in all ages, an additional culprit was identified: man himself. This was so because he was unable to restrain his passions, his appetite, and his intrepidity. In addition, he began to associate in larger and larger groups and tardily devised or insufficiently adhered to beneficial rules of social conduct. He did devise, or was advised on, rules of conduct to which the term "morals" has been applied. Implementation of morality would have provided a bulwark against many of the plagues of mankind. But it was ignored then, just as it is now. And so, as succinctly summarized by Dr. Roy Porter,[4] some of the ancients began viewing disease as a consequence of civilization, thus necessitating the field of

---

[1] To which Galen responded, "Whatever the whole world confirmed, Asclepiades contradicted." Many consider Aesclepiades of Bithynia to have been little more than a hugely successful but very lucky charlatan, and one of his principal methods in achieving success was to ridicule other physicians. The quotation is from the *New York Medical Journal*, 9:410, 1869, which cites the *London Quarterly Review*.

[2] Comprehensive textbooks of surgery and of other specialties can be equally long.

[3] The ICD-9-CM, *International Classification of Diseases - 9th revision - Clinical Modification*, is used to code diagnoses for statistical and reimbursement purposes. It is a version of the ICD produced by the World Health Organization, but it is published with the Clinical Modification by the federal government for use in the United States.

[4] Porter, R., *The Greatest Benefit to Mankind*, II, p. 15.

medicine.

The idea that diseases occur because of moral lapses is an old one; in the Golden Age portrayed in Greek mythology, as in the Garden of Eden, disease was unknown. But simply analyzing today the serious diseases and the causes of death of today's popular personalities is quickly convincing of a strong etiologic association with imprudent behavior and of the wisdom expressed in the Ten Commandments and in famous Greek axioms.[5, 6] As the 17th C English proverb stated: "Diseases are the tax on pleasures." For morality indeed provides a great survival advantage, to the individual, his posterity, and his society. The major categories of imprudent behavior in today's society include violence, illicit drug use, alcoholism, poor eating habits, tobacco use, and venery. In ancient Greece the categories for adults were, except for smoking and "illicit" drug use, probably similar. The list is small, but the number of distinct diseases directly or indirectly associated with each entity is great in both quantity and variety.[7]

In interpreting the consequences of what a society has determined to be immoral behavior, religion need not be invoked, although some would argue there is no morality without religion. But the fact remains, most of man's serious illnesses are inflicted by himself or by another person of his society. This was obvious to the early Greeks. Pythagoras (d. 497 BC) or one of his followers commented that mankind's sufferings are self-inflicted.[8] Plato attests that the proliferation of Athenian law courts and places to care for the sick was a consequence of licentiousness, idleness, and lifestyle in a city where diseases were occurring that had been unknown to the Asclepius of Homer.[9]

What can now be said about gods or goblins being the cause of man's diseases? In the ancient Greece of Hippocrates that idea was dying out and was doing so prior to

---

[5] The author tabulated discharge diagnoses of 420 consecutive admissions to his medical service in one month at a large municipal hospital in 2002. Most admissions involved more than one diagnosis, but the cause underlying the diagnosis of that particular admission was determined. Of the 420 admissions, 185 (44%) were for preventable health problems attributable to risky or intemperate behavior or to a problem imposed on them by another person exhibiting such behavior. A higher percentage was reported for deaths in 1993, as listed under *Actual Causes of Death in the United States*: McGinnis and Foege concluded that, of 1,757,216 deaths from the ten leading causes of death as assigned by pathology, 1,060,000, or about sixty percent, were the consequence of tobacco use, diet, alcohol, firearms, sexual behavior, drug use, motor vehicles, and certain infections and toxic agents. (*J. Amer. Med. Assoc.*, 270:2207-2212, 1993.)

[6] μηδὲν ἄγαν (meden agan), "nothing too much" – attributed to Solon (638-558 BC), the father of Athenian democracy; μέτρον ἄριστον (metron ariston), "moderation is best" – Cleobulus, one of the Seven Sages of 6th C BC Hellas. The Hippocratics agreed: τὸ δὲ κατὰ μικρόν, ἀσφαλές ("little by little is safest"); *Aphorisms*, II, 51, translation by the author.

[7] For example, *alcohol* and *alcoholism* produce, promote, or contribute to, among other things, convulsive seizures, delirium tremens, dementia, diarrhea, liver cirrhosis, cancers of the esophagus, stomach, oropharynx, liver, and rectum, hypertension, cardiomyopathy with heart failure, gastritis, hepatitis, hypoglycemia, hypomagnesemia, hypophosphatemia, fetal malformations, bleeding, ketoacidosis, anemia, thrombocytopenia, pancreatitis, stroke, neuropathies, Wernicke-Korsakoff syndrome, and many deficiency states, not to mention social dereliction, psychiatric disorders, and physical injury to the alcohol drinkers themselves and to others.

[8] "You'll learn that men have ills which they themselves bring on themselves, for harm comes to each of them through themselves, and they go astray through their own impulse and are harmed by their own purpose and determination." Cited by Aulus Gellius (125-180 AD) in *Attic Nights*, 7.2.12, translation from the Latin version by John C. Rolfe, 1927, for the *Loeb Classical Library*.

[9] *Republic*, III, 405, d; Asclepius, in the *Iliad*, was taught medicine by Cheiron and was the father of the two so-called "physicians," Machaon and Podaleirius.

Hippocrates.[10] If man blatantly induced his own diseases then clearly the gods did not cause them. It logically followed that the gods were less likely to be interested in curing problems they themselves had not caused. It was up to man to do so, and the ancient Greeks proceeded as follows.

B. The Peripatetic Physician

The developing greatness of 6th C BC Athens and other Greek cities prompted a desire to have a properly prepared citizenry to maintain that greatness and to teach the upcoming generation. In the century before Hippocrates, teachers of the youth were brought into Greece from the fringes of Greek settlement. They were itinerant and were the original Sophists,[11] learned instructors bearing both classical knowledge and new ideas who were hired to "teach young men the wisdom of life."[12]

Sophists were not the only peripatetics. At a time when population density was low and communities small, tradesmen and artisans moved from town to town to seek an outlet for their products and services. Physicians at the time of and preceding Hippocrates were similarly itinerant, even as Hippocrates himself was said to have been. Itinerant physicians were implied in the 8th C BC Greek world of Homer in *The Odyssey*,[13] and they were also to be found in contemporary Babylonia.[14]

The sojourns of Hippocrates and his colleagues were in response to invitation as well as personal wanderings with an eye to employment. Some medical itinerants would be temporarily hired under contract as City Physicians, being paid to provide specified medical services to the general community for a specified period, positions that were desirable but were not sinecures. Therefore, in the early days of Greece, and well into its democratic era, mobility was a prominent feature of Hellenic medicine.[15]

---

[10] But it was the Hippocratics who formally "distinguished causes dependent on external events, like climate, season, etc., from those subject to human will, like the diet," thereby removing further the list of earthly afflictions caused by the gods. See: Windelband, W., *History of Ancient Philosophy* (translation by H. E. Cushman), New York, 1910, p. 107.

[11] "Sophist" as defined in *Webster's Third New International Dictionary* (1966): "One of a class of teachers of philosophy and rhetoric in ancient Greece who became prominent about the middle of the 5th C BC and .... were the first to offer anything approaching systematic education beyond the elementary branches, and argued for the natural equality of men, but taught also the art of successful living and partly by virtue of their unorthodox opinion and their acceptance of pay for instruction gradually fell into disrepute."

[12] Dr. William Boyd describes the difference between the early peripatetic and the later indigenous sophists, the latter forming permanent schools of higher education, the first one in Athens being founded by Isocrates, followed by Plato and others. Boyd, W., *The History of Western Education*, London, 1947, 4th edition.

[13] Homer's *Odyssey*, Bk 17, 386: οὗτοι γὰρ κλητοί γε βροτων ἐπ᾽ ἀπείρονα γαιαν· ("For these men are invited all over the boundless earth.") This is a reference to important strangers from abroad, which included prophets, healers, and masters of some public craft. (Translation of A. T. Murray, *Loeb Classical Library*.)

[14] Elgood, C., *A Medical History of Persia and the Eastern Caliphate*, Cambridge, 1951, p. 17.

[15] At least this is received opinion, but as a stimulus for further investigation of the matter, see the interesting possibility raised briefly by Dr. L. Dean-Jones, (Dean-Jones, L., *Literacy and the Charlatan in ancient Greek Medicine*, in *Written Texts and the Rise of Literate Culture in Ancient Greece*, Cambridge, 2003, chapter 5, H. Yunis, editor, p. 117), namely that the Hippocratic work, *Decorum*, suggests that many sophistic itinerants were, when compared to established

Effects that can be laid to a spontaneous system of medical care in which the physicians were never at rest included the following: (1) there would have been the absence of entrenched medical interests within local communities; (2) few opportunities would exist for collegial interaction; (3) the practice of medicine could evade authority, and with the city-state unable, or unwilling, to shoot at a valuable moving target, the itinerant physician could argue his own terms of practice with potential patients, doing so with an eye to emoluments and to competitors waiting in the wings; (4) physicians had this advantage as well, that if a patient treated by a previous physician improved while under the care of his replacement, the new physician might receive the credit. On the other hand, if a patient did not fare well under his care, the blame and its consequences might never catch up with him. This pessimistic perspective is, in fact, counterbalanced by the benefit of new eyes and ears brought to bear on a patient's problem by the entrance of a new physician, a practice employed in many teaching hospitals even today, as Resident Physicians and Attending Physicians are periodically rotated from ward to ward.

As time passed physicians, like the Sophists, became less peripatetic, the traveling physician a disappearing way of life. For, as the city-states grew and prospered, it was no longer necessary for traveling tradesmen and artisans to seek out their clients town by town. They now could settle permanently in one place and let clients come to them. In medicine, therefore, itinerant physicians were fewer and the established local clinician emerged. How much this change would affect the profession is unknown, but it must have been important.

There is no mention in Hippocratic works, however, of continuity of care beyond the occasional case of acute illness that had a delayed resolution or late complication necessitating serial visits over weeks. No family physician, as now understood, has been described in ancient writings. The peripatetic physician's life would not permit it. It is probably for this reason that the consequences of many acute illnesses in the *Hippocratic Corpus* remain unidentified. A clinical vignette declared "resolved" in a Hippocratic work may not have resolved at all; a relapse or a complication may have occurred after the physician left the city. Equally important, a physician who knows a patient only over a matter of days or weeks will rely on history and hearsay in attempting a full description of an illness, whereas it is only with the familiarity of years that the physician can see, with the evidence of his own eyes, the entire scope of a patient's illnesses and the subtleties of disease expression.

It is impossible at this point not to repeat the words of the eminent clinician, Francis W. Peabody, MD (1881-1927), a practical and homely description that is matched neither in ancient nor in most contemporary medicine:

"The truth of the matter is that the practice of medicine is intensely personal and no system or machine can be substituted for the personal relationship. The proper interpretation of symptoms involves not only a comprehension of the causes of symptoms but also of the person in whom the symptoms arise. Every experienced physician knows that when one of his patients complains of a pain in the stomach it is probably a very trivial matter and when another makes apparently the same complaint it is probably a very serious matter.

"professionals" living in a city, to be considered frauds. Medical itinerants were not specified as being included in this lot, but as *Decorum* is oriented to physicians one wonders if, by focusing on the itinerant practioner, we are missing an important part of the picture of early Greek medicine, the established practitioner. Although Hippocrates is sometimes identified as an itinerant physician, factual information of his life is almost nonexistent, and perhaps the various cities supposedly visited by him were purposeful relocations rather than anecdotal perambulations.

It all depends on the type of patient, and the better the physician knows his patient the better will he be able to decide on the proper treatment. .... He knows the patient from childhood up- his physical health, the nervous and mental strain to which he has been subjected, the conditions of his social, business and domestic life, and, more even than this, he may have the same detailed knowledge of the patient's parents and of the circumstances of their lives. Now all this kind of information, which is difficult to obtain except as the result of years of intimacy, has an infinitely important bearing on the question of health and disease."[16]

This is the very antithesis of the peripatetic physician, who is not missed.[17]

C. The Physician-in-training; The Role of Society

In some regions of pre-Hippocratic Greece, such as Cos and nearby Cnidus, the competence and reputation of a practitioner reflected on his family, including its other physician members. A scion of an Asclepiad family of physicians had a duty to the family's profession because it supported the family and was a source of pride. It was not necessary that there be any other prod to performance such as special interest or aptitude in the care of the sick or appreciation of the adventure of biological discovery. Like the wisdom of the arranged marriage, the handing down from father to son of the family profession provided longitudinal stability for society and family. But this arrangement would not have been particularly conducive to medical progress, for any discovery of a new clinical sign or a more effective therapy would likely have been viewed only as utilitarian, not exciting, and sharing of information with others was limited because the family's interests might be compromised.[18] All this is reminiscent of aristocratic European families when, as special interest groups, they provided most of the talent of society. Occasionally one of their well-bred and well-educated progeny would stand forth as a giant, a Wellington or a Lavoisier or a de Tocqueville, and become, justifiably, a source of societal self-congratulation. But for the most part aristocratic families merely permitted their own special interests to be first in line for centuries, the many defects of such a system being vividly described by Thomas Paine. But such elitism disappeared in medicine when, apparently through the good offices of Hippocrates, the profession was opened to those outside the Asclepian families and, in a word, became democratized.

Although Hippocratic physicians were at home in their society by virtue of both training and inclination, this does not mean that they were representative of society at large. There has always been a favorable aura attached to those in the medical profession, and once persons outside those families gained admittance to it the aura would attach to

---

[16] Peabody, F.W., *Doctor and Patient*, NY, 1930, p. 23.

[17] He may not be missed, but the ancient peripatetic physician has his counterparts in today's emergency-rooms, in busy clinics where patients are randomly assigned to available physicians and seldom see the same one twice, in *locum tenens* practices, and in teaching hospitals, to name a few locations. Physicians practicing in these locations are responding to need and are not the problem, indeed are a Godsend for their patients.

[18] A more recent example of how sequestration of medical knowledge can inhibit progress occurred in the Chamberlen family which, over several generations, failed to disclose the nature of the obstetrical forceps the senior member had invented in the 16th C, thus delaying for perhaps more than a century the incorporation of this valuable tool into general practice. The medical profession at the time responded harshly to this selfish behavior.

them as well. It is true that the newly admitted were unlikely to have come from impoverished or uneducated families, for they had been able to purchase their Hippocratic affiliation. On the other hand, the medical *techne*, being a profession requiring hands-on labor, would have been unappealing to the well-to-do or to the aristocrat as Athens and other city-states prospered, although it was pointed out earlier that up through the Periclean Age (460-429 BC) physical work was not despised to the extent that it later would be. In the Hippocratic Oath the financial assistance to be rendered by a physician to his colleague, should he come to need it, is testimony that physicians as a group were not invariably, or even usually, wealthy, and that for a physician to become needy was not a rare event. Many writers have used the example of Democedes (see footnote p. 139) to argue that ancient Greek physicians were often highly paid and internationally esteemed, quite a jump of faith when, in fact, most physicians were paid at a standard laborer's rate.[19] Beyond this, not only was the Athenian physician included among the city's "craftsmen," but most Athenians could not have afforded the services of an expensive physician. It has been proposed that even a lower "upper class" Athenian citizen had little disposable wealth, based on the annual returns of his estate and investments (*e.g.*, slaves). These citizens, termed Liturgists, numbered less that 4,800 in 4th C Athens, and therefore those with disposable income and able to be beneficent to their physician would have been far fewer.[20]

Prof. Nutton reviews recent scholarship on the subsequent status of physicians in Hellenistic and Roman times, a "station in the lower middle class."[21] Dio Chrysostom (40-120 AD) listed physicians with traders, farmers, soldiers, builders, lyre-players, and "not inferior to joiners," and Prof. Rostovtzeff classified them as "petty bourgeoisie," along with money-changers, salaried clerks, and minor municipal officers.[22] Schmeling affirms that in the novels of the Greco-Roman period few "learned professions," including medicine, receive mention.[23] And, while it may have been fashionable for an aristocrat to have an amateur's knowledge of medicine, the actual practice of the profession for a wage was menial.[24] Finally, Prof. Max Laistner reviews classical Greek writings on political economy and markets, and, except for the passing use of the physician as a philosophical metaphor for a specialist, there is no mention of medicine in an economic context.[25] Medicine as a career was not sought by the wealthy, nor was it sought for wealth.

What enticement existed, then, for the practice of medicine beyond obtaining a modest livelihood? The reasons would have been the same that entice students into medicine today: a humanely useful, meaningful career, one holding a lifelong intellectual

---

[19] Zimmern, A. E., *The Greek Commonwealth* (Oxford, 1915), Part III, chapter 7, p. 271.

[20] Casson, L., *The Athenian Upper Class and New Comedy*, in *Trans. and Proc. Amer. Philol. Assoc.*, 106:29-59, 1976, in which Casson makes the following statement: "Only the very rich, the members of the Three Hundred, had no financial worries."

[21] Nutton, V, *The Fatal Embrace: Galen and the History of Ancient Medicine*, in *Science in Context*, 18:111-121, 2005. A similar assessment is presented by H. W. Pleket in *The Social Status of Physicians in the Graeco-Roman World*, in *Clio Med.*, 27:27-34, 1995.

[22] Rostovteff, M., *The Social and Economic History of the Roman Empire*, Oxford, 1957.

[23] *The Novel in the Ancient World*, Boston, 2003, chapter 6 by A. Billault: *Characterization in the Ancient Novel*, p. 123, Schmeling, G., ed.

[24] Austin, M.M. and Vidal-Naquet, P., *Economic and Social History of Ancient Greece*, California, 1977, pp. 11-18, 159-78.

[25] Laistner, M. L. W., *Greek Economics*, London, 1923.

challenge and filled with daily examples of the wonders of existence.[26] These provide a mighty and attractive draw, despite many daily activities of the physician, which, then and now, can be technically difficult, dangerous, depressing, distasteful, and at times a bit disgusting.[27] Other reasons for the attractiveness of medicine as a career include:

1) There has been an element of pride and an appreciation of the good opinion of the public on becoming a physician. There is also a sense of honor attached to careers that protect the public, such as law enforcement and firefighting. After all, the police and fire-fighters must bargain vigorously to extract a dime more from the public purse, but the public continues to expect the policeman and fireman to risk death on behalf of total strangers. This leap from civil servant to saint cannot be explained in solely economic terms; the role of pride and honor make paltry such a consideration. And so it was, is, or should be, in medicine. Plato felt the distinctive mark of a "true doctor" was concern for the welfare of his patient, not the making of money.[28] As far as this is a comment on pride rather than altruism, Plato was correct. The importance of pride cannot be overstated, for Hippocratic physicians were not born elite, but it was in their best interest to appear elite, and this they did by earning the right to be viewed as elite.

2) There is a natural curiosity about nature and man's own body. Every man, should he be unencumbered, is a researcher, a seeker after things new or better. In medicine, research can be assigned to one of three categories: epidemiological, basic, or clinical:

(a) *Epidemiological research* is for the most part research in the third person and is heavily weighted towards data collection and statistical analysis. There is often a clinical datum under investigation but the research process itself is intellectual rather than clinical. Over the last century the complexity of statistical methods has made the statistician the critical component of this research team.

(b) *Basic research* is also non-clinical, although it is always the basic researcher's hope that information derived from his work will ultimately have clinical relevance. But the questions asked and the techniques used in basic research make the person with special knowledge, the scientist, the critical person on the basic research team. And, as exciting as it is to have a foot in both the clinical and basic research fields, it is the rare clinician-scientist of today who can justify doing so, although many try. Basic research, more than

---

[26] The author hereby acknowledges that more than fifty years ago in his medical school class of 140 graduates whom he knew personally during a rigorous four years there was not a single comment in private conversation or in public that even hinted that handsome remuneration was even a minor enticement to enter the profession. And the reason, he asserts, is not because such mention would have been viewed as unseemly, but, knowing his colleagues well, that the idea never entered the doorway of their mind. But then those were the days when the State medical association had decreed to its membership that the letters in a physician's sign outside his office should not be greater than [six] inches high so as not to be viewed as an unseemly method of competition for acquiring patients. (The exact measurements have long since been forgotten by the author, but they were modest.)

[27] The Hippocratics put it more eloquently: ὁ μὲν γὰρ ἰητρὸς ὁρῇ τε δεινά, θυγγάνει τε ἀηδέων, ἐπ' ἀλλοτρίῃσί τε συμφορῇσιν ἰδίας καρποῦται λύπας· ("For the medical man sees terrible sights, touches unpleasant things, and the misfortunes of others bring a harvest of sorrows that are peculiarly his; ..." *Breaths*, I, 6-8, *Loeb Classical Library*, *Hippocrates*, II, translation of W. H. S. Jones.) And for a first-hand account by an ancient practitioner of a commonly encountered medical problem (an anal fistula) and the physical nature of its management, read the Hippocratic work, *On Fistulas* (περὶ συριγγων), as found in the *Loeb Classical Library* series on Hippocrates.

[28] Plato, *Republic*, I, 342, c.

any other type, builds on a foundation of knowledge acquired by earlier investigators, sometimes on information amassed over centuries. From this base of knowledge hypotheses are derived and then scientifically tested. To be a basic research scientist one must have academic credentials that often come from years of study relevant to the area to be researched. The clinician can rarely justify an expenditure of such time without jeopardizing his primary mission of patient care.[29]

(c) *Clinical research*, in contrast, requires only standard clinical training, although the clinical researcher's credentials become more valuable as clinical experience is accrued. Furthermore, this type of research does not utilize complex statistics, nor does it require academic credentials of a non-clinical nature. What it does require is objectivity, curiosity, ingenuity, careful observation, and what is now described as clinical acumen, or, more simply, clinical judgment, or, in the age of the Hippocratics, προγνοστικον (prognostikon), facility in prognosis. As prognosis is involved in every aspect of clinical care (see below), those most adept at clinical care will be those most likely to advance clinical research.

In conclusion, from these descriptions of research it should be obvious that clinical research, while not identified by name, was a real option for the Hippocratic practitioner and a natural attractant for the medical entrant, for the materials, techniques, and justification were always at hand, were, in fact, part of his daily task and a way of improving his effectiveness, just as they are now. Every day brings today's clinician some new aspect of disease that is inadequately addressed in a textbook, some new idea for better management, some new experience to be learned from and brought into play for the benefit of some future patient.[30]

In the time of Hippocrates, the attachment of the new apprentice-physician to his clinical teacher presumably was as described in the Hippocratic Oath. The view of some historians and ethicists that the Oath describes an incestuous aspect of the medical profession carries no force when placed in the context of the master-pupil relationship described above. The relationship was not unnatural, the apprenticing of a young man to a master craftsman being a normal pathway for advancement in many crafts and trades into modern times. And yet the new physicians were sympathetic practitioners by virtue

---

[29] The quantitative deficiencies imposed on most people who seriously pursue disparate interests was recognized by the ancient Greeks, who advised a soldier not to waste his time on nonmilitary enjoyments such as becoming adept at playing a musical instrument. They had little praise for a "Renaissance man." And Plato, in *Laws* VIII, 12, noted that "Hardly any human being is capable of pursuing two professions or two arts rightly." (Translation by B. Jowett.)

[30] A wonderful example of the general practitioner's value as a researcher is found in the saga of Dr. Lawrence Craven of Glendale, California. The story of his discovery of the usefulness of aspirin in preventing myocardial infarction and stroke, a usefulness that at one time or another has probably benefited every family in America today, is recounted by Miner and Hoffhines in: *The Discovery of Aspirin's Antithrombotic Effects, Tex. Heart Inst. J.*, 34:179-186, 2007. And it does not always take a physician. In 1975 Polly Murray accumulated a list of children who recently had evidence of "arthritis" in and around her community of Lyme, Connecticut. After submitting her observations to the State Health Department, epidemiological investigations by Dr. Allen Steere led to a newly described tick-borne entity, Lyme arthritis. (See, for example, Steere, A. C., *et al.*, *Erythema chronicum migrans and Lyme arthritis*, in *Ann. Intern. Med.*, 86:685-698, 1977.) Society even defines disease. R. A. Aronowitz has described the traditional workings of "symptom-based" diagnoses in a discussion of *When do symptoms become a disease?* (*Ann. Intern. Med.* 134:803-9, 2001), noting that a cluster of symptoms, being patients' descriptions, can at times define a disease for the medical profession, thus indicating the importance of social influence in the process.

of birth, training, and self-interest. The relevant Greek expression at the time was, "The city is the teacher of man."[31] Society's daily interactions played a role in shaping the physician then as now, but it did not do so by legislative coercion.

D. The Practicing Physician: Physicians' Practices

Most specific historical references to practitioners concern the City Physician and another type of physician described by the German term, Leibartz,[32] a private physician to royalty or to otherwise prominent individuals or families. As for the average practitioner there are anecdotes such as the one by Plato that differentiates physicians for free citizens from those who served the slave population.[33] It is curious, therefore, that ἰατρός (iatros), routinely translated as "physician," was also applied to physician assistants who served as slave practitioners. This suggests that the generic "health care provider" might be a more appropriate translation of the Greek "iatros."[34] On the other hand, in modern times "doctor" is not only applied to physicians but often to those assisting a physician, and in military service the medic or corpsman is usually called "doc" by his Company.

But the authentic setting of Hippocratic medical practice remains inferential. Physicians of Hippocratic Greece were often peripatetic, and apprentices or slaves who

---

[31]"πόλις ἄνδρα διδάσκει (polis andra didaske)," Simonides of Ceos (556-469 BC), 95 *Lyra Graeca* vol. 2. Simonides, a poet and man of learning, was a champion of the morality of moderation.

[32] The role of City (or "Public") Physicians has been long debated, some favoring the view that they represented a Greek version of socialized health services that moderns would do well to copy and others who interpret their role as involving public health matters and perhaps a free clinic but distinct from the bulk of physicians who were in private practice. There are, however, few references to City Physicians in the 6th and 5th centuries, and only in the Hellenistic period are sufficient epigraphical findings available to better define their practices (see: Cohn-Haft, L., *The Public Physicians of Ancient Greece*, in *Smith College Studies in History*, Vol. XLII, Massachusetts, 1956). Public physicians, employees of their respective cities, were able to collect fees from patients, and their job description, principally the guarantee of a resident physician, is recognizable well into the age of Imperial Rome. In contrast, the Leibartz is a term for general use rather than one identifying a specific category of physician, retaining its original German sense of "personal physician to a prominent person." A prominent Leibartz was Dr. Theodor Morell, personal physician to Adolph Hitler.

[33] Plato, in *Laws* IV, 720a, makes the distinction thus: "There are some we call 'physicians', and [then there are] some who are supervised by those physicians, but these are nevertheless being called 'physicians.' " (Translation by the author.)

[34] This definition of "iatros" was retained by the Roman Empire as indicated by the Roman jurist, Ulpian (170-228 AD), in Book VII of *On All Tribunals*: "Anyone understands a physician to be one who promises a cure for any part of the body or relief from pain, as, for example, an affection of the ear, a fistula, or a toothache; provided he does not employ incantations, ..." (Translation of S. P. Scott, *The Civil Law*, Cincinnati, 1932.) And two centuries later Eunapius (347-414 AD), a Greek historian, *despite no medical training*, told ἰατροί (iatroi) to incise the veins of the elderly philosopher, Chrysanthius. This they did, suggesting their role was that of a technician and probably similar to that of the barber-surgeon. The patient died. See Eunapius, *Lives of the Sophists*, *Loeb Classical Library*, p. 562. The equating of the modern physician with a medical practitioner of the ancient world would, except for the Hippocratic physician, be a very loose translation at best and usually highly misleading.

worked intermittently with the physicians may have been at times the permanent local practitioners, being instructed periodically by a physician as conditions permitted and, making periodic follow-up visits, relaying new information about a patient to the physician. But it is not unreasonable to suggest that there were sufficient physicians to provide for everyone. Assuming the population of ancient Greece was approximately 3,000,000,[35] and there was one physician for every 1,000 persons, 3,000 active physicians would have been required. And if the average professional career spanned thirty years, then 133 physicians would need to enter practice each year to maintain that physician density, not such an extraordinary number, and, relative to population size, the total annual output of all American medical schools today approximates one-tenth that.[36]

Bits and pieces of evidence, gleaned from writings of ancient philosophers, poets, and playwrights, have been integrated into believable, but still fictional, practice scenarios, such as Becker's *Charicles*.[37] To better understand the Hippocratic physician's world, therefore, it is more accurate to focus on specific aspects of medical practice than to imagine the overall event, to concentrate on elements of the pattern rather than speculate on the yet-to-be-completed garment. These can be examined under the following headings:

1) The physician's office:

Although physicians' offices, called ἰατρεῖα (iatreions), existed, all examinations of the patients described by Hippocratic physicians in the *Epidemics* took place in patients' homes. As sixty percent of those patients died, the seriousness of their illnesses indicates that office visits were for the less sick and more mobile patients. By staying home in bed to receive medical attention patients were, in effect, admitting themselves to a hospital. Physicians apparently made home visits not for patients' convenience but because of patients' necessity. House calls for what might be termed routine outpatient problems were probably viewed as a luxury, except in those circumstances where the physician's task and time were valued less than the patient's.

Becker has provided an entertaining social perspective of the ancient Greek physician and his office in *Charicles* (*ibid.*, on p. 281*ff*). The Hippocratic work, κατ' ἰητρειον (*In the Surgery*), addresses primarily the technical aspects of dressing various types of wounds, the title indicating an office setting. It describes a surgical procedure as requiring "the patient, the operator, assistants, instrument\s, lights and their proper placement." There is a discussion of natural vs. man-manipulated lighting, both direct and oblique, as well as the comfort of the operator and adequate visibility of the object to be operated, noting that "the operator will in this way get a good view and the part treated not be exposed to view" to either the patient or the public. The patient should assist in positioning himself so as to prevent movement during the procedure. Temperature of the water to be used is to be tested by pouring some on the operator's own hand, the physician's fingernails "neither to exceed nor come short of the finger tips." His objective

---

[35]This is the estimate in *Atlas of World Population History*, 1978, Harmondsworth, C. McEvedy and R. Jones. It does not indicate the percent that were slaves.

[36] For the year 2011, the total U. S. population was 311,000,000 and medical graduates numbered 17,364.

[37] For example, Becker, W.A., *Charicles or illustrations of the private life of the ancient Greeks*, (trans. F. Metcalfe), London, 1845: "Scene the Eighth"; Davis, W. S., *A Day in Old Athens*, Boston, 1914: Chapter X, *The Physicians of Athens*.

in the performance of procedures, including bandaging, is "to obtain ability, grace, speed, painlessness, elegance and readiness."[38]

The Hippocratic bench for reduction of dislocations of the skeletal system, called the "scamnon," has received much attention, and several attempts have been made to portray it, two of which are illustrated in the *Loeb Classical Library* series on *Hippocrates*, vol. 3. It is current opinion that the Hippocratic works on fractures, joints, and dislocations are likely to have been composed contemporaneously with Hippocrates, and perhaps many a physician's office had such a device.

All in all, the physician's office in later Hippocratic times would seem familiar to today's physicians, with this caveat: it is primarily the Hippocratic writings that are the source of this information. Non-Hippocratic practitioners, those outside the professional boundaries of Coan medical services, may have had quite different procedures and venues.

2) Physician's bag:

There is no Hippocratic era physician's "black bag" that has been discovered. A box containing instruments and drugs has been described by Mary Beard, the instruments including scalpels, hooks, forceps of various types, specula for internal examination, cupping vessels, probes, scissors, spatulas, instruments for lavaging, bone drills, sounds and metal catheters found in the ruins of Pompeii, buried by the eruption of Vesuvius in 79 AD, and instruments of an equivalent antiquity were portrayed in wall engravings of the temple of Kom Ombo in late 2nd C BC Roman Egypt.[39] It is likely that similar physicians' instruments were used by Hippocratics, as suggested in a Hippocratic writing called *Decorum* (VIII, X):

> Translation: [Bring with you] lint, gauze, bandages, essentials for stabilization of an injury, medicines for wounds and for the eyes and related things, and carefully plan in advance for necessary instruments, devices, knives, and the like;
>
> You should carry with you another, auxiliary, medical case for house calls, one that is easily managed and accessible.
>
> And prepare in advance all types of emollients.

3) The combined practice of medicine and surgery:

The two great divisions of the medical profession from its earliest days have been surgery and internal medicine. Surgery traditionally has dealt with visible structural, or anatomic, abnormalities, the consequences of either external forces causing injury or internal physical disruptions leading to organ dysfunction. The attempt to physically rectify the abnormality is the realm of the surgeon. Some of man's earliest medical

---

[38] Translations from *In the Surgery* by E. T. Withington, *Loeb Classical Library*, *Hippocrates*, vol. III.

[39] Beard, M., *The Fires of Vesuvius*, Cambridge, 2008, and Nunn, J., *Ancient Egyptian Medicine*, Norman OK, 1996, p. 165. But see also: Bliquez, L., *Roman Surgical Instruments*, Mainz, 1994. Bliquez notes that while instruments were found in twenty-seven sites, perhaps only four sites were locations where surgery was performed, the remainder probably being for the personal use of families.

records are of a surgical nature, such as the Smith papyrus (1550 BC; see p. 495*ff*) and the *Susruta Samhita* (? 400 AD; see p. 88, the Bower manuscript). Wonderful discoveries in the techniques of empirical wound management have been made over the centuries. It seems extraordinary, therefore, that those who are expert in surgical treatments that have proven eminently useful, intellectually challenging, physically demanding, and, as their results are often promptly beneficial, profoundly satisfying, have held over the ages a social status inferior to practitioners of internal medicine.

Internal medicine deals with all the rest of medicine, that which is not surgical, although in recent times certain specialties have become so unique in methodology that it seems they belong to neither internal medicine nor surgery or to both. The natural tendency of the body to heal itself is equally observable in surgical and medical illnesses. Most surgical wounds will heal satisfactorily by "primary or secondary intention"[40] given time and limited expectation, and many acute internal medicine (medical) disorders, such as pneumonia, measles, and cholecystitis, often or usually resolve, at least in the short term, satisfactorily on their own given time and with no outside interference. So what is it that led to this apparently undue esteem for those engaged in management of "internal diseases" as compared with their surgical colleagues.

There are four reasons. One is that practitioners of surgery were deemed effective on the basis of technical rather than intellectual skills.[41] With proper instruction many were capable of being the local expert in setting fractures, applying poultices, searing wounds, or extracting arrows. It was not an exclusive art, and it called more for verve and nerve than reserve.

The second reason is that, in requiring technical skills, surgery did not appeal to the higher socioeconomic or intellectual classes. Because physical work, often distasteful, was involved, surgery was held far inferior to soldiering or managing estates and akin to carpentry or making pottery.[42]

A third reason is that an illness without a visible cause invited explanation. Invoking a demon or divine intervention therefore satisfied curiosity, and the tyranny of the "priest physician," and later the cleverness of the charlatan, exploited this. The natural tendency of most illnesses to improve spontaneously by means of antibody formation or local inflammatory responses, led to four out of five illnesses resolving, at least in the short term, a success story for any type of ancient practitioner. Failure could be explained away as due to flaws of the victim or tardiness of the consultation, scapegoats that remain in force today. In contrast, a knife wound from battle required no speculation as to cause.

Lastly, the exaggerated appeal of mystical healing was due to fear of the unknown. An illness given a name, said to be understood, or claimed to have been previously encountered gave, and still gives, relief to the severely ill patient and his family, even when there is no hope of cure. This relief is not a respite from pain, suffering, or sorrow; it is relief from the dread of the unknown. It means that the patient is not alone, that he has not in some unknown way been selected to undergo a personal affliction

---

[40] Primary intention: the wound edges are apposed, perhaps using sutures or tape; secondary intention: the wound is allowed to granulate in from the periphery of the wound and naturally seal the injury site.

[41] Edelstein, L., *Ancient Medicine*, Baltimore, 1967, p. 26-27, a section referring to the procedure of lithotomy in which this prejudice is put forth as an explanation for its proscription by the Hippocratic Oath.

[42] Examples of the persistence of this early perspective of surgical practice include the barber surgeons in the Western world and the formal address of "Mr." for British surgeons to this day.

previously unencountered by others, and in this there is always the hope that something observed in previous cases may help him. The physician, the priest, and the charlatan, if sufficiently convincing, were all able to assuage those fears.

Montaigne (1533-1592) recognized the objective nature of surgery, in contrast to the incredible conjectures of internal medicine.[43] But man is a peck of rationality in a bushel of emotion, and true is the old adage that mankind reverences most what it least understands. Practitioners thought to understand and to deal effectively with the unknown were therefore held in higher esteem than those who dealt with the obvious. To be held in higher esteem, of course, does not mean to be better liked. The ancients may have loved their local surgeon, but they were in awe of the palace "internist" and courted his attentions with flattery and enticements not provided to their neighbor, the drainer of abscesses down the street.

And so it is that the history of surgery has been consistently useful and distinguished by skill, ingenuity, and practicality, whereas the history of internal medicine has been, until recently, a tale of mountebanks, rhetoricians, and philosophers. Except, of course, for the Hippocratics.[44] And it may have been some early neighborhood surgical practitioner, perhaps Hippocrates himself, who realized that, if natural philosophers were satisfied that they could explain natural phenomena without invoking deities, then why could not the same apply to nonsurgical illness? Indeed, it might be argued that the Hippocratics pulled the formerly mystical and subjective internal medicine into the objective world of surgery. If this is so, then Hippocratic medicine finds its roots in surgery, which would explain its rationality, in contrast to the prattle of the shaman or priest medicine.

Perhaps to Hippocrates must go the honor for this great innovation. With one stroke he elevated surgery to an esteemed profession, and, by denying the mystical nature of epilepsy,[45] he brought internal medicine down to earth. And sad it was when this conjunction, so fruitful to the profession, came asunder during the next few centuries. It could even be argued that the schism between surgery and internal medicine was, in fact, an important contributor to the disappearance of Hippocratic medicine. The Roman

---

[43] "and 'tis thence that I conclude surgery to be much more certain, by reason that it sees and feels what it does, and so goes less upon conjecture; whereas the physicians have no *speculum matricis* by which to examine our brains, lungs, and liver." *Essays of Michel de Montaigne*, chapter 2.37, translation of Charles Cotton.

[44] Greek physicians retained these two faces of medicine down to the time of Galen, who stated, "Surgery is but a method of treatment." But by the 12th C medical students in Paris were required to renounce manual labor in the practice of their new vocation, and the Western Church worked actively to inhibit the practice of surgery. What had once been merely detached from the profession of medicine was now on its way to extinction in the West. The study of anatomy was subsequently to benefit by studies from the Renaissance, but surgery, except for its military aspect, remained in the hands of non-professionals. As recently as 1905, long after the invention of modern anesthesia and the professionalization of surgery, important physicians' organizations still rendered the two branches of medicine utterly distinct. For a scholarly review of the schism between internal medicine and surgery see: Allbutt, T. C., *The Historical Relations of Medicine and Surgery*, London, 1905.

[45] This refers to the famous book of the *Hippocratic Corpus*, περὶ ἱερῆς νούσου (Concerning the Sacred Disease), in which the writer indicates there is a natural rather than divine causation of epilepsy.

writer, Celsus, described the schism two thousand years ago, noting that five hundred years earlier Hippocrates had promoted the practice of surgery by general practitioners.[46]

In summary, Hippocratic physicians took the view that both internal medicine and surgery were but aspects of the same profession. In the public's eye effective and skilled surgical attention by the physician must have made his often ineffective efforts in treating non-surgical disease seem less a personal defeat or error and therefore easier to forgive and to bear. It may well be that some future history of internal medicine will be subsumed by the history of surgery, relegated to a branch of the tree of clinical medicine, the trunk of which will represent surgery.

4) Definition and significance of "prognosis:"

Much has been written concerning the use of prognosis by early Hellenic physicians. It has not all been flattering. The historian, Dr. Erwin Ackerknecht, considered prognosis a consequence of the "unprotected social position of the Greek physician."[47] Professor Owsei Temkin agreed, stating that the physician's interest in prognosis "stemmed neither from exclusively therapeutic nor from purely scientific interests. It was largely motivated by the doctor's need to protect himself from suspicion and accusations in case of an unfavorable outcome." Facility at prognosis, he wrote, enhanced a physician's reputation and resulted from "social motivation."[48] One should be cautious, however, about attributing motives to the actions of others, for this sometimes sheds unflattering light on motives of the attributor. Another proposal is that prognosis implied a link to religion, for prediction was the work of oracles and soothsayers, and perhaps physicians were also adepts.[49] And, again, "They took on the guise of rhetors in order to obscure the manual aspects of their discipline" is another explanation for the sophistic nature of early attempts at prognosis by some Hippocratic physicians, one that, like the others above, misunderstands, ignores, or seeks to impune Hippocratic motivation.[50]

But clinicians work with prognosis every day. The estimable Dr. Mirko Grmek noted that prognosis "offered an immediate way to verify the professional know-how of an itinerant practitioner," but its "main role" was to give the physician "a simple and effective way to distinguish and articulate typological regularities in the jumble of a still

---

[46] Autem cum haec pars sit vetustissima, tamen exculta-est magis ab illo parente omnis medicinae Hippocrate, quam a prioribus: deinde, posteaquam diducta ab aliis, coepit habere suos professores, ... ("Now this branch [surgery], though it be the most ancient, yet has been more cultivated by Hippocrates, than by his predecessors. Afterwards being separated by its other parts, it began to have its own professors,..." Celsus, *De Medicina*, Book VII, Preface, translation of J. Grieve, Edinburgh, 1814.) "Professor" is better translated as "teacher" or "schoolmaster."

[47] Ackerknecht, E. H., *A Short History of Medicine*, New York, 1968, p. 61.

[48] Temkin, O., *Hippocrates in a World of Pagans and Christians*, Baltimore, 1991, p. 11.

[49] Withington, E. T., *Asclepiadae* in *Studies in the History and Method of Science*, vol. ii, Oxford, 1921.

[50] Horstmanshoff, H. F. J., *The Ancient Physician: Craftsman or Scientist?*, in *J. Hist. Med.*, 45: 176-197, 1990. It would have been difficult to disguise manual procedures, for effective therapies such as draining an empyema, returning a ball-and-socket joint to its proper position, relieving acute urinary obstruction with a catheter, or draining a perinephric abscess, would have been gratefully praised by the patient, no matter how the procedure was rhetorically couched to others. And why would anyone want to disguise something that they would have been justifiably pleased and proud to have accomplished, the relief of someone in acute distress?

very crude nosological taxonomy."[51] In other words, it functioned for the Hippocratics in part as a primitive surrogate for diagnosis. But beyond this, from clinical evidence physicians anticipate the course of events in the short term (should the patient be intubated?; will he benefit from transfer to the ICU (Intensive Care Unit)?; will intravenous adenosine be safer than electrical cardioversion?), in the intermediate term (should a medication be changed?; when can the patient be safely discharged?), and in the long-term (what can prevent a recurrence?; when is the best time for the next appointment?) All of this is prognosis in action, not diagnosis. If things look hopeless the physician may elect to do nothing. If signs and symptoms suggest forthcoming improvement he may decide to not change the treatment plan. If a new sign is detected consistent with a poorer prognosis he may add a new medication. *In medical practice prognosis is everything; it is a part of every clinical decision made, all day and every day; wherever there is choice there must be an estimate of prognosis. It is, in a word, clinical judgment.* The only difference between "prognosis" for Hippocrates and for the modern physician is quantitative; now there are many more choices with which to contend. Compared to the ancients, prognosis is no less important, just more complex. Prognosis is not studied to "show off," to "wow" the public, to guard against criticism, advance socially, or identify frauds. It is instead the buttress upon which all clinical decisions depend, for choice is the occasion for knowledge of προγνωστιχον ("prognosticon"; prognosis). This is the reason it was so studied by the Hippocratics, and it is odd that over the centuries such varied guises have been devised at great effort to otherwise explain the obvious.

Prognosis is also a critical element of the physician-patient relationship. At its most basic, it is an important reason for visiting the physician in the first place. A person has a particular symptom and wishes to know what it means, what will happen if something is or is not done, and what will be the long-term consequence. Aeschylus (525-456 BC) had Prometheus point out this concern in *Prometheus Bound*: "To the sick 'tis solace clearly to know beforehand what pain still awaiteth them ...."[52] The desire for a prognosis is natural, and to receive a prognosis from a Western physician has, at least for 2,500 years, been expected by the patient because, with few exceptions, the sick, including the sick physician, will want to know, "What will happen to me, doctor?" In many parts of the world the truth, if it is unfavorable, is often withheld from the patient, perhaps at the request of the family or a friend. But in the United States the next statement of the patient will likely be, "Please tell me the truth." And in the United States that is what the patient will hear, for in an educated society the physician and patient equally share in decisions, and a democratic koinon of two demands honesty from both parties.[53]

---

[51] Grmek, M. D., *Diseases in the Ancient Greek World*, Baltimore 1991, paperback edition of a translation by M. Muellner and L. Muellner of the 1983 work, p. 293.

[52] Aeschylus, *Prometheus Bound*, 698. Translation of H. W. Smyth, in vol. 1 of the *Loeb Classical Library* series of Aeschylus, p. 277.

[53] The fine Internist, Dr. Saul Radovsky, provided a practitioner's experience with this approach in: *Bearing the News*, in *New Engl. J. Med.*, 313:586-588, 1985. Dr. Radovsky was merely repeating the advice of an early Hippocratic physician: "It is not correct to portray [to the patient] a disease in any way other than it is, for example, a serious one as being a minor one, or a minor one as one that is serious. It is also not correct to represent to a patient a non-fatal illness as being fatal, or a fatal illness as one from which he will recover." *Works of Hippocrates, Loeb Classical Library*, vol. 5, *Diseases* I, 6, translation by the author. In consonance with this see: Jackson, J., *Truth, Trust and Medicine*, Philadelphia 2001.

Finally, there is great value of prognosis in furthering medical knowledge. Once the usual course taken by a particular disease has been defined, deviations from that prognosis can be noted and possible explanations considered. Also important would be the effect of treatments, for, knowing the usual course of an illness, a better idea could be had of whether a particular treatment was good, bad, or ineffective. Generalizations were less likely to be made on the basis of one or a few observations, thereby minimizing the effects of statistical sampling error and wishful thinking.

There is no doubt that the ability to accurately forecast the course of a disease added to the reputation of the early physician. His use of prognosis probably did puff up his pride and image. But in the greater picture, the prognostication of the Hippocratics placed them ahead of other practitioners for a reason: their data collection provided a better statistical base from which to make decisions. This gave them a competitive edge. Is it fair, or even sensible, to deride a proud professional who is better than all the others in doing his job? The Hippocratics recognized the all-embracing importance of prognosis, the heart of scientific medical practice.

5) Techniques:

If the Hippocratics were scientific, why were their therapies for medical illness apparently no further advanced than those of other societies? After all, phlebotomy, cupping, and purgatives were not unique to the Greeks. The reason is that Hippocratic medicine was a work in progress, not fully evolved. Its evolution was cut short, ending before important new treatments could replace traditional therapeutic ones. Left alone, cupping would have found its true place in Hippocratic therapeutics, for its utter ineffectiveness would have been uncovered.[54] Suspicion as to the limited usefulness and unknown risks of many popular therapies was the basis for the caution displayed by the Hippocratics. Their limited pharmacopoeia, for example, has been ridiculed and compared unfavorably with the vast array of drug treatments in other societies, for it supposedly indicates show inadequate was their knowledge and how little they could affect the course of disease (see p. 345*f*). But therapies multiply in the absence of effectiveness, and the real reason for their restricted pharmacopoeia was that most available medicinal treatments were probably recognized by them to be ineffective or dangerous.

Nevertheless, it would have required much more time and great discrimination before they would have realized the full clinical significance of phlebotomy. Ridiculed by moderns as an archaic procedure that somehow managed to survive into the 19th C,

---

[54] Techniques of cupping were known to the ancient Egyptians, as mentioned in the Ebers papyrus of 1550 BC. The earliest documentation in Asia is found in the writings of the 4th C AD philosopher Ge Hong. Interestingly, the latter advised its use in treating pustular lesions, and therefore it conceivably may have hastened the drainage of superficial abscesses. But cupping is a visually dramatic yet utterly useless procedure that merely causes local superficial vasodilatation in the skin by the application of vacuum. Nevertheless, it was recommended as an adjunct to diuresis in chronic renal failure as recently as 1938 in a pediatric textbook (J. Griffith and A. Mitchell, *The Diseases of Infants and Children*, Philadelphia, p. 802). There are variations in technique that permit blood extravasation from abraided or punctured skin ("blood cupping"). Numerous theories have been advanced to support the use of cupping, such as the removal of toxin-laden blood, alterations in the flow of body energy (qi) and decreasing blood stagnation by increasing local blood flow. It was discredited in American medicine in the 19th C but remains extremely popular worldwide. The modern persistence of cupping vividly documents man's uncontrollable desire not to do nothing.

there have been, and are, many reasonable indications for phlebotomy, the removal of blood from a large vein. At the beginning of the 18th C Boerhaave noted these:

1. It prevents "too great a Resistance to the Force of the Heart." And, again, "When the Blood is too thick, so that it cannot easily pervade the pulmonary Artery, it is there accumulated, and resists the Contraction of the right Ventricle of the Heart. Hence arise those frequent Palpitations..."
2. The "Fullness of the Vessels" is lessened.
3. Some use phlebotomy, even in patients over seventy years of age, to treat "plethora," although he recommends this only when unavoidable.
4. It "restores the over-distended Vessels to their former Contractions and Elasticity."
5. Phlebotomy decreases "Redundancy" of the blood, *i.e.*, excesses, either of total blood volume or blood components.

6. Relief from excessive "Blood and Humours" is needed when there is "Palpitation of the Heart, and great Turgescence of the Veins."[55]

At the beginning of the 21st C are found the following indications for its use:[56]

1. Pulmonary edema – Although no longer used for this manifestation of severe congestive heart failure, those who have seen the effect of acute removal of sufficient blood from a patient *in extremis* will not forget how immediately it relieved respiratory distress and returned a moribund patient, however briefly, to an alert and communicative state. Phlebotomy did not cure any cardiac disease, but on occasion it prolonged life until some other measures could be instituted. This is the basis for use of tourniquets to acutely decrease effective circulating blood volume by restricting venous return to the heart in an emergency setting.
2. Polycythemia vera – This uncommon but by no means rare disorder of malignant overproduction of red blood cells is still treated by phlebotomy in most instances, with the removal of blood from a plethoric patient capable of improving mental status, preventing strokes, and reversing heart failure, visual disturbances, phlebitis, paresthesias, and other distressing symptoms. Phlebotomy is the long-term management of choice for this disease, extending life expectancy in many patients with polycythemia vera to normal.
3. Porphyria – Phlebotomy can ameliorate the cutaneous manifestations of porphyria cutanea tarda.
4. Cyanotic heart disease – The increase in blood viscosity associated with the overproduction of red blood cells in chronic hypoxemic states can aggravate heart failure and its symptoms. Phlebotomy can temporarily improve symptoms by decreasing blood viscosity.

---

[55] These comments are taken from the sections on "The Symptoms of Diseases" and "Of Phlebotomy" found in volume 6 of *Dr. Boerhaave's Academical Lectures on the Theory of Physic*, London, 1757, 6 vols.

[56] Phlebotomy, which in the Greek means the cutting of a blood-vessel, was a form of medical therapy throughout the ancient world. Cutting an easily visible distended vein releases continuously flowing blood until the process of coagulation seals the cut with a blood clot, whereas cutting an artery releases blood under high pressure. The former bleeding is easily controlled with slight local pressure, and so venous phlebotomy has been used for bloodletting.

5. Hypoxemic lung disease – Smoking cigarettes has made chronic lung disease a common health problem. But chronic lung disease of many types can lead to overproduction of red blood cells as the body attempts to compensate for poor tissue oxygenation. When blood viscosity reaches high levels because of overproduction of red blood cells, phlebotomy may be necessary to control symptoms.

6. Multiple myeloma and related disorders of overproduction of plasma proteins are not rare, especially in the elderly, and increased blood viscosity is a frequent complication, producing problems relating to bleeding, strokes, and heart failure. Phlebotomies for plasma removal can usually control symptoms until chemotherapy has taken effect.

7. Hypervolemia of any cause – In advanced renal failure the circulatory congestion attendant to acutely or chronically decreased urine output can be immediately eased by phlebotomy. Acute renal failure is common in severe septicemias, and most patients would not have survived in pre-antibiotic days. But some might have, and if they had been phlebotomized it would have been easy to attribute survival to this symptom-easing procedure.

Given the many situations in which phlebotomy has been proven to be useful and to have a solid basis in physiology, it is not surprising that in medicine's early days there might have arisen a theory of its general usefulness, even as a preventive medical procedure.[57] And it may be that *distention* of veins (or "turgidity," as Boerhaave called it) provided one of the clinical clues to the Hippocratics as to the patient most likely to benefit from the procedure, for distended veins are characteristic of the blood volume overload of congestive heart failure and of renal failure, uncontrolled polycythemia vera, pulmonary heart disease, and hypervolemia and hyperviscosity from any cause.[58] It would have taken only a few patients who appeared to respond to bloodletting to convince the practitioner of its value. And this does not include the psychological benefits a rather arresting procedure might induce in those who anticipate improvement, the infamous *placebo* effect, and who for the most part would suffer no serious consequences. Even in situations where the risk was real the perceived benefit might prevail, as, for example, in the use of phlebotomy to remove sufficient blood so as to impair consciousness for the purpose of anesthesia prior to an amputation.

---

[57] Although the Hippocratics did not use leeches for removal of blood, that procedure was popular in many other societies. Indeed, it is increasing in popularity today, although the therapeutic value of the leech is now thought to reside primarily in its saliva. See: Michalsen, A., *et al.*, *Effectiveness of Leech Therapy in Osteoarthritis of the Knee*, Ann. Intern. Med., 139:724-730, 2003.

[58] *The Natural State of Medical Practice: Hippocratic Evidence*, Maitland, (FL), 2019, p. 27*ff*, discusses neck vein distention as a marker of circulatory congestion. Phlebotomy was used to reverse aphasia or aphonia that occurred in an otherwise healthy person (*Regimen in Acute Diseases*, Appendix, 4-6); a 17th C physician advised the same, commenting that in one case at autopsy "the blood was found to be so coagulated, that one might draw it out of the Veins, as if it had been a solid body," concluding that in such cases bleeding was essential. And the term παρ᾽ οὖς which has been interpreted as "by the ear" may actually refer to jugular venous distention "up to the ear," an everyday clinical description heard in hospitals, and therefore the statement "He [Alexander of Tralles] lays down a very good rule in relation to a Parotis, (*i.e.*,) at first to be sure to bleed, before any discussing or drawing applications be made: that those who have been forward in doing this without bleeding, have been the instrument of strangling their patients." [sic] See: Freind, J., *The History of Physick, from the time of Galen* ..., London, 1726, 3rd edition, vol. 1 (of 2), p. 102*f*.

But there can be complications from phlebotomy, and well into the 19th C practitioners uncritically used the procedure in conditions where it was of no value.[59] It was being widely used in the 17th C when Dr. Thomas Sydenham observed that excessive phlebotomy promoted "weakness of the blood."[60] Dr. Herman Boerhaave, in his *Theory of Physic* recommended plebotomy "within *Bounds*, so as not to diminish the Strength."[61] And it was Louis who finally presented statistically analyzed evidence against the use of phlebotomy in certain situations, his publication first translated into English as recently as 1836.[62] There followed a distinct retreat from its use, for at the beginning of the 20th C textbooks of medicine do not even mention the procedure, and yet the obvious clinical benefits of phlebotomy for certain indications was noted by contemporary physicians such as Dr. Austin Flint. Modern texts again acknowledge it usefulness in a variety of situations.[63] It is remarkable that in recent centuries authoritative opinion on the risks and benefits of phlebotomy has been so varied, but for many centuries it did not vary, and this invites an excursus:

Excursus on the Appeal to Authority
(*Argumentum ad verecundiam*)

The function of logical argument involving "appeal to authority" is well described and the fallacies to which an appeal to authority is susceptible are well known. In modern medical matters the appeal to authority frequently is not fallacious, however, for areas of medical expertise are well defined and their practitioners can reasonably comprehend the full scope of available knowledge in their respective areas. Thus, for example, an appeal to authority regarding Crohn disease, if the authority is a gastroenterologist, is usually valid, and an appeal to a medical authority is often essential in law courts. In recent

---

[59] But to be fair to those practitioners, even after a critical review of published data, Sturges and Coupland (*The Natural History and Relations of Pneumonia*, London, 1890, 2nd edition, chapter XIX) could not determine the effectiveness of phlebotomy in treatment of pneumonia, the reasons being (1) the great number of variables possibly affecting outcome, (2) adequate assessments of various treatments required "many observers of a wide stretch of time," and (3) "every advocate of a particular remedy finds numbers on his own side." As a consequence, phlebotomy for treatment of pneumonia retained its popularity in many circles throughout the 19th C, but it was not from lack of questioning its effectiveness.

[60] *The Works of Thomas Sydenham, MD*, London, 1850, vol. 2, translated from the Latin by R. G. Latham, MD, p. 164. As the phrase was used in a discussion of "dropsy" it is likely that he was describing anemia as "weak blood," for severe anemia can result from the iron deficiency induced by repeated phlebotomies and from chronic renal disease, one of the causes of anasarca, or "dropsy."

[61] *Dr. Boerhaave's Academical Lectures on the Theory of Physic*, London, 1766-1773, 3rd edition in six vols., vol. 6, p. 420.

[62] Louis, P., *Researches on the Effect of Bloodletting in some Inflammatory Diseases....*, Boston, 1836.

[63] Dr. Austin Flint (1812-1886) was a prominent American clinician and teacher whose name is associated with a cardiac murmur. He wrote: "The time will come (and that ere long, for it is now foreshadowed) when it [phlebotomy] will have its proper rank among therapeutic agencies." He understood that, "A remedial agent can have but little value if it be not capable of acting injuriously as well as usefully. ... to secure their good and avoid their evil effects lies the secret of true success in the practice of medicine." This is found in a prescient little volume by Dr. Flint: *Medicine of the Future*, New York, 1886, p. 19.

medical practice the explosion of knowledge in many areas has been so great that one might even appeal to an authority on Crohn disease directed only to those gastroenterologists that deal primarily with that and related intestinal disorders, whereas a specialist in another area of gastroenterology, for example liver disease, a "hepatologist," would not be the best person from whom to seek advice for management of Crohn disease. An appeal to authority is a form of inductive logic, for the likelihood of a true conclusion will reflect the likelihood that the authority is correct rather the axiomatic correctness that is the foundation for deduced logic.

In earlier centuries learned professors in medieval universities were the authorities on most academic matters. Their word went unchallenged, at least openly and by those whose advancements depended on a good word from such an authority, and professors were held in high regard. But in medicine a different situation existed. During the Dark Ages lay medical practioners, primarily found among the clergy, had attempted to fill the void previously occupied by the Greek ἰατρός and the Roman *medicus*, and during those dark years there would have been no medical authority to whom to appeal. But lay involvement by the Church then declined with the advent of the "physician" of the medieval period as copies of recovered Greco-Roman medical writings were now claimed as authoritative and experts on their exposition were acclaimed as authorities. Thus, an appeal to authority was not an appeal to someone with knowledge of the currently evolving status of a particular area of medicine; it was, instead, an indirect appeal to ancient practitioners who had lived many centuries earlier. The cachet of those ancient authorities had somehow carried over to the medieval professors, not because of the professors' erudite and new contributions to medicine but to their knowledge of ancient literature. In reading the works of the early encyclopedists of medicine the citing of Galen or Hippocrates and other famed early clinicians is incessant, their names even being preceded at times by adjectives such as "the divine" or "the great." Thus, the legitimacy of an appeal to third person authority was stretched to the limit, and the weaknesses, fallacies, and harm of appeal to authority were fully operational. The intrinsic weakness of such an authoritative system was apparent as well in the study of mechanics. The French scholar Rene Dugas has summarized the doleful effects of undue veneration of Aristotle's *Problems of Mechanics* (μηχανικὰ προβλήματα) as follows:

> "The prejudices of the Schoolmen [*i.e.*, medieval educators], whose authority in other fields was undisputed, restricted the progress of mechanics for a long period. Annotating Aristotle was the essential purpose of teaching throughout the Middle Ages."[64]

---

[64] Dugas, R., *A History of Mechanics*, New York, 1955, translated by J. R. Maddox, p. 11. Dugas, lecturer at the Ecole Polytechnique near Paris, continues: "Not that the mediaeval scholars lacked originality. Indeed, they displayed an acute subtlety which has never been surpassed, but most often they neglected to take account of observation, preferring to exercise their minds in a pure field. Only the astronomers were an exception and accumulated the facts on which, much later, mechanics was to be based." Astronomy was also affected by a scholastic inability to ponder new explanations for observed events, and while data continued to be collected throughout the Middle Ages it remained the universe of Plato and Claudius Ptolemy (2nd C AD) into which those data were fit until the Copernican revolution (1543). Dugas also cites the writings of John (Philiponus) of Alexandria (490-570 AD), the first and only voice to question the work of Aristotle until the Renaissance and a far superior scientist than the much later Paracelsus who was to be the first to renounce Galenism in medicine (see p. 345). It is to be noted in passing that there is still scholarly

In the appeal to ancient authority that cited Galen, the problem was not with Galen. Indeed, Galen seldom appealed to any authority other than himself and Hippocrates. Whatever his errors, they were not the result of faulty logic based on appeal to authority. It was, instead, the reverence subsequent medical educators had for Galen and his writings, sometimes called "Galenolatry," that was a problem, namely their apparently unquestioning confidence in ancient knowledge. But was that really the limit of their problem? Or did they truly have so little confidence in their own medical prowess that it was thought best to rely on ancient authority, not because they were confident that it was better but because it was remote, untouchable, and, as an inviolable source of medical knowledge, a basis for decision-making, and, if matters went awry, a way of camouflaging their ignorance? This seems likely, and how similar this all is to medicine by committee in authoritarian bureaucracies. There the authority is also distant, impersonal, and arbitrary. The committee's actions can then be diffused by those in positions of influence or power so as to provide direction for policy and yet be positioned in the process to permit circumvention of new ideas or observations that might be considered undesirable or irreverent and also to avoid any personal liability that might result from a committee's actions. While it is true that a form of appeal to authority can include appeal to consensus, a point commonly addressed in committee debates, it is the inductive nature of the logic involved and its probability of error that cautions unquestioning acceptance of decisions, committee or otherwise, based on consensus.

No less a brilliant thinker than Jeremy Bentham (1748-1832) discussed at length the subject of argumentation. Although primarily directed at legislative bodies he commented the following about *Argumentum ad verecundiam*, which he also termed "the wisdom of our ancestors" or the "Chinese argument."[65] He wrote: "What, then, is the wisdom of the times called old? Is it the wisdom of gray hairs? No; it is the wisdom of the cradle." For it is obvious that experience is gained with the passage of time, and what is called the "old times" should more accurately be termed the "new times." Even the Tibetan Buddhists, he pointed out, while revering an infant, had the satisfaction of knowing that their selection for the new Dalai Lama had had the experience of prior existences. The ideas of an earlier society, however ingenious, were a product of their age, and to think that linearly succeeding generations should be more ignorant would be anomalous and overvalue "the wisdom of untaught inexperienced generations" of the past. Bentham also points to the reverence for the dead; "A dead man has no rivals," and, as the ancient authorities had long since departed, "the principle in which imagination is the sole mover," a form of idolatry, took the place of reason.

But the principal point to be made is not the method of faulty logic of the medical Schoolmen of medieval times, but why they, being intelligent, would choose to accept it as true. Bentham gives four possible reasons: sinister self-interest, interest-begotten prejudice, authority-begotten prejudice, and self-defense against counter-fallacies. Which of these applied to medieval medical academics? It would be unjust to consider sinister self-interest as the motive of the appeal to ancient and long-departed authority. Although some may have had sinister motives, it is likely, given the charitable and devout

---

debate as to authorship of μηχανιχὰ προβλήματα (Problems of Mechanics), some considering it to be Archytus of Tarentum (428-347 BC).
[65] See: *The Works of Jeremy Bentham*, Edinburgh, 1838-1843, J. Bowring, editor, vol. 2 (of 11), Chapter II: *The Wisdom of Our Ancestors; or Chinese Argument* – (ad verecundiam).

tenor of the times, that most were honorable men. It would also be unfair to blame their Galenolatry as an attempt to counterattack fallacious arguments, for they had none that threatened. Authority-begotten prejudice is unlikely because the Schoolmen claimed authority for themselves and had no way of receiving personal dispensations from the ancients, and it appears that Galenolatry was, throughout Europe, virtually a unanimous sentiment. It is, therefore, of Bentham's four choices, interest-begotten prejudice that fueled their attachment to the arcane medicine of Hippocrates and Galen, rather than infatuation with it. Because of self-interest they were easily deluded into veneration. What were the particular aspects of self-interest that appealed to them? Perhaps it was the ease of accommodating those ancient ideas, for it spared them considerable intellectual inquiry, laborious examination and data collection, and probing interrogation by peers. Perhaps, not knowing the Hippocratic methods, they simply did not know how to proceed. Thus, it was far easier and more reliable to join with their peers in espousing unassailable authority than to create a new one. And in such an environment it is also easy for a personal issue to take priority, namely one that provides a means by which personal responsibility can be averted, not to mention one that requires much less work. Thus, motives of convenience prompted medical "authorities" and "Schoolmen" in the West over a thousand or so years to illogically profess the superiority of the arcane.

One might argue that the shift from the Classical age to the Medieval was not linear, that the Dark Ages represented such a reversion to ignorance that the idea of Classical age superiority was sincerely considered to be superior, as indeed it was, and represented something that contemporary physicians needed to catch up to before they could make their own advances. This is unlikely. The accumulated knowledge of the ancients, although acquired over decades and perhaps even a century or two, could have been assimilated within a few years. Modern medical students successfully assimilate in four years vastly more data in their training than Hippocrates, Galen, and other ancient medical scholars could even begin to imagine.

In view of the preceding discussion, therefore, it is now pertinent to note that the Hippocratics had no earlier authorities to whom they might appeal. Perhaps this was their strength. Perhaps it contributed to their great leap forward to scientific medicine: they were unconstrained, not only by civil authorities but also by venerable ones. Clinical objectivity was not clouded by established assumptions.

To conclude, there is no attempt here to disparage the great value of expert opinion, but it is a note of caution to realize that the term "authority" is derived from the Latin *auctoritas*, its meanings including: an opinion, command, cause, will, and authority to act. The authoritative nature of the term was strengthened in medieval times to imply authority to enforce, a principal definition of the word today and one of great concern as centralized bureaucratic medicine on a national scale becomes operational and the national threat of physical coercion of the individual is overwhelming. But such authority is inappropriate in intellectual discourse, and in that setting any appeal to authority is always to be questioned. Indeed, in the spirit of hopefulness, one need only to accompany an Attending Physician on ward rounds in a teaching hospital in the United States to see such skepticism healthily displayed by medical students and residents. These precious few will not easily give up their sovereignty to the authoritarian.

End of excursus

Purgation is a globally used technique about which any textbook on the history of medicine abounds. This is understandable, for giving purgatives was one of the few ways that physiologic effects could be predictively induced, although their dangers were pointed out by the Hippocratics. Plato himself was generally opposed to the idea. For the Hippocratics, however, the purpose of purgatives was καθαίρειν ("to cleanse") or, more explicitly, "to clear out so as to make room for more."[66] But there is a more important aspect of purgatives, particularly those that induce emesis and catharsis of the bowel: botanicals typically have many effects, any particular effect being a consequence of dose of the botanical and the nature of its preparation. A particular salutary effect of one preparation may, therefore, be mistakenly attributed to another, detrimental but more immediately obvious, effect. Thus, the Hippocratics used white hellebore for gout, but since the most obvious effect of the hellebores upon ingestion is vomiting and diarrhea, subsequent relief from the pain of an attack of gout could logically be attributed to the vomiting and diarrhea, *i.e.*, purging, the cleansing of some harmful substance from the body. Of course, all this is further complicated by the difficulties in differentiating gout from other, particularly acute, arthridites, although the Hippocratics did this with greater accuracy than did 17th and 18th C Europe, where the range of symptoms and signs attributed to gout was beyond remarkable. [67] But to be fair, insofar as gout can be associated with arthritis, kidney stones and their complications such as infection and urinary obstruction, subcutaneous nodules, and is often a secondary complication of many other disorders including lead poisoning, psoriasis, and hematological diseases, it is not surprising that a wide and confusing range of signs and symptoms have been attributed to the single diagnosis of "gout," long known to be the consequence of an abnormality in purine metabolism with uric acid crystals being precipitated within an affected joint. In contrast to Renaissance and Enlightenment physicians, Hippocratic physicians were not confused on this point, perhaps because they limited their clinical diagnostics to the more clinically consistent and confirmable "podagra" (ποδαγρα, classical gout), rather than any anecdotal clinical association that included a bout of arthritis.

Purgatives included not only laxatives and emetics, but also diuretics, and were these categories of medicines to be removed from modern medical practice there would be a large and dangerous void. Diuretics are used for hypertension, heart failure, chronic renal failure, and many edematous and ascitic states; emetics are found in every emergency room to manage specific toxic ingestions; and proof of the usefulness of laxatives is obvious in every bathroom cabinet and every pharmacy. There are also less common but specific indications for use. Certain types of diuretics help manage hypercalcuria in patients with calcium renal stones, hypercalcemia, acute renal failure, alkalinization of the urine, acute mountain sickness, diabetes insipidus, and, from the methylxanthines, control of asthma. Specific laxatives may help neurogenic bowel problems, irritable bowel syndrome, diverticular disease of the colon, and optimizing glucose and cholesterol levels. Even agents that induced sneezing or coughing might be

---

[66] See the Hippocratic works *Nature of Man* 6, *Aph.* 5.4 and *Prenotions of Cos* 554, the former two in volume 4 of the *Loeb Classical Library* series on *Hippocrates* and the latter in the recently released volume 9 of the same series. Also see the Wordlist entry in the Appendix of: Adams, W. H., *The Natural State of Medical Practice: Hippocratic Evidence*, Maitland (FL), 2019.

[67] See, for example: Porter, R. and Rousseau, G. S., *The Patrician Malady*, New Haven, 1998, for a scholarly and entertaining account of gout through the ages.

used to purge the head.[68]

Scarification is a procedure involving disruption of cutaneous blood vessels. This causes exudation of serum, the liquid phase of blood minus some coagulants, rather than plasma plus the cellular blood components of whole blood. It is, in theory and if done assiduously, a modification of phlebotomy. In extensive skin injury, as with second and third degree burns or in diseases such as pemphigus, the exudation of serum can lead to serious blood volume depletion. When cutaneous scarification is applied to a very limited in area, as it would have been when used as a therapy, it is hard to imagine that anything other than a risk of infection could result. On the other hand, Oribasius (320-400 AD), using deeper and more extensive incisions, recommended it as an alternative to phlebotomy, estimating that he bled himself "two pounds" (roughly two pints) of blood, thereby protecting himself from the plague then taking place.[69] He also may have assumed that this procedure, unlike phlebotomy, would cause little loss of the red component of blood (red blood cells) and therefore was an improvement over whole blood removal, a logical assumption.

Incision and drainage of collections of pus was commonly performed. It is the nature of focal infection anywhere in the body to tend to spontaneously drain externally by eroding or tunneling through tissue to the surface. This is the body's way of ridding itself of a deep infection or other inflammatory focus. A focus of infection that remains loculated continues to be a source of problems, including fever, septicemia, and metastatic abscesses, although tunneling can be lethal when the erosion extends into a vital area. When the timing is appropriate, drainage can be lifesaving or can markedly shorten the course of illness. Collections of pus include the common "boils," carbuncles, empyemas, pelvic or abdominal abscesses, and brain or kidney abscesses.

To summarize this section, Hippocratic therapeutic techniques were useful. Poor Aesclepiades, who is quoted at the beginning of this chapter, blatantly exposed his incompetence and confirmed the suspicions of his detractors by impuning the Hippocratics. Within the context of their age they were not idle bystanders to misery. To a certain extent this can also be said of some empirical medical practices in other societies, but the Hippocratics were able to make wiser therapeutic choices because they had an accumulation of shared observations that helped them avoid dangerous ones and made them more aware of effective ones. They may not have understood why a particular choice improved their patient; that would be centuries in coming. But if a particular measure worked in one situation it could be tried in others until a level of certainty about indications for its use was determined. And so the uselessness of cupping would in time have been proved, the indications for phlebotomy would have been refined, and the indications for various types of purgation clarified. To uncritically condemn their apparent preoccupation with bleeding and purging is to confuse the early days of ancient science with 17th C ignorance.

6) Dietetics:

The Greek term, δίαιτα (deeaita) commonly translated as "regimen," means one's "way of living" or "way of life." But included in one's way of living is one's way

---

[68] Wootton, A.C., *Chronicles of Pharmacy*, London, 1910, available in a reprint by USV Pharmaceutical Corp., Tuckahoe, NY, 1972, topic of sternutatories, agents that induce sneezing.
[69] Freind, J., *The History of Physick, from the time of Galen* ..., London, 1726, 3rd edition, vol. 1 (of 2), p. 16.

of eating, and the Hippocratics wrote much about the diet, for diet was the preferred method of intervening in an illness, taking priority over the more hazardous pharmaceutical and surgical approaches.

Presumably the human early diet was composed of what was readily at hand, and, if there was a choice, that which had gustatory appeal. It has been proposed, for example, that meat-eating resulted from salt-craving. Even a canine licks its master's face because perspiration contains salt. But at some point food supplies became sufficiently varied and abundant that preferences could be based in part on things other than availability and taste, observation of the effects of diet were made, and the branch of study called dietetics was begun. The *Handbook of Nutrition and Food*, as published in 2002, had 1533 pages, indicating the prominence of dietetics in modern life.[70] And the full story is far from known. Many today feel modern dietetics remains deficient in many profound truths. They are correct.[71]

Egyptian diets are portrayed, along with scenes of banqueting, farming, and hunting, in many contemporary paintings going back to almost 3000 BC, all suggestive of a good and varied diet. Sumerian diets were also described in some detail and were varied. Then, with the increasing aridity of Egypt and the salinization of the fields of Sumer, dietary changes were necessary. But at issue here is not the nutritional status of the population as a whole but the role of diet in combating individual illness, and in Egyptian writings little of relevance can be found. There are admonitions about eating certain items, presumably because they could produce illness, as is briefly mentioned in the Insinger Papyrus and dated to the 1st C AD, and Herodotus reported in Book 2 that the pig was an abominable animal and that beans were disparaged, perhaps for social reasons. Medical applications of diet are not listed.

Diet treated as a science is found in the *Hippocratic Corpus*. In earlier translations the terms "slops" and "uncompounded" or "crude" foods make it difficult to analyze Hippocratic diets. And yet, consider this passage from *Ancient Medicine*: "As such patients were thought to need weaker nutriment, slops were invented by mixing with much water small quantities of strong foods, and by taking away from their strength by compounding and boiling."[72] The "slop," or broth, thus produced may well have been the equivalent of the "chicken soup" folk remedy for many illnesses treated at home today, its virtue being in its fluid and electrolyte replacement, something very useful in managing volume depletion in those with dehydration, poor oral intake, or fluid loss from diarrheas.[73]

---

[70] *Handbook of Nutrition and Food*, C. D. Berdanier, editor, New York, 2002.

[71] As a simple example, juiced pomegranate in a palatable form is presently a popular drink, and yet never in human history has such a large amount of pomegranate been part of the daily ration over prolonged periods by a sizeable population. The results of this unintended human experiment now under way will be of interest to all.

[72] ἀσθενεστέρου δὲ δή τινος οἱ τοιοίδε ἐδόκεον δεῖσθαι, εὗρον τὰ ῥυφήματα μίξαντες ὀλίγα τῶν ἰσχυρῶν πολλῷ τῷ ὕδατι καὶ ἀφαιρεόμενοι τὸ ἰσχυρὸν τῇ κρήσει τε καὶ ἑψήσει. (*Loeb Classical Library, Hippocrates*, vol. I, translation by W. H. S. Jones, *Ancient Medicine* V, 21-25.)

[73] Chicken soup has been occasionally recommended as oral replacement therapy for diarrheas, based on observations from cholera research, although with some cautions. See: Starshak, R. J., *Fluid Overload Following Chicken Soup Rehydration for Gastroenteritis: The Demything of a Therapeutic Legacy*, in *Clinical Pediatrics*, 25: 527-528, 1986.

It is difficult, given incomplete understanding of ancient Greek terms for many dietary components such as grains and other foodstuffs, to confidently attribute any particular benefit to their use. Difficulties in attribution also arise in attempts to judge the effect of a particular diet, for a reasonably healthy-looking person might harbor a significant nutritional deficiency. Looks can be deceiving. A healthy-looking person might have had subclinical rheumatic heart disease or insipient renal failure unknown to the practitioner, and therefore the patient's clinical response to a diet may have been modified by unrecognized disease or deficiency rather than by dietary idiosyncracy. It would have taken many dietary experiments to permit rational food choices, for Hippocratics were aware that diet could cause, as well as cure, disease: "...some [diseases] being somatic, some dietary, and some from the nature of the disease [itself]..."[74] Finally, toxicities, deficiency states, and bacterial food poisonings that could affect outcome must have been frequently encountered, and thereby confounding any assessment of effectiveness.[75]

With individual variables including size, age, gender, allergies, psyche, and anatomic and metabolic proclivities on the one hand and the infinite variety of foodstuffs and methods of preparation, each with its own range of toxic or discomfiting effects, on the other, to which must be added the distinctive features of the great number of diseases and their effects on gastrointestinal function, it is a miracle that any dietary regimen could ever be scientifically devised. Nevertheless, devise they did, but with the following always in mind: "...I think a physician must know, and be at great pains to know, ... what man is in relation to foods and drinks, and to habits generally, *and what will be the effects of each on each individual* (italics added)."[76] Understanding the metabolic basis for varied responses to diet was to wait for the 19th C studies of Magendie (1783-1855) and Liebig (1803-1873).

Specific dietary recommendations are now available for patients with renal failure or insufficiency, diverticular disease of the colon, Crohn disease, and on and on. Hospitals typically can offer thirty or forty different diets for adult patients. Examples of current dietary variations commonly useful in treatment or prevention of disease include diets low in salt, high in protein, low in protein, low in carbohydrate, high in carbohydrate, high or low in potassium, high or low in fiber. There are diets for specific food allergies or metabolic abnormalities, diets that are minced, pureed, soft or cruditee; there are diets for peptic ulcer, esophageal reflux, constipation. Dietetics is as important today as it was in ancient Greece, and its appeal to the Hippocratics suggests effectiveness. Their preoccupation with diet, unique among ancient civilizations, may be viewed as a nascent science that, after thousands of years, continues to be exploited.

7) Medical theories:[77]

---

[74] ...τά ἀπὸ τῶν διαιτημάτων, καὶ καταστάσιος τῆς νούσου, ... *Humours*, XII, 4-5, translation by the author.

[75] For a scholarly historical review of dietary manipulations in the Mediterranean region see: Giugliano, D., *The Way They Ate: Origins of the Mediterranean Diet*, Naples, 2001.

[76] *Loeb Classical Library Hippocrates*, vol. I, translation of W. H. S. Jones, *Ancient Medicine*, XX, 17-23.

[77] A modern definition of terms is useful: a *theory* has "considerable evidence in its support," whereas a *hypothesis* represents an earlier phase of reasoning, but, while inadequately supported by evidence, can be used, by inference, as a basis for further investigation.

Man's natural impulse is to explain the unexplainable and to interpret facts to fit theory. This confounds his attempts to accurately ascribe causation.[78] The Hippocratics knew this: "I am aware that most physicians, like laymen, if the patient has done anything unusual near the day of the disturbance ... assign the cause to one of them, and, while ignorant of the real cause, stop what may have been of the greatest value."[79] The opening lines of *Ancient Medicine*, one of the earliest works in the *Hippocratic Corpus* and one often attributed to Hippocrates himself, declare against theoretical constructions: "All who, on attempting to speak or to write on medicine, have assumed for themselves a postulate as a basis for their discussion – heat, cold, moisture, dryness, or anything else that they may fancy- who narrow down the causal principle of diseases and of death among men, and make it the same in all cases, postulating one thing or two, all these obviously blunder...."[80] Brilliant insight.

There has been a modern preoccupation with the theories of disease proposed by the ancients such as that of the four humors. It has been suggested that these theories guided the clinician's efforts, and that the pedantry surrounding them was required for a successful practice. This is highly unlikely in Hellas. Attributing importance to the theory of disease produced by imbalances in yellow bile, phlegm, black bile, and blood is overlooking the primary function of the clinician, who does not, and, in ancient Greece did not, dwell in an ivory tower.[81] When considered in literal translation the average Hippocratic clinician might have wondered what in the world could be the utility of such irrelevancies. But, if "phlegm" is equated with tissue fluid (extracellular fluid), "bile" is equated with greenish material associated with a variety of septic disease states, especially those with greenish pus, "blood" as blood, and "black bile" as digested blood or blackish urine such as can be seen in, respectively, gastrointestinal bleeding and hemolytic anemia or biliary disease, then one may suspect that the terms were more descriptive than hypothetical, and suggesting they were a metaphor for inflammation.[82]

---

[78]In the words of Francis Bacon, "Wherefore, if there be any humility towards the creator, if there be any reverence and praise of his works; if there be any charity towards men and zeal to lessen human events and human suffering; if there be love of truth in natural things, any hatred of darkness, and desire to purify the understanding; men are to be entreated again and again that they should dismiss or at least for a moment set aside those inconstant and preposterous philosophies which prefer theses to hypotheses, which have led experience captive..." See: Farrington, B., *Francis Bacon: Philosopher of Industrial Science*, New York, 1949, p. 149.

[79] *Loeb Classical Library*, *Hippocrates*, vol. I, *Ancient Medicine*, XXI, 5-12, translation of W. H. S. Jones.

[80] *Loeb Classical Library*, *Hippocrates*, vol. 1, *Ancient Medicine*, I, 1-8, translation of W H. S. Jones.

[81] The prominent medical historian, Dr. Sigerist, comments on the practical irrelevance of theorizations in Hippocratic works such as *Decorum* and *Precepts*. And yet it is obvious to all who deal in complex fields that rough schemata can aid in memorization and recall, even if they serve no other purpose. Furthermore, having a particular theory of physiology might be useful in approaching problems not previously encountered, and there may be value in theories insofar as they provide a backdrop on which to hang disparate facts until better ideas are forthcoming. In some theorizations, no matter how rudimentary, will be found elements of truth. It has been a commonplace in dermatological teaching that, in general, a moist skin lesion should be kept dry and a dry one moistened. This axiom, while being a hazardous generalization from an earlier age, is often correct. See the following footnote. As an aside, a "modern" theory of the Hare Krishna sect assigns disobedience to Nature and an imbalance of air, bile, and mucus causing disease.

[82] See: Adams, W. H., *The Natural State of Medical Practice: Escape from Egalitarianism*, Maitland (FL), 2019, Appendix B.

E. Disease Patterns in Ancient Greece

Life expectancy at birth in England/Wales in 1838 was 40.4 years for males. One hundred and forty years later, in 1978, it was 70.3 years in Wales, a gain of 29.9 years. But the life expectancy of a 60-year-old man in 1838 was 13.6 years and in 1978 it was 15.9 years, an increase of only 2.3 years.[83] It is mortality early in life that makes average life expectancy difficult to interpret in a standardized yet meaningful way. Studies of life expectancy in early Greece note that accounts of elderly persons abound. Prof. Timothy Parkin estimates that about 7% of the population of Rome in its heyday was sixty years of age or older, about what it was in the United States around 1900, and perhaps the same held true for Hippocratic Greece.[84, 85] But the pattern of disease must have differed, and the statement is made in *Regimen in Acute Diseases* that "...acute diseases cause many times more deaths than all others put together," whereas the modern internist deals mainly with chronic diseases into which acute events are interjected. [86]

But the long-term consequences of what were once thought to be "acute" illnesses have become much clearer. The end-stage renal disease that can follow, by many years, persistent but low-grade kidney infections, the cirrhosis and ascites in adults that result from childhood infections by certain hepatitis viruses, the cirrhosis that follows years of alcoholism, and the congestive heart failure in middle age arising from valvular heart disease initiated by rheumatic fever acquired as a child, all have acute manifestations as a late event in what are clearly "chronic," but for many years clinically quiescent, diseases. This knowledge has been painstakingly acquired, and the distinction between an *acute* and a *chronic* disease now becomes much less obvious. [87]

Finally, the human body has limited ways in which to respond to injury. Systemic iron overload, viral hepatitis, the parasitic worms of schistosomiasis, certain hepatotoxic substances, right ventricular heart failure, alcoholism, and many other pathologic processes damage the liver by different mechanisms, but they all can result in end-stage damage known as liver cirrhosis, which is manifested by extensive scar tissue throughout the liver. The scarring caused by these disparate diseases can appear grossly similar, and the late stages often follow a clinically similar downhill course. It is not surprising, therefore, that attempts to diagnose, in retrospect, the diseases of the ancients has met with limited success.

---

[83] These figures are from Lancaster, H.O., *Expectations of Life*, New York, 1990. It has also been noted, for example, that the population in the United States has increased over the past century by a factor of three whereas the number of those greater than 65 years of age has increased by a factor of eight. This relative increase, as striking as it is, is due less to better medical care for the elderly than it is due to an increasing number living through childhood and thereby able to reach a venerable age. See: Hine, D., *Demography and Epidemiology of Old Age*, in *Geriatric Medicine, Problems and Practice*, London, 1989, M. S. J. Pathy and P. Finucane, editors, chap. 2, p. 15-30.

[84] Angel, J. L., *World Archeology*, 4:66-105, 1972.

[85] Parkin, T. G., *Old Age in the Roman World*, Baltimore, 2003, p. 36-56.

[86] From vol. 2 of the *Loeb Classical Library* Hippocratic work: *Regimen in Acute Diseases*, V, 10-12, translated by W. H. S. Jones.

[87] For example, the well-known rheumatic heart disease is caused by a prior infection, usually pharyngitis, with β-hemolytic streptococcus. Despite centuries of isolated observations, the association of sore throats followed by valvular heart disease many years later was identified for the first time only in 1935, three years before the birth of the author of the present volume. (See: Coburn, A. F., *et al.*, *Studies on the Immune Response of the Rheumatic Subject and Its Relationship to Activity of the Rheumatic Process. IV*, in *J. Clin. Invest.* 14:755-762.)

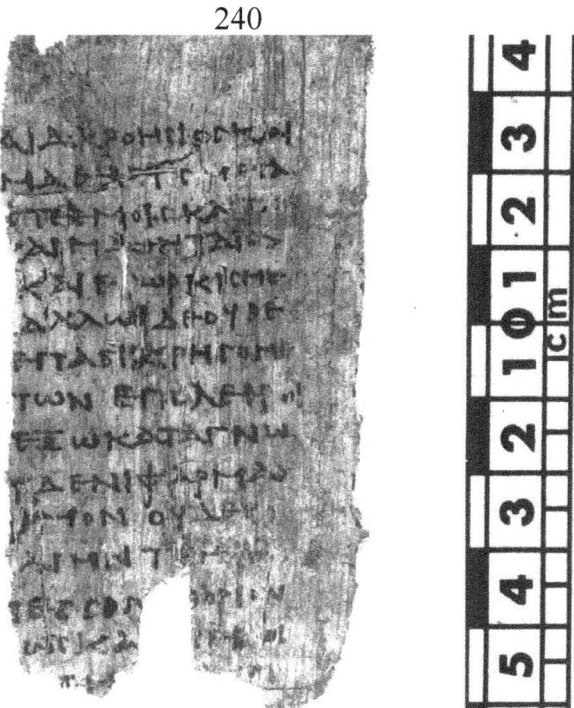

Line 1	[παραγγελίης τε] καὶ ἀκροήσιος καὶ
2	[τῆς λοιπῆς ἁπάσης] μαθήσιος, μετα-
3	[δοσιν ποιήσασθαι υἱοῖς] τε ἐμοῖσι καὶ
4	[τοῖσι τοῦ ἐμὲ διδάξαντος] καὶ μαθηταῖσι
5	[συγγεγραμμένοις τε] καὶ **ἐφωρκισμέ-**
6	[νοις νόμῳ ἰητρικῷ,] ἄλλῳ δὲ οὐδε-
7	νί. διαιτ]ήμασί τε χρήσομαι
8	[ἐπ᾽ ὠφελείῃ καμνόν]των **ἐπ᾽ ολεθρος**
9	.... εξω κατὰ **γνω-**
10	**μεν** [ἐμήν **δὲ καὶ ἀδικίη εἱρξειν.** οὐ δώσω δὲ ο]ὐδὲνὶ φάρμακον
11	[οὐδενὶ αἰτηθεὶς θανάσ]ιμον οὐδὲ ὑφ
12	[ηγήσομαι συμβου]λίην τοιήνδε
13	[ὁμοίως δὲ οὐδὲ γυναικὶ] πεσσὸν φθόριον
14	[δώσω. ἁγν]ῶς (δὲ) καὶ ὁσίως
15	[διατηρήσω τὸν βίον ἐμὸν καὶ] τέχνην ἐμήν[?].

Fig. 10: A papyrus fragment, located at the Wellcome Institute in London and dated to *ca*. 275 AD, contains the earliest extant copy of part of the Hippocratic Oath. The text of the papyrus is superimposed below on a standard version (*Loeb Classical Library* series on *Hippocrates*, vol. 1), with the missing words in brackets, diacritics added, and variant words in the fragment being bolded. The bolded and italicized clause may not have been included, based on length of the line. The "εξω" in line 9 is deemed to be from παρέξω ("I will furnish") by Barns.[1] Photo: Wellcome Images, London, under Creative Commons Attribution Only license CC International 4.0.

---

[1] Barns, J. W. B., *The Hippocratic Oath: An Early Text*, in *Brit. Med. J.*, 2(5408):567, 1964.

CHAPTER FIFTEEN

HUMANENESS AND HELLENIC MEDICINE

Οὐτὲ ἱεροῦ βωμὸν, οὔτὲ ἐκ τῆς ἀνθρωπίνης φύσεως ἀφαιρετέον τὸν ἔλεον.
"Neither the altar of the temple nor the nature of man can be estranged from mercy."

Phocion (Stobaeus, *Florilegium*, I, 31)[2]

There are profound limits on the assistance that a person can expect from a stranger unless society establishes, by custom or by laws, a form of compensation for the stranger. Compassion, as a modern "virtue" and viewed as commanding some vague form of intrinsic emotional compensation and one traditionally identified with medicine, holds no special place in that profession, and can at times be counterproductive, a problem identified by the Hippocratics. More important by far is humaneness. This was a component of many ancient philosophical doctrines, but it expressed the thinking of but a few individual philosophers who, living in authoritarian societies, devised those doctrines and wished to inculcate humaneness into their followers. In contrast, Greek humaneness became a component of daily life concurrently with individual liberty. Although no discoverer of this virtue, the Greeks elevated humaneness from philosophy to action. The reason, of course, is that virtue is impossible in the absence of freedom of choice. It was, therefore, the Greeks that injected humaneness into medicine. The Hippocratic Oath was not intended to mold a physician into the perfect man; it was a humane working document outlining the physician's obligations, and its enforcement was based on trust.

A. Introduction: The Physician's Compensation

Dr. Johann Zimmermann (1728-1795) opined, in his *Solitude*, that if a man wandering alone in the wilderness encountered another human's footprints he would follow those tracks with a hope of finding comradeship and intelligent conversation. But the Age of Reason had earlier witnessed Thomas Hobbes defining human nature as individual, nonsocial, competitive and aggressive, and Hume declared that "there is no such passion in human minds as the love of mankind...."[3] Two hundred years after Zimmerman's passing and in light of greater knowledge of human history, an analysis of his stalker would likely predict that rape, robbery, or enslavement would be the probable consequence of any meeting up. What, then, can be reasonably expected of a stranger who encounters someone in distress? What should that stranger be willing to give up, what risk be willing to take, what effort expend, what burden bear? At first glance it appears that the person in distress should be grateful for any assistance whatsoever. Indeed, it may be enough just to have avoided being victimized by that stranger. If "physician" is substituted for "stranger," it is unreasonable to view any proffered

---

[2] Phocion, a 4th C BC Athenian statesman described by Plutarch in *Parallel Lives*, was nicknamed "The Good."

[3] The famous statement by Hobbes, found in Chapter 13 of Leviathan, is "...the life of man solitary, poor, nasty, brutish and short," referring to a mankind short of necessities and direction. The full statement of Hume is: "In general, it may be affirmed that there is no such passion in human minds as the love of mankind, merely as such, independent of personal qualities, of services or of relation to oneself." (*A Treatise of Human Nature*, Bk III, part 2, sect. i.)

assistance as a privilege or an obligation, because any privilege or obligation consequent on the assistance would accrue to the person in distress who accepts that assistance, not the benefactor. The truth is that most people, despite the popular rhetoric and given an impersonal and anonymous choice, will shun, and some even further victimize, the victim. But when other factors, such as shared societal values, compensation, or notoriety are brought to bear, this response is modified.

It has long been assumed that human nature, whether compassionate or not, whether social or nonsocial, has been unchanging, at least since the dawn of history; mankind can progress but man himself remains unchanged. And so it seems remarkable that there has evolved, over many centuries, sectors of Western society dedicated to the care of others to the point that they now nearly dominate modern life, the field of medicine being the foremost example. For Western man has unquestionably progressed in humaneness. Indeed, anyone seeking evidence of virtuous progress of mankind can look to the history of the West, to a society now steeped in humaneness, where are to be found large segments of that society that knowingly and willingly disregard their own welfare under the banner of humaneness. Whether humaneness is compatible with survival of a society in an authoritarian world is a question for others to answer or experience to enlighten.

But, leaving humaneness for the moment, economic enticement permits a legally binding enlistment of the labor of another individual. What can it command? Certainly it can command effort, physical or intellectual, an exchange easily reducible to a quantitative economic equation. A fixed rate of reimbursement, therefore, can compensate for effort.

Salary also compensates for purchasing such necessary goods and services that, while most can provide for themselves, physicians might acquire with difficulty because of time spent being on call, studying, learning from others, and the like, in addition to filling the required working hours. It is, after all, rather silly to expect a physician to take several hours repairing and cleaning the gutters of his house rather than hiring someone to do it so that he can attend to his professional activities, unless, of course, in that household chore he takes pride or pleasure. This is a simple and obvious example of why physicians are paid more, and must be paid more, than many in other employments, although the hourly rate may not actually be increased.[4] Common sense says it is in society's interest that as much of a physician's time as possible be focused on implementation of his complex professional tasks rather than on such mechanics of daily living. Indeed, since the very first society this has been the whole point of specialization.

Salary also reflects trust, according to Adam Smith: "The wages of labour vary according to the small or great trust which must be reposed ...," whereas profits are unaffected by trust. He implied that such trust was commensurate with the importance of the thing being entrusted: "We trust our health to the physician.... Such confidence could not safely be reposed in people of a very mean or low condition. Their reward must be

---

[4]An example of immoderate expectation occurred in 1976 when a prominent U. S. Congressman broke both arms falling from a ladder while repairing his roof. Taxpayers certainly would prefer to approve a salary for Congressional representative sufficient so that they can hire others for such tasks should they wish it, thereby preserving their efforts for the national interest. As for the hourly rate of recompense for a hospital-based and salaried physician of Internal Medicine whose time was spent on ward coverage, subspecialty coverage, and being on home call at night, the author estimates his take-home hourly rate during the year 2002 to have been approximately $20, currently the average hourly wage for a salaried plumber.

such, therefore, as may give them that rank in society which so important a trust requires."[5] This linking of financial benefit to social status seems no longer relevant, if ever it was, for it has always been the practice of ordinary people, a social grouping that includes physician clinicians, to be wary of those of high social status and influence.

Other demands are not so readily quantified, appropriately reimbursed, or conveniently extracted. They include: 1) risk - how can salary be adjusted for the risk of a job. It could be affected by the communal value placed on altruism. But in medicine only the physician can be expected to knowledgably estimate the personal risk involved in providing medical assistance; (2) sacrifice – this term in the present context implies irreversibly giving up something of value, for example, time or family pleasures. While being subject to public opinion or expectation, in medicine it is again the physician who will determine the acceptable degree of personal sacrifice; (3) burden - in medicine the burden is responsibility, the burden of anxiety over outcome, and the burden of sadness when an outcome is adverse. This is an unavoidable part of the physician's job. But, again, only the physician can feel, on a daily basis, and then only vaguely quantify, its effects.[6] These demands apply as well to those in the military, to police and firemen, and to those with similar, often hazardous, responsibilities. It is remarkable, indeed a blessing, that careers are made of such activities. Equally remarkable, important volunteer work in these endeavors occurs throughout our nation, whereas few become volunteer plumbers or hairdressers.

Acceptance of risk, sacrifice, and burden must come willingly from the individual and it necessarily bears on the nature of his personality. The motives that prompted entry into the medical profession in early Greece are unknown. Religion was not the explanation, and this would remain so until the arrival of Christianity. Altruism was not a factor, for altruism was no virtue of Athenians.[7] The ancient Greek's acceptance

---

[5] Adam Smith, *An Inquiry into the Nature and Causes of the Wealth of Nations*, Dublin, 1785, 4th edition, Bk. I, chapter 10, p. 106.

[6] Some years ago, in a moving lecture on the role of the physician, Dr. Franz Inglefinger, the great teacher who helped establish the subspecialty of Gastroenterology, described the profound relief that followed his decision to cease directing his own care for his esophageal cancer, instead handing that responsibility over to a medical colleague. With that decision he removed the anxiety of indecision, letting his worries now be borne by his physician. Some may feel that any "burden" is not unique to medicine, that "burden" is to be expected in life and is a part of any position of responsibility. To this it may be responded that there are different types of burden. In the first place, the physician will have his own life burdens with which to cope. Secondly, recall that trite admonition to "drive carefully," for "The life you save may be your own." Surely most people realize the superficiality of this warning, which fades to insignificance when compared to participation, even accidentally, in the death of another innocent human being. "The life you save may be someone else's" may be metrically flawed but it is a more appropriate banner. The physician's burden lies not only in the struggle to help his patient regain health; it also involves constant vigilance against missteps on the part of himself or his patient that would make that goal unobtainable, a burden indeed.

[7] And yet Hobbes viewed altruism as disguised self-interest, and self-interest is normal. Eric Cassell (*The Nature of Suffering*, Oxford, 1991, xi) defines altruism as action on behalf of another based on trust, and adds that there is no suggestion of self-sacrifice (Blum, L. A., *Friendship, Altruism and Morality*, London, 1980). But the more disingenuous modern definition, "devotion to the welfare of others" (*Webster's New Collegiate Dictionary*) has been, in Western culture, implied as a necessary element, perhaps even part of the definition, of a profession; see Saks, M., *Professions and the Public Interest*, London, 1995, especially Chapter 1. The danger of this definition of altruism as applied to government has been exposed for what it is by C. R. Badcock (*The Problem*

of the physician ethic must have been the consequence of a high opinion of the profession by the general public. Compensation was to be based on effort and perhaps on the quality of the delivered product. But risk, sacrifice, and burden were not to be quantified in drachmas. The less tangible element(s) associated with service was intangibly recompensed. What shall that element be called?

B. The compassionate physician

Attestations through the ages indicate that the Western physician has been, deservedly or not, generally well regarded. One reason is, as a colleague of the author has said, the physician is viewed as a "compassionate medical scholar." This is an elegant phrase, but whence comes this compassion?

Excursus on Compassion

Is compassion a virtue? Compassion is not one of the theological, God-oriented, virtues, which include Faith, Hope, and Charity. It is not included in the ancient Egyptian virtues listed in "The Instruction of Ptahhotep": "self-control, moderation, kindness, generosity, justice and truthfulness tempered by discretion."[8] Nor is it one of the pagan virtues of classical Greece, the predominant ones being Justice, Prudence, Fortitude and Temperance. Nor is it Aristotle's favorite virtue, which was wisdom. Aristotle, defining vices as the consequence of excess or deficiency, considered observance of the mean as a virtue.[9] And Adam Smith described the three virtues of a citizen as Propriety, Prudence, and Benevolence. None of these include compassion.

A standard definition of compassion implies both pity for another's sufferings plus an urge to help; as Prof. Blum writes, "An active regard for another's good," sympathy plus action.[10] It is derived from a Latin, not a Greek, root, cum + patior, "to suffer or endure with."[11] It is more a sentiment, or a passion, than a virtue, the latter being defined as

---

of Altruism, Oxford, 1986): "...societies based on induced altruism exploit deception to an unprecedented degree (for example, in trying to persuade the majority that things are done in its interest) and fall back on the one psychological tendency that can be exploited – the projection of aggression against outsiders. This tends to make such societies not merely bureaucratized and heavily internally policed but also paranoid in their foreign relations and militaristic to a high degree." The deception that institutional altruism imposes is usually successful because we do not have the integrity to admit to our personal inadequacy or lack of courage to do something on our own. We soothe our feelings, therefore, by praising institutional altruism, fooling ourselves into thinking that that altruism is ours. Instead, by this means we fraudulently usurp the genuine and justified altruism of others.

[8] Lichtheim, M., Ancient Egyptian Literature, vol. 1, The Old and Middle Kingdoms, California, 1973, p. 61ff.

[9] "...the mean is both an excellent and proper virtue." Translation by the author; Aristotle, Eth. Nich. II, 6, 1107a, 2-3, the Bywater edition, Oxford, 1894.

[10] Blum, L., Compassion, in Explaining Emotions, Berkeley, 1980, A. O. Rorty, ed., pp. 507-517.

[11] Adam Smith also wrote of "sympathy," which James Wilson (The Moral Sense, New York, 1993, p. 30) defined as "the human capacity for being affected by the feelings and experiences of others."

"conformity to a standard of right."[12]   A virtuous medical scholar need not be compassionate to do his job.[13]   Nor is it one of the emotions, which are short term psychological states.

Is compassion a behavioral characteristic limited to the human species, one that can be considered as desirable in that it is a requirement for excellence of character? Is it a characteristic innate or acquired? If acquired can it be instilled, and if it can be instilled can it be demanded?[14] If innate, might it in the 21st C be selectively propagated?

In a cage containing ten mice which are then removed one at a time, the anxiety of the remaining mice increases with each mouse removed.[15] The remainder are clearly in sympathy with the departed mice, although that sympathy seems manifestated as fear rather than pity, sympathy being a "relationship between persons or things wherein whatever affects one similarly affects the other."[16] There is no evidence of compassion in the cage of mice in that there is no evidence of a protective response of one mouse for another.

Man is different, at times. Although prehistoric evidence of compassion is elusive, biblical translations refer to compassion as an attribute of God and as a basis for an ethical obligation of man to respond to a neighbor in need. The concept of compassion is thought to be identifiable in ancient Greek writings, including several citations in the *Iliad*, although in that poem it assumes more the connotation of mercy.[17] Compassion has been

---

Here again it is the "active" regard that distinguishes compassion from sympathy. Adam Smith, however, added another dimension in that he noted sympathy can be either for or against someone. The full thrust of compassion is "for," not "against," someone. There is also an imitative component in compassion. Spinoza wrote that, in contrast to "compassion," if the imitation was of desire rather than pain the response was termed "emulation." It was the actual appearance of the affected person that prompted one or the other of these two responses; a person's appearance inspires either emulation or compassion, indicating a large emotional, rather than rational, component in compassion.

[12] *Merriam-Webster's Collegiate Dictionary*, 10th ed.

[13] A modern virtue is "humility," at which the ancient Greeks would have chuckled, as did Aristotle: "Hence all flatterers are mercenary; and all humble men are flatterers." (*Nich. Eth.* Bk. IV, chapt. 3, translation of Thomas Taylor, *The Rhetoric, Poetic, and Nicomachean Ethics of Aristotle*, London, 1818, vol. 2.) Pythagoras, who identified a long list of virtues, did not include humility among them, and it will not be considered one herein.

[14] R-Z Qiu has commented, in *Cultural Dimensions in Medical Ethics*, (Frederick, MD, 2000, 2nd edition, R. M. Veatch, editor, Chapter 5, p. 336), that Chinese medical ethics has always stressed humaneness, and as a consequence *"cultivate the heart of humaneness in medical personnel by rectifying themselves."* (Italics added.) This suggests an attempt by the Chinese government to instill, and perhaps demand as a prerequisite for entry into the profession, that which is herein described as humaneness.

[15] Presumably they fear some hazardous event is affecting the departing mice. It is not yet settled that nonhumans benefit from consciousness in the sense that they can regulate their own behavior in response to mental images of themselves in that particular situation. But this example and the familiar whining of a dog outside a store when its master goes inside to shop suggest it is so.

[16] *Webster's New Collegiate Dictionary*, 1979.

[17] In the *Iliad* 22:76, 23:548, and 24:516, for example, the word οἰκτείρω is translatable in various grammatical forms as "pity." The objects of that pity are, respectively, the elderly Priam who, anticipating his death, pities it because of its circumstances, Achilles is considered to pity the loser of a chariot race, and Achilles pities the consequences of aging in Priam. None imply compassion.

analyzed by many philosophers, and perhaps it is not hyperbole to state that the vagueness of the origin of compassion the deed is exceeded only by the vagueness of compassion the word. And it would be hazardous to translate an ancient Greek term, such as οἰκτίρμων ("oiktirmon," meaning "mercy") from the Septuagint, as "compassion," knowing that no term equivalent to "suffer with" existed at the time.

It is interesting that the ancient Greeks make no mention of compassion as a desirable attribute of a physician or, indeed, of anyone. They pointed out that the physician should be clean, well-dressed, carry himself well, and maintain what was later called by Sir William Osler, *aequanimitas*, the Latin for "calm composure," and "imperturbability," even though he felt that "this precious quality is liable to be misinterpreted, and the general accusation of hardness, so often brought against the profession, has here its foundation." Despite this, he continues, "a callousness which thinks only of the good to be effected, and goes ahead regardless of smaller considerations, is the preferable quality," namely, preferable to an excess of "keen sensibility." [18] The ancient Greeks would have agreed and must have viewed the sharing of sufferings of the patient as useless, even dangerous. Certainly the Stoics, who have included Seneca the Younger, Marcus Aurelius, and, more recently, Henry David Thoreau and W. B. Yeats, would have thought so, for they, as a group, had a strong bias against a passionate basis for any action; emotionally triggered decisions were inferior to cool-headed ones. To ancient Stoics emotions served no useful purpose whatsoever. The Greeks did have a term for sympathy, συμπαθεία (sympathia):

δίοτι συμπάθησις ὑπὸ λύπης ἐοῦσα ὀχλεῖ, ἐξ ἑτέρου συμπαθείης τινὲς ὀχλεῦνται. "Because having sympathy for [another's] distress is disturbing, being sympathetic for another can be the source of troubles." *Precepts* of Hippocrates, 14

In conclusion, for the Hippocratics there were words for pity, ἔλεος (heleos) and οικτος (oiktos), but, as an emotion or sentiment, "to purposely suffer with" was not a word.[19] Even in mid-18th C Samuel Johnson commented in his famous dictionary that "compassion" was ". . . a word scarcely used."

End of excursus

---

[18] Every medical student should read the great Osler's Valedictory Address, *Aequanimitas*, given at the University of Pennsylvania, May 1, 1889, both for the importance of its topic and the irrelevance of some of its corollaries. See also the footnote on *Against Aequanimitas*, p. 191 of this work.
[19] συμπάσχω means "I suffer together.., am affected with the same thing," and, when used with the dative, Lidell and Scott Grek-English Lexicon, abridged edition, reads it as "I sympathize with" rather than "I have compassion for." The critical element in deriving the Greek word for "compassion" is missing, which is that the element be an active, or potentially active, one. ξυμπονέουσι, strictly "to labor or suffer with," is used in περὶ αδενων ουλομελιης ("Glands" II,3, *Loeb Classical Library, Hippocrates*, vol. VIII), but here it is used to describe the systemic effects of "glandular" diseases: "seldom, though, do they *ail in sympathy* with the body," by which is meant they tend to represent localized, rather than systemic disease. (Translation of P. Potter, italics added.) The term refers more to a "part of the whole." The term οἰκτιρμὸν as used in the Septuagint (Zach. 7:9) has been translated as "compassion," but the context is, again, rather one of "mercy," whereas in Pindar's *Pythian Odes*, 1, 164, it is "pity."

The Encyclopedia of Bioethics[20] devotes nearly half of its monograph on compassion to its various manifestations in medicine. This tying of compassion to the medical profession, seeing as how the term is, patently, more a sentiment than a virtue, implies that adherents of the profession are expected "to suffer with" their sick patients.[21] To apply this notion while assessing and treating twenty to forty patients per day, each with a unique list of problems and priorities, and each expecting, properly, personal commitment by the physician, seems quite a remarkable requirement.[22] It is, of course, ludicrous.[23] But Plato liked the idea. Drawing an analogy between midwifery and the birth of a young man's new idea, Socrates says that barren women should not be midwives because "human nature cannot know the mystery of an art without experience;... ."[24] And elsewhere Socrates comments on the desirability of physicians having once had themselves the diseases they treat, surely a nearly perfect manifesto for "compassion."[25]

Plato's unrealistic demands concerning compassion in medicine are consistent with the unworldliness of the author's *The Republic*. The fact is that humans desire not to be sick, and to try to "suffer with" a patient is utterly opposed to reason. Secondly the act would promptly incapacitate the clinician even if performed. Thirdly, even if it were possible to perform, it would be absolutely the wrong thing to do, for objectivity and rationality in decision-making is critical for any clinician and is in the best interests of the patient. It is for this reason that there are age-old injunctions against a physician treating himself or his family.[26] For most people have compassion, although in varying degrees,

---

[20] *The Encyclopedia of Bioethics*, first issued in 1978 (New York) in five volumes, is now a standard medical library reference and has been periodically updated.

[21] Is compassion in fact just an emotion? A psychologic definition of "emotion" is "any short-term evaluative, affective, intentional psychological state, including happiness, sadness, disgust, and other inner feelings." A list of the more core emotions and their corollaries does not include compassion. Perhaps compassion is better termed a "sentiment." A sentiment is a complex combination of feelings and opinions used as a basis for action or judgment, says the *Encyclopedia of Bioethics*. This seems more to fit the everyday concept of compassion. But since there is an emotional content to a sentiment, can it be instilled or must it be already in place for an individual to be compassionate? All mankind seems to share the same spectrum of emotions, but the degree of compassion may vary from one person to the next. In fact, an emotional intelligence index has been developed to quantify it. See: Schutte, N. S., and Malouff, J. M., *Measuring Emotional Intelligence and Related Constructs*, Lewiston, 1999.

[22] The hazards of requiring compassion to be a "standard of excellence" for the clinician has been discussed by Dr. Howard Brody (*The Healer's Power*, Yale, 1992), who points out that "the art of compassionate medicine, then, will require of the physician an openness to the wounding power of a patient's vulnerability," a "shared" vulnerability.

[23] But such is the expectation as expressed by many present-day writers on the subject, based on their personal experience with an individual clinician. They seem to have few qualms about imposing their unavoidably narrow world perspective on everyone else.

[24] Plato, *Theaetetus,* 149 c, translation of Benjamin Jowett.

[25] "The cleverest doctors are those who, in addition to learning their craft, have had contact with the greatest number of very sick bodies from childhood on, have themselves experienced every illness, and aren't healthy by nature, for they don't treat bodies with their bodies..."; Plato, *The Republic*, 408e, translation of G. M. A. Grube (revised by C. D. C. Reeve), as printed in *Plato, Complete Works*, Indianapolis, 1997, J. M Cooper, editor. This idea as expressed by Plato is so bald-faced as to indicate irony.

[26] "A physician who treats himself has a fool for a doctor," as the Oslerian aphorism goes. Aristotle agreed: "To be treated from the book is mediocre, rather it is preferable to be treated by those who

and when excessive it can be disabling and even destructive.

Nevertheless, compassion has been invoked as a highly desirable, even a primary, goal for the physician-in-training. But it was Christianity that stamped compassion on medical rhetoric, and the word itself can be traced back only to late Latin.[27] This bears on the reasons for selecting Greek medicine as a focus in the search for the natural state of medical practice. Hippocratic medicine was notable for the objective recording of medical observations. But concurrent with the advent of Christianity objectivity in medicine was lost, for the Hippocratic battalions were no longer in the fray. Once again it would be God or gods who inflicted man with diseases, and medical nihilism would return in full flood. Compassionate clinicians would have little to offer patients over the next 1500 years but their condolences. It is only natural that marketable compassion would be viewed as important during this period of scientific abstinence.[28]

Now whether one sect, political candidate, nation, or even profession, is the more compassionate is debated in the daily newspapers. But personal observations prompt the view that within a few years of adolescence, and probably much earlier, human personalities are set, and set permanently. If compassion is in part an emotional commitment required for a profession, it is surely asking the impossible for an adult to develop an emotion that has been subjectively considered deficient since birth.

It is time to cut through the fog on this subject. Compassion is an intrinsic and universal characteristic of man, one that sets man apart from other species, if not qualitatively, then at least quantitatively. It is a form of passion, a sentiment. And it is a sentiment easily overruled by self-interest, but, as with emotions, it in turn can dominate common sense. It is expressed daily in a myriad of ways. It is bred into man, and although it may vary quantitatively it cannot be taught to him and nor impressed upon him. Any such attempt may make one *act* as a compassionate but it will not make one *be* compassionate. In the modern bureaucratic world, in television advertisements, and in liberal debate where, with a degree of hyperbolic rhetoric never dreamed of by the Ancients, even entire governments or nations can be declared compassionate, there is no distinction between the two, but, as individuals, every thinking person knows how disparate "acting" and "being" truly are.

Physicians have no greater claim or obligation to compassion than any other segment of society, nor should that be expected. And, perhaps most to the point, recent experience has shown that the greatest human expression of compassion as popularly understood had nothing whatever to do with the medical profession.[29]

---

are the professionals, for they never act contrary to principle from motives of friendship..." *Politics,* Bk. III, 16, 1287; translation by the author.

[27] The *Oxford English Dictionary*, however, traces its origin to the late Latin of early Church fathers, including St. Jerome (340-420 AD).

[28] The reasoning of Aristotle, Philo, the Stoics, and many others had concluded that passions were to be moderated or suppressed. But in subsequent centuries displacement of objectivity by subjectivity raised the currency of emotional appeal, an important characteristic of the approaching Dark Ages.

[29] September 11, 2001, in America was the day that witnessed the most satanic act in history. Unexpectedly, without any affront, with no declaration of hostilities, and in complete innocence of any subsequently purported reason for the act, 3,000 dear people of all ages and ethnicities were murdered by fellow humans, many burned to death in full view of their families. For those familiar with human savagery in all its forms, the scale of barbarity on 9/11 may seem relatively diminutive, but the wantoness, the randomness, and the joyous acknowledgement of human life being as meaningful as an asteroidal rock, the very imprimatur of terrorism and its apologists, will never be

C. The Humane Physician

More relevant than compassion to the role of physician is being "humane."[30] The Barnhart Dictionary states: humanitarian = humanity + arian, or "promoter of humanity." This term, in 1819, had a religious connotation. Then it acquired a disparaging connotation: excessively humane principles. By 1844 it meant one who devoted himself to human welfare, a philanthropist. But, as now considered, "humanitarianism" blends philanthropy, which is love of mankind, and zoophily, or kindness to animals.[31] This is in line with the opinion of Dr. Ludwig Edelstein who cited Aristotle's definition of φιλανθροπία (philanthropia) as the emotion of friendliness towards "members of the same species" except that the same friendliness has now been extended to other species as well.[32] This distinction is not at odds with the present focus for there were veterinarians as well as physicians during the classical period, and Greek speculations regarding the soul did not necessarily restrict it to man, as tends to be true of several modern religious interpretations.[33] Pythagoras (6th C BC), who espoused reincarnation, forbade the killing of animals, except for those that harmed man. Aristotle considered even plants to have a variety of soul.[34] Humaneness, therefore, requires a "recognition of the kinship of all sentient life," and it is expressed in acts of kindness and mercy. Humanitarianism as a philosophical concept is "organized humaneness."

---

sufficiently captured by our literati. In a contrast so stark as to also defy description, 343 firemen, 60 policemen, 15 emergency medical technicians and an unknown number of others who knowingly raced into the unknown to the rescue of thousands of complete strangers facing imminent destruction were also killed. Their loss will forever represent the zenith on a scale of humaneness in which the murderers will forever be identified with its nadir.

[30] Plutarch used τό φιλανθρώπευμα to mean a humane act (Plutarch, *Sol.*, 15), but earlier Isocrates (Ep. 5.2, letter to a young Alexander the Great) used φιλανθρωπία in the sense of "love of mankind," as did Hippocrates (*Precepts*, 6). It is derived from φιλέω, "I love or regard with affection," and ἄνθρωπος, a generic term for "man," and from which is derived *philanthropy*. The love of mankind is not the equivalent of love of self, one's family, or members of one's tribe. It represents a more general ideal, a perception based on an appreciation of the common strengths and weaknesses, needs and hopes, of all humans, and, according to the Oxford English Dictionary, a "disposition or active effort to promote the happiness and well-being of one's fellow man." Edelstein (*The Ethics of the Greek Physician*, p. 319, in *Ancient Medicine: Collected Papers of Ludwig Edelstein*, Baltimore, 1967) translates the term not as love of man but as a friendliness of disposition, dignified, willing to accommodate the patient's ability to pay. And W.H. Jones translated it as "kind to all," in contrast to μισάνθρωπος, or "unkind." In recent linguistic evolution philanthropy has come to represent the long-term expression by a wealthy individual of love of his fellow man through sustained munificence.

[31] See: *Encyclopedia of Religion and Ethics*, Edinburgh, 1908-1927, J. Hastings, editor, volume 6. A modern version is available from internet sources.

[32] See: *Ancient Medicine: Collected Papers of Ludwig Edelstein, Baltimore, 1967*, O. Temkin and C. L. Temkin, editors, p. 322, note 7.

[33] Furthermore, Humane Societies for the relief of animal suffering abound world-wide.

[34] ὑπάρχει δὲ τοῖς μεν φυτοῖς τὸ θρεπτικὸν μόνον, ("Plants possess the nutritive faculty only: ..." Aristotle, *de Anima*, 414b,32-33, translation of R. D. Hicks, Cambridge, 1907). By this is meant that the plant soul has limited "psychic power" compared to higher organisms, but it has, by virtue of being a living thing, some. The range of "powers" includes the nutritive, the appetitive, the sensory, the locomotive, and the power of thinking, the latter being at the extreme of the hierarchy.

Humaneness is considered a virtue.[35] Showing kindness and mercy solely to one's family and friends or one's tribe is not humaneness.

A realization of humaneness seems to have been formally brought forward to general consciousness in several regions of the world about the 6th C BC as man began to see beyond tribalism. In *Jeremiah 7:22* the irrelevance of pagan animal sacrifice to God was recorded,[36] although an earlier injunction by God against labor on the seventh day extended to the labor of domestic animals.[37] Buddhism, the teachings of one man that one's soul was destined to enter innumerable cycles of existence until release from the wheel of life was finally attained, presented existence in a negative light. Earthly existence and its suffering were something unavoidable and to be borne because it held the means by which Nirvana could be obtained. It was not an end; it was merely a beginning. The Hebrew prophets, on the other hand, were concerned with the proper social development of a single lifetime of opportunity, the ultimate goal on earth being, not release, but perfection of action. Both the allegiance of the individual and the reason for aiming at personal perfection were to glorify God. In Greece, ethical perspectives were derived in a relatively open society, and it was the Pythagorean message that the goal of man's efforts was to become god-like himself, and ultimately even to dwell with the gods, a goal for later Christians as well. It is unclear whether the religious doctrines of Pythagoras contributed to scientific advancement. Still, one might have expected his philosophy to have a ripple effect on a wide range of interests within society, more so than the self-dampening doctrine of Buddhism and the other-worldliness of Judaism, for Pythagoras stressed differences between opinion and knowledge, considered philosophy an intermediate step between earthly existence and life with the gods, and used reason and observation to understand how "divine cosmos" brought the soul closer to God.[38]

---

[35] Peterson, C., and Seligman, E. P., *Character Strengths and Virtues*, Oxford, 2004.

[36] "nor commanded them in the day wherein I brought them out of Egypt, concerning whole-burnt offerings and sacrifice; but I commanded them this, saying , Hear ye my voice ....," Jeremiah 7:22-23. The translations of all Old Testament passages are from the diglot Septuagint version as published by S. Bagster and Sons, Ltd., London, *ca*. 1884. New Testament translations are from the King James version, the original of 1611 as edited in 1769.

[37] "Six days shalt thou do thy works, and on the seventh day there shall be rest, that thine ox and thine ass may rest, ...," *Exodus* 23:12, KJV.

[38] Pythagoras founded a religious brotherhood in 530 BC that was austere, communistic, and authoritarian. He left his home island of Samos during the tyranny of Polycrates, perhaps because the authoritarian nature of his cult was not consistent with the democratic nature of the general population. He then founded another oligarchical commune in Croton, one that again instigated a "democratic revolt" by the local population, this time a violent one. This brotherhood was known for its taboos on eating certain beans and on killing any animal that was not dangerous to man. The scientific doctrines associated with the Pythagorean school surely do not reflect the insight of one man nor the consequence of open scientific enquiry but must have mirrored the general desire for knowledge that was emerging throughout the Greek world. His doctrine that numbers were fundamental to all things was supported by his development of a system of harmonics in music, which he extended to include the music of celestial spheres. Much Pythagorean mathematical and geometrical doctrine was added by later adherents, and it is remarkable that Copernicus acknowledges this sect as giving him the notion of a heliocentric solar system. Even today the idea of "number" being intrinsic to the cosmos is very much alive: "In the pure mathematics we contemplate absolute truths which existed in the divine mind before the morning stars sang together,..." wrote Edward Everett (1794-1865), and G. W. Hardy (1877-1947) noted: "I believe that mathematical reality lies outside us, ...," in *A Mathematician's Apology*, Cambridge, 1941, p. 63. As mystical as the cult was, scientific speculations of the Pythagoreans were exposed to proofs.

Humaneness can be found, therefore, in Taoism, Buddhism, and Jainism in Asia, Zoroastrianism in the Middle East, and in the Pythagorean philosophy of the West because several, including the latter, advocated reincarnation.[39] These philosophical movements may merely have exposed a latent humaneness, but it is notable that they developed at the time the common man was first countering privileged authority. Now it has come to be a mark of a proper society, at least in name.

But the more authoritarian the society, the fainter is the face of humaneness. There will be disagreement over which societies are the more humane, the arguments coming with particular vigor from authoritarian ones that wish to disguise their lack of humaneness, and so the definition of "humaneness" as recognition of "kinship of all sentient life expressed through kindness and mercy" must be closely adhered to. For Confucianism the highly important word *jen* has been translated as "humaneness," but that word has been considered to encompass "love, benevolence, humanity, human heartedness, virtue, perfect virtue, true manhood" and "the ideal relationship between people."[40] Therefore, this broad and vaguely defined term as translated may not satisfy the definition of "humaneness."[41] Eclectic Hinduism includes features of most religions, but the essential features of Hinduism, certainly in prior ages, have been (1) correct living within the caste system, and (2) reverence for revealed moral guides. The former has been the Asian subcontinent's pillar in sustaining an authoritarian society; it is an essential ingredient of Hinduism. And the "moral guides" are merely relative guides as expressed

---

Pythagoras is often mentioned in connection with transmigration of the soul as though that concept is derived from his studies. But transmigration of the soul is a common concept of societies worldwide, whether ancient, primitive, or modern. Pythagoras died around 480 BC and the brotherhood, politically unpopular, disappeared in the 4th C, although it was resurrected with modifications over the next few centuries.

[39] Some aspects of humaneness may be difficult to identify. Jainism's five vows to liberate the soul from its karma encompass honesty, chastity, detachment, and no destruction of life. For Buddhism, the average person (*i.e.*, not a monk or nun) must refrain from killing of animals, stealing, libel, and use of drugs or alcohol, and the temples are to be supported. But neither mention mercy or kindness. The renunciation of the killing of animals is based in part on a threat of no happiness in the hereafter, rather than invoking respect for all living things. But vegetarianism is not a Buddhist requirement in many regions, and it is reported that the Dalai Lama is not a vegetarian. There is also no requirement for kindness. Likewise, the concept of reincarnation, a common feature of Eastern religions, implies a selfish rather than humane facade to the avoidance of killing. In final analysis, while we may applaud the humane attention and platitudes concerning other species as proof of modern man's moral superiority over the ancients, the emergence of this respect for all sentient life can be attributed not to any moral epiphany of our evolving species but to such an abundance of comestibles, the product of commercialism, that we as a society now have the time for the malignant nature of maltreatment of animals to be recognized. This is not a moral epiphany; it is an uncovering of a morality long hidden by circumstance. The march from a peaceful Eden has been difficult not only for mankind.

[40] In recent usage its meaning has been extended to include respect for animals, except for those that are harmful to man. This is according to the translation, by Laurence Thompson, of *Ta T'ung Shu, the One-World Philosophy of K'ang Yu-Wei*, London, 1958, in which the love encompassing this philosopher's utopian "one world" extends *jen* to animals.

[41] Tsai, D. F-C., *The Bioethical Principles and Confucius Moral Philosophy*, in *J. Med. Ethics*, 31:159-163, 2005. Confucianism came face-to-face with the anti-authoritatianism of Taoism, but both began as philosophies, only later emerging as state religions/philosophies of China. That Taoism remains topical in an authoritarian world, see the Letter to the Editor, *Wall Street Journal* of Saturday, June 1, 2013 (Vol. CCLXI, No. 127): *Lao Tzu and Leaving People Alone*.

through the wise ruler. Hinduism's late competitor, Buddhism, countered that moral behavior came from the individual based on an analysis of whether suffering or pleasure was the consequence of one's action. Kindness was expanded to include a kinship with all living things, an unambiguously humane philosophy.

In ancient Greece matters were different. The evolution of democracy was associated with a need to fill the vacuum left by the disappearance of a palace economy, authority, and religion that hitherto had controlled human interactions in Hellas. New guides to behavior were needed, and in a relatively open society public debate occurred on matters such as truth, goodness, and morality. Along with his new liberties the individual citizen acquired the intellectual autonomy necessary for being humane.[42] Francis Rowley offered a paean to the humaneness of ancient Greece in his evocative little volume on Humane Societies.[43] On this point Milton has been contrasted with Thomas Hobbes: "He [Milton] argued for free speech precisely because he believed that the public could not become virtuous in the presence of a state that would make moral decisions for them, and because no group of leaders could be virtuous enough to be conscience for all."[44] Unquestionably, humaneness and freedom go hand in hand, just as the great undercurrent of freedom has been deemed necessary for man's decency to be displayed in other ways. Frederick Douglass declared, "There can be no virtue without freedom," and President G. W. Bush stated that there is "no justice without freedom."[45]

Previously, in Greece as elsewhere, medicine had been guided by group dynamics under authoritarian governance and cults; humaneness was not a social force. Kindness had a role only within the limits of one's small social circle. Grassroots humaneness did not suddenly grip entire societies. Even in 4th C Athens Aristotle did not view lower animals as having rights and worthy of justice, and killing of animals for study was not an issue, although Edelstein felt that in the latter half of that century matters in Greece began to change, and he credits the Hippocratics for first introducing morality into medicine.[46] Later, Celsus (25 BC-50 AD), the Roman medical writer, recorded public opinion on vivisection of criminals in his work *On Medicine*, "Nor is it, as most people say, cruel that in the execution of criminals, and but a few of them, we should seek remedies for innocent people of all future ages." Galen, of all the great names in medicine, was merciless in his view of the importance of dissection and vivisection of animals. And while a few individuals expressed kindness and sympathy for all life, blood sports were a

---

[42] Democracies exploit this luxury. Today there are tens of millions of Americans who rush to the aid of the underserved, the victims of misfortune, and the threatened species, whereas in the 6th C BC among the tens of millions of inhabitants of the Asian subcontinent such behavior was acknowledged to be the legacy of but one man, Gautama Buddha, a compliment to both Buddha and democracy.

[43] Rowley, F. H., *The Humane Idea*, Boston, 1912.

[44] Morehouse, I. M., *Areopagitica: Milton's Influence on Classical and Modern Political and Economic Thought*, in *Libertarian Papers*, 1, 38, 2009.

[45] Foner, P. S., editor, *The Life and Writings of Frederick Douglass*, New York, 1950, in 5 vols., vol. 2, pp. 182-183, and the State of the Union address by President George W. Bush, January 20, 2005. With a broader compass D. D'Souza wrote: "Without freedom there is no virtue: A coerced virtue is no virtue at all." See his *Letters to a Young Conservative*, New York, 2002, p. 16.

[46] Edelstein, L., *Ancient Medicine*, Baltimore, 1987 (paperback edition), p. 322, which references the contrast between φιλανθρωπία and μισανθρωπία, and see its p. 335 for a discussion of Hippocratic morality, which he says was found in no other "medical sects." Of course, the translation of φιλανθροπία is central to an accurate understanding of the issue.

perennial favorite in authoritarian Rome.[47]   Christianity was labeled by Rowley, cited above, as "indifferent" to lower animals. Other societies, therefore, had little basis for accommodating a humane profession; the practitioner was either a State functionary or a person of little official consequence. This is not to deny the existence of humane practitioners elsewhere. But authoritarian rule is by decree, not consent, and humaneness is therefore unnecessary for the functioning of its component systems. This concern is central to the great debate over the nature of governmental health care, under which medicine will march where it has been told, not where it will. Humaneness and individual freedom distinguish a democratic medical profession from an authoritarian medical craft. In Hippocratic Greece was to be found a truly humane medical profession:

ἢν γὰρ παρῇ φιλανθρωπίη, πάρεστι καὶ φιλοτεχνίη.
"For where there is love of man, there is also love of the art."
Hippocrates, Precepts, VI[48]

In summary, humaneness can exist only in a free society.[49] Hippocratic medicine was raised on a latticework of freedom and humaneness, which in Greece was chronologically associated with a developing democracy.

D. The Ethical Physician[50]

Some consider ethics to have formally begun when man acknowledged moral codes such as the Ten Commandments. One goal of the Vedic hymns from around 1500 BC was to urge fulfillment of one's moral duty. Devotees recognized a "moral" order proper to the Universe, the goals of life being prosperity, satisfaction of desires, liberation

---

[47] These humane individuals included Seneca (4 BC-65 AD), the historian Plutarch (46-127 AD), in his *Moralia*, and the philosopher Porphyry (234-305 AD).

[48] Translation is by W. H. S. Jones in the *Loeb Classical Library* series of *Hippocrates*. But, not to overstate the case, φιλωνθρωπίη (philanthropia) was not listed as a virtue by the Greeks.

[49] A tyranny, whether of one man or a council of the proletariat, may provide, for example, access to medical care for all (as pointed out on page 152, "a contented proletariat is a condition of the tyrant's tenure of power"), but this is an arbitrary decree and compliance will by necessity ultimately be backed by threat of physical force initially disguised as an economic jeopardy. A "humane" decree is rarely an act of humaneness; it is an arbitrary act of political savvy. Nevertheless, there are as many who take pride in such a humaneless system as there are those who do not know the difference.

[50] The word "ethical" is derived from the Greek adjective, ἠθικός (ethicos) meaning "of or for morals," moral, ethical. It, in turn, comes from ηθος, "an accustomed place," or, "custom, usage, habit." The latter term *implies no right or wrong*, indicating, rather, that which is usual. Plutarch stated, "Morality is nothing but long-established habit" (τὸ ηθος ἔθος ἐστι πολυχρόνιον, translation of T. B. Harbottle, *Dictionary of Quotations (Classical)*, London, 1902). Its modern sense is far more noncommital: "A principle of right or good behavior," with no reference to what is right or good (Webster's II New College Dictionary). "Moral," the adjective, is derived from the Latin *moralis*, which had been itself derived from ἠθικός by Cicero (see the Oxford English Dictionary), and now means "...concerned with principles of right and wrong..." Often used interchangeably, "ethical" tends to refer to implementation of that which is "moral"; society recognizes moral vs. immoral behavior, whereas a profession devises a code of ethical conduct which finds its basis in society's notions of morality.

from a finite existence, and moral duty.[51] Morals/ethics generally have religious connotations, for early interpreters were priests and prophets.[52] Secular application of a moral code was historically asserted in Egypt of 1000 BC, where instruction for self-improvement was given to its scions, namely, that they should treat courteously those of an inferior social station.[53] The Mosaic laws and the Hebraic admonition to "love thy neighbor as thyself" disclosed moral principles.[54] Tithing to aid the needy and eschewing harm to the defenseless were components of Hebrew law, just as protecting the defenseless may have reflected on the personal morality of Hammurabi. The Edict of Cyrus the Great, a declaration made upon Persian occupation of Babylon in 539 BC, has been interpreted as the first expression of principles of human rights.[55]

It was noted above that in ancient Greece the switch from an agrarian monarchy to commercial and industrial democracy prompted ethical inquiry. People who were maintained as uneducated serfs in a rigid authoritarian society attended by traditional gods needed not think on such matters as the soul, but when elements of self-regulation became necessary to fill the vacuum created by loss of authoritarian control, man resumed his natural inquiry into the nature of things. New rules of conduct were necessary, and Socratic teachings included many ethical issues. In elucidating them Socrates often used analogies involving the medical profession. Physicians and ethics have a long association.

The ethical is more historically traceable than the humane, for self-preservation is an implied part of moral/ethical systems that evolve from living together, whereas the humane is a general notion of behavior befitting man that even transcends speciation. In ancient Greece Pythagoras and the early sophists concluded that goodness and justice were relative to the customs of each society, and thus were up to man to determine. In contrast, Socrates and Plato thought an objective basis for goodness could be derived, applicable to all situations. With regard to physicians, therefore, are customary standards of conduct to be applied in a relative or absolute way? If Platonic, physicians might be expected, or even be required, to be more "good" than other people. Or, if sophistic, physicians can merely be as good as everyone else. This is germane to modern medicine.

Except for the Oath, there is little written on clearly ethical issues in the

---

[51] Jhingran, S., *Aspects of Hindu Morality*, Delhi, 1989, a detailed and complex analysis.

[52] The *Code of Hammurabi*, 1754 BC, preceded the Ten Commandments, but contained no principles of justice. Scholars have noted that the laws of Ur-Nammu, written some three centuries earlier, were actually more advanced than those of Hammurabi for, instead of demanding "an eye for an eye" type of justice, or *lex talionis*, they provide monetary compensation for injury.

[53] These are found in the *Instructions of Ptah-hotep*, composed by a 5th dynasty (2494-2345 BC) vizier of that name.

[54] *The Religion of Moses*, by A. Moses, Lexington, 1894, p. 102.

[55] On receiving a jubilant welcome on his entry into that city, however, Cyrus may have just been expressing his appreciation for the submission of his new subjects, rather than implying an ethical code to be followed with all subjugated populations. He had just won the battle of Opis, 47 miles away, slaughtering, some say "massacring," its army and citizens, thus leaving little in the way of defensive options for Babylon. (See the *Nabonidus Chronicle*, probably composed in the 6th C BC, the extant copy from several centuries later.) Cyrus also was harsh in dealing with revolts among Greek cities. Successful diplomacy was key to his victories, and it is easier to be magnanimous when an adversary submits without a pitched battle. Nevertheless, this did not prevent the Secretary General of the United Nations, U Thant, from thanking His Imperial Majesty and the people of Iran and praising "Cyrus' desire to establish peace...," a statement made in 1971, the 2500th anniversary of the founding of the Persian Empire.

Hippocratic Corpus. There were probably many such issues, but, at least in medicine, most were likely handled by the physician and patient in private deliberation, neither requiring nor seeking outside intervention. And perhaps the Greek way was best: "The constant prattle about medical ethics is something to be deplored. There are no special medical ethics. Ethics are ethics. An ethical man is one who would act toward his patient exactly as he would like to have the patient act toward him if the patient were a physician and he the invalid."[56] A less likely explanation is that the Greek physician preferred not to argue with the patient, or vice versa.

Just how closely the average Hippocratic physician came to approximate the ideal physician is not known, and it is likely to never be known, for the Hippocratics were practitioners, not sophists, and would not have wasted their time on a useless exercise in the ideal. On the other hand, society's expectations would be difficult to oppose, given the competition among the various types of healers contending for public popularity. It is likely, therefore, that the opinions expressed by society must have contributed not only to the form of the medical organization and to the methods of its practitioners, but to their ethics as well. Dr. William Durant has listed the characteristics of Athenian morality during the classical age. He noted that infanticide was approved for population control, a perceived need to prevent a "pauperizing fragmentation of the land." Athenians were nevertheless hospitable, charitable, and, although women were cloistered, family oriented. Men looked after external affairs, but women were responsible for the home. Honesty was not observed, but this may have differed from the present day only in that the Athenians paid less lip service to it. Athenians were vain and loved wealth, admired manliness, worshiped beauty and freedom. There was loose sexual morality but there was also religious toleration. Their moral perspective was tribal.[57] What, if any, were the ethical implications for a medical practice embedded in a society with the attributes described by Dr. Durant. Indeed, what, if any, are the implications for medical practice anywhere? Since ethics is a reflection on the "customary standards of conduct," are there socially diverse normative values from which ethical guides can be derived for the peculiar association between physician and patient? Or is there a universal, absolute, Platonic basis for judging conduct?

If the answer is Platonic, each society through its laws, whether ordained by religion or the State, would have the right to regulate the ethics of its professions, including physicians. Therefore, the modern physician in China who carries out a state regulation and sterilizes a resisting woman or terminates a desired or late pregnancy is to be judged "ethical" in that society, that is to say, can force his technical expertise on a patient against that patient's will.[58] This is consistent with Plato's valuation on the overweening importance of the State, the role of an expert as the unchallenged authority, and his assertion that, should a patient decline a physician's treatment, the physician has

---

[56] Porter, L., *Thesis and Antithesis in Medical Philosophy*, 500 copies privately printed, 1946, last paragraph.

[57] Durant, W., *The Life of Greece* (Vol. 4 in *The Story of Civilization*), New York, 1939.

[58] In 1980 the Chinese Communist Party inaugurated a single-birth policy that required birth permits for a first child, mandatory IUD placement to prevent future births, and forced sterilization and severe economic punishment in event of a second child. Its "womb police," third trimester abortions, and public postings of womens' menstrual cycles have received global attention. The program has been very effective. And see a recent article by Leslie Chang in the Wall Street Journal: *China Tries Easing Once-Brutal Approach to Family Planning*, Feb.2, 2001.

the authority to enforce that treatment.[59] Another notorious example occurs in societies where female "circumcision" is commanded. To justify such an approach requires that the State determine moral certainties.

Excursus on Authoritarian Ethics

The nature of morality has probably been debated from the time of man's first societies. "Probably" is warily used here, for any such early debate must have been limited and most times nonexistent, for strict authoritarian governance fulfills society's moral needs: there is no higher authority, moral or otherwise, except as permitted by the authority itself. As discussed elsewhere in this chapter, the debate became a significant intellectual issue when the authoritarian's grip loosened in the Greek city-states. In the 19th C the era of Darwinism saw its complex social implications propel moral issues to the forefront of popular discourse, and in the 20th C West a profound fear of moral authoritarianism occupied the space usually reserved for society's discussions of morality.

Authoritarianism, whether secular or religious, is authoritarian first, all else being a distant second, a point understood by all. But it is in concerns about target selection that the true nature of the debate is frequently missed. As the substance of the present work involves individual and group freedom in an increasingly authoritarian world it is important to examine the effects of authoritarian governance on morality in individuals or segments of society rather than society as a whole. Two perspectives can be briefly mentioned. (1) John Ladd, who studied the ethics of Navajo Indians, has accurately defined certain attributes of authoritarian ethics: moral obligations are controlled by a command figure, most people "are ethically incompetent" and need to obey the "ethically competent authority," and the authority itself is not restrained by its own code of ethics.[60] (2) But in the more philosophical realm quite a different idea of morality/ethics is discussed in the eminent Dr. James Q. Wilson's book, *The Moral Sense*, in which he argues that there are innate moral values that all humans share that help guide man's social interactions, but they are easily susceptible to repression and are shared unequally.[61] Given equal voice and free discussion among its members, a community, if left to its own devices, would identify certain actions that are morally correct and others that are morally wrong, and if the debate occurred in several disparate communities the ultimate decision as to what was right or wrong would tend to be similar among them all. Relevant to the first perspective, those who have committed an arguably immoral act might claim "I was just doing my job," by which assertion the responsibility for any immorality is passed to a higher authority. The Chinese physician who forcibly carries out an order to terminate a pregnancy could use such an argument. Being morally right or wrong is not an issue under authoritarian governance, for the little voice that might have led to a truly moral action is coercively silenced. But if the moral sense is strengthened by appropriate teaching and if the authoritarian bludgeon is restrained the Wilsonian flame will brighten and the sham morality of the authoritarian, as unearthed by Mr. Ladd, will be recognized for what it is.

---

[59] Plato, *Statesman*, 293a-c.
[60] Ladd, J., *The Structure of a Moral Code*, Cambridge, 1957, p. 188.
[61] Wilson, J. Q., *The Moral Sense*, New York, 1993.

Authoritarian morality, which comprises that which is convenient for the authority in controlling society and for which the authority is not answerable, is not the equivalent of moral authoritarianism, in which morality derived from within society, whether total or partial, is selected or drafted as a guide for that society. In the latter instance the goal is a better life *for* society; in the former it is better control *of* society, even though it may be pitched as the path to a better life. But both are susceptible to dangerous implementation. The better approach occurs in a free society where seeking agreement among all individuals in the society as to what constitutes right or wrong action permits individual conscience to surface and to help guide decisions. A society may not be entitled to be defined as "virtuous," but it can assist the moral character of its members by the nature of the laws it adopts, as long as those laws reflect the considered opinions of a free society and thereby consistent with natural law.[62]

End of excursus

To conclude this section, at the level of a profession or other cohesive group the membership's covenant represents the profession's ethical views reflecting its interaction with its clients. Prof. T. H. Marshall has pointed out that "Ethical codes are based on the belief that between professional and client there is a relationship of trust, and between buyer and seller there is not."[63] The concept of trust in this picture is critical, for it provides an anchor in the midst of an individualistic, and therefore inevitably selfish, society; the study of society's interactions has been said to be the art of mistrust.[64] To trust is no virtue, for blind trust can be foolish or misplaced. To be trustworthy, however, is a virtue. To be ethical in most societies one must be trustworthy, but to whom? For the medical profession the Hippocratic Oath provides an answer.

E. The Hippocratic Oath

The medical profession in the Greece of Hippocrates, representing local membership, did not compel its members to be other than they already were except when they were acting on behalf of their profession. They were not exhorted to be brave, faithful, obeisant, prudent, temperate, or compassionate. The membership evidently was not inclined to insert a list of often impossible standards into personal affairs. But when about their job they were expected to observe those obligations specified in the Oath. The Oath was a working document, not merely one about which to feel good.

The Hippocratic Oath has elicited unceasing commentary, some eulogizing,

---

[62] Much more on this issue and the concept of natural law is found in chapter 36 of this work.

[63] Marshall, T. H., *The Recent History of Professionalism in Relation to Social Structure and Social Philosophy*, in *Can. J. Econ. and Pol. Sci.*, 5:325-340, 1939. This is a classic paper on the professional in society amidst contemporary change that included a greater number and variety of professionals and the tendency for them to work in organizations rather than a solo practice.

[64] Berger, P. L., *Invitation to Sociology: A Humanistic Perspective*, Garden City, 1963, in which Berger quotes Nietzche on this point.

some demeaning.[65] It has undergone many translations.[66] The earliest extant complete version is in the 11th C *Marcianus Venetus* 269 manuscript.[67] Perhaps the closest to consensus regarding the date of the Oath's composition is the 4th C BC, less than a century after Hippocrates, although some think it predates Hippocrates himself. An Asclepiad oath from a similar early date has been uncovered at Delphi, but its role was apparently to protect religious privileges of the extended family of Asclepiadae rather than to serve as a clinical avowal.[68]

The Hippocratic Oath, as a statement of the commitment of physician to patient, has remained Western medicine's guide for 2400 years. Prof. Temkin says the Oath was much esteemed by 1st C Christians and that it retained its "pagan form" through the 4th C, at which time references to pagan deities were removed.[69] St. Jerome honored it in a letter written to a fellow clergyman in 396.[70] The Oath of Asaph the Physician and Yohanan ben Sabda, composed by Asaph Harofe in the 6th C AD and intended for Hebrew physicians, contain much of the content of the Hippocratic Oath plus an extensive religious statement. In contrast, the medical oath of a graduate from a medieval university of about 1350 AD included no mention of a commitment to the patient, being instead a statement of professional protectionism.[71]

Variations in the text of the Oath have been noted, and Dr. W. H. S. Jones considered the oldest Greek texts to be the best versions. Two of the earliest are from the 11th and 12th centuries, but it has also been noted that all versions are post-Christian, an association that has raised questions of authenticity. But a fragment of the Oath that has been dated to 275 AD is presented in Fig. 10. As discussed by Barns, two or three words that would imply an Ionic dialect source of the Oath are replaced by *koine* terms of later Greek, but that seems to have been merely a contemporary alteration to better its local understanding rather than to change its meaning. Scholarly criticism of the versions of the Oath has produced a sizeable literature. But to the more casual reader it may seem remarkable that a roughly 250-word document would, after 2400 years during more than three-quarters of which every copy was written by hand, in a variety of languages, and sometimes penned by persons who, if not illiterate, might have had a personal interest and perspective on the text's content, and transmitted contemporaneously with institutional histories that over many centuries would have included much social upheaval, have

---

[65] For example, the Oath is trivialized by Bulger and lionized by Pellegrino in: Bulger, R. J., *In Search of the Modern Hippocrates*, Iowa, 1987, chapters three and four. This book has an excellent discussion of medical ethics.

[66] For a modern discussion see: Tallis, R., *Hippocratic Oaths: Medicine and Its Discontents*, London, 2004. Tallis is an English physician and philosopher.

[67] The *Marcianus Venetus* 269 manuscript, which includes the *Oath,* is one of the most esteemed copies of the *Hippocratic Corpus*. The earliest extant copy of the *Oath* is but a fragment (Fig. 10).

[68] Jouanna, J. *Hippocrates*, translated by M. B. DeBevoise, Baltimore, 1999, p. 50

[69] See Temkin, O., *Hippocrates in a World of Pagans and Christians*, Baltimore, 1991, p. 182.

[70] "Let it therefore be your duty to keep your tongue chaste as well as your eyes. Never discuss a woman's looks, nor let one house know what is going on in another. Hippocrates, before he will instruct his pupils, makes them take an oath and compels them to swear obedience to him. That oath exacts from them silence, and prescribes for them their language, gait, dress, and manners. How much greater an obligation is laid on us who have been entrusted with the healing of souls!" Letter LII, 15, "To Nepotian"; see *Loeb Classical Library* series, *Select Letters of St. Jerome*, translation of F. A. Wright. The Hippocratic Oath does not, of course, extort obedience from the new physician for personal advantage to the Oath-giver.

[71] Riesman, D., *The Story of Medicine in the Middle Ages*, New York, 1936, p. 159.

survived in such a cohesive form. This is suggested in the fragment shown in Fig. 10, p. 240, for most of the confidently identifiable words of the fragment, penned 600 years after the original, are identical to the same text from a copy (*Marcianus Venetus* 269) of a completely different provenance made after a further 900 years.

The arbitrariness of translation is also found to be minimal when comparing different translated versions of the oldest copies of the Greek Oath. Three versions of lines 21-22, including the 1849 translation by Francis Adams, MD, the 1923 translation of Dr. Jones, and 2006 translation by the author, are examined side-by-side below, and demonstrate this. The opening lines (1-5 in the *Loeb Classical Library*, *Hippocrates*, vol. I, p. 299) represent the avowal. Then follows (lines 5-15) a commitment of the apprentice to his master, one fully consistent with contemporary apprenticeships in other trades and crafts. Lines 16-32 specify obligations of the physician to and protections of the patient. The final section, lines 32-36, gives the consequences of keeping or breaking the Oath.

There are five *obligations* of the physician: to help the sick, to avoid inflicting injury, to give way to those more expert, to abstain from wrongdoing, and to maintain strict privacy regarding the affairs of patients and others. The *protections* for the patient are three in number and include prohibitions regarding the malicious administration of dangerous drugs, interference with pregnancy, and salacious activity. There is only one brief comment that might contain a moral message:

ἁγνῶς δὲ καὶ ὁσίως διατηρήσω βίον τὸν ἐμὸν καὶ τέχνην τὴν ἐμήν.
Lines 21-22

Variability in translation:

a. "In a pure and holy way I will guard my life and my techne'."
Translation of Heinrich von Staden

b. "But I will keep pure and holy both my life and my art."
Loeb Classical Library translation
by W. H. S. Jones.

c. "With purity and with holiness I will pass my life and practice my Art."
Translation of Francis Adams, MD[72]

d. "I will honorably and conscientiously pursue my life and my profession."
Translation by the author

Morality is suggested if "holy" or other words with a divine implication are used in translation. But ἁγνῶς and ὁσίως need not be translated as "holy," and furthermore they are adverbs. Hyperbole detracts from credibility. With this in mind the Oath can be seen not so much as a moral guide, but rather a high-minded statement that has an ethical foundation, one that reflected from its first writing the thinking of medical professionals within a humane society. Although physician-generated and physician-specific, it is society-wide in the appropriateness of its tenets insofar as they represented the ethical preferences and expectations that society impressed on its professionals.

Dr. Jones, the translator of the Oath for the *Loeb Classical Library*, asks, in his

---

[72] Volume 2, pp. 278-280, of *The Genuine Works of Hippocrates*, translated by Dr. Francis Adams, New York, 1929, reprint of the Sydenham Society's 1849 publication.

opening statements regarding the origin of the Oath, "What binding force had it beyond its moral sanction?"[73] In a very practical sense the Oath could be considered a mission statement that came out of a strategic planning session of the Hippocratic koinon on Cos. And if the resulting internal regulation of the physician in an open society is based on personal and professional pride, there is no need for moral sanction. True, the Oath does invoke divine animosity in the event of transgression. But the alpha and omega of the Hippocratic Oath is personal commitment, a commitment that pride does not allow to be controverted, and a commitment not to society but to the individual. And it is society's trust that the physician will adhere to the Oath, a trust based on the physician's sense of pride and honor rather than organizational mandate that has protected the Hippocratic Oath over so many centuries. It has survived virtually unchanged[74] amidst innumerable organizations, from guilds to nations to international movements, most of which have saturated their memberships with mandates. That this important instrument has not been distorted into a meaningless generalization regarding some greater good of society suggests that it was an early accretion to the *Hippocratic Corpus*, and much credit must be ascribed to its copiers over many centuries who recognized that any changes would degrade it.[75]

The Hippocratic physician was compassionate because he was human, humane because he was free, and ethical because he was proud. He was the unswerving advocate of his patient and his profession. The succinctness and clear focus of the Hippocratic Oath as regards commitment to the patient is unequalled by any other statement of medical doctrine. It is certainly a document for the ages.

---

[73] Jones, W.H.S., in the *Loeb Classical Library, Hippocrates*, vol. I, p. 291.

[74] The evidence for little change in the Oath's statement is based on existing copies and copies of copies. There are arguments, however, that there was significant change from the original, as deduced from ethical and philosophical perspectives of the earlier societies, especially ancient Greek. As cogent as the arguments are, they have little factual support, and the original form of the Oath remains unknown.

[75] This is solely the opinion of the author.

CHAPTER SIXTEEN

DISAPPEARANCE OF HIPPOCRATIC MEDICINE

Nuper erat medicus, nunc est vespillo Diallus;
quod vespillo facet, fecerat et medicus.

"Diaulus, who was once a surgeon,
Now assists an undertaker,
Here at length he finds the office
To which alone his skill is suited."

Martial (40-104 AD), *Epigrams*, I, xlvii
(translator unknown)

With the decline of Greek city-state democracies, a process that began in the 4th C BC, Greek medicine came under increasing criticism, and over the next two centuries a declining number of physicians were identified with the island of Cos, presumed home of Hippocrates. Concurrently in ascendant Rome scientific medicine never became an established vocation. As Rome embraced the Mediterranean, its medicine was for the most part provided by alternative practitioners, often Greek, a process well advanced as the Common Era opened and virtually complete shortly thereafter.

A. Introduction: The Passing of a Profession

Prof. Toynbee wrote that the decline of the Roman Empire was but the most obvious manifestation of the decline of Hellenic civilization, which decline he felt began with the Peloponnesian War (430-404 BC) and factional and class warfare.[1] Edward Gibbon's famed history of the decline of the Roman Empire commences after the Age of the Antonines in 180 AD and concludes in 1453 with the fall of Constantinople.[2] But the course of medicine during so many turbulent centuries is not reflected in the grand sweep of these historians, neither of whom even mentioned the term "medicine" or "physician" in the indices to their works.[3] Such omissions accurately represent the status of the medical profession as western civilization entered and traversed the Dark Ages. Any expectations that should have attended the Greek invention of scientific medicine and the natural state of medical practice were to be disappointed, as consequences of vast scale were wrought by withholding knowledge already accrued and waiting to be improved upon. But the extent of loss can only be pieced together in retrospect from the accumulated misery of subsequent ages. In fact, when viewed at the time of its happening, the passing of scientific medicine was not at all newsworthy; it was a nonevent. In contrast, the momentous decline of Hellenic civilization, or, if one prefers, the Roman Empire, ushered in a new society. Perhaps that new society was merely the offspring of the old, but however one might argue its worth at least Greco-Roman civilization was

---

[1] Toynbee, A. J., *A Study of History*, Oxford, 1934-1961, 12 vols.
[2] Gibbon, E., *The Decline and Fall of the Roman Empire*, London, 1776-1788, 6 vols.
[3] Toynbee mentions Hippocrates and Galen only once (*op.cit.*, vol. 10, p. 134, footnote) and then only as a comment on medieval translations of Greco-Roman works.

honored with a replacement. The calamity of scientific medicine was that no substitute came forward. Until its rediscovery many centuries later the medicine of hope and compassion was all that the sick in Western civilization could avail themselves, but for all of society's esteem for those qualities they were no substitute for what had been lost.[4] Matters relevant to that loss are found in the works of Gibbon, Toynbee, and many other scholars, even though medicine itself is only nominally addressed. This chapter briefly examines the status of medicine in the early years of Greco-Roman decline.

It has been said that the fall of the Roman Empire was the greatest tragedy in world history, for a "world-civilization" regressed in "spiritual and material, political and economic, life," a "dissolution of civilization."[5] The search for a culprit to explain its demise would lead to many accusations, the targets being identifiable events or people or things, such as Roman hedonism, the Gothic barbarian, or the Christian Church. But the Hippocratic koinon, having no specific name or address or edifice, a koinon of action rather than ceremony, would vanish without notice, just as a magazine whose subscription is not renewed.

Of medicine's three pillars, two would remain. One was the "art" of medicine.[6] That essential of the physician-patient relationship had been captured in descriptions during Hippocratic times from the *Decorum, Physician*, the *Oath*, and other Hippocratic works that described the obligations and comportment of the attentive physician. This, plus the humane face of Hippocratic medicine, easily outlived its inventors.

The second pillar of Western medicine, the "science" of medicine, was also retained. It was the theories of medicine that were revered by Plato, not its practitioners, an opinion only a healthy person could hold (he lived to the age of eighty-one years).[7] For a while new information was added by Greek physicians in Alexandria and other Greek enclaves, and preservation of this knowledge was guaranteed by ancient medical writers *seriatim* well into the new millennium: by Celsus (25 BC – 50 AD),[8] Aretaeus (1st C AD),[9] Galen (129- *ca.* 200 AD),[10] Oribasius (320-400 AD),[11] and Aetius (502-575

---

[4] Shakespeare (1564-1616) wrote "the miserable have no other medicine but only hope." *Measure for Measure*, Act III, sc. i.

[5] Nilsson, M. P., *Imperial Rome*, New York, 1926, translated by Rev. G. C. Richards.

[6] See Excursus on τεχνή, p. 196*ff*, for definitions of the art, science and profession of medicine.

[7] Plato admired the intellectual and theoretical aspects of medicine more than its empirical discoveries and their implementation. His opinion of medicine, therefore, is of limited value, for he did not recognize the cumulative wisdom attainable from empirical observations scientifically confirmed and analyzed. Thus, he remained a theorist concerning medicine as well as in politics.

[8] Possibly a physician, A. Cornelius Celsus wrote *De Medicina* (On Medicine), a Latin work in eight books. It can be found in the *Loeb Classical Library*, Cambridge, 1938, translation by W. G. Spencer.

[9] The only surviving works of Aretaeus are: *On the Causes and Symptoms of Acute and Chronic Diseases* and *On the Treatment of Acute and Chronic Diseases*. The standard English translation has been that of Francis Adams, MD: *The Extant Works of Aretaeus, the Cappadocian*, London, 1856.

[10] Galen wrote extensively, and, although some of his works were destroyed early on, many survive, including περὶ φυσικῶν δυναμέων (*On the Natural Faculties*), translated by A. J. Brock in the *Loeb Classical Library*, Cambridge, 1916.

[11] Oribasius, a sophist who later learned medicine under Zeno, himself an "iatrosophist" with no clinical experience, was in charge of the library of Emperor Julian, and wrote his συναγωγε ιάτρικη (*Collection of Medical [Writings]*) while in that position and at the command of Julian. Some twenty books survive, and in them are his transcriptions of other ancient medical writers.

AD).[12] In the short term, knowledge assembled by Hippocratic physicians passed through many hands and may have suffered somewhat in translation, but it was not lost.

Perhaps, therefore, scientific medicine of the Hippocratics, in the words of the Hippocratics, ἐφθίσε (epthisei), simply "wasted away." The ability of the apprentice will sometimes be inferior to that of the master. And efficiency in transmitting skills through generations can decrease with each passage; something is forgotten, something remains unused, errors accumulate, each incident tending to diminish the effectiveness of the original skill. As for writings, they sustain their value only if copied precisely, translated accurately, and interpreted correctly. And so, over several generations vigorous practices can become enfeebled by imperceptible degree. The further removed in time, the less likely a retrieval of past excellence will be realized. But there is nothing to suggest that Hippocratic medicine suffered such an asthenic demise. Celsus (25 BC-50 AD) was an advocate of Hippocratic medicine and much of his writing is based on or is a restatement of Hippocratic writings. Galen considered his own work an extension of Hippocratic thinking, and Galenic medical writings and commentaries, the basis of medical tracts for centuries to come, were a paean to Hippocrates. Even the first Latin translations of the writings of Hippocratic physicians, made in the 5th C AD, were true to their authors.[13] Their message, the second pillar of medical knowledge, did not "waste away." Here, therefore, is the prelude to the story of the lost third pillar of medicine, ἡ τεχνή (techne), the *profession*.

B. Contemporary Events and Status of Medicine up to the Fall of Rome

The disappearance of the Hippocratic clinician was not apocalyptic. Dr. Dean-Jones notes that in Aristophanes' *Plutus*, the prize-winning play of 388 BC, Athenians at the beginning of the 4th C still preferred the physician as the first consultation in event of illness.[14] This was despite the physician's apparent ineffectiveness during the Athenian plague in 428 BC, following which there was the introduction of the popular mystical

---

There is a recent translation by Mark Grant of the first four books: *Dieting for an Emperor*, Illinois, 1998. Some contemporaries referred to Oribasius as "Simia Galeni" (the ape of Galen), claiming that he added nothing to Galen's writings except notes on salivary glands. See: Freind, J., *The History of Physick, from the time of Galen* ..., London, 1726, 3rd edition, vol. 1 (of 2), p. 13. Some consider Oribasius' tutor, Zeno, to have been a charlatan.

[12] Aetius wrote βιβλία ἰατρικά ἑκκαίδεκα (*Sixteen Books on Medicine*), in which he cites the work of earlier medical writers, especially those relating to obstetrics and gynecology. See: *The Gynecology and Obstetrics of the VIth Century A.D.*, Philadelphia, 1950, translated from a later Latin edition by J. V. Ricci. Aetius himself included incantations and spells in medical practice.

[13] Soranus (1st C AD and a follower of the Hippocratics) wrote, among other things, an important treatise on obstetrics and gynecology, a history of Hippocrates, and treatises on acute and on chronic diseases that refer to Hippocratic writings, works that were translated from Greek into Latin by Caelius Aurelianus, a Roman physician from North Africa, in the 5th C.

[14] Bl. - Must we not go and seek a physician? Cr. - Seek physicians at Athens? Nay! there's no art where there's no fee." Aristophane's *Plutus*, lines 406-8 translation as originally published by the Athenian Society, London, 1912. The poor salaries of Athenian physicians apparently implied an inferior product. But the point is that, for the problem with vision for which they considered seeking aid, they were not on their way to an Asclepian temple.

healing cult of Asclepius into Athens in 420 BC.[15] Dr. Dean-Jones also states there is no evidence before the 4th C BC of impostors in medicine, speculating that it was the appearance of impostors that prompted a decline in the reputation of medicine.[16] This is probably true. In the 4th C Hippocratic work, *Regimen in Acute Diseases*, there is this statement: "Yet the art as a whole has a very bad name among laymen, so that there is thought to be no art of medicine at all."[17] And *Law* (νομός, Nomos), also part of the Hippocratic Corpus, begins with a statement about the low esteem of the profession: "Medicine, of all the arts, is the most distinguished; but because of the ignorance of practitioners of it, and [the ignorance] of those who recklessly judge them, of all the arts it is now left far behind. The chief reason for this error seems to me to be this: medicine is the only art which our states have made subject to no penalty save that of dishonor...."[18] *Law* is thought to have been composed *ca.* 400 BC, and the authorship is unknown. There should have been little reason to contemplate state penalties if the profession were properly maintaining the quality of membership. A change in society's opinion of its practitioners was also on display on Hippocrates' home island of Cos where an Asclepian temple of healing was erected in 366 BC.

A diminishing public esteem for the profession occurred over several centuries, with Cicero indicating the presence of some good physicians in the 1st C BC, whereas inferior practitioners were the rule by the time of the Marcus Aurelius (121-180 AD). Although Aurelius was a friend and admirer of Galen, cynical comments about physicians characterize the learned writings of this self-effacing emperor as well as in those of Galen himself. This was with good reason, for mysticism had firmly reinstated itself into medical practice. Amulets, introduced from the East about 50 AD, were used not just to prevent disease, but "to cure almost every physical ailment," usually being hung around the neck or arm. The worship of Asclepius was popular during the time of Aurelius, and magical medical poetry was being composed by two prominent nearly contemporary physicians, Marcellus of Sida (*fl.* 150 AD) and Quintus Serenus Sammonicus (*fl.* 240 AD). But Aurelius recognized the difference between the medicine of Galen and these, Galen's competitors. Thus, the road to the medicine of the Dark Ages was paved long before the Roman Empire "fell." Before the cause is analyzed, social changes and their medical consequences up to the time of relocation of the seat of Imperial government to Constantinople must be reviewed. East-West distinctions justify separate assessments.

1) The Western Empire

Rome, founded in 753 BC, became a republic in 509 BC, reached its greatest

---

[15] Wickkiser, B. L., *Asklepios Medicine, and the Politics of Healing in Fifth-Century Greece*, Baltimore, 2008.

[16] Dean-Jones, L., *Literacy and the Charlatan in ancient Greek Medicine*, in *Written Texts and the Rise of Literate Culture in Ancient Greece*, Cambridge, 2003, chapter 5, H. Yunis, editor.

[17] *Regimen in Acute Diseases*, VIII, 17-19, *Loeb Classical Library*, *Hippocrates*, vol. II, translation of W. H. S. Jones. There is, however, an implication of "false accusation" in διαβολή, that suggests some of the problem was public perception rather than professional delinquency. Dean-Jones considered Hippocrates to be the writer, which would imply 5th C or early 4th C BC for this composition. Note that Dean-Jones uses the word "art" for the translation of τεχνή, rather than "profession," as discussed in the Excursus herein, p. 196.

[18] *Law*, I, 1-4, in vol. 2 of the Hippocratic works in the *Loeb Classical Library*, translation of W. H. S. Jones.

geographical extent under its emperors, and was reduced to a cohesive state in name only by 423 AD, a 1,200 year dominion. A tottering of the State was suspected early on by Seneca the Younger (4 BC – 65 AD) as he considered the deficiencies of Roman Emperors.[19] Ultimately, some fifty different explanations would be offered for the fall of the Roman Empire, including the institution of slavery and a "top-heavy" minority civilization,[20] moral degeneracy of Roman society, the Antonine plague, and loss of the highest leadership due to heritable or toxin-induced mental debility.[21] Petrarch blamed Julius Caesar, who had destroyed the liberty of the people, and Machiavelli blamed barbarians and decadence. Voltaire selected two: the barbarian invasions and the rise of Christianity. Gibbon agreed: "I have described the triumph of barbarism and religion." Spengler gave no reason but considered it inevitable.[22] The true reasons are still debated.

But in 146 BC Rome was growing rapidly, extending its military control after the complete destruction of Corinth in 146 BC to include all of Greece. There then followed a movement of Greek medical practitioners to Rome, where the Greek term, *iatros,* was replaced by the Latin *medicus*, both currently translated as "physician." But the *medicus* himself remained a Greek, or at least not Roman.[23] Early Roman writers commented negatively on the Greek practitioner, their bias reflecting the scorn conservative upper-class Romans had for Greek society, just as centuries later the conquering Normans would scorn the culturally superior Anglo-Saxons.[24] Practical experience fed this bias, for most Greek "physicians" in Rome were not Hippocratic physicians, were in fact slaves or freed slaves who had merely acquired some degree of practical medical proficiency in Greece and then sought their fortunes in the Imperial City.[25] Nevertheless, several Greek physicians appearing in Rome between 200 BC and

---

[19] Lactantius, *Divine Institutes,* VII, 15.

[20] Walbank, F. W., *The Awful Revolution: The Decline of the Roman Empire in the West*, London, 1969, p. 108. (First published in 1946.)

[21] The potential role of lead poisoning was recently reviewed by Nriagu, J. O., *Lead and Lead Poisoning in Antiquity*, New York, 1983. The symptoms and signs of lead poisoning were well known to the Romans.

[22] The rise and fall of some twenty-three civilizations described by Dr. Toynbee in *Study of History*, (Oxford, 1934-1961, in twelve volumes) would add to Oswald Spengler's argument as expressed in *The Decline of the West* (translation from the German by C. F. Atkinson), New York, 1926. For example, Dr. Spengler, in his chapter 2, compares the course of mathematics in the Classical Period, beginning with Pythagoras (6th C BC), to that of recent Western mathematics, beginning with Descartes (1596-1650), describing their conception, flourishing, and dissolution, a conclusion that coincides with the end of their respective civilizations. But Dr. Spengler gave no particular reason for the inevitable decline of civilizations. His theory was based on a personal perspective of history colored by the First World War. While skilled in mathematics and other areas, he has been considered by most scholars a dilettante in philosophy and history; his ardent supporters included Allen Ginsberg and Jack Kerouac. It is difficult to credit Spengler's work in the absence of a stated explanation, but it might apply if each civilization that arises were to return to its basal state, a tenet seriously considered in the present work.

[23] Well over ninety percent of named physicians in Roman Italy were not Roman. See: Nutton, V., *The Medical Profession*, in: *From Democedes to Harvey: Studies in the History of Medicine*, London, 1988, p. 258.

[24] Cato the Censor (234-149 BC) warned against the effects of Greeks on the intellectual development of Romans. As Pliny says (*Nat. Hist.*, 29, viii), "it is quite sufficient to dip into the records of Greek genius, without becoming thoroughly acquainted with them."

[25] An overview relevant to this point is found in: Vogt, J., *Ancient Slavery and the Ideal of Man*, Cambridge, 1975, translated by T. Wiedemann, pp. 114-121.

200 AD were popular and became well-known from their own writings or from the writings of others (see Table 7, p. 267). Pliny the Elder (23-79 AD) wrote that Romans gave credit to anything in medicine if it was Greek, even though Romans had done well for centuries without any physicians, relying instead on their own traditions and common sense.[26] He flatly stated that no Romans learned medicine: "Medicine is the only one of the arts of Greece, that, lucrative as it is, the Roman gravity has hitherto refused to cultivate."[27]

But there was this most important consequence: the influx of Greeks into Italy in the years following the fall of Corinth was met with a determined effort to keep the newcomers dispersed so as to prevent local concentrations of Greeks from posing territorial, commercial or intellectual threats to Roman society.[28] Greek genius, therefore, remained an import under Roman stewardship. That the Greeks were not the sole object of repression is seen in the perennial attitude of the Roman government toward indigenous guilds (collegia) of virtually all trades and arts, although for a different reason. Government concern was not about capitalist motives or strikes. The issues initially were that guilds were sometimes a cover for what was considered seditious disruption, and, being relatively homogeneous in membership, guilds tended to vote in blocs. Political leaders, therefore, attempted by bribes and other subtleties to acquire large blocs of guild votes. An emperor whose supporters had something to lose by these voting blocs could proscribe the guilds.[29] Most of the time, therefore, guilds of any kind, manifestations as they were of private and generally plebeian sympathies, were unwelcome among the aristocratic Romans.[30] And yet it was unlikely that medicine would have generated a

---

[26] In Book 29 of *The Natural History* of Pliny the Elder, probably published in 78 AD shortly before his death from the Mt. Vesuvius eruption, is found a rash of complaints about medicine: "barren of charms," "lucrative ... beyond all the rest"; about Greeks: "a most iniquitous and intractable race," "conspired among themselves to murder all [of us] with their medicines," "we are impelled onwards by the puffs [flatus] which emanate from the ingenuity of the Greeks"; and about physicians: they purchase celebrity "at the downright expense of human life," "For what profession has there been more fruitful in poisonings, or from which there have emanated more frauds upon wills, and then, to what adulteries have been committed, in the very houses of our princes even!"

[27] Pliny, *The Natural History of Pliny*, XXIX, 8, 4.

[28] The interesting conflict between Roman guilds and aristocracy is briefly reviewed in: *Trade Guilds of Europe*, Wash., D.C., 1885, U. S. State Dept. publication, J. T. Dubois, editor, p. 5.

[29] The Greek equivalent of a collegium, ἑταιρεία, existed in Periclean times, and was usually of a religious or political character. Even then guilds were sometimes socially disruptive. Roman Collegia, or "guilds," plebeian in membership, also existed in earliest Rome, supposedly instituted by Numa (ruled 715-672 BC) when he wished, according to Plutarch, to diminish the polarity of social contention in Rome by diffusing society's energies and loyalties among a variety of suborganizations. Interestingly, Plutarch calls such organizations "koinonia." Roman Collegia began to come under State control in the 1st C BC to curb their political influence. Over several centuries they would come to be unofficially incorporated into the functioning of the State, with membership in the trade collegia being hereditary, mandatory, and nontransferable, basically State monopolies. They became, in effect, an extension of State power, particularly useful in manipulation of smaller cities throughout the Empire. Fowler and Charlesworth (*Rome*, London, 1947, 2nd edition, p. 145) concurred that "illegal association was a serious crime" and early Christian communities apparently labored under suspicion just as had earlier Greek immigrant organizations. Also see citations in: Durant, W., *The Story of Civilization*, vol. 3, *Caesar and Christ*, NY, 1944.

[30] Around the contemporary Roman world, North Africa had very few guilds, for the region was primarily agricultural with small towns and little worth exporting. Near Eastern trade guilds, however, were numerous, but no mention is made of a medical guild. Likewise, in Asia Minor

Table 7: Prominent Medical Personages and Their Ethnicity during the Roman Republic and Early Empire (none on this list were slave practitioners or freedmen.)

Name	Dates	Origin
Archagathus	219 BC	Greece
Hailed by the Roman Senate and given citizenship.		
Aesclepiades of Bythnia	120-70 BC	Greece
Galen called him a charlatan; he repudiated Hippocrates, declaring physicians cured disease.		
Themison of Laodicea	1st C BC	Asia Minor
Prominent empiricist, but butt of Juvenal in satire 10.221: "as many sick folk as Themison has killed in a single autumn."		
Scribonius Largus	1-50 AD	Sicily
Wrote Compositiones, a small compendium of drug therapies. He makes the earliest reference to the Hippocratic Oath.		
Heliodorus	1st C AD	Greek
Surgeon, devised methods of treating dislocations		
Dioscorides, Pedanius	41-ca. 90 AD	Greek
Composed the great pharmacopoeia called De Materia Medica, used well into the Renaissance.		
Celsus, Aulus Cornelius	fl. 14-37 AD	Roman ?
Perhaps a physician, he primarily updated Hippocrates.		
Andromachus, the Elder	1st C AD	Crete
Physician to Nero 54-68 AD.		
Archigenes	75-129 AD	Syrian
Surgeon		
Soranus	fl. 98-138	Ephesus
Wrote major work on obstetrics and gynecology		
Rufus of Ephesus	ca. 110-180	Ephesus
Anatomy was his forte.		
Antyllus	2nd C AD	Greek
Surgeon famed for discoveries in amputations, ligation		
Galen	129-200 AD	Pergamon
Prolific Hippocratic physician		
Aretaeus	fl. 140 AD	Cappadocia
Practiced in the Hippocratic tradition, adding new clinical descriptions, but received no recognition in his day.		

strong guild, or collegium, for, being composed of mere physicians, and foreign at that, its organizations were devoid of any economic authority. Neither "medicine" nor "physicians" are mentioned in the scholarly works of either Prof. Toutain or Dr. Tenney Frank on economic life in the classical world, including that of the Hellenistic age, even though they specify guilds of many kinds and acknowledge their place in the economic

where guilds were numerous because there was little slavery, no medical guild is mentioned among the ninety-seven listed by T. R. S. Broughton in: *Roman Asia Minor*, the final section of volume 4 of *An Economic Survey of Ancient Rome*, T. Frank, editor, Baltimore, 1938.

structure of the time.[31] Freda Utley (1899-1978), in her thesis *Trade Guilds of the Latter Roman Empire* (London School of Economics, 1925), lists some eighty guilds/collegia, but one for the *medicus* is not included.

There were other factors. Romans often had their ills treated by their own slaves or local healers as the need demanded rather than pay for the services of medical envoys of a degraded culture.[32] Furthermore, Roman tradition had vested medicine in a mantle of altruism. Requiring payment for medical assistance was anathema. One might wonder which was the more important factor, the aristocratic early Roman's sense of cultural superiority or his stinginess. The call for ambitious young Romans to enter a profession based primarily on altruism would surely find few respondents. A short list of well-paid physicians, some notorious, was employed by ruling families. And there were city physicians hired by cities as commanded by Rome to provide municipal services, presumably to the poor. But it was easier and cheaper for most to go to the nearest herb-gatherer (*rhizotomi*), bath attendant (*iatroliptae*), medical slave (*servi medici*), or salve-dealer (*unguentarii*) than to seek out a more expensive foreigner. Finally, the younger male Roman citizen could gaze on far brighter horizons for a career. In the military and civil service the expanding empire needed competent applicants for staffing important governmental and military positions. As a result, the increasing size of and need for the equestrian class, an important source of business entrepreneurs, would have attracted those most likely to have considered a medical career had they had not had such opulent options.

Given the size and longevity of the Roman Empire and the extensive and detailed records of its administration, remarkably little remains to document the nature or even the existence of an indigenous medical establishment. This is reflected in the histories of Rome published in recent times; virtually nothing on this point is found in the accounts of Gibbon, nor in Prof. Martin Nilsson's *Imperial Rome* (New York, 1926), the great Theodor Mommsen's *The History of Rome* (three volume edition, London, 1862-1866), Prof. A.H.M. Jones' three volume *The Later Roman Empire (284-602)* (Oxford, 1964), Dr. Max Cary's *A History of Rome Down to the Reign of Constantine* (London, 1975, 3rd ed.), or in Prof. Rostovtzeff's *Social and Economic History of the Roman Empire* (Oxford, 1957, 2nd ed.), all standard scholarly works. In the extensive *Corpus Inscriptionum Latinarum*, there are only fifty-one inscriptions referring to "physicians," and many of these were Greek freed men, *i.e.,* former slaves, while others were government appointees, the *archiatri*.[33] [34] Caches of Roman medical instruments can be examined in

---

[31] Toutain, J., *The Economic Life of the Ancient World*, London, 1930, Part II (The Hellenistic World), translated by M. R. Dobie. Dr. Toutain mentions baggage-porters, masons, donkeymen, second-hand dealers, felt-makers, wool-carders, embalmers, grain-crushers, and quarryman, to list a few, but not medical practitioners. In T. Frank's *An Economic History of Rome* (London, 1927, 2nd edition), wages are given for many services and crafts, even including 32 cents/day for a painter and 11 cents/day for an unskilled workman, but there is no mention whatever of medical practitioners of any sort. T. R. S. Broughton (see previous note) also noted that in Roman Asia there was no information available concerning either private or "city" physicians' incomes, with the exception of a few atypical physicians attached to Emperors or engaged in charlatanry.

[32] Garrison, F. H., *An Introduction to the History of Medicine*, Phila., 1921, 3rd edition, for a discussion of Greco-Roman medicine, p. 96*ff*.

[33] Scarborough, J., *Roman Medicine*, London, 1969, Chapter VIII.

[34] The *Corpus Inscriptionum Latinarum* presently comprises seventeen volumes and over 180,000 entries, being the repository of ancient public and private inscriptions collected by classical scholars since its inception in 1853 by Theodor Mommsen. It was examined for occupational names, and

modern museums, but they often belonged, not to a physician, but, perhaps following the advice of Pliny, to Roman families who retained their own stock of medical supplies and instruments for personal use.[35] Objective descriptions of Roman physicians and their patients are absent. Historical statements on medical personnel in the Roman army, on the obstetrics of midwives, on public works that improved sanitation, and on local practitioners who purportedly performed specified medical procedures find their place in history books, but the theater of action of the "compassionate medical scholar" in the Roman world was not described.

Had a Roman medical establishment been created that merely copied that of the Hippocratics like the Romans copied Greek sculpture, an irretrievable eclipse of the medical profession might have been averted. Alternatively, had a few Romans apprenticed their sons to experienced Greek physicians, that experience might have passed into sufficient Roman hands to sustain a medical profession. For the eclipse of scientific medicine cannot be ascribed to the decline in population or population centers. In the earlier years of Imperial Rome cities around the Mediterranean and beyond grew in number and size. Business was booming, industry was specializing, and guilds were proliferating. Simultaneously, Roman intellectual life itself was stirring. Literacy rates as high as twenty percent have been suggested, although in large portions of the citizenry it must have been very low, whereas in the military and in the upper classes it would have been much higher, the latter often being bilingual. In poetry and the arts, in philosophy and jurisprudence, the 1st C saw a new face of Rome. As Sir John Mahaffy has stated it, "The Romans were, indeed, imitators and pupils; but what pupils!"[36] Why did they not imitate Greek medicine? Certainly a critical mass of educated people was present in many cities, enough to promote exchange of ideas in medicine as the Greeks had done. Both private support of education and professional services for private tutoring were popular. The bankrolling of the medical profession should have been easily accomplished had it been deemed desirable. Time was not wanting. Had there been some small and scattered foci of Hippocratic medical practice in Roman lands any threat of Greek organization to Roman security and identity might have been irrelevant, and they would, therefore, have been less likely than a single insular Greek one to be overwhelmed. But society sets expectations by which entrepreneurs gage their strategy for success. A society that is used to little will settle for little. In medicine the Romans received not that for which they could pay, but that for which they were willing to pay, which was very little, a feeble inducement to potential Roman medical initiates.

---

only 51 "medici" were identified, along with 4 (female) "medicae." See: Carcopino, J., *Daily Life in Ancient Rome*, New Haven, 1940, p. 201. The archiatri designated "*archiatri sancti palatii*" were senior physicians in the medical hierarchy who tended emperors and prominent individuals. They would be more likely to inspire inscriptions than the "archiatri populares," the modest city physicians elected and salaried by the people to care primarily for the poor. See: Nutton, V., *Archiatri and the Medical Profession in Antiquity*, in *Papers of the British School at Rome*, 45:191-226, 1977, and Smith, W., *Dictionary of Greek and Roman Antiquities*, 2nd edition, Boston, 1870.

[35] Another advocate of "amateur medicine" was Gargilius Martialis who in the 3rd C AD was a writer on horticulture. Gargilius' works frequently were to find their way into medieval manuscripts used for medical teaching. See: Wallis, F., *Signs and Senses: Diagnosis and Prognosis in Early Medieval Pulse and Urine Texts*, in *Social Hist. Med.* 13:265-278, 2000.

[36] Mahaffy, J.P., *The Silver Age of the Greek World*, Chicago, 1906. But they were pupils nonetheless, or, as stated by Marquardt, "Bei den Griechen ist jedes Handwerk eine Kunst; bei den Romern jede Kunst ein Handwerk." ("With the Greeks every handicraft is an art; with the Romans every art a handicraft.") Marquardt, J, *Das Privatleben des Romer*, Leipzig, 1882, p. 589.

But by 200 AD only ten percent of the Roman Empire's population was urban. While rural areas bore the burden of empire, dissolution of empire was brewing in the cities. Previously Roman opulence had been acquired by imports from the East and paid for by exports to the West. But as western cities began to produce their own goods, tributes to Rome from conquered lands came to be the main support for an ever increasing military and civil service budgets. In addition, principle cities were along the Mediterranean coast, and they thrived as long as inland supplies could be delivered to them. Therefore, when barbarian tribes began to more effectively counter the Roman Legions and when Romanized tribes established their own principalities, borders of the Western Empire began to constrict. Cities became less well supplied with necessities and their populations rapidly dwindled beginning in the 4th C AD.[37] Beyond Rome those citizens of poorer backgrounds now found themselves able to take up public office and to acquire properties once belonging to the wealthy. Rome itself became less and less the hub of Empire for there now were provincial leaders interposed between the people and Roman leadership.

The West was breaking up, becoming increasingly rural and dependent on local economies. It came under the hegemony of local lords who were supported by local taxation. The independent man disappeared. During the time of the emperor Theodoric (454-526 AD) there was a transient improvement in public opinion regarding medicine, for the profession was highly valued by that emperor. Perhaps the esteem for the Hippocratic Oath prompted this revival in public opinion, the Oath being so consistent with the themes of Christianity which Theodoric embraced. Unfortunately, scientific medicine did not benefit from this resurgence, for it had long since ceased to exist. Like oil and other international commodities, reliance on external suppliers is risky business.

2) The Eastern Empire

In reviewing the final years of the Roman Republic (1st C BC), scholars note that Rome had yet to define its policies dealing with matters outside of Italy. It was only when suddenly faced with empire that Rome was pushed to learn how to deal with its windfall, whether in the abundance of luxury, in the press of international affairs, or in the integration into Roman society of large numbers of immigrants and slaves from conquered territories, which included Greece.

Emigration and the loss in local hegemony of the city-state had unsettled Greek society beginning in the 4th C BC. The Hellenistic period that followed (323 – 30 BC) was one of revolution, a time when traditional fraternal ties of the city-state and the tribe disintegrated. By 250 BC the citizens of once famous Sparta numbered only seven hundred. On the Greek mainland the mines and forests had become depleted. Farms grew in size as land was acquired by the wealthy, but there were few left to farm them. The population of Athens and environs, estimated at 172,000 citizens in 431 BC, declined to about 100,000 freemen with 21,000 male citizens by 320 BC, if the census of Demetrius of Phalerum is to be believed. There are no good estimates of its population in the 3rd C,

---

[37] Discussed by Brown, P., in *The World of Late Antiquity*, New York, 1971. There is even some scholarly debate as to whether true cities remained in the West after the 3rd C AD and in the East from the early 7th C AD.

but the historian Polybius (200-118 BC) describes early 2nd C Greece in gloomy terms.[38] The Roman victory at Corinth in 146 BC and the razing of Athens by Sulla in 87 BC proved the end of Greek freedom. Calamity was magnified when, to more efficiently control newly conquered territories, Roman authorities supported local puppet governors in exchange for promises of military support. Power, wealth, and land ownership became concentrated into fewer and fewer hands. Democratic institutions and democratic sympathies ceased. A few powerful aristocrats, guided by self-preservation as much as by enrichment, served as minions of Rome. As in other Roman provinces, inhabitants of Greece became as Romans. Survival for much of the population required that they remove themselves to the countryside and adapt to an agricultural existence, one of hardship and deprivation rather than the bucolic state portrayed by early poets. Many emigrated to the more prosperous colonies,[39] and it was in places such as Alexandria and Pergamon where Hellenic identity persisted.[40]

Even in Roman and in Greek provinces not subject to Rome there was resistance to Hellenism as provincial forces began to replace, rather than integrate, those elements of Greek society that for so long had remained isolated and aloof in their midst, implants of a culture that deigned neither to accept local customs nor to impose Greek customs or language. Overall, Greek influence was quickly fading in the 2nd C BC. This applied as well to Alexandria. This Greek colonial city would remain highly regarded as an intellectual center well into the new millennium, but its contributions to contemporary clinical medicine, to be discussed in the next chapter, were inconsequential.

Also in the East was the island of Cos, the home of Hippocrates. Cos had received recognition and visits in the 4th C BC by Alexander the Great and subsequently by members of the Ptolemaic dynasty that ruled Egypt, at which times its training of superior clinicians was acknowledged by those in highest authority.[41] And yet Cos has been described in the 1st C BC as having physicians sufficient only for the local population, even though a rate of one newly trained physician every two or three years would have easily sufficed for its small population.. No natural disasters of a magnitude that could have explained a decrease in physician training occurred on Cos prior to the earthquake of 27 BC. And after this date there is little mention of Cos, although Tacitus confirms a Coan physician for the Emperor Claudius (ruled 41-54 AD), the infamous

---

[38] "In our own time the whole of Greece has been subject to a low birth-rate and a general decrease of the population, owing to which cities have become deserted and the land has ceased to yield fruit,..." Polybius *Histories*, 36, 17, 5 (translation of W. R. Paton, from the *Loeb Classical Library*).

[39] They settled in cities belonging to the kingdoms that emerged following the death of Alexander the Great, the "cities of the Diadochi," which included Rhodes, Alexandria, Pergamon, Antioch, Seleucia, Ephesus, and Miletos. A quantitation of the emigration from Greece during Hellenistic times is not available.

[40] Pergamon became a kingdom in the 3rd C BC and reached its zenith as a commercial and artistic center in the 2nd C BC, a century after Alexandria. Its famed commercial production of parchment, made from the scraped stretched skins of goats and calves, is postulated to be in response to Ptolemy V who restricted the supply of papyrus from Egypt to the rest of the ancient world. Two hundred thousand books from its magnificent library purportedly were given by Mark Anthony to Cleopatra in 40 BC. It had an Asclepeion, grandly replaced in the 2nd C AD, that was so famed for temple healing that Prof. Sarton (Sarton, G., *Galen of Pergamon*, Kansas, 1954, p. 12) has likened it to Lourdes. This was also the city of Galen.

[41] Alexander the Great had a Coan physician, as did Roxana, his wife.

Xenophon.[42] If there were a want of new Coan physicians at the close of the millennium the cause is not obvious. It is far more likely that there never had been more than a few Coan physicians being trained there at any given time, and that the decline in their representation throughout the Empire represented not a decrease in size of a "graduating class" on Cos itself but a decrease in physicians outside Cos who could obtain the benefits of a professional affiliation with the koinon of Hippocratic physicians, if it still existed.

It remained, therefore, for Rome to rescue Greek colonies from oblivion. Whatever the disdain of the Romans for Greek morality and inconstancy, Greece was still Rome's Mediterranean neighbor and far superior to the people of transalpine Europe, Asia, and Africa. In the face of barbarism Greek cities and colonies were not permitted to perish. In fact, by 350 AD Athens was again, albeit temporarily, a great city for scholars, primarily due to the largess of wealthy Romans.

The course of events in the western and eastern parts of the empire was different. In the early centuries of the Common Era, the West fragmented when overrun by tribal societies having admiration for Rome but no common culture. This eroded material support for the large cities, and the West became more rural. In the East, however, city governments strengthened. The East, now with Constantinople as the seat of Empire, maintained a common Hellenic tradition and had a *lingua franca*, the Greek language. In contrast, the West, struggling for survival, retained nothing of a Greek legacy. The decline in the West produced a concentration of power in the hands of local lords, whereas in the East the emperor Constantine strengthened his hold on his subjects, that tether now including a powerful new component, the State religion of Christianity. In the West the independent man was vanishing, and in the East such entrepreneurship as could be controlled and directed by central government remained in force. In such disparate worlds how could the medicine of Hippocrates have come to similarly disappointing ends? The answer is provided in the next chapter.

---

[42] This was Xenophon of Cos, a favorite of Claudius. The fortunate Coans were thereby exempted from paying tribute to Rome and permitted to rule themselves. See Tacitus' *History*, XII, 61.

CHAPTER SEVENTEEN

DISAPPEARANCE OF HIPPOCRATIC MEDICINE: THE CAUSE REVEALED

"While we breathe and move, while we imagine and invent, we ourselves are laying up new stores for the ridicule of posterity."

Lord Lytton (1831-1861)

Possible reasons for the loss of Hippocratic medicine are presented, but only one seems adequate to the task. Early in the 1st C BC Roman guilds (collegia) became increasingly regulated by the State that frowned on plebeian organizations in general and Greek organizations in particular. Thus, although there was a diminishing number and status of Coan physicians concurrent with a declining Greece, the proximate cause of the loss of scientific medicine was the profession's inability to sustain, within the Roman world, the medical koinon, or venue of common council, as a source for medical excellence. The medical koinon would have provided a focus for public esteem and, thereby, recruitment. In its absence medical attrition was quantitative rather than qualitative, but it was complete. Furthermore, it occurred before the Common Era, which explains why, in response to the question posed at the end of the preceding chapter, practitioners of Hippocratic medicine were not to be found in either the Eastern or Western Empires. Whereas the Caesars and their successors were replaced by a theocratic bureaucracy, nothing filled the void produced by the disappearance of the Hippocratic clinician as the Dark Ages approached.

A. Disappearance of the Hippocratic Clinician: Arguments Concerning the Cause

Hippocratic medicine was admired in its day, perhaps influencing medical practice as far away as China. Fifteen centuries later its resurrection would be acclaimed. There has been a universal appeal in Hippocratic thinking. But something extinguished it during its early development, something that, as Prof. McNeill wrote, replaced the naturalism and rationalism of 5th C BC Hellenism with the transcendentalism and mysticism of the 5th C AD.[1] Ancient Mediterranean civilization was unable to retain what it had been fortunate enough to gain. In the latter days of Hippocratic medicine impostors came to assume the place of the scientific clinician. This was not because the impostors were better, but because they were available, whereas the Hippocratic clinician was not. Many considerations bear on this tragic outcome. Possible causes and comments on their plausibility are as follows:

1. Greed

The modest income of the physician and his humble position not only in 5th C Greek society but in subsequent centuries make it unlikely that either a scion seeking an avocation or an entrepreneurial son of the middle class seeking a vocation would see in the profession a preferable venue for avarice, except for those few atypical practitioners who performed for the rich and powerful. The average physician was not a recipient of

---

[1] McNeill, W., *The Rise of the West*, Chicago, 1963, p. 27.

the prosperity of Classical Greece, and thus that prosperity should have negatively influenced neither him nor the profession.

2. Disappearance of the Greek City-State

Despite the misfortunes of mainland Greece the resilience of Greek society should not be underestimated. There was an emigration of physicians from the Greek mainland and islands to the city they hoped would be the new center of power and scholarly life, and it was there that the Alexandrian medical community would make contributions to anatomy and physiology. The city of Pergamon, famous as the home of Galen in the 2nd C AD, developed in Hellenistic times and was not a preexisting Greek city-state. But unexpected wealth allowed what was merely a mountaintop temple and guardpost in the 4th C to become a wealthy city under the Attalid dynasty (281 BC – 133 BC) and ultimately the capital of Asia for a brief period under the Romans. It benefited much from immigration from Hellenistic Greece, and its library was second only to that of Alexandria. Rostovtzeff concluded as well that there were no important changes in the financial organization or constitutions of the scattered Greek cities during Hellenistic times.[2] From the point of view of medicine, an alternative to the city-state had been found, even Cos island itself retaining its medical reputation for two centuries.

3. Decline of Hellenism

A relevant opinion has been put forth by Prof. Muller, who noted that Rome's "great contributions to civilization" came "after it had been corrupted. If we had only its Golden age it [Rome] would reflect only valor and public spirit, not the arts, literature ...." One explanation he offers is the delay between an original observation and its widespread acceptance, the time required for confirmation, discussion, and dissemination, and for displacement of earlier opinion.[3] Another explanation is that much of the later flowering of the Greek intellect reflected the greater regional influence of Hellenism subsequent to the conquests of Alexander the Great (356-323 BC). Finally, recall further that additions to the Hippocratic Corpus were made throughout the 4th C BC. Dr. Baas lists forty-two named 4th C BC physicians or persons with scientific interests in areas relevant to medicine.[4] This underscores the prominence of the medical profession in post-Classical Greece, to which the later Roman entries are so meagerly compared. It is evident that the socio-economic decline of mainland Greece was not paralleled by a decline in the spirit of Hellenism. This, however, does not address the physician-patient relationship that was central to Hippocratic medicine, for the following reasons:

Excursus on Alexandrian Medicine and the Physician-Patient Relation

It is relevant to this work that, in contrast to physicians identified with Cos, there are no honorific inscriptions for contemporary practitioners trained in Alexandria. Fraser noted

---

[2] Rostovtzeff, M. I., in *The Social and Economic History of the Hellenistic World*, Oxford, 1953, vol. 3, p. 1304.

[3] Muller, H. J., *Uses of the Past*, Oxford, 1967, p. 211.

[4] Baas, J. H., *Outlines of the History of Medicine and the Medical Profession*, New York, 1889, H. E. Henderson, translator, pp. 94-143.

that as Ptolemaic Alexandria aged, productivity in medical science persisted but originality decreased. It has been stated that the truly productive years of Alexandrian ingenuity lasted but a century, although its reputation lasted ten times that.[5] The ingenuity and the barbarism of some of the researchers of Alexandria are routinely dwelt upon in modern histories of medicine. But where were the practitioners of Alexandria, what were their office routines, where are their case histories?[6] Medical science, on the other hand, found a home in Alexandria, and physicians who made ingenious discoveries in anatomy and physiology became justly famous, although just how far their contemporary circle of fame extended is unknown.

A feature of Alexandrian medical advances is that they required little organizational framework, for their scope of investigation was narrow and well-defined, capable of being managed by one or a few individuals. In contrast, a network was needed for clinical discoveries such as had characterized the koinon of the Hippocratics because observations of many patients were required in order to draw useful conclusions. Detailed observations of a singular patient's problem can surely advance medical knowledge on a wide front if the nature of that problem has broad application or implication. It is for this reason that today's major medical institutions often have "metabolic" or "research" units for studying unique medical problems of select patients in exhaustive detail. But in ancient times almost any confirmable clinical observation would have been a significant advance, and dissemination rivaled original observation in determining the importance of an invention or discovery. Deciphering the riddle of an irregular pulse on one patient might have had immediate relevance to many other patients. And so the value of Alexandrian discoveries cannot be minimized. But it must be admitted that they form a category unto themselves. That they were new, were sometimes profound (in retrospect), and had the potential to push back further the ignorance and mysticism of that age cannot be denied. But from the practical standpoint this had happened before. They were akin to the primitive identification of jaundice, of edema, of fever, although at a more complex level. What, for example, did the discovery of narrowed blood vessels in the livers of Egyptian patients with cirrhosis, first described by Erasistratus and insightfully given as the cause of ascites, mean to practitioners of that age? Galen disobligingly ridiculed it.[7] Erasistratus' description of liver cirrhosis is surely relevant to modern medicine. But it had to be rediscovered anew by Bilharz in 1852 before its significance could be clarified, namely the pipestem fibrosis and portal hypertension of schistosomiasis. Until that rediscovery the observation regarding the vascular status of the liver identified by Erasistratus remained just a curiosity, one that was generally ignored. For contemporary physicians in Alexandria it may have been a scientific advance but it was not a clinical one. It did not prevent or cure a disease, it did not alter an outcome. In time it would, but not for two

---

[5] So durable were Alexandrian intelligentsia that that city was still considered a center of medical learning in 642 AD when conquered by the Arabs, a span of almost a thousand years.

[6] Fulgentius (late 5th C AD grammarian), in the Introduction to his *Mitologicae*, claimed that in his time there were "more surgical butcher stalls than dwelling places" on some Alexandrian streets, an unsustainable claim according to modern historians.

[7] Remarkably, Erasistratus accurately described *portal vein* fibrosis, *i.e.*, blood flow was inhibited *before* entering the liver. Galen wrote: "For, does it not show the most extreme carelessness to suppose that the blood is prevented from going forward into the liver owing to the narrowness of the passages, and that dropsy can never occur in any other way?" Galen, *On The Natural Faculties*, II, viii, 109, p. 170, translation of A. J. Brock in the *Loeb Classical Library*.

thousand years. It did not assist the practitioner in Rome, in Athens, in Miletos. And it surely did not secure the future of Hippocratic medicine. Without practical application, no discovery, however brilliant, would have excited patient, patron, or practitioner. For this reason the medical centers of Alexandria and Pergamon were unable to achieve a reputation for clinical excellence. Polybius (203-120 BC) railed at the clinical ineptitude of Alexandrian practioners in his *Histories*.[8] There was no forum for enticing others into pursuing further the clinical significance of their findings, no *Annals of the Pergamon Center for Medical Excellence*, no *Milesian Medical Quarterly*, no *Alexandrian Journal of Medicine*.

An important factor in determining the course of Alexandrian medicine was the chasm separating Alexandrian Greeks and their minions from the general population of Egypt, for Egyptians considered Alexandria a Greek, not Egyptian, city. The population of freemen in Alexandria in Hellenistic times is thought to have been as low as 75,000, rising, according to Diodorus Siculus, to 300,000 under Roman hegemony. But for whatever reason, the great intellectual metropolis of the Hellenistic era and subsequently the city second only to Rome in importance within the Roman Empire would hold a distant second place in the history of medicine when compared to the little island of Cos. Despite their brilliance, apparently the scientific researches of Alexandrian physicians were little known, little appreciated, or viewed as of little importance when compared to the clinical acumen of Coan clinicians, a marked contrast with the modern perspective of the medical profession in which scientific discoveries, often prematurely optimistic, are front-page news and the everyday practitioner is considered a person who has settled for a humdrum career, a substantial inversion of reality.

In summary, the emigration of medicine from Greece to Alexandria was by individual physicians, not the koinon. Thus, the Coan network for clinical data collection, once disrupted, remained so, and the flow of ageless clinical Hippocratic commentary ceased. Some historians, including Dr. J. H. Baas, date the decline of Hippocratic medicine with the death of Hippocrates, although others cite the passing of the first prominent Alexandrian physicians, Herophilus and Erasistratus (280 BC and 250 BC, respectively).

End of excursus

---

4. Roman intellectual intransigence

Perhaps the Romans thought that scientific curiosity and hypotheses, often an outgrowth of a search without a practical goal, was an impractical mechanism for enrichment. But the Roman public into the 1st C AD admired Greek medicine, as noted by Pliny.[9] Public libraries were founded under Augustus, and teachers were patronized by the great and the wealthy. Alexandria saw a great economic and intellectual revival during the reigns of the early Roman Emperors. Hadrian (ruled 117-138 AD) founded an imperial system of education. Cities were required to maintain a certain number of physicians, grammarians, and "sophists" (who taught philosophy, rhetoric, and civic virtues). Hadrian also fostered a renaissance of learning in Athens that spread throughout

---

[8] Polybius, *Histories*, Frags. of Book XII, 25d.
[9] Pliny the Elder, *Natural History*, Bk. 29.

the Greek-speaking world, including the founding of the Athenaeum, a school of Hellenism, in Rome itself. The popularity of Athens would last for a century and, ironically, would be avidly sought by early Christian leaders in preference to established Rabbinical schools of the Near East, a change guaranteeing that studies of physics, geometry, and other sciences would survive in the Greek-speaking East, if not in the Latin-speaking West. Greek learning was also honored by Marcus Aurelius (121-180 AD) with university endowments to Athens. Aurelius, author of the famed *Meditations*, Galen, his contemporary, Ptolemy, famed mathematician and astronomer (87-150 AD), and Diodorus Siculus, the historian from Sicily, wrote their works only in Greek, and there were no contemporary translations into Latin, and commerce outside of Italy was also carried out in Greek. Even masses of the Catholic Church were not in Latin until later in the 4th C. Finally, while some Romans resented medicine of the foreigner, "medical schools" were proliferating around the Empire, including those of Pergamon, Smyrna, Laodiceia, and Ephesus, although just how these so-called schools functioned is uncertain.[10] Over several centuries, therefore, there may have been Roman intransigence to Greek culture, but not to Greek knowledge or language.

5. "Narrowness" of Roman vision

It is remarkable that, given the propensity of great civilizations to incorporate new and useful ideas encountered through either mercantile or mercenary expansion, Rome failed to incorporate an effective and esteemed profession already in existence within its new borders. Lord Macaulay[11] wrote that the Romans admired only themselves and the Greeks, and that "narrowness and sameness of thought" was likely to lead to a "tottering, driveling, paralytic longevity" but for the fortunate eruption onto the scene of a barbarian invasion and Christianity that would invigorate it. Roman leadership had been from the very beginning oligarchic, despite the great pride shown for its Senate. [12] If "narrowness and sameness of thought" characterized its authoritarian leadership, its goals might have been similarly tightly focused, and it has been stated that the Roman Empire represented the mastery of the State, Greece the mastery of the individual.

But Romans wished for their society to shine throughout history, and, like the Greeks before them, wealthy citizens raised monuments to the glory of Rome and to themselves. Boyd notes that when, in the 1st C BC, Roman education under Quintilian recognized Latin literature, that system, while remaining Greek in form, finally became

---

[10] For example, here is Strabo (63 BC – 24 AD): "Between Laodiceia and Carura is a temple of Men Carus, as it is called, which is held in remarkable veneration. In my own time a great Herophilian school of Medicine has been established by Zeuxis, and afterwards carried on by Alexander Philalethes, just as in the time of our fathers the Erasistrateian school in Smyrna was established by Hicesius, although at the present time the case is not at all the same as it used to be." Bk. 12. 8. 20, translation of W. Falconer in *The Geography of Strabo*, London, 1892. The term διδασκαλεῖον (didaskaleion) is used, which does indeed imply a "school." But von Staden notes that, except for Strabo's comment and for two coins showing Zeuxis' name, "We are therefore left with one laconic geographer and two four-word bronze coins as our only sources for Zeuxis the Herophilean." (von Staden, H., *Herophilus: The Art of Medicine in Early Alexandria*, Cambridge, 1989, p. 531.)

[11] Lord Macaulay's essay, *History*, published in 1828.

[12] Mommsen, T. *The History of Rome*, New York, 1895, translation of W. P. Dickson, vol. 3 (of 5), p. 16-17. A recent justification of Mommsen's opinion is presented by Ward, A. M., *How Democratic was the Roman Republic?*, in *New Engl. Classical J.*, 31.2:101-119, 2004.

Roman in content. [13]   There were Roman innovations in education, including a School of Law.   In Republican Rome books and libraries had been found only among private citizens, but under the Empire public libraries were endowed, greatly favoring the book trade and attracting authors to Rome, which began to rival Alexandria as a literary center.[14]   Roman poets and historians assumed places of honor in Roman society along-side Greek ones.   Roman architecture assumed eloquent forms rather than massive ones. Schools of philosophy were supported.   All these points and more do not suggest a "sameness of thought" or restricted vision as to the future of Rome.

Even the healing arts had not been ignored in the seat of the empire.   Early on there had been the *Lex Aquilia* (287 BC), "private" laws which provided for compensation for injuries to property, including the consequences of negligence by physicians when treating slaves by either surgery or the prescribing of medicines.   Later came *Lex Cornelia* (82 BC) which provided punishment for making, selling, and using poisonous drugs. Julius Caesar (100-44 BC) admitted Greek medical practitioners to Roman citizenship, a rise in status that further stimulated their immigration and thereby may have rendered doubtful any attempt by Romans to develop an indigenous medical profession.   Augustus Caesar gave all physicians who served in the military the rank of "Knight," making them all citizens, and relieved them of paying taxes.   Hadrian (76-138 AD) released physicians from jury duty and military service.[15]   There was also the occasional constitutional approval for guilds and colleges such as the *Scholae Medicorum*.   Antonine Pius (86-161 AD) mandated a specified number of salaried physicians in eastern cities of the Empire, and the institution of the *Archiatri*, or "chief physicians," was put in place, a system that specified those physicians hired by the State or local government to attend agencies of the emperor, municipalities, and the poor.[16]   Severus Alexander (reigned 222-235 AD) issued laws regulating training and certification of physicians, the *medicus a republica probatus* ("certified state physician.")   Emperor Valentinian in 368 AD created a College of Physicians for Rome, although it comprised only fourteen physicians.   The *Codex Theodosianus* of 439 AD regulated first Eastern, then Western physicians of the Empire.[17] Finally, the *Codex Justinian* of 528 AD (especially Codex X, 53, 1-6) had extensive references to physicians.   Medical practitioners of all sorts did not, as a class, suffer from Roman "narrowness,"

6. Insufficiency of the Latin language

There is, of course, the nature of the language itself, for von Ranke viewed the Greek language as "the most elaborate and best fitted to express in adequate terms the natural logic of the human mind."   If true, Latin was at an immediate disadvantage.   But

---

[13] Boyd, Wm., *The History of Western Education*, London, 1966, 8th edition, chapter 2, The Disperson of Greek Education, p. 61.

[14] L. Casson, *Libraries in the Ancient World*, New Haven, 2001, chapter 6.

[15] Cited from Modestinus (*fl.* 250 AD) in the *Digesta*, XXVII.1.6.1-8 of the *Justinian Code*.

[16] J. H. Baas, in *Outlines of the History of Medicine and the Medical Profession* (New York, 1889, H. E. Handerson, translator), mentions that all appointed Roman physicians (those named to positions within the Imperial court system and the municipalities) were comprised within the *Collegium Archiatrorum*, which functioned as a state guild. Replacing a deceased Archiatrix under the Justinian Code required the approval seven guild members.

[17] Promulgated under Theodosius II (401-450 AD), this Code also outlawed infanticide, proscribed the bloody entertainment of the gladiators, closed pagan temples, and made Christianity the religion of the Empire.

Greek had become the language of the Roman intellectual, even at times being mandated in the education of the upper classes. The subjugation of Greece in 146 BC facilitated the spread of Greek into Rome, not Latin into Greece, and not only the Greek language, but also Greek authors. And in the early centuries of the new millennium Greek prevailed over Latin in the Eastern part of the Empire. It is noteworthy, therefore, that the attrition of Hippocratic medicine occurred while the Greek language was widely popular.

7. The new religion, Christianity

Temkin concluded that the techniques, the science, and the ethics of medicine not only were maintained throughout Hellenistic times in Alexandria, but persisted well into the Christian era.[18]

8. Arrival of the Barbarians

Then came the barbarians, both from the fringes of the Empire and within the walls of Rome. This resulted in stewardship of the West passing into the hands of a culture unfamiliar with learning and science, as is proved by the fact of the Dark Ages, a time of ignorance that could only represent a legacy of ignorant forebears. But the *desire* to learn did not regress. By the time the Visigoths under Alaric arrived in Rome they had already been influenced by Greco-Roman learning and tradition.[19] Learning may not have been held in high esteem, but that does not mean it was held in low esteem. There merely may have been a shuffling of priorities, with learning relegated, temporarily, to the background. For the "barbarians" were admirers of the Empire and sought to partake of its culture. A letter of Bishop Sidonius (430-489 AD) to a friend stated: "...because the imperial ranks and offices now have been swept away, through which it was possible to distinguish each best man from the worst, from now on to know literature will be the only indication of nobility."[20] Learning was actively pursued, and literary achievements were prized.[21] There is little reason to think that the new rulers of the Empire, having assimilated so much else, would selectively disavow medicine, especially as they had nothing to put in its place.

9. Internecine competition

---

[18] This is the overall message of the book by Owsei Temkin, *Hippocrates in a World of Pagans and Christians*, Baltimore, 1991.

[19] Alaric I, who under Roman rule had been a commander of *foederati* (troops from peripheral realms under Roman leadership), attempted to "Romanize" aspects of Visigoth culture even before he sacked Rome in 410 AD. It also is felt that the destruction of Rome's buildings, monuments, and especially the churches (the Visigoths were considered Arian Christians), and the savaging of its citizens was restrained, although it was nonetheless savage. Subsequent near-contemporary writings of Sidonius (430-489 AD), Bishop of Auvergne, reveal that even in the face of a "wreck of Roman power" there remained an intellectually flourishing Gaul supporting many authors and scribes, with many country estates containing fine libraries.

[20] *The Letters of Sidonius*, Oxford, 1915, translation of O. M. Dalton, vol. 2, Book VIII, Letter 2, p. 139.

[21] Dales, R. C., *The Intellectual Life of Western Europe in the Middle Ages*, Washington, D.C., 1980, especially chapter 3. "Barbarians" and Christians in turn attempted, in the midst of social chaos, to retain and even to build on the Roman intellectual literary base, even as the Greek language was disappearing from the West. The result, however, was a qualitative decline in learning.

The competition included dream-interpreters, old women (*graes*), oculists, aurists, surgeons, dentists, astrologers, aroma therapists, uroscopists, phlebotomists, specialists in catheterizing and the giving of enemas, herb-doctors, milk-doctors, gynecologists, movement-curers, venereal disease specialists, specialists in fistulae, cosmeticians, hair-doctors, wine-doctors, and hernia-doctors. Orosius (4th C AD historian and priest) noted that at the time of Caesar Augustus the physicians were but slaves.[22] Galen himself made the comment that "There is no distinction between robbers and physicians, except that the former commit their misdeeds in the mountains, the latter in Rome."[23] The definition of "physician" among the general population of ancient Rome was much like the droll modern definition of "art": "something sold in an art shop."[24]

There may have been intrinsic competition as well, either between practitioners themselves or among the different schools of medical thought that arose from time to time. The Methodists, the Dogmatists, and the Empiricists were some of those "schools," and, while it may seem that they represented new ideas or trends in medicine, it is more likely that they resulted from lack of professional cohesion.[25] And a traveling physician from India, home to many centuries-old centralized guilds of medical professionals, might have viewed Roman medicine as quite consistent with rumored European populations that, in battle, painted themselves blue and charged stark naked at the enemy, a chaotic system with every man for himself.

But Hippocratic medicine had always competed with other medical practices in

---

[22] He comments: "And therefore in the forty-eighth year of Caesar Augustus so fearsome was the famine in Rome that he proceeded to drive out from the city the mercenaries used for the public games, all aliens, and a great many slaves, doctors and teachers excepted." - Orosius, *Historiae Adversum Paganos*, 7.3.6, translation by the author. The Latin is: "itaque anno imperii Caesaris quadragesimo octauo adeo dira Romanos fames consecuta est, ut Caesar lanistarum familias omnesque peregrinos, seruorum quoque maximas copias, exceptis medicis et praeceptoribus, trudi urbe praeceperit.

[23] Cited by Baas in his *Outlines of the History of Medicine,* p. 150. The author has unsuccessfully sought the original citation.

[24] Legal definitions of medical practitioners were equally vague. See: Nutton, V., *Murders and Miracles: Lay attitudes towards medicine in classical antiquity*, in: *From Democedes to Harvey: Studies in the History of Medicine*, London, 1988, pp. 23-53.

[25] Celsus defined some of the schools as follows (from the Prooemium to *On Medicine*, translated by W. G. Spencer, from the *Loeb Classical Library* series on Celsus):

1. Dogmatists: These were practitioners "endeavouring to go more deeply into things, claimed for themselves also a knowledge of nature, without which it seemed that the Art of Medicine would be stunted and weak." They "profess a reasoned theory of medicine,.....a knowledge of hidden causes involving diseases..." They valued the study of anatomy, and considered Hippocrates as the initiator of their sect.

2. Empirics: "... those who are called 'Empirici' because they have experience, do indeed accept evident causes as necessary; but they contend that inquiry about obscure causes and natural actions is superfluous, because nature is not to be comprehended." Anatomical study was considered by them as futile.

3. Methodists: They "maintain that medicine should examine those characteristics which diseases have in common. .... they are unwilling that the Art [of medicine] should consist in conjecture about hidden things, and ... they think that in the observation of experience there is little of an Art of Medicine."

4. Pneumatists considered diseases an alteration of πνεῦμα, which was inspired and incorporated throughout body systems. There were also the Eclectics, a syncretic school of medical thought that selected preferred medical opinions from the various philosophical perspectives.

the marketplace. There was no organized activity among them that might have been considered purposefully fractious. The unpredictable nature of illness or consequences of treatment have always lent a helping hand to the physician's competitors. It was amidst this array of competing practitioners and quacks that rational medicine, and then scientific medicine, arose in the first place.

After all, the eternal attraction of quackery is based on the gullibility of an individual, especially for his own hypothesis, which in turn finds its basis in fear of the unknown and the hope that one's personal search will reveal "something out there that we do not understand" that will "beat the system."[26] It is normal and as old as mankind.[27]

Excursus on Charlatanism and the "K'ang Yu-Wei Syndrome"

Definition: charlatan – a pretender to medical knowledge.
Webster's Seventh New Collegiate Dictionary

There is the desire in each person to have control over his own health and fate. Rather than admit a personal inadequacy in knowledge or method, the preference is to manage a health problem in one's own way, to devise a logic that explains one's choice, especially if in doing so it can help avoid the inconvenience, discomfort, embarrassment, and expense of a visit to the physician. There is nothing abnormal in this. What is undesirable is the person who promises the easy but untested cure to others; that is the problem, that is the charlatan. The displacement, by easy acceptance of fanciful personal theories, of true knowledge acquired by a profession based on centuries of careful observation can, of course, be a sign of intellectual confusion. But the charlatan may offer a remedy or restorative consistent with one's own hypothesis or one that has some particularly attractive feature, and an illness or event may appear to respond favorably. The consequences of a particular medical treatment are far from being invariably predictable: the course chosen may be wrong, but, because of unknowable or unforeseeable events, the outcome may be good; alternatively, the course chosen may be right, but, for similar reasons, the outcome may be bad. The first assures the success of the charlatan and the

---

[26] See the letter of M. J Sergeant, M. D. in *Ann. Intern. Med.*, 132:675, 2000. Also see F. H. Garrison's *On Quackery as a Reversion to Primitive Medicine,* in *Bull. N. Y. Acad. Med.* IX, 601-612, 1933: "The success of the quack is due, then to the suggestibility of his victims (pithiatism), to the *mundus vult decipi* ('The public likes to be humbugged'), to a primitive craving for the supernatural which is ever latent in man; and here folk-medicine and quackery are at one. '*To folk-medicine,*' as Allbutt stated in *Greek Medicine in Rome* (London, 1921, p. 21), '*doubt is unknown; it brings the peace of security.*' [Italics added]. Rationalism abides on lonely heights, "where those who have scaled them live alone"; but the mental processes and self-deceptions of average humanity are irrational and therefore unpredictable. But let us bear in mind the perpetrator as well as the victim. Swindling, whether in medicine, finance or other business, will always be with us, keeping with Schiller's dictum that the gods themselves can do nothing for stupidity. The Hippocratics recognized the debt of the quack to luck, time, and the wealth and ignorance of his patients. See παραγγελιαι, or *Precepts*, vii, a Hippocratic work.

[27] See for example Lucian's *Lie-Fancier* (p. 87, v.1, of *Lucian of Samosata*, as translated by W. Tooke, 2 vols., London, 1820) which reveals similarities between his time and the present day regarding religious mysticism, ghosts, magnetizers, and magic, except that Lucian even poses a bronze statue of Hippocrates as a god requiring sacrifices.

second is the plague of the physician.[28] The two taken together will, in the minds of the ignorant, the impressionable, and the wishful thinkers, blur the distinction between physician and charlatan. And the scaffolding for all this is twofold. First, most acute illnesses comprise self-limited episodes and therefore have been a fine source of reputation and income for both physicians and quacks throughout the ages. Francis Bacon (1561-1626) in his 1605 publication *The Advancement of Learning* put it well: " …the physician…hath no particular acts demonstrative of his ability, but is judged most by the event, which is ever but as it is taken: for who can tell, if a patient die or recover,…whether it be art or accident? And therefore many times the impostor is prized, and man of virtue taxed. Nay, we see weakness and credullity of men is such, as they will often prefer a mountebank or witch before a learned physician."[29] And "For in all times, in the opinion of the multitude, witches and old women and impostors, have had a competition with physicians." The Hippocratics were well aware of the role of nonserious disease in the promotion of the charlatan:

> "There are many bad health care providers that treat patients having no serious problem and from which the greatest of errors present no dangers – many are such diseases and they occur more frequently than the serious [diseases] – and in these instances any errors in treatment are not apparent to the layman."   *Ancient Medicine* IX

The modern physician also is well aware of this aspect of self-limited disease, as Dr. H. L. Trott wryly noted in his captivating autobiography: "I have enjoyed much credit in treating maladies relieved by time."[30] But not all blame should be directed at the charlatan, for there is the second prop, the K'ang Yu-Wei syndrome. K'ang Yu-Wei (1858-1927), a philosopher and self-styled sage admired by Mao Zedong, recognized the great benefits of modern technology and modern medicine, even expressing concern that its practitioners could become a political force. His one-world philosophy therefore proscribed political organizations. As for the medical practitioner, "The physicians will be awarded decorations by the government for their accomplishments.... Physicians who by making mistakes are responsible for the death of a patient will be severely punished: they will be deprived of their right to practise, disgraced, and possibly imprisoned for a time," reminiscent of the days of Hammurabi's version of *Lex Talionis*, surely one reason for the lack of progress of the medical profession in authoritarian hands. K'ang was profoundly ignorant of even the most elementary aspects of human responses to disease. It was K'ang's fantasy that daily examinations by a "physician" would be able to prevent not just a disease, but all disease. This extraordinary testimonial merits inspection. Even though he was an outspoken proponent of technology, he had bizarre expectations for a profession that in his time and place had no diagnostic tools and few effective therapies. It must be assumed, given the high regard and critical acclaim accorded him by many, including the Chairman of the Chinese Communist Party, Mao Zedong, that K'ang did

---

[28] This plague affects not just the physician; it is universal, as Solon wrote: "...and none knoweth, at its begining, which way an undertaking will turn. One man, though he is trying to acquit himself well, falleth unaware into great and dire misfortune. Another, who playeth his part ill, is blessed with good luck by the gods and granted release from his folly." Stobaeus *Eclogae* iii 9 (περὶ διαιοσύνης), 23: Σόλωνος. Translation of I. M. Linforth in: *Solon the Athenian*, Berkeley, 1919, p. 167.

[29] Translation of B. Montagu as published in the first complete American edition of Bacon's works, Philadelphia, 1842, p. 202.

[30] Trott, H. W., *Campus Shadows*, Hemlock, NY, 1946.

not suffer from some form of mental aberration and that he therefore had a rational basis for expecting a successful implementation of his extraordinary plan for physicians. In fact, K'ang had been duped by charlatans, namely his countrymen's physicians or those who spoke for physicians.[31]

For K'ang was susceptible to the charlatan's message. In the first place, living, as it might have seemed to him, a healthful life, he reasoned that if others would but do the same they would be as healthy as he. And thus we often advise others, based on the apparent success of our personal experience. Indeed, we may have even momentarily considered the idea that others should be required to live according to our apparently successful personal lifestyle. K'ang described his famous "One World" ideas when he was in his late twenties and healthy. If he could be healthy, so could anyone else. Who among us has not expressed to others some aspect of our daily regimen as a source of our wellbeing, some testimonial regarding our personal lifestyle choices about which we feel confident despite the fact that the statistical sample on which that confidence is based numbers only "one." This all ends, of course, when the inevitable serious illness strikes. Secondly, there was his ignorance of the issue at hand, in this instance, medicine. He was unfamiliar with the infinite number and manifestations of illnesses that affect humankind, and he had no conception of the pathobiology of disease. This is, to varying degrees, a universal phenomenon, for no one can comprehend the totality of medical knowledge, and even if he could much of that knowledge would soon be out-of-date or found to be patently incorrect. But, in general, the greater the degree of ignorance the greater the susceptibility to the charlatan's claim. As Prof. Philip Lindsley noted in 1829, an era rife with charlatanry, "Well informed men cannot be easily imposed on by any species of charlatanry...." Despite his many accomplishments, K'ang was utterly uninformed about medicine. He had somehow been persuaded that the medical profession in China at that time was remarkably effective. But this was not done by means of cure-all nostrums or snake-oil. Since there were few effective therapies in China in those years his view of the physician's effectiveness lay in disease prevention. K'ang was duped. He concluded that if the effectiveness of physicians lay in prevention rather than treatment, it is only logical that daily examinations would provide the best health care. The importance of prevention has a strong tradition in Chinese medicine despite a lack of scientific understanding of mechanisms of prevention. So strongly did he feel about his theories that he advised the leadership of a great nation of hundreds of millions on its implementation. Thus, the bigger problem is this: those who can be made to believe absurdities can also be made to commit atrocities.[32]

The collection of preconditions described above are the basis for what might be called the K'ang Yu-Wei syndrome. It is on display in the victims of charlatanism. The components of this syndrome are, to some degree, common to all, but when present in excess are the basis for the success of the medicine-man and the charlatan. They are, briefly, 1) ignorance of the subject at hand, 2) a desire for the simple solution, 3) undue confidence

---

[31] For details on K'ang's life, his political activism, and his ideal world see Thompson, L. G., *Ta T'ung Shu, The One-World Philosophy of K'ang Yu-Wei*, London, 1958.

[32] Voltaire (1694-1788): Certainement qui est en droit de vous rendre absurde est en droit de vous rendre injuste. ("It is certain that whoever can make you absurd can make you unjust.") From *Questions sur les Miracles* (1765). It is relevant to review Dr. Weissmann's statement in the final paragraphs of chapter 1 of the present volume.

in one's weakly founded personal theories, and 4) wishful thinking. The charlatan is the natural competitor of the physician, but the physician is the source of inspiration for the charlatan. The two will always reside together as long as there exists the K'ang Yu-Wei syndrome, *i.e.*, an ignorant population on which the charlatans can feed. The population that acclaimed K'ang Yu-Wei join him at the opposite end of the spectrum from the intelligent audience that acclaimed the genius of Aeschylus.

End of excursus

---

10. Inadequate supply of physicians

If the Mediterranean population of the Empire were twenty million, an annual output of perhaps a thousand physicians might have been adequate to further the progress of scientific medical practices. Furthermore, inland Roman provinces had their own culture with their own peculiar medical practices that the Romans would have felt no obligation to replace. A thousand physicians per year should have been a number easily attainable by the apprenticeship method if applied in a few of the great cities of the Empire. Therefore, the capacity for physician training would seem to have been sufficient to look after the health of the Empire.

To summarize this section, at some undetermined date the scientific medicine of Hippocrates began to disappear, perhaps as early as the 4th C BC. As the process unfolded there is no evidence of medical leadership that would have provided cohesion within an administrative structure, and cohesion provides stability. A foundering Greece was unable to provide that leadership and cohesion, and an ascendant Rome did not realize its necessity, apparently assuming an inexhaustible supply of medical resources lay in its conquered provinces.

B. There Was No Decline

The ultimate causes of failure of man's social adventures can be divided into those that derive from defeat, from transformation, or from indifference. In applying these to Hippocratic medicine, it is difficult to postulate a defeat for scientific medicine in the absence of a proclaimed adversary. Alternatives to scientific medicine such as fanciful biological speculation or attempts to manage one's health via the family garden hardly represented a frontal assault on established Hippocratic medicine. There were no legal or physical threats, no organizational menacing, from these perennial competitors. Hippocratic medicine was not proved wrong. It was not defeated.

The second possible cause, transformation, can be willful or imposed. John Dewey assessed the interrelation of philosophy, science and the arts. He held that the separation of knowledge from practice leads to "evils" in education and in other fields. He would say that mankind long ago discovered the arts, and that these were the isolated observations from which the Greeks developed science and thereby an understanding of causes.[33] The Hippocratics applied art and science into a philosophical unity, combined

---

[33] Dewey, J., *Philosophy and Civilization*, New York, 1931, pp. 299-301.

the "mind and body" of medicine. When Galen defined the position of the medical profession six hundred years later there clearly had been no significant change in its philosophy or content. The merits and indeed the very words and ideas of the Hippocratics are often repeated in the writings of Galen, just as they were by Celsus, Soranus, Aretaeus and other medical writers. And Galen's eminence in the generations that followed him was not so much due to the excellence of his personal effort as it was due to the fact that he was the last Hippocratic left standing.[34] It is necessary, therefore, to consider the third possible cause, indifference.

System errors can affect entire societies, and it has been suggested that Roman indifference to Greek medicine and science represented a lack of curiosity. Perhaps the Roman educational system was at fault. Natural curiosity has often been praised as the mark of a superior student and a deciding factor permitting success. But curiosity is primarily an organic function, based on an instinctive desire to inquire after the unexpected. When something happens time after time and then does not happen, the natural response is to explore this unusual event. How such a response might promote survival in a species is beyond the present subject, except to note that all animals exhibit curiosity about the new or unexpected, whatever sense is involved. But intellectual it is not, nor is it persistent.[35] If the unexpected event were to happen several more times, it would no longer incite curiosity. But success in life is not found in curiosity; it is found in motivation, the impetus to action, rather than merely reacting to the unexpected, the unusual, or the unexplained.

There simply was insufficient motivation in ancient Rome to take up a medical career. The desire for wealth is a powerful motivator. Expanding Roman domination vastly increased the flow of riches into the empire. Furthermore, expanding trade and commercial capitalism created additional wealth, and with an extensive and, for the most part, peaceable world surrounding the Mediterranean, opportunity for a better life abounded in the neighborhood of the great cities. As population, wealth, and travel increased, so did a desire for luxury. Where was a young man to go to get his share of the wealth? Not to medicine, surely. Remuneration was paltry except for those few physicians lucky enough to find a niche in society's higher echelon and clever enough to remain there. The early days of scientific medicine had no great attractions to those without great vision. The people saw no "magic bullets" such as antibiotics, no technical masterpieces like magnetic resonance imaging, no electronic monitoring. The scientific physician was in competition with the non-scientific, and the one's results were often not demonstrably superior to the other's. The public, ignorant of the reason for successes of scientific medicine, often chose its alternative. Solomon knew this phenomenon well: "If it befall to me as befalleth to the fools, why should I labour to be more wise?"[36] As

---

[34] This explains why Galen was so free with his criticism of medical practitioners. Perhaps he was unduly egotistical, but the dearth of *bona fide* Hippocratic physicians and the shortcomings of virtually all contemporary practitioners would have justified his exalted opinion of self-worth.

[35] Nevertheless, a "scientific" curiosity has been postulated, as "when the philosophic brain spots an inconsistency, or gap, in its knowledge." This is an individualistic response and an interesting and important subject. It includes, for example, curiosity and anxiety as antagonistic drives to motivation. A variety of such opinions are presented in: *Motivation: Theory and Research*, O'Neill, H., and Drillings, M., editors, New Jersey, 1994.

[36] This is Sir Francis Bacon's paraphrase of the following Greek of *Ecclesiastes* II, 15-16: "And I said in my heart, As the event of the fool is, so shall it be to me, even to me; and to what purpose have I gained wisdom? I said moreover in my heart, This is also vanity, because the fool speaks of his abundance. For there is no remembrance of the wise man with the fool for ever; forasmuch as

medicine in the Soviet Union would so perfectly demonstrate, the "labourers" understood Solomon's message far better than did their bureaucratic overlords (see footnote, p. 440).

Prof. Abraham Maslow[37] described five hierarchical levels of motivation, which may be defined as "the drive that produces goal-directed behavior."[38] Importantly, levels essential to survival should be fulfilled before proceeding to gratifying ones. They are:

Table 8:   Levels of Motivation (from Maslow, *op. cit.*)

Relative value	Hierarchy of motivation	Characteristic
ESSENTIAL	1. Biological drive	Averts imminent threats to survival
	2. Safety	Averts long-term threats to survival
INDULGENT	3. Belonging	Pleasure/benefits of association with a group or an individual
	4. Esteem	Individualistic
	5. Self-actualization (being all one can be)	Intrinsic and persisent

There are also modifiers of motivation, such as initiation, direction, and intensity. The teacher may spark an interest, direct it, and motivate the student to achieve a successful conclusion or seek improvement, whether the student is a child or a professional. But the levels of motivation effected by a teacher are refined ones. The more basic are instilled by nature, family, friends, and personal experience, and how those goals of motivation are achieved is less important than that they be achieved.

Money, for example, can represent economic "safety," the second most essential in the above list. Sufficient income might have been an absolute requirement for those who were not independently wealthy, its insufficiency a deterrent. Medicine offered no guarantee of sufficiency, so the choice lay elsewhere. But assuming quackery was no more remunerative than a Hippocratic practice, it would not explain the selective disappearance of the latter. As neither were high paying it is unlikely that aspirants were preferentially repelled by a Hippocratic practice because of insufficient compensation.

Moving down the scale, therefore, the young person seeking to affiance himself to a practitioner of Hippocratic medicine rather than an alternative practitioner may have been greatly affected by esteem. Esteem, an "indulgent" motivator, is motivational fine-tuning. The esteem attached to being a Hippocratic practitioner had, in earlier centuries, assured a source of motivated apprentices and respected public and private physicians.

The importance reputation is expressed at the end of the Hippocratic Oath:

> "Now if I carry out this oath, and break it not, may I gain for ever reputation among all men for my life and my art; but if I transgress it and forswear myself, may the opposite befall me."[39]

---

now in the coming days all things are forgotten: and how shall the wise man die with the fool?" The translations of all Old Testament passages are from the diglot Septuagint version as published by S. Bagster and Sons, Ltd., London, *ca.* 1884.

[37] Maslow, A. H., *Motivation and Personality*, 2nd edition, New York, 1970.

[38] *Encyclopedia of Psychology*, R. J. Corsini, editor, New York, 1984, 4 vols., see "motivation."

[39] The *Oath*, lines 31-36, from *Hippocrates*, *Loeb Classical Library*, vol. 1, translation of W. H. S. Jones.

A favorable social valuation, esteem, depends in part on a professional's ability to do something better than others. Going to a physician for an illness is seeking a better way of managing that illness than one is likely to do for oneself. If a physician is the only option the choice is relatively easy. But if there are multiple options the lay person has a more difficult decision. Affordability, palatability, and accessibility are but a few of the considerations now before him. And, most important, the more limited his education and his knowledge of science and the scientific method the less likely it will be that he will distinguish among a list of alternatives those practitioners who are the most qualified.

If a small vial containing a tiny amount of the radioactive element ^{241}Am (Americium; this isotope is used in smoke detectors) drops by accident from a delivery van onto a street and someone sees the HAZMAT sign and yells "Watch out, it's radioactive!," all in the immediate area will instantly distance themselves and seek help from any source.[40] If a knowledgeable person examines the vial and says "It is but a miniscule dose of an alpha emitter, so do not worry, for it is virtually harmless as it is," the uninformed will still not approach, for everyone knows from the cinema and popular media how insidious and exceedingly dangerous radiation is, and, after all, why did the knowledgeable person say "*virtually* harmless"? Some may then feel they could have received a dangerous dose of radiation and seek an opinion. The expert would say there was virtually nil exposure and nothing whatever to worry about, whereas another who considers himself expert will say that even if the "exposed" person feels fine he may have suffered unseen genetic damage that could affect his future children, or that he has possibly suffered damage to his immune system that could increase his chance of cancer. To the uninformed both persons claim or seem to be expert, so which should he believe? Since he can not be certain, the uninformed person makes the assumption that they each have an equal chance of being correct, and therefore his perceived chance of getting the best advice is "50-50." The newspaper reporter, who shares his ignorance, will try to be "fair" and will also equate the two opinions in his reporting of the event on page one, thereby compounding the problem by disseminating his own ignorance to tens or hundreds of thousands. All this will happen despite the fact that one of the "experts" is a radiation physicist having several university degrees to support his claim of being an expert in handling radioactive material, and the other, who has carefully read the relevant section in an encyclopedia, has talked to friends about the problem. The former is almost certainly correct, the latter almost certainly incorrect. But a friend of the latter happens to be an attorney, and matters now become more complex as the layman, for whatever reason, chooses the attorney to advise him. In the public's eye decisions on matters of which they are ignorant become a throw of the dice. In an uneducated society that seeks certainty this is the daily fodder of the media, whether the Grey Lady or Hollywood. What, then, is the benefit of being a professional if only those who graduated with degrees in radiation physics agree with you? There is little esteem there. Better to be an attorney for the radiation-exposed. At least there you are appreciated by your client, who, by the way, will have a personal interest in your being adequately compensated for your time.

Thus, society plays an enormous non-legislative role in shaping the functioning of its components, including the motivation of groups or individuals. A free society permits the expression of individual genius, and on page 451 Newton and Locke are identified as inherent expressions of a free society. But there is this other factor: society's competence in either recognizing the genius of a Newton or, among those unversed in the

---

[40] An episode with similarities to the triggering of this fictional event shut down a circumscribed area near the Boston neighborhood of Jamaica Plain in the 1980s.

calculus, valuing the reasoning of those that do. As Plato noted, "Do you not know that the measure of the speech is with the listener, not with the speaker?"[41] The reclusive Newton was free, therefore, both to pursue his studies and to have his work judged by others held in esteem by society, namely, the Royal Society. Conversely, society's limitations, whether in education or fealty, limit its components.[42] Another limitation is institutional veracity, and scientific malefaction, as a consequence of either outright fraud or as a justification for a particular societal objective, can be a source of appalling societal harm.

Also needed was the esteem generated by a collegial network, a koinon, a group of clinicians that could analyze collected clinical observations and thereby improve an individual physician's ability in prognosis.[43] For example, had such a clinical network existed in ancient Egypt and had it observed pipestem cirrhosis, ascites, and blood in the urine to be far more common in persons tending fields irrigated by canals and ponds extending from the Nile than in those with non-agricultural employments or from other regions of Egypt, a feature of environment might have been implicated, a corrective applied, and some measure of control over the disease of schistosomiasis put in place. No microscopes and no laboratory tests would have been necessary for such epidemiological discoveries, for Hippocratic physicians often made note of occupation or location of residence of their patients. But the integration of useful clinical information had ceased, because, alas, it was no longer being collected. There was no Alexandrian koinon (see excursus, p. 274). Indeed, von Staden states that there were no records of the actual general practitioners in Egypt or Alexandria during the Alexandrian years.[44] Whether Hippocratic medicine's decline began in the 4th C BC or the 3rd, the absence of the koinon

---

[41] Stobaeus *Florilegium*, III, 79e, translation of T. B. Harbottle, *Dictionary of Quotations (Classical)*, London, 1902.

[42] Here there is a political corollary to the medical quandry: the survival of a free state, just as with scientific medicine, is not guaranteed by democratic institutions alone; it requires a body politic able to formulate optimal democratically-arrived-at decisions. That body must be both educated and dedicated. Pliny the Younger realized that in a democracy equality is a different matter than equity. He also knew that democracies were courting disaster "...so long as men have the same right to judge, but not the same ability to judge wisely." (*Letters and Panegyricus*, Pliny the Younger, Bk. II, 12, translation of B. Radice in the *Loeb Classical Library* series on Pliny.) A great attribute of a democracy lies in the ability of its people, after deliberation, to choose the likely best course, but, in voluntarily agreeing to pursue it unanimously, the "likely" can often be made a "certainty." *Constancy* in society's attachment to the tenets of democracy is essential because in contentious decisions arrived at by democratic process the losing side must voluntarily support the winning side in implementing that decision. If this does not happen there is chaos, the losing faction risking being accused of undermining the democratic process, a potentially treasonous action. A democracy steered by emotions and ignorance is doomed; universal suffrage becomes a joke as the incompetent become putty in the hands of the rhetorician. All this being said, matters are worse in authoritarian society where an otherwise intelligent and educated public can, in important matters, be maintained in utter ignorance, the illusional world of propaganda.

[43] For medicine to advance there must be an amalgamation of scientific analysis and clinical observation. This was true for the Hippocratics and, as Dr. William Castle taught, remains true for modern medicine. One cannot supplant the other, for individually one is a pot-pouri of theories and curious findings without relevance and the other is a menagerie of observations without cognition. The early Alexandrians were close: Erasistratus associated fibrotic liver disease (now identified as cirrhosis) with ascites, but it was never discerned as a complication of what is now called schistosomiasis, common in the Nile river valley.

[44] Von Staden, H., *Herophilus: The Art of Medicine in Early Alexandria*, Cambridge, 1989, p. 23.

can be offered as a valid reason for the wanting of a clinical reputation of Alexandrian physicians.

The crux of the matter is this: Rome, although relying on health care providers from Greece and elsewhere, excluded Greek medical organizations from a population that had little prejudice against them. Despite occasional gratuitous acknowledgements of guilds, the central government inadvertently fostered a state of perpetual medical ignorance. The problem had not been regulation of the individual. It was, instead, regulation, in this case prohibition, of the organization. It was the arbitrary proscription of guilds in general and Greek organizations in particular. No infringement was made on individual transfer of trade or professional wisdom. Eusebius (263-339 AD) records that even at the close of the 2nd C Galen was of sufficient reputation that an early churchman could write about those "atheists" who preferred the sciences, including medical science, to study of the Holy Scriptures:

> "Some of them are smitten by the measurements of the earth by Euclid, others revere Aristotle and Theophrastus, and similarly some of them virtually prostrate themselves before Galen."[45]

Admirers and compilers of medical writings were not seditious. But group dynamics were unable to freely come to bear on trades and professions. This was the opening gambit in a process that would see subsequent generations of Roman workers increasingly become State chattel and contribute to the mighty Empire's fall. The immediate consequence to medicine, however, was the inability to assemble a "common council," or koinon, whether or not the Romans could grasp its nature and significance, and they probably could not. The individual physician may have been relatively unhindered and a senior physician might have a train of apprentices following him on rounds as Martial (40-102 AD) satirically describes, but the advantage of many interacting minds freely motivated and applied to common problems was lost.

There is a final Roman dousing of the flame of Hippocratic medicine. The early Greek guilds for artisans were small affairs, for cities were small, and therefore inhabitants did not support or need large numbers of professionals in any one area. But, as time passed, guilds grew in number and variety, and their membership increased as cities enlarged. In some trades an increase in population is a mighty spur to entrepreneurship, and a guild dealing with exportable goods could expand its influence beyond city or regional boundaries.[46] But for other trades, such as bakers and butchers, their area of influence was necessarily local. The physician, of course, performed his duties locally. No economic benefit was to be derived from intercity expansion of a guild from which no portable product was produced. Thus, the final blow was demographic. Greek culture was quantitatively overwhelmed when the population of the Greek Mediterranean empire, estimated at seven to nine millions, was incorporated into a Roman Empire estimated to contain as many as one hundred millions, with Italy itself containing

---

[45] *Eusebeii Caesariensis Opera*, Leipzig, 1890. *Historiae Ecclesiasticae* V, 28, 14. Euclid, Aristotle, and Threophrastus (Aristotle's successor) lived in the 4th C BC, Galen in the 2nd C AD.

[46] In medieval times there were occasionally violent efforts to resist the tendency for the heads of some city guilds to become, in effect, capitalists managing a trade's production and profiting from external sales of a particular product. Karl Marx, in chapter 1 of his *Communist Manifesto*, calls guilds "Die bisherige feudale oder zunftige Betriebsweise der Industrie..." ("The earlier feudal system of industry...")

fifteen to twenty millions.[47] The tenfold increase in population controlled by the Romans would diminish that which had been distinctive within the smaller Greek society. Who of Rome's one hundred millions knew anything of Hippocrates?

C. Conclusion

In setting and enforcing standards for the profession, a professional organization provides a mechanism by which public esteem and confidence can be maintained. Consulting a physician is then preferred to the unknown dangers of self-treatment or alternative practitioners. The situation is analogous to the baseball umpire. His is not a "team" effort. He stakes his reputation on his competence. Should he have a personal interest in the game's outcome, his decisions may be swayed by that interest. The fans would be much more rebellious over marginal calls were there no Professional Baseball Umpires Corporation that vetted its members and their training, thereby providing a bulwark against the deceitful referee and the unfair critic. It oversees quality by being selective in membership, responding to criticism, and maintaining standards.

And so, with no physician's association to attract membership and to maintain professional reputation, the Hippocratics became numerically depleted; it did not waste away, it did not "decline." Its demotion was relative and quantitative, not qualitative. The natural state of medical practice is not a willy-nilly affair, a notion that can be adapted to just any setting. First, like democracy, it must be chosen, not imposed. Second, it must be responsive, not authoritarian. Third, it must be sustained by an organization that is, and is perceived as, the source of the best medical care. Fourth, as it is a social endeavor, society must be capable of knowing the difference. Greeks did; Romans did not.

Esteem and pride are to individualism what gratitude is to collectivism. Which is the more motivating factor? It has been duly noted that "Gratitude is merely the lively expectation of favours yet to come."[48] With no organizational base to instill and maintain professional pride, Rome failed to provide an environment that would motivate new practitioners to enter into rigorous and modestly paid careers in helping the sick. Competitors stepped in to provide care that was often easier, cheaper, more convenient, and more satisfactory to the psyche than going to a physician.

The possible contributors to the loss of the Hippocratic clinician were many. But Hippocratic training became sought by so few among a population become so vast that no replenishing of the lists of scientific physicians was possible. Romans indeed settled for little. The march of history, which can be so exciting in its retrospective, can seem, from the perspective of a point in time, almost monotonous. No one can date the end of Hippocratic medicine, although it was for the most part complete by the time of Christ. This culmination, one of the greatest calamities of history, was unassociated with violent cataclysm and it was therefore not memorable. What was the cause? It was loss of the apparatus for common council, for an earlier Pan-Hellenic medical organization, a koinon [purportedly] located on the little island of Cos, had shown what was possible. The doleful consequences will now be exposed.

---

[47] See: *The Cambridge History of the Greco-Roman World*, Cambridge, 2007, Scheidel, W., Morris, I., and Saller, R., editors, for the basis of these estimates and the factors affecting ancient population density.

[48] A translation of Francois de la Rochefoucauld's Maxim 298: "La reconnaissance de la plupart des hommes n'est qu'une secrete envie de recevoir de plus grands bienfaits."

CHAPTER EIGHTEEN

THE PROFOUND DARKNESS OF THE DARK AGES

"My opinion is that leaders led the people into the dark ages, and that the people finally had to lead themselves out, after much unnecessary suffering and trouble."

> Ed Howe, in the Dayton, Iowa, *Review*
> Feb. 2, 1933

Absent the rediscovery of classic authors there is little to recommend the Dark Ages (400-1000 AD) and High Medieval period (1000-1300 AD), at least in the field of medicine. This is vividly shown by a timeline of medical discovery covering the period from the age of Hippocrates through the Renaissance. It was in the Renaissance that there was a burst of individualism as select individuals, invariably under the sponsorship of patrons, offered a glimpse of the potential for genius that lay concealed for 1500 years. This chapter focuses on the dearth of medical discovery of the Dark Ages and the Medieval period, and the following chapter explains it.

A. An Age Well-Named

The Dark Ages (*ca.* 400-1000 AD) and High Medieval period (1000-1300 AD) are increasingly portrayed not as a time of abysmal ignorance, misery, and poverty but as a time of progress, slow perhaps but progress nonetheless, evidence being the occasional insight, invention, or discovery in a wide range of human endeavors that preceded the Renaissance.[1] It is undeniable that political structures that would support the Renaissance were taking shape, such as the 11th C Italian communes that would lead ultimately to independent city-states and the monopolistic guilds that presaged great universities.[2] But long before the Medici came to power the philosopher and revolutionary Abelard (1079-1142) and the poet Petrarch (1304-1374) had in their hands manuscripts of the ancients, or copies thereof, an indication that not all of past learning had been lost, or that some that had been lost was being sporadically reclaimed. And the oldest Hippocratic writings available to us have been dated to the 9th C *Vindobonensis med. IV* manuscript presently residing Vienna. In consequence, many ideas attributed to intellectuals in the Dark Ages represented reflected glory of the Ancients, not the spontaneous generation of new ideas.

---

[1] See, for example, Landes, David, *The Wealth and Poverty of Nations*, Norton & Co., 1998, p. 29, where he contends the Middle Ages represented "one of the most inventive societies that history had known," citing a number of key inventions. There are, of course, others who favorably view medieval society as locally self-sustaining, free from nationalism and national boundaries, under careful religious tutelage, protected from wayward thought, and focused on spiritual aspects of life and beyond, an approximation of ideal society.

[2] Some European universities can trace their origins to monastic schools. See: Riche, P., and Contreni, J., *Education and Culture in the Barbarian West: From the Sixth through the Eighth Century*, Columbia (SC), 1976, translation of 3rd edition, but guild connotation, via designations such as *universitas magistorum,* were assigned to them in later centuries, or at their founding, as shown by the University of Glasgow, designated as a guild of scholars (*universitas scholarium*) by Pope Nicholas V in 1451. The status of "guild" or "corporate cartel" for the university is still debated; see: *Perspective – Disrupting Education*, in *The Freeman* issue of Feb. 27, 2013.

Attempts to portray the Dark Ages and Medieval Period as times of medical progress will also not succeed. There were occasional flashes of discover and invention, but the obvious is repeatedly discovered, no matter what the nature of underlying society. An analysis of several lines of clinical discovery will reveal the profound absence of scientific thought in medicine between approximately 400-1400 AD. A number of useful ideas and procedures will now be placed in chronological context during the long march toward modern medicine through an age that for a thousand years or more did so little to advance it.

B. Timeline of Medical Discovery

Several lines of clinical thought are explored below. Descriptions are provided of relatively simple but important discoveries and inventions spanning the period from 400 BC to the 17th C, including the basis for each discovery and some relevant precedent observations.

1. Therapies and procedures -

a. Thoracentesis

The Hippocratics provided an excellent discussion of the technique of thoracentesis for removing fluid from the pleural (chest) cavity.[3] The procedure was subsequently mentioned by other Greco-Roman writers. Armand Trousseau (1801-1867) reviewed the history of thoracentesis, and described its reemergence as a valuable clinical technique in his *Lectures on Clinical Medicine*.[4] He considered it to have been forgotten after the early Greek physicians until again discussed by several 17th C practitioners.

Comment – Almost 2000 years of disabling and often lethal emypemas and pleural effusions had to be suffered by an inestimable number of patients before relief could again be provided by Western physicians employing a Hippocratic technique now in daily use in hospitals around the world. As for the technique itself, it is performed much as described in Hippocratic writings, the next significant improvements in managing pleural infection being the discovery of X-rays in the 19th C and the development of antibiotics in the 20th C.

b. Tracheotomy/intubation

Intimations of the procedure of tracheotomy are found in ancient Egyptian drawings, although some authorities consider the drawings as evidence of sacrificial killing. But it was Aesclepiades who is credited in the 1st C BC with performing the first

---

[3] For a translation see: Adams, W. H., *The Natural State of Medical Practice: Hippocratic Evidence*, Maitland (FL), 2019, p. 97*ff.* Many translations to follow are to be found in that reference.
[4] A. Trousseau, in *Lectures on Clinical Medicine*, Phila., 1871, vol. 1., Lecture 22, pp. 556-565, translation of Drs. Cormack and Bazire. Trousseau was a prominent French physician, one of his eponymic contributions being the Trousseau sign, an indication of latent tetany in hypocalcemia.

elective tracheotomy.[5] Caelius Aurelianus (*fl.* 5th C AD) wrote that the Hippocratics had recommended it as a measure of last resort in upper airway obstruction, but then later argued against its use, citing difficulties in healing of the tracheal wound. There are no citations in the extant *Hippocratic Corpus* that support the latter statement. The Hippocratics did, however, describe the performance of both tracheotomy and intubation.[6] Paulus of Aegineta (625-690 AD), a Byzantine physician, gives the remarkable description of tracheotomy as described by Antyllus, a 2nd C AD Greek surgeon who preferred a transverse incision between the third and fourth tracheal rings.[7] The wording of procedure suggests it was effectively performed by Antyllus, although there is no way to know if other physicians attempted it. There are a few mentions of tracheotomy over the next thousand years, especially as the writings of Paulus influenced Arabic medicine, particularly Albucasis (936-1013 AD), but there is no evidence in the Middle East that the procedure was ever used on humans. During the Dark Ages in Europe the tracheotomy and intubation were not mentioned by medical writers.

Although Baillou in 1578 considered the option of tracheotomy for upper airway obstruction and Fabricius (1537-1619) described the technique and its value, it was Antonio Brassavola in 1546 who first reported a successful outcome, publishing his result.[8] He does not mention any earlier attempts at the procedure by others. A few years later Severino used a trocar to percutaneously enter the trachea and bypass obstruction during a diphtheria epidemic in 1610. The tracheotomy was then rediscovered by Santorio in 1614. Intubation was not mentioned during this period.

Comment – The "windpipe," or trachea, is the channel by which air enters the lungs and is an obvious anatomic entity in the neck obvious to everyone. A method of bypassing upper airway obstruction by surgically opening the trachea in the neck below the level of obstruction occurred during Hippocratic times and was employed by Aesclepiades in the

---

[5] Aesclepiades (124-40 BC), a Greek "physician" whose reputation was made in Rome, is cited by Galen; only a few fragments of Aesclepiades' writings remain.

[6] From the Hippocratic work *Dis*eases III, 10, the following extract can be interpreted as a tracheotomy for reasons given in the author's Comment section on p. 87*f* of *The Natural State of Medical Practice: Hippocratic Evidence*, Maitland (FL), especially for justification of translating the trachea as the tube to be incised and the τιτθόν as the laryngeal prominence rather than nipple of the breast:

τούτων φλεβοτομέειν χρή μάλιστα μὲν ὑπὸ τὸν τιτθόν· συνακολουθεῖ ταύτῃ ἐκ τοῦ πλεύμονος θερμὸν πνεῦμα· ("It may be necessary to cut into the [air] channel of these patients, particularly below the thyoid cartilage, and warm air flowing from the lungs promptly follows this." Translation by the author.) The performer of the procedure thus knows when it has been successfully completed. In contrast, a chest incision with free air entry will collapse the lung.

Also described in *Dis*. III, 10, when faced with a suffocating pharyngeal abscess the physician must τοὺς αὐλίσκους παρῶσαι ἐς τὴν φάρυγγα κατὰ τὰς νγάθους. ὡς ἕλκηται τὸ πνεῦμα ἐς τὸν πλεύμονα ("insert tube into the throat behind the jaws, in order that air may be drawn into the lung," *Loeb Classical Library* translation by P. Potter in vol. VI of *Hippocrates*, or "...bypass with a tube into the pharynx below the [level of the] jaw. Thus air may be sucked into the lungs ..." translation by the author.) While this cannot be technically termed an intubation of the trachea, this "supraglottic" intubation would be similar in function.

[7] Paulus Aegineta, *De Res Medica Libri Septem*, Bk. VI, 33, as translated by Francis Adams in *The Medical Works of Paulus Aegineta*, London, 1834, vol. 2.

[8] Brassavola, Antonio Musa: *In libros de ratione victus in morbis acutis Hippocratis & Galeni commentaria & annotationes*, Venice, 1546.

1st C BC and by Antyllus in the 2nd C AD. The argument that tracheotomy (or "bronchotomy") was avoided by Hippocratic physicians because of poor healing of the tracheal rings is unlikely to have been valid or even stated by them. Modern tracheostomy sites routinely heal over within a week or two after cannula removal, and infection and impaired healing should have occurred no more frequently after tracheotomy than any other surgical procedure.[9] Furthermore, (1) Antyllus indicated it might be sufficient to transect the membrane connecting two tracheal rings by a transverse incision, thereby avoiding injury to cartilage, (2) it is likely that ancient cannulas, if they were used to temporarily maintain an open ostomy site, would have been made of silver, which has antimicrobial properties, and (3) openings might have been cut through the cricothyroid membrane rather than the trachea, thus avoiding cartilage altogether. Tracheotomy was "rediscovered" as an effective procedure during the Renaissance by Brassavola. There is no evidence that the procedure was actually employed in treating airway obstruction in humans during the interval between its use by the ancient Greek physicians and then by Brassavola as reported in 1546. The elapsed time from Antyllus to Brassavola was 1400 years during which time the various causes of pharyngeal occlusion, including diphtheria, were permitted to strangle their innumerable victims, predominantly children.[10] It is insufficient to blame two or three ancient writers for that lapse merely because they expressed concern over complications. There is some deeper problem that prevented use of tracheotomy for all those years, for the potential lifesaving value of opening a small hole in the anterior neck into the trachea to avoid suffocation is immediately obvious to anyone with minimal medical training when faced with upper airway occlusion.

c. Urinary tract surgery

The Hippocratics described very concisely the method for surgical drainage of a perinephric abscess, indicating that one cause of the lesion was occlusion of urine flow from the kidney by renal stones, and that after surgical drainage of the abscess stones can sometimes be flushed out by increasing urine flow.[11] Kidney function as manifested in the urine was also assessed by the Hippocratics, including urine color, viscosity, volume, precipitates, and particulate matter. They also distinguished between various causes of lower urinary tract obstruction, and perineal surgery for removal of bladder and urethral stones and urethral catheterization were used. Aretaeus explained how urine was removed from the blood by the kidneys[12], and Celsus (25 BC to 50 AD) gave a detailed description

---

[9] For a dramatic recounting of this fact see: *A Letter from Dr. William Musgrave to Dr. Sloane, being an argument for the more frequent use of laryngotomy urged from a remarkable cure in chirurgery; performed by Mr. John Keen of Roch in Cornwal*, in *Phil. Trans.* 21:398-405, 1699.

[10] Fear of the procedure persisted much longer, permitting the death of President George Washington in 1799. It is presently concluded that Washington was suffocated by either a peritonsillar abscess ("quinsy") or, in view of the rapid course of his illness, acute epiglottitis, and phlebotomy was used in his management rather than tracheotomy. He may have died, therefore, from hemorrhagic shock. For one of many articles on the subject see: Cohen, B., *The Death of George Washington, (1832-1899) and the History of Cynanche*, in *J. Med. Biogr.*, 13:225-231, 2005.

[11] See *Internal Affections* (*Loeb Classical Library* series on *Hippocrates*, vol. VI), where four clinical scenarios are presented in sections 14-17, three of which suggest renal or perinephric abscess. No. 14 is referred to here. Presumably the kidney itself was not knowingly incised.

[12] "In shape they [*i.e.*, the kidneys] resemble the testicles, but are broader, and, at the same time, curved. Their cavities are small and like sieves, for the percolation of the urine; ...", translation of

of lithotomy for bladder stones through the perineal approach.[13]

It was not until the anatomical studies during the Renaissance and Vesalius, Bellini, and Morgagni, the latter through his autopsy studies and use of the microscope, that knowledge of renal structure and function resumed. It is Pierre Franco (1505-1578) who is credited with inventing the suprapubic cystotomy. The Marian lithotomy, or median raphe approach, was first performed by Jacques de Beaulieu (1651-1720).

Comment – During the centuries following the Hippocratics and their encyclopedists such as the 7th C practitioner Paulus Aegineta there was little mention of surgery on the urinary system. In its place "uroscopy," the gross observation of a urine specimen, was the focus of medical training on renal matters during the Dark Ages and, especially, during the medieval period. That procedure became increasingly complex but no more meaningful. Theophilus Protospatharius in the 7th C provided a standard academic work on uroscopy for clinical management of urinary tract disease that was in use up to the Renaissance.[14] A 14th C manuscript from Serbia gives a typical detailed description of uroscopic technique, urinary symptoms, and Hippocratic theory on renal function, but surgery is not mentioned.[15] Perhaps one reason physicians conveniently declined to perform the procedure was because it could be argued that it was proscribed by the Hippocratic Oath (p. 432f). Surgery was also proscribed by the Fourth Lateran Council (1215). Histories of medicine mention but provide no literary citation concerning practitioners who performed stone removal. The excruciating pain of urinary lithiasis and its associated symptoms would have prompted someone, indeed anyone, to attempt stone removal. But physicians were not involved, for had they performed such operations there would have been documentation of it. Instead, stone removal was left to the ingenuity and intrepidity of laymen even into the Renaissance, as graphically described by Dr. Harry Herr. It took about 1500 years before crude lithotomy techniques were improved and the procedure re-entered the realm of an evolving "professional," the barber surgeon.[16]

d. Podalic version

The massaging of the abdomen of a woman in the midst of difficult labor is probably a universal response to the urgency of the moment. Hippocratic writings went further, their purpose being to instruct on external manipulation of the fetus prior to delivery so that the fetal head would be first to present (cephalic version), as is the usual case in an uncomplicated delivery. Celsus in the 1st C AD discussed both cephalic and podalic version, although no version was recommended for a living child. It was Soranus in the early 2nd C AD who preferred podalic version for abnormal fetal presentation, instructing the physician or midwife to grasp the feet of the fetus and gently guide it foot-first through the birth canal. His description, as translated by Prof. Temkin in consultation

Francis Adams, from Bk. II, chapter 3, of Aretaeus, *De Causis et Signis Acutorum Morborum*, in *The Extant Works of Aretaeus, the Cappadocian*, London, 1851.

[13] Celsus, *De Medicina*, Book 7, section 26.

[14] For an overview of uroscopy see: Wallis, F., *Inventing Diagnosis: Theophilus' De Urinis in the Classroom*, in DYNAMIS, *Acta Hisp. Med. Sci. Hist. Illust.*, 20:31-73, 2000.

[15] The Serbian manuscript is discussed by G. S. Gorgieva in *Kidney Disease in Medieval Serbian Manuscripts from the Chilandar Monastery*, in *J. Nephrol.*, 19 Supp. 10, S30-37, 2006.

[16] Herr, H. W., *"Cutting for the Stone": The Ancient Art of Lithotomy*, in BJU, Feb. 2008; https://doi.org/10.1111/j.1464-410X.2008.07510.x.

with obstetricians, is wonderfully clear.[17] The text of Soranus, and perhaps another contemporary, was available to Aetius of Amida (5th-6th C AD) who repeated their earlier recommendations, although podalic version may have been reserved for the dead fetus.

The technic of podalic version then goes unmentioned until Ambroise Pare (1510-1590) reintroduced the technique in 1549.[18] There was a book for midwives published by Eucharius Rosslin (the *Rosengarten*, Wurms, 1513) that hinted at podalic version, but that work was a compilation of contemporary expertise of midwives rather than a medical treatise by physicians.[19]

Comment - From extant writings it took fourteen centuries for the ancient procedure of podalic version to be rediscovered and employed. During that interval it is incomprehensible how much agony, anguish, and death from obstetric delivery, especially in young women with their first pregnancy, was the consequence. It is germane that Pare acknowledged that he knew the technique not from familiarity with ancient writings but from discussions with two other Parisian barber-surgeons who were using it.[20] His candid statement is a peek into the unwritten history of mankind, for rediscovery of the obviously important is the natural way of things. The tendency to associate an important discovery with a singular individual subsequently declared to be a person superior in one way or another ignores the work or good fortune of innumerable other discoverers of whom nothing is ever to be known. Pare's barber-surgeon friends or Stearns' "ignorant Scotch woman" who advised him of the usefulness of ergot or Withering's elderly Shropshire herbalist and her botanical mixture that included foxglove, the source of digitalis, all of whom are fortunate enough to be vaguely remembered, are the stagehands who change the scenery for the great names of the day who are on stage. Those "stagehands" are perennially present, but there is no one to tell their stories unless one of the great names is honest enough to mention them (and to their credit, most do). Thus, this book, as an ancillary feature, has attempted to mention their stories. Their unrequited efforts relieved rhe suffering of innumerable persons. But the medical "profession," even if it can be considered to have existed in the Dark Ages, gets no share of that credit.

2. Physical examination -

a. Percussion

An important physical examination technique taught to every medical student is

---

[17] *Soranus' Gynecology,* O. Temkin, editor, Balitimore, 1956, Book IV.

[18] Pare's writing, *Briefve collection de l'administration anatomique,* was primarily an anatomical work, but it included a description of podalic version, a technique explained in greater detail in a later publication. Pare's writings were translated into English by Thomas Johnson: *The Works of that Famous Chirurgion Ambrose Parey,* London, 1634.

[19] An English version was published in 1540, Raynalde's *The Byrthe of Mankynde,* in which it is stated that if it is impossible to turn the fetus to a "normal" position the midwife may be forced to deliver the child by traction on the feet.

[20] The two surgeons, friends of Pare, were Thierry de Hery and Nicole Lambert, the latter his godfather, as cited in Dr. Francis Packard's *The Life and Times of Ambrose Pare,* New York, 1921, a publication which includes Packard's translations of some of Pare's works.

percussion, in which the body surface over the region of interest is tapped, directly or indirectly, with a finger or hand. The sound of the tap will vary according to the density and extent of underlying tissue or substance. In a patient with an abdominal ileus and gaseous distention there is a tympanitic sound upon percussing the abdominal wall, whereas a fluid-filled abdomen will have a severely dampened or dull sound. It is likely that the Hippocratics recognized this as a diagnostic tool, although its earliest written descriptions come from Aretaeus (1st C AD)[21] and Alexander of Tralles (6th C AD).

Percussion next comes to notice in the 17th C. Cowherds, to determine if an intracranial cystic mass (now known to be caused by *Echinococcus granulosa*, the dog tapeworm) was the source of an animal's illness, used percussion by tapping a small mallet on the cranium and assessing the resulting sound to investigate a sick bovine. If there was a "cracked-pot" percussion sound, which suggested separation of the cranial sutures, trephining was performed and the fluid aspirated out of the cyst, sometimes successfully.[22] This method of identifying internal pathology was recorded by Dr. Gerhard van Swieten (1700-1772), a physician trained in Boerhaave's famous medical school in Leiden. He, in turn, obtained his information from a Swiss physician's publication of 1658.[23] The elapsed time between Aretaeus' description and Dr. van Swieten's publicizing of the percussion by cowherds was about 1600 years; from Alexander of Tralle's descriptions to van Swieten's was 1100 years.

Comment - Whether percussion was first a tool of the Hippocratics or Alexander of Tralles is irrelevant here. What is relevant is that for about fifteen centuries thereafter it was an unexploited tool. And when percussion was discovered to have been reinvented by cowherds as recorded in the 17th C, it was a *de novo* invention, not a residuum of Hippocratic medicine. It is to be admitted that the "cracked pot" sound of separated cranial sutures as sought by the cowherds depends on tissue density only in part, and thus the analogy with Aretaeus' and Alexander of Tralles' percussion is not entirely accurate. Nevertheless, the technique is similar, using an external procedure to determine internal pathology, and the cowherds applied it to the heads of their animals rather than the limited abdominal percussion of the Hippocratic physicians, indicating a broader use for the procedure. Furthermore, they used a small mallet to produce the sound, a process similar to that which would be elicited by the pleximeter and, ultimately, the modern reflex

---

[21] Aretaeus, *Chronic Diseases*, Bk. II, I, translation of Francis Adams. "Tympanites may be recognized, not only from the sight of the swelling, but also by the sound which is heard on percussion. For if you tap with the hand, the abdomen sounds; neither does the flatus (pneuma) shift its place with the changes of posture; for the flatus, even although that which contains it should be turned upwards and downwards, remains always equally the same; but should the flatus (pneuma) be converted into vapour and water (for Ascites may supervene on Tympanites), it shifts its form, indeed, the one half running in a fluid state, if the conversion be incomplete." The author concurs with "percussion" as the translation of Aretaeus' word δονέων in context, although "shaking" may be more literal. The tapping of the hand confirms he used percussion, and by repositioning the patient, abdominal fluid relocates, a sign called "shifting dullness."

[22] For this and other relevant information given here see: Schiller, F., *The Reflex Hammer: In Memoriam Robert Wartenberg (1887-1956)*, Med. Hist., 11:75-85, 1967.

[23] Dr. Johann Jakob Wepfer (1620-1695) reported in his *Historiae Apoplecticorum* (Amsterdam, 1727), p. 64: "close to the horns some unnatural cavity is present under the skull, the Swiss cowherds immediately trephine the place just hit. They introduce a tube through the hole, extract the fluid, and so empty the cysts." (Translator not specified; see: Schiller, F., *The Reflex Hammer*, in *Med. Hist.*, 11:75-85, 1967.)

hammer. Rediscovery of percussion and its exploitation in physical examination could have occurred at any time between Tralles and Dr. van Swieten, but it apparently did not. In today's medicine effective percussion is becoming a lost art because modern imaging techniques are so excellent. But like any "art" successful exploitation relies on practice. In urgent situations and when imaging is unavailable, competency in percussion can be lifesaving still, especially in chest disease. And it would have been a life preserver many times over had it been available for the fifteen centuries preceeding its 17th C reinvention, not to mention its usefulness in assessing organ size, fluidity and location of effusions, and distention of body cavities, and thereby contributing to knowledge of the pathophysiology of disease as well as directing therapy.

b. Auscultation

This topic and pertinent references are discussed in detail on p. 390*f*, but the essential clinical point for present purposes is that the Hippocratics applied an ear directly to a patient's chest to listen for sounds that were clues to the nature of the underlying disease process. This technique has been termed "immediate auscultation," whereas with a stethoscope it would be called "mediate" auscultation. The sound heard by applying the ear directly to the chest after shaking a patient with fluid in the chest has been termed *succussio Hippocratis*, or a succussion splash. It is likely that the Hippocratics also heard some heart murmurs, but the first mention of this is found in the works of Aretaeus (1st C AD), who noted the πάταγος τῆς καρδίης, translated by Dr. Francis Adams as "a bruit of the heart," a clinical detail obtainable only by placing the ear on the chest.[24]

Throughout the Dark Ages and into the medieval period immediate auscultation is not mentioned in the West, although a few early Byzantine physicians mention the Hippocratic technique. The next reference to "immediate auscultation" for detection of internal chest pathology is found in writings of Renaissance era physicians, including William Harvey and Ambroise Pare.

Comment - The additive value of percussion and auscultation in providing a perspective on internal pathology in the living patient would have served as a stimulus to improved treatment, techniques, and knowledge in Roman and post-Roman European medicine just as they would in early 19th C Europe. Furthermore, the physical examination, having been made more effective by their use, would have made it less likely that uroscopy and pulse assessments would have assumed their undue prominence. The lack of effective physical diagnosis was for perhaps 1500 years an enormous loss to virtually every patient during those intervening years, which means virtually every person. There has been scholarly discussion as to why there was slow acceptance of methods of physical diagnosis even into the 18th C, and it has been surmised that it was the physical contact necessary for such examination procedures that was not appreciated by medieval practitioners.

c. Body temperature

Fevers described by the Hippocratics included high and low ones, fevers that were continuous, remittent, intermittent, irregular, periodic, and relapsing or recurring.

---

[24] Adams, F., *The Extant Works of Aretaeus*, London, 1856, p. 271. The Greek term refers to the sound of two objects colliding with one another or the splashing of a wave.

These distinctions were made by estimating body warmth with the hand placed on the body surface. Herophilus (335-280 BC) devised a method of timing the pulse in an attempt to quantify subtle temperature elevations, for the frequent association of a rapid pulse with fever had been noted. Thus, there was a focused interest in an accurate measure of body temperature. But the most important discovery of the Hippocratics was the association of various fever patterns with distinctive clinical syndromes and outcomes.

There were no known Western attempts to exploit fever as a diagnostic tool over subsequent centuries until quantitating fever was attempted by Dr. Santorio Santorio who, in 1614, devised an early thermometer, the thermoscope.[25] Some think that instrument found its origin in Galileo's observation, in 1592, that the volume of air in an inverted long-necked glass vessel, when the neck was immersed in liquid, contracted or expanded as it was cooled or heated, causing the liquid to rise or fall in the vessel's neck, an experiment that may have been suggested by Galileo's reading a few years earlier of the *Pneumatica* by Hero of Alexandria (10-70 AD).

Comment – Surely in the centuries separating the Hippocratics and Galileo someone could have followed up Hero's observations on thermal contraction and expansion of gases and liquids, from which some earlier Santorio could have recognized in that observation a potential clinical tool and devised a clinical method that would help clarify causes of fever. The ease of doing so is exemplified by Jean Rey (1583-1645) who, trained in medicine, also invented a thermoscope, which he described as a container with a long thin neck filled with water that, when held by a person with a fever, raised the water level in the neck of the container higher than when fever was absent. Had that happened the confusing periodicities of fevers frequently cited in Hippocratic writings might have been explained, musings on malaria and other pestilences in ancient times partially untangled, and investigations initiated into the association of foci of inflammation with fever. It is true that estimating fever by feeling the patient's skin with the hand is often accurate to within one degree, and for many clinical purposes this is sufficient for decision-making. But with a convenient mechanism for assessing fever patterns much useful information relevant to epidemiology and nosology of disease would have been acquired and would have provided insight into mechanisms of disease. This is exactly what happened in the 19th C when the clinical thermometer was popularized (p. 374*f*). The relevance here is that the elapsed time between fever assessments by the Hippocratics and the focused attempt by Dr. Santorio to understand fever was 1800 years. Ignorance concerning fever during this period was an easily obviated void.

d. Air vs. bone conduction of sound (hearing)

The Hippocratics provided early descriptions of the ear, including the tympanic membrane, which was likened to a spider's web. Its usefulness was in detecting sound in the air.[26] But there is little evidence of exploitation of sound conduction through solids.

---

[25] Santorio, S., in *Commentaria in Primam Fen Primam Libri Canonis Avicenna*, 1625. Dr. Santorio was a careful observer, but he was prone to devising idiosyncratic theories. His studies on insensible perspiration, so carefully performed, were not done to improve on methods of fluid balance in patients. Instead, he used them to develop a comprehensive theory of disease in which perspiration was claimed to be similar to gastrointestinal and renal excretions.

[26] In the *Loeb Classical Library* volumes of *Hippocrates*, see *Fleshes*, XV, for mention of the thin, spider-web-like skin inside the ear that, by virtue of being "dry," is specially designed to transmit

In Pliny's *Natural History* (XVI, 73) there is a description of sound being used to ascertain the presence of defects in long board planks, performed by putting the ear to one end of the board and listening to the quality of the sound elicited by striking the board at its far end. Aristotle, however, had described in the 4th C BC what can be interpreted as wave conduction of sound in air, and Vitruvius, in his 15 BC work, *De Architectura*, chapter V, considered sound to be carried in waves based on analogy with ripples on water and sound transmission in water. [27]

Dr. Girolamo Cardano (1501-1576) reported in 1550 that the pitch of a sound produced by a metal rod was sensitively detected when the rod was held between the teeth and caused to vibrate.[28] Dr. Hieronymi Capivacci (1523-1589), by attaching the rod to a musical instrument as a source of vibration, was able to differentiate nerve deafness from middle ear deafnss, the complete inability to hear the sound indicating nerve deafness. His work was published in 1603.[29] This was the first advance in knowledge of the mechanism of hearing in 1800 years.

Comment – The Hippocratics and near contemporaries established an early anatomical basis for hearing by air conduction, and a theory of sound wave propagation through air and water was proposed. Much later, Drs. Cardano and Capivacci differentiated sound transmitted via air conduction from bone conduction. Superior sound conduction through solids has been common knowledge, and by putting one's ear to the ground distant low frequency sounds could be detected by the conduction of sound traveling through the solid earth and thence through the bones of the cranium to the cochlea. The transmission of sounds through the air to the tympanic membrane is also followed by transmission of energy to the cochlea. As normally activated, air conduction is more sensitive than bone conduction. It has been stated that the study of audiology, a science dealing with hearing and balance, had its beginnings when bone conduction of sound was differentiated from air conduction of sound, but early Greco-Roman observations had already established a theoretical framework for investigation. [30] In the intervening fifteen centuries the mass of the deaf and near-deaf with disabled linguistics skills were viewed as invalids and defective, unable to learn, with no attempt on record of a medical professional to ascertain the cause or alleviate effect of their hearing loss.

---

sound to the brain. τὸ δὲ δέρμα τὸ πρὸς τῇ ἀκοῇ πρὸς τῷ ὀστέῳ τῷ σκληρῷ λεπτόν ἐστιν ὥσπερ ἀράχνιον, ξηρότατον τοῦ ἄλλου δέρματος. ("The skin from the ear when it is near the hard bone [the petrous portion of the temporal bone, the most dense bone in the body] is thin like a spider's web and dryer than other skin." Translation by the author.) Also described next to the bone was a cavernous hollow, perhaps meaning the intraosteal portion of the Eustachian tube.

[27] Aristotle, *On the Soul*, 420b, 11-12: καὶ τοῦτ᾽ εὐλόγως, εἴπερ ἀέρος κίνησίς τίς ἐστιν ὁ ψόφος. ("It is logical, since sound is a certain movement of the air." Translation by the author.) And see: Vitruvius, *De Architectura*, V.

[28] H. Cardano , *De Subtilitate*, Nuremburg, 1550.

[29] H. Capivacci, *Opera Omnia Quinq Section Comprehensa*, Venice, 1597.

[30] North American Indians were able to detect a herd of buffalo by "listening" with their ear to the ground. And bone conduction of sound has been the basis for certain aids to hearing. In 1879 Richard Rhodes, who had developed air conduction deafness, invented a hearing aid device using a sound collecting diaphragm attached to an appliance held in his teeth, from whence sound vibrations were transmitted via the teeth and boney structures to the cochlea. This idea occurred to him after he had noted that he could hear his watch tick if held in his mouth. It is unexplained as to why ear trumpets or other hearing devices were not devised in medieval times. Perhaps there were, but the deaf and near-deaf were unlikely to write about themselves.

3. Syndromes of Disease -

a. Proteinuria, a common problem

The foaming of urine on shaking was known by the Hippocratics to indicate a kidney problem, often one that was protracted.[31] They also recognized generalized edema as a sometime consequence of kidney disease. Rufus of Ephesus, writing *ca.* 100 AD, indicated the association between renal sclerosis, or hardening, and edema in his περὶ σκλεριας νεφρον (On Hardening of the Kidneys).[32]   In some patients cloudiness in heated urine was noted by Theophilus Protospatharius (7th C AD).[33]

Chemical testing of the urine received no further attention until Paracelsus (1493-1541) noted cloudiness upon adding vinegar to urine, although clinical utility did not result. By either of the simple expedients of heating the urine or adding a drop of vinegar, Dekkers, in 1674, noted the formation of a sweetish milk-like coagulum in the urine of some emaciated patients, a coagulum that he thought looked like serum similarly treated.[34] Usually the abnormally increased protein in urine in kidney disease is primarily albumin, a component of serum proteins. The elapsed time from the Hippocratic observation of bubbles in urine and from Protospatharius' mention of urine heating to Dekker's discovery that urine from an anasarca patient developed a white precipitate on heating or adding vinegar was 2000 years and 1000 years, respectively, each a century shorter if Paracelsus' testing is used as the endpoint.

Comment – Visual inspection of urine became increasingly popular during the centuries that lapsed between the Hippocratics and the Renaissance, so much so that it superseded even the pulse and the physical examination of patients in perceived diagnostic importance. This legendary but for the most part useless technique, first promoted by Magnus of Nisibis, a physician and orator from Antioch in the 4th C AD, and known as "uroscopy," was far more complex but no more useful than Hippocratic visual inspection of the urine. Uroscopy was finally laid to rest by the *Pisse Prophet*, a book published by Thomas Brian in 1637. But with just looking at surface bubbles of freshly passed urine (by the Hippocratics, 4th C BC) or with some heating of the urine (by Dekkers in the 17th C and described as the first ever clinical laboratory test) the understanding of proteinuria was poised for a great advance: once excessive bubbles or a precipitate was identified the ancients could have found it to correlate with certain types of kidney disease, with the clinical course, and perhaps with some its causes, which might have included exposures to toxic compounds. It would have been a small step to semiquantify protein in the urine, thereby devising an important prognostic test. This was recently proven by Diskin, who showed a correlation between visual estimation of urine bubbles and the amount of protein in a urine specimen, confirming the plausibility of usefulness of even the Hippocratic

---

[31] "Bubbles floating on the urine surface indicate kidney disease and a prolonged illness." *Aph.*, VII, 34, translation by the author; see p. 398 and footnote for commentary.

[32] See: *Rufi Ephesii; de renum et vesicae morbis*, in *Corpus Medicorum Graecorum/Latinorum*, Berlin, 1977, Kidneys and Bladder, III, 34-35, edited and translated into German by A. Sideras.

[33] Theophilus Protospatharius wrote several medical works, for the most part a reworking of Galen and Hippocrates, but his book *De Urinis* was popular for centuries.

[34] See: Dekkers, F., *Exercitationes Practicae Circa Medendi Methodum,* Leiden, 1694, chapter 5 on purging, p. 338 in the cited edition.

observation.[35]   Many descriptions of disease and death made in the days of medical ignorance were of, or were superimposed on, chronic kidney failure and its metabolic consequences that were unknown to their writers. Many symptoms and signs, like the sluggishness of advanced hypothyroidism and the frenzied state of hyperthyroidism, would often have been ascribed to emotional states or a "nervous problem." Such errors, physically and psychologically hurtful, might have been allayed had a better categorization of diseases been developed. Simple testing of the urine for a protein precipitate would have been a big advance in this regard.

b. Diphtheria

A clinical delineation of diphtheria (the "cough of Perinthus") was made by the Hippocratics, including their observations on its neurological complications. This is described in some detail on p. 206*ff.*

The next association of neurological abnormalities with clinical diphtheria occurred in the 19th C, when Brettoneau was one of several physicians commenting on the palatal paralysis of diphtheria, although even then ciliary muscle paralysis escaped their notice.

Comment - A first step in scientific understanding of a disease is to define its usual clinical manifestations so that it can be identified when it occurs elsewhere. The Hippocratics did this, and with perspicacity they identified the neurological features of diphtheria, although they did not provide the disease a name. The time between the Hippocratics and Bretonneau was 2200 years. Earlier characterization of the disease, of which the sign of ciliary muscle paralysis would have been an important observation, might have resulted in a better understanding of its epidemiology and perhaps its management and control even without knowledge of its bacterial origin. Diphtheria is an epidemic disease, but one that evolves slowly and can even encircle the globe, most of its victims being children. Suffocation by obstruction of the airway in the neck is one way it causes death. Despite the initially hopeful characterization of the disease, its human toll in a wretched death and misery over 2200 years is impossible to estimate.

c. Lead poisoning

Nikander (2nd C BC), author of a poetical pharmacopoeia, has been credited with an early description of lead poisoning from lead carbonate, or cerussa, one use being a skin-whitening agent for women. His poem is convincing, and his attribution of symptoms to the source was a remarkable revelation. A Roman architect, Vitruvius (1st C BC), also described, in an extraordinary passage in his classic book on architecture, a causal association between workers making lead pipes and symptoms of plumbism.[36]

---

[35] Diskin, C. J., *et al.*, *Surface Tension, Proteinuria, and the Urine Bubbles of Hippocrates*, in: *Lancet*, 355:901, 2000.

[36] 10. "Water conducted through earthen pipes is more wholesome than that through lead; indeed that conveyed in lead must be injurious, because from it white lead is obtained, and this is said to be injurious to the human system. Hence, if what is generated from it is pernicious, there can be no doubt that itself cannot be a wholesome body. 11. This may be verified by observing the workers in lead, who are of a pallid colour; for in casting lead, the fumes from it fixing on the different members, and daily burning them, destroy the vigour of the blood; water should therefore on no

Dr. Samuel Stockhausen published, in 1656, a small tract describing the causative relation between symptoms now attributable to lead poisoning with lead glazing and with dust and fume exposure in lead mining in what is now Lower Saxony.[37] Written in Latin, it included an addendum in German so that mining engineers would be alerted to the problem. In 1696 a Swabian edict against adulterating wine with a lead-contaminated sweetener was based on similar observations of Dr. Eberhard Gockel.

Comment – Forgotten or ignored after Greco-Roman times, lead toxicity was rediscovered in its entirety in the 17th C. Seventeen hundred years had to pass before the ancient warnings of Nikander and Vitruvius would be duplicated. Their early discoveries found only a niche in a poem and in a book on architecture. Centuries of enormous morbidity and mortality from lead poisoning induced by lead salts as sweeteners, lead pipes and containers, and other substances and articles containing lead were therefore permitted, although the comments of Vitruvius indicate that among those who themselves worked with lead the injuriousness of its salts was sometimes known, thus being another "peek into the unwritten history" of medicine (p. 296*f*).

4. Physiology and Epidemiology -

a. Circulation of blood

The *Hippocratic Corpus* contains statements that some suggest indicate an understanding of the pulmonary circulation and an appreciation of a driving force for blood moving around the body.[38] Herophilus and Erasistratus differentiated arteries from veins *ca.* 300 BC.[39] Sir William Osler considered Plato to have described motion of the blood for systemic nourishment, as from a fountain.[40] Galen considered the heart to be a pump. It does appear that the pre-Galenic idea that arteries primarily carried air or pneuma (the life spirit) and not much blood to tissues was a theoretical stumbling block

---

account be conducted in leaden pipes if we are desirous that it should be wholesome. That the flavour of that conveyed in earthen pipes is better, is shewn at our daily meals, for all those whose tables are furnished with silver vessels, nevertheless use those made of earth, from the purity of the flavour being preserved in them." Vitruvius, *De Architectura*, VIII,.6,10-11, translation of J. Gwilt, *The Architecture of Marcus Vitruvius Pollio*, London, 1826.)

[37] Stockhausen, S., *Libellus de lithargyrii fumo noxio morbifico, ejusque metallico frequentiori morebo vulgo dicto die Hutten Katze oder Hubben Rauch*, Goslar, 1656.

[38] R. Kapferer, in his controversial translation of *de Corde*, (*Die Werke des Hippokrates*, Stuttgart, 1939, part 16, *Des Herz*, p. 59) goes further, stating (in translation): "In other words, the author clearly recognized that blood circulated from and to the heart. Thus the circulation of the blood was already known prior to 400 BC." There is also the statement in the Hippocratic work, *Places in Man*, 3, that "And all blood vessels communicate and flow into one another, some uniting with another, but some [unite] with stretched-out blood vessels coming from [other]vessels, some [vessels] nourishing the tissues, then connecting with each other." Translation by the author. The "stretched-out vessels" likely refers to much smaller vessels. But the overall meaning can be viewed as implying a complete network of interconnected blood vessels throughout the body.

[39] Claudii Galeni, *De Placitis Hippocratis et Platonis*, Leipzig, 1874, edited by Iwan von Mueller, p. 552, Bk. vi. The text is in Greek with Latin translation.

[40] Osler, W., *Physic and Physicians as Depicted in Plato*, in the *Boston Med. and Surg. Journal*, 128:129-133 (part 1), 1893.

to a comprehensive theory of blood circulation,[41] but it is simply inconceivable that that theory would have been maintained for long. Any practitioner cutting, purposely or not, an artery will immediately know that the artery carries blood under considerable pressure rather than air, and Galen did show this. Finally, there is a distinction between pneuma and air, the former being the source of life found in the air that might now be considered a metaphor for oxygen and carried in small packets.[42]

The next event relevant to corporeal circulation occurred when Pare devised the tourniquet about 1550. Then Dr. William Harvey (1578-1657) began lecturing in 1616 on his new insights concerning the circulation of blood, work that was published in 1628, *Exercitatio Anatomica de Motu Cordis et Sanguinis in Animalibus.* He had pondered reasons why, over a matter of minutes, the output of blood from the beating heart should be far greater than that contained in the entire body. He then described the effect of a tight tourniquet, which cut off all blood flow into the extremity under study, and a "medium tight" one, which permitted distal arterial pulsation but prevented return flow of blood via the veins, one result being the far greater flow of blood during phlebotomy of a vein than was seen without application of the "medium tight" tourniquet. Finally, he showed, by finger pressure over the course of veins, that blood had directional flow assisted by valves inside the veins themselves.[43] Erasistratus had, of course, shown in about 300 BC that cardiac valves also permitted only unidirectional flow.

Comment - Harvey's studies were careful and logical, fastidious but not complex. It has even been argued that he merely rediscovered, but more accurately described, what had been first discovered by Erasistratus and Herophilus in 3rd C BC Alexandria, an argument that still finds supporters. He began his investigations on many other animal species and backed up his observations with his clinical experiences in treating humans. Beyond this, the application of a tourniquet would be seen by some as but common sense and demonstrating a mechanism for directional blood flow in veins of the arm is a parlor trick. Herophilus and Erasistratus were on the right track about 300 BC, the anatomy of the heart was well-described,[44] and a reasonable theory of blood circulation should have appeared soon afterward. Had that happened, its seminal value in the understanding of human physiology might have propelled medical discovery in the 3rd C BC in the same way it it did in the 18th C, promoting a cornucopia of information with ramifications in all branches of medicine, including intravenous therapies, that would have been of benefit at some point in the life of everyone. Dr. Herman Boerhaave's estimation of the great significance of Harvey's work is cited on p. 367. Instead, there was a 2000-year period of ignorance. The ancient observations of Herophilus and Erasistratos were lost for centuries. Even Dr. Girolamo Fracastorius (1478-1553) declared that the motion of the heart was to be understood by God alone. The case was reopened by Dr. Harvey, who

---

[41] Harris, C. R. S., *The Heart and Vascular System in Ancient Greek Medicine,* Oxford, 1973. In chapter 9 Harris describes how close Erasistratus was to a correct and comprehensive description of the circulation, and he then proceeds to analyze Galen's opinions in like manner.

[42] Erasistratus explained arterial bleeding as an aspiration of venous blood into the artery because of the vacuum that resulted from loss of air (pneuma).

[43] The anatomist, Hieronymus Fabricius (1537-1619), had already noted a system of valves in the veins, as had Erasistratus in the 4th C BC.

[44] *De Corde,* perhaps written after 300 BC, was by an unknown author. It is not considered a Hippocratic work.

cites no prior investigator in the field except for Galen, whom he proceeds to discredit.[45]

To further explain the significance of this and other discoveries relevant to human physiology, comment is needed regarding historiography and ancient medicine:

Excursus on Historiography and Medicine

Historiography, the way of writing history, can be defined as the study of "the principles, theory, and history of historical writing." In present context it is especially the "principles" as they apply to primary sources of information relevant to the history of medicine that are the focus of this excursus. A list of hierarchical principles of historiography has been developed,[46] and an important one is that the credibility of an item is greatly enhanced if there are two independent citations that are in agreement, and this is especially true when working with fragments of manuscripts or third person descriptions.

It is a fact that most ancient medical writings to come into modern hands were unique works in their final state, but that final state may postdate the original by 1000-2000 years, as is the case with the manuscript tradition of Hippocratic works, and sometimes several versions of a Hippocratic work can be traced back to a single manuscript made centuries earlier and of which they were but copies. Such copies do not represent "independent citations that are in agreement." In fact, they represent only the common copy from which they all are derived, plus any clerical errors or emendations as may have occurred in the interim. In the context of a history of medicine, a definitive edition of an ancient work is often presented historically as representing a point on a graph, and when works of Hippocrates, Diocles, Herophilus, Celsus, Aretaeus, Galen, Orobasius, Paulus, and others are strung together like data points in a narrative there is a suggestion of coherency, cause and effect, and perhaps even progress over the centuries. But the works of each of these writers cannot be likened to a battle, a coup d'etat, or an election, singular events that often have specific dates, winners, and consequences. Ancient medical works, in contrast, contained many facts, each fact having its own specifications as to technique, effectiveness, and side effects. Each of those works, therefore, was no singular large fact of medical history; rather each was a mass of particulars, each particular detail with its own unique provenance.

These masses of particulars synthesized by earlier medical authors and encyclopedists into a unity that have come into our hands tend to be viewed by the historian as a single fact among the many facts surrounding the society that is the focus of the historian's interest, and it is fitted snugly into that society's intellectual image. But consider this perspective: the time between the purported birth of Hippocrates (460 BC) and that of

---

[45] Details of directional flow were added by the early physicist, Giovanni Borelli, in his *De Motu Animalum* in 1680. It is relevant to note that Harvey, in his work *On Animal Generation*, cites the ideas of Empedocles (490-430 BC) regarding the generation of life and the four humors, but Empedocles, despite his concepts on blood flow and the heart and lungs, is not mentioned in *de Motu Cordis*, the inference being that Harvey's theory of the circulation of blood was not based on ancient ideas, although he does mention a 3rd C BC late Hippocratic work by an unknown author, *de Corde,* in its reference to the heart as a muscle.

[46] Gustafson, Carl, *A Preface to History*, New York, 1955.

Aretaeus (1st C AD) approaches 500 years. The author, at the time of this writing, is 75 years of age. He is also American. Thus, the author has witnessed, however closely, virtually one-third of the existence of the great Republic, including an era of unprecedented international turmoil and previously unimaginable advances in medical knowledge and therapy. All this occurred in one-sixth the time that passed between the ages of Hippocrates and of Aretaeus. How, then, can one justify inferring some sort of collegiality in thought between Hippocrates and Aretaeus, even with the help of the intervening Herophilus and Erasistratus, especially in an age with limited libraries, only scribal facilities for publication, factiousness, social turmoil, natural disasters, and no gasoline engines? It almost seems ludicrous to imagine Aretaeus as some sort of Hippocratic disciple when his age is separated from his master's age by little less time than separates our own age from Columbus' discovery of the New World. Would we spend as much time looking for wisdom in the *Badianus manuscript*? (See p. 102.) Aretaeus may have been a scholar aware of Hippocratic writings, but he was not a disciple. It seems, therefore, that the works of the various early masters and encyclopedists of medical history might be better viewed not so much as representating their times and part of continuum of knowledge but as extraordinary coincidences in manuscript survival; not so much a peep into a continuum, a continuous succession describing the evolution of medical practice, as an indication of the thinking of one perceptive and, on occasion, superior mind.

Thus, arrives the main point of this excursus, namely the significance of what Herophilus (*ca.* 335-255 BC) and Erasistratus (*fl.* early 3rd C BC) did in contrast to what they might have done had they been given a few more years of productive work. Surely they would have agreed with Aristotle's statement that if someone cannot confirm one of his (Aristotle's) explanations, that explanation should be appropriately changed (p. 199, with footnote). There seems to be, therefore, no *a priori* reason why the stated conclusions of the studies of Herophilus and Erasistratus, as cited by subsequent writers, should be considered their final opinions on a matter, especially when their actual words are not extant. Surely their opinions were in a state of flux or at least receptive to new data and interpretation just as are those of the true scientist of the present day. There is no reason to accuse them of being "scientists with their minds made up," a study in vested interest that is the antithesis of science.[47]

The careful observations of Erasistratus on cardiac valves, his understanding of the heart as a pump, and his postulation that there were connections between the arterial and venous systems should have been the stimulus for his, or another's, further experimentation.[48] He had many followers. But that experiment apparently did not happen, although perhaps it did and no record of the event survived. Nevertheless, historical events are not isolated

---

[47] As expressed by a true scientist, a friend of the author, the excitement of science to the individual scientist comes not when he checks his testtubes or culture plates and cries "Eureka!" It occurs instead during the intellectual challenge of devising the next experiment. The recording of the results of an experiment, whatever its outcome and regardless of its inferred significance, is merely one of several necessary steps in scientific procedure, a dispassionate collection of new data upon which another intellectual challenge will be erected. How many modern scientists believe this?

[48] Dobson, J. F., *Erasistratus*, in *Proc. R. Soc. Med.* 20:825-832, 1927. This well-focused article provides many citations to Galen, who was responsible for preserving what little still existed of Erasistratus' work.

and static, and but for interfering incidents an accurate concept of blood circulation could have been revealed in those early years, perhaps by Erasistratus himself. It is untenable to consider that the world had to wait 2000 years before only one person as brilliant as William Harvey could come along to enlighten an entire profession with his genius. This is the answer, therefore, to those who would argue that it was the ignorance or narrowness of vision or prejudice of some of medicine's great early names that thwarted critical insights that might have speeded up medical progress. That it is almost presented as fact that Erasistratus was wedded to his idea that blood flowed through veins and air (or "pneuma") flowed through arteries is especially perverted in that there is not a single word of his that has been handed directly down to us, and neither his dates of birth and death are known nor is it certain that he even had a direct association with Alexandria.[49] Everything is a work in progress. An image of Erasistratus pondering air-filled arteries being presented to generations of readers of the history of medicine as an example of "close but not close enough" (to discovering the circulation of blood) is less demeaning to Erasistratus than it is to medicine's reporters. It is without question that the solution to an understanding of the circulation of blood in ancient Greece was close at hand but for some "interfering incidents," and an understanding of those incidents is, of course, one reason for this book.

End of excursus

---

b. Petechial hemorrhage

Early clinical descriptions by the Hippocratics included a form of intradermal bleeding now called "petechial hemorrhage" in which a low blood platelet count, sometimes caused by severe infection, produces a punctate, red, non-elevated skin rash that does not blanch when pressed..

Lazarus Riverius (1589-1665) associated petechial hemorrhages with febrile illnesses, bruising, and a bleeding diathesis, and he indicated "capillary veins" as the source of the skin lesions.[50] There are many other descriptions of small skin lesions, exanthems, that probably were petechial, usually in association with severe infectious diseases, but the characteristic persistence of the lesions despite compression is not mentioned until 1829.[51] The delayed accurate recognition of petechial hemorrhage, from the Hippocratics to 1829, was 2,200 years. It may have been that, because the role of bleeding into the skin was felt to be obvious, there was no need of further characterization.

---

[49] Fraser, P. M., *The Career of Erasistratus of Ceos*, in *Instituto Lombardo*, 103:518-537, 1969. But see the discussion on liver cirrhosis on p. 275 of the present work, where Galen's recounting of autopsy findings by Erasistratus is consistent with schistosomiasis. This disease, at least in modern times, is more often found in the region supplied by the Nile than adjacent to the Orontes river near the site of ancient Antioch where Erasistratus is known to have worked, although schistosomiasis occurs there. Whether this epidemiology applied in Hellenistic times is unknown.

[50] Riverius, L., *The Practice of Physick in Seventeen Several Books*, London, 1655 (translated by N. Culpepper).

[51] The hemorrhagic nature of petechiae and purpura was probably assumed for centuries. There is an 1829 description of "petechial scurvy" in which a petechial rash is differentiated from flea bites. In the latter there is a central punctate lesion where the bite occurred, but, in contrast to petechiae, the surrounding redness blanches under pressure. See: Bateman, T., *A Practical Synopsis of Cutaneous Diseases*, London, 1829, 7th edition, pp. 152-153.

But it is its noncompressibility that separates a hemorrhagic rash from the myriad of other types of skin rashes characterized by small red lesions, including systemic illnesses like measles or roseola infantum and even typhoid fever. Riverius is singled out for mention here, 2000 years after the Hippocratic description of petechiae, merely because medical historians have selected his description of petechiae as particularly notable, despite the fact that even he did not comment on their incompressibility.

Comment - Petechial hemorrhages often are a clue to a very low platelet count,[52] an important aspect of many serious diseases, and the clue to petechial hemorrhage is the noncompressibility of its punctate rash, *i.e.*, pressure applied by a finger does not make the punctate rash blanch, for the blood has broken out of the tiny vessel and has bled into the skin itself. Blood platelets themselves would not be discovered until late in the 19th C, for they are much smaller than the cellular components of the blood. But their clinical relevance would have been discoverable without knowledge of platelets themselves. Petechial hemorrhages have been selected for discussion here because of their association with certain clinical syndromes. Thus, the peculiar, and relatively specific, nature of petechiae would have helped differentiate many diseases, thereby adding information on which to base prognosis. Petechial hemorrhages in smallpox are a bad prognostic sign, and the rash and epidemiology of epidemic typhus (at one time called "petechial fever") might have been better comprehended. Nosology would also have been furthered by such distinctions, and from that the epidemiology and other aspects of some diseases could have been recognized. While not as dramatic in clinical application as a magnifying lens or the speculum, improvements in prognostication and a better understanding of the epidemiology of diseases would have been most valuable had clinicians of the Middle Ages had access to information such as those clinical situations in which petechial hemorrhages could be identified.

c. Contagion and the implication of microorganisms

In the Hippocratic work *Nature of Man* can be found the statement: "But when an epidemic of one disease is prevalent [settles down on the people], it is plain that the cause is not regimen [way of life] but what we breathe in, and that this is charged with [emits] some unhealthful exhalation...the place should be moved as far as possible from that in which the disease is epidemic [established]."[53] The historian, Thucydides, wrote that the plague of Athens was thought to be a λοιμός (loimos, "pestilence"), not a λιμός (limos, a famine) that, arriving from Ethiopia and thence spreading from the Athenian port of entry, the Peiraeus, claimed its victims without regard for age or status. Aristotle considered phthisis, ophthalmias and a type of skin disease as contagious.[54] Varro (116-27 BC) clearly stated the existence of invisible microorganisms: "Like precautions must be taken against swampy places for the same reasons and particularly because as they dry, swamps breed certain animalculae which cannot be seen with the eyes and which we

---

[52] As is true with virtually everything in medicine, exceptions, not being discussed here, are neither rare nor easily explained.

[53] *Nature of Man*, IX. The translation is by W.H.S. Jones from the *Loeb Classical Library* series of Hippocrates, the brackets containing alternative translations of the author.

[54] Aristotle, *Problemata* VII, 8.

breathe through the nose and mouth into the body where they cause grave maladies."[55]

The next scholarly commentary on contagion was by Dr. Fracastoro (1484-1553), who divided contagions into three types: ". . . the first infects by direct contact only; the second does the same, but in addition leaves fomes, and this contagion may spread by means of that fomes...clothes, wooden objects, and things of that sort, which though not themselves corrupted, can, nevertheless, preserve the original germs of the contagion and infect by means of these; thirdly there is a kind of contagion which...infects at a distance; for example, pestilent fevers...."[56]

Comment – The spread of a contagious acute illness among a population is unlikely to escape a layman's observation, comment, and attempts at causal association in any community. It was no medical advance, therefore, when Isidore of Seville (560-636 AD) wrote the following: "Pestilence is a contagion that as soon as it seizes on one person quickly spreads to many. It arises from corrupt air and maintains itself by penetrating the internal organs. Although this generally is caused by powers in the air, it never occurs without the consent of Almighty God."[57] He does not suggest minute living organisms as a cause of disease. Thereby followed centuries of reliance on astrology and superstition as the means to escape a plague. Official quarantine for the plague was then recommended by a 14th C Italian physician, Raimondo da Vinario. The serious suggestions of disease-causing miasms and microorganisms by the Hippocratics and Varro and the 14th C quarantines were separated by 1500 years. Further observations along the lines established by the Hippocratics and contemporaries would, without technology, have led to considerations of airborne disease, fomite-dependent transmission of disease, the importance of crowding and of isolation, the role of sanitation and masks, and isolation/quarantine. Thus, some earlier Vinario had the potential to limit the destructiveness of Dark Ages plagues even without knowledge of microorganisms.

d. Central nervous system: Crossed association

The central nervous system was identified as the locus of consciousness in the Hippocratic work *On the Sacred Disease*,[58] and the ability to associate the focality of a seizure after trauma to the opposite side of the head was also identified by the Hippocratics.[59] They also noted some head wounds were associated with paralysis of the

---

[55] Varro, *Rerum Rusticarum de Agri Cultura*, Bk. I, 12, 2: "Note also if there are swampy places, both because of the same reason and because miniscule animals grow there that are impossible to detect with the naked eye, and through the air they enter inside the body through the mouth or nose and cause serious disease." Translation by the author. Translation in the text is by Fairfax Harrison, from his *Roman Farm Management*, New York, 1913.

[56] Fracastorius, *De Contagione et Contagiiosis Morbis et eorum Curatione, Libri III*; Bk. I, chapter 2, as translated by W. C. Wright in *Hieronymus Fracastorius*, New York, 1930. Note that the translated term "fomes" is a "fomite," an inanimate object that can passively transmit infectious particles.

[57] Isidore of Seville: *Etymology*, 4.6.17 (translation of Barney, S., Lewis, W., Beach, J., and Berghof, O., in *The Etymologies of Isidore of Seville*, Cambridge, 2006.

[58] "Therefore I declare the brain to be the vehicle of consciousness." *On the Sacred Disease*, XX, 1-2, translation by the author.

[59] "And a convulsion usually seizes one side of the body; should the injury be to the left side of the head, the convulsion seizes the right side of the body; but should the injury be on the right side of

opposite side of the body.[60] Herophilus (335-280 BC) differentiated sensory from motor nerve trunks. Aretaeus, in 140 AD, formally recorded that some neurological functions crossed from one side to the other via the spinal cord.[61] Aretaeus also distinguished central from peripheral causes of neurological paralysis. At about the same time, 140 AD, the notion of hemispheric specialization was put forth.[62]

In 1707 Valsalva (1666-1723) noted in postmortem studies that contralateral paralysis accompanied cerebral strokes, a crossed association some have termed the "Valsalva doctrine."[63] In describing his findings he does not refer to ancient authors.

Comment – The concept of crossed association, an indispensable tool for localizing central nervous system injury or disease, had it become common knowledge after its recognition in Hippocratic times, would have been such an intriguing observation to an interested clinician that its usefulness would have been promptly realized. Lateralizing signs related to the pupil of the eye, speech, and muscle weakness should have quickly followed. Had this happened there would have been two consequences: (1) many distinct neurological disorders would have been identified, and (2) the organic basis for many neurological disorders would have been substantiated, thereby lessening social stigmata as a consideration from innumerable patients in ensuing centuries. The elapsed time from Hippocrates to Valsalva was 2100 years.

5. Medical Technology -

---

the head, the convulsion will seize the left side of the body." *On Wounds of the Head*, XIX, 21-27, translation by the author.

[60] "and for some [there is] flacidity, and should the lesion be on the right side [of the head], the left; but should [it] be on the left, the right.) *Epidemics* VII, 35, translation by the author.

[61] "If, therefore, the commencement of the affection be below the head, such as the membrane of the spinal marrow, the parts which are homonymous and connected with it are paralyzed: the right on the right side and the left on the left side. But if the head be primarily affected on the right side, the left side of the body will be paralyzed: and the right if on the left side. The cause of this is the interchange in the origins of the nerves; for they do not pass along the same side, the right on the right side, until their terminations; but each of them passes over to the other side from that of its origin, decussating each other in the form of the letter X." Aretaeus of Cappadocia, *On the Causes and Symptoms of Chronic Disease*, London, 1856, translation of Francis Adams, MD, for the Sydenham Society, Book I, Chapter 7. The most obvious X crossing on gross inspection of the brain is that of the optic chiasm, not the motor tracts, and so it is not likely that Aretaeus was referring to the decussation of the pyramids in his discussion of crossed association. If he were, however, it would have been a brilliant observation.

[62] Lokhorst, G-J. C., *The First Theory about Hemispheric Specialization: Fresh Light on an Old Codex*, in *J.Hist. Med. Allied Sci.*, 51:293-312, 1996. Hemispheric specialization of the brain indicates a functional asymmetry, such as intellectual function being on the dominant side and perceptivity on the other. Lokhorst refers to the following passage in *De Semine*, a 12th C manuscript that transmits a 2nd C AD work by an unknown author: "That with which we understand is namely different from that with which we perceive. There are accordingly two brains in the head. The one gives us our intellect, the other provides the faculty of perception. That is to say: the brain on the right side is the one that perceives, whereas the left brain is the one which understands." The translation is by Lokhorst.

[63] Valsalva's important contribution was described in his *De Aure Humana Tractatus*, chapter 5, first published in 1704, and subsequently referred to in Morgagni's (1682-1771) classic work of 1761, *De Sedibus et causis morborum per anatomem indagatus*, III, 13.

a. Image magnification

Observations on the optical magnifying properties of water, glass, and crystal were made by the ancients. Opaque glass for decorative purposes was known in Egypt in the 15th C BC. Recent archeological finds have included a magnifying lens from Assyrian excavations at Nimrud dated to the 7th C BC and Cretan quartz lenses thought to be from archaic Greece (750-500 BC), one example being 8 mm in diameter and 4 mm thick, with an approximate magnification of 20X and a focal length of 12 mm,[64] and in the Archeological Museum in Rhodes are found a series of crystal lenses dated to the 6th C BC that have graded focal lengths engraved on their metal frames (Fig. 11). The burning of distant objects by focusing light on them by means of concave mirrors or of transparent spherical crystals or glass filled with water are well-described, even by Aristophanes in mid-5th C BC.[65] It has been proposed that the "microscopic" fine impressions in early Greek coinage probably required a magnifying visual aid. Also, during Hippocratic times there is mention of the "spyglass."[66] Magnifying mirrors were used, one for a notoriously salacious purpose mentioned by Rosenbaum in which a finger appeared as big as an arm.[67] Biconvex lenses had been made. There is a suspicion of the existence of lenses used in telescopes in the 1st C BC. Sidon and Tyre were Phoenician cities on the Mediterranean famous for glass production because of certain qualities of the sand available there. The invention of glassblowing and new molding processes permitted clear and transparent glass articles. In Rome, Seneca reported reading aids of glass balls filled with water. Although eyeglasses have not been identified, artificial glass eyes were used in ancient Rome. It is possible that the similarity of the crystalline lens of the eye was noted as homologous to a biconvex crystal.[68]

Reading glasses, which would have magnified objects, were first mentioned in *Lilium medicinae* by Bernard de Gordon in the 13th C, although "reading stones," quartz hemispheres, were used by monks with poor eyesight in the 11th C, indicating, not unexpectedly, the usefulness of magnifying instruments for poor vision was of perennial interest. But it was not until approximately 1600 that observations were made that again suggested further usefulness for magnifiers. The use of more than one lens in sequence, thereby permitting greater magnification, was carried out in Holland by the Jansson family. Optics in medical science were advanced with the work of a German Jesuit, Athanasius Kircher (1602-1680), who invented, among other things, a projector of still images and an early compound microscope with a 32X magnification with which he examined the blood of plague patients, although even a simple microscope (*i.e.*, one using only a single lens) was able to provide a magnification of 270X in the hands of Antonie

---

[64] Sines, G., Sakellarakis, Y. A., *Lenses in Antiquity*, in *Amer. J. Archeol.*, 91:191-196, 1987.

[65] Strepsiades: "At the pharmacist's have you seen this stone, lovely and clear, from which they ignite a fire? Socrates: "Do you mean the crystal lens?" and the following statements. Aristophanes, *Clouds*, vv.765-772, first performed in 423 BC.

[66] Alcaeus, frag. 53, οινος γὰρ ἀνθρώποις δίοπτρον ("Wine is a spy-glass through which we may view man as he is." (Translation of T. B. Harbottle, *Dictionary of Quotations [Classical]*, London, 1902.) And a 4th C fragment of Greek pottery showing a man looking through a tube has suggested use of an early telescope.

[67] Rosenbaum, J., *The Plague of Lust*, Paris, 1901, translation by "an Oxford M.A."

[68] Most facts collected here are from *When Glass Matters, Florence*, 2004, edited by Marco Beretta, especially chapters by G. di Pasquale and by M. Baretta, and William Locy, 1922, *Primitive Microscopes and some early Observations*, in *Transactions of the American Microscopical Society.*

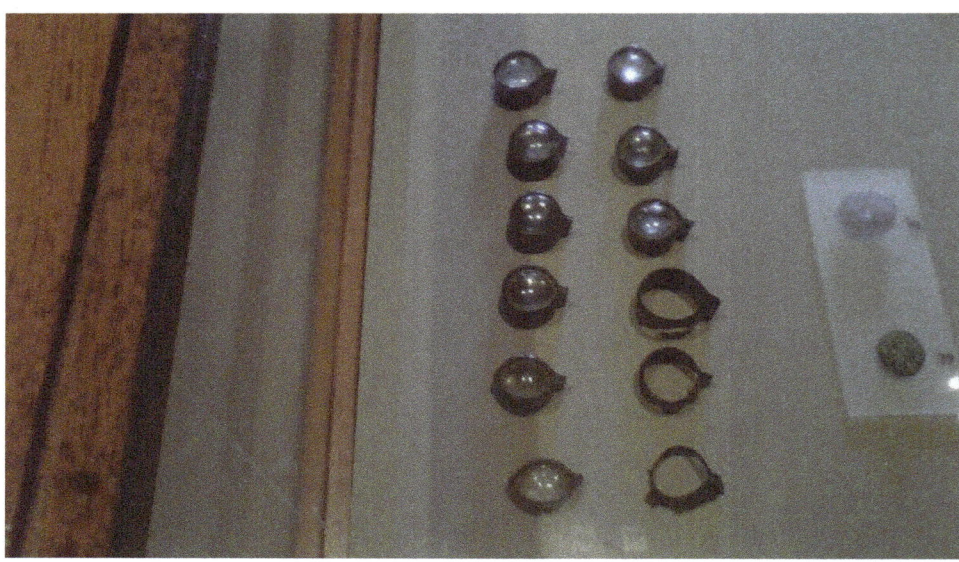

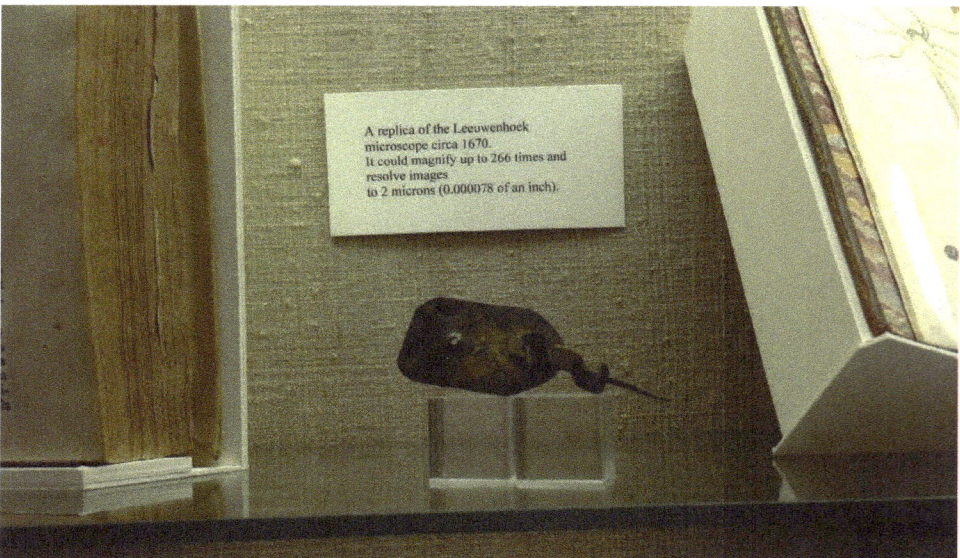

Fig. 11: Top - Quartz crystal lenses with graded focal lengths engraved on their frames. They were used for making fine jewelry in the 6th C BC on the Greek island of Rhodes, where they are now exhibited in the Archeological Museum. Photograph by the author.

Bottom - This replica of a single lens microscope measuring 2 inches long and 1 inch wide was built by Leeuvenhoek and was capable of 266X magnification, with which he was able to see bacteria. Human red blood cells are biconcave discs 7 μ in diameter, whereas common bacilli are thin rods 1-2 μ in length and cocci are spheres usually 0.5-1 μ in diameter. The resolution of this microscope is about 1 μ. The lenses were tiny droplets of glass, *i.e.*, biconvex, thus magnifying objects similar to that of a transparent round container of water. Photograph by the author.

van Leeuwenhoek a few years later.[69] The time between the early jeweler's lenses in the Rhodian museum (Fig. 11) and Kircher's look at a plague patient's blood was 2100 years.

Comment – The modern compound microscope with its series of lenses is the complex offspring of the single lens. With a single lens van Leeuwenhoek was able to see individual cells and bacteria (Fig. 11, bottom). From a clinical perspective, mere visual inspection of spinal fluid can reveal turbidity due to only a slight increase in cellular content, and such observations are made more sensitive with a mere 10X hand lens. The ability to see blood cells moving through capillaries in the web of a frog's foot can be made with a single lens of 50X. A theory of optics was developed by Euclid in the 3rd C BC. All the requirements for microscopic examination of tissue were available in Hippocratic times with the exception of the use of dyes to selectively stain tissues for better analysis. With but modest magnification, even as little as 10X by a small hand lens, small increases in cellular content of a clear fluid can be detected, or at least the fluid can be declared to not be clear and to contain suspended particles. The same magnification permits accurate identification or characterization of many dermatological lesions. The urine sediment would have quickly yielded up information on cells, casts, and crystals to relatively low magnification. But the Dark Ages and Medieval period did not see beyond uroscopy. Although local discoveries capable of magnifying images have occurred in most societies at one time or another, it was not until the Renaissance that a renewal and rediscovery of the science of optics could occur in the West, a 1600-year lapse.

b. Specula

In the Hippocratic work περὶ συριγγων (*Concerning Fistulae*, III, 331) there is mention of anoscopy as useful for directing treatment of anal fistulas, ulcerations, and papillomas. Procedures for curing the fistulas are carefully described, some aspects of which are still employed. There is also mention of a bivalved nasal speculum. Apparently, the earliest western vaginal speculum is one recovered from Pompeii, the city destroyed in 79 AD, although it is only logical that such an obvious and useful instrument would have been in use earlier by the Hippocratics. Indeed, the house where the speculum was found is thought to have belonged to a Greek surgeon. Greek terminology differed for the anorectal and the vaginal specula, indicating a specific nature to their designs. Several Greco-Roman trivalve specula in known.[70]

There is mention of various forms of speculum examination in the works of Aetius (5th C AD), Paulus Aegineta, and other early Byzantine writers, but much of this was a rewriting of Galen, Orobasius, and Soranus (2nd C AD). The application of their writings on the subject to contemporary practice of medicine is unlikely, and it appears that examination using various forms of specula, especially vaginal, virtually ceased in

---

[69] Kircher, in his *Scrutinium Physico-Medicum*, Rome, 1658, wrote "but not until after the wonderful invention of the microscope was it found that all putrid substances swarm with an innumerable brood of worms which are imperceptible to the naked eye, ...," and later reported seeing them in tissues of plague victims. It is debatable as to whether he actually visualized bacteria, but he could have. Kircher, a polymath in the early days of modern scientific discovery, resided most of his career in Rome and worked under the patronage of the Vatican.

[70] Longfield-Jones, G. M., *A Greco-Roman Speculum in the Wellcome Museum*, in *Med. Hist.*, 30:81-89, 1986.

the West until the 16th C, an exception being a small speculum for examining the nose and ears as described in 1363 by Guy de Chauliac.[71]

Comment: The extraordinary value of the speculum for pelvic examination in managing gynecological disease was lost to the West for at least 1200 years. The ignorance resulting from the lack of such a useful instrument propounded the enormous physical suffering to women during those years. Common disorders that would have been more effectively managed would have included abscesses, uterine vs. vaginal bleeding, tumors and polyps. Tragedies of the rectovaginal and vesicovaginal fistulae, the complications of birth trauma, rape, and inflammatory disease that commonly do not spontaneously heal, could have been moderated by curative surgical techniques had surgical procedures using specula been pursued, for the Hippocratics had already mastered the management of anal fistulae. The anoscope would have been very useful, but in terms of mortality and suffering its value pales beside the vaginal speculum.

c. Syringes

Bulb syringes for injection and extraction were used by ancient Egyptians in the course of mummifying, and they were widely available for enemas, douches, and for cleansing wounds and reachable internal purulence, including compound fractures and uterine lesions. In the Hippocratic work, *Fistulae*, (περὶ συγιγγων), section 6, it is stated: "Make this injection by tying the quill of a feather to a bladder and introducing it into the fistula. Continue to inject in this manner; ...."[72] Hollow tubes attached to the bladder of a pig could be used to force infusions into a cavity, so the concept of a syringe was common knowledge. Ctesibus (3rd C BC) invented a piston and cylinder mechanism (also reported by Hero of Alexandria in Section 57 of his *Pneumatica* of the 1st C BC and capable of injection and aspiration), and its clinical use was the aspiration of purulence. A translation of the term for the syringe of Celsus was "pus-puller," and he also used it for lavaging ears and for urological procedures (*de Medicine*, Bk. 7, chapters 26, 27 for urinary use, Bk. 5, chapter 28 for fistulae). Ctesibus is said to have been similar to a barber-surgeon, but was able to become, because of royal patronage, an inventor and ultimately was in charge of the famous Alexandrian library.

The use of syringes in the medieval period is suggested in some writings, although evidence of their existence is rare.[73] But a piston syringe was used by Hieronymus Brunschwig, in the 15th C,[74] and Abroise Pare (1510-1590) mentioned that syringes were a standard medical instrument. `

---

[71] Ricci, J. V., *The Development of Gynecologic Surgery and Instruments*, Philadelphia, 1949, especially chapter 6. Going forward, there are a few suggestions of vaginal instrumentation in the Dark Ages and Medieval Period. This is not surprising, for the practical importance in acquiring better visibility during examinations would occasionally inspire an involved person to try some ingenious method of doing so. It is, however, a combination of the religious and the modest that may explain the virtual absence of physical evidence of metallic vaginal speculum between Greco-Roman times and Renaissance.

[72] This is the translation of P. Potter in the *Loeb Classical Library Hippocrates*, vol. VIII, p. 397.

[73] Egan, G., *Material Culture of Care for the Sick*: *Some Excavated Evidence from English Medieval Hospitals and Other Sites*, in: *The Medieval Hospital and Medical Practice,* Burlington, 2007, B. Bower, editor, (chapt. 5, pp. 65-76).

[74] *Dis ist das buch der Cirurgia*, 1497.

Comment – The removal of substances from and the injection of substances into cavities and orifices was familiar to the Hippocratics and the piston syringe was available to Celsus. But until the 16th C the latter appears to have been a forgotten medical tool. Aspiration and injection in healing and in prevention was lost for more than 1000 years.

Eighteen areas of medicine have now been reviewed for brief discussions of their importance and the consequences of their absence during medieval times. Some, like internal podalic version, had relatively prompt and harmful consequences, and it can be confidently stated that as a result of the denial of its widespread application millions of women in the West over approximately 1500 years, primarily those in their younger childbearing years, would die from obstructed delivery of their fetuses, painfully and in anguish in the inevitable milieu of sorrow, and millions more would have complications of delivery.[75] With percussion, auscultation, and accurate measurements of temperature a more accurate clinical assessments of disease in living patients would have inspired a revolution in diagnosis and treatment. Lastly, a mature explanation of the human circulation, once realized, may have led to a scientific revolution within two centuries.

The problem was not that one or other of the eighteen items did or did not develop, and had they done so the course of medicine would have been dramatically altered. The problem also is not a lack of ingenuity to develop them, for ingenuity is an integral redundancy built into societies. The problem, instead, is that all eighteen were unable to maintain or regain relevance for more than a thousand years.

One can look on the Dark Ages as part of a natural progression of mankind but merely cyclical rather than a continuum. And the fact that modern life for many in the West has been, apart from the destructiveness of human agencies, so pleasant to an extent unimaginable in other ages, instills in moderns a tendency to think that the "more than a thousand years" was a necessary prelude to modernity, a poor period, perhaps, but bearing the seeds for a brighter tomorrow. It surely was not so. The cycle of degeneration predestined for societies as predicted by Plato was, in the West, fulfilled, most of its human consignment being the inescapable innocent victims of its collapse, not contributors to the cause.

---

[75] Podalic version can be performed externally and internally, and it is the latter that was described by Soranus, Celsus, and Aetius. The procedure is not always effective or appropriate for obstructed deliveries, and its use would certainly not have prevented all maternal and fetal morbidity and mortality resulting from obstructive delivery, but it would have saved many. Obstructed delivery in modern times affects perhaps one in twenty-five, or 4%, of term pregnancies. The development of forceps delivery and then caesarean section has vastly superceded internal podalic version in importance, but it remains a useful procedure, especially in areas with limited medical care.

CHAPTER NINETEEN

MEDICAL PRACTICE IN POST-ROMAN EUROPE

There is no fool, what'er the sex or grade,
Monk, barber, Jew, comedian, or old maid,
Soap-boiler he, or poor alchemist,
Bath-keeper, forger, or poor oculist,
But has his name among wise Doctors placed,
And thus through greed the Healing Art's disgraced.

Translation of John Ordronaux (Phila.,1870)
From the *Regimen Sanitatis Salernitanum* of 1480

Clinical medicine is the focus of this chapter. Hippocratic medical practice in the Eastern Roman Empire was never established, and in the West the Greco-Roman physician was replaced by the lay practitioner. Much Hippocratic learning was preserved, however, by 6th C Nestorians in Gondeshapour (Jondi-Shapur), passing in subsequent centuries into Persian and Islamic hands and then reentering Europe by the 11th C. Later, with a growing population and the creation of independent European city-states, medical practitioners organized through guilds and university faculties. But, instilling the words rather than the concepts of Hippocratic medicine, they produced, even through the 17th C, only the facade of a profession.

A. Introduction: Unforeseen Consequences

What is already known about the field of medicine is so vast that even if medical advances were to cease totally the world has in hand the necessary ingredients, if not the recipe, for a healthy global population. Recall, however, that rational medicine may have existed in Old Kingdom Egypt (*ca.* 3000 BC) but subsequently disappeared. And scientific medicine existed in ancient Greece (*ca.* 400 BC). It too disappeared. Therefore, at a time when the finding of water on Mars enlivens man's perception of his cosmic presence and self-importance, it is provocative to consider what may be in store for mankind and for the medical profession in the approaching centuries, in view of what has happened in the West once, and probably twice, in the past. For very likely the rational Egyptian practitioner of 3000 BC, having made such interesting clinical observations and treatments, would never have believed that his place would be taken by Pharaoh's priest, nor the scientific Hippocratic physician of 400 BC by Bishop Isidore of Seville (p. 309 and footnote) and medieval "leeches."[1] But as a prelude to such a consideration it is necessary to understand how the Hippocratic physician, after a hiatus of two millennia, resumed his rightful prominence.

---

[1] Definition of "leech": 1. *archaic*: physician, surgeon (Webster's Seventh New Collegiate Dictionary). It was only in the 18th C that "leech" began to mean blood-sucking annelid worms of the class Hirudinea then being used by physicians for purposes of limited phlebotomy. The etymology of the word has been traced to Anglo-Saxon and earlier, with a meaning akin to "healer" or "enchanter."

B. Clinical Practice after the Fall of Rome (5th - 10th C)

1. The East

In the Greco-Roman Middle East Hippocratic medical practice never did establish a foothold. Greek hegemony in the East was truncated by the western expansion of a new Persian (Parthian) dynasty (247 BC – 224 AD) and resurgent Persian culture, and by a disruptive eastern expansion of the Roman Empire. To put the quietus to any Hippocratic medicine remaining in the Near East, the next Persian dynasty was the Sassanid (226-651 AD) with its rigidly stratified Zoroastrian society under strong monarchical control. This succession of social cataclysms, therefore, is the likely reason that Hippocratic medical practice failed to gain a hold in the East at the time that it was vanishing in the West. A local exception was a university established in 271 AD in Gondeshapour, western Iran. When, in the 6th C AD, some Nestorian Christian scholars fled Byzantine religious persecution, they strengthened Greek learning in Gondeshapour, where, favored by the Sassanid monarchs, the university played a major role in the survival of many ancient Greek writings. The expatriated scholars and their students ultimately held many important positions within the university, and the arts and sciences are thought to have flourished. In the non-Byzantine East, therefore, Gondeshapour would provide the forthcoming Islamic Empire with the means for a promotion of learning that might be likened to later events in Florence and Padua upon their medieval and Renaissance reception of ancient Hellenic writings.

In the Islamic Middle East, the maturing of Islamic culture affected Eastern medicine in several ways. One of consequence was the transition in the 9th C of the hospital into an institution for curing as well as for caring. The hospital was also recognized as a place of medical learning. The famed Persian physician, Al-Razi (865-925), has been credited with founding a hospital in Baghdad, and some of his medical contributions derived from clinical observations made there.[2] Al-Razi was apparently a jeweler, lute-player, and alchemist before he decided to learn medicine at age thirty. He recorded some nine hundred case histories, and he urged young physicians to keep similar personal records. From his observations he concluded that the writings of Galen were often incorrect, even writing a book of the subject, *al-shukuk ala Jalinus* ("Doubts about Galen"). It is unclear if another prominent Persian physician, Avicenna (980-1037), had an association with a hospital, and his reputation as a clinician is in dispute, although he was an acknowledged expert physician by age eighteen years, having begun his studies on his own, it is said, but two years earlier.[3, 4] Ibn al-Haytham (965-1040) was another

---

[2] In addition to well over one hundred books on medicine, Abu Bakr al-Razi wrote many works on astronomy, alchemy, mathematics, philosophy, and theology. A fundamental work is adjudged to be *Kitab al-tajari*, a recording of his case histories, personal data perhaps unique in ancient Eastern medicine. He died at age sixty years, thus accomplishing all this within the span of thirty years even though in his later years he is said to have become blind. Al-Razi was highly esteemed in the West, even the learned Maimonides (1135-1204) quoting from al-Razi's philosophical writings in his *Guide for the Perplexed*.

[3] Famous for his *Medical Canon*, Avicenna carried forward the ideas of Hippocrates, Aristotle, and Galen. His work was studied and taught in the West for five hundred years.

[4] C. A. Millan, in *The Case Histories in Medieval Islamic Medical Literature: Tajarib and Mujarrabat as Source*, in *Med. Hist.*, 54:195-214, 2010, p. 195, notes an inclination by Avicenna

profound medical thinker who wrote his most famous work, *Book on Optics*, while in prison when he was about fifty years old. He also authored commentary on many works of ancient Greek authors, including those on geography, the cosmos, mathematics, and philosophy, adding some personal observations to his critical analyses. It has been pointed out with pride that those Muslim physicians of renown were also philosophers, mathematicians, and scientists.[5] A few physicians, however, do not a profession make. When, in the 7th C, Arabic culture came to dominate the Near and Middle East, learning was restricted to the elite, for the Koran alone was thought sufficient for the masses.[6]

In the Byzantine Empire on the other hand government/municipal physicians were civil servants in a system of socialized medicine, salaried by taxation, in return for which they were "preferred" to serve the poor.[7] Termed *Archiatri*, merit probably meant little for advancing within a byzantine bureaucracy. In 335 AD pagan temples had been abolished by order of Constantine the Great, who had recently embraced Christianity, and some were requisitioned for use as hospitals. These institutions were principally a charity for the poor, a detached facility for lepers, and a site where the presumed contagious could be housed. They were staffed by religious orders. The term "hospital," derived from the Latin *hospes* meaning "guest" or "host," indicates how their original function differed from the modern hospital.[8] Baas suggests the function of "physicians" was limited to that of a military medic or corpsman, sometimes even being paid per wounded soldier taken from the battlefield, a task that had been similarly assigned to medical attendants of the Roman Legions.[9] Furthermore, the non-military practitioner, eschewing surgery, was very much an economic captive of his ability to popularize his particular proprietary remedies:

---

and several other Islamic medical authors, but not including al-Razi, toward the self-promoting "scientific rhetoric" of Galen.

[5] This is seen in the history of medicine composed by Ibn Abi Usaibi (1203-1270 AD), for that work, although specifically addressing physicians, is considered a comprehensive masterpiece on Muslim science. See: *A History of Muslim Philosophy*, Weisbaden, 1966, M. M. Shariff, editor, vol. 2, for the section on medicine.

[6] O'Leary, De Lacey, *How Greek Science Passed to the Arabs*, London, 1949, especially chapter 2, where he states science and philosophy were greatly circumscribed under the patronage of the royal courts, philosophy being viewed as close to heresy, that "the inspired Qur'an was well adapted for the spiritual life of the unlettered and simple....," and that such scholarship "was confined to one privileged coterie."

[7] For a description of duties see: *The Theodosian Code and Novels and the Sirmondian*, Princeton, 2008 (10th printing, translation by C. Pharr), especially Book XIII, 3, 12.

[8] Here the concept of hospital must be distinguished from the *pandocheion*, an eastern Mediterranean institution that functioned as a hostel for travelers. With Christianization of the Roman Empire (4th C AD) there emerged from the *pandocheion* the *xenodocheion* as a "charitable hostelry" that sometimes became a hospital and was popular in the West and, with a change of name, under Islam in the Middle East. See: Constable, O. R., *Housing the Stranger in the Mediterranean World*, Cambridge, 2003. D. Riesman, in *The Story of Medicine in the Middle Ages*, New York, 1936, chapter 33, comments that later medieval hospitals were not so much places for treatment as a place to pass time until well enough to return to work. As centuries passed they became more prominent in communities as feudal lords displayed their munificence, the statement being made that the high-and-mighty paid handsomely to build personally glorifying edifices of healing that they had done so much to fill.

[9] Baas, J. H., *Outlines of the History of Medicine and the Medical Profession*, New York, 1889, H. E. Handerson, translator, p. 213.

"What must have been the general condition of medicine in that day may be judged from the fact that frequently the sole and extensive reputation of a Byzantine physician depended singly and solely upon some nostrum invented by him." (*ibid.*, p. 214)

During the Byzantine domination in the East, which lasted from 395 to 1453 AD, Garrison lists but four practitioners who merit historical attention: Oribasius (326-403), Aetius of Amida (6th C), Alexander of Tralles (525-605), and Paulus of Aegineta (625-690).[10] Writings of Galen were available, but Hippocratic works were rarely seen, although Hippocrates is mentioned by the 7th C physician, Theophilus, famous for his treatise on uroscopy. The status of Byzantine medicine, as expressed by a modern writer, seems remarkably similar to Asiatic medicine as interpreted from the *Huang Ti Nei Ching Su Wen* and the *Charaka Samhita* (see chapters 4 and 5 of this work).

"Overall, Byzantine medicine is characterized as a holistic therapeutic method for the body and soul, a prophetic and preventive science, a free function, an art of peace, philanthropy and justice, a divine science with a humane perspective and treatment-working miracles."[11]

And so it was that the legacy of Byzantine medicine during Europe's Dark Ages would amount to nothing, an opinion implied by several prominent historians of the Byzantine State, who make no mention whatever of the profession of medicine in their works.[12] Byzantium could hardly bequeath to subsequent generations something it had never really acquired. The backdrop of all this was a precipitous decline in urban life that occurred throughout the Byzantine Empire during the 7th and 8th centuries.[13] Although two centuries had to pass, it took the arrival of Islam to do what Byzantium did not.

In those eastern regions formerly under Greek hegemony it had been a feature of Hellenistic culture to ally itself with the upper classes, not commoners. In Egypt, for example, no effort was made by the Greeks to Hellenize the average Egyptian. As the Greek language was thought difficult for the Egyptians to master, even ordinary commerce of the marketplace was carried out in Egyptian. Therefore, given the rigidly authoritarian governance throughout the East, benefits of Greek learning were restricted to a privileged few. The noxious effect of this on the profession would be documented in the public opinion of later Byzantium:

". . . and the constant upbraiding and mockery of doctors as incompetent, negligent, failures, providers of counterfeit medicines, and greedy professionals charging exorbitant fees."

---

[10] Garrison, F. H., *An Introduction to the History of Medicine*, Phila., 1921, 3rd edition, pp. 82-85. For a more extensive list, along with biographical sketches and assessments of accomplishments, see: Prioreschi, P., *A History of Medicine*, volume IV – *Byzantine and Islamic Medicine*, Omaha, 2001, Chapter 4.

[11] Eftychiadis, A. C., *Byzantine Nephrology*, in: *Amer. J. Neph.*, 17:217-221, 1997.

[12] G. Ostrogorsky, *History of the Byzantine State*, translated by J. Hussey, rev. edition, New Brunswick, 1969; A. A. Vasiliev, *History of the Byzantine Empire*, 2nd edition, Madison, 1952; W Treadford, *A History of the Byzantine State and Society*, Stanford, 1997.

[13] Islamic conquests in the Near East and North Africa removed the source of great wealth from the Byzantine Empire that previously had supported what was for some an opulent way of life. For a modern perspective of events of this era see: Browning, R., *The Byzantine Empire*, Washington, D. C., 1992 (revised edition), section on "The New Order."

There appear to have been few physicians and no physicians' organizations, and even government must have considered it a waste of time for the State to control them. [14]

2. The West

In the early Dark Ages there appear to have been few, if any, true physicians in the West. Baas quotes an unidentified source who states "Physicians for the so-called common people" were "for the most part monks."[15] There was also a fatalistic view of disease, so prevalent in those dark times and earlier expressed so clearly by Cyprian (d. 258 AD) in his work *De Mortalitate*, written at the time of a great plague:

> "That now the bowels loosened into a flux exhaust the strength of the body, that a fever contracted in the very marrow of the bones breaks out into ulcers of the throat, that the intestines are shaken by continual vomiting, that the blood-shot eyes burn, that the feet of some or certain parts of their members are cut away by the infection of diseased putrefaction, that, by weakness developing through the losses and injuries of the body, either the gait is enfeebled, or the hearing impaired, or the sight blinded, all this contributes to the proof of faith. What greatness of soul it is to fight with the powers of the mind unshaken against so many attacks of devastation and death."[16]

No more dramatic tribute to therapeutic nihilism has ever been penned.

The Church consistently dissuaded clergy from practicing medicine, especially outside the monasteries. Early hospitals were not for medical instruction, for they functioned, as in the Byzantine East, more as almshouses or places to put those with frightening or presumed contagious diseases such as leprosy. The local medical practitioner was usually an unlettered, self-taught successor to itinerant empirical practitioners. Perhaps what was lacking was a medical St. Jerome. Jerome (340-420 AD) was partial to medicine, considering its knowledge and practice in no way inconsistent with religious tenets. It was Jerome who collected, selected, and compiled historical evidence for the Church, thereby bracing it against future assaults. But medicine is not dogma; it is constantly changing and infinitely more complex, and it is based on facts rather than faith. Still, Jerome provided, in part, what medicine lacked: a respected and renowned authority. But it takes many minds to manage a complex profession, keep it on track, and protect it from attack. This is what the Hippocratics had managed to do and what Romans and Byzantines failed to do.

There had been, early on, the *archiatri*, medical officers hired to provide

---

[14] Much documentation is cited by G. C. Maniatus in: *The Domain of Private Guilds in the Byzantine Economy, Tenth to Fifteenth Centuries*, Dumbarton Oaks Papers, No. 55, pp. 339-369. The cited quotation is from pp. 350-351, and it in turn references several additional citations. It is debatable as to whether or not a valid medical profession even existed. This is also suggested in Dumbarton Oaks Papers #38, *Art, Medicine, and Magic in Early Byzantium*, a monograph by Gary Vikan detailing the overwhelming importance of magic, astrology, and religious icons in that earlier Byzantine age for seeking cures and in preventing disease. Nevertheless, by the 12th C medicine had been purged of magic by the Byzantine Church. See: Duffy, J., *Reactions of Two Byzantine Intellectuals to the Theory and Practice of Magic*, in *Byzantine Magic*, (Dumbarton Oaks), Washington, D. C., 1995, H. Maguire, editor, pp. 83-97.

[15] Baas, J. H., *Outlines of the History of Medicine and the Medical Profession*, New York, 1889, H. E. Handerson, translator, p. 322.

[16] *Thasci Caecili Cypriani de Habitu Virginum*, Washington, D.C., 1932, translation by Keenan, A. E. St. Cyprian, *De Mortalitate*, Bk. 14.

inexpensive health services to the poor and to supervise municipal medical practices in cities. These tax-exempt positions, a Roman version of the earlier Greek office of public physician (the δημιουργός, demiourgos), had been strictly limited by Rome and were obtained by public competition.[17] But by the 7th C AD Greek and Roman institutions of higher learning had been superceded by monastic schools, and the *archiatri* and other public institutions of Roman cities were no more. This was anticipated by Cassiodorus (*ca.* 485-585), who indicated the Church's place in fulfilling this need in his "*On Monks Having the Care of the Infirm.*"[18] And beyond the depopulated European cities frequently lay the tribal and mystical medicine with which this book opened its first chapter.

And so it was that monastery schools came to fill the educational void left by collapse of Western cities and their institutions, maintaining and copying manuscripts, a process well under way by the 9th C.[19] There was, however, not much to work with. It has been calculated that the inventories of all German libraries from the 9th to 12th centuries included but fifty-five medical manuscripts.[20]

To conclude this Section, in the West medical practice in the Dark Ages was caught up by the dismantling of society. It is to the credit of religious institutions that some attempt was made to fill the vacuum thus created, and the clergy were literate. But, lacking both knowledge and method, the task was far too great, and they could not qualitatively supplant the scientific practitioner. In the East the course of medical practice in Byzantium was one to be expected if Hippocratic medicine had failed to take hold in the first place, and so it was and it never changed. Only later were Hippocratic writings adopted and expanded by some Islamic physicians who then proceeded to model their medical practices accordingly, at least in their writings.

---

[17] Nutton, V., *Archiatri and the Medical Profession in Antiquity*, in *Papers Brit. School at Rome*, 32:191-226, 1977.

[18] A. Cassiodorus, *De Institutione Divinarum Litterarum*, chapter XXXI, De monachis curem infermorum habentibus. As for the medical capability of monasteries themselves, the famous Fountains Abbey in England, founded in 1132, had a sizeable infirmary run by the *infirmarius* who served as guardian and nurse ("doctor, nurse, and spiritual adviser") for sick monks and monks "who had been professed fifty years." There was a "lay-brother" infirmary at the opposite end of the monastery that was in charge of the *cellarius*, the person responsible for the community's food and care of guests; St. Benedict (*cap.* xxxi) had ruled "Let him have the charge of everything." The Abbey also had two *hospitia*, or "guest-houses," not hospitals, also under care of the *cellarius.*" That was the extent of medical care available to an elect group of people of that era. What must have been available to the others? (This information is from: Oxford, A. W., *The Ruins of Fountains Abbey*, Ripon, 1967.)

[19] Beccaria, A., *I Codice di Medicine del Periodo Presalernitano*, Rome, 1956, cited by V. Bullough in *Universities, Science and Medicine in the Medieval West*, Burlington, 2004, Chapter I, *The Study of Medicine and the Medieval University*,

[20] Streeter, E. C., *Mediaeval Libraries of Medicine. 500 A. D. to 1500 A. D., Bull. Med. Libr. Assoc.*, 10:15-20, 1921. Only with the invention of the printing press can any quantities of medical books be identified in private and public libraries. There were also no known medical book-lists from the cathedral schools, from Salerno, or from Monte Cassino. "It can only be surmised that some classical medical texts were available." Compare this with the library of the father of Quintus Sammonicus Serenus, a 3rd C AD writer and poet who composed a long treatise on medicine and magic; that library purportedly contained 60,000 volumes.

C. Clinical Practice in the High Medieval Period and Early Renaissance

A surge in capitalism throughout most of Europe consequent to distant travel and trade was associated with development of guilds in the 11th and 12th centuries, and population increased from about twenty million in the 5th C AD to sixty million in the 14th C. The increasing population and prosperity of this period, however, proved not to be a stimulus for advances in medical practice, and two important scholarly works on the economic history of medieval Europe do not mention a single word relevant to the medical profession.[21]   Thus medicine and the newly devised medical guild were economically irrelevant even though society experienced what Adelson has called the "commercial revolution" of 1100 to 1348.[22] Once again medical progress and the natural state of medical practice are found causally unassociated with either prosperity or capitalism.

Monastic orders in the West provided both the copying and the libraries necessary to retain rudimentary scholarship. In the East monastic libraries were small, perhaps containing one hundred books, and even the famous monastery in Patmos had, in 1201, only 330 books, an "exceptionally large" collection.[23] Furthermore, virtually all were religious works. But it was with the founding of a university in Bologna in 1088 that free-standing institutions of learning began appearing in the larger European cities. As these universities acquired more traditional features there are many descriptions of schools of medicine, of courses taught, of teachers' fees, of oaths at graduation, and of feuding student collectives. Control of the universities lay with the Church, and ancient texts, including medical ones, were subjects of religious glosses.[24] Those texts must have been well-worn, for Putnam writes that even in 15th C Paris there were no independent booksellers.[25] Early universities were similar to trade guilds and may have been derived from them.[26] Medical training was incorporated into curricula, and by the 13th – 14th centuries Compayre states that there were at least thirty European cities that had centers of medical education.[27] Once medical schools were established medical training was treated as a serious matter, the course of study taking up to nine years, even twelve years at Oxford University. The training of barber-surgeons, surgeons, and pharmacists involved a educational pathway of apprenticeships rather than university courses, although similar long periods were required for apprenticeships.[28] University instruction "was a literal interpretation of hallowed texts" (*ibid.*, p. 252), done under religious guidance to ensure that health of the soul took precedence in patient management.

---

[21] Pirenne, H., *Economic and Social History of Medieval Europe*, translated by I. E. Clegg, New York, 1939, chapter 5; Adelson, H. L., *Medieval Commerce*, Princeton, 1962, Chapter 6.

[22] Adelson, H. L., *Medieval Commerce*, Princeton, 1962, p. 69.

[23] L. Casson, *Libraries in the Ancient World*, New Haven, 2001, p. 142.

[24] Baas, J. H., *Outlines of the History of Medicine and the Medical Profession*, New York, 1889, H. E. Handerson, translator, Section Second, second period, *History of Medieval Medicine*, for his detailed description of medicine during this period.

[25] Putnam, G. H., *Books and Their Makers in the Middle Ages*, New York, 1896, vol. 2.

[26] The term "university" is derived from the Latin *universus*, meanings including "all in one" and "association." It has also been suggested that medical colleges were the outgrowth of the singular and popular center at Salerno (see p. 336*f* for its history).

[27] Compayre, G., *Abelard, and the Origin and Early History of Universities*, New York, 1893, p. 242. Compayre was a prominent French professor and theorist of education.

[28] Bullough, V. L., *Training of the Nonuniversity-Educated Medical Practitioners in the Later Middle Ages*, in *J. Hist. Med. and Allied Sci.*, 14:446-458, 1959.

Remarkably, the first book on anatomy to be based on dissection of a human cadaver, written in 1316, was not even published until 1478, at which time it helped establish anatomy as part of the medical curriculum.[29] In contrast to university training, surgeons, barber-surgeons, and pharmacists were exposed from the very onset of training to the naïve but frequently useful empirical practices of practitioners who had to deal with the daily realities of clinical practice, experiences that often placed the practice of apprentices ahead of university graduates. This explains why the barber-surgeon and pharmacist guilds grew in importance and were viewed as a threat by traditional medical guilds.

Nevertheless, organization of any sort profited medical professionals, if not the patient, and, as the medieval period progressed, more named practitioners are recorded and medical writings appear and multiply. This would seem like progress. Instead, "Every idiot, priest, Jew, monk, actor, barber, and old woman, fancy themselves physicians."[30] This quotation, while an indication of the indiscriminate nature of medical practice, implies the existence somewhere of true physicians. Another medieval opinion was "*ubi treis medici, duo athei,*" and it set Sir Thomas Browne to write his famed *Religio Medici* to counteract that trend. It is to be expected, given the occasional stance of the Church against complicity of its devotees in practicing medicine, that atheists would be more often found among medical practitioners than otherwise, but the ratio of two out of three practitioners being atheists is arresting. This proverb also implies the existence of practitioners distinct from those listed in the opening sentence of this paragraph. Where were these freethinking physicians to be found, and what were their practices like?

Monastic libraries had a few medical books. Here is a list of the categories and quantity of books and manuscripts in several 15th C monastic libraries[31]:

Divinity	175
Scholastic	89
Epistles, controversial literature	65
History	54
Arts, mathematics, astrology	31
Philosophy	13
Law	6
Biology	3

The Benedictine Order in particular retained an interest in Hippocrates and Galen, but both Dr. George Coulton and Dr. B. L. Gordon viewed the ultimate culprit in medicine's decline to be the Church.[32] As the above list suggests, however, medicine was not a

---

[29] The work of Mondino de' Luzzi (1275-1326), *Anathomia*, is not considered a strategic advance in medical knowledge. It represents, instead, an example of the sad state of medicine, both in 1316 and in 1478. Likewise, the *Tractatis de Herbis*, Salerno, *ca.* 1280-1300, was the first book in the West to include botanical drawings illustrated from nature, another example of diffident progress, given that the herbal of Dioscorides (40-90 AD) defined five hundred botanicals and served as the basis of pharmacology for fifteen centuries. It is not known, however, if that work, *De Materia Medica*, was originally illustrated.

[30] Cited by: Benham G., in *Benham's Book of Quotations*, London, 1949, 579a, a restatement of the quotation opening this chapter.

[31] Putnam, G. H., *Books and Their Makers During the Middle Ages*, New York, 1896, 2 vols., p. 142 of vol. 1.

[32] Coulton, G. G., *Medieval Panorama*, New York, 1938, p. 447; Gordon, B. L., *Medieval and Renaissance Medicine*, New York, 1959, see Introduction.

preoccupation of 15th C clerics. Dr. Gordon discusses true practitioners, noting that their existence must for the most part be inferred. There were, after all, schools at "Alexandria, Constantinople, Berytus, Caesarea, Laodicea, Pergamon, Antioch, Athens, Rome, Athenaeum, Ravenna, Marseilles, Autun, Bordeaux, Treves, Toulouse, Poitiers, Lyons, Narbonne, Arles, Vienna and Besancon."[33] But the objects of study were the Seven Liberal Arts. Derived from Varro (116-27 BC), these now included arithmetic, geometry, astronomy, music, grammar, dialectic, and rhetoric. Varro's "architecture" and "medicine" had since been relegated to the technical rather than scholarly subjects, and not worthy of inclusion among the liberal arts.[34] Those trained physicians for whom there is substantiation involved themselves primarily with legal matters such as expert testimony in courts of law. Others were physicians to emperors, princes, and popes.

Still, motivation and curiosity were active among entering medical students, for at personal risk some obtained cadavers for dissection. The Church, in the Fourth Lateran Council of 1215, prohibited clergy of major orders from procedures that shed blood, a Council of Rheims in 1131 forbade the practice of civil law and medicine, and the Council of Tours (1163) forbade clergy from study of "worldly laws," including healing "bodies of sick brothers."[35] It also separated "internal" medicine from surgery and took the latter out of clerical hands, an important boost to the barber-surgeons, and it prohibited students from practicing medicine prior to graduation unless that practice was pursued outside the city walls. Early in the 13th C paid practitioners are described who periodically visited infirmaries, overseeing the purchase of herbs and other medicines, and diagnosing and prescribing treatments for the sick.[36] There was also the reappearance of practitioners hired by cities, a practice not recorded in the West for six centuries.[37] Dr. David Riesman paraphrases a 1441 AD oath made by new physicians at the University of Paris[38]:

> 1. To observe faithfully the secrets, honor and practice, customs and duties of the Faculty with all his power and no matter what may happen, never to go against them.
> 2. To render honor and respect to the Dean and to all the masters of the Faculty.
> 3. To aid the Faculty against any one who undertakes anything whatever against the statutes or the honor of the Faculty and especially against those who practice illegally and to submit to the punishments inflicted by the Faculty in case of default.
> 4. To be present in academic costume at all masses ordered by the Faculty, to arrive at the latest before the end of the epistle and to remain until the end of the office, be it even a university mass for the dead, under punishment of an ecu, and likewise under a similar penalty to be present every Saturday at the mass of the school, vacation time excepted.
> 5. To be present at the exercises of the Faculty and at the arguments of the school during two years and to maintain a thesis upon one question of medicine and hygiene, and finally to observe always peace and good order and a decent mode of argumentation in the scientific discussions prescribed by the Faculty.

---

[33] *Ibid.*, Chapter IV.

[34] Abelson, P., *The Seven Liberal Arts, A Study in Medieval Culture*, New York, 1906, p. 60.

[35] This and related restrictions on the clergy are what moved the lowly barber-surgeon into a place of prominence well into the 18th C. See: Seigworth, G. R., *Bloodletting over the Centuries*, in *N. Y. State J. Med.*, 80:2022-2028, 1980; also: Kjeldsen, A., *The Origins and Reception of the "Medical Canons" of the Fourth Lateran Council*, Apr., 2009, http://voxindeserto.wordpress.com/

[36] Ridyard, S. J., editor, *Death, Sickness and Health in Medieval Society and Culture*, Univ. of the South Press, 2000, p. 16-19.

[37] Sistrunk, T. H., *The Function of Praise in the Contract of a Medieval Public Physician*, in: *J. Hist. Med. Allied Sci.*, 48:320, 1993.

[38] Riesman, D., *The Story of Medicine in the Middle Ages*, New York, 1936, p. 158.

The exclusivity of this oath was one reason, in addition to guild monopoly and the prestige of the university, that the medical profession, despite the inadequacy of its canon, was able to insulate itself from competition and thereby to increase its valuation without increasing its value.

The day-to-day practice of trained practitioners became better defined as literacy improved. It is clear, therefore, that whereas the Medieval Period can be viewed as a successor to the Dark Ages, in medicine there was no such advance to a higher orbit. The importance of astrology, the enormous pharmacopoeia and the often disgusting contents of its preparations,[39] incantations, bezoars and amulets to protect against poisons and plagues, prayers, patron saints of all and sundry diseases along with the relics assigned to them, all these were important techniques of practitioners who flourished in the later medieval period, techniques that found their precursors in the Dark Ages.[40] The field of surgery was not exempt from developmental paralysis. The surgeon, Guy de Chauliac (1300-1368), wrote his *Chirurgia* in Latin in 1363. It was then printed in French in 1478, and with little competition the 68th edition was being published in 1683.

There was little, if any, difference between the contemporary "medicus" and the charlatan except that the former had official recognition, perhaps by a university, perhaps by guild membership, perhaps by a purchased local license. The miserable status of medicine led to the first licensing of physicians in 1140 by Roger II of Sicily: "The spurious medicine of the time, as practiced under the sanction of the Holy See had raised up a herd of ignorant and mercenary ecclesiastical charlatans. These operated by means of chants, relics, and incense; and their enormous gains were one of the chief sources of revenue to the parish and the monastery, and a corresponding burden on the people."[41]

---

[39] For an eye-catching list of popular remedies, such as that described by Mercier, C. A. in *Astrology in Medicine*, London, 1914, p. 89: "An awful and characteristic combination is the following: Pounded earthworms, ants' eggs, asses' dung, urine of a bull or of a virgin, vipers' fat, the water that had been used washing a corpse," see: Riesman, D., *The Story of Medicine in the Middle Ages*, New York, 1936, chapter 29.

[40] In contrast, the Byzantine East had by this time developed an antipathy to magical devices, and indeed outlawed them. See: *Duffy, J., Reactions of Two Byzantine Intellectuals to the Theory and Practice of Magic*, in *Byzantine Magic*, H. Maguire, editor, (Dumbarton Oaks) Washington, D. C., 1995, chapter 5.

[41] Scott, S. P., *History of the Moorish Empire in Europe*, London, 1904, vol. III, p. 26. The grandson of Roger, Frederick II (1194-1250), who became Holy Roman Emperor, extended further the autocratic hand to include the managing of cities and schools, including the medical school in Salerno, an action coincident with the decline in the latter's popularity, just as he was prominent at the time of the decline of the medical reputation of Monte Cassino (see footnote, p. 332). Frederick II's laws, proclaimed in 1240, were well-considered and were to protect against charlatans, costliness, collusion with pharmacists, and poor medical teaching, even stipulating that, in the University of Naples, surgery should be included in the study of medicine and receive equal attention, a stipulation others would have been wise to follow (see: JAMA, Oct. 26, 1907, and for a translation of Frederick's law, plus an effusive commentary on its value to society, see: Walsh, J. J., *The Popes and Science*, New York, 1911, Appendix III, p. 419-423). But the deeper problem lay in what was being taught and practiced rather than who was teaching and practicing. The laws specified the use of 1200-year-old textbooks, namely Hippocrates and Galen, required three years of preliminary training in "logic," that being the liberal arts, and an examination in "legal form." Otherwise the medical training was the usual apprenticeship, although under the aegis of the university. Frederick's legislation may have indeed inhibited the work of charlatans, but it also (1) codified the grossly inadequate existing medical knowledge of the time, thus stamping it with a royal imprimatur, and (2) threatened local non-charlatan empirical healers who might have

After this condemnation sanctions against poorly prepared or covetous practitioners appeared in major cities throughout Europe, and within a century licensing was commonplace.

Yet public opinion was appropriate for this profession of presumptive healers. Petrarch (1304-1374) quoted a popular proverb of his time, "You lie like a physician" (*Mentiris ut medicus*). He wrote a pamphlet denigrating the profession: *Contra Medicum quendam Invectivae* (Invectives against a Physician):

> "But suppose - I shudder to think it! - that the pope had paid his debt to nature. Even the vicar of immortal God is mortal. What great and unresolved discord there would have been among you concerning his pulse, his humors, his critical day, and his medications. Ignorant of the real cause of his illness, you would have filled heaven and earth with dissonant cries. Wretched are the sick who trust in your aid!"

Petrarch's opinion is carried forward ably by Montaigne (1533-1592), who did not go to physicians, for "they just prop you up temporarily." There is little, therefore, to be gained; if it's time to go, go! Or, as he put it, "We ought to let diseases take their course...," judging nature's remedies superior to the physician's. He recognized that good outcomes were often independent of the physician's efforts, and therefore he avoided physicians' potions until he was better, just as some physicians themselves "seldom used medicinal drugs." Nevertheless, he recognized the difficult situation of the internist, who could not actually see the problem with which he had to deal, and "that there is no physic which has not something hurtful in it," an undeniable pharmaceutical fact of life. He counted as important the patient's confidence in his physician as more important than treatment from a learned and experienced physician with whom he is unacquainted. But overall this 16th C wit and moralist had a poor opinion of the profession, for he assigns a major reason for medicine's good reputation to "the fear of death and of pain." Furthermore, "each physician seems to alter what another physician prescribed," indicating they were more concerned about reputation and income.[42] Chaucer (1343-1400) chose to be less indignant with practitioners of his day, for there were none like his Doctor of Physic "for he was grounded in astronomye," colluded with the apothecary so that "for each of them made other for to wynne," and therefore, not surprisingly, "he loved gold in special."[43] Dante (1265-1321) made few comments, none negative, but then he had earlier received some medical training.[44] A practicing physician, Heinrich Agrippa, wrote in 1530 that there was more danger in the practitioner and his medicine than in the sickness itself, and that medicine was the "art of manslaughter," although it was allowed

---

discovered improved therapies or patient management. The laws also required two visits daily to see a sick patient, which would have restricted to the extreme the number of patients capable of being seen per day by the physician. Let this be a warning for those who feel quality can be legislated. It is probable that the laws were ignored for the most part and that village/rural life went on after those laws much as it had before. The evidence for this is the dismal course the medical profession followed for the next five hundred years.

[42] *The Essays of Michel de Montaigne,* translation of Charles Cotton, chapter 2.37.

[43] Chaucer's physician has also been characterized as a "secular cleric": Ussury, H., *Chaucer's Physician*; Tulane Studies in English, No. 19, Tulane, 1971.

[44] In his *Purgatorio*, Canto XXIX, Dante describes [St. Luke] "as one of the disciples of that great Hipppocrates, whom Nature made for those living creatures whom she holds most dear [the human race]." Vernon, W. W., *Readings on the Purgatorio of Dante*, New York, 1907, vol.2.

to pass for philosophy.[45] But even Agrippa, as a true representative of his age, was part of the "occult Renaissance," his major work being *De Occulta Philosophica*.[46] The advice of Gaspard de Tavannes (d. 1573) to Duc d'Orleans on how gentlemen should best spend their time was to study theology or jurisprudence, but not to learn an "ignoble profession" such as medicine. Matters were no better in England. Thomas Hobbes (1588-1679), in 1637 wrote ". . . and namely in Physick, fallacies are pernicious."[47] Moliere (1622-1673) in France could have made a living on his medical satire. The physician, John Locke (1632-1704), wrote: "He that in Physick shall lay down fundamental maxims and from thence drawing consequence and raising dispute shall reduce it into the regular forme of a science has indeed done something to enlarge the art of talking and perhaps laid a foundation for endless disputes."[48] Shakespeare (1564-1616) avoided the topic altogether.[49] A member of the Royal Society, eminent diarist, and the architect of British naval power, Samuel Pepys (1633-1701) relied heavily on a hare's foot for good health.[50] On developing a fever with a pruritic red papular rash, he went not to a physician but "by the Apothecary's advice I am to sweat soundly." The Republican herbalist and popularizer of the *London Pharmacopoeia*, Nicholas Culpeper (1616-1654), wrote "A physician without astrology is like a pudding without fat."[51] Lastly, by 1700 in London there were five times more apothecaries than physicians. From these examples it is clear that not only were common people exempted from medical advances; the ingenious medical discoveries of the 16th and 17th centuries described in preceding chapter found little relevance in the life experiences of even prominent persons of that age.

The medical profession considered its knowledge privileged and not to be shared, quite unlike the openness of Hippocratic knowledge to the citizenry of ancient Greece. Sequestered knowledge protected the physician of ignorance in medieval society, contributing to the opinion of Erasmus (1466-1536) that "What the priest is to our souls, the physician is to our bodies," and that the medical profession was as a "parent, nurse, guardian, and protector of life, second only to God." His medical opinions, while mostly

---

[45] Modified from: Pender, S., *Examples and experience: on the uncertainty of medicine*, Br. J. Hist. Sci., 39:1-18, 2006. The author provides a penetrating review of several 16th C scholars.

[46] *De Occulta Philosophica* was in part an attempt to justify magic, as observed via astrology, demonology, and humanistic intellectual approaches, and in part a derision of medieval superstition. Its author, Heinrich Agrippa (1486-1535) is known to occasionally have practiced medicine, but his training is unknown. He was a well-known but controversial intellectual, and his attempt to synthesize a singular philosophy from ancient and "modern" thought was not unique for the time. The occult was very real.

[47] Hobbes, T., *A Brief of the Art of Rhetorick*, chapt. xvi.

[48] Locke, J., *De Arte Medica*, 1669.

[49] "By medicine life may be prolonged, yet death will seize the doctor too." *Cym.* 5, 5, 29-30; "I will not cast away my physic but on those that are sick." *As You Like It*, 3, 2, 358-9; "Striving to better, oft we mar what's well." *King Lear*, 1, 4, 346. – see: Yearsely, M., *Doctors in Elizabethan Drama*, London, 1933.

[50] Cited in his diary entry for Feb. 9th, 1663. Also valuable to his apparent good health was the taking of a pill of turpentine every morning and the not wearing of a nightgown: *Diary and Correspondence of Samuel Pepys*, Esq., F. R. S., New York, 1884, 12 vols. There is no indexing in Pepys' diary of Sydenham, Boerhaave, John Locke, or "physician" for the period covering the diary (1660-1669), although his government work brought him into contact with several local physicians. He seems otherwise to have been totally insulated from the medical establishment, and even during his several entries commenting on the plague outbreak of 1665-66 there is no mention of a physician.

[51] Culpeper, N., *Semeiotica Uranica*, London, 1671, 4th edition, p. 75.

of an ethical nature, also revealed an undemocratic bias characteristic of his age, for it has been pointed out that Erasmus considered the physician-patient relationship "as a friendship between extreme unequals."[52] Otherwise, he often disparaged the actions of some physicians and the effectiveness of their medicine, and he wrote regarding astrology, "the fatal application of inexact knowledge can often produce a fatal remedy."[53] His contemporary, Martin Luther, was more direct: "Medicine makes sick patients, for doctors imagine diseases, as mathematics makes hypochondriacs and theology sinners." Dr. Garrison states that Luther "despised" physicians.[54]

The medieval West and the Renaissance represent little in the history of the physician-patient relationship and nothing in the history of the profession of medicine. Even with the resurrection of ancient medical writings by the Islamic East and the esteem of Western practitioners for Eastern practitioners such as Avicenna, Maimonides, and Al-Razi, the deplorable state of western medical practice remained unchanged. At the close of the medieval period, its appalling nature can be inferred from the final paragraph of Chapter XXIX of *Medical Treatment in the Middle Ages* by Dr. Riesman:[55]

> "Human blood as a remedy is very old; during the later Middle Ages it came into sporadic use for kings or popes who alone could afford the risks of killing the donors. Louis XI of France (1461-1483) drank the blood of several infants in the vain hope of gaining health; and Pope Innocent VIII is supposed to have received the blood of three young boys who died soon after they were bled."

There is a discontinuity of over fifteen hundred years between the disappearance of Hippocratic medicine and the age to be discussed next. While the Islamic East can be credited for preserving what it had, the same cannot be said for the Holy Roman Empire, which may be dated from 800 to 1806 AD. North of the Alps it was an authoritarian surrogate for the Roman Empire, but even though it "closed against none of its subjects the path of honorable ambition," its medical ambitions were in no way superior to those of its predecessor. [56, 57]

---

[52] Albury, W. R., and Weiss, G. M., *The medical ethics of Erasmus and the physician-patient relationship, J. Med. Ethics, Medical Humanism*, 27:35-41, 2001.

[53] Quoted by Pender, S., *Examples and experience: on the uncertainty of medicine*, in *Brit. J. Hist. Sci.*, 39:1-28, 2006.

[54] Garrison, F. H., *The Evil Spoken of Physicians and the Answer Thereto*, in *Bull. N. Y. Acad. Med.*, V, 1929, p. 51.

[55] Riesman, D., *The Story of Medicine in the Middle Ages*, New York, 1936, p. 304. The chronicler, a historian and lawyer, writing in 1516 of events in the life of Innocent VIII, is considered unreliable by the Catholic Church, but that has not prevented the cited incident from being interpreted as the first attempt at blood transfusion, and there are three independent accounts supporting its veracity. The event of Louis XI was recounted by Robert Gaguin in 1514, Gaguin being an associate of Erasmus.

[56] Bernard Lewis has explained the significance of the "Arabisation" of other cultures that played such a prominent role in the expansion of Islam. He stresses the importance of the Arabic language: "… a literature where the impact of words and form counted for more than the transmission of ideas." Arabic culture developed a synthesis of foreign ideas with Arabic words, an acceptable compliment to both the conqueror and the conquered. Prof. Lewis, in *The Arabs in History* (New York, 1960 [paperback edition], chapter 8: Islamic Civilization) stresses the importance of the language by devoting more time in the cited chapter to Arabic poetry than to science and medicine.

[57] This quotation and a sympathetic review of Imperial Rome's replacement are found in: Bryce, J., *The Holy Roman Empire*, London, 1889.

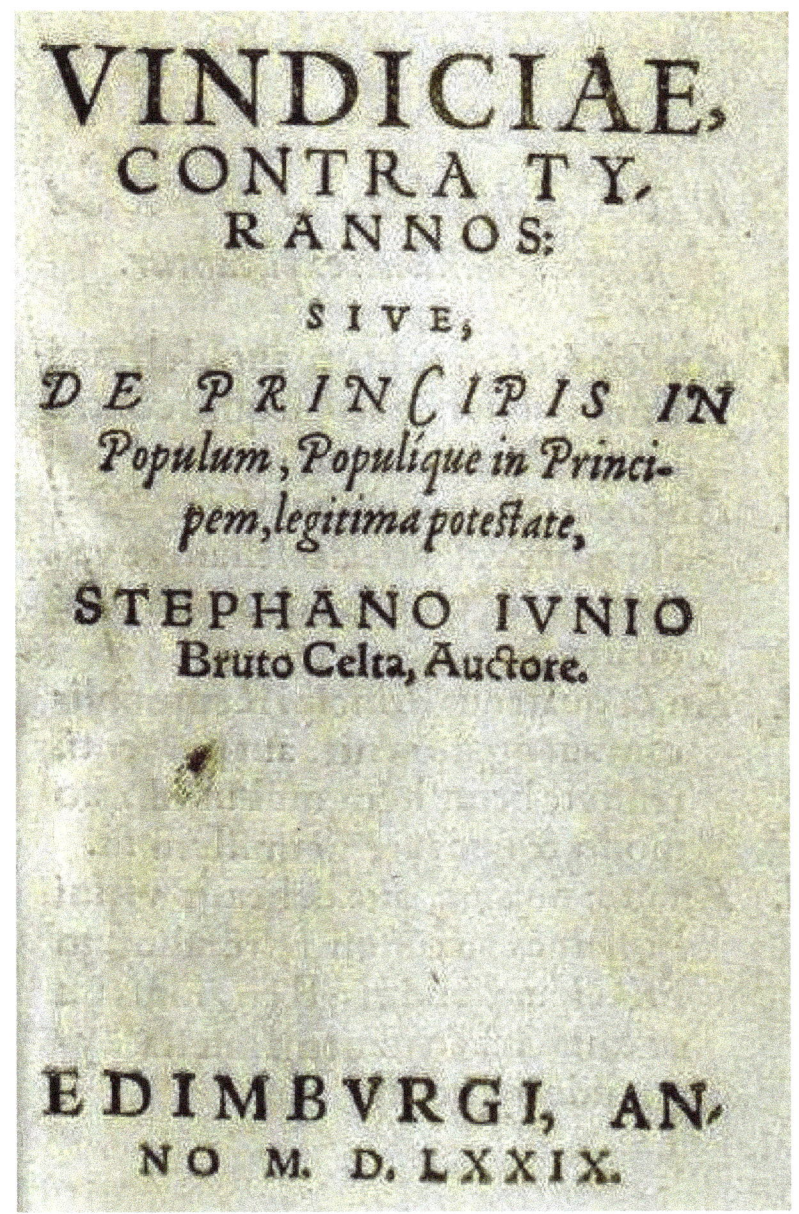

Fig. 12: Title page of *Vindiciae, contra Tyrannos* ("A Defense of Liberty against Tyrants," although more literally it might be read as: "Legal Redress, Against Tyrants"), a Huguenot tract of uncertain authorship published in 1579 in Basel (not Edinburgh), the legal authority being primarily the Old Testament. Photograph is in the public domain.

CHAPTER TWENTY

POST-ROMAN (MEDIEVAL) AND RENASCENT EUROPE:
REDISCOVERING THE INDIVIDUAL

"For arbitrary power's so strange a thing,
It makes the tyrant and unmakes the king:..."

The True-Born Englishman, Part II
Daniel DeFoe, 1701

"... Calvinistic theology develops a liberty-loving people. Where it flourishes despotism
cannot abide."

Loraine Boettner, in *The Reformed Doctrine of Predestination*
(Grand Rapids, 1951, 7th edition, p. 422)

With the fall of the Western Roman Empire and the onset of the Dark Ages in Europe medicine became the work of the layman. This explains the dearth of invention described in the preceding two chapters, for the medical professionals had become extinct. Humanists then reopened the books of ancient scholarship, but this would have led to little had not medieval Europe retraced the political steps of ancient Hellas, passing sequentially through feudalism, aristocracy, and then tyranny in the guise of the Italian Renaissance. The vast abyss that was the medicine of the Dark Ages had been traversed, and over several centuries knowledge again moved from the mystical to the questioning and, finally, to the observational. The resurgence of individualism was reflected in the 16th C Reformation and the 17th C separation of Church and State.

A. The West Again without Physicians

Cassiodorus (490-585 AD), historian and statesman of the Ostrogoths in Rome, was the "hero and restorer of science in the sixth century."[1] Cassiodorus advised that Hippocrates and Galen be studied even by monks who cared for the infirm. The emperor Theodoric (474-526 AD) had his own Greek physician, Anthimus, famous for dietary medicine, and Pope Gregory I valued, employed, and recommended secular medicine in

---

[1] Flavius Magnus Aurelius Cassiodorus Senator straddled the factions of Rome, the Goths, and Byzantium, and tried to establish a common intellectual ground for the clergy. He preserved from unintended destruction by barbarians much secular and religious correspondence and many manuscripts, founded a monastery in which monks were given to copying important manuscripts, and he himself wrote several historically important works. His high position in the civil service of Rome uniquely positioned him for this task. It was Cassiodorus who preserved the oral instructions of Theodoric the Great (474-526 AD) to physicians, as expressed in his *Institutiones divinarum et saecularium litterarium*: "Among the most useful arts which contribute to sustain the faith of human nature, none can be placed above or on an equality with medicine; it ever assists the sick with material benevolence, it banishes our pains." (Translation from the Latin as recorded by D. Riesman in *The Story of Medicine in the Middle Ages*, New York, 1936, p. 12.)

preference to spiritual and mystical healing techniques.[2] But by the time of Cassiodorus the West had for centuries been relying on prayer rather than science for therapeutic benevolence. Even the publication of books became a province of the Church as the Empire was disrupted, George Putnam noting that an author's patron was now God rather than a secular power.[3] North of Italy Hippocratic medicine was never introduced to those distant people whose traditional and shamanic practices therefore had no competition. There is no named educated medical practitioner prior to an Icelandic named Hrafn Sveinbjarnarson (d. 1213) who some think displayed an acquaintance with medicine as taught in Salerno (see p. 336*ff*).[4] Indigenous cultures in England and Scotland retained their peculiar magical theories of disease, although wherever Roman Legions had been sent there could be found elements of Greco-Roman medicine, and at least the Anglo-Saxons were to some extent familiar with herbal remedies described by writers of antiquity.[5]

Into the most remote areas the word of Christianity was soon to command, whereas medicine as a profession diminished, coinciding with the shrinking of cities and territories controlled from Rome. Medicine thus became, except in the Eastern Empire and to a limited extent along the Mediterranean in southern Europe, the domain of the lay practitioner and the priest.

In medicine an example of the absence of anything new and a preoccupation with things past are apparent in the writings of Stephanus of Athens, a 7th C physician (although some identify him as a philosopher and polymath) who explicated selected Hippocratic and Galenic works. Sometimes taking pages to explain a one-sentence aphorism, he was fully seized with a desire to understand in infinite detail the great truths expounded by Hippocrates, both practices and theories.[6] Stephanus adds to them nothing new of his own, although in one of his (presumed) writings, *On the Signs of Virginity*, he popularizes the Egyptian observation that virginity is proven when peas, on which the woman in question has deposited urine, germinate, surely a test that needed no help in being popular. Those points on which he disagrees with Hippocrates can for the most part be explained by vagaries of translation or by his desire to appear a worthy critic of the Master. It is apparent as well that he anticipates nothing new in the future. He is fully satisfied with insights of the past, with medical knowledge now a thousand years old. Whether or not Stephanus was a physician, the fact of the great barrenness of Egyptian medicine over thousands of years becomes fully believable in light of the similar course taken by post-Hippocratic medicine and its expositors. It did not take Pharaoh to command convention; medieval practitioners would prove themselves quite capable of a

---

[2] Thorndike, L., *Medieval Europe*, London, 1920, p. 154.

[3] Putnam, G. H., *Books and Their Makers During the Middle Ages*, New York, 1896, 2 vols., especially the preface, the introductory matter, and chapter 1 of the first volume covering the period of 476-1600 AD.

[4] Larsen, Th., *Medicine and Medical Treatment*, in *Medieval Scandinavia*, P. Pulsiano, editor, New York, 1993.

[5] Grattan, J. H. G., and Singer, C., *Anglo-Saxon Magic and Medicine*, London, 1952.

[6] *Stephanus of Athens: Commentary on Hippocrates' Aphorisms*, text and translation by L. G. Westerink, Berlin, 1998, 2nd For example, Stephanus takes almost five pages to explicate Aphorism I, 3, which is translated by Westerink (pp. 50-59) as: "In cases of disturbance of the belly and spontaneous vomiting, if the matter purged out is of the right kind, this is beneficial and easily tolerated; if not, the contrary."

disabling veneration of the archaic on their own.[7]

In the centuries accompanying the decline of the Roman Empire there was no prejudice against learning or medical knowledge. Instead, the "curse of written tradition," so apparent in the writings of Stephanus, revealed features of the final common pathway that resulted from the loss of the natural state of medical practice. Perhaps this is too great a burden to place on Stephanus, for he was but one practitioner among many. Still, his perspective may accurately reflect the medicine of his time. Just as a poor teacher is more likely to produce the failing student and an inspiring teacher the scholar, absent the scholarly interactions of expert practitioners there was finally produced the archetypal tenured medical sycophant represented by Stephanus, the consequence rather than cause of mediocrity.[8]

Particularly relevant to medicine at this time was a Europe powerfully affected by religious institutions. This occurred not by Vatican decree, but because the vacuum in specialized services created by the ruralization of Roman Europe, which included medicine, was of necessity filled by literate members of religious orders. St. Benedict (480-543) promoted the care of the sick at Monte Cassino, and a medical center developed at that site which historians maintain dominated European medicine for centuries.[9] Other medical centers followed, although their libraries contained only a few poor copies of the works of early Greek physicians. Prominent clergy promoted medicine: Bishop Isidore of Seville (560-636) wrote an *Etymologiae* which included a section on medicine, and the venerable Bede (674-735), a monk from Jarrow, put his medical opinions down on parchment.[10] Stephanus of Athens, mentioned above, may have explicated Hippocratic aphorisms, but he saw an analogy that linked prognosis and prophecy, and in this analogy prognosis as used in medicine was "a divine attribute that linked the physician to God."[11] The opinions of such men were not based on knowledge of or interest in medicine. The eminent Sevillian Bishop embodied a Western view of the universe not unlike that of the

---

[7] The term "Galenolatry" has been applied to a specific form of veneration of the archaic, the uncritical lionization of Galen. Garrison noted that Galen adopted the Roman system of codifying and systematizing, applying it to medicine. Thereby he sought "why" rather than "how" and sterilized medicine for 1700 years (Garrison, F., *Medicine as an Agency in the Advancement of Science, Art and Civilization,* in *Bull. N.Y. Acad. Med.,* Apr., 1929, p. 20). The problem, of course, lay not with Galen but with those who blindly followed him. The ancient Greeks expressed a similar phenomenon in their veneration of not only the words, but also the ideas, found in the writings of Homer, which has been referred to as their "bible."

[8] The author extends his apologies to Stephanus of Athens should it be determined that he (Stephanus) had no training as a physician.

[9] Monte Cassino, some eighty miles from Rome, did not become truly prominent in medicine until the end of the Dark Ages when Latin translations of Arabic medical works were made by Constantinus Africanus (1018-1085). In the 13th C with Frederick II and the unsettled social conditions of the age the monastery precipitously declined, as did its prominence in medicine.

[10] Isidore of Seville composed an influential encyclopedia of general knowledge. In his *Etymologiae* the section on medicine recounts Hippocrates, the humoral theory, and ancient lore such as: "So too in man's head the air passages and the veins produce a windiness from the resolving moisture and make a whirling in his eyes whence vertigo is named." (Translation of Brehaut, E., in *An Encyclopedist of the Dark Ages,* Columbia Univ. Press, 1912, p. 34); Bede the Venerable, who wrote some sixty historical, biographical, and scriptural works, included comments on medical topics in some of his writings, although none solely addressing medicine.

[11] See Temkin's note 66, p. 192, in his *Hippocrates in a World of Pagans and Christians,* Baltimore, 1991. Stephanus was easily deluded or he was bordering on prevarication, for it is hard to imagine a more self-serving marketing tool for a medical practitioner.

ancient Far East: man and his universe were an amalgam, and therefore there was no real distinction between natural and supernatural, between the material and the insubstantial. Indeed, the insubstantial took precedent over the material, the latter an "emanation" of the former. The famous physicians, Paul of Aegina (Paulus of Aegineta) (625-690) and Alexander of Tralles (525-605),[12] were exceptions in that objectivity was retained in most of their writings, but both resided in the eastern empire (Asia Minor and Constantinople) where residual Greek learning still existed.

In summary, the earlier loss of Hippocratic medicine produced a vacuum increasingly occupied by faith-based medicine. Religion itself did not cause the problem, but it could not reverse it. The Roman Empire had, inadvertently, knocked medicine down, and its replacement, the Christian Church, was unable to help it back up. Sadly, because it had no organizational guidance or common standard, no koinon, the profession had no motivation to get up on its own. The professional disappeared, being replaced by lay practitioners with the name but not the merit of "physician." But events of a different nature were to change this, for Western society, ever restless, began to follow a path the Greeks had taken a thousand years earlier.

B. The Dark Ages, *ca*. 400-1000: Feudalism

In looking back over the Dark Ages and thence into the Medieval period and on into the Renaissance there is a parallel between the social history of Europe and that of ancient Hellas.[13] In the early centuries of the Dark Ages Western society was organized into a feudal, manorial system. Power had become concentrated in the hands of a few Romans or Romanized surrogates, vestiges of a disintegrating Roman government. Villeins of a region coalesced around local authority for protection.[14] Many, former slaves or their descendants, were now better off having been raised to the status of serfs, but dependency of serfs on a local lord was absolute.[15] Freemen also required security,

---

[12] Paulus Aegineta (625-690) was a medical encyclopedist and physician who wrote in Greek his *Praecepta salubria*, a seven-part work. He is considered the "last major representative of Byzantine medicine." An experienced and highly regarded surgeon, he gets little credit for originality from F. H. Garrison, in *An Introduction to the History of Medicine* (Phila., 1921, 3rd edition, p. 85), who cites his apologetic tone that acknowledged no advances from the days of Hippocrates. Alexander of Tralles, of a prominent and wealthy family, wrote a *Practica*, a twelve-book encyclopedia that is thought to include some sound clinical observations of his own. He described both direct percussion of the abdomen and the use of colchicine for gout. Despite his preeminence among Byzantine physicians he considered it a sin to omit charms and spells if a treatment was not working, and he required incantations in the preparation of his many herbal remedies.

[13] For present purposes it is convenient to divide the years 400-1300 AD into the Dark Ages (400-1000) and the High Medieval Period (1000-1300), although both terminology and dates are arbitrary.

[14] "Villein" (and therefore "villain") is derived from medieval Latin "villanus" and in turn from the Latin "villa," a country estate. It comprised the peasant population attached to the land, whether free or serfs. Other regions had their counterparts. See the brief but comprehensive work on the subject by Charles Seignobos, Professor, University of Paris: *The Feudal Regime*, translated by E. W. Dow, New York, 1926

[15] This was not new, for peasants, under an institution known as a "colonate," had been permanently secured to the land by the emperor Diocletian (245-313) in the same way that Roman trade and craft guilds had become State monopolies, a temporarily helpful but ultimately disastrous State planning.

and these, too, flocked to the local protector. As commercial and military ties with Rome evaporated, assistance from a powerful distant government was unavailable. Self-sufficiency in local production was necessary and achievable, but there was no excess production and therefore little stimulus for trade. National boundaries were impractical because geography, like society, was held in fiefdoms. All this bears a resemblance to Homeric descriptions of the age of Mycenaean kings,[16] of Agamemnon and Nestor, the time of the Trojan war (12th C BC). Society was agricultural, there was subservience to the local prince, and labor was organized to support the requirements of the palace.[17]

The status of medicine in those brutal and impoverished times can be estimated from a history of 6th C Gaul. Cures were attributed not to medicine but to omens, charms, and other religious devices in a mixture of traditional demonology and Christian theology. During a terrible plague witnessed by Gregory of Tours, a Bishop and later a Saint who had acquired some medical knowledge of the age, he displayed the nature of his medical knowledge as he documented, in four Books, Saint Braga's miraculous cures. Gregory even reported in Book III his own cures: "Whenever a headache comes on or a throbbing in the temples or a dullness of hearing or a pain attacks some other part, I am cured at once when I have touched the affected part on the tomb [of St. Martin] ...." Physically touching a "virtuous" object was thought to be particularly important in affecting cure. When a servant of Gregory contracted the plague, the servant recovered "by drinking a potion of the sacred dust."[18] Gregory, of elite parentage (his father was a Senator), related to numerous prominent personages, and would live in Tours, a commercial hub, would have had access to the best medical care and knowledge as existed at that time.

C. The Medieval Period, *ca.* 1000-1300: Aristocracy Redux

After several centuries the European population expanded, generating new towns and cities and a need for more arable land, the Medieval Period. More efficient social organization was required. How would this be managed? The Roman aristocracy that had once enjoyed an easy life during the later days of the Empire had disappeared except for those fortunate enough to have assumed high positions within the Christian church. As a consequence, leadership, which heretofore had centered solely on the king or lord of the manor, began to be distributed to those on whom the king or lord most depended for support. Thus, a second, non-theocratic, aristocracy was formed. It was composed of those who had land, those who were given land in return for their support,

---

See: Adelson, H. L., *Medieval Commerce*, Princeton, 1962, p.13. It is the author's opinion that it was this rigid State-regulated socialistic economy, unable to adapt to changing circumstances, that was the ultimate cause for the fall of the Roman Empire. It should be noted that the rigid caste system of Hinduism has been equated with the occupational guilds of the Roman Empire in the 4th C AD, forced labor within a familial structure (see *Eight Decisive Books of Antiquity* by F. R. Hoare, London, 1952, chapter 5). One difference, of course, is that the Roman system disappeared whereas Hinduism and the caste system has not.

[16] The Homeric princes were considered the equivalent of feudal knights by J. P. Mahaffy (*Social Life in Greece*, London, 1898), except that he considered them "second-rate" because they talked back to their lords.

[17] Chadwick, J., *The Mycenaean World*, Cambridge, 1976, chapter 5.

[18] Dill, S., *Roman Society in Gaul*, London, 1926, p. 258*ff*. Dill's description of the horrors of the plague and the status of medical practice at the time are chilling.

and those who had wealth or dealt in wealth, including money changers, for the expense of construction and defense was great, not to mention the cost of military expeditions to reclaim the Holy Land. Perhaps two or three percent of the population belonged to this aristocracy, which had within it varying degrees of nobility or entitlement, the path to a more noble status being the one that would best benefit the king. While it was sometimes hereditary, this aristocracy would increasingly include wealthy commoners.[19]

But as the kings exchanged personal power for financial support there were far-reaching consequences. First, serfdom gradually but inexorably disappeared as serfs became able to purchase their freedom, and even cities could purchase their way out of servitude. Second, kingships became more dependent on aristocrats, who in turn became less dependent on their kings. A king's dominions may have been extended, but not necessarily his personal power. Third, the rumor of mass discontent became a political force, just as it had been in Archaic Greece, permitting the aristocrat to effect political change. Lastly, the new aristocrats found that they must tread gently with commoners; otherwise, uprisings might occur or the population might simply disperse and join with another lord or aristocrat who offered better terms of employment. A sense of the "individual," a distinguishing feature of Western society, was reemerging.[20]

The outlook for medicine, however, was not helped by the Church. Clerical domination, moderate at the beginning, was increasing: St. Bernard (1090-1153) advised against consulting the physician because God was in charge of matters; man should not interfere. The eminent Roger Bacon (1214-1294) wrote extensively on the sciences, yet entered a Franciscan friary, was subjected to rigorous censoring, including imprisonment, by the Church, and believed alchemy to be linked to salvation. Bartholomew Anglicus, a 12th C Franciscan monk, wrote *De proprietatibus rerum*, a popular text in which Book VII is devoted to medical practice. John of Gaddesden, *Prebendary of St. Paul's* in London, in 1314 wrote the famous *Rosa Anglica practica medicine a capite ad pedes*, a treatise on medical practices, and the surgeon, Guy de Chauliac (1300-1368), who took holy orders, composed his *Chirurgia magna* in 1363. Secular medical champions had yet to appear who could lead medicine into a new age, and thus responsibility for health of parishioners remained clinging to clerical robes. Religious sanctions based on the sacredness of the human body continued to impede advances in anatomy and surgery, but in fairness those who would have been able to profitably untake such studies were few or nonexistent.

With the re-emergence of cities, however, medicine became an apparent beneficiary in two ways:

1. Medical guilds: Patterned after other trade guilds, and ranked among them, medical guilds appeared in the 12th C as growing towns needed more practitioners. The guild organization provided members with protections and afforded them a mechanism for

---

[19] Of the various definitions of "aristocracy" found in *Webster's New World College Dictionary* (4th edition, 1999), the one that best fits here is "a privileged ruling class; nobility."

[20] Colin Morris, in *The Discovery of the Individual*, (Toronto, 1987) states that during the period between 1050-1200 AD the ancient Greek saying, γνῶθι σεαυτόν ("Know thyself"), was one of the most frequently quoted injunctions, coinciding with the early popularity of autobiography, personal portraits, psychology, and satire, activities also reflecting discovery of self. "Know thyself" is attributed to the 6th C BC Spartan sage, Chilon. A major work of the great philosopher, Pierre [Peter] Abelard (1079-1142), was *Ethica: Seu Liber Dictus: Scito Te Ipsum*: "Ethics, or the book called: Know Yourself."

internal regulation. For member physicians, the public face of their profession needed to be maintained. Therefore, in the area of ethics and comportment the guild provided at least a semblance of worth even though underneath all was conformity, not quality. Medical guilds grew in number and size over the next three centuries, and the number of practitioners and their incomes did as well:[21]

> They came in throngs to court,
> From doctors of the highest fee
> To nostrum-quacks without degree.
> Jean de La Fontaine[22]

2. Medical schools: The first medieval school of medicine was begun in Salerno, probably in the 9th C, from vague origins. Founded in an attractive cosmopolitan region near Naples that was home to a Greek-speaking population, it was made popular by its reputation as a health spa, a place frequently visited by the wealthy and by returning Crusaders for the purpose of rest and relaxation. The Salerno school may have begun as a nidus of Hippocratic learning that had managed to subsist despite the decline of Rome. Its good reputation had preceded the arrival of Constantinus Africanus (1018 – 1085).[23] The names of the physicians Urso and Maurus, active in the school *ca.* 1160-1200, are identified with the peak of Salerno's popularity.[24] Salerno may be viewed, therefore, as a recrudescence of the medical koinon of Hippocrates that is postulated to have existed on the island of Cos.[25]

But by the 13th-14th C Salerno had changed and was no center for excellence; its physicians now were members of a medical guild (under Frederick II), and medical guilds were no reincarnation of the medical koinon of Cos. A medieval guild, which comprised

---

[21] In the 5th and 6th centuries tradesmen were often itinerant, teachers and empirical medical practitioners (to be distinguished from clerical practitioners in Church facilities mentioned earlier) among them. But as population and demand for services increased, permanent residence was established. Then arose the earliest trade unions, comprising both masters and lower level workers. Later, economic factors led to domination by the latter, as the evolving pyramidal structure of the trades permitted fewer individuals to reach the level of master. As long as the medieval guilds existed their purpose was primarily to regulate their particular commodity or service, if possible to the point of monopolization, thus differing from the ancient Greek guilds that were mainly social gatherings.

[22] Jean de La Fontaine (1621-1695), French Fables, Book VIII, 3, *The Lion, the Wolf, and the Fox*, as translated by Elizur Wright, 1882.

[23] Constantine Africanus was, as far as can be determined, a Carthaginian merchant and nonphysician who brought many Arabic manuscripts to Europe. After some time in Salerno where he apparently learned or taught some medical skills, he became a Benedictine monk at Monte Cassino, thereafter spending many years making *Latin* translations of *Arabic* translations of *Greek* medical writings. This contributed to the school's fame.

[24] See Dales, R. C., *The Intellectual Life of Western Europe in the Middle Ages*, 1995, chapter 11, especially pp. 212-214. These physicians introduced new translations of Hippocrates and Aristotle to their colleagues, but much of their writing was based on personal experience rather than an exposition on Greek writings.

[25] One theory suggests that the "school" in Salerno can be traced to an influx of Greek physicians from the nearby city of Velia, earlier a Greek city of Magna Graeca, at the time of the Gothic invasions of the 5th C AD. (For argument *pro* and *con* this proposal see: Nutton, V., *Velia and the School of Salerno*, in *Med. Hist.*, 15:1-11, 1971.) Salerno was even known as the *Hippocratica Civitas*, the "city of Hippocrates.".

all engaged in a particular craft, maintained "the dynamic of a pressure group."[26] Guilds arose in the 11th and 12th centuries as freely associated craftsmen that promptly came under public (municipal) regulation. Pirenne states this is because "the regulative character which had dominated the whole economic legislation of the Roman Empire did not disappear...," and so it was to be expected that regulatory efforts were increasingly "perfected by communal authority."[27] It is no coincidence, therefore, that the decline in influence of Salerno, which in the 8th C AD had escaped the wide grip of Charlemagne, can be dated to the political control, both of the city and its schools, by Frederick II, the Holy Roman Emperor of the Hohenstaufen dynasty who came to power in 1194 AD and established the first centralized European state, an absolute monarchy, in 1231. Despite his seemingly salutary and frequently praised introduction of physician licensing and the overseeing of pharmaceutical practices, Salerno's days in the sun were over.[28] No longer the creation of a local consortium of involved and motivated practitioners with no rigid institutional structure, the conformity imposed by Frederick II (he "reduced the University of Salerno to a state medical School, ..."[29]) removed any uniqueness of their efforts, and his attempt to locate a medical school in nearby Naples further detracted from its reputation, although competition from other developing medical centers around Europe has usually been stated as the cause of the Salerno school's decline. Another explanation is the sack of Salerno by forces of Henry VI of France, vividly described in poetry by Aegidius (Gilles de Corbeil), a physician educated at Salerno in the late 13th C. Whatever the reason for its decline, no longer being a voluntary association of colleagues, the Salerno "school" assumed the characteristics of a guild.[30]

Characteristics of the internal workings of craft guilds included complete power over 1) their associates, originally a necessary protection against arbitrary feudal power, 2) their workplace, as a means of controlling production, and 3) their market and its relation to the State. All this amounted to economic monopoly. The individual guild member was subject to regulation "of quality and quantity of his products, of the price which he should charge to the consumer, and of his relations to his journeymen and apprentices."[31] Guilds grew in size and importance, and by 1350, for example, the *Arte dei medici e speziali* comprised more than a thousand members in Florence.[32] An examination was necessary for entry into the guild, but, once a member, there were no taxes and the commune provided a horse and an attendant for the Florentine practitioner. There were also salaried practitioners for the poor, for prisoners, and for those criminals

---

[26] Black, A. *Guild and State*, New Brunswick (NJ), 2009, 4th printing, p. 7.

[27] Pirenne, H., *Economic and Social History of Medieval Europe*, translated by I. E. Clegg, New York, 1939, p. 179.

[28] In the first volume, chapter three, of H. Rashdall's *Universities of Europe in the Middle Ages* (Oxford, 1895) it is stated: "Salerno remains a completely isolated factor in the academic polity of the Middle Ages. ..... it remained without influence in the development of academic institutions."

[29] Thompson, J. W., and Johnson, E. N., *An Introduction to Medieval Europe 300-1500*, New York, 1937, p. 722.

[30] The postulated reason for the decline of the Salerno school as presented here is the opinion of the author. The sack of Salerno occurred almost forty years prior to the regulatory laws of Frederick II.

[31] Renard, G., *Guilds in the Middle Ages*, London, 1918, translated by D. Terry, edited by G. D. H. Cole..

[32] That number included many in socially equivalent trades, for in 1282, haberdashers were added. Membership was also extended to painters, for many paints were made from substances sold by apothecaries who were also members of the guild. See: Walton, G. L., *The Medical Saints Cosmo and Damian*, in *The Proceedings of the Charaka Club*, vol. IV, 1916, p. 19.

who had been injured from their punishments. A practitioner's fee was one florin, whereas an astrologer received only one-half that sum. So prominent were guilds that every citizen endeavored to enroll: "Through the guilds, and only through them, could a man hope either to share in ruling the city or to make his fortune: to be a citizen you had to belong to a guild."[33] Guild membership, therefore, was tantamount to a civil service position.[34]

As for medical schools, Hippocratic writings were increasingly incorporated into medical education, but the objective inquiry on which those writings were based was not part of the curriculum.[35] The writings and not the methods were the object of veneration, perfectly analogous to Egyptian veneration, by Late Kingdom priests, of Old Kingdom medical tracts. The origin of the university was probably the guild, which did not represent entrepreneurs. Society saw evolve, therefore, nothing but a more sophisticated version of a lay medical practice, not a descendant of Hippocratic medicine. The new practice was privileged, self-serving, condescending, and, in its mystical methods and rote learning, reflected medicine-man, more than Hippocratic, roots. And society knew no better, for fictions of medical knowledge were now masked by robes of academia.

Notable features of medieval medicine included polypharmacy from a pharmocopoeia rivaling that of ancient China and Egypt. Medical procedures such as enemas, blistering, and phlebotomy were done under astrological or religious guidance, and medical "science" concluded that the latest diagnostic tool, uroscopy, had value beyond limit.[36] Alternative practitioners abounded. Barbers and phlebotomists in some cities were required to attend anatomical dissections. Medical recipes in rhyme, pamphlets on the technique of phlebotomy, instructions on inspecting the urine, and ways to avoid or treat the plague were increasingly written for laymen in their common language rather than in Latin. Herbals became popular among the laity for their medicinal value. This enlightenment for the layman, however, did not enlighten him as to the latest

---

[33] This statement and much related information on Italian guilds come from *The Merchant of Prato*, by I. Origo (New York, 1957), a unique account of contemporary life drawn from the diaries of Francesco Datini (1335-1410), a merchant.

[34] A broad characterization of the anticapitalist grasp of medieval city guild can be found in K. Morrison's book, *Marx, Durkheim, Weber*, London, 2006 (2nd edition), with a summary statement on p. 18.

[35] Dr. Singer described the situation thus (Singer, C., *A Short History of Medicine*, Oxford, 1928, p. 69): "This Arabic-Latin literature is generally characterized by the qualities most often associated with the words *medieval* and *scholastic*. It is extremely verbose and almost wholly devoid of the literary graces. And immense amount of attention is paid to the mere arrangement of the material, which often occupies its author more than the ideas that are to be conveyed. Great stress is laid on argument, especially in the form of the syllogism, while observation of Nature is entirely in the background. Above all, there is a constant appeal to the authority of the ancient masters, especially Aristotle and Galen. Lip-service is often paid to Hippocrates, but his spirit is absent from these windy discussions."

[36] Riesman, D., *The Story of Medicine in the Middle Ages*, New York, 1936, chapter 30. Uroscopy, the practice of visual examination of the urine, often in specially adapted transparent containers, was, of course, performed in Hippocratic times, as described in the Aphorisms and Coan Prenotions of the *Hippocratic Corpus*. But it grew to be a "science" unto itself in the hands of Byzantine practitioners such as Magnus of Nisibis (?5th C AD) in his *De Urinis*, and then Stephanus of Athens (6th-7th C AD) in *Peri Ouron*, and Theophilus Protospatharius (7th C AD). Whereas the Hippocratics used it as an objective tool for managing urinary tract problems, the Byzantines extended it to explain causation of systemic disease, including interplay with bodily humours. The technique included assessment of urine color, consistency, and position of particulate matter in a standing urine specimen.

in medical discovery. Instead, the new medicine was but the translation into the vernacular of treatises from centuries just past.[37] The statement that "Not only medical but natural science flourished in this period" reflects the power of the pen, not science.

With dismal professional prospects and given one centralized and dominant religion and one social system as described by Dr. Riesman, one may question why a medical priesthood did not develop in Europe.[38] Although the Dark Ages had included the mystical medicine of the Druid priests of the Celts and the medicine-men of the Teutons and Anglo-Saxons,[39] it was the feudal clerics who taught medicine in monasteries throughout Europe. As a consequence, Dr. Riesman comments that each disease became associated with a different saint. He concludes, however, that medicine remained but an avocation of the clerics. Only one area of medicine was systematically proscribed by religion's aristocrats, that being dissection for the purposes of studying anatomy or determining cause of death. In later centuries religious restrictions were imposed on universities, but overall the Church infringed less and less on medicine as time passed, and an established caste of priest practitioners did not develop. Perhaps the Church did not appropriate medicine because European priests obtained adequate and secure sustenance from their communities. Their survival did not depend on dispensations of a Pharoah, a central administration, and they therefore did not need to justify their position within the Church by other dealings, evidence that it was not religion itself that posed a risk to medical progress. Rather it was the nature of the political structure to which religious practices were affixed that was the danger.

In any event, of the medieval aristocracy, neither its newly rich and nor its newly anointed came to be associated with medical progress.

D. The Renaissance, *ca*. 1300-1650: Reemergence of the Tyrant

Other animals have limited patterns of response to environmental variation, and changes in species accord with changes in nature. But man has the ability to adapt as an individual, not just conform genetically. He can thereby tolerate circumstances that he cannot control and, in a changing world, improve his chances of survival. It is impossible to conceive of an ancient Egypt governed by Pharaoh and his minions as representing the proper state of things. It was, for most Egyptians, a deplorable place.[40] Yet it survived

---

[37] Bennett, H. D., *Chaucer and the Fifteenth Century*, Oxford, 1947, Chapt. 7, Fifteenth Century Prose.

[38] Riesman, D., *The Story of Medicine in the Middle Ages*, New York, 1936, opening of chapt. 35.

[39] Such variations on shamanistic medicine were, and are, a global phenomen. Even Odin is viewed as a "shamanistic god." He was "the patron and the divine prototype of seers and magicians, especially those who (like shamans in Arctic Europe and Asia in modern times) undergo terrifying initiations and communicate with other worlds in ecstasies and mediumistic trances." (Simpson, J., *Everyday Life in the Viking Age*, London, 1971, p. 215.)

[40] Recent discoveries reinforce this conclusion, such as a study reported by Rose, J. C. and Zabecki, M., in which a commoners' cemetery of the New Kingdom (*ca*. 1300 BC) provided paleopathologists with specimens indicating a predominance of trauma and degenerative joint disease consistent with "hard physical labor," anemia due to iron deficiency and probably folic acid deficiency in 83% of juveniles and 19% of adults, 52 % of the interred being between five and twenty years of age, and a "faunal analysis indicating very low meat consumption." (Presented at the 34th annual meeting of the *North American Paleopathology Association* in 2007.) Nunn (Nunn, J. F., *Ancient Egyptian Medicine*, London, 1996, p. 22) relates the arithmetic mean of life

thousands of years, not because the administration of the kingdom was good, but because it was tolerated. And it is in the context of enduring that human societies have evolved in disparate ways, whether the limits of tolerance find their basis in fear or impotence.

It is easier to tolerate than to chance or change. And so, until the development of democracy, it was easier for men to tolerate powerful authoritarian forces than attempt to change them, easier to join with their preferred authoritarian than to avoid them altogether. And it was exactly those societies that were most most commanding of subservience and uniformity that succeeded in garnering the blessing of survival.

But that success came at a price. Thus, Pharaonic Egypt, the Emperors of Asia, Agamemnon, and oligarchy of the Spartiatae share a prize of debatable worth. This was obvious to some 2500 years ago, for in the *Hippocratic Corpus* a clear statement on the debasing effects of authoritarian governance can be found:[41]

> Wherefore Europeans are more warlike, and also because of the institutions, not being under kings as are Asiatics. For, as I said above, where there are kings, there must be the greatest cowards. For men's souls are enslaved, and refuse to run risks readily and recklessly to increase the power of somebody else. But independent people, taking risks on their own behalf and not on behalf of others, are willing and eager to go into danger, for they themselves enjoy the prize of victory. So institutions contribute a great deal to the formation of courageousness.

And the point was not missed five hundred years later, for Pseudo-Longinus, in περὶ ὕψους (*On the Sublime*), has a philosopher-friend describe a popular sentiment thus: [42]

> "A world-wide sterility of utterance has come upon our life. Must we indeed accept," he continued, "the *well-worn cliche that democracy is a good foster mother of greatness, that great speakers flourished when she flourished and died with her*? [italics added for emphasis] Freedom, they say, is able to nurture the thoughts of great minds and to give them hope; with it comes eagerness to compete and ambition to grasp the highest rewards. Because of the prizes available in free cities, the natural talents of speakers are trained, sharpened, polished as it were by practice, and they shine forth in the free handling of affairs. In our own day," he said, "we learn righteous slavery as children, we are all but swaddled in its customs and practices while our minds are still tender; we have never tasted of the most beautiful and most creative spring of language. By this I mean freedom," he said, "and so we turn out to have genius except for flattery."

Humans seem able to tolerate about anything and even be cheerful in the process, if

---

expectancy was thirty years in predynastic and thirty-six year in dynastic Egypt, and Baines cites a life expectancy for those who were fortunate enough to reach 14 years of age to be 29.1 years in Roman Egypt (J. Baines, *Society, Morality, and Religious Practice*, in *Religion in Ancient Egypt*, Ithaca, 1991, B. E. Shafer, editor, p. 133).

[41] *Airs, Waters, Places*, xxiii, 34*ff*. The translation is that of W. H. S. Jones as found in the *Loeb Classical Library* series of the Hippocratic works.

[42] Little is known of the author of περὶ ὕψσος, which is usually translated *On the Sublime*, although it could also be translated as a variation on *Concerning the Very Best*. He is thought to have lived *ca.* 1st-2nd C AD, and his work, a classic on style in writing, remains influential. This translation, by G. M. A. Grube, Indianapolis, 1991, is taken from Section 44 of περὶ ὕψος as edited by Otto Iahn, Leipzig, 1890. This and the preceding quotation, despite their lengths, are given in full as they represent important insight into ancient Greek political thinking apart from the traditional assemblage of philosophers.

repression is sufficiently unrelenting. Among the most hospitable populations on earth today will be found the most subservient. But the cheeriness must reside mainly in the belief that in subservience utter destruction has been thereby avoided, or that at least one's lot is not as miserable as the next person's.[43]

It is no wonder, therefore, why centuries may pass without progress when external threat is a more formidable force against change than internal motivation is in promoting it. The operative survival of the Ebers papyrus, the Hammurabic Code, the *Huang Ti Nei Ching Su Wen*, and the *Charaka Samhita* is a monument not to human inquisitiveness but to the lack thereof. Not surprisingly, therefore, the feudal and aristocratic phases of medieval Europe saw no medical advances, just as did the feudal and aristocratic ages of ancient Greece. And even the *Hippocratic Corpus* would not have survived had not the West received a second chance at deliverance. What was that second chance? Gottfried interestingly suggested that it was the infectious plagues of the 14th C that killed off the old style practitioners of medicine, killed off Latin-speaking medical faculty of the universities, thereby introducing the vernacular in medical texts, killed off so many "physicians" in fact that the laity came to pay more attention to the field of medicine, and killed off so many people overall that hospitals became increasingly prominent and legislative restrictions on movement led to early "boards of health."[44] But perhaps that second chance was the Renaissance.

Medieval European civilization ended with a terrible period of "contraction and decline," the consequence of calamitous wars and plagues.[45] But then followed another transition as greater productivity recurred. Trading centers developed as a result of an enlarging economy and population. In emerging towns, the arts, crafts, and guilds began to flourish as urbanization proceeded. Another feature of the age was the emergence of nationalism as a counterbalance to the influence of the Church. And now the aristocratic system encountered its competition and would meet its match. A new political force was on the rise: alongside a developing capitalistic commerce appeared powerful, independent, city-states. Indeed, it is estimated that Europe contained more than five hundred "states," many not more than cities, by the year 1500.[46] This occurred earlier and most prominently in Italy where the Alps provided some protection from northern invasions and where a mountainous geography promoted independent city-states. Here again recall Archaic Greece around 700 BC when a new social organization, the city-state, began to trade and colonize, to provide venture capital, to accumulate wealth for both the city-state and the individual. Dr. Muller wrote: "The rise of Western civilization, as of Greek culture, was inseparably connected with the rise of commerce and industry."[47] And those were also the ages, both in ancient Greece and in Renaissance Italy, of tyrants,

---

[43] In G. Frier's curious *The Masters and the Slaves, A Study of the Development of Brazilian Civilization*, (New York, 1946), a recounting of the Portuguese colonization of Brazil, an African lad is described who lightheartedly carries, in a basket on his head, the brimming latrine slops of his Portuguese master's household. The boy is a happy one, purportedly satisfied with his lot because he felt himself treated as a racial equal by the master. This seems an unlikely explanation, a contention supported by the description of the horrors of slavery witnessed by Charles Darwin in Pernambuco, Brazil, misery profound enough that he felt compelled to include it in his classic. See: *Journal of Researches into the Natural History and Geology*, 2nd edition, London, 1845, pp. 499-500.

[44] Gottfried, R. S., *The Black Death*, New York, 1985, esp. chapter 7 (paperback edition).

[45] Adelson, H. L., *Medieval Commerce*, Princeton, 1962, Chapter 7.

[46] Cited by Zakaria, F., *The Future of Freedom*, New York, 2003, p. 36.

[47] Muller, H. J., *The Uses of the Past*, Oxford, 1952, p. 239.

those leaders who courted rather than commanded the support of their communities and who have been associated with the rebirth of classical ideas.[48]

One family that came to prominence was the Medici. Of peasant origin, some of its members moved to Florence in the 12th C, where their businesses prospered, particularly banking.[49] By the 15th C the family was wealthy and powerful, patronizing the arts, and politically active. Cosimo the Elder (1389-1464) became the "uncrowned monarch" of Florence, appointing trustworthy friends to important city positions, and restricting civil liberties to maintain his privileged status. He therefore became the counterpart of the familiar tyrant of the Greek city-state. In this he joined the company of other tyrants such as F. Hohenstaufen (1194-1250) in Sicily, C. Scala (1291-1329) in Verona, the Visconti and M. Sforza (1369-1424) in Milan, and on and on. The Renaissance saw the proliferation of such leaders. It was, at least in Italy, an Age of Tyrants, even in those States belonging to the Roman Church, although the definition of "tyrant" may not have been as narrowly defined as in 6th C BC Greece.[50] In fact, the Renaissance recovery of Greek and Roman writings describing ancient republics led some to conclude that popular tyrants protected freedoms threatened by the monarchies and oligarchies.

But indigenous medicine in the Age of the Tyrants was not particularly admired. Petrarch (1304-1374) described his physicians in a letter:

> "The physicians came running. Having disputed at length, as they are wont, they ordained that at midnight I would be dead;.... Their orders were not carried out, for I have always besought my friends...to do just the opposite. Wherefore I spent the whole night in a deep sweet sleep...[and] was discovered by the physicians, when they came back on the morrow, writing."[51]

His concerns were well-founded, for here is a letter of a favored physician regarding the ailing wife of a prominent Florentine merchant:

> "If she would be healed right speedily, let three sage-leaves be picked at morn before sunrise, and let the man who picks them, be on his bended knees, saying three Paternosters

---

[48] There is even a vague analogy between the Italian city-states of Florence and Venice and 6th C BC Athens and Sparta. Venice in its earlier centuries was a strict oligarchical society, as was Sparta. Its geography preserved it from Church interests, as well as from politics and threats by other city-states. Self-contained, self-confident, and scorned, it grew to control a vast commercial empire. Freedom of expression was not fostered, although this proved but a small hazard inasmuch as its patriotic citizenry very much thought uniformly. Florence, on the other hand, was the *alter ego* of Athens, a birthplace of liberty and a cauldron of political schemes, some tyrannical, some democratic. To this freedom, or forceful assertion of dissent, can in part be attributed its preeminence in arts and letters and its central position in the Renaissance.

[49] One of several explanations for the balls on the Medici coat of arms is that they represent cupping glasses or pastilles (troches) signifying the family's medical past.

[50] The Greek tyrant, τύραννος, a leader who was granted unlimited power and unencumbered by law, tended at first to refer to the way by which power had been obtained, *i.e.*, it was granted by the people. Later, it represented the often fraudulent courting of the masses to achieve the same end. Still later, and into modern times, it referred to the way power was used, usually the brutal use of absolute power. See: Burckhardt, J., *The Civilization of the Renaissance in Italy*, London, 1878, wherein is described, century by century, the grossness and brutality of Renaissance tyrants and the fragile coattails on which those who depended on their patronage hung.

[51] Petrarca, *Lettere Senili*, vol. II, libro XIII, lettera VIII.

and three Hail Marys in honour of God and the Holy Trinity, then send the leaves here in a letter, and I will write divers words on each. And as the fever approacheth, let her say a Paternoster and a Hail Mary, and then eat a leaf, and so for each one of the three. And when she is done with eating them, she will be rid of the fever. But she must have faith, for if she has not, they will be of no avail."[52]

The year of the woman's illness was 1396. And here is an example from an English medical herbal of 1440:[53]

256. For deliverance of a dead child. Take leek blades and scale them, and bind to the womb about the navel; and it shall cast out the dead child; and when she is delivered, take away the blades or she shall cast out all that is in her.

Further east, however, works of ancient authors had been preserved in Islamic lands. Greek manuscripts had been transferred by Nestorian scholars from Edessa to the "university" in Gondeshapour (in present-day Iran) where they had fled to avoid persecution by the Byzantines at the end of the 6th C. There the texts would be translated into Aramaic, Syriac, Persian, and later into Arabic. Centuries later the wisdom in them was admired by Islamic scholars, and in the Middle East further observations and attempts at clarification were added to those texts.[54] It was the ability of Arabic scholars to synthesize from preexisting concepts of the East and the West, primarily those in Greek and Sanskrit, rather than to conceive them, that led to the prominence of Persian, Christian, and then Islamic scientific writings in the centuries following Islamic conquests.[55] From their careful work some of those writings were reintroduced into

---

[52] Origo, I., *The Merchant of Prato*, New York, 1957, p. 337.

[53] Dawson, W. R.: *A Leechbook of the XVth Century*, London, 1934. This is the text of manuscript No. 136 as transcribed from contemporary English by Dawson. It includes two sections on "unlucky days." The literary structure of the medical advice is similar to that of translations of Egyptian medical papyri, except, of course, that here there is no issue regarding accuracy of translation. Note that the same statement with identical wording has been attributed to the wife of Edward III of England (1327-1377), as cited by R. S. Gottfried in his book, *The Black Death*, New York, 1953, p. 120 (paperback edition).

[54] Many works by Hippocrates and Galen were translated into Syriac by Greek and Syriac scholars in the 5th and 6th C in Gondeshapour and the translations were the basis for subsequent Arabic translations in the 8th and 9th C. See: Browne, E. G., *Arabic Medicine*, Cambridge, 1921, Lecture I, p. 19*ff.* As regards the quality of the translation, Browne argues that it is translations into Latin that pose the biggest problems. In part this is because Arabic did not lend itself to development of compound words that might express a new scientific thought, and so it was by use of paraphrase that new concepts might be expressed. Insurmountable difficulties in subsequent translation are therefore predictable.

[55] Prof. George Sarton noted as well that the translations from Greek and Sanskrit were by non-Muslims and often non-Arabs, especially Syrian Christians and Jews, but, being a strong advocate of Arabic science, he felt Arabic influence was far undervalued. See: Sarton, G., *Arabic Scientific Literature*, Ignace Goldziher Memorial Volume, Part I, Budapest, 1948. Another example of Arabic synthesis is found in *The Arabian Nights*, as translated by Richard Burton in 1885, for the dialogues of the 449th and 451st nights, which discuss, among other things, medical theory under Islam, are remarkably similar in style and hypothesis to the dialogue between the mythical Chinese Emperor and his physician/minister, Ch'i Po, of the *Huang Ti Nei Ching Su Wen* of early Chinese medicine (see p. 71*ff*). In other ways medicine does not come off well in this collection of tales from *ca.* 1000 AD, as revealed by the beheading of forty physicians who attempted but failed to cure the madness of a king's daughter (Night 193). In fact, references to physicians and medical

Europe in the 11th C by Constantinus Africanus. Three centuries later, when Arabic science had begun to decline, the westward flight of eastern Christendom from Islam put more Greek and Arabic manuscripts into European hands, from which copies of Latin translations were made by monks in European monasteries. Some Latin translations were from Greek translations of Syriac translations of Arabic works or translations, and there has been serious debate about intended meanings of those translations at each step.[56] Despite this literary renewal and in contrast to the enthusiastic reception of Greek writings by Arab intellectuals, Europeans may have used the copying of Latin manuscripts more as a means of controlling the enterprising spirit of monks and nuns than a purposeful perpetuation of knowledge.[57] On the other hand, famous Eastern physicians such as Avicenna, Al-Razi, and Albucasis were esteemed by European practitioners.[58]

Then, in 1445 came the printing press. Medical textbooks were put into type, anatomical drawings could now be engraved, and multiple copies of these works could be run off a printing press for wide distribution. But often the text was redundant and the marvelous intaglios more ornamental than academic. Efficient duplication led more to standardization of medical ignorance than progress. This contrasted with intellectual movements throughout Europe whereby the printed word efficiently transmitted new ideas and fostered change. Veneration of archaic medicine maintained its hold. Thus the end of medieval medicine has been dated not to the invention of the printing press, but

---

practice in this classic are rare, which is surprising in view of the broad regional and chronologial span of its anecdotes. Even the legal systems of Muslim nations are derived to a great extent from the Roman. "If Aristotle supplied the Arabians with their logic, it was Basil, Leo and their Greek commentators who supplied them with their law." See: Amos, S., *The History and Principles of the Civil Law of Rome*, London, 1883, p. 409.

[56] This was the sequence with Al-Razi's famous treatise on smallpox, of which the early translators are unknown and which was translated into Greek about 1060 by order of a Byzantine Emperor. In the early Arabic translations of Greek works, literal translations were of little value, for there was no equivalent technical vocabulary in the language of an Arab society emerging from isolated tribalism. Translators, therefore, tried to imagine what they thought was the point under discussion, and from this they fashioned their "translation," although it should more accurately be described as an interpretation. (For more on this point see: *A History of Muslim Philosophy*, Weisbaden, 1966, M. M. Shariff, editor, vol. 2, for the section on medicine.) And as Arabic translators had no personal experience with what they were attempting to translate, how accurate could any Latin translation have been? Even when the disease of smallpox had been personally observed, accuracy remained an issue. al-Razi, in his descriptions of smallpox and measles, wrote that of the symptoms of the two diseases there was more back pain in smallpox but more inquietude, nausea, and anxiety in measles. (See chapter 3, first paragraph, of the *Treatise on the Small-Pox and Measles*.) He also made this statement, as translated by Greenhill: "The Measles are more to be dreaded than the Smallpox, except in the eye." (Morbillis autem est majoris timoris quam variolae, nisi in oculo.) See *Divisio Morborum*, cap. 149, para.6, in the Sydenham Society publication of al-Razi's work, *A Treatise on the Small-pox and Measles*, London, 1848. The translation from the Arabic into Latin was by Gerard of Cremona in the 13th C. Had patients with smallpox and measles been observed side-by-side such statements would be quickly judged as ludicrous. They surely would not have represented the intent of al-Razi were he a competent clinician.

[57] G. H. Putnam wrote that "the principal and most constant occupation of the learned Benedictine nuns was the transcription of manuscripts." (*Books and Their Makers during the Middle Ages*, New York, 1962, vol. I, p. 52.)

[58] Early Arabic-speaking practitioners benefitted not only from their discovery of the Greek classics, but Al-Razi and others may have had access to Indian Sanskrit classics. Thus was Islamic medicine introduced into Europe in the 17th C, and it has even been proposed that in this sense European medicine in the Middle Ages was based on Indian, rather than Islamic, medicine.

almost a century later with the writings of Paracelsus (1493-1541), who was first to break with the tradition of Galen. It will be shown below that this dating was premature.

There was one medical area that continued to grow, although more in complexity than effectiveness; that was the pharmacopoeia. Some have viewed the enormous lists of drug remedies of the ancients as evidence of their great knowledge, a vast cornucopia of good things that gave a wide selection of choices for any particular problem. The opposite, of course, was true; the vast majority was utterly useless or dangerous. The Hippocratic pharmacopoeia, in contrast, had been unique in that it was small. And it was small for a reason: scientific observations by Hippocratic practitioners did not verify the usefulness of many, or the safety of some, medications. They had learned to refrain from using those agents. Perhaps Prof. Iain Lonie's perspective is the best: "If we exclude diet, therapy in Hippocratic texts reduces to a few simple formulae for purges and emetics. The one exception to this generalization is offered by the gynecological texts."[59] It was then, and is now, better for a physician to know well a limited number of effective drugs than to sporadically use many, the side-effects of which can be so varied and unpredictable. There is no other way to explain the ancient *Materiae Medicae* of Egypt: 811 prescriptions;[60] of India: in the *Charaka Samhita*, 2000,[61] and in the *Susruta Samhita*, 760; of China: 2000, with 16000 variations; of Dioscorides in 1st C Rome: 1000;[62] of Pliny's *Natural History*: 1700; of Marcellus Empiricus of 5th C Roman Gaul: 2500;[63] of 17th C England: 1,960 (p. 362); and of the Hippocratics: 130.[64]

Returning to the subject of the tyrants as they vied for power, segments of the population benefited from the tyrant's most effective weapon, his patronage. And this is one distinction between tyrants and hereditary monarchs. The necessity of patronage permitted selective liberties for selected individuals and groups, particularly those that might lead not just to greater pleasure for the tyrant but also to greater wealth and fame. Thus evolved one facet of the patron's security. In the pages to follow there is a striking

---

[59] Lonie, I., *Literacy and the Development of Hippocratic Medicine*, in Lasserre, F., and Mudry, P., *Formes de Pensee dans la Collection Hippocratique*, Geneva, 1983, p. 153.

[60] See: *Ancient Egyptian Medicine*, Chicago, 1974, translation of papyrus Ebers by C. P. Bryan and first published in 1930; Michael Parkins cites "over 900 specific drugs" named in the Ebers papyrus in *Pharmacological Practices of Ancient Egypt, Proc. of the 10th Annual History of Medicine Days*, pp. 5-11, 2001. Also see: Von Staden, H., *Herophilus: The Art of Medicine in Early Alexandria*, Cambridge, 1989, p. 19.

[61] Kothare, S. N. and Pai, S. A., *An Introduction to the History of Medicine*. Please note that the author has been unable to relocate this reference. Dr. Pai provided an eloquent obituary on the passing of the eminent Dr. Kothare in 2004. See: *Nat. Med. J. India*, 18 (2), 2005. This information is provided to support the authenticity of the reference and the information from it.

[62] Dioscorides of Anazarbus wrote *de Materia Medica* about 70 AD. It is one of the most famous catalogs of botanicals ever written, remaining an authoritative pharmacopeia well into the 17th C and containing some 4740 medicaments derived from approximately 500 botanical species.

[63] Marcellus Empiricus was *magister officiorum* to Theodosius I. He composed an extensive work on pharmacology, *de Medicamentis* (410 AD), that included about 2500 recipes heavily influenced by magic and *dreckapotheke*, the latter being the use of "offensive" human or animal excretions or parts in treatment of disease (although it is now thought that in some instances they were actually codes for botanicals that the profession wished to keep secret).

[64] Riddle, J. M., *Dioscorides on Pharmacy and Medicine*, Austin, 1985, xviii, although Wootton (Wootton, A. C., *Chronicles of Pharmacy*, London, 1910, available in a reprint by USV Pharmaceutical Corp., Tuckahoe, NY, 1972, p. 78) provides Le Clerc's list of 195 drugs. Recent publications cite many more Hippocratic "recipes," but more than eighty percent are from gynecological texts, although Totelin enumerates 285 non-gynecological recipes.

relation between the great names in the arts and sciences of the Renaissance and wealthy and aristocratic patrons, an association that would extend into the Enlightenment, for it was through its patrons that ancient learning reemerged in the West.[65] With publication of the works of ancient authors, renewed interest in biology began to bring the state of science back to where it had been 1500 years earlier.[66] Admiration for Greek thinkers led not only to emulation. Discoveries such as the anatomical studies of Vesalius were made, inspired by the findings of the ancients, that were advances over those of earlier days. The University of Padua, protected by Venice and shielded from the Church and its censorship, attracted many brilliant students.[67]

The reason for recovery from the Dark Ages was political change and population growth, and these occurred primarily in those cities not under feudal control. Such a process, under way by the 11th C, was best seen in Venice, Florence, Lucca, Bologna and Milan, city-state republics of a contested Italy rather than in those of a still feudal Europe. It is no surprise, therefore, that important medical discovery first reappeared in Italy. The encyclopedic historian of clinical medicine, J. H. Baas, lists fourteen prominent physicians of the 14th C, thirteen of whom were Italian, and the fourteenth ended up in Albano, Italy.[68] For the 15th C he lists twenty-nine, of which twenty-two were Italian, Italian-trained, or resided in Italy. As for the University of Padua, its students and teachers included Copernicus (1473-1543), Vesalius (1514-1564), Galileo (1564-1642), William Harvey (1578-1657), and Morgagni (1682-1771). In Renaissance discoveries listed in the next chapter, the earlier ones were predominantly made by Italians. Medicine and science generally are indeed indebted to Italy, its tyrants, and to Venice, more than to any other aspect of the Renaissance. The consequences of patronage provided by tyrants are described in the next chapter.

---

[65] The patron exists in many guises, and modern medical researchers usually receive patronage, although it more often comes from Government than from a wealthy individual or other private source. As it happens, however, Government patronage, in the form of grants, is more restrictive than that of the Renaissance tyrant. The latter provided (1) subsistence so that the tyrant's favorite could fully devote himself to his work, and (2) rewards for a satisfactorily completed commission, whereas Government patronage provides limited subsistence and, far more importantly, specifies what work is to done. The tyrant rewarded success, whereas modern medical grants reward adherence to process. That process is a subtle one in which the person seeking a grant crafts his application in a way he thinks is most likely to meet with approval of granting committees. The idea that patronage in democratic Governments (1) reflects the power of the people, (2) pertains only to traditional political appointments, or (3) is an efficient mechanism for progress, is naïve.

[66] The *Editio princeps* of Galen's works was published in 1525 (five volumes), that of Aristotle in 1495-1498 (five volumes), and that of Hippocrates in 1526, all from the Aldine Press in Venice.

[67] In 1405 Padua had been incorporated into the Republic of Venice where it can be argued that its university made Padua the equivalent in science to what Florence was in art. The academic freedom permitted to university students under the protection of Venice brought it applicants from all over Europe, and there was even a flourishing trade in books, especially medical ones. Whereas Catholic graduates received their diplomas from the Church, non-Catholics could obtain them from from representatives of the Holy Roman Empire. Post-mortem dissections were permitted. See: Andrioli, G. and Trincia, G., *Padua: The Renaissance of Human Anatomy and Medicine*, in *Neurosurg.* 55:746-755, 2004. The Republic of Venice ended in 1797 with its occupation by Napoleon's forces.

[68] Baas, J. H., *Outlines of the History of Medicine and the Medical Profession*, New York, 1889, H. E. Handerson, translator, p. 286*ff.*

E. Postscript and Prelude: Religion and Medicine in the West

The roles of monarchs, tyrants, patrons, and the Church as they affected the course of medical practice during the Dark Ages and early recovery therefrom have now been briefly discussed. But profound contemporary events unrelated to the Renaissance were occurring in regions outside Italy. These events, more than the Renaissance, would shape the course of medicine in subsequent centuries. In preparation for the dramatic changes to come, it is relevant at this point, given the chronological association of religious change with the Renaissance, to review how religion and medicine have been entwined in the West.

Excursus on Religion and Medicine in the West; Classical and Modern Times Compared

Religion:
> 1. "Belief in and reverence for a supernatural power accepted as the creator and governor of the universe." *Webster's II New Riverside University Dictionary*
> 2. A complex belief that involves the following:
>> a. belief in god(s)
>> b. distinction between sacred and profane
>> c. ritual
>> d. moral code
>> e. religious feelings
>> f. prayer
>> g. a world view
>> h. the individual's place in that world view
>> i. society's place in that world view
>>> *Encyclopedia of Philosophy* (New York, 1967)

There is nothing in either a simple or complex definition of religion that places it in opposition to medicine. This is also apparent from the paths followed by religion and Hippocratic/Western medicine:

A. The Classical Age[69]

1. The earliest form of Greek religion was mysticism, and it expressed regional idiosyncracies. The famed Greek oracles can be traced back to an origin such as this. Medicine then was empiric/ shamanistic.

2. The successor to this state has been termed "Olympian," for it now included the pagan gods described by Homer, gods who conquered the earlier reigning deities of the cosmos. Some date the commencement of the Greek classical age not with Pericles, but with Peisistratus (607-528 BC) who facilitated the incorporation of the Ionic Olympian divinities such as Zeus and Apollo into the culture of Athens. It is the opinion of some

---

[69] This sequence of religious change among the Hellenes is derived from Gilbert Murray's *Five Stages of Greek Religion*, London, 1935.

that the Olympian gods were a reaction to a changing social situation. These new gods, human in their desires, were no longer tribal, and at that time Greek society was losing its tribal identities. Much gory ritual was then removed from religious practices and replaced with less "vulgar" sacraments. Thus, the Classical Age could be dated from the late 6th C BC, and it would encompass rational, pre-Hippocratic, medicine.

3. With regression of authoritarianism and the expansion of many variant democratic city-states, individualism percolated not only into politics and commerce, but into religion as well. The collapse of the pagan's Olympians that followed was reflected in (1) the rise of the great schools and philosophers of the 4th C BC who sought "truth," and (2) a longing of the individual for a personal association with some universal presence. There was a desire to feel that, despite the injustices of the present world, an ultimate arbiter of justice in the next would soothe the wounds of injustice and deal appropriately with the unjust. It was now that Hippocratic medicine became prominent, and it, the schools, and the philosophers would survive for several centuries. At this point the phenomena were still somewhat local.

4. Then came the great upheavals of society around the Mediterranean as Macedonian and then Roman influences inexorably extended. Left with a pagan religion that increasingly lacked credibility, mysticism and pessimism became a dominating presence, at least until the time of Christ. It was during this period that Hippocratic medicine diminished in importance.

5. The subsequent remarkable attraction of Christianity promoted a universal Church and prompted a reaction by the pagan world. The Roman emperor, Julian (331-363 AD) attempted to reverse the Christian orientation of the State, and Neoplatonism and Gnosticism are examples of philosophical sects that had risen prior to Jerome's Christianity. There developed a "national" spirit aroused by the appeal of the ancient gods. But Christianized pagans successfully resisted this "counter-reformation," and Christianity became all-embracing. Hippocratic medicine had by this time vanished.

It has been argued that it was religious dogma that retarded medical progress in those early centuries. From the above, however, the following can be proposed:
1. The naissance of democracy, the concept of a personal God, and the birth of scientific medical practice in ancient Greece were events reflecting the same social upheaval, a displacement of earthly authoritarianism,
2. Similarly, what engulfed the course of Hippocratic medicine was not religious fervor or doctrine but reassertion of that earthly authoritarianism as initiated by Macedonian and Roman territorial conquests. The zenith of Hippocratic medicine had coincided with democratic city-states and colonies, its nadir with disappearance of the Hellenic freedoms that had tolerated the presence of autonomous groups motivated by self-interest and thus predating Christianity.

B. The Modern Age -

Christianity then followed a sustained upward curve during the Dark Ages, becoming ever more important, global, and comprehensive. Medicine, in contrast, lay mired. Why?

As the early Christian Church evolved its doctrine it also evolved a hierarchy. This was necessary to maintain consistency in its message in response to strong convictions to alternative theological interpretations as described below. In addition to centralization of power within the Church that predictably would occur, there arose, from small pockets of devout and relatively isolated adherents, early monastical orders that would enlarge and spread as the Church's local representation throughout Europe and beyond, assisting local populations in not only matters of faith but also in learning, production and marketing of necessities, and interaction with feudal authority. Thus integrated into daily life throughout the continent, the Church's influence was enormous. What had begun as a sodality, or informal association, became a focus of influence that was, in effect, what has been termed a kinship sodality. Much effort of the members of this "kinship" was oriented toward preserving and improving the Church, and thus it flourished.

The medicine of the Hippocratic physicians could not benefit from these changes, for it had already disappeared. But why could not a true medical practice start anew? Requirements for initiation of human progress are the subject of Part II of this volume, but parameters include a population center of sufficient size and decentralized governance with commercial activity. Another requirement is shedding the obligations and responsibilities attendant to the egalitarian kinship, thus freeing up the individual to join with other like-minded persons to exploit an idea for personal benefit. To the extent that early medieval communities understandably focused on necessities for survival and on the activities and needs of the prominent institutions that enfolded them, *i.e.* the Church and feudal authorities, the resulting obligations and responsibilities made any entreneurial enterprise with another focus an unlikely event. But the opportunity finally presented itself.

It has been astutely argued that early democratization in a renascent Europe was reflected in and propelled by the great religious movement termed the Reformation as represented in the famous 16th C Huguenot treatise *Vindiciae, contra Tyrannos* (see Fig. 12), which Prof. Harold Laski (1893-1950), the prominent socialist, wrote "was the real starting point of democratic ideas."[70] It was at this point that medical science resumed, albeit sporadically at first. This freeing up was not a consequence of relief from Christianity. The latter had, if anything, continued to gain in importance and popularity. The recommencement was associated instead with a relief from authoritarianism. What had happened? In the 4rd C Christian doctrine was at last being analyzed and codified. The Gnostic Gospels, for example, were considered by some to be a menace to the formation of a cohesive Christian church or indeed any organized church at all. The early divines, scholars, and Church Fathers were, therefore, convened in Nicaea to resist this fragmentation, and from this the canon of the Catholic Church would ultimately emerge. That Church, despite the writings of St. Augustine, became progressively authoritarian with the passing centuries, just as had Hinduism in the hands of the Brahmins and Judaism in the hands of the Pharisees. Much as Buddhism and Jainism had been responses to the

---

[70] Discussed in: Nichols, J. H., *Democracy and Churches*, Philadelphia, 1951, Chapter 1. Harold Laski wrote the *Historical Introduction* to this reprinting of the first English translation of the 1579 work, *A Defense of Liberty against Tyrants* (London, 1924). John Calvin (1509-1564) was one of the spokesmen for the reform movements of the 16th C, and by the spread of Calvinism in its various forms, including Puritanism, the analogy would be brought westward to the New World. Laski was a prominent English Socialist committed to liberty and equality.

Brahmins and Christianity the alternative to Judaism, the Reformation would be a reaction to the Vatican.

If one person were to be selected to represent the theological dynamism that prompted political change based on the principle of equality of all men before God it would be a Frenchman, John Calvin (1509-1564). Reared as a devout Catholic, he subsequently became fully committed to Protestantism while a young man, and, finally attaining a safe haven in Geneva, he taught and wrote extensively on the absolute sovereignty of God in all matters, a teaching now generically termed "Calvinism." From his writings the eminent British jurist, James Stephen, summarized the four principles of what he termed a "spiritual republic,"[71] namely:

1. The will of the people was the sole legitimate source of the power of their rulers.
2. That power was most properly delegated by the people to their rulers by means of elections.
3. In ecclesiastical government the clergy and the laity were entitled to an equal and co-ordinant authority.
4. That between the Church and the State no alliance or mutual dependence, or other definite relation, necessarily or properly subsisted.

The political consequences of the concept that no priest, king, or president is more important that any other man and that an elected leader who disobeys God's law in flouting his electorate justifies his removal became manifest in vigorous clamor against State infringement on individual freedom. Much has been written about *Vindiciae, Contra Tyrannos*, but, relevant here, its deepest meaning is unequivocally stated at the beginning of the author's "3rd question" exposition, "The Whole Body of the People is Above the King." He continues: "No truly, but it is said in regard of all people, …," thus assuring its general applicability to humanity.[72] Despite the stern public aspect attributed to Calvinists and associated sects, their uncompromising demand for political and religious liberty led the French Huguenots, the English Puritans, the Scottish Covenanters, and the Protestant population of the Netherlands to be in the vanguard of political reform and the struggle against contemporary tyranny. As regards America, George III declared the American Revolution a "Presbyterian Rebellion," and the great French historian, Hippolyte Adolphe Taine (1828-1893) declared "They founded Scotland, they founded the United States."[73] The great German historian, Leopold von Ranke (1795-1886), expressed a similar opinion.[74] Alexis de Tocqueville wrote of the importance of the

---

[71] Stephen, J., *Lectures on the History of France*, New York, 1875, Lecture XV, p. 415.

[72] Translation of Wm. Walker, London, 1689.

[73] Taine, H. A., *History of English Literature*, Edinburgh, 1871, vol. 2, translated by H. Van Laun, p. 472. Taine was a prominent French historian and literary critic.

[74] Ranke wrote: "Es ist sehr bemerkenswert, dass ein Auslander, ein Franzose, von Avignon, welcher jedoch, von Zwingli bekehrt, in Luthers Schule von der evangelischen Lehre durchdrungen worden, diese Ideen so weit ausbildete. Es sind spaterhin gegrundet worden, von denen man wohl sagen kann, dass das Dasein, die Entwickelung von Nordamerika auf ihnen beruht. Sie haben eine unermebiche, welthistorische Wichtigkeit. Gleich bei idem ersten Versuche traten sie auf; eine kleine deutsche Synode nahm sie an." (" It is very remarkable that the man who worked out these ideas into so complete a scheme of church government, was a foreigner – a Frenchman of Avignon – who, converted by Zwingli, had become deeply imbued with evangelical doctrines in the school of Luther. The ideas are the same on which the French, Scottish, and American churches were

religious and civil underpinnings of early Anglo-American settlers such as the Pilgrims as the basis for the great experiment in democracy that he saw under way that would inevitably propel America to the pinnacle of nations; "Puritanism was not merely a religious doctrine, but it corresponded in many points with the most absolute democratic and republican theories."[75] And the historian, John Fiske, wrote of Calvin, "The spiritual father of Coligny, of William the Silent, and of Cromwell must occupy a foremost rank among the champions of modern democracy."[76] The critical reason for this evolution from what, on its face, would be considered an intolerant sect was its absolute separation of temporal from secular authority and its basic premise that all men were equals before God, regardless of wealth or power or "ecclesiastical jurisdiction."[77] Also relevant to religion in the West, the purely economic importance of Calvinism was discussed in a book by the sociologist, Prof. Max Weber, who argued that the basis for modern capitalism was to be found in the Protestant movements of northern Europe.[78] There is also scholarly support for an important role of Puritanism in promoting scientific study in Great Britain, for there was a flourishing of discovery from 1640-1660, the years of

---

afterward founded, and indeed on which the existence and the development of North America may truly be said to rest. Their historical importance is beyond all calculation. We trace them in the very first attempt at the constitution of a church; they were adopted by a small German synod." Whether Ranke was correct or subtly attempting to secure a nationalistic hold on the origin of Calvinism via a "small German synod" is not the issue. The significance of the "Frenchman," Francois Lambert, and the synod called by the Landgrave Philip of Hesse in response to early advice from Martin Luther were indeed important events, although Lambert's idea included a church constitution that was highly authoritarian with the head of state given charge of its implementation. But it is Ranke's conclusion about the incalculable importance of such a doctrinal discipline as he opined in the development of North America that is the point, and it is Calvinism. It is for this reason the extensive quotation from von Ranke's book has been provided. See: Von Ranke, L., *History of the Reformation in Germany*, London, 1905, translation of Sarah Austin, p. 461. The first edition was in German: *Geschichte im Zeitalter der Reformation*, Berlin, in 6 vols., 1839-1847.

[75] *Democracy in America*, New York, 1838, translation of Henry Reeve, 2nd American ed., p. 15.

[76] *The Beginnings of New England, or the Puritan Theocracy in Its Relations to Civil and Religious Liberty*, Boston, 1899, p. 58. A concise but authoritative interpretation of predestination and its role in shaping political thought can be found in the final chapter of Loraine Boettner's *The Reformed Doctrine of Predestination*, Grand Rapids, MI, 1932. A related phenomenon, and one that provides some underpinnings for Boettner's interpretation, is found in studies that associate the Reformation in general, and, as a more specific example, the Scottish reformation, with a marked increase in literacy that some scholars associate with the Reformation in northern Europe. See p. 350 of the present work.

[77] A scholarly explication of this important subject can be found in: Lamber, F., *The Founding Fathers and the Place of Religion in America*, Princeton, 2003. Even Adam Smith, in his *Wealth of Nations,* was able to see the value of competition among religions as a basis for tolerance and religious development, just as he saw the value of competition in his economic and commercial theories: "…zeal must be altogether innocent where the society is divided into two or three hundred, or perhaps into as many thousand small sects, of which no one could be considerable enough to disturb the public tranquility. The teachers of each sect, seeing themselves surrounded on all sides with more adversaries than friends, would be obliged to learn that candour and moderation…." See: Smith, A., *Wealth of Nations*, 4th editor, Dublin, 1785, Bk. 5, chapter 1, Part III - *Of the the Expense of public Works and public Institutions*, Art. III - *Of the Expense of the Institutions for the Instruction of People of all Ages*, p. 310.

[78] Weber, M., *The Protestant Ethic and the Spirit of Capitalism*, New York, 1958, translators P. Baehr and G. C. Wells, a work judged the fourth most important book on sociology of the 20th C.

Cromwell, as well as the beginnings of the Royal Society.[79]   But the return of the monarchy was associated with a profound reaction to Commonwealth ideals and stigmatized any further effort along those lines for over a century, thus extinguishing a nascent flame of scientific discovery.   Some of the preceding ideas as they bear upon Puritanism and the evolution of the "American character" are perceptively critiqued by the prominent historian, Prof. Richard Schlatter.[80]   Finally, the prominent sociologist, Prof. R. A. Nesbit, proposed that it was the amalgamation of Greek and Judeo-Christian worldviews that promoted the idea that man himself could not only better the hardships of life, but could establish a goal, over time and beyond mere existence, one that would better the lives of future generations.   This spur to progress toward that goal thus became, for 3000 years, the unique treasure of Western culture.[81]   The famous phrase "Protestant work ethic" considered any job to be important if it was of value to one's fellow man, and the importance of work in acquiring self-sufficiency and wealth is reminiscent of the importance of the work ethic in the early years of Classical Age Greece.

The force of a religion in promoting individual freedom has now been reviewed in the context of the Reformation, but the inhibitory role of religion also needs addressing. Blame has been placed on the Roman Church for impeding medical progress, and it has been pointed out that when the printing of books in Renaissance Italy was suppressed by Church censorship the number of presses decreased from 125 to 40, upon which the publishing industry relocated itself to a Protestant-oriented France, and when that country espoused Catholicism, the industry again relocated, this time to Holland.[82]   But in fact there were few medical books to be printed, for divinity, scholastic, epistolary, and historical writings comprised more than ninety-five percent of the holdings of any monastical library. The Church leadership had not employed its might to direct the course of medicine.[83] The relocation of great publishing houses was not done to liberate medical writings. The force of the Church had been directed, instead, against individualism. It militantly protected an obeisant congregation against a lone, freethinking individual. This

---

[79] For a critical assessment of this issue see: Raab, T. K., *Puritanism and the Rise of Experimental Science in England*, Neuchatel, 1962, an offprint of *Cahiers d'histoire mondiale*, 7:1, 1962.

[80] Schlatter, R., *The Puritan Strain*, in *The Reconstruction of American History*, New York, 1962 (paperback edition), John Higham, editor, pp. 25-45.

[81] Nisbet, R. A., *History of the Idea of Progress*, London, 1980. Nisbet pointed out (1) the Jewish concept of millenarianism in this life was consistent with Divine values and thus a driving force for progress, and (2) with regard to Christianity (p. 341 of the cited work), "at no point did the Church Fathers dismiss the Greek criterion of progress; that is, advancement of knowledge of [about] world and society." Progress as an expression of "Providential design" thus both preceded and superceded the Greek concepts, although the syllogistic arguments were similar. This interpretation Nisbet supported with an aphorism from Thomas Aquinas' *Summa Contra Gentiles*, Bk. 3-1, chapter 3, noting that Aquinas was "Greek to the very essence" in that aphorism (p. 93). The author has no argument with the importance of the accumulation of knowledge in promoting progress, but as fascinating as Nisbet's proposal is regarding the Judeo-Christian concept of progress, the author respectfully disagrees. The Dark Ages and the Medieval West are his argument, as will be put forth later in the present work.

[82] Putnam, G. H., *Books and Their Makers During the Middle Ages*, New York, 1896, vol. 2, p. 384.

[83] H. M. Malkin, for example, argues that it was the Church that caused medicine to lag behind other arts and sciences, in part because study of pathological anatomy was impossible because of proscriptions on autopsies. See his *Out of the Mist* (Berkeley, 1993), an enlightening review of anatomical discoveries in pathophysiology which have been so important to medical progress.

action was not religion speaking. This was a secular juggernaut in a cowl with its survival in the balance; on the one hand a vision of peace and redemption, on the other an authoritarian menace. The innocence of religion itself in deleteriously affecting the course of medicine is vividly proven by the pitiful, even criminal, status of medical care in recent decades in Russia, Cuba, and China, atheistic states forcibly interned by atheistic principals. In their attempts to make religion the scapegoat for society's inadequacies, religion's critics have attributed its failings to doctrinal rather than institutional policies. Yet it is clear that at least for medicine it has been the command structure of religious institutions rather than religion *per se* that has posed obstructions to progress, and even this was of limited significance.[84]

End of excursus

As Church and State parted company, confusion bred by the conundrum of choice of Christian doctrines became compounded by the proofs of Copernicus in 1543 that the earth was not the center of the universe. Dr. Hugo Engelhardt has surmised that there was now a competition among philosophies, one consequence being that governments began to withdraw their allegiances from the Church, thereby permitting new ideas to emerge.[85] New ideas, in the hands of a few of the tyrant's favorites, could now flourish in niduses of individualism.[86] Medicine was not so favored, however, for, unlike art, architecture, and other vocations, it had little to offer to the tyrant. But embers of science were to be fanned in the Renaissance by the patron.

---

[84] The same argument can be made for science. As more evidence has accrued, for example, it is certain that Galileo was admired by many in the Church, and his apostasy was related more to the nature of "what is true" rather than "what is [at] the center of the universe." Theological principles rather than observable facts were the disputed issues. This is not surprising. St. Augustine considered scientific knowledge of the natural world as consistent with God's gift of reason and free will to man. St. Thomas Aquinas had no qualms with scientific process or its conclusions as long as a distinction between theory and fact was maintained. The advent of scientific process into medieval thinking has been attributed to Robert Grosseteste (1175-1253), Bishop of Lincoln, whose analysis of Aristotelian writings is thought to have influenced positively the subsequent course of Western scientific method, although it may have been more his translations and his embrace and popularization of ancient Greek thinkers than original discovery on which his significance lies. (See: Crombie, A. C., *Robert Grosseteste and the Origins of Experimental Science 1100-1700*, Oxford, 1953.) None of the great names of the Church mentioned in this paragraph offer any evidence of off-hand dismissal of scientific discovery for the purpose of maintaining Church prominence.

[85] Engelhardt, H. T., Jr., *The Foundations of Bioethics*, Oxford, 1986. An exceptional response of this type was resistance of a Calvinist Netherlands against Spanish occupation and its Catholicism, whereby the Pilgrims were able to obtain haven in Leiden and would later be given priority for the introduction into America of many institutions and traditions of freedom, liberty, and equality that they observed during exile in the Netherlands, most of which were nonexistent in contemporary England. See: Campbell, D., *The Puritan in Holland, England and America: An Introduction toAmerican History*, New York, 1893, 2 vols.

[86] One of the most individualistic of man's endeavors has been art, and many are the inspired artists whose legacies were assured by the largess of a Renaissance tyrant, without whom the beauty of the Western world would be greatly diminished. Paul Strathern has pointed out, in his *The Artist, the Philosopher and the Warrior* (London, 2009), that certain Renaissance popes should also be included under the rubric of "tyrant."

CHAPTER TWENTY-ONE

INDIVIDUALISM AND DISCOVERY: ROLE OF THE PATRON

Patron: ". . . a wretch who supports with insolence, and is paid with flattery,"
Samuel Johnson
Author of *Dictionary of the English Language*
(London, 1745)

There was a flourish of medical discovery during the Renaissance that a preceding chapter revealed to be independent of ancient physicians and natural philosophers. The source of Renaissance rediscovery was, instead, the work of a few individuals who were able to initiate studies of their own design. Consistent with the social pattern of the age, fine arts, architecture, music, and science were supported by the patron, a wealthy or prominent individual who afforded both protection and support for his favorites, expecting in most cases some public acknowledgement and secondary gain from his benevolent wisdom. Thus, the patron was a vital force in Renaissance discovery.

A. Individualism and Discovery

Preceding chapters documented, for the practice of medicine, a frightening ineptitude during the Dark Ages and Medieval Period. The absence of medical discovery between the age of the Hippocratics and the Renaissance was exposed. The consequences of that hiatus in discovery operate on two levels:

1. Patients and their posterity - Medical discoveries that should have been available prior to the advent of Christianity were not acquired for approximately another 1500 or more years. Thus, there was withheld a vast store of practical information potentially useful to the health of every human born during those intervening centuries of ignorance, information that would in turn have formed the basis for further discovery.

2. Society in general - On an even grander scale, one might reflect on the sentiment that all other sciences owe their origins to medical science. This, in fact, was the opinion of Hippocrates: "I also hold that clear knowledge about natural science can be acquired from medicine and from no other source."[1] The reason for this seemingly pretentious statement is that Hippocratic medicine was the only objective discipline within the framework of ancient Greek natural philosophy. The atomism of Leucippus and Democritus, the planetary notions of Philolaus, the theory of contagion of Varro, and other theories now supported by scientific proofs were, among the ancient "scientists," ingenious thoughts only, supported by imagination and insight but not fact. They entered the realm of science in recent centuries only after confirmation by observation and experiment. Thus, had Hippocratic medicine and its scientific method not disappeared, the scientific revolution of the Enlightenment might have occurred sooner, the Rise of the West would not have been delayed by the Dark Ages, and, with evidence of the successes of liberty visible to

---

[1] *Ancient Medicine* XX, translation of W.H.S. Jones in vol. 1 of the *Loeb Classical Library* series on Hippocrates. *Ancient Medicine* has traditionally been attributed to Hippocrates himself. φυσις is interpreted as "nature," not the "nature of man."

all, authoritarian wars might now be behind us, but a painful reminder of the consequences of the close association between ignorance and authoritarianism.

Why, once having disappeared, did it take scientific medical discovery 1500 years to re-emerge in the West? Although the Hippocratics had no exotic instrumentation, subsequent experience has confirmed that to be unnecessary for significant medical progress. Assuming that men over the next fifteen hundred years were no less intelligent than the ancient Greeks, the same or similar observations could have been made at any time. The answer is that such observations almost certainly were made, for it is likely that potential Galileos and Santorios have always been around, perhaps even in abundance. But there existed no mechanism by which their ideas could accumulate and be propagated throughout society. How could some of that genius be allowed to surface?

B. Role of the Renaissance Patron

A clue to the answer of the question posed in the preceding paragraph is as follows: there was a window of opportunity for a few individuals in Renaissance and Enlightenment Europe to follow ideas with action. That window was opened by the tyrant in his role as patron.

Excursus on Patronage

Patronage: the support or influence of a patron.
Patron: a person chosen, named, or honored as a special guardian, protector, or supporter.

Webster's New Collegiate Dictionary, 1979

Although Samuel Johnson, in his dictionary, defined a patron as "a wretch who supports with insolence, and is paid with flattery," patronage has always been an important and integral component of social life. Indeed, as the patron is characterized as one-half of the ἀνισολογιζομένος ("that which is being reasoned by unequals"; p. 127), he has directed human affairs for over 10,000 years. For in matters between unequals the patron is the more than equal; you and I represent the lesser.

There is an ancient Greek term, εὐεργετής (euergetes, "benefactor"), that has been translated as the equivalent of "patron." Two forms of *euergetes* were described by Aristotle, one being a benefactor of the community and an expression of the benefactor's nobility. The other was of a personal nature and had this distinction: the benefactor was ashamed to receive benefits and, when in receipt of a gift, returned a benefit of greater value, a mark of the "great souled" man.[2] Neither type of euergetes conforms with Samuel Johnson's definition of "patron," which for present purposes refers to those who dispense patronage so as to entail influence, service, or reputation of another. Nevertheless, the

---

[2] "and whenever he does good, he is ashamed to have the favor returned, for the one act is elevating but the other is to be outdone." Aristotle, *Nicomachean Ethics*, IV, iii, 24-26, translation of the author. A sense of pride, not an effort to control, here seems to be the overweening principle.

latter form of patronage even in classical Greece must have been a fact of life, for the aristocrat and the tyrant both survive by patronage, and both were publically prominent prior to Greek democracy.

Prof. David Hahm has noted that in 3rd C BC Rome, "A priesthood was normally bestowed, not as a reward for meritorious service, but as a form of patronage to promising young men who were aspiring to political office."[3] But some consider the Romans to have formalized the patronic system during the Augustan Age. Prior to this time it had been a selective attachment to a Patrician that provided the Plebeian with both security and access to social benefices in return for his fealty and services rendered, an often contractural arrangement that was sometimes intergenerational. But with formal recognition through Roman law called *Clientela* it became a political tool as well, and in time it came to regulate affairs between governor and governed, between a general and his troops, and between central government and other regions or states. Patronage also provided an economic advantage through its use of friendships whereby financial transactions were more expeditious and allocations adjusted with greater precision. It is not surprising, therefore, that with the decline of the Roman Empire there emerged in its place the rights and obligations of the Catholic Church as a patron. This was formalized in the *uis patronatus*, a highly detailed system that guides relations and gifts from the Church to highly select benefactors.[4] On a more mundane level, the political patronage in the earlier years of the United States was known as the Spoils System, in which most political appointments were promised to those who had helped a particular candidate obtain office. This system generated sufficient opprobrium that it was for the most part replaced by a Civil Service, in which "what you know" (merit) was thought to be more important than "who you know" in hiring and promotion, although there have been many who question the honesty of that distinction or who prefer the stability and loyalty the Spoils System provided.

The process of patronage, when it pervades society, becomes the accepted custom and a network that can promote community stability, development, and accord. On the other hand, it is both a consequence and a perpetuator of inequality, and, except for a few lacunes in history, it has kept democratic contenders at a distance. And so, with the Medici's, Tammany Hall, Joseph Stalin, or modern politics, patronage has always been with us, its consequences being both good and bad, for patronage makes social inequality palatable by creating a unique type of "middle class," a group that, while under obligation to the patron, can feel superior to those unfortunates with *no* patron. In some instances patronage provided its own bondage: writers during the Renaissance often wrote effusive works about their patrons, not because of their patrons' just deserts but because of financial necessity. Works of artistic inspiration they were not. On the other hand, patronage freed the ingenuity of the occasional gifted individual by providing sustenance and protection.

To conclude this excursus, it is important to be reminded that the patron, the controlling force of the ἀνισολογιζομενος, need not be an individual. In the Dark Ages and the Late

[3] Hahm, D. E., *Roman Nobility and the Three Major Priesthoods, 218-167 BC*, in *Transactions and Proceedings of the American Philological Association*, 94:73-85, 1963.
[4] Verboven, K.: *The Economy of Friends. Economic Aspects of Amicitia and Patronage in the Late Republic*, Brussels, 2002.

Medieval Period the patron often was the Church, and it was the Church that was the beneficiary rather than secular leaders. Perhaps this accounts for much of the wealth, prestige, and power acquired by the Church during those centuries. The resulting magnificence permitted the Church, during the Renaissance, to distribute its munificence for objects of luxury. An important goal of this patronage was to increase the splendor of Rome as a center of magnificence appropriate for the organizational center of the Church, although there was also a desire to add to the glory of the Church and its message. Now it is the Modern State in its role as patron that through its political machinations and by its grants and awards directs to a major extent the course of collective intellect within many disciplines. It is also important, in the history of medicine, to understand the role of the patron in civilizations other than the West. The famed Al-Razi, who decided to learn medicine at age thirty years, died at age sixty, and in the intervening years wrote hundreds of books on many subjects, including medicine, pharmacology, alchemy, philosophy, and even music, had as his patron the Samanid prince, Abu Sajih Mansur,[5] which probably explains his prominent hospital appointments. The historian of medicine, Ibn Abi Usaibi (1203-1270 AD), was in the service of the Emir of Sarkhad. Even hospitals were within the purview of the patron. The famed Bimaristan al-Nuri in Damascus and the Mansuri hospital in Cairo were established by sultans, and to maintain practice standards specified employees were sent to check on patients and to report back to authorities if any physician was found neglecting his responsibilities. Dr. Cristina Alvarez Millan noted the following: "A quick look at the history of medieval Islamic medicine shows that virtually all theoretical treatises – particularly those which had a major impact on the western medical tradition – were written by medical authors working for governors or princes. In other words, while rulers undertook intellectual and artistic patronage to help extend their hegemony and the cultural influence of their courts, on the authors' side there was a practical concern not only for medical scholarship, but also for making one's name known in political and social circles as much as in the professional sphere."[6] But the client-patron relationship in Islamic states was always an integral part of existence, a manifestation of a kinship system that preceded the Prophet. To the overarching significance of the patron must be attributed all the intellectual successes and failures of early Islam.[7]

End of Excursus

It was because of the largesse and protection of patrons that many Renaissance artists, philosophers, and scientists were granted the opportunity to realize their inventions

---

[5] The Samanid dynasty (819-899 AD) revitalized the Persian Empire, and one of its Emirs, Abu Sajih Mansur, has been identified as Al-Razi's patron and presumably to whom his work *Liber ad Almansorem* was dedicated.

[6] Millan, C. A., *The Case Histories in Medieval Islamic Medical Literature: Tajarib and Mujarrabat as Source,* in *Med. Hist.*, 54:195-214, 2010.

[7] "All regimes were built upon the loyalties of slaves, clients, and retainers to their masters and patrons." See: Lapidus, I. M., *A History of Islamic Societies*, Cambridge, 1990, p. 188. The work is replete with examples of this sort.

Table 9: Patrons of Prominent Renaissance/Enlightenment Individuals

Beneficiary	Dates	Patron(s)
Raphael of Urbino	1483-1520	Pope Julius II
Servetus, Michael	1511-1553	Hugues de la Porte, Symphorien Champier
Lonicer, Adam	1528-1586	City of Frankfurt, Count Phillipp of Nassau; Dedicated his *Kreuterbuch* to the Count
Fabricius, Hieronymus	1533-1619	various Aristocratic families
Harvey, William	1578-1657	Primarily family and personal wealth and earnings, but his *de Motu Cordis* was dedicated to Charles I, whom he accompanied in travels
Borelli, Giovanni	1608-1679	Royal Court: Queen Christina of Sweden, Aristocracy, Leopoldo de Medici,
Cassini, Giovanni	1625-1712	Louis XIV
Pare, Ambroise	1510-1590	Gen. Montejan, Duke de Vendome, Charles IX; poor, could not afford licensure, became a military surgeon
Vesalius, Andrea	1514-1564	Charles V
Paracelsus	1493-1541	Ecclesiastical and aristocratic patrons; Froben (publisher)
Galileo	1564-1642	Cosimo de Medici, Ferdinand II
Santorio, Santorio	1561-1636	Court, Venetian nobility
Willis, Thomas	1621-1675	Thomas Iles, Archbishop Gilbert Sheldon
Fracastoro, Girolamo	1478-1553	General Alviano, Cardinals Farnese and Pietro Bembo; Bishop Giberti
Valsalva, Anton	1666-1723	Senate of Bologna; unlike many, did not seek patronage.
Cardano, Gerolamo	1501-1576	Church (Pope Gregory XIII), Sen. Filippo Archinto, Marquis D'Avalos
Malpighi, Marcello	1628-1694	Court: Berdinand II; Giovanni Borelli
Dubois, Jacques	1478-1555	Court: Henry II
Boyle, Robert	1627-1694	Court: Charles II; Boyle was independently wealthy through inheritance.
Descartes, Rene	1596-1659	Cardinal Beroulle, Princess Elizabeth; Descartes was wealthy by inheritance, and his patronage was primarily important for his protection.
Shakespeare, William	1564-1616	3rd Earl of Southampton
Kircher, Athanasius	1602-1680	Vatican; came from poor family, was a Jesuit priest.
Hooke, Robert	1635-1703	Court; Robert Boyle
Wren, Christopher	1623-1723	Royal Court; Wren's father had been Chaplain to Charles I and was wealthy.
Linnaeus, Carl von	1707-1778	Dr. John Rothman, Dr. K. Stobeus

and discoveries. As Sir Richard Jebb stated, "Augustus was to Virgil and Horace, what Lorenzo de' Medici was to members of the Florentine Academy."[8] Patrons usually were wealthy prominent individuals, although there was some group patronage. A contractural arrangement was common. The patron, therefore, provided select individuals with financial assistance and independence, within limits, to exploit their individual interests and abilities. Thus, patrons played a permissive but critical role in scientific advances, and for this they should receive praise. Contemporaries did praise them, and artists and others usually dedicated their works to their patrons. Table 9, p. 358, is an attempt to redress the historical anonymity of some of them, for it is they who guaranteed that the scientific revolution would occur in the West rather than the East. Many of their beneficiaries were investigators mentioned in chapter 18.[9]

But in medicine the quality of knowledge does not always guarantee the final product, for the final product is not manifested in the laboratory of the scientist, the *laboratorium* of the Church or the laboratory of public opinion. As identified by the physician, Francois-Joseph Broussais (1772-1838):

> "The real physician is the one who cures: the observation, which does not teach the art of healing, is not that of a physician, it is that of a naturalist."

And beyond that we have the words of Dr. J. C. Spence (1892-1954): [10]

> "The real work of a doctor is only faintly realized by many lay people. It is not an affair of health centres, or public clinics, or operating theatres, or laboratories, or hospital beds. These techniques have their place in medicine, but they are not medicine. The essential unit of medical practice is the occasion when, in the intimacy of the consulting room or sick room, a person who is ill, or believes himself to be ill, seeks the advice of a doctor whom he trusts. This is a consultation and all else in the practice of medicine derives from it. The purpose of a consultation is that the doctor, having gathered his evidence, shall give explanation and advice.... It is not difficult to realize something of the intimacy, the courtesy, and the understanding which is required in this work."

That work, the τεχνή (*techne*, "the profession") of medicine, is explored in the next where chapter where it will be shown that, *had the Renaissance and its patrons never happened,* modern medicine could easily have been where it is today.

---

[8] Jebb, R. C., in *Bacchylides*, Cambridge, 1905, p. 201, in his introduction to Ode 5, composed in 476 BC and describing the patronage of Hieron, tyrant of Syracuse

[9] An excellent source of relevant biographical information, including patrons, is provided on the Internet via the Galileo Project in the work of Richard S. Westfall, *Catalog of the Scientific Community in the 16th and 17th Centuries*, which contains biographical information on more than six hundred prominent scientists.

[10] Spence, J., *The Purpose and Practice of Medicine*, Oxford, 1960, chapter 18. But the Hippocratics were well aware of this: πρὸς δὲ ἰητρὸν οὐ μικρὰ συναλλάγματα τοῖσι νοσοῦσίν ἐστι· ("The intimacy also between physician and patient is close;" From *Physician*, translation of P. Potter, *Loeb Classical Library* series, *Hippocrates*, vol. VIII.)

CHAPTER TWENTY-TWO

RETURN OF THE KOINON AND THE NATURAL STATE OF
MEDICAL PRACTICE

"... *in science, the credit goes to the man who convinces the world, not the man to whom the idea first occurs.*"

Francis Darwin (1848-1925)
Eugenics Review, April, 1914, p. 9,
from text of the first Galton Lecture

Subsequent to the Renaissance and concurrent with the emergence in Europe of elements of democracy, as manifested in 18ᵗʰ C parliaments, a *bona fide* medical practice appeared, just as it had 2300 years earlier in Greece. Western Europe and Great Britain were the sites for this reincarnation of the Hippocratic koinon of Cos. Autonomous professional organizations and medical journals improved the work of the profession. Discoveries would now be vetted by the new koinons, and physicians began to successfully compete with the medicine-men of their day. It was the unencumbered physician and his organizations, not the Renaissance, that would bring about a second approximation to the natural state of medical practice.

A. Clinical Practice and the Renaissance

With the Renaissance began a period of medical progress that many think has continued to the present. Dr. Baas, in his *Outlines of the History of Medicine* (specifically, Second Section, third period, "*History of More Modern Medicine*") has uniquely explained this transition.[1] First, he has the Modern era fall immediately on the coattails of the Medieval. Secondly, he characterizes the medical profession of the medieval period as unregulated, with unlimited license of its practitioners to practice as they pleased. From this he implies that great harm was done to the profession. Thirdly, in the 17ᵗʰ C and on into the Age of Absolutism (see below), when the State was all-powerful, he noted that the profession became regulated, licensed, and policed so that fraud, antisocial behavior, and greed could be controlled. From this regulation he concludes that the reputation of the profession benefited and medical progress ensued. To Baas it appears that the key to medical progress was not so much the Renaissance with its innovative ideas as it was a firm authoritarian hand, a dangerous and myopic opinion commonly held today as centralized governmental control of medicine is courted. Neither was the case.

Quite a contrary interpretation can be put on Dr. Baas' theory. In the first place, it should not be surprising to learn that Western efforts at regulation derived from the authoritarian world of Islam and its long-established tradition of licensing.[2] Second, there were no scientific physicians in the Dark Ages and medieval times. Dr. Fielding Garrison lamented that in the Dark Ages the state of surgery throughout Europe, Italy excepted,

---

[1] Baas, J. H., *Outlines of the History of Medicine and the Medical Profession*, New York, 1889, H. E. Handerson, translator.
[2] Campbell, D., *Arabian Medicine and Its Influence on the Middle Ages*, London, 1926, I, p. 119. Also note Roger II and his licensing of physicians in 1140 (p. 325 of the present volume).

was worse than had existed at the time of the Trojan War almost 2500 years earlier.[3] Perhaps the modern definition of profession was indeed fulfilled by medieval practitioners: "A vocation requiring advanced education and training; collectively, the members of such a vocation."[4] But medicine-men are not professionals, even though they might study hard, pay annual dues, and attend the annual meeting of medicine-men. When in medieval times medicine became a recognized vocation of the learned, medical education was a self-serving mixture of archaic theory and religion. State regulation of such practitioners accomplished nothing except to render their systems canonical and remunerative because, from the varied mass of practitioners, a designated special class of practitioner was declared, thus clearing the way for higher income for those in that class.

That modern medical *science* can be attributed to the Renaissance is highly questionable, and Prof. Jerome Buckley has characterized Renaissance discovery as primarily an act of personal fulfillment.[5] Other important events were occurring in the 17th C. One was the separation of church and state, so that by the end of that century direct clerical influence on medicine had declined even further and a secular aristocracy had taken charge of secular affairs, of which discovery, fame, and fortune characterized the released curiosity and covetousness of the age. This impetus for change produced a flood of new information, much of it arriving from the New World. An astonishing vista of new peoples, flora, and fauna invited inquiry and documentation. Universities were not equal to the task: "The universities were incapable of adapting themselves to the requirements of the new age. - Hence the great need for societies...."[6] Universities were not the research institutions they are today. Scientific societies, therefore, arose, first in Italy, then throughout Europe and the British Isles.[7]

It is also debatable whether modern medical *practice* can be ascribed to the Renaissance. The London College of Physicians, founded in 1518, at its outset required candidates to pass comprehensive examinations on Hippocrates and Galen, knowledge two thousand years old. As a university-trained profession, medicine remained a field that attracted few students, and Dr. Baas records that the University of Strassburg had only thirteen medical students between 1612 and 1631, and he cites other schools as well, although he notes that the Thirty Years' War was in progress.[8] The schism between internal medicine and surgery would continue to have baneful effects for another two centuries, although there were increasing numbers of surgeons who, on their own, sought new knowledge in the fields of physiology, pathology, and pharmacology. And it took some time before the residua of the preceding age's practitioners faded away, for in the 17th C the pompous but useless "proper physicians" were still consulted. The circumstances at that time were reminiscent of the *asipu* and *asu* of ancient Babylon 4000 years previously, for two classes of doctors coexisted, the *Medici puri* and the *Medicus*.

---

[3] Garrison, F. H., *An Introduction to the History of Medicine*, Phila., 1913, 1st editor, p. 113. Surely the state of internal medicine was even worse than was surgery.

[4] Black's Law Dictionary, 7th edition, 1999; *Webster's New World College Dictionary*, 4th edition, adds "and involving intellectual skills..."

[5] Buckley, J. H., *The Triumph of Time*, Cambridge (MA), 1966, chapter 3, a brief but excellent analysis of the subject in its modern context.

[6] Tannery, P., *Memoire Scientifique*, Paris, 1912-1950, vi, p. 394.

[7] These societies included: *Societas secretorum naturae* (Naples) 1560, *Accademia de lincei* (Rome) 1603, *Royal Society* (England) 1662, *Academie des Sciences* (France) 1666, and *Society of Sciences* (Berlin) 1700.

[8] Baas, J. H., *Outlines of the History of Medicine and the Medical Profession*, New York, 1889, H. E. Handerson, translator, p. 554.

The former, of which a *Physicus* was an example, was an official city or state physician, and the *Medicus*, of lower grade, a common practitioner or perhaps a local barber-surgeon. Medical degrees could be purchased. The full range of practitioners, the lithotomists, the astrologist-physicians, the barbers, the bathkeepers, herniotomists, oculists, itinerant practitioners and surgeons, midwives, apothecaries, and even hangmen and miracle-workers to name a few, were in competition for a living through ministrations. While the salaries of some credentialed physicians for prominent persons are known, the common man had to deal with a quite different sort of practitioner, although it is difficult to say that he was worse off because of it. The University of Paris in 1437 decreed that an astrological almanac was required by physicians and surgeons in order to practice. The pharmacopoeia of London, in 1618, comprised 1,960 treatments, including oil of ants, vipers' flesh, and butter made in May. Editions of 1650 and 1677 showed no improvements.[9] Discoveries and inventions in medical science of the 15th and 16th centuries did not improve medical practice of the 17th or early 18th centuries. Even Casanova (1725-1798), the brilliant gigolo and expert on imposters, wanted to be a doctor, for it was "a profession in which charlatanism takes you even further than it does in the legal profession."[10] But change was on the door stoop.

B. The Enlightenment, *ca.* 1650-1800: Absolutism and the Evolution of Democracy

It is amazing but true that the compilation and lexicography of the works of Hippocrates by Foes published in 1595 remained, in effect, the basic textook of medicine well into the 19th C.[11] Indeed, in 1862 the physician-scholar, Littre, completed his translation into French, after twenty-three years labor, of all the Hippocratic works, just in time to realize that Hippocratic writings had become "of interest only to medical historians."[12] The harbinger of that change had been Francis Bacon (1561-1626). This

---

[9] Garrison, F. H., *An Introduction to the History of Medicine*, Phila., 1921, 3rd editor, pp. 219-220. And in 1664 the fourth edition of Sir Kenelm Digby's book ("*A Late Discourse on ......,*" London) still included the "powder of sympathy" which "cured wounds by being rubbed on the weapon that inflicted them... It worked by a combination of occult and natural powers, that is, by attraction and by the small material particles given off by all objects."

[10] See his biography, *Casanova*, by J. Masters, New York, 1969, p. 15.

[11] The works of Foes, considered among the earliest and greatest of "modern" editions of Hippocrates, were: *Oeconomia Hippocratis alphabeti serie distincta*, Frankfort, 1588, and *Magni Hippocratis medicorum omnium facile principis opera omnia quae extant in VIII sectiones*, Frankfort, 1595. Francis Adams (*The Genuine Works of Hippocrates*, translated by Dr. Francis Adams, New York, 1929 reprint of the Sydenham Society's 1849 publication) frequently cites Foes regarding translations and authenticity of Hippocratic works.

[12] Paul-Emile Littre (1801-1881) was a French lexicographer, famous for his *Dictionary of the French Language*. He had a medical degree as well as an extensive education in linguistics, but it is unclear whether he was ever in medical practice. His *Oeuvres completes d'Hippocrate* was published in ten volumes between 1839 and 1862. Dr. Horstmanshoff was of the opinion that Hippocratic works had become, by that time, of no interest except as part of a Classics library. And yet technical advances have not outdated the procedures of medical inquiry, nor has society arrived at a point where it need inquire no further. It is important that the Hippocratic works continue to bear the standard of clinical medicine as its first and finest, not to say the most economical, example of scientific thought.

man recognized that understanding natural processes would lead to the development or exploitation of things that made life easier and more enjoyable, and that this, rather than the mere acquisition of knowledge, was a proper goal of study. He stated that if science were made a Vestal Virgin one should not expect her to bear fruit. Improving the improvable was, to him, of far greater importance than seeking to know the unknowable, and susceptibility to improvement is essential for progress to occur. Galileo had advanced scientific observation by adding to it the objectivity of calculation, its full expression emerging with Isaac Newton. The ability of man to understand the workings of his world and the universe released a flood of invention in Europe that would lead to the Industrial Revolution. This age, which also involved a reassessment of man's relationship with God, has been called the Enlightenment. Analogy has been drawn between Enlightenment and Aristotelian thought of 4th C BC Greece, with science again in the vanguard.

In Italy the Renaissance tyrant was embattled. Elsewhere, however, reinstatement of the divine right of kings found a prominent proponent in Jacques-Benigne Bossuet (1627-1704) who advanced time-honored biblical arguments that royal authority was sacred and absolute. As a consequence, the Enlightenment has been identified with the "Age of Absolutism." Struggles among aristocrats, legislatures, and monarchs led to centralized governments with a large civil service, precursors of modern nation-states. But at the same time men began to apply scientific reasoning not only to mechanical things but also to society and to man himself.

In ancient Athens it had been the press of class hostility and economic disparity that led to the appeal of the tyrant and his ultimate replacement by democratic assembly. A different path was pursued in ancient Ionia, whereby Hellenic democracy was less forced as privileged land ownership gradually blended into a commerce-based society.[13] In contrast to both of these, the Renaissance advanced a form of republicanism rather than democracy. Thereby governing power was nonmonarchical and theoretically in the hands of the people, but stability was provided by a structured commercial class society that assumed the masses were unequal to the task of self-government, the perennial authoritarian argument.[14] North of Italy larger and more complex centralization of authority occurred, spurred by the disastrous wars of the 16th and 17th centuries. Thus, neither in Italy nor in most of Europe was democracy promoted.

But seemingly out of nowhere came John Locke (1632-1704), himself trained as a physician, who propounded the morality and benefits of individual liberty, an idea that would resonate throughout the Old World and the New and provide the philosophical basis for the American Constitution.[15] By 1700, well into the Enlightenment, the Dutch Republic had been declared, England's Glorious Revolution had occurred, and Williamsburg and New York in the New World were flourishing under their locally elected councils. Even the Thirty Years War (1618-1648) might be considered a

---

[13] Discussed in: Emlyn-Jones, C. J., *The Ionians and Hellenism*, London, 1980.

[14] Bartlett, K. R., *A Short History of the Italian Renaissance*, Toronto, 2013, chapter 6, especially the discussion of the Ordinances of Justice, a constitutional document imposed in 1293 by commercial (guild) efforts.

[15] John Locke apparently had a limited practice in Oxford, submitted medical articles to journals, and was the "physician" who traveled with Lord Shaftsbury. He received a Bachelor of Medicine degree, but not a Doctor in Medicine. See *Locke and Sydenham* by John Brown, MD, Edinburgh, 1858. A Bachelor of Medicine, Bachelor of Surgery (MBBS) in England at the present time is the equivalent to the American MD degree, the Doctor of Medicine being reserved for those with additional distinguished research careers.

consequence of "individualism" at the national level as member states resisted the international authority of The Holy Roman Empire. And it is the increasing acceptance of representative government, whether through republicanism, democracy, or advisory assemblies, that most likens this period to Classical Greece, the age of Pericles and of democratic city-states, although it was the Swiss Cantons, being virtually independent and many being democratic, that would best approximate those polities.[16] Increasing democratization was driven by a desire for personal liberty, and it permitted increasing interactions among those individuals having similar interests. There were two corollary developments. One was been expounded by Dr. Friedrich Hayek. It describes the value accruing to society of personal freedom that sanctions, through the marketplace, the free interactions of men with others unknown to them throughout society and thus to better the personal condition of each, with the larger consequence being that the conjunction of ideas and efforts so released leads to better services for the community at large. This is, by virtue of its vastness, an abstract theory of economics that is nevertheless supported by much objective evidence and to which the term "catallaxy" has been applied.[17] But the other development of the desire for liberty that led to democratization is the focus of this book: the value of the small group freely entered into and based on principles of equality among its members, i.e., the koinon. This is not an abstract idea, and the successes in the West of the physician-patient relationship and of the multitude of medical societies have documented for all time a parallel phenomenon to catallaxy, namely, the inestimable value of individual liberty released within a sympathetic group in promoting progress outside the marketplace. While great difficulties of the Dark Ages were now past, other difficulties remained. But Prometheus was again unbound, and some of the consequences of his release are the subject of the remainder of Part I of this volume.

C. Return of Democracy, a Modern Hippocrates, and Clinical Medicine

A momentous development within the Dark Ages was the university, and one of the great legacies of the medieval university was that matriculation existed as an option for rich and poor alike. Dr. Riesman has pointed out that few of the nobility became scholars in either ancient Greece or medieval Europe.[18] On the other hand, a poor lad, if admitted, could become a prominent scholar or, in medicine, a wealthy doctor. And, comments by Petrarch and Montaigne notwithstanding, the university-trained medical man could be a member of high society. But during the Renaissance centuries of university affiliation had promoted medicine's popularity rather than its development. It

---

[16] In fact, some Swiss cantons were self-sufficient democracies as early as the 13th C, protected by geography and viable because of their small size and uncomplicated political issues. See: Clarke, M.V., *The Medieval City State*, London, 1926, especially chapter 8. It may not be by chance that the famed physician, Paracelsus, considered the first to break with the medicine of Galen, was born in the canton of Schwyz in 1493. Arguably far more important to modern medicine was the selection by John Calvin of the safe haven of Geneva for his home, from which he was able to spread the Protestant banner under which the Huguenots, Puritans, Covenanters, Pilgrims, and the Protestant Netherlanders would descend on tyranny and propel forward the message of civil liberty (see p. 350*ff* and Fig. 12 on p. 329).

[17] The derivation of "catallaxy" is from the Greek καταλάσσω (katalassow), meaning "to give in exchange," in this case not only goods and services, but their associated ideas.

[18] Riesman, D., *The Story of Medicine in the Middle Ages*, New York, 1936, p. 376.

was only in the 18th C that patients were finally getting closer individual attention while alive, in contrast to the meticulous anatomical studies of the Renaissance centuries past that were obtained from postmortem dissection. After all, knowing the details of the course of anterior tibial recurrent artery, the *nervus cutaneous brachii posterior*, and the *transversus perinei superficialis* muscle, is, like *Goethe's bone*, relevant to the daily life of very, very few.[19] This was apparent to none other than John Locke who wrote that anatomical discoveries amounted to little more than "more superficies...to stare at."[20] There began to take place important changes in medical curricula. Interestingly but not surprisingly, this change did not occur in any of the ancient universities of Europe; rather, it began in a relatively new one in Leiden. For it was there that an emerging Dutch Republic founded its first university in 1575 (The University of Orange-Nassau, later University of Leiden). Under its motto, *Praesidium Libertatus* ("Stronghold of Freedom"), and linked to freedom of speech and religion, the University of Leiden promptly produced many great names in continental scholarship. The event of the University of Leiden is reminiscent of that of Padua, mentioned earlier. The latter was one of the oldest institutions of learning in Europe, founded in 1222, but, protected by the Republic of Venice, it was known for its academic freedom and brilliant graduates, attracting students from other universities. Its motto, a harbinger of that of the University of Leiden, had been *Universa universis patavina libertas* ("The freedom of Padua is complete for everybody").

Did the Enlightenment have its "Hippocrates" as did the Greece of Pericles? In Thomas Sydenham (1624-1689) some think it did. But rather than discover Hippocratic method, he but redeployed it. Known as the "English Hippocrates," Sydenham has been admired for his accurate clinical observations and attention to detail, producing works of clinical importance, including writings on epidemic disease, fevers, and gout. Hippocrates was his hero and scientific method his method. Although Sydenham formed theories of disease he did not let them guide his treatments. He espoused new ideas if they worked, including cinchona bark for certain fevers. But he presided over no medical organization, and his efforts represented only his own and his patients' interests. He was unable to shake off the still prevalent nihilistic view of medical progress: ". . . the cause[s] of disease...are the invisible and insensible spirits that govern, preserve, and disorder the economy of the body.... We are still ignorant, and likely to remain so, of the true essential causes of diseases, their manner of production, forms, and ways of ceasing." He gave the

---

[19] Discovered by, among others, Johann Wolfgang Goethe (1748-1832), the *intermaxillary* bone is, except for some plastic surgeons, of little or no interest to physicians, but it is of considerable interest to Darwinians because of its presence in other mammalian species.

[20] Locke, J., *Anatomie*, 1668. John Locke (1632-1704), the famous English philosopher, was a physician with a special interest in pediatrics. He became attached to the household of Lord Shaftesbury as personal physician. In the midst of his political writings he retained an active interest in medicine, as this particular reference shows. It has even been suggested that Locke's legacy in individualism and government can be traced to his interest in Hippocratic principles, although more commonly it is suggested that Spinoza was its source. See Coleman, W. O., *The Significance of John Locke's Medical Studies for his Economic Thought*, in *History of Political Economy*, 32:711-731, 2000. That similar political opinions were percolating in England at that time and previously, please consult Henry Care's *English Liberties* (1680) and Christopher St. Germain's *Two Dialogues in English* (1528). And when encomiums are raised to the great anatomist, Andreas Vesalius (1514-1564) and his masterpiece, *De Humani Corporis Fabrica*, considered one of the "greatest treasures of Western civilization," it should be noted that he was in no way an accomplished clinician, despite the high offices he was given.

famous opinion to Sir Hans Sloane: "Anatomy and botany, nonsense."[21] Baas describes him as a "reluctant author,"[22] although one of his books was a popular text for many years.

But neither Sydenham nor his European contemporary, Friedrich Hoffmann (1660-1742), were contenders for the title of an Enlightenment Hippocrates.[23] The new Hippocrates, twenty-one years of age at the time of Sydenham's death, was Hermann Boerhaave (1668-1738). Born near Leiden, one of nine children and with very modest prospects, Boerhaave anchored his early studies on Hippocrates, "the original source of all medical knowledge" and thus a contemporary statement on the value of Hippocratic thought on the development of the medical profession. Observation rather than imagination was his method, and thus he was freed from superstition and the restrictions of philosophy, which Sir Thomas Browne could not do,[24] yet open to modern inquiry, which Sir Thomas Sydenham did not do. Reminiscent of Hippocratic thought in *Ancient Medicine,* Dr. Boerhaave, as described by Samuel Johnson, vigorously opposed "arrogant philosophers" in medicine, those who "possessed with too high an opinion of their own abilities, rather choose to consult their own imaginations, than inquire into nature, and are better pleased with the charming amusement of forming hypotheses, than the toilsome drudgery of making observations."[25] Hermann Boerhaave did what had been done once before, whereas the Hippocratics had no template. Nevertheless, Boerhaave did indeed lead medicine into its modern era, and Dr. Johnson granted him "second place among those which are of the greatest benefit to mankind."[26]

---

[21] Sydenham's full statement, responding to a letter by Robert Boyle, was: "…Anatomy, Botany – Nonsense! Sir, I know an old woman in Covent Garden who understands botany better, and as for anatomy, my butcher can dissect a joint full as well; no, young man, all this Stuff: you must go to the bedside, it is there alone that you can learn disease." The letter contains some career recommendations for a young Dr. Hans Sloane. Sloane (1660-1753) was a talented Irish scientist and a physician whose extensive collections, when donated, were the foundation for the British Museum. From: De Beer, G., *Sir Hans Sloane and the British Museum*, Oxford, 1953, p. 25. Sloane completed his medical training at the University of Leiden, subsequently the academic home of Hermann Boerhaave.

[22] Baas, J. H., *Outlines of the History of Medicine and the Medical Profession*, New York, 1889, H. E. Handerson, translator, p. 504.

[23] Friedrich Hoffmann has been styled as the German Hippocrates because of his success in organizing the important new medical school at Halle, his brilliant teaching, concern about medical ethics, and the importance he attached to moving away from the humoral and vascular theory of physiology and disease toward a more mechanistic and quantitative approach, especially in the area of neurology. He was a member of the Royal Society in London.

[24] Nevertheless, Thomas Browne (1605-1682), a physician remembered more for his literary skill than for medicine, attended the universities in both Padua and Leiden, and it is, therefore, not surprising that he discussed hereditary features as "All which mutations, however they began, depend upon durable foundations, and such as may continue forever," two centuries before Mendel (1822-1884). This is apparently the first use of the term "mutation." See his *Pseudodoxia Epidemica*, Bk. VI, chapter 10, "Of the Blackness of Negroes." Dr. Boerhaave would have been fourteen years old when Browne died.

[25] Johnson, Samuel, in *Herman Boerhaave*, first printed in *The Gentleman's Magazine*, 1739. Johnson's eulogy represented public perception and published accounts rather than personal experience with Boerhaave.

[26] Having described Boerhaave in such a positive light, it is appropriate that a somewhat different opinion be offered, and for that see: Cook, H. J., *Boerhaave and the Flight from Reason in Medicine*, in *Bull. Hist. Med.*, 74: 221-240. That well-presented and referenced perspective of Boerhaave states, however, that "it was the viewpoint of Dutch medicine, which Boerhaave happened to be in

It was at the University of Leiden that Dr. Boerhaave came to be the quintessential academic physician. He was a teacher and a scientist prominent in the fields of botany and chemistry, but most importantly Boerhaave was an advocate of clinical medicine. As the most prominent envoy of the Leiden School he saw it become the first center of clinical training, the first authentic medical school in history, profoundly influencing Western medicine. He introduced bedside teaching to 18th C Europe, one of his students being Dr. Anton de Haen, who became the first clinical teacher in all of Germany.[27] And so it was in 1708 in Leiden that Dr. Boerhaave published his textbook *Institutiones Medicae*.[28] This book, comprising his series of lectures to medical students, became the dominant medical text for almost a century. In the republican atmosphere of the new Dutch states entrenched medical authority that had so unquestioningly followed Galen no longer had a hold. Dr. Boerhaave boldly stated that all works on physiology before the time of Dr. William Harvey became outdated with the appearance of *De Motu Cordis*, a truism said to be not in the least apparent to Dr. Harvey himself.[29] Even though Boerhaave did not introduce new scientific concepts or pursue major clinical research, Johann Baas, the medical historian, reported that his fame as a clinician was such that there was no lecture hall at the University of Leiden large enough to accommodate his audiences. Known worldwide, he was able to make the Russian Czar, Peter the Great, wait to see him, making the point that all patients equally deserved his attentions. Dr. Boerhaave was, for many years, chairman of the Surgeons' Guild of Leiden, although it is not known if the latter functioned as a true koinon.

As a description of the condition of medical practice at the end of the 17th C, it is essential to repeat this statement of Boerhaave:

"If we compare the good which a half dozen true sons of Aesculapius have accomplished since the origin of medical art upon the earth, with the evil which the immense mass of doctors of this profession among the human race have done, there can be no doubt that it

---

the position to communicate, that made him famous, rather than his character or intellect." We are all products of our times. It is indeed the principal argument of the author that individual and group freedom has been the linchpin for medical progress. For whatever reason, therefore, Boerhaave was a product of the new freedoms occurring in western Europe, and he did not fail to bear the responsibilities and fulfill the duties of his profession. Perhaps the greatest attestation that he did that well is found not in modern rethinking of his writings but in the great contributions of his students. He was cited by Haller as "communis Europae praeceptor," the "common teacher of Europe."

[27] The earliest reintroduction of clinical bedside teaching actually occurred in Padua, where the famed Giovanni de Monte (1498-1551), Italy's "second Galen," took his students on rounds in a hospital in Padua. Citations on this point are found in P. F. Grendler's *The Universities of the Italian Renaissance*, Baltimore, 2001, p. 342*ff*. After his death de Monte's lecture notes were published in Venice by a student, V. Lublinus, in 1556: *Consultationum Medicinalium Centuria Prima*, and a *Centuria Seconda* in 1559. These were clinical cases.

[28] In 1707 *Institutiones Medicae* was published in Leiden, a text of physiology for students that included a review of writings of many medical authors that were melded into a combination of theory and practice. It saw many editions throughout the 18th C

[29] In Dr. Boerhaave's words: "...consequently, everything that has been written before is not only useless but also pernicious." Cited and translated by A. M. Luyendijk-Elshout: *The Anatomical Illustrations in the London Edition (1741) of Part I of Herman Boerhaave's Institutiones Medicae*, in *Boerhaave and His Time*, Leiden, 1970, G. A. Lindeboom, editor, p. 83.) Dr. Harvey himself apparently had little interest in the development of scientific societies and was not a "modern" Hippocrates (see *Comenius in England*, R. F. Young, editor, Oxford, 1932, p. 5).

would have been far better if there had never been any physicians in the world."

His opinion mirrors that of a Hippocratic writer:

> "Medicine is the most distinguished of all the arts, but through the ignorance of those who practice it, and of those who casually judge such practitioners, it is now of all the arts by far the least esteemed. ... Just as these have the appearance, dress and mask of an actor without being actors, so too with physicians; many are physicians by repute, very few are such in reality."[30]

Historians of medicine have been consistent in their praise of Boerhaave,[31] although, as Dr. Lindeboom wrote, he was "more a transmitter and transmuter that a creator, more a road builder than a pathfinder."[32] William Osler would agree that the "credit," from the opening quotation of this chapter, goes to Dr. Boerhaave. If a Hippocratic surrogate is to be named, it must be Boerhaave, Professor of Medicine and Rector of the University of Leiden, the man who made it the first true medical school and the most progressive medical institution of Europe, of the West, indeed, of the world.

D. Return of the Medical Koinon: A Consequence of Political Change in Western Europe, not the Renaissance

Subsequent to Boerhaave, scientific botanical investigations began to reap benefits as Dr. William Withering (1741-1799) identified an active principle by isolating the leaves of *Digitalis purpurea* from a mixture of herbs mentioned to him by an elderly woman in Shropshire, an herbalist, and thereby confirming the usefulness of the foxglove, discovering the source of digitalis alkaloids, and determining the optimal preparation to be administered, along with quantifying effective and toxic doses. Poor sanitation and overcrowding in public facilities were being institutionally addressed. Prof. Friedrich Hoffmann published his *Medicus politicus*, a treatise on medical ethics. Advances in medical science increased the reputation of the profession, and Fielding Garrison stated that the 18th C physician came to be as highly regarded as physicians were when he published his highly regarded *Introduction to the History of Medicine* in 1913. The popularity of the profession produced a unique social twist: for the first time the upper classes, who had no financial motive for embracing a profession, desired to enter it, so much so that a sliding scale of tuition was instituted in some universities to assist talented applicants from the the lower classes.

A telling feature of reemerging western scientific medical practice in the 18th C was geographic: its epicenter was in western, rather than eastern, Europe, with England, Scotland, and the Dutch Republic having an inordinate representation among prominent clinician-scientists. Boerhaave, Withering, the Hunter brothers, Smellie, Pott, Cullen,

---

[30] *Law*, I, translation: W. H. S. Jones in the *Loeb Classical Library* series of *Hippocrates*, vol. 2.

[31] Dr. Charles Singer wrote, in his famous history of medicine, the following: "Taking one thing with another, considering his influence as a teacher, his clinical acumen, his power of inspiring younger workers, his wide learning, his balanced vision, his eagerness for new knowledge, his sanity, his humanity, his generosity, and his prophetic power, Boerhaave must be regarded as the greatest physician of modern times." (*A Short History of Medicine*, Oxford, 1928, p. 140, 142.)

[32] Lindeboom, G.A., *Boerhaave and His Time*, Leiden, 1970, p. 36.

Heberden, and Jenner were but a few of the prominent Western clinicians at this time. And of other great names in European medicine some, like Marcello Malphigi of Bologna (1628-1694) and Antoni van Leeuwenhoek of Delft (1632-1723), published their findings in the *Transactions* of the newly formed Royal Society in London. Indeed, most of Malpighi's research publications were printed in the *Transactions*, and he became the Society's first Italian member in 1668, only a few years after its founding. Benjamin Franklin, despite his part in separating America from England, was also a member, even being honored by the Society for his role in protecting the explorations of Capt. James Cook from American cruisers during the War of Independence. The international reputation of the Royal Society in London reflected the increasing population and political significance of cities in the west. Eastern Europe was far more rural. A greater concentration of interested clinicians, therefore, may have been the natural consequence of urban growth. Paris, however, with a population of about 600,000, was among the largest of cities and yet French medicine of the 18th C was marked with a level of medical discovery no greater than most of Europe. R. A. Houston provides a "bold geographic summary" of modern historical European literacy: "If Europe was homogeneous in terms of its restrictive literacy at the end of the Middle Ages, it had three massive cultural zones by the end of the nineteenth century; a literate, economically developed (and largely Protestant) north; a center with pronounced regional variations, notably France; and a less literate, underdeveloped (Catholic and Orthodox) south and east. The 1900 distribution was itself the result of four centuries of more robust advances in literacy in the northern parts of Europe than elsewhere."[33] Some scholars have stressed the importance of the Reformation for advances in literacy, others stressing regional socioeconomic differences and urbanization. All these factors were probably in play and fed one another.

But there is a more fundamental explanation for the disparity between eastern and western Europe, namely the greater urban autonomy that was associated with the freedoms attendant to western parliaments. This contrasted with the dependent rural and village populations further east, populations that were only slowly breaking with the monarchical institutions that characterized the Age of Absolutism, a process just beginning. The independence of the Royal Society in London contrasted with the dependence on government of similar societies elsewhere.[34] In Vienna it was left up to Maria Theresa who, in mid-18th C and recognizing that Vienna was a medical backwater, looked to western Europe and persuaded Dr. Boerhaave's student, Gerhard van Swieten, to vitalize Austrian medicine. This he did, in part by ridding the Empire of its academic patronage system and by introducing clinical teaching and formal examinations.[35] The first medical school in Scotland was founded in 1726, and its initial faculty was composed entirely of physicians trained in Leiden. Scotland's medical schools were immediately to be in the forefront of medical progress. In Germany, it was Dr. Boerhaave's student, Anton de Haen rather than prominent German physician, Friedrich Hoffmann, who received his medical training at the University of Jena (see footnote, p. 366), who introduced the clinical teaching championed by Boerhaave.

The democratic tendency in the West was apparent as well in medical publishing. The 1640s saw in England, at the time of its civil war, a collapse of censorship as Puritans

---

[33] See the entry *"Literacy"* in the *Encyclopedia of European Social History*, 5:391-406, Detroit, 2001.
[34] The Royal Society was able to refrain from receiving government largesse until 1850.
[35] Kidd, M., Modlin, I.M., *Van Swieten and the Renaissance of the Vienna Medical School*, in *World J. Surg.*, 25:444-450, 2001.

and other sects disseminated thousands of pamphlets and books in their quest for religious freedom. This was the time of Milton's *Areopagetica*. A major achievement was the translation from Latin into English of the *London Dispensatory*, the pharmacopoeia of licensed apothecaries. By this translation, and despite much criticism, Nicholas Culpeper in 1649 opened to public inspection the mysterious remedies of the pharmaceutical establishment.[36] It has also been proposed that the spirit of Puritanism was a major factor that for a brief span, 1640-1660, propelled British science to eminence, only to see that effort fail with the Restoration. The democratizing of science was greatly enhanced by the great role played by a new publication: the *Philosophical Transactions of the Royal Society*. This powerful instrument for disseminating scientific discovery commenced publication in 1665,[37] and in science and medicine it was the prototype for all subsequent journals, the reason being obvious from the "Advertisement" printed in every issue up to recent times:

> "It is likewise necessary on this occasion to remark, that it is an established rule of the Society, to which they will always adhere, never to give their opinion, as a Body, upon any subject, either of Nature or Art, that comes before them."

How it is wished by many that today's scientific organizations would follow such a course and in their medical journals refrain from endless editorializing on issues irrelevant to or antithetical to the clinical discourses of clinicians.[38]

Then came Dr. William Buchan's *Domestic Medicine*.[39] This was probably the most widely read nonreligious book in English after its publication in 1769.[40] Just as in the age of Hippocrates, when "there [were] many books by physicians,"[41] discussion and explanations of contemporary medical thought was, via Dr. Buchan's book, available to an increasingly literate lay population. As a Hippocratic venture, the book made it easier for the physician to be an educator, which in turn may have increased his effectiveness.[42] Dr. Buchan was critical of the medical profession's practice of secrecy, and in the Introduction to his book he stated: "Medical authors have generally written in a foreign language, and those who were unequal to the task, have even valued themselves upon

---

[36] Culpeper, N., *A Physicall Directory, or, A Translation of the London Dispensatory*, London, 1649.

[37] It was the same year, and two months earlier, that the first European scholarly journal was published, *Journal des scavans*, a Paris weekly of 12 pages that was of source of current literary, legal, and scientific writings, although its editor was not a scientist.

[38] The week this paragraph was proofread the cover of the esteemed *New England Journal of Medicine* (May 7, 2015) listed a total of sixteen subject headings, of which only six were clinical, the other ten being discourses on German health care, Medicaid block grants, foreign language, Medicare and hospice costs, interhospital variation in outcomes (two articles), same-sex marriage, commercial-academic interface, improving nursing home terminal care, and industry-physician relations. One of the five letters of correspondence was on bullying of sexual-minority youth.

[39] Buchan, W., *Domestic Medicine*, Edinburgh, 1769. It subsequently went through about one hundred editions. For a convenient biography of Dr. Buchan and his book see: Lawrence, C. J., *William Buchan: Medicine Laid Open*, in *Med. Hist.* 19:20-35, 1975.

[40] See Rosenberg, C. E., *Explaining Epidemics 2*, Columbia, 1992, p. 32*ff*.

[41] Or, as in the *Loeb Classical Library* translation, "medical treatises make a large collection." The Greek is: πολλὰ γὰρ καὶ ἰατρῶν ἐστι συγγράμματα. Xenophon, *Memor.*, iv, 2.10.

[42] Ludwig Edelstein, in *Ancient Medicine*, Baltimore, 1967, p. 100, footnote 20, writes that the Hippocratic work *On Affections* is probably a treatise directed at the laiety, and if so it suggests a similarity to *Domestic Medicine* of Buchan.

couching, at least, their prescriptions, in terms and characters unintelligible to the rest of mankind." Dr. Buchan knew there was a place for lay practice, although it was not to take the place of a knowledgeable physician. The book helped unite the physician and the patient, for this democratic innovation provided common terms of understanding, common frames of reference.

The 18th C, whether viewed as the Age of Enlightenment or of Absolutism, was a time when speculation was being replaced by observation (see Table 10, p. 414). To what, specifically, could this remarkable change be attributed?

It has been charged that modern civilization has been the consequence of the replacement of slave labor by machines, a European invention, not a Renaissance discovery.[43] For it is proposed that in Greco-Roman civilization, as in every other society from time immemorial, the convenience of slave labor precluded invention and fostered a "universal cleavage of society into freeman and slave." Thus, when slavery was first declared, by moral argument, to be wrong and to be outlawed, a replacement was required.[44] Thus was invention liberated and modernity invented. Slavery, however, was not an element of medical progress, nor were machines. However one may view the spark that led to the power loom or the steamboat, neither medical invention nor the natural state of medical practice has owed anything to slavery, its emancipation or otherwise, or to mechanization.

In another perspective, Arnold Toynbee wrote that "the essence of the Industrial Revolution is the substitution of competition for the mediaeval regulations which had previously controlled the production and distribution of wealth."[45] As the Industrial Revolution in England has been dated from the ascendancy of George III (1760), this might suggest that 19th C medical progress was its consequence. It has been pointed out, however, that there was a sophisticated measure of capitalism and industrialization already existing even into 17th C England.[46] Futhermore, the East India Company was chartered in 1600, its stockholders being private and commercial interests, as was the Dutch East India Company in 1602, New Netherland, and the Dutch West India Company in 1621. It impossible to chronologically associate medical progress with wealth acquired through capitalism and such flagrant but primarily nongovernmental commercial enterprises.

It is also certain that change in medicine did not originate in the universities, for clinical medicine must be taught by experienced clinicians, and prior to Herman Boerhaave the teaching faculty of medical schools was clinically inadequate for the ranks

---

[43] Farrington, B., *Greek Science*, Harmondsworth and Middlesex, 1944, in the Forward to Part II of the book, p.151.

[44] It is to be expected that the universality of the practice of enslavement should meet its match in the West, the birthplace of freedom as a concept of existence. As Aristotle noted in *Politics* I, iii, "Others affirm that the rule of a master is contrary to nature, and that the distinction between slave and freeman exists by law only, and not by nature; and being an interference with nature is therefore unjust." (Translation of Benjamin Jowett in his *The Politics of Aristotle*, Oxford, 1885.) Orlando Patterson noted that most non-Western societies had no word for "freedom" except as it might be used to define licentiousness or equivalent escapes from social molding. See Patterson, O., *Freedom in the Making of Western Culture*, Cambridge, 1982. For an ancient opinion on the value of freedom see p. 340 of the present work.

[45] Toynbee, A., *The Industrial Revolution*, London, 1894, 4th edition, p.32.

[46] Redford, A., *The Economic History of England* (1760-1860), London, 1931, chap. 1.

of new apprentices who would reestablish the good reputation of physician.[47]

To repeat the question, what brought about the revolution in medical practice? In Hippocratic medicine the instrument for good reputation had been its common council, the professional koinon. And so it was that in the 18th C the newly founded professional society became the resurrection of that koinon. Presaged by the Royal Society of London, many professional societies would ultimately be functionally independent of government. They included in France the *Societe de Chirurgie* in 1731 and the *Academie Francaise* in 1795; in England the *College of Barbers and Surgeons* in 1745 and the *Royal College of Surgeons* in 1800; in Prussia the *Collegium-medico-chururgicum*; in Austria the *Medicinisch-chirurgische Akademie*; and in Denmark the *Royal Academy of Surgery*, to name some of the societies that addressed the various fields of surgery. In internal medicine it was the pioneering work of Linacre to lead the effort to obtain a charter from Henry VIII for the founding of the *College of Physicians* in 1518 in London, and then came the *Royal Faculty of Physicians and Surgeons of Glasgow* in 1599, the *Royal Medical Society of Edinburgh* in 1737, the *Medical Society of London* in 1773, and the *Societe de medecine de Paris* in 1796. There also appeared independent schools of medical training distinct from those in the universities, often privately funded and usually affiliated with the large hospitals. Independent educational activities also sponsored publications, such as the *Transactions of the Royal College of Physicians* in 1786, and the *Medical Repository of New York* in 1797. State medical societies in the United States were organized near the end of the 18th C, for example the *Massachusetts Medical Society* in 1781 and the *Medical Society of New York City* in 1769.[48]

Moreover, the Societies listed above were not called into existence by the discoveries of Harvey or those of any other Renaissance investigator. There is no question that the occasional singular invention by an individual can be sufficient for a great advance; one person might, by concluding that the potential of steam energy could power an engine, unite theory with achievement. One person, by inventing moveable type, could provide a vehicle for great changes in society. But medicine is different, for it is a broad profession of infinite complexity and it is useful throughout society; it is continually being modified, and it copes with an endless variety of illnesses expressed in an endless variety of hosts as described by writers of endlessly variable proficiency. Thus, even Dr. Harvey's scientific method, as expressed in his famed *De Motus Cordis* of 1628, did not come into broader use for almost a century, and the validity of some of his findings was still being debated in 19th C. No one man can say that he has invented "medicine." The best he can do is to add his smidgeon of knowledge to the contemporary pile. It was, therefore, not for Harvey or other great names, but for the koinons of the 18th and 19th centuries to provide places where discovery could be debated, vetted, popularized, and ultimately made relevant to clinical practice throughout society, just as in Hippocratic times it had

---

[47] Apprenticeship remained the principal entry into medical practice throughout the 18th C and well into the 19th C, despite the attention and importance historians assign to medicine's schools and academics.

[48] It is notable that Dr. Baas, in *Outlines of the History of Medicine and the Medical Profession*, New York, 1889, H. E. Handerson, translator, p. 791) writes that "Medical arrangements in America have been from the outset similar to those of England, but continued until a short time since entirely unregulated, practice free, etc., and without the English *self-government* [italics added]. The latter is now just beginning to show itself, so that quackery in the United States has overgrown reputable practice." Another opinion, however, cites the resistance of European charlatans to transfer to the New World because of its rigorous life and limited recompense of colonial practitioners.

been the professional organization, the koinon with its dispersed membership, rather than the individual practitioner or primordial biologist, that promoted scientific advances throughout its membership. Desire for anesthesia, antisepsis, and control of contagion stimulated empirical endeavors throughout history, but only in the mid-19th C did those three ancient concepts finally acquire a scientific basis and a foundation for advancement. The *Boston Medical and Surgical Journal* in 1846-47 announced the successful demonstration of ether for surgical anesthesia,[49] the *Lancet* in 1865 was the venue for disseminating Lord Lister's magnificent achievements on antisepsis,[50] and the *Zeischrift d. k. k. Gesellshaft der Aerzte in Wien*, 1847-49, published the first observations by Semmelweis on puerperal sepsis, to be followed by his book on the subject in 1861.[51] Manson and Laveran announced their observations on the cause and transmission of malaria in 1879-1880.[52]

There is, therefore, this confusing aspect of medical discoveries of the Renaissance. Should they not be considered the key to the return of a true medical practice and all the benefits of modern medicine? This is unlikely. Michael Servetus (1509-1553) is now praised as being in the vanguard for modern understanding of the pulmonary circulation, but in his lifetime as a devout divine his insight into biology came to nothing, and he ended his life as a martyr for his religion. Of the few copies of his book *Christianismi Restitutio* in which his anatomical discovery was described, only three escaped incineration, and it was not until almost 150 years later that any notice was given to his biological speculations, and another century before his work was actually printed for the medical profession.[53] In the 13th C Ibn Nafis described the pulmonary circulation. Six copies of his manuscript were made, and his work was not recognized until the 20th C.[54] Famed 12th C manuscripts on women's diseases, the compilation of some being called *The Trotula*, was not printed and available to medical professionals until 1544.[55] The careful sketches of Leonardo de Vinci in 1498, so relevant to anatomy and physiology, were not available to the scientific world until they were discovered in the

[49] *Boston Med. Surg. J.*, 35:309; 379, 1846-47.

[50] *Lancet*, 1865, i: 308, 335, 362.

[51] *Ztschr. d. k. k. Gesellsch. d. Aerzte in Wien*, 1847-48, iv, pt. 2, 242; 1849, v, 64, and *Die Aetiologie, der Begriff und die Prophylaxis des Kindbetfiebers*, Pest, Wien und Leipzig, 1861.

[52] Manson: *J. Linnaean Soc.*, xiv, 304-311, 1879; Laveran: *Compt. rend. Acad. d. Sc.*, xciii, 627, 1880, Paris.

[53] Servetus' *Christianismi Restitutio* contained his description of the pulmonary circulation, but only three copies of his work survived his burning at the order of Calvin. Notice of it was made by the theologist William Wotton in 1697, but it was not reprinted, from one of two copies extant, until 1790 in Nuremburg.

[54] See: Whipple, A. O., *The Medical School and Hospital of Gondi-Sapor and Its Influence on Arabian Medicine*, in *Proceedings of the Charaka Club*, 9:109, 1938.

[55] Earlier *Trotula* manuscripts were not rare, and Prof. Monica Green states that there are almost 200 extant copies, both Latin and vernacular, some previously possessed by monks and royalty. For there to be 200 copies spread over 300 years does not suggest a concerted effort at publication for medical professionals at a time when the estimated population of Europe in 1300 AD was at least 80,000,000. Granting that many manuscripts must have been lost, there is no evidence of multiple copies emanating from a single source and time. Chaucer may have been aware of "Trotula," as mentioned in his *Wife of Bath's Prologue* in *The Canterbury Tales*, but evidence does not suggest that "physicians" other than those associated with certain circles of popular society were aware of the texts as educational treatises. The purpose of this footnote is not to belittle Trota or the *Trotula*, but to point out that, if anything, it did not, or was not allowed to, receive the attention it deserved. For a current assessment of the *Trotula* see: Green, M., *The Trotula*, Phila., 2002.

Royal Library at Windsor and elsewhere and published around 1900. The prescient Antonio Benivieni (1440-1502), in the course of his dissections for anatomy didactics, made notes on over 150 patients, his brother publishing, in 1507, a selected one hundred and eleven case histories, some with autopsies to determine cause of death, but clinical and professional relevance of autopsy findings was not achieved until Morgagni published his own careful work on the subject in 1761.[56] The writings of Paracelsus (1493-1541) concerning occupational diseases of miners was probably composed around 1525 but was not widely available until well into the 17th C.[57] Bartolomeo Eustachi (Eustachius, 1500-1574) completed a series of anatomical engravings in 1552, and, although judged less artistic than those of Vesalius (1514-1564), they were sometimes more accurate. Yet they remained unpublished until 1714 when they were discovered in the Vatican Library.[58] It has been stated that if the works of Eustachius had been published and popularized at the time of their composition the progress of medicine would have been expedited by two centuries. Then there was Raymond Lully in the 13th C who described a "sweet vitriol" that is now called diethyl ether, Valerius Cordus (1515-1544) who invented "sulphuric ether" in 1540, and Paracelsus who noted that if chickens ingest the sweet-tasting agent they fell into a sleep from which they awakened unharmed. Subsequently his was the first recorded use of ether for human sedation.[59] Both ether and chloroform were explored in the 18th C search for "pneumatic therapies," including management of asthma, not to mention the popularity of their euphoric effects. But it was not until, in the Ether Dome of Massachusetts General Hospital in 1846, that Drs. Morton and Warren publicly demonstrated the practical benefit of ether anesthesia and thereby provided the stimulus for its prompt and widespread use.[60] The invention of the thermometer can be dated to the days of Galileo (p. 299), but the thermometer's early developers, one of whom was Santorio, were acquaintances of Galileo; they were a close circle of comrades, not representatives of the medical profession at large. Even with the advice of Elisha North (1771-1843) regarding the potential usefulness of a clinical thermometer in his book on meningitis in 1811, it was not until Dr. Wunderlich's 1868

---

[56] Benivieni, A., *De abditis nonnulis ac mirandis morborum et sanationum causis*, Florence, 1507. Benivieni, whose patients included the Medicis, was of noble birth. The famed Morgagni mentions Bienvieni cases in his *De Sedibus et Causis Morborum per Anatomen Indigatis* of 1761.

[57] Rosen, G., in *Paracelsus, Four Treatises*, (ed. H. Sigerist), Baltimore, 1941, p. 45. Rosen translated the work from the German and provided the Introduction. The German version, *Von der Bergsucht und Anderen Bergkrankheiten*, was first published posthumously in 1567 by S. Zimmermann, and it seems only thirty copies, rather than the expected 350, were delivered by the printer. See: Sudhoff, K., *Bibliographica Paracelsica*, Berlin, 1894, #88. Paracelsus did become widely popular after his death, but it was primarily because of his reputation in chemistry and, in medicine, as an alternative to Galen.

[58] Eustachius, *Tabulae anatomicae .... editio Romana altera*, Rome, 1728.

[59] For a review of these three prominent names in the history of ether see: Pagel, W., *Paracelsus*, New York, 1982, p. 373 (2nd ed.), and Chauncey Leake's *Valerius Cordus and the Discovery of Ether*, Weissenbruch, 1925, p. 22-23.

[60] The tragedy of the late exploitation of earlier discoveries was recognized outside the circle of physicians. In *The Future Independence and Progress of American Medicine in the Age of Chemistry* (written by a committee of the American Chemical Society, New York, 1923) is found the following statement, reminiscent of the Introduction of the present work: "For instance, ether had been discovered in the thirteenth century, but its value as an anaesthetic was not definitely recognized until 1846. During the intervening five or six hundred years untold suffering resulted from lack of knowledge of its application..."

clinical publication on fevers that this valuable tool was popularized among his colleagues.[61] And Fracastoro in 1546 may have been prescient in describing patterns of contagion and their invisible causes, but it was not until Prof. Louis Pasteur (1822-1895) that the nature of infectious disease and wound infection was clarified, and, with the use of carbolic acid by Lister as published in *The Lancet* in 1865-67, its practical management realized.[62] The earlier discoverers and inventors revealed their successes to their patrons and to a small group of colleagues through Gutenberg's new invention. But, in contrast to the Reformation, which burgeoned immediately upon the invention of the printing press because of its prompt employment by Martin Luther, medicine did not begin to flourish for two more centuries.[63]

No, the key to the ultimate triumph of medical discovery and invention lay not with the Renaissance but with the modern professional organization, the koinon. An organization that communicates to its members rather than among its members may be fraternal, but it is not a koinon. The secret is not *fraternite*. It is, instead, *liberte* and *egalite*, a common council free to pursue self-interest. Individual autonomy and equality were the essence of the koinon, and its vital role in medical practice was now to unfold. With resumption of activities of the koinon, a natural state of medical practice was now reestablished. Spurred by competitive medical disciplines, unleashed curiosity about biology, and close scrutiny of diseases, all under the humane cloak of the Hippocratic Oath, new clinical observations were made, old ones rediscovered, and the power of the koinon was focused on them. The result was the medical progress of the 19th century, a century of medical and biological achievement that towers over the history of mankind like a colossus. Although it is popular to trace the origins of "modern" discovery as far back as possible, this often introduces a bias that gives credit where little credit is due. It is also often unfair in that it can devalue the genius and effort of modern discoverers. There is no justification for false humility. And the reason for this is that virtually all of those 19th century achievements referred to above would have occurred had there never been a Hippocrates or a Renaissance, as will be proved in the next chapter.[64]

---

[61] Wunderlich, C. A., *On the Temperature in Diseases*, a publication of the New Sydenham Society, London, 1871, translated from the German by W. B. Woodman.

[62] It has been pointed out that criticism of Semmelweis' work on controlling infection came from European sources that greatly impeded acceptance of his recommendations. This sad state of affairs has been attributed, rightly, to an authoritarian legacy apparent in Rudolph Virchow (p. 22*f*) and many other prominent 19th C magisterial professors. J. H. Baas, in *Outlines of the History of Medicine and the Medical Profession*, New York, 1889, H. E. Handerson, translator, p. 1083, has perfectly described the process: "... the discoverers of truth now are no longer crucified, but their names are simply written upon the proscription-list of the *lease-holders of science*." [italics added] Lease-holders of science were, gratefully up to the early 20th C, least evident in America. Today, of course, the lease-holder of science has reemerged: government.

[63] A variety of factors limited the availability of early medical books. One was the size of a new edition, which was based on anticipated sales in a generally illiterate populace. Thus, in the 15th C printings of new works averaged perhaps two hundred copies.

[64] A somewhat similar conclusion was reached by Benjamin Farrington, but for different reasons. In his work, *Greek Science* (Harmondsworth [UK],1944), he viewed modernity as the consequence, not of democracy, but of the replacement of slavery with machines. Modernity, therefore, was a "European invention" rather than a "Renaissance rediscovery."

CHAPTER TWENTY-THREE

THE VALUE OF THE KOINON AGAIN REVEALED: DISCOVERY
VS. REDISCOVERY

*"Don't misunderstand me, my boy. I'm not belittling your discovery. Most discoveries
are made regularly every fifteen years; and it's fully a hundred and fifty since yours was
made last."*

Sir Patrick in Act I of *The Doctor's Dilemma*
by George Bernard Shaw, 1906

This chapter offers support for the assertion in the previous chapter that modern medicine would
have progressed to its present point even without Hippocrates or the Renaissance. The conclusion
is that in each of three eras (Greco-Roman, Renaissance, and Modern) equivalent discoveries were
not only made, but were made for the most part without sophisticated technology and independent
of any prior discoveries. A logical corollary is that seminal discoveries and inventions of the 18th
and 19th centuries could just as well have been made prior to the Common Era.

A. The 19th Century and Science

Matters now moved quickly. Just as the century following Hippocrates saw a
proliferation of named physicians and medical discoveries, especially from Alexandria,
so, too, the century that followed Herman Boerhaave saw many exciting discoveries,
many by physicians who had trained under Boerhaave, such as Albinus, von Haller,
Robert Whytt, and John Monro. Sir D'Arcy Wentworth Thompson described a sequence
of Golden Ages.[1] He placed the Age of Pericles far above the Age of Plato and Aristotle
a century later. But the Golden Age for science he places in the 18th and 19th centuries,
predominantly the latter. His witnesses included Faraday, Lister, Darwin, Bruce,
Bernard, Ross, Einstein, Pasteur, and Ehrlich. The abrupt appearance of these scientists
may be likened to the scientific flourishing around the Hellenistic Mediterranean.
Subsequent technological advances in modern times have been startling, but in many
ways the advances of the 20th and early 21st C have been but embellishments on the
discoveries of the 19th C, the Golden Age of modern medicine, the Golden Age of Science.
Are there similarities between the two eras? Is there a perennial capacity for a Golden
Age?

B. Discovery vs. Rediscovery

In the examples that follow, both ancient and Renaissance/Enlightenment
medical inventions and discoveries are compared to similar inventions and discoveries
made in the late 18th and the 19th centuries. Specific techniques and famous individuals

---

[1] See Thompson's essay, *The Golden Ages*, in *Science, Medicine and History*, London, 1953, E. A.
Underwood, editor.

are cited as are the circumstances surrounding their discoveries, but this is not intended to dismiss collateral investigators that comprised the scientific milieu in which those discoveries were made, for they could have been made in many instances at any other time and by any of a large number of observant and motivated investigators. There are two purposes behind this appraisal. One is to show that there was equivalent interest and ingenuity directed at the topics selected for examination in the three eras, Hippocratic, Renaissance/Enlightenment, and modern. The second is to illustrate many aspects of modern medicine that were within reach of Hippocratic practitioners and that Western medicine and perhaps scientific endeavor in general might have produced their "modern" miracles in that early age, or soon afterwards, thus averting a 1500 year history of medical ignorance.[2] Seven categories of medicine have been selected for review: pharmacology, physiology, technology, physical examination, diagnostics, clinical procedures, and basic sciences.

1. Pharmacology

a. Colchicine

Colchicine may have been known to early Egyptian practitioners, although this inference is based on the description of a plant extract in the Ebers papyrus (transcribed *ca.* 1550 BC) rather than any described clinical effect. The Hippocratics used white hellebore for gout, attributing the salutary effects to the purging action of the drug, and white hellebore is related to *Colchicum autumnales*. But it was Alexander of Tralles (525-605 AD), writing of the effects of colchicum for gout, who was able to dissociate the diarrheal effect from the rheumatic effect of the botanical. It is thought he used "hermo-dactyl," a subsurface component of *Colchicum autumnale*. This botanical was described by Dioscorides (*ca.* 40-90 AD) in his *De Materia Medica*, but this author ascribed its usefulness to being a cure for mushroom poisoning, not gout. In the 13th C *Compendium Medicinae* of Gilbertus Anglicus, a physician mentioned by Chaucer, there are several remedies for gout, and some probably included *C. autumnale* as a component, but it was not singled out as the active principal. He also noted that some preferred binding a frog's foot to the patient's foot, although it was important to use the right foot of the frog if the gout troubled the right foot of the patient. Sydenham, by not recommending *colchicum* because of its toxicities, contributed to its continued irrelevance as a gout therapy. Then a modification of *Colchicum* reemerges in 1763 when *eau d'Husson*, a patent medicine marketed by a Frenchman, Lieutenant Husson, was advocated for gout. This medicine

---

[2] Had a scientific revolution occurred in the early centuries following Hippocrates the course of history would have been dramatically altered, and unknowable is whether it would have been for the better or for the worse, even though medical care would have vastly improved. Thus, any conjecture of less suffering has no factual support. Everyone's life is afflicted by suffering, and perhaps a certain quantity of suffering is part of every person's destiny. But having that quantity of misery spread over 75 or 80 years rather than compressed into 5 or 15 or 25 years of existence is surely a benevolent gift of the past to the present, not to mention the often remarkable easing in most medical situations of the suffering that does occur. For those born in the West during the last half of the 20th C the daily load of misery burdening most persons in centuries past cannot be imagined, for modern therapies, analgesics, and preventions seem the normal run of things. They most certainly are not. Absent our atrocities to each other, modern Westerners have been blessed, to say the least.

contained opium and herbal agents, but the specific ingredients were kept secret for many years. *Eau d'Husson* became a popular therapy. When in the 19th C it seemed likely that the active ingredient was from *Colchicum* its popularity spread and similar elixirs were marketed. The reason Husson selected *Colchicum* is unknown, but it may have been part of popular lore at the time.

Comment – Colchicine was rediscovered in the 18th-19th C rather than being in continual use by professionals since the days of Alexander of Tralles and probably many undocumented times as well, and used for a variety of clinical illnesses, probably including gout. But if all the collected clinical experience from a mélange of empirical trials over many centuries had never happened prior to Lt. Husson's *eau*, the first specific anti-gout therapy would still be on the shelf in our pharmacies today and used for prevention and therapy of acute gout, as a highly effective treatment of familial Mediterranean fever, and for valuable symptomatic relief of viral pericarditis.[3]

b. Ergot

Knowledge of ergot, a growth of fungus (*Claviseps purpurea*) found on corn and grains, especially rye and wheat, has been inferred for practitioners in ancient China, Greece, and Persia,[4] although more recent studies find little support for this opinion. Between the first written description in 1582 of the use of ergot as an oxytocic agent to stimulate uterine contractions at parturition and its next mention in an English book in 1667 ergot was probably used by midwives in much of Europe, for 18th C apothecaries often carried *pulvis ad partum*, their designation for "ergot," for obstetrical use. In 1787 ergot was first described in a journal.[5] But it was Dr. John Stearns (1770-1848) who, in 1807, reported on the effectiveness of a substance obtained from rye that initiated uterine contractions.[6] He later published a fuller account in which he attributed his discovery to an "ignorant Scotch woman" who advised him on the properties of the material.[7] The

---

[3] A confusing point about therapy of the confusing disease of gout is that *Colchicum* in its various forms was denigrated and even warned against by many prominent names over the centuries, including Pliny, Dioscorides, Hildegard of Bingen, Dr. Anton Storck, and Thomas Sydenham, and such criticism may have contributed to the disappearance of *Colchicum* as a therapy since the days of Alexander of Tralles. It was, however, the side-effects of *Colchicum* when used as a diuretic and as a purgative that prompted that criticism, not any inadequacy in the treatment of gout. Dr. Sydenham decried its use because of the severe diarrhea that sometimes occurred.

[4] See brief comments in: Ainsworth, G. C., *Introduction to the History of Medical and Veterinary Mycology*, Cambridge, 1986, pp. 123-124, with references.

[5] *Neues Magazin fur Aerste* (New Magazine for Physicians), 1787. See G. Barger's *Ergot and Ergotism*, (London, 1931), chapter 1, for a well-researched early history of ergot.

[6] Dr. Stearns published a letter in the *Medical Repository of New York* in 1807 in which he attributed the effect to a "spurious growth of rye," especially rye that had been grown in a particularly moist season. The other citation is found in *J. Med. Rec.* V, 1822. The material described by Stearns was in powder form, *pulvis parturiens*, and it was more from his publications than midwifery use that notice of the drug came to the attention of the European medical profession, the reason likely being that he provided both quantitation of the substance to be administered and detailed descriptions of its clinical indications.

[7] The American reference for this is: Stearns, J., *Observations on the Secale Cornutum, or Ergot; with Directions for its use in Parturition*, in *The New-York Medical and Physical Journal*, vol. I, pp. 278-286, 1822.

important toxic effects of ergot alkaloids were discovered to be associated with a fungal infestation of rye by Louis Tulasne in 1853. But it was the wide distribution of the Stearns article that led to scientific evaluation by the medical community of the usefulness and toxicities of the ergot alkaloids that would over the next century become so important in several areas of medicine, including control of uterine hemorrhage and therapy of disabling migraine headaches.

Comment – Ergot may have been known to ancient medical practitioners (although this point is not certain), then lost, then rediscovered at the time of the Renaissance, again lost to practitioners, and rediscovered anew by physicians in the late 18th C and early 19th C. In the meantime, folklore and midwifery either kept shadowy knowledge of ergot alive or regularly rediscovered it in rural Europe and probably around the world. But unfortunate it was for many pregnant women during those centuries who had no access to but might have benefited from the uterine effects of ergotamine. The medical "profession" was no help. Rediscovery of the drug by Dr. Stearns was not dependent on its ealier Renaissance recognition. It was, instead, a gift of folklore that he would then scientifically investigate.

c. Antimicrobial therapies

There were numerous Hippocratic therapies that were used to aid healing, the mechanism in many cases now known to be antimicrobial activity. In περὶ ἑλκων (*Concerning Ulcers* [wounds]), sections 12-13 make mention of honey, flower of copper (hydrated salt of copper), a form of finely ground lead, copper ore (cuprite), Melean and Egyptian alum (hydrated aluminum salts), a salt of "red copper" (copper oxide), verdigris (usually copper carbonate), flower of silver (lead oxide), and myrrh (a tree resin) and many other botanicals. Even utensils and containers made of copper or silver were thought to improve healthfulness of their contents, and there is reason to think this was at times correct.

Molds from various sources have been used for wound care. Examples include moldy soybean curd in ancient China, moldy bread in Egypt in the 17th C BC, and moldy bread and jam in early 20th C England.[8] In 1928 Alexander Fleming made the chance observation of lysis of bacterial colonies in the presence of a fungal contaminant on bacterial culture plates. The story of the subsequent development of penicillin and related antibiotics is a story of ingenuity and scientific method.

Comment - The use of honey, molds from a variety of sources, and many other agents were the focus of unending trial-and-error search by laymen and practitioners alike for empirical therapy of wounds. In this sense the fortuitous discovery of penicillin by Fleming was a rediscovery. But, unlike all previous observations on the salutary effects of molds on wound healing, the discovery of penicillin by Fleming was serendipitous and made possible only because of a contaminated culture plate that probably resulted from a laboratory worker's poor technique, whereas in earlier centuries the use of mold to control local infection was based on observation of the response of actual wounds following

---

[8] Methods for the production of penicillin from food molds at the home is available on the internet, along with extensive disclaimers about its use and effectiveness. Nevertheless, see: Wainwright, M., *Moulds in Ancient and More Recent Medicine*, in *Mycologist* 3:21-23, and the article's references.

empirical attempts at therapy. The latter, therefore, can be considered more scientific than Fleming's discovery, for discovery by trial and error is more scientific than a chance observation, even if made by a superb scientist.[9] But beyond this, a French medical student, Ernest Duchesne (1874-1912), observing that visible growths of molds and bacteria tended to proliferate in different environments, postulated that they may possess mutually antagonistic mechanisms. It was proposed, therefore, that some molds might have antibacterial activity, and such was suggested by his subsequent intravenous inoculation of guinea pigs with broth cultures of selected pathogenic bacteria and/or *Penicillium* sp. Survival from the bacterial injection was associated with *Penicillium* injection, although he acknowledged that confirmation was necessary.[10] Thus the usefulness of mold-contaminated substances as a topical therapy described by ancient sources was rediscovered twice in the modern era, although this time with systemic application. Penicillin is extracted from cultures of the mold, basically aqueous solutions, and it is conceivable that the ancients, once they were confident of the therapeutic properties of molds by topical application, might have found some method of aqueous extraction or concentration that would have permitted oral administration.

d. Salicylates

A source of salicylates is the bark of the willow tree, which is mentioned in the Eber's papyrus from ancient Egypt and in a tablet from Ur III of ancient Sumer, although indications for its use are uncertain. Many other botanicals contain salicylates, but not in the high concentration of willow bark. A mixture containing willow leaves was recommended by the Hippocratics for use as a fumigant to expedite delivery of either fetus or placenta, but not for any anti-inflammatory properties.[11] Celsus (2nd C AD) mentions willow bark extract for treatment of anal prolapse (*De Medicina*, Bk. VI, 18, 10), and Dioscorides (40-90 AD) in his *Material Medica*, part I, lists its external use in earache, gout, warts, and cataracts. Despite the apparent usefulness of the willow tree as a source of medicaments in ancient times, there is little mention of willow bark or leaves

---

[9] Late 19th C investigators tried to fabricate an antimicrobial substance that would concentrate in specific tissues and thereby both direct its effects more efficiently against microorganisms in those tissues and also decrease systemic toxicity. Dr. Paul Ehrlich used dyes known to concentrate in tissues to study the problem. His efforts and those of others led to the discovery of trypan blue as a trypanicidal agent, but one that was impractical for clinical use because it tinged its subjects blue. Later, Bayer 205 was invented, a related but colorless agent useful in treating human and animal trypanosomiasis. Ehrlich also was critical to development of other chemotherapeutic agents, including Salvarsan, an arsenical, for syphilis. The work of Ehrlich and other investigators of the late 19th C was scientific method rigorously applied, and it provided a path into modern antimicrobial therapy.

[10] A summary of Duchesne's thesis for his medical degree and a description of its logic is provided by Jean Pouillard: *A Forgotten Discovery: the Doctoral Thesis of Dr. Ernest Duchesne (1874-1912)*, in *Hist. Sci. Med.*, 36:11-20, 2002 (in French). The author has been unable to confirm the anecdotal association of Duchesne's learning of anti-infective activity of molds by observing Arab stable boys applying fungal scrapings from old saddles to skin lesions on horses.

[11] See the Hippocratic work, *Diseases in Women*, Book I, chapter 78, as translated by K. Whiteley for her Master thesis at the University of South Africa, 2003. Although the idea of therapeutic vapors penetrating the genitalia seems preposterous to moderns, aromatherapy is popular today for it delivers volatile plant oils via inhalation or skin absorption that are intended to be systemically therapeutic.

in medieval writings, and Hildegarde von Bingen's *Physica* of the 13th C notes that the willow "is not good for medicine."[12] It is not mentioned as a treatment in Gaddeson's *Rosa Anglica* of 1317. Culpeper's *The Complete Herbal*, published first in 1653, notes that the beneficial effects of the willow tree "are so well known that they need no description. I shall therefore only shew you the virtues thereof." He goes on to list many marvelous properties, but none imply its systemic use for inflammation and fever, in which reside its proven medicinal value. In his *Pharmacopeoeia Londinensis* of 1659 it is stated:

> "Salix: Willow leaves, are cold, dry, and binding, stop spitting of blood, and fluxes; the boughs stuck about a chamber, wonderfully cool the ayr; and refresh such as have Feavers; the leaves applied to the head, help hot diseases there, and Frenzies."

In an ancient Chinese pharmacopoeia the willow is mentioned under the name Liu Hua, its uses being for jaundice, scab sores on horses, and expelling pus.[13] In the pre-Columbian *Badianus manuscript* the willow in mentioned once in relation to parturition (chapter 11). Nothing of substance is mentioned in all these sources that conforms to modern knowledge of the systemic action of salicylates. Thus, despite many modern commentaries on the popularity of the willow over the ages, documentation for specific systemic use is sketchy at best. The reason may be that the effects of the salicylates in willow bark, depending on the source, may be of an extractable concentration that would require an impractical quantity for ingestion to produce analgesia, anti-inflammatory activity, or interference with platelet function. Then in 1764 Edward Stone, a vicar, reported in a letter to the *Transactions of the Royal Society* that a preparation of willow bark given every four hours promptly reduced fever, based on his observations after giving the extract to about fifty patients.[14] This he did after noting, accidentally, that the bark of the willow tree was exceedingly bitter, a characteristic of the febrifuge, cinchona bark. He first, however, searched the literature for prior experience with willow bark by others, and finding nothing of significance, he proceeded with his studies. No one continued Stone's work, however, until Joseph Buchner and then Henri Leroux each obtained small quantities the active principal by extracting it from willow bark, Buchner naming it "salicin."[15] The reason for their search also was the similarity in the bitterness of willow bark to that of cinchona bark, although in scientific terminology the two trees belong to separate Orders. In a Materia Medica of 1846 Jonathon Pereira gives its use as a substitute for cinchona, indicating some European scientists were aware of the association in taste and perhaps aware of Stone's first report on it.[16] It was a generation later when Maclagan, reasoning that species of willow were found in locations where "rheumatic fever" was more common, used preparations of salicin from willow bark for

---

[12] Throop, P., *Hildegarde von Bingen's Physica*, Rochester (Vermont), 1998, p. 127. There is a translation of the *Rosa Anglica*, but there is no mention of a use for any part of the willow.

[13] *The Divine Farmer's Materia Medica* (a translation of the *Shen Nong Ben Cao Jing* by Yang Shou-zhong), Boulder (CO), 1998, p. 108. It is considered a compilation of local lore completed about 200 AD. The author(s) is unknown.

[14] Stone, E., *An Account of the Success of the Bark of the Willow in the Cure of the Agues*, in *Philosophical Transactions*, 53:195-200, 1763

[15] Leroux, H., *Rapporte*, in *J. de Chimie Medicale*, 6:340-341, 1830 (the discovery was reported by Guy-Lussac and Magendie).

[16] Pereira, J., *The Elements of Materia Medica and Therapeutics*, Phila., 1846, 2nd Amer. edition, p. 156. It first appeared in 1839-1840.

treatment of that type of fever and reported it efficacious in 1876. This time the discovery was popularized among professional organizations, which greatly increased its commercial value, a major factor leading to the synthesis of the valuable acetyl derivative known as aspirin.[17]

Comment – The report of Rev. Stone's discovery was possibly the stimulus for attempts by Buchner and others to purify a therapeutically active component of willow bark, for quinine had just been isolated from cinchona bark a few years earlier. Thus, some relatively pure salicin was on chemists' shelves for MacLagan's use. Shortly after he reported his results he received a letter from South Africa stating that similar benefits had been noted by the Hottentot (presumably referring to the Khoikhoi tribe, formerly a pastoral people in southern Africa) and used by them and the Boers as a treatment of fever, in which the writer specified "rheumatic fever." Thus a compound from the bark and leaves of the willow, said to be useful by the ancients yet abandoned for the most part during the Middle Ages was rediscovered by several individuals, each in unique circumstances, and evaluated as a medicine because of its taste and its environmental setting in nature, not because of a history of therapeutic usefulness in earlier ages. All this may seem relatively unimportant from the perspective of history, but in 2005 it was estimated that 20% of all adults in the United States were taking daily or alternate day aspirin for cardiovascular prophylaxis, a number that does not include the vast number of adults who take it for the occasional fever, pain, or inflammation.

e. Drug therapy of severe depression

Recent studies of neurotransmitters have suggested that scopolamine, an antimuscarinic agent, may have a significant role in future management of depression, and clinical trials support this conclusion. It is relevant, therefore, to review a Hippocratic's comment on the subject in *Places in Man*, 39:

> For severe (acute?) depression with suicidal ideation give mandrake root each morning, but in a dose smaller than that used for managing severe delirium.

Comment - Mandrake root is a time-honored herbal medicine with a great variety of effects, some salutary, some dangerous. Pharmacologically active ingredients include scopolamine, atropine, and hyocyamine. Its soporific and anesthetic properties have been of particular value to man. The Hippocratics recognized its value in severe depression. Whether it had been previously known to have specific value in depression is unknown, for a necessary preliminary would have been the ability to distinguish the suicidal ideation and other symptoms of severe depression from other psychiatric diagnoses or even ordinary sadness. In the Middle Ages mandrake root was used for many disorders, including neuropsychiatric ones, but severe depression was not specifically identified, although this does not rule out the possibility that some practitioners were aware of its usefulness in such situations. Angelo Sala (1576-1637) has been credited with espousing another antidepressant, St. John's wort, a yellow flower with legendary qualities, the psychiatric effects being attributed now to several components, the most important being hyperforin. But modern medicine may reinstate antimuscarinics as a psychiatric tool. The value of scopolamine as a rapidly acting antidepressant has been rediscovered, as

---

[17] Jeffreys, D., *Aspirin*, New York, 2004

indicated in a recent medical study. Importantly, that drug was included in a test system designed to "evaluate the role of the cholinergic neurotransmitter system...." The authors stated the following: "In a pilot study ..., we unexpectedly observed an antidepressant response to scopolamine in depressed patients." Because of that unexpected finding the authors proceeded to confirm it in a second study.[18] Although the modern role of scopolamine in treatment of severe depression remains to be determined, its reentry into contemporary psychiatric thinking appears unrelated to Hippocratic wisdom, as well as that of unknown empiricists in other ages who recognized the usefulness of mandrake root in psychiatric disorders.

f. Digitalis

Squill, the "sea onion" (*Urginea maritima*), has an ancient medical bibliography said to include the Ebers Papyrus of 1550 BC. It was listed among drugs used by Hippocratic physicians, and Dioscorides (*ca.* 40-90 AD) identified one of its uses as being a diuretic: (squill can be used) "when you desire to stimulate urination, and against ascites with regurgitation in which [undigested] food is obvious, and against jaundice, in those with [abdominal] colic, chronic coughing, labored breathing, and in those bringing up (phlegm?, pulmonary edema?)"; *de Materia Medica*, Bk. 2, 171, translation by the author), an opinion repeated by Pliny (23-79 AD) in his *Natural History*, 20.39, in which it is specifically stated that the passing of urine is for management of "dropsy," an edematous state.

Albertus Magnus, a 13th C German philosopher, theologian, and teacher of Thomas Aquinas, included among his many works on botany. In it he discusses squill as a pharmaceutical agent whose uses included management of hydrops/dropsy: Et confert hydropisi, et icteritiae et provocat urinam... ("And it opposes hydrops, and jaundices and it stimulates urine [production]..."; *de Vegetabilibus*, VI, 2, 17). Squill is mentioned in the 1542 herbal, the *De Historia Stirpium* of Leonard Fuchs, but it is merely a version of that of Dioscorides.

In 13th C Wales the physicians of Myddfai were using foxglove for medicinal purposes, the preparation of poultices for swellings. It is also mentioned in the above 1542 herbal on p. 891, plus engraved figure. The discovery of the flower, foxglove (*Digitalis purpurea*), as a component of an herbal preparation also useful for dropsical patients was made, however, by an herbalist in Shropshire, England, but, after inquiries about those components, the singling out of that particular botanical and subsequently assessing its toxicities, effectivess, methods of standard preparation, and dose was the great accomplishment of Dr. William Withering (1741-1799).[19] The generic term, digitalis, has been applied to the cardioactive principal in foxglove, and for almost two hundred years "digitalis" in various forms was a mainstay in cardiac care.

Comment – The class of chemicals to which digitalis belongs has been termed "cardiac glycosides," and a variety of glycosides are found in botanicals other than foxglove. One

---

[18] Furey, M. L. and Drevets, W. C., *Antidepressant Efficacy of the Antimuscarinic Drug Scopolamine*, in *Arch. Gen. Psychiatry*, 63:1121-1129, 2006.

[19] A recent recounting of the discovery of foxglove as an herbal therapy and an admission that the name of the Shropshire woman who successfully used it remains unknown is found in: Kahn, R. J., *William Withering's Wonderful Weed*, in *Clio in the Clinic: History in Medical Practice*, Oxford, 2005, J. Duffin, editor, pp. 189-200.

of those is the sea onion, or squill (genus *Scilla*), and another is found in the genus *Strophanthus*. The value of cardiac glycosides in treating "dropsy" is found in their ability to improve heart function and/or rhythm so that fluid retention from heart failure is reversed. The increase in urine output that often results is the consequence of improved heart, rather than kidney, function, and the easing of breathlessness is the consequence of ridding the lungs of fluid by controlling heart rate or failure rather than treating asthma due to allergy or other cause. But fluid retention can be a consequence of kidney disease, liver cirrhosis, and other causes, in none of which are cardiac glycosides effective. The inability to distinquish among the many causes of edema (fluid retention, "hydrops," "dropsy") limited the ability of ancient practitioners to define the parameters within which a botanical now known to contain cardiac glycosides would work. Squill, if it is even mentioned as a treatment for fluid retention, is referred to as a diuretic, which it is not. Nevertheless, it and the other cardiac glycosides have apparently been effectively used to treat heart failure, even though the postulated mechanism was incorrect. There is no apparent connection between the work of Withering and the knowledge of Dioscorides, for the botanicals involved were from different genera even though their mechanism of action was similar if applied to cardiac causes of fluid retention. Albertus Magnus, although of great learning, was not a medical practitioner, and the source of his information on squill is unknown, although the writings of Dioscorides were known to some throughout the Dark Ages. Physicians of Myddfai used foxglove preparations in poultices for swellings, and it is known that toxic systemic levels of topical glycosides are obtainable, although it is not apparent that they used it for edematous states. But the conclusion is that the effectiveness of cardiac glycosides found in some botanicals was discovered at different times and places even though the mechanism of their effectiveness was unknown. The modern valuation of effectiveness digitalis stems from the work of Dr. Withering, whose research, *An Account of the Foxglove* (Birmingham, 1785), was unrelated to any prior discovery.

2. Physiology

a. Circulation of blood

The observations of the Hippocratic physicians and then Herophilus and Erasistratus concerning factors relevant to blood circulation were described earlier (p. 303*f*). No further knowledge of the circulation accrued until William Harvey's lectures in 1616 and his publication, in 1628, of his findings on the circulation of blood. Harvey's work permitted, among other things, Christopher Wren's attempt at intravenous administration of drugs and it stimulated interest in blood pressure measurements.

Comment – Dr. Harvey's work illustrates the difficulty in positing arbitrary groupings of historical events, for it straddles the Renaissance/Enlightenment era and the modern era. His publication was definitive in its interpretation of the circulation.[20] Receiving widespread acknowledgement in the century after its publication in the 17th C, it could not be "rediscovered" in the 19th C. It is mentioned here because Harvey exemplifies 18th-

---

[20] This did not happen quickly. In *Aubrey's 'Brief Lives'* (Oxford, 1898, edited by Andrew Clark, vol. 1) the author relates Harvey saying that, after publishing his famous work (1628), "all the physitians were against his opinion, and envied him…"

19th C researchers rather than the Renaissance era researchers whose circumscribed discoveries were often the consequence of patronage. Harvey did have a Royal patron, Charles I, but his discoveries preceded this association and any patronage was not one of material support but as recompense for services rendered to aristocratic families and the King. Furthermore, his discoveries transformed medical thinking and ushered in the era of "modern" medicine. The elucidation of the circulation had been on the door stoop of medicine in ancient Greece and, as discussed in the excursus on p. 305*f*, when completed it likely would have transformed the understanding of human physiology within a century just as it did modern medicine.

b. Contagion

Although the work of Fracastoro on contagion (p. 309) has been praised as a prescient and important Renaissance work, he made no experiment nor used any special devices to develop or prove his theory. It was an inference based on epidemiological observation alone, and to his contemporaries it was not an improvement over prior miasmic theories. His theory was enveloped by theories already in existence and never popularly recognized as a new idea that would support a germ theory of contagion.[21] He was not even mentioned by Dr. Tytler's polemic against the concept of contagion delivered to the Medico-Botanical Society of London in 1834: it [the concept of contagion] was "a grievous error [that] has been allowed to creep into our science, and to corrupt medicine to its very core, destroying and polluting the fountains of the healing art...."[22] But in 1795 Dr. Alexander Gordon had published his observations on puerperal fever, noted similarities with wound infection, and stated that the disease was transmitted by persons attending women at delivery. Others confirmed and extended his work, and it is the 1847 report by Semmelweiss that has been given the greatest acclaim by posterity.[23] Comment - Fracastoro did not acknowledge any obligation to the ancients for his theory of contagion, although he was familiar with the writings of Thucydides, Hippocrates,

---

[21] Nutton, V., *The Reception of Fracastoro's Theory of Contagion: The Seed That Fell Among Thorns*, in *Osiris* 6:196-234, 1990.

[22] Tytler, R., *Refutation of the Doctrine of Contagion*, in London Medical and Surgical Journal, 1834, p. 553-559. Tytler had spent thirty years in Bengal as a physician and arrived at his conclusions from personal observations on cholera, which he attributed to deteriorated rice.

[23] Gordon, A., *A Treatise on the Epidemic Puerperal Fever of Aberdeen*, London, 1795. Subsequently Dr. Oliver Wendell Holmes, upon hearing a discussion of local cases of puerperal sepsis, collected medical reports that appeared to confirm Dr. Gordon's conclusions, publishing them in a medical journal in 1843. His paper included a list of procedures that he thought would prevent the devastating disease. The journal in which his work was published was new, transient, and little known, as was his essay. The work of Semmelweiss on antisepsis soon followed and was first reported by an acquaintance in a medical journal in 1847, but the reason for its effectivess in preventing puerperal fever was not understood by him. Nevertheless, his careful documentation and his use of an antiseptic solution set his work apart. Henle (1809-1885) wrote *On Miasms and Contagia* in 1840, a clear description of contagion caused by living microorganisms. It was Louis and Henle's student, Dr. Robert Koch (1843-1910), who proved the matter beyond doubt. Pasteur, who, having described the process of fermentation as a product of bacterial action, later declared the microorganisms he cultured from a woman with puerperal fever to be the likely cause of the disease. See: Pasteur, L., *Septicemie Puerperale*, in *Bulletin de L'Academie de Medicine*, 1879, p. 271.

Aristotle, Galen, and Lucretius.[24] In the dedication of his book *De Contagione, Contagiosis Morbis et eorum Curatione* in 1546 he states "Hippocrates, however, did touch on the subject of contagion, when he discussed maladies current among the people, but rather as an observer than as one who records their essential nature. And Galen, coming later, wrote much on this subject, but he and his follower, Paulus of Aegineta, and Aetius of Amida and other ancient writers have omitted much that greatly needed investigation."[25] Likewise, in Gordon's 1795 monograph on puerperal fever there is no mention of Fracastoro, and Hippocrates and Galen are mentioned only in the context of phlebotomy which they recommended as an occasional treatment for fevers in general, not for patients with what would now be called puerperal fever. It is a particularly melancholic endeavor to read Gordon's 124-page account of the epidemic of puerperal fever that he observed, inasmuch as his report included autopsy findings, the result of his poignant task of performing postmortem examinations on women who had died from puerperal fever, some of whom he personally had attended, had previously known, and presumably was the inadvertent cause of their deaths. This face of medicine, with the ineffable depth of feeling that accompanies the solitary practitioner who answers as best he can when duty calls and attends to the final details of such human tragedies is rarely seen by others and cannot be put into words.

The relevance of the story of puerperal sepsis is that its identification and resolution were the consequence of contemporary clinical and epidemiological observations, not an embellishment on Hippocrates, who described what some think was puerperal fever (endometritis),[26] or on Fracastoro, who postulated the cause of contagions. Furthermore, it did not require technology for purposeful clinical action, although the biological processes involved were later identified using instruments unavailable to the early writers. Had there been no Hippocrates or Fracastoro the 19th C discoveries could have taken place as they did, although the clinical settings would have been quite different inasmuch as there were no or few hospitals in ancient times, probably rendering puerperal sepsis as seen by modern physicians an uncommon disease, becoming epidemic only in the 17th C.

c. Crossed association

The ancient Greeks had identified the brain as the locus of consciousness, observed the phenomenon of what is now called crossed association in both brain and spinal cord, differentiated sensory from motor nerves, and distinguished between central and peripheral paralysis (reviewed on p. 310*f*). It now appears that in mid-2nd C AD functional asymmetry of the brain had been described.[27] In 1707 Valsalva (1666-1723)

---

[24] For a highly detailed discussion of Lucretius and other ancient writers and how their writings must have contributed to Fracastorio's thinking, although the authors note unique features of Fracastorio's theories, see: Singer, C., and Singer, D., *The Scientific Position of Girolamo Fracastoro*, in *Ann. Med. Hist.*, 1:1-34, especially p. 29*ff*.

[25] Fracastorius, *De Contagione et Contagiiosis Morbis et eorum Curatione, Libri III*, as translated by W. C. Wright in *Hieronymus Fracastorius*, New York, 1930, p. "B," located between the Roman numeral and the Arabic page enumeration.

[26] Hippocrates, *Epid.* I, case 4, and *Epid.* III, case 14, might qualify for non-epidemic puerperal sepsis, but they were not identified in Hippocratic texts as unique to pregnancy or delivery.

[27] Lokhorst, G-J. C., *The First Theory about Hemispheric Specialization: Fresh Light on an Old Codex*, in *J.Hist. Med. Allied Sci.*, 51:293-312, 1996.

described the contralateral paralysis and other symptoms that accompanied cerebral strokes, a crossed association some have termed the "Valsalva doctrine."[28] Importantly, he supported the clinical picture with postmortem findings. He also noted that the association was not rare, and he did not refer to ancient authors. At about the same time Domenico Mistichelli 1709 and Francois du Petit in 1710 separately published their anatomical studies in which the pyramids of the upper medulla were stated to be the site of the crossing over, the pathway connecting lateralized lesions with contralateral effects. Mistichelli had noted the Hippocratic clinical observations and considered his observations regarding the pyramids as explaining the Hippocratic texts, but he based his conclusions on clinical cases of "apoplexy." Du Petit (1664-1741) does not mention the ancient observations.

The idea that the two cerebral hemispheres were, in terms of function, not mere mirror images but that each had specialized capabilities was a 19th C rediscovery by a French neurologist, Marc Dax, who wrote a relevant paper on it in 1836. Importantly, his conclusions were solely clinically based rather than supported by anatomical dissection. Paul Broca is therefore given priority as the definitive discoverer of the neurological basis of aphasia in 1861.[29]

Comment – The concept of crossed association, an indispensable tool for understanding and localizing central nervous system injury or disease, was identified during Hippocratic times and improved on by Aretaeus and others. It can also be argued that hemispheric specialization was realized not long after Aretaeus. Then crossed association was rediscovered in the 18th C by Valsalva, now supported by anatomic correlations. It would be placed into an integrated system for localizing neurological functions and lesions in the 19th C.[30] Importantly, the discovery of Dr. Dax in 1836 that a deficit in crossed association could reveal differences in hemispheric function was a purely clinical deduction, unassociated with any earlier investigators, ancient or recent. Thus the discoveries concerning crossed association in all three time periods were unrelated.

3. Technology

a. Ophthalmoscope

The ophthalmoscope, first made in 1849 by Helmholtz from a small lens and some glue and cardboard, did not require electricity. The direct ophthalmoscope familiar

---

[28] Valsalva's important contribution, including autopsy correlations, was described in his *De Aure Humana Tractatus*, chapter 5, first published in 1704, and subsequently referred to in Morgagni's (1682-1771) classic work of 1671, *De Sedibus et causis morborum per anatomem indagatus,* III, 13.

[29] For a discussion of that priority and a reprint of a 1964 paper by Joynt and Benton that provides a translation of Dax's memoir of his discovery, see: Benton, A., *Exploring the History of Neuropsychology*, New York, 2000, *The Memoir of Marc Dax on Aphasia*, pp. 167-174.

[30] See a brief historical review: Rezende-Cunha, F. and Oliveira-Souza, R., *The Pyramidal Syndrome and the Pyramidal Tract*, in *Arq. Neuropsiquiatr.* 69: 836-837, 2011. The authors note that D. Mistichelli (1675-1715) even postulated that the anatomical site of the crossing over occurred in the pyramids of the medulla. For a fuller review of the subject, however, see: Thomas, H. M., *Decussation of the Pyramids – An Historical Inquiry*, in *Bull. Johns Hopkins Hosp.,* 21:304-311, 1910.

to all is a specialized microscope that permits visualization, through the pupil of the eye, of the retina. The necessary ophthalmoscopic magnification of 10X-15X was already available. But perhaps more pertinent to present discussion is the *indirect* ophthalmoscope, which in its simplest form is but a lens about two or three inches in diameter that is held in the hand and through which the retina of the eye can be assessed at arm's length. Using a bright light source (*e.g.*, light reflected from a handheld mirror) held near the eye of the patient and directing it toward the eye, a low-power lens held in the other hand will permit visualizing the ocular fundus. In 1823 Jan Purkinje reported that he was able to visualize the fundus of his dog's eye merely by using biconcave eyeglasses, the light behind the dog being deflected into the eye by the eyeglasses.[31]

Comment – Given a hand lens it is a natural desire to look at small things in an attempt to see what was previously inapparent. Faced with eye disease, any clinician given a hand lens would look closely at his patient's eyes and try to see inside the pupil. It would not have taken a theory of optics to stimulate clinical interest in a better understanding of eye diseases. The ophthalmic instruments described above were within the grasp of the Hippocratic physician, for quartz lenses were used in making fine jewelry (see Fig. 11, p. 312). Subtleties of eye examination included pupillary paralysis in diphtheria (see p. 209) and the corneal light reflex.[32] By the use of lenses new information on systemic diseases and eye diseases would have been uncovered, and an understanding of the proper role of the lens, cornea, and retina in light reception soon would have followed. As for perceived awkwardness of application to humans, indirect ophthalmoscopy by the method described above is routinely used for veterinary eye examinations. Although miosis (a small pupil) and focusing the light from the mirror present technical obstacles, these were but details that could have been overcome by the Hippocratics. Mydriatic (pupil-dilating) drugs were available to the Hippocratics, including Galen, as stated in his *Methodus Medendi*, namely botanicals with atropine-like qualities, examples being mandragora and hyoscyamus from *Solanaceae* family. It is commonly cited that Cleopatra VII used an extract of henbane for producing dilated pupils to increase her attractiveness, although the original citation for this has eluded the author. But just as relevant for present discussion is the use of belladonna leaf and its effects on the pupil as first described by John Ray in 1686.[33] As reported by R. Kobert, the mydriatic effect of certain botanicals was rediscovered six more times by unrelated investigators before Runge happened upon its effects, in a most curious anecdotal account,[34] and the perennial usefulness of the operative compounds then followed.

---

[31] As reported by R. Weale, *On the Invention of the Ophthalmoscope*, in *Documenta Ophthalmologica*, 86:163-166, 1994: "Moreover, I chanced to examine by the appropriate method also the region of the eye occupied by the vitreous body; furnished with glasses worn by myopes, I inspected the eye of a dog in order to discover the cause of the brilliance spreading frequently from the eyes of dogs and cats. The illumination was provided by a candle shining from far behind the animal. Lo and behold! when I examined the puppy's eye from a given direction, a very bright light kept appearing till I found as its source light deflected into the eye and, in turn, reflected from the vitreous chamber." Dr. Weale's translation from *Commentario de examine physiologico organi visus*, Purkinje's thesis published in 1823.

[32] See: Adams, W. H., *A Case Report from the Ancient Past*, in *Amer. J. Case Rep.*, 20:1907-1914, 2019

[33] Ray, J., *Historia Plantarum*, London, 1686, (in three vols.) vol. 1, p. 680.

[34] Kobert, R., *Discovery of the Mydriatic Action of Solanaceous Plants*, in *The Chemist and Druggist*, 29:279, 1886. This is abstracted from the original article in the *Therapeutic Gazette*.

b. Endoscopy

With lenses, quartz crystal, and glass already available, with metallic tubes and specula already in use for gynecologic and proctologic investigations in Hippocratic times, it is but a natural progression to enhance lighting and adding magnification for better visibility. All components were at hand for development of more advanced forms of endoscopy by the Hippocratics. Pierre Borel (1620-1671) is cited as first using a concave lens to permit better lighting through a tube being used for internal visualization. In 1806 Bozzini (1773-1809) introduced his "lichtleiter" for internal examinations, an instrument lit by an internal candle.[35] In his first publication on the lichtleiter he described its construction and noted it could be used for examining ears, nose, mouth, male and female urethras, rectum, and vagina, and even considered for use as a laparoscope. It was soon modified for use in cystoscopy by M. Segalas, and improved models were being produced as late as 1868 when Philip Wales described his urethroscope, all before the availability of electricity to power a light source.

Comment – The components for endoscopy, an advance over the speculum, were in the hands of Hippocratic physicians, Renaissance physicians, and modern physicians, all prior to the availability of electricity, each situation independent of the others, although, as with the postulated ophthalmoscope, the Hippocratics did not have the time to develop such a technique. Many new diagnoses and therapies would have resulted, and deeper visualization into the body via orifices, fistulae, and wounds would have revolutionized the practice of medicine and surgery in whatever era they developed.[36]

c. Percutaneous injection

Invented by Ctesibus in the 3rd C BC and used medically by Celsus (25BC-50AD), the piston syringe was familiar to the later Hippocratic physicians. Pare (1510-1590) mentions a syringe as a physician's tool. It appears to have been a piston syringe, but its use at that time was for administering enemas. It was Sir Christopher Wren (1632-1723) who is credited with performing an intravenous injection for the purpose of studying systemic pharmacological effects of a variety of agents in experimental animals.[37] His needle was a quill, and the infusion was driven by gravity. Others used

---

[35] Bozzini, P., *Lichtleiter, eine Erfindung zur Anschauung innerer Teile und Krankheiten, nebst der Abbildung*, in *J. pract. Arz. und Wundarz*. 24:107-124, 1806. In the article he describes its ability to assess the bladder meatus, cervix, rectum, pharynx, and perhaps even intra-abdominal organs: "...the cavity of a drained abscess, the abdominal cavity after removal of ascites, could perhaps become counted among them. Translation by the author.

[36] While admittedly stretching the point, the ability of electricity to make this and many other ancient inventions practical may not have been totally out of reach of the ancient scientists, for the "Baghdad battery" from 100 BC is touted by some to have been used for electroplating, although scholarship considers that as untenable. An alternative use, however, also involving electric current generation, has been proposed; see: Keyser, P. T., *The Purpose of the Parthian Galvanic Cells: A First-Century A. D. Electric Battery Used for Analgesia*, in *J. Near-Eastern Studies*, 52:81-98, 1993.

[37] The collaborative experiment, performed by Wren on a dog provided by Robert Boyle, confirmed that intravenous opium acted far more rapidly than when it was given *per os*. The many facets of the ingenious Wren are described by L. Jardine in *On a Grander Scale*, New York, 2002. For the cited experiment see R. G. Frank's *Harvey and the Oxford Physiologists*, Berkeley, 1980.

this procedure in attempts at blood transfusion and the injection into blood vessels of agents that permitted their accurate anatomical localization. Wren cites no earlier work for his invention, implying it was made possible not by advancing ancient ideas but by the discoveries on the circulation by his somewhat older contemporary, William Harvey. The uses to which Wren and a few other investigators put intravascular injection in the 17th and 18th centuries were not pursued and were for the most part forgotten. Then Dr. Thomas Latta (1796-1833) in Edinburgh read of Dr. O'Shaunessy's suggestion that fluid loss in cholera was "serum." Concluding that a serum substitute given intravenously might be of value, Dr. Latta devised a weak saline solution that he infused, via "Read's patent syringe" (which was used for enemas and gastric lavage) to which he attached a thin silver tube, into a moribund patient during a local outbreak of cholera. The result of his 1832 effort is dramatic reading, and, upon reporting the experience, his procedure was duplicated and the results in part confirmed and discussed in the literature within months.[38] Over the next twenty years Drs. Francis Rynd of Ireland, Alexander Wood of Scotland, and Charles Pravaz of France, working separately and apparently unaware of Latta's work, each invented his own device for injection of drugs, Wood for the purpose of local injection of an anesthetic.[39] A calibrated modern syringe was promptly patented by Charles Sage (1843).

Comments – It was clinical need for subcutaneous or intravenous delivery of therapeutic substances that in modern times led four unrelated investigators, each for his own purpose and with the stimulus of necessity rather than precedent, to invent a form of syringe for parenteral use, with medical journals then providing a wide audience of clinicians who would soon realize the great potential of parenteral injection. But the mechanics of a piston syringe were know to Ctesibus, mentioned by Hero, used by Celsus, and considered a standard tool for 16th C physicians by Pare. Indeed, both the syringe and the Alexandrian studies of the circulatory system occurred in the 3rd C BC, just as Harvey's discovery of the circulation and Wren's intravenous injections belonged to the 17th C. It is apparent that the syringe was discovered in ancient times and was used for parenteral injection in the 17th C and 19th C, the circumstances of its discovery being unique at each point. Subcutaneous, intramuscular, and intravenous therapies, like the discovery of circulation of the blood, were on medicine's door stoop in ancient times, and the ancient syringe's subsequent incarnations in Renaissance and modern times were unrelated to technical inventions in Hippocratic times or to each other.

4. Physical examination

a. Auscultation

The technique of direct auscultation, in which the examiner's ear, in order to hear internal sounds, is placed directly against the patient's chest wall or elsewhere on the body

---

[38] Latta, T. A., *A Letter to the Secretary of the Board of Health, London, affording a view of the rationale and results of his practice in the treatment of cholera by aqueous and saline injections*, in *Lancet* 1831-32, ii:274-277. Failure of some attempts at this type of therapy plus the ending of the cholera epidemic dampened enthusiasm for the procedure for some time.

[39] The Rynd, Wood, and Pravaz citations are, respectively: *Dublin Med. Press*, xiii, p. 165, 1845; *Edinburgh Med. and Surg. J.*, 82:265-281, 1855; *Compt. rend. Acad. d. sc.*, xxxvi, pp. 88-90, 1853.

surface, assisted the Hippocratics in localizing pleural effusions.[40] With this technique they also recorded rales and pleural, and perhaps pericardial, friction rubs, noting associations with pulmonary pathology.[41] Abdominal complaints may also have been so examined for that would have been a logical extension of its value in examination of the chest, although increased bowel sounds were described without mention of placing the ear against the abdomen; they were audible at a distance from the patient.   Direct auscultation was not improved on until 2300 years later when Dr. Rene Laennec (1781-1826) invented indirect, or mediate, auscultation with his version of the stethoscope. Laennec cited Hippocratic observations on succussion in his epochal publication in 1819, but they were not the stimulus for his discovery. Dr. Laennec based his invention on the increased conductivity of sound by solids rather than the amplification produced by concentrating sound waves, even though it was at this time that the ear trumpet was becoming popular with the hard of hearing. In 1816, desiring to listen to the chest in an overweight young woman with heart disease, he recalled "the augmented impression of sound when conveyed through certain solid bodies, - as when we hear the scratch of a pin at one end of a piece of wood, on applying our ear to the other." He reached for a rolled up quire of paper. He found her heart sounds more distinct than usually heard when placing the ear directly against the chest, and at the same time he avoided embarrassment to his patient.[42] The new invention was, however, not solid wood. It was a tube, and at the distal end there was a wooden stopper, and with this in place he could better hear the heart sounds and variations in transmission of the voice, whereas with the plug removed, *i.e.*, there being a column of air between the patient's chest wall and the examiner's ear, it was the breath sounds that were clearer.

Comment – The importance of listening to sounds emanating from internal organs was realized by the Hippocratics, by Renaissance/Enlightenment physicians such as William Harvey, and by the inventor of the stethoscope.[43] Importantly, there was no evolution in technique of auscultation between the time of the Hippocratics and Laennec that made the invention of the stethoscope more likely to be his discovery than theirs. Dr. Laennec's instrument was an uncomplicated device with no moving parts, and the superior conduction of sound through solids and liquids vs. air is a common observation.

And yet many of the diagnoses by stethoscope could also have been made by placing the ear directly on the affected and surrounding area. The usefulness of direct

---

[40] προσέχων τὸ οὖς ἀκουάζῃ πρὸς τὰ πλευρά ("in listening by placing the ear on the chest wall"); Hippocrates, *Diseases* II, 61. This and the following translations are by the author.

[41] καὶ τρίζει οἷον μάσθλης ("it squeaks like leather"); *Diseases* II, 59, referring to a pleural friction rub.

[42] Laennec, R. T. H., *A Treatise on the Diseases of the Chest*, London, 1821, translated by J. Forbes, MD, p. 281*ff*. The original was *De l'Auscultation Mediate*, Paris, 1819.

[43] The concentration of sound by means of the ear trumpet might have suggested to someone a way to improve on direct auscultation, for cupping one's hand behind the ear to improve auditory acuity is no modern discovery. Instruments for improving auditory acuity over great distances have an ancient history among mariners, and ear trumpets were first mentioned in 1624. Kircher determined that a megaphone of sufficient size could carry a voice for several miles. Improvements on the stethoscope would include its evolution into an instrument that relies solely on transmitting amplified sound waves via air through tubing. The Jesuit, Jean Leurechon, (Henrik van Etten, *Recreations Mathematiques*, sixth edition, Lyon, 1627) describes the use of tubes to conduct sound for purposes of overhearing conversations of others (Problem 59). The Leurechon work also displays an engraving of an early thermometer.

auscultation is shown by the fact that some clinicians were slow to accept Laennec's invention because they did not view it as a significant improvement, and certain benefits of "immediate" auscultation have been recently pointed out.[44] A critical component of Dr. Laennec's work was his description of chest and heart sounds in relation to symptoms, other signs, clinical outcome, and internal anatomy as detected at postmortem examination or some surgical procedure. Hippocratic (especially Alexandrian) and Renaissance practitioners, had they the opportunity to correlate direct auscultatory with anatomic findings as did Laennec and his stethoscopic findings, would, therefore, have identified many forms of valvular heart disease, the acute abdomen, categories of pulmonary infection, and incipient diseases of all sorts in those early years *with or without* the benefit of a stethoscope.[45]

b. Body temperature

Ctesibius (285-222 BC) and Philo of Byzantium provided a mechanism demonstrating that heating of air caused it to expand, an observation further developed by Hero of Alexandria. These instruments, however, were not intended for clinical use. Galileo's experiments relevant to the thermometer (see p. 299) were of local interest at the University in Padua, where he and others exploited the knowledge exposed by the recent publication, after some 1500 years, of Hero's writings, Hero perhaps being the amanuensis of the great inventor, Ctesibius (285-222 BC), especially in matters dealing with air pressure and siphons.[46] Santorio quantified fever in 1614 by means of an early "thermoscope." Early in the 18th C Drs. Boerhaave and Anton de Haen (1704-1776) evaluated the clinical oral thermometer in healthy and sick subjects, the latter publishing his results.[47] "Contemporaries were unimpressed."[48] Dr. Thomas Allbutt produced, in

---

[44] Puddu, V., *Immediate Auscultation – An Old Method Not to be Forgotten*, in *Circulation*, 52:526-527, 1975.

[45] Important advantages of the new stethoscope were ease of physical performance of the procedure and and its convenience, for modesty and cleanliness were, and are, important associated issues of physical examination. Dr. Laennec announced his 1816 discovery of mediate auscultation and invention of a stethoscope to the Academy of Science in 1818 and published his book on the subject in 1819. Within ten years the practice was widespread, in part because of a brilliant marketing decision with his second edition that could include the stethoscope itself, and mediate auscultation was available to medical students throughout Europe and in America. Before the development of X-ray imaging it was percussion and auscultation that permitted a glimpse of the internal manifestations of disease in a living patient and a more knowledgeable grasp of its management.

[46] The *Pneumatica* of Hero of Alexandria was published first in Italian in Bologna (1547). The more widely read Latin version was published in 1575. Galileo's dates are 1564-1642, so Hero's ideas would have been available to him. Also to be considered as inventor of the thermometer is Philo of Byzantium (280-220 BC), from whom Hero of Alexandria may have received the idea of heating causing expansion of gas volume.

[47] De Haen's findings were interspersed throughout the fifteen books of his *Ratio Medendi in Nosocomio Practico* (Vienna, 1759-1770), and perhaps few would have read this extensive work closely enough to realize the thermometer's value.

[48] For references see: Pearce, J. M. S., *A Brief History of the Clinical Thermometer*, in *Q. J. Med.* 95:251-252, 2002. Interest in temperature and the nature of heat was prominent among 18th C scientists, and animal heat was an interest of physiologists. Thus, a Scottish physician, George Martine (1702-1741) first published accurate measurements of the temperature in human subjects in 1740, but the purpose for using his apparently ungainly instrument was scientific calibration and investigation of the heat of "bodies" rather than clinical use. George Fordyce wrote of his theories

1868, a convenient clinical thermometer.[49]   But the pivotal event relevant to the thermometer can be ascribed to Dr. C. A. Wunderlich who, in 1868, reported accurate serial temperature measurements in 25,000 episodes of febrile illness, and from his millions of observations a fine tuning of the tactile method was widely popularized.[50]

Comment - The practiced hand can detect one degree of fever above a normal Fahrenheit temperature of about 98.6 degrees (a sensitivity that does not apply to distinguishing between 102 and 103 degrees), and no thermometer is needed to distinguish among no, low, moderate, or high fever if care is taken to adjust for cutaneous vasoconstriction and other variables. For many patients this alone can be adequate in diagnosis and treatment. Even in 1836 a French physician noted "the hand to be the only proper instrument to determine it [fever]" (*ibid.*, p. 28). It is understandable, therefore, why contemporary physicians would be in no hurry to replace their time-honored method with an apparatus invented by Ctesibus even if there might be a more precise body temperature measurement. And yet it was Herophilus' interest in more accurately measuring fever that led him to develop his water clock mechanism (p. 299*f*). The clinical value of the thermometer lies as much in the ease of repeated measurements as in its precision, although it does away with interobserver variability, a point that Dr. Allbutt repeatedly stressed. Dr. Wunderlich himself stated ". . . if they [temperatures by thermometer] are to be of any use at all, it is essential that the results obtained should be continuously recorded." He went on to describe the utility of graphed values. At last the physician was able to accurately associate the several fever patterns, such as intermittent, remittent, and biphasic or relapsing, with clinical syndromes. Dr. Wunderlich was merely repeating the observations of the Hippocratics. The difference was a simple device, one based on the observation that heating causes gases and liquids to expand. The 3rd C BC discoveries of Ctesibus and the small container of water used by Renaissance physician, Jean Rey (p. 299), had finally been incorporated into a convenient device for measuring body temperature.

The expansibility of certain liquids on heating was no new observation, nor was the apparatus for measuring that expansion. They had been available to the Hippocratic, Renaissance, and modern physicians. All that was needed was a convenient clinical

---

and experience with fever in 1815 and included was a description of an oral thermometer that required only four minutes to equilibrium. But its readings he thought represented the "apparent heat" of a body rather than clinical fever. Like pulse rate, tactile sensation of heat, and other variables, he concluded that there was no precise way to determine or quantitate fever. Southwick Smith, physician to the London Fever Hospital, published an extensive work on fever in 1830 in which ambient temperatures were correlated with mortality and other factors, but there is not a single word regarding use of a thermometer for documenting a patient's fever. A thermometer is also especially clinically useful in gauging a subnormal body temperature, as is its ability to quantify extreme values.

[49] Allbutt, Thomas Clifford: *Medical Thermometry*, a two-part article highly praising the work of Wunderlich, to which Allbutt added observations of his own. *British and Foreign Medical-Chirurgical Review*, 45:429-441 and 46:144-156, 1870.

[50] Wunderlich, C. A., *On the Temperature in Diseases*, a publication of the New Sydenham Society, London, 1871, translated from the German by W. B. Woodman. Chapter II gives an exhaustive history of the development of the thermometer. It is a measure of the wide acceptance and obvious great value of Wunderlich's studies that the Sydenham Society, which published classics such as translations of Hippocrates and Aretaeus, chose to print in its entirety a translation of Wunderlich's work only three years after its first appearance in German (*Das Verhalten der Eigenwarme in Krankheiten*, Leipzig, 1868).

mechanism or opportunity for its exploitation. It could have been devised in Hippocratic times, but the often satisfactory method of feeling for fever with the hand probably removed any urgency for development of such an instrument, just as it did in the 19th C. Put another way, if Dr. Wunderlich in the 19th C had personally assessed by hand every four hours or so the fevers of all his 25,000 patients and correlated the results with clinical outcome, the quality of the data, while distinctly inferior to those obtained with a thermometer, would still have been of great clinical value to the profession and therefore to patients. Correlations of palpatory assessment of fever with clinical outcome was available to any practitioner, whether Greco-Roman, Renaissance, or modern. The diagnostic and prognostic importance of a patient's fever characteristics correlates directly with the quality and quantity of available clinical information. Without clinical input the clinical thermometer has little value, and clinical input was what Wunderlich provided. And it was the ease in measuring body temperature that permitted Wunderlich to take a million observations of body temperature over a matter of years rather than several lifetimes.

In a sense it is similar to the situation with magnifying lenses; the important 19th C advances in magnification, in measurement of body temperature, and in other areas, were to a great extent due to clinical application rather than just discovery or rediscovery. As such it was the clinician's elaboration on and use of discoveries that determined a discovery's value. It is likely, therefore, that similar elaboration on and use of those same discoveries would have been successfully undertaken by Hippocratic physicians given a bit more time, a comment relevant to the next item.

c. Percussion

Percussion as a clinical tool must have been familiar to the ancients, although its first known descriptions are from Aretaeus (1st C AD) and then by Alexander of Tralles in the 6th C AD. Thereafter it seems to have been forgotten. But percussion of the cranium of sheep was used by 17th C shepherds to diagnose hydatid cysts, as noted by van Swieten (p. 297 and footnote). Modern concepts of percussion can be traced to Dr. Josef Auenbrugger (1722-1809), who described a method of tapping on the surface of the body in such a way that the subsurface density can be estimated.[51] As a child he had watched his father, an innkeeper, tap on the sides of wine casks to determine their fullness. In 1753, after becoming a physician, he applied the same method to examination of the chest and found he could differentiate consolidation, effusion, and pneumothorax by carefully assessing the sound and tactile vibration produced by the tapping on the chest wall. After seven years of correlating percussion findings with clinical course, surgery, or autopsy findings, he published, in Latin, a 95-page description in 1761.

Comment – Dr. Auenbrugger acknowledged no other description or work on percussion antedating his discovery, the opening sentence of his publication stating: "I here present the Reader with a new sign which I have discovered for detecting diseases of the chest." He therefore was unaware of Alexander of Tralles' use of percussion of the abdomen in

---

[51] Auenbrugger, L., *Inventum Novum ex Percussione Thoracis Humani ut Signo Abstrusos Interni Pectoris Morbos Detegendi* (New Invention to Detect Diseases Hidden Deep Inside the Chest), Vienna, 1761, the translator of the English version, *On Percussion of the Chest* (London, 1824) being John Forbes. The quotation cited near the beginning of the next paragraph begins the Preface of Auenbrugger's work.

assessing ascites, a process similar to the percussion of a partially filled cask of wine, and apparently he was also unaware of the 18th C report on the use of percussion of the skulls of bovines suspected of having intracranial cystic masses, although the sound produced by percussion of the latter was based on separation of cranial sutures rather than varying density of the underlying tissue. Dr. Auenbrugger's percussion was indeed an *inventum novum*, unrelated to either ancient or Renaissance age observations. As a common sense observation and because of its simplicity in execution a formal description of Auenbrugger's percussion could have occurred in any age, including that of the Hippocratics and the Renaissance, and to a certain extent it did. But what made Dr. Auenbrugger's invention monumental was his correlation of percussion results with clinical outcome, surgical and postmortem findings, and related observations, and then publishing his findings. It should be more apparent now, given these examples, of the importance of the clinician's touch in turning a device, simple or complex, into a touchstone for medical science. It can be stated, in fact, that *it was the inventing clinician's attention to his patients rather than his invention that was the great event* that led to many a famous physician's prominence, and that, relevant to the analysis in this volume, the option of a clinician's attention was available in all three eras.

d. Audiology

Hippocratic observations relevant to hearing are mentioned on p. 299*f.* Dr. Cardano, in 1550, had identified bone conduction of sound, a discovery made clinically relevant by his fellow physician, Heironymus Capivacci. Clinical experimentation, carried out by Prof. Gunther Schelhammer (1649-1712) who published his findings in 1684, reaffirmed Capivacci's work and furthered an understanding of air and bone conduction of sound, making its application more practical. But Dr. Schelhammer's work was not applied to clinical practice. The next notable event occurred after the tuning fork had been invented for musical purposes. In audiological investigations in 1834 by Drs. Ernst Weber, by E. Schmalz in 1846, and by Heinrich Rinne in 1855, the physiology of air and bone conduction of sound was made clinically relevant, although some write that it was Dr. Johann Lucae whose 1870 book was essential to the widespread clinical use of the tuning fork.[52] It is relevant that Rinne does not indicate why he chose a tuning fork for his experiments, but Weber's description is similar to that of Sir Charles Wheatstone's description in studies of resonance in 1827, for Wheatstone discussed the louder sound of a tuning fork placed on the cranium when heard on the side of an occluded ear.[53] Neither Wheatstone nor Weber refer in their papers to Renaissance discoveries by Capivacci on this point.

Comment – Tests of air and bone conduction of sound are part of any thorough neurological examination, primarily as a screening test for narrowing the differential diagnosis. But the distinction between the two mechanisms has also been important in stimulating further work on sound, the speed of sound, hearing, and ways to improve hearing. The reality of sound transmission unrelated to the auditory apparatus used for

---

[52] E. Schmalz, *Erfahrungen uber die Krankheiten des Gehores und ihre Heilung*, Leipzig, 1846; A. Rinne, *Beitrage zur Physiologie des menschlichen Ohres*, in *Vierteljahrschrift fur die praktische Heilkunde*, 45:71-123, 1855; C. Wheatstone, *Experiments on Audition*, 1827; E. Weber, *De pulsu, resorptiene, auditu et tactu: Annotationes anatomicae et physiologicae*, Leipzig, 1834.
[53] *The Collected Papers of Sir Charles Wheatstone*, London, 1879, p. 31.

air conduction is easily tested by occluding one ear and then speaking, for a louder sound will be detected on the side of the occluded ear, and everyone has made the observation of increased internal sound transmission when ears feel "blocked" by physical changes brought on by the common cold virus. The vibrations of rods, strings of musical instruments, and even kitchen utensils (Capivacci used a metal kitchen fork held between the teeth for his tests) have always been known to induce or magnify sound. An analogous mechanism, the tuning fork, was invented in the 18th C for use in music. Nineteenth century discoveries were, therefore, unconnected in any way to the Renaissance discoveries of Cardano and Capivacci. While the circumstances of the discovery of the distinction between bone and air conduction of sound by Dr. Weber were "modern," the mechanisms were age-old, had been discovered in the Renaissance, and could just as easily have been, and maybe were, noted by Hippocratic physicians and their contemporaries.

5. Diagnostics

a. Diabetes mellitus

Polyuria, the passing of excessive urine, was mentioned by the Hippocratics, and Aretaeus is credited with the first description of diabetes mellitus, at that time a "rare disease" according to Galen. Dr. Matthew Dobson (1732-1784), in 1776, described the vinous smell of standing diabetic urine, and concluded there had been sugar in that urine because he knew that sweet liquids, including wine, tended to form vinegars as they fermented. Dr. Dobson's next step was to taste a bit of the patient's blood, and, finding it sweet, concluded that the kidneys did not themselves generate sugar into the urine. Instead, it was circulating in the blood and cleared by the kidneys into the urine.[54] Clinical clues to diabetes mellitus have been discovered repeatedly over the centuries because polyuria and other associated symptoms can be such striking findings.

But the outstanding discovery relevant to diabetes mellitus, one that immediately made most previous investigations of the problem obsolete, was by Minkowski and von Mering who, in 1889, reported the consequences of extirpation of the pancreas in the dog: it was noted that the animal developed all the signs found in human diabetes, beginning with marked polyuria.[55] Their study was intended solely to determine the function of the

---

[54] This was reported in *Medical Observations and Inquiries*, London, 1776, vol. V, p. 298. In his case studies he records the smell of acetone in the urine, indicating the patient was in a state of ketoacidosis, and he also notes opalescent serum, indicating the presence of hyperlipidemia often seen in uncontrolled diabetes mellitus. Dr. Adolph Kussmaul reported in 1874 a form of diabetes mellitus to be associated with air-hunger breathing, a sign, in the absence of treatment, of often lethal diabetic acidosis. The motivation for Dr. Dobson's study was nine patients who had polyuria and sweetness of the urine, and in his report he makes no mention of work by any prior investigator. He proceeded to characterize the urine and blood by heating and by evaporation, thereby adding further important observations, and he reasoned that sugar was cleared from the blood into the urine and that the emaciation that can result from untreated diabetes mellitus was the consequence of loss of that sweet nutrient. One direct consequence was the therapeutic recommendation by some physicians in the 19th C of a diet with a large proportion of meat and little sugar. Thus, tasting and heating diabetic urine allowed useful clinical conclusions to be drawn.

[55] v. Mering, J. and Minkowski, O., *Diabetes Melitus nach Pancreas Extirpation*, in *Arch. f. exper. Path. u. Pharmakol.*, XXVI:371-381, 1889-1890. Interestingly, this publication was preceded by

pancreas; they were not investigating the cause of diabetes mellitus, which can be defined as a metabolic disorder resulting from a deficiency of, or impaired utilization of, insulin that is produced in the pancreas, and they had no idea that pancreatic extirpation might produce such a result. Thus, all prior observations of diabetes mellitus and which include the remarkable 1840s observations by Claude Bernard on glucose production by the liver and Paul Langerhans' 1869 discovery of pancreatic islet cells were eclipsed by the profound discovery of Minkowski and von Mering.

Comment - To place the work of Prof. Hermann Minkowski and Dr. Josef von Mering in historical context, human and animal dissection and even vivisection were familiar to ancient medical investigators. Aristotle and Herophilus, both of whom mention the pancreas,[56] had no qualms about studying anatomy and physiology in living animals, and Galen did many experiments on animals, including tying off ureters to show that urine in the bladder was produced by the kidneys. Several sources suggest knowledge of the consequences of removal of the spleen: Aristotle – *Metaphys.* IV, 27, 1024-1028; Pliny – *Nat. Hist.*, XI, 205; Sammonicus – *Liber Medicinalis*, XXII, 29; Celsus – *De Medicina*, V, 26, 24c, 1.[57] Extirpation of selected organs for the purpose of learning their function was an obvious path to knowledge of the body. Pliny commented that removal of the spleen from dogs is compatible with survival, and the systemic effects of castration were well known, so why not apply extirpation to the pancreas. Even the name, pancreas, is of Greek origin: παν (pan) – all; κρέας (kreas) – meat, flesh, muscle. Surgical removal or cannulation of the pancreas in an animal, done with or without sedation, was certainly within the grasp of ancient Greek investigators as was shown by Dr. Regnier de Graaf (1641-1673) who cannulated the pancreatic duct of a dog with a goose quill,[58] although pancreatic extirpation with survival of the animal admittedly is not easily performed. But the point is, the extirpation of an organ and subsequent inferences on its biological significance was a process familiar to Hippocratic physicians as well as modern physicians, and probably to many others over the ages. It would not have been a surprise if Herophilus or some other Alexandrian investigator had performed a pancreatectomy on a dog to see what would happen and then noting the resulting polyuria.

b. Proteinuria

The Hippocratics had noted the increase in bubbles in the urine in patients with renal disease, and Theophilus Protospatharius (7th C AD) noted cloudiness of some urines when heated. These findings can be explained by protein in the urine, as could the observation of Paracelsus when he added vinegar to urine and noted cloudiness.

---

thirteen years by a publication of E. Lancereaux, a French physician who noted the association of diabetes with a diseased pancreas, from which he concluded that an abnormality of pancreatic function was the likely the source of diabetes mellitus. See his *Note et Reflexions sur deux cas de diabete sucre avec alteration du pancreas*, in *Bull. Acad. Med.* 2e series, VI:1215, 1877. Even earlier a French pharmacist, A. Bouchardat, was advising dietary management of diabetes mellitus and had suggested the pancreas was the source of the problem.

[56] Aristotle: *Historia Animalium*, Bk. III, 4; Herophilus: Potter, P., *Herophilus of Chalcedon*, in *Bull. Hist. Med.* 50:45-60.

[57] See also the excellent reviewe by Fabre, A-J., *Splenic Surgery in Antiquity?* (title in English translation) in *Histoire des Sciences Medicales*, 36:255-266, 2012. Numerous Latin citations are appended.

[58] De Graaf, R., *De Succi Pancreatici Natura et Usu Exercitatio Anatomica Medica*, Leiden, 1664.

Subsequently, Prof. Domenico Cotugno (1736-1822) described, in 1775, "for the first time," the coagulation of urine from an edematous patient when it was heated, a coagulum he likened to egg albumin. Thus, it was 18th and 19th C physicians, not those earlier investigators who brought proteinuria and its relation to disease to the attention of clinicians.[59]

Comment - It is a nice piece of irony that Dr. Charles Diskin could report, in 2000, a quantitative correlation between bubbles on the urine surface and the concentration of protein in the urine (p. 301).[60] The Hippocratics had noted the association between persisting bubbles in shaken urine and kidney disease.[61] It would have been technically simple at any time from the Hippocratics forward to develop a semiquantitative test for proteinuria, either by the degree of bubble formation on shaking of the urine as did Dr. Diskin, heating the urine (mentioned by Theophyllus in the 7th C AD), or adding a small amount of acidic substance such as vinegar and observing the precipitate (as did Paracelsus in the 16th C). In each of these eras there was knowledge available to semiquantitate proteinuria and thereby more closely follow the course of kidney disease patients who had proteinuria and observe their responses to dietary manipulations, even today an important component of therapy for many renal disorders, although it was especially valuable prior to the invention of kidney dialysis in the 1950s.

6. Clinical Procedures

Some modern procedures known to the Hippocratic era practioners are described elsewhere in this volume and thus thoracentesis, urinary tract surgery, and podalic version are not discussed here.

a. General anesthesia

Methods for diminishing pain from trauma or surgical procedures have been sought and found throughout the ages and in many societies. Plato (428-348 BC) describes, in *The Republic*, 488c, the benumbing of a ship's captain by a crew using mandragora, a genus of plants containing hallucinogenic and hypnotic alkaloids. Methods have included topical application of something cold to induce superficial numbing of the skin, induction of unconsciousness by various techniques including extensive blood removal by phlebotomy, induction of analgesia by nerve compression, alcoholic inebriation, and ingestion of opiates and other mind-altering agents. It is

---

[59] In 1806 Dr. William Wells reported in a journal his studies of urine on post-scarlet fever edema, and in 1811 he described studies of hematuria and proteinuria not due to scarlet fever. These reports brought the clinical significance of proteinuria to the notice of many practitioners. Dr. John Blackall (1771-1860) nicely correlated proteinuria, as determined by heating or adding nitrous acid to a urine specimen, with anasarca, as described in 1813. In addition, in the hospital next to Dr. Wells was Richard Bright, who would become famous for his investigations of nephritis and proteinuria, the latter now known to usually represent albumin.

[60] Diskin, C. J., *et al.*, *Surface Tension, Proteinuria, and the Urine Bubbles of Hippocrates*, in: *Lancet*, 355:901, 2000. Every now and then an enlightening paper is published relevant to Hippocratic medicine, and they often affirm the correctness of ancient observations.

[61] *Aphorisms* VII, 34.

reported that a Chinese practitioner had developed an oral anesthetic in the 3rd C AD. In 1805 a Japanese physician, Seishu Hanaoka, formulated his own oral anesthetic after years of study, one that was thought to be similar to the earlier Chinese one. Its primary active ingredients were hyoscyamine and aconitine. He confirmed its effectiveness on more than 150 patients and developed dose-response curves and other scientifically derived data to improve its safety and effectiveness.[62] It is inconceivable that 1,500 years had to pass before an effective anesthetic was reintroduced in Asia. Far more likely it is that pharmaceuticals were repeatedly discovered in villages throughout China and around the world that would produce, to some degree, the desired effect. The reason no standard anesthetic was developed and used throughout ancient China despite knowledge of it in the 3rd C AD had nothing to do with discovery. It had everything to do, however, with its propagation among the region's practitioners. And it is recorded that when Seishu Hanaoka became a prominent Japanese physician he was a member of a "medical school" that kept his anesthetic agent secret, thus preventing other "schools" from duplicating his results. And so his technique was never to become a standard for general use.

The use of sponges impregnated with narcotics, dried for storage and, when needed, moistened in water, were used in 13th C Europe for inhalation anesthesia by Drs. Hugh of Lucca and his son, Theodoric, although the technique has also been identified in a 9th C manuscript from the monastery at Monte Cassino, suggesting that the idea of a soporific sponge had been been around at the time of Imperial Rome.[63] This would have been a remarkable accomplishment of "aromatherapy." Theodoric, also a champion of antisepsis, described the anesthesia in his *Chyrurgia*, a manuscript written about 1250 and translated into Catalan, but only when it was published in 1498 in Venice did it become available to a larger audience, a delay of 250 years.[64] During the Renaissance Valerius Cordus (1515-1544) discovered "sulphuric ether," and Paracelsus observed that it put chickens to sleep from which they awakened unharmed after its oral administration,[65] and both ether and chloroform were explored in the 18th C search for "pneumatic therapies," including management of asthma, not to mention the popularity of their euphoric effects. But it was not until 1846 that inhalation anesthesia with ether and later chloroform was introduced in the West and immediately came into use worldwide (p. 374 and footnote), although Sir Humphry Davy in 1799 had suggested nitrous oxide for surgical anesthesia based on his research on biological effects of gases, a field of science known as "pneumatic chemistry."

Comment – Moderns tend to date general anesthesia from the 1846 demonstration by Morton of ether inhalation for surgery, but inhalation of soporic or mind-altering drugs was available in the ancient world. Herodotus recounts the effect on Scythians of vapor baths in which the smoke of hemp seed was used to induce a state of euphoria. It has even been recently proposed that the Delphic Oracle was, for many centuries, a

---

[62] Stevens, J E., *Anaesthesia in Japan: past and present*, in *J. Royal Soc. Med.*, 79:294-298, 1986.

[63] Carter, A. J., *Narcosis and Nightshade*, in *Brit. Med. J.*, 313:1630-1632, 1996.

[64] The retrograde nature of medieval medicine is displayed in Theodoric's 1267 manuscript, despite a few inspiring insights such as his soporific sponge. It is noteworthy that the book was sponsored by a cleric, and Theodoric himself was a cleric. More remarkable is that 250 years after his manuscript was written the same text was met with applause and went through many editions into the 16th C. See: Zimmerman, L. M. and Veith, I., *Great Ideas in the History of Surgery*, Baltimore, 1961, chapter 10 (*Theodoric*).

[65] Pagel, W., *Paracelsus*, Basel, 1982, 2nd edition, p. 276f.

manipulation of ethylene that naturally escaped from vents in the Oracle's cave. Inhalation of opiates was used in the 9th C and 13th C and may have been available in Roman times, and ether was produced in 1540 and subsequently shown by Paracelsus to be harmless in chickens. There is no evidence for inhaled anesthesia by Hippocratic physicians, but inhaled aromatics, vapor baths, and fumigations were popular, indicating that the use of aromatic medicines to induce pharmacological effects was an accepted approach to therapy. Three points can be considered. (1) One explanation for limited spread of any newly devised method of gaseous anesthesia is the necessity of acquiring a quantity of the desired gas, thus limiting gaseous agents to those released from volatile liquids. (2) In earlier times the need for surgery, and therefore anesthesia, tended to be acute: a wound in battle, an injury while working, a kidney stone, a dental abscess. Hospitals were either unavailable or were not places where the sick received much medical care, especially surgery, until the Renaissance. Furthermore, someone who had an effective anesthetic near at hand and who was competent to surgically manage a serious surgical problem would have been exceedingly rare in rural Europe, and illiterate practitioners would have had no access to the knowledge of Theodoric's book about his soporific sponge. Whether it was in Seishu Hanaoka's Japan, in Theodoric's Italy, in Paracelsus' Switzerland, or in any part of the globe, procedures for pain management, especially by use of botanicals, have been commonplace, but implementation of those ideas on anything beyond local use has been exceptional. (3) As for the method of discovery, alchemy and chemistry were necessary for discovery of ether, impossibilities in Hippocratic times. It is, nevertheless, possible that aromatic agents capable of inducing equivalent hypnotic effects were known and would have been employed by them, just as Theodoric did in the 13th C. In addition to cannabis, opiates and hyoscyamine have a long history of inhalation use. Interestingly, there has been the relatively recent development of inhalational naloxone to reverse opiate toxicity.

b. Tracheotomy/intubation

These two procedures, known to Hippocratics (p. 293f) but forgotten until the Renaissance, were occasionally attempted as the Enlightenment approached, but often failed to preserve life. Only twenty-eight known attempts at tracheotomy had been documented up to the time Dr. Pierre Brettoneau, in 1825, used the procedure in patients with "croup"/diphtheria. He was successful in a number of cases, and his report in 1826 made his procedure known to many practitioners.[66] That some form of the procedure was already practiced is indicated by a paper by Dr. H. G. Jameson read before the Medical Society of Maryland in 1822.[67] Brettonneau's pupil, Dr. Armand Trousseau, then amplified the findings by studies of his own reported in 1833 in the *J. Connais. Med. Chir.*, and tracheotomy rapidly became an acceptable practice. But the dangers and poor outcomes of tracheotomy done in patients *in extremis* were still formidable, and this prompted Drs. William MacEwen of Scotland and Joseph O'Dwyer of Cleveland, Ohio,

---

[66] D. Guthrie, *Early Records of Tracheotomy*, in *Bull. Hist. Med.*, 15:59-64, 1944; Brettoneau, P., *Des Inflammations speciales du tissu muqueux et en particulier de la diphtherite, ou inflammation pelliculaire*, Paris, 1826.

[67] Jameson, H. G., *A Memoir on Bronchotomy*, in *The American Medical Recorder*, VI: 151-168, Philadelphia, 1823, *viz.* "Such are the number and respectability of authorities in favor of this operation, that the only difficulty seems to be, how a judicious selection shall be made." See p. 152 of that paper.

to separately develop a new technique to bypass upper airway obstruction. Dr. MacEwen used a flexible tube passed through the mouth into the trachea for managing anesthesia[68] whereas O'Dwyer, over several years beginning in 1880, invented an instrument used for nonsurgical intubation of the trachea in cases of upper airway obstruction due to diphtheria.[69]

Comment – The logic of making an emergency opening in the trachea to bypass upper airway occlusion and thereby prevent suffocation is so obvious to even untrained observers that use of a legendary ancient procedure (tracheotomy) as has been surmised from 1st dynasty Egyptian drawings and the Rig Veda is almost believable. Surgical procedures in the neck, however, are prone to technical difficulties and the underlying disease process may pose additional local complications, so this may have hindered its application and its popular acceptance. It required a series of patients undergoing tracheotomy to prove that survival following use of the procedure was better than no procedure, and it was under the fearsome threat of imminent death by suffocation of children with diphtheria that prompted Bretonneau to record his experience with such patients. Once he showed that tracheotomy probably improved survival, advances in technique could begin. It took verve and desperation, not sophisticated instrumentation, to proceed as he did, for techniques of the procedure had been previously described, including those of Antyllus (2nd C AD) and Fabricius (1537-1619), the latter recommending, but not attempting, a vertical incision into the trachea.

Verve, knowledge of anatomy, and sharp scalpels were available in ancient Greece, and the Hippocratics described tracheotomy and a primitive intubation of the upper airway. The logic of the 19th C attempts at tracheotomy, so apparent to some Renaissance physicians and to many 19th C ones, had already been recognized as a method in critical care by the Hippocratics. But intubation received no post-Hippocratic description until the 19th C when Drs. MaEewen and O'Dwyer, the latter unaware of any previous attempts at intubation, each developed a mechanism that proved successful to the point that it is now in routine daily use around the world. O'Dwyer's invention was, in effect, a *de novo* invention, but a version had been described by, and presumably used by, the Hippocratics, namely, intubation of the supraglottic region of the pharynx. MacEwen's tracheal tubes may also have been of his own invention, although, as his own review of the literature pointed out, there had been several prior investigators in Europe who had attempted, and accomplished to varying degrees, intubation of the larynx or trachea in the preceding fifty years. Tracheal intubation should, therefore, be considered a multifocal invention.

As a summary statement, the concept of tracheotomy has been common

---

[68] Wm. MacEwen, *Clinical Observations on the Introduction of Tracheal Tubes by the Mouth instead of performing Tracheotomy or Laryngotomy*, in *Brit. Med. J.*, 2:163-165, 1880 (the second part of a two-part article, but useful for his review of prior attempts by others using related techniques).

[69] J. O'Dwyer, *Two Cases of Croup Treated by Tubage of the Glottis* in *NY Med. J.*, 42:146-151, 1885. He had previously published in 1885 a discussion of the features of his invention, and prior to his publications he also personally gave instructions on its use to other physicians, including F. E. Waxman, who performed an emergency intubation in April, 1885 as recorded in *Intubation of the Larynx, with Personal Reminiscences*, in *J.A.M.A.*, 36:1109-1110, 1901. O'Dwyer himself said he was unaware of any previous attempts at intubation and that the stimulus for his invention was the record of poor outcomes reported for tracheotomy.

knowledge among, or repeatedly discovered by, practitioners for at least 2500 years. Like common botanicals, honey, and cathartics, it did not have to be rediscovered; it just needed to be implemented and critically evaluated by clinicians. That happened in the 19th C.

7. Glimpses into the basic sciences

Three examples tangentially related to the basic sciences are provided below, the first suggesting that it may be possible to avoid toxic effects *in vivo* by *in vitro* study, the second being a metabolic hypothesis that implies a gaseous nutrient, a designation in modern times sometimes applied to oxygen, and the third indicating that practical preventive measures resulted from observing the resistance of previously infected persons to subsequent exposure by the same infection, suggesting preventive immunological measures might have been taken by Hippocratic clinicians had they had prior experience with epidemic infectious diseases of a type now known to be viral in origin.

a. *In vitro* testing

Evidence of chemical change is seen in the fermentation associated with winemaking and the production of other alcoholic beverages, with production of vinegar, and with various methods of food preservation. Some of this would have been noted in all ancient societies. The Hippocratics, however, went a step further, implying in the work *Ancient Medicine* that the product of chemical change might have predictable effects relevant to the original substance, and that this could be a guide for selection of agents used for treatments.[70] A further discussion of this point is provided in volume 2 of the unabridged edition of this work.[71]

> Concerning the metabolic effects of various liquids and which one is liable to be tolerated by a person and the relation they have to one another, as it was stated previously, I say the following: if a sweet liquid should change into another form, not from being mixed with something else but by some intrinsic action, what might it first become, bitter or salty or sour or acidic (tart)? I think, acidic. Therefore an acidic liquid should be more unsuitable for the person than the others if a sweet liquid were the most unfit of all. And so, if someone is able to be accurate in such *in vitro* investigations, then he will always be able to select the best of all [the possibilities.]

Comment - Most ancient societies were familiar with fermentation, and evidence of winemaking has been identified from 7000 years ago. Consider the liquid in the preceding example to be apple juice. On standing it will ultimately become tart, or acidic, as acetic acid is produced by the metabolic action of certain aerobic bacteria.[72] For discussion here

---

[70] See the writings of *Hippocrates* , in the *Loeb Classical Library*, vol. 1, *Ancient Medicine* XXIV. In the translation provided here it is argued that translation of δύναμις as "metabolic activity" is appropriate.

[71] Adams, W. H., *The Natural State of Medical Practice: Hippocratic Evidence*, Maitland (FL), 2019, p. 68*f.*

[72] There is an intermediate step, for environmental yeasts produce ethanol (familiar to United States devotees of "hard" cider) that is in turn, in the presence of oxygen, metabolized to acetic acid. As for taste, pure undenatured ethanol would have been impossible for the ancients to acquire. In high

it is not relevant whether apple vinegar is fit or unfit for a person in whom apple juice causes some sort of problem. The point is that the Hippocratics were attempting to improve on simple empirical selection, and, recognizing that what is now termed biochemical change can occur in nutriments, suggested it might be used as a guide. The writer also suggests (line 12 of the citation) that *in vitro* (ζητέων ἔξωθεν, "studying outwardly," *i.e.*, "outside the patient"), as opposed to *in vivo* ("in the patient," literally "in the living body"), investigation could lead to improved choices of medicines. In fact, this approach to biochemical study would not be improved on until the 19th C, when Dr. Louis Pasteur identified microorganisms as the cause of fermentation.

b. Metabolism

Essential to cellular respiration and oxidative metabolism is oxygen, for the enzymatic reactions of cellular metabolism release energy by means of oxidation. Some experts consider it appropriate to consider oxygen as a nutrient.[73] Controlled oxidation is the basis for cell viability, and one product of that metabolism is heat. A mammalian characteristic is a constant body temperature, one maintained by the continuous production of energy by cellular metabolism. The Hippocratics thought that body warmth was a characteristic of life maintained by inspired πνεῦμα ("pneuma") from the air. In the absence of pneuma, tissues lose warmth and the various body organs lose their ability to function. In a sense the Hippocratics recognized some basic facts of cell survival, even though they knew nothing about oxygen or cells. Pneuma was carried throughout the body by the blood. Thus, pneuma, a force inspired from the air, carried in blood vessels, and necessary for life and for production of body heat (*i.e.*, one consequence of metabolism) was acknowledged to exist even though not understood, its nature a detail to be worked out later. It is known now as oxygen.

Comment - Hero of Alexandria (10-70 AD) reported an experiment by Philo of Byzantium demonstrating that when a burning candle was placed inside a jar and the jar was placed upside down in water, the water rose to a certain level in the jar before the flame extinquished, just as medical cupping causes the skin to be pulled up into the cupping apparatus.[74] Hero concluded that the burning consumed or altered a component of the air. Could the pneuma be required for burning just as it was necessary for maintaining body heat? It is now known that the cited experiment was not an enclosed system, and the using up of a gaseous component, or pneuma, did not explain the rise in water level into the jar and therefore would not permit quantitation of the oxygen content

---

concentrations it is very injurious to tissues, and its perceived taste seems to be related more to a potentiation or diminishing of tastes of other substances. Thus, the Hippocratic citation must refer to the vinegar taste, termed acidic. Some might describe the taste as sour, but sourness is more a feature of lactic acid production, as in sauerkraut. Aristotle discusses tastes in detail in his *de Anima*.
[73] Forster, R. E. and Estabrook, R., *Is Oxygen an Essential Nutrient?*, in *Annu. Rev. Nutr.*, 13:383-403, 1993.
[74] Woodcroft, B., *The Pneumatics of Hero of Alexandria*, London, 1851, p. 3-4, although Philo of Byzantium (280-220 BC) was the likely discoverer. The statement by Hero in Greek is: "for the basic explanation is that the fire in it [the cupping glass] destroys [consumes?] and attenuates [lessens the compression of] the air in it, ..."; translation by the author. There are variant interpretations attendant to different manuscripts of Philo's "*Pneumatica.*"

air.[75] But the pertinent point is that such an experiment was performed and a hypothesis for the result presented. Furthermore, the candle flame was extinguished, an indication that something in air was (1) necessary for combustion, and (2) that substance was finite. Merely placing an animal in a small closed container would over time lead to the animal's death (as oxygen was used up) and the leftover air does not support a flame. This experiment was performed by John Mayow (1643-1679). Such simple experiments as described by Hero would have led to a more scientific characterization of the "pneuma" and thereby a more scientific view of metabolism.

c. Immunization

A prominent ancient testimonial to the ability of the body, having recovered from an attack by a contagious disease, to resist subsequent attacks is described in Thucydides' history of the plague of Athens, a pertinent section being translated on p. 140f. One of the infectious diseases often suggested as the cause of that plague is smallpox.[76]

Contagiousness of certain diseases has been common knowledge, and isolation of individuals suspected of having contagious disease has been common practice in many societies. But the earliest documentation of purposeful immunization against disease in the West is found in writings of the medical community of 11th C Salerno:

> "In order that variola may not produce death among tender babes, put into their veins a favorable variola. Better still they should avoid touching the contagium of the disease; the sick person, the breath of the sick, the clothes, the coverings, the garments and such clean bodies he may have infected with his hand."

> Translation of A. C. Klebs, in his article *The Historic Evolution of Variolation*, in *Bull. Johns Hopkins Hosp.*, 24:69-83, 1913[77]

The procedure described from Salerno is known as "variolation," the purposeful

---

[75] For a scientific discussion of the experiment see: Vera, F., *et al.*, *Burning a Candle in a Vessel, a Simple Experiment with a Long History*, in *Sci. and Educ.*, 20:881-893, 2011.

[76] For a recent consideration of the cause of the Athenian plague see: Cunha, B. A., *The Cause of the Plague of Athens: Plague, Typhoid, Typhus, Smallpox, or Measles?*, in *Infect. Dis. Clin. N. Am.*, 18:29-43, 2004.

[77] A translation alternative for first line might be "those not robust" rather than "tender babes." For the verse, Klebs cites: S. de Renzi, *Flos Medicinae Scholae Salerni*, Naples, 1859, p. 90. The *Flos Medicinae* was not written for physicians even though it became a part of the medical curriculum for centuries. See: Stelmaschuk, A., *The School at Salerno: Origin of the European Medical University*, in *Proc. of the 10th Annual History of Medicine Days*, p. 65-71, 2001. It has been suggested that several ancient tribes existing at the time of the early Roman Empire (*e.g.*, the Psylli and the Marsi) purposefully immunized themselves against snake venoms and were therefore able to be known to antiquity as experts in manipulating snakes. But few dangerously toxic snakes are now present in the region formerly occupied by the Psylli. Modern opinion is that purposeful immunization was not attempted, although this people sometimes exposed infants to a snake bite as a test of legitimacy, and survivors, considered legitimate offspring, might inadvertently have developed some active immunity. The possibility of immunization against some pestilences is mentioned by Fracastoro (1476-1553), the terms he used for "immunity" being "adsuescere" and "consuescere," both meaning "to adapt to" or "to become accustomed to." Their context makes clear he meant some form of innate acquired resistance that is the consequence of prior exposure.

inoculation of a healthy person with infectious material from a patient, thus passing on the infection, but with the hope that it would be clinically mild. If this occurred and the immunized person survived, he would then be resistant to a naturally acquired infection of the same type. The introduction of variolation into Europe has traditionally been credited to the letters from Turkey of Lady Montague (1689-1762). The East has always been considered the source of the variolation technique,[78] and smallpox may have been introduced into Europe in the 6th-7th C AD. Nevertheless, variolation for the prevention of lethal smallpox was an old story for Europe when a chance clinical observation introduced into medicine one of the greatest life-preserving discoveries of all time. Dr. Edward Jenner (1749-1823) had noted the association of a previous infection in humans by cowpox with (1) resistance to smallpox infection and (2) inability to respond to variolation using infectious smallpox material from smallpox patients. After more than twenty years of collecting and recording these occasional associations he reported them to the Royal Society which declined to publish his paper. He therefore published them himself in a small booklet in 1798.[79]

Comment - The basic observation of protection provided by prior infection, the foundation of immunology, was duly noted by Hippocratic clinicians and by the Athenian population, having been brought to their attention by a terrible epidemic. It has even been proposed that the "plague" of Athens as described by Thucydides was the earliest description of an epidemic,[80] in which case his was also the earliest description of specific immunological protection provided by prior infection. The protection would have been difficult to detect without a significant cluster of cases with similar clinical presentations. The Athenians, crowded as they were from an influx of those fleeing a Spartan offensive of the Peloponnesian War, were able to make that important observation, one that would be made with increasing frequency as global populations and crowding increased.

Isolation of persons with certain disorders considered contagious was practiced by the ancient Hebrews, but immunological prevention of infection is the issue here. The physicians of Athens had no opportunity to evaluate that possibility during the Athenian

---

[78] Virtually every reference that includes the history of variolation states its origin as China or India, although some also suggest Africa. Nevertheless, documentation of these claims is poor, and the earliest conclusive statement is the 11th C Salerno statement given above. One argument for the Far East being the site of earliest variolation is that its areas of high population density might have provided the best opportunity for the contagion to recognized.

[79] E. Jenner, *An Inquiry into the Causes and Effects of the Variolae Vaccinae, or Cow-pox, a Disease Discover in Some of the Western Parts of England, particularly Gloucestershire, and Known by the Name of Cow Pox,* London, 1798.

[80] Martin, P., and Martin-Granel, E., *2,500-year Evolution of the Term Epidemic,* in *Emerging Infectious Diseases,* 12:976-980, 2006. Despite the implication of uniqueness to the Athenian plague, biblical recounting of the Philistine capture of the Arc of the Covenant and the subsequent "plague" of "emerods" in the 9th C BC raises the question of just what is an "epidemic." Circumstances suggest the plausibility of a Philistine plague, given that rodents were mentioned as part of the phenomenon, for the latter may have spread the plague. In a similar vein, it has been proposed that epidemic smallpox did not appear in China until localized populations reached a size that supported the development of an epidemic, perhaps the 1st or 2nd centuries AD. Alternatively, R. Chamseru, in the 18th C, postulated that some "epidemics," *e.g.,* the "cough of Perinthus" (p. 206*ff*) were in fact the concurrence of several diseases rather than a single contagion, and others have considered this as a possibility for the Athenian "plague." See: Chamseru, R., in *Memoirs de la Societe Royale de Medecine,* 8:130-178, 1786.

plague. But how difficult is it to institute such a preventative? It is appropriate to review here the circumstances of smallpox.

Who and where variolation was first tried is unknown, and probably it was of multifocal origin. That there was knowledge of variolation in 11th C Salerno seems fairly assured. The idea of giving a "tiny amount" of material from a lesion in a person sick from an observed contagion to induce a "tiny amount" of disease in a healthy individual that might protect him against a serious form of the disease seems logical, and it has been suggested that variolation in its various forms is a classic example of the common sense of laymen as opposed to the impractical theories of the learned. "This indebtedness to the intuitive genius of popular reason and procedure is strikingly illustrated in the reports of early practice of variolation."[81] Variolation had been popular in some areas of India in the 18th C and probably much earlier, and it remained popular even after the introduction of smallpox vaccination, for its effectivess was considered by contemporary society to be equivalent to the latter technique.[82] Oral history suggests nasal insufflation of powdered crusts of smallpox lesions was used in ancient China to protect against smallpox, but the approximate dates of the origin of this procedure are conjecture. The eminent scholar, Joseph Needham, has proposed it was in use during the Song Dynasty in China (960-1279), but the earliest objective verification of variolation in China is 1695.[83] Forms of variolation have also been described in various sites in Africa, although it is unknown if they were of indigenous origin or introduced by the Mamelukes in Egypt. The Caucasus region was the home of many of the Mamelukes, slave soldiers that over several centuries became masters of many Islamic regions, including North Africa. And if that were the case it has been suggested that their knowledge of variolation was Circassian in origin, for variolating infant girls not only protected the girls against smallpox, but also led to a great decrease in subsequent disfiguring scars in those that survived the inoculation compared to those who survived the natural disease. This contributed to the high opinion of the beauty of Circassian women, for they were sought out by many prominent rulers in Ottoman society, a fact that brings little honor to the Ottoman rulers and the Circassian men.[84]

Moving forward in time, circumstances leading to the invention of vaccination began when Dr. Edward Jenner heard a paper read by John Fewster in 1765 at a medical society meeting in London. It was an unpublished case report on the inability of a person with a history of cowpox to develop a typical reaction to Mr. Fewster's attempt at variolation. Dr. Jenner, in his 1798 publication on prevention of smallpox does not give any credit to Fewster, even though Fewster was personally known to him and provided him with clinical observations on other patients that Jenner included in subsequent reports. Also, the association of cowpox, a zoonosis found in England and parts of Europe, with a decreased risk of smallpox was a commonly acknowledged local

---

[81] A. C. Klebs, in his article *The Historic Evolution of Variolation*, in *Bull. Johns Hopkins Hosp.*, 24:69-83, 1913, p. 70.

[82] The correctness of that opinion has been difficult to verify. See: Arnold, D., *Smallpox and Colonial Medicine in Nineteenth Century India*, in *Institutions and Ideologies; A SOAS South Asia Reader*, Richmond (Surrey), 1993, D. Arnold and P. Robb, editors, p. 224-244. As for the origin of variolation in the subcontinent, it is unknown, the earliest clear description being the early 18th C.

[83] Leung, A. K. C., *"Variolation" and Vaccination in Late Imperial China, Ca 1570-1911*, in *History of Vaccine Development*, S. A. Plotkin, editor, New York, 2011, pp. 5-12.

[84] *The Works of Voltaire, A Contemporary Version*, vol. 19 (Philosophical Letters), New York, 1901, translated by W. Fleming, p. 19*ff*.

observation unrelated to variolation. Indeed, a farmer named Benjamin Jesty, being familiar with local lore in Dorset, also in the West of England, had infected his family with cowpox material in the face of a smallpox outbreak in 1774, and they did not contract the disease. This was an unpublished observation. The significance of the association between cowpox (now classified as an orthopoxvirus) and protection against smallpox was also apparent to another earlier discoverer of vaccination, Mr. Peter Plett in northern Germany, also an endemic focus of cowpox, who reported his experiences in vaccination in 1790. His findings were not published by his University. The control of smallpox by vaccination, therefore, may be considered a multifocal *de novo* discovery, the critical component being the presence of cowpox rather than any prior writings by ancient or medieval practitioners. And once immunization was recognized by the medical establishment to be an effective control of smallpox it opened the vast field of immunity for study.

While Hippocratic physicians may have been the first to clinically describe the problem of contagion and the acquisition of innate resistance, they were not part of any solution. Perhaps this is because a deadly contagion in a sizeable confined population had not previously been encountered in the region. But it is the contention of the author that the purpose of this book is not to lionize any particular ethnic population. It is, instead, to praise that form of social structure that permits the expression of ingenuity to surface and to provide evidence that such expression is desireable in all human societies. And it is for this reason the author has dwelled on smallpox even though there is nothing in the Greco-Roman age to suggest its clinicians had progressed to the stage of developing immunologically-based preventive measures for contagions.

C. Conclusion

This chapter has tediously described twenty inventions or areas of discovery found to be of great value in modern medicine. Importantly, the invention or discovery was made significant when their inventor or discoverer provided clinical or anatomic correlations that made those inventions or discoveries worthwhile, *i.e.* significance lay less with inventions of the inventors than it did with the clinical associations that those inventors acquired in applying the inventions. If this is so, the three ages of medical insight resulted not from the freeing up of inventiveness. Indeed, the inventions were generally quite simple and more the product of common sense than genius.[85] Their importance resulted instead from the liberation of clinical talents of practitioners. The answer as to why the Dark Ages were so tragically barren of knowledgeable medical care is not explained by lack of inventiveness. It was, instead, due to a lack of clinical physicians. This is consistent with the repeated observation in earlier chapters of this work that there were few true physicians in ancient Rome, none in post-Roman Europe, almost none in Byzantium, none in the medieval universities, and almost none in the Renaissance. So important were clinical correlations by authentic physicians that without

---

[85] This is not to deny true genius and its value to progress, although it is questionable whether the word "genious" has any real meaning. A good salesman can easily turn a common sense finding into a work of genius. Such distinctions are arbitrary. The ultimate arbiter of a product of value (or "of genious") is the freedom of the society in which both exist. Perhaps a functional definition might be that the product of genius is something new and bold; the product of common sense is something good.

them inventions would have been curiosities of little value. There are, therefore, two important inferences. (1) Hippocratic clinicians, having already acquired much important clinical knowledge, and, more importantly, using a method of scientific discovery that could be applied to future medical advances, would have promptly seized on more convenient and accurate ways to identify pathology and improve prognosis had they had more time to take advantage of such discoveries made by them or presented to them. Had this happened a scientific revolution would have occurred in Greco-Roman times. (2) More importantly, it highlights the critical role of the practicing clinician in determining events that promote medical progress. It also argues for individual and group freedom as the all-important permissive event. Dr. Augenbrugger's fame for inventing percussion is explained by his freedom to work on his own to clinically correlate anatomical and physical examination findings and by a social environment that had a mechanism for communicating his ideas to others who had similar interests, in the present instance that mechanism being his book. His discovery was not a work of genius; it was merely the consequence of unfettered common sense. And so it is: medicine's progress is attributable to the freeing up of common sense, not to gifted genius.

Henri Huchard, a French physician, felt "that the revival of the Hippocratic methods in the seventeenth century and their triumphant vindication by the concerted scientific movement of the nineteenth, is the whole history of internal medicine."[86] But, from the foregoing examples, basic and simple clinical discoveries capable of triggering an explosion of medical progress can occur in just about any place and age if there is the appropriate social milieu. There is no need to seek the origin of modern medical progress in Hippocratic tracts any more than there is to imply a logical progression of scientific discovery over the ages where none exists. Indeed, there is a reason not to do so. For if Huchard's position is successfully argued it means that all that mankind requires to sustain and promote progress in medicine is scientific method. This is blatantly and dangerously in error. Gladstone's pronouncement is accurate: "...the great fact [is] that liberty is a great and precious gift of God, and that human excellence cannot grow up in a nation without it."[87]

---

[86] Garrison, F. H., *History of Medicine*, Phila., 1913, p. 66. Huchard (1844-1910) was a prominent French cardiologist who wrote on vascular disease and hypertension.

[87] Gladstone is cited by F. Gribble in *The Romance of the Oxford Colleges*, Boston, 1911, p. 225. Gladstone referred to institutional reticence in attributing a role of society in fostering greatness.

CHAPTER TWENTY-FOUR

THE MAGIC OF THE KOINON

> *"The true rate of advance in medicine is, however, not to be tested by the work of single men, but by the practical capacity of the mass."*

S. Weir Mitchell, MD[1]

The role of medical journals in the history of medicine has received inadequate attention, for it is the medical journal, as the mouthpiece of the koinon, that brought back the natural state of medical practice. Whereas the Renaissance inventor and his patron relied on distribution of a relatively small number of books, usually written in Latin, to a relatively small number of friends, associates, and prominent persons, the democratic and vernacular medical journal was available to professionals in all reaches of society, the phenomenal result being that koinons now had an international reach and were thereby internationally productive to the benefit of all mankind.

A. The Medical Journal: Mouthpiece of the Koinon

Dissemination of clinical discovery among a small group of friends and academicians with a common interest is not sufficient for the comprehensive education required by a profession dispersed throughout a society. It has been argued herein, therefore, that the Renaissance was irrelevant to subsequent progress in the West, at least in medicine. After all, what proportion of the general population in Linnaeus' day would have had any interest in the definitions of "genus" and "species"? There is a tendency to assume that the correspondence among great men of the Renaissance and Enlightenment reflected the general knowledge of the time, that if Linnaeus had walked into an English pub he would immediately have been the center of attention, that Copernicus had a popular following throughout Europe that had a sympathetic resentment of religious leaders who derided his theories. No, few of the general population knew of his quandary, fewer cared, and with great caution he published his work in 1543, the year he died, some of the 400 or so copies of the first edition remaining unsold. The heliocentrism proposed by the book remained on the Catholic Church's *Index of Forbidden Books* until 1758 and the book itself finally removed from the *Index* in 1835. Although reprinted several times, it was not widely read. Dr. Ludwik Fleck described the problem thus: "Such scientific exploits can prevail only if they have a seminal effect by being performed at a time when the social conditions are right... Had Vesalius lived in the twelfth or thirteenth century he would have made no impact... The futility of work that is isolated from the spirit of the age is shown strikingly in the case of that great herald of excellent ideas Leonardo da Vinci, who nevertheless left no positive scientific achievement behind."[2] This distinctly

---

[1] An address before the Second Congress of American Physicians and Surgeons, Sept. 23rd, 1891, entitled *The Early History of Instrumental Precision in Medicine*, New Haven, 1892, p. 24. Mitchell, a remarkable man, was President of the Congress at the time.

[2] Fleck, L., *Genesis and Development of a Scientific Fact*, Chicago, 1979, translated by F. Bradley, p. 45. Fleck's comments as selected from his book by G. Weissmann in *Wood's Hole Cantata* (New York, 1985) ring with plausibility, his thesis being that the real value of da Vinci's work would

was not the case with 19th C medicine, for the reason now to be described.

If one were to identify the most overt expression of the koinon that propelled modern medical practice forward it would be the medical journal. Prior to the commonplace medical journal there was the relatively uncommon published book, one often written entirely by the medical man himself, perhaps the only publication of his lifetime, often describing but a single discovery of limited interest to most medical professionals, an unvetted publication representing solely the author's judgment of the value of his work, and published, often in Latin, in an edition of only a few hundred copies that would be distributed to a few friends, professors, patrons and other prominent personages, or interested parties who could afford them.[3] Such were the medical books of the 16th, 17th, and much of the 18th C. For example, Auenbrugger's important 95-page treatise on percussion, published in 1761, was known to several prominent medical persons. But Auenbrugger had no patron, which probably explains the poor quality of the paper of his book and the limited number of copies printed. Smith, noting the fifty years between the date of Auenbrugger's publication and the general acceptance of its message in 1808, was unable to determine the cause for the delay.[4] A repetition of these circumstances, and an example of how a profound chasm between the original observer and his pertinent reading public can resurface even today, is admirably included in Dr. Barry Marshall's book, *Helicobacter Pioneers*, in which Chapter 7 is a recounting of the regrettable events that impinged on the discoveries of Dr. John Lykoudis regarding the cause of most gastroduodenal ulcer disease.[5] In neither instance did a medical journal

---

have been realized only if he had some contemporary colleagues to carry on his work. But the reason is not so simple. Da Vinci was idolized by his contemporaries and after his death his manuscripts were recognized for their genius. They were in great demand, being purchased from his friend, Melzi, and from his family by a variety of collectors, royal and private. What scientific mind that might build on the great man's work could afford such one-of-a-kind treasures? The manuscripts, therefore, were, over three centuries, closeted, dispersed, disassembled, lost, or destroyed so that it was only in the late 19th C that inexpensive copies of some manuscripts became available. The problem was not the lack of potentially enthusiastic colleagues; it was the lack of a way to notify them, to share knowledge with them.

[3] There was great variability in "runs" for printed editions. Prior to the 16th C Woolf states edition sizes in Europe tended to range from 200-1000 copies (see: Woolf, D. R., *Reading History in Early Modern England*, Cambridge, 2000), and G. H. Putnam, in *Books and Their Makers During the Middle Ages*, New York, 1896, 2 vols., chapter 3 of the first volume, writes that the average run in 15th C Italy was 200, with volume being limited by anticipated sales. The house of Plantin-Moretus in 16th and 17th C Amsterdam averaged about 1000 copies per run, and in 18th C England runs were often in the range of 1000-2500 but could be as few as 25, depending on anticipated sales or the number of subscriptions. But this sort of information from publishers is difficult to acquire for individual titles and is affected by many variables. Auenbrugger's publication, probably paid for by himself as he includes no Dedication and, except perhaps for some presentation copies, printed on thin, cheap paper, might have been no larger than a few hundred. Even Laennec's epochal 1819 publication on the stethoscope, when translated into English with the first printing of 500 copies being sold out in 1823, its translator, John Forbes, said the popularity of the book was "unprecedented."

[4] Smith, J. J., *The Inventum Novem of Joseph Leopold Auenbrugger*, in *Bull. N. Y. Acad. Med.*, 38:691-701.

[5] In 1958 Dr. Lykoudis made the astute clinical observation that a certain antibiotic therapy, given for an unrelated reason, appeared to cure peptic ulcer disease. Despite evidence of its effectiveness in thousands of patients he was unable to get his results published. He therefore privately published them in 1966 in a booklet entitled *The Truth about Gastric and Duodenal Ulcer*. This publication

disseminate essential information, and, while reticence of the profession to acknowledge or accept a new idea was perhaps a factor in the delay, more important was the limited audience that received the initial report.

Particularly important was the vetting by members of the professional organization of articles published in its journals. The ordinary medical journal was immediately, frequently, regularly, and economically available. A book on the other hand had not only a limited number of copies for distribution, but often years would pass before a second edition updated the first, and if the author had evoked any professional enmity that second edition might never come to publication. To acknowledge the role of the koinon in advancing medical practice and progress, rather than apportioning medicine to eras such as the Renaissance, the Enlightenment, the Golden Age, or Modern, it is more accurate to consider medicine as either pre- or post-journal.[6] The journal's essential feature, from the early clinician's perspective, can be captured in a passing comment by Prins and Bastiaanse:[7]

> "Schenck von Grafenberg [1530-1598] may still be credited as being the first author who implicitly made a distinction between a disorder of language (aphasia) and a disorder of speech (dysarthria), thus appreciating the essential nature of aphasia. ...
> The idea that aphasia is not caused by a paralysis did not become generally known, however, *and this fact would be 'rediscovered' time and again during the following centuries* [italics added]."

And that is the great value of the koinon: once new knowledge is available and scrutinized by the koinon it promptly becomes the common property of all in the koinon, and this makes it less likely that new knowledge will need to be "rediscovered time and again," less likely that it will disappear. It is resilient knowledge. Dr. Johnson recalled the words of Cicero that "not to know what was transacted in former times, is to continue always a child."[8] Journals removed this threat from the profession. Freedom of the press is as critical to medicine as it is to the greater society. The editorial process must remain openly accessible to all members. Given its incalculable importance as an expeditor of the work of the koinon it is odd that a scholarly generic history of the medical journal has yet to be published.

B. Renaissance and 19th C Medicine Compared

---

was in Greek. Encountering local resistance, his scientific breakthrough was ignored and the medical profession remained ignorant of its significance until, through a different circumstance and venue, the story of *Helicobacter pylori* became known. See: Rigas, B, and Papavassiliou, E. D., *John Lykoudis*, Chapter 7, in Dr. Barry Marshall's book, *Helicobacter Pioneers*, Victoria, 2002, and see also footnote, p. 410, of the present work.

[6] The Hippocratics had, to our knowledge, no medical journals, although the case histories probably served that purpose in some small way, and the population of physicians to be kept up to date by the Hippocratic koinon of Cos was relatively small. Importantly, however, the success of the Hippocratic koinon in the absence of journals indicates that they play a supportive rather than permissive role for the voice of the koinon. Journals exploit the magic of the koinon, but they do not produce it.

[7] Prins, R, and Bastiaanse, R., *History of Aphasia, The early history of aphasiology: From the Egyptians surgeons (ca. 1700 BC) to Broca (1861)*, in: *Aphasiology*, 20:762-791, 2006

[8] Samuel Johnson, in *The Rambler*, No. 154, London, 1751.

Avidly seeking ways to improve effectiveness, physicians, through their professional organizations, quickly integrated new ideas and new technologies into their practices, and the benefits of 18th and 19th C Western medicine were then showered on 20th C Western society, flowing around the world. There are those who would argue that it was diffidence within the profession that delayed implementation of earlier discoveries and insights. But within the profession no skullduggery was involved, no criminal intent. Although there were differing opinions on what was progress, no evidence suggests anyone hid earlier results so as to prevent progress. The fact is that there was in those earlier years no organization through which open discussion could shed light on otherwise obscure discoveries, no debate that would disclose a foolish opposition. What must be realized is that the genius associated with memorable names of medical science in the 16th and 17th centuries represented local insight fortunate enough to have been documented by a patron and thereby preserved for posterity; but it was only a portent of progress rather than progress itself. One can argue that, in the greater picture, Galileo, Santorio, Floyer, Cardano, Carpivacci, Fracastoro, Servetus, and other great names were irrelevant to the development of modern medicine, for all clinically meaningful advances had to be discovered anew in the late 18th and the 19th centuries. Only when Western societies continued their march toward democratic governance did a true medical profession emerge. Santorio's discoveries in 1614 did not initiate two hundred years of gradually increasing fruitful cogitation and experimentation on the thermometer. Santorio's work is remarkable and admired not because it proved valuable but because it was clever and it was first. It was indeed those things, but it then disappeared. Then in 1868 Wunderlich applied the thermometer, which had been adapted for bedside use after its value in meteorology was shown, to a clinical setting. This was the great advance for medicine. And it seems unfair: whereas the third edition of the 1614 book by Santorio (the first edition is unavailable) can be bought for $4000, $200 will buy a first edition printing of Wunderlich's masterpiece.

An interesting perspective on Renaissance discovery is apparent in Freind's history of medicine, the earliest review, in English, of medicine from ancient times up to the 16th C.[9] Most of the investigators mentioned in the preceding chapter are not mentioned in Freind's book, including Santorio, even though Freind's book was first published in 1723, and of the few that are mentioned most are barely mentioned, except for William Harvey (1578-1657).[10] Finally, the same delay and likely for the same reason afflicted sciences other than medicine. Copernicus (1473-1543) had his famous work, *De Revolutionibus Orbium Coelestium*, published in 1543, but it was one-and-a-half centuries before there was scholarly acceptance of his heliocentric solar system, and

---

[9] Freind, J., *The History of Physick, from the time of Galen ...*, London, 1726, 3rd edition, vol. 1 (of 2), p. 233*ff.*

[10] In fairness it must be pointed out that Freind intended his history of medicine to conclude with the end of the 15th C, a convenient cut-off inasmuch as his sources comprised primarily manuscripts. And yet had he bothered to make his book more current it should have been easy to include discoveries of his near contemporaries by the time of the 3rd edition. Since he does provide a personal critique of existing therapeutic practices as they relate to similar practices by the ancients, and since he mentions a number of 16th and 17th C persons, the conclusion is that, as a medical historian, only limited information on Renaissance/Enlightenment medical discovery was available to him, even by 1726 (the 1st edition is dated 1723). This is not surprising, for even Harvey's great discoveries that were first presented in 1616 were in part misunderstood by Laennec two centuries later. See: McMichael, J., *History of Atrial Fibrillation* 1628-1819 Harvey – de Senac – Laennec, in *Br. Heart J.* 48:193-197, 1982.

another generation before it was taught in the great universities.[11] And Galileo published his *Siderius Nuncius* in 1610, but in the "new" edition of *Philosophia juxta Inconcussa Tutissimeque Divi Thomae Dogmata* (Cologne, 1764), a work of the prominent 17th C philosopher Antoine Goudin, Galileo is mentioned only briefly in one sentence and that is in reference to his discovery of the rings of Saturn.[12]

A new idea in archaic times would for the most part wither on the vine, but a new idea at the close of the 19th C was promptly placed before its judges and proclaimed. Even such an intangible and previously unimaginable concept as an invisible stream of miniscule wave-particles able to penetrate solid objects became household knowledge within days after an article on the X-ray by Dr. W. C. Roentgen (1845-1923) in 1895, and within three years X-ray films were used to diagnose injuries during the Spanish-American War, the same year that knowledge of radioactive elements was proclaimed by M. Curie.[13]

The period between ancient discoveries and their modern usefulness as described in this and the previous chapter, a span of about two thousand years, was not a time of graded progress. During those intervening centuries there were no ruminations on how to improve upon Hippocratic observations, there was no testing, no formal confirmation of earlier investigations. Eighteenth/nineteenth century discoveries burst forth as fireworks rather than the final chapter of an Ian Fleming novel with an exciting but predictable conclusion. It is worth noting, furthermore, that none of the discoveries and inventions mentioned in the previous chapter and referred to above depended on findings at autopsy, although in some instances that study greatly enhanced their significance. Thus, while it is appropriate to acknowledge the genius of those early discoverers of the Renaissance and Enlightenment, it is to the "magic of the koinon" and to those who dwelled within its ranks that the greatest honor is due. There are, of course, contributory events: concurrent developments that might have promoted 19th C discovery included the printing press, large population centers, and separation of church and state. But three centuries separated invention of the printing press in the West from flourishing 18th-19th C European medical science, whereas other disciplines in the arts and letters promptly claimed popularity and prominence after Gutenberg and shaped the course of society. The populations of Paris, London, Naples, and Constantinople around 1550 were 210,000, 75,000, 209,000, and 660,000, respectively, similar to cities in 430 BC: Athens was 155,000 (excluding slaves), Syracuse was 125,000, Babylon was 200,000,and Memphis

---

[11] Mizwa, S. F., *Nicholas Copernicus*, New York, 1943. The Copernican work was published in Nuremburg in 1543. Approximately 400 copies were printed. (See: Gingerich, O., *The Book Nobody Read*, New York, 2004, chapter 8.) It was indexed among prohibited books by the Catholic Church in 1616, and was ridiculed by leaders of the Protestant Reformation, but these facts are not likely causes of the delay in acceptance. It is stated that the the book was purposefully so technically difficult that it was understandable to relatively few, primarily sophisticated, astronomers. Copernicus was, among other things, a physician, having studied medicine at the University in Padua from 1501-1503.

[12] First composed by 1670, Goudin died in 1695. The reference to Galileo is in Book III, p. 54, of the 1764 edition. The problem, of course, was not Goudin's book and its seemingly facile handling of Galileo. The problem was, instead, a dearth of other options for disseminating the news.

[13] Roentgen, W. C.: *Eine Neue Art von Strahlen*, in *SitzungsBericht der Physikalisch-Medzinischen Gesellschaft zu Wurzburg*, 137:132-141, 1895; Curie, M: *Sur une nouvIelle substance fortemente radio-active, contenue dans la pechblende*, in *Comptes rendus de l'Academie des Sciences*, Paris, 127:1215-1217, 1898.

was 100,000.[14] As for the Church and State, there was the Enlightenment in the 17th-18th centuries immediately preceding the Golden Age of Science, but, with expulsion of Absolutism of the Church by the Absolutism of the Monarch, one ruling caste merely replaced by another. Instead, the emergence of medical discovery in 18th-19th C Europe coincided chronologically and geographically with devolvement of political freedom, linking both the natural state of medical practice and scientific medicine with a free society. This European advance, as its ancient Greek precursor, can be viewed thus:

Table 10: Reemergence of Classical Western Society in New Attire

Social milieu	Ancient Greece	Europe	Type of knowledge
Kingdoms	Mycenaean	Dark Ages	Mystical (*e.g.*, charms)
Aristocracies	Early Archaic	Medieval Period	Questioning (*e.g.*, alchemy)
Tyrants	Late Archaic	Renaissance	Observational (*e.g.*, astronomy)
Democracies	Classical	18th-19th C	Analytical (*e.g.*, stethoscope)

It is a central tenet of this work that the natural state of medical practice preceded 19th C clinical discovery, not the other way around. This was the sequence as well in the Greece of Hippocrates, and it underscores the critical role of the natural state of medical practice in promoting medical progress:

group freedom ⟶ natural state of medical practice ⟶

accumulation of shared knowledge ⟶ scientific method and invention

The importance of the platform of the koinon, both its meetings and its publications, whether on papyrus, vellum, or paper, cannot be overstated. The 19th C was awash with discovery and invention, in the large cities and in small towns, in all branches and levels of medical science, in the clinic and the laboratory. True, it was also awash in opportunists, charlatans, and theories later to be proven incorrect. But medical and scientific journals, with each article reviewed by peers of the discoverers and vetted by its respective koinon, brought benefit beyond measure to all mankind.[15] With this valuable tool, looking over the vigorous attempts and ultimate success of the medical profession to decide its own interests after centuries of having them decided by others, medical associations came to be the modern face of medicine and the common council of the Hippocratic koinon. This was the catalyst, not the Renaissance, that made the 19th C the Golden Age of medicine.[16]

---

[14] Chandler, T., *Four Thousand Years of Urban Growth*, New York, 1987.

[15] Dr. Baas, in his *Outlines of the History of Medicine and the Medical Profession* (New York, 1889, H. E. Handerson, translator, p. 854), remarks that in 1878 there were 78 distinct medical journals being published in Germany alone.

[16] The names of many of the organizations mentioned in this Section were extracted from the remarkable work of Dr. J. H. Baas mentioned in the preceding footnote, pp. 730-790.

C. The Physician and His Competition

To focus again on the koinon of two, namely the physician and patient, the sick in the 19th C were the object of competition from a great variety of healers that textbooks of medical history describe in detail because charlatanry was brash, garishly recorded, and could be indiscrimantly applied to any practitioner or group. But family physicians that could provide continuity of care were now becoming available to smaller communities, for a sufficiency of physicians reflected the growing number of medical schools that could more efficiently educate physicians than could the apprenticeship. The medical schools, in turn, reflected a greater number of those desiring a career in medicine. The stethoscope, the popular journals, and the rising reputation of physicians were doing their magic. The quality and nature of those medical schools varied greatly and they were in competition for fame, fortune, and students. At the onset of the 19th C their treatments would not have been so very different from those of the Hippocratics. Phlebotomy was still in vogue, diet and clean air were staples in managing illness, and important medicines were the cathartics, emetics, diuretics, and analgesics that would have been familiar to the Hippocratics. There was also increasing awareness among physicians of the Hippocratic notion that for many illnesses nature was often best left alone. Despite this limited ability to actively assist the diseased body, the popularity of the physician was increasing. Furthermore, the 19th C was also characterized in the West by a vast improvement in literacy of the general population and by a fascination with scientific discovery. Educational opportunities and a free press could make anyone an expert in something, at least in his own mind. Thus, to the purveyors of patent medicines, the charlatans, the faith healers and other perpetual rivals of physicians were now added practitioners of new disciplines based on what was interpreted by the public as scientific method.[17] Schools and sects of healers, including osteopathy, Chiropractic,[18] Christian Science, hydrotherapy, homeopathy and others attracted their own professional and lay following. Competition indeed flourished, and to survive traditional scientific medicine needed to become more competitive.

The popularity of "alternative" medicine, then and now, reflects a natural desire

---

[17] A wonderful example of the competition was Lydia Pinkham's Vegetable Compound, composed of Unicorn root, Life root, Black cohosh, Pleurisy root and Fenugreek seed, suspended in 19% alcohol as a "preservative" and then filtered, some more alcohol being added to further assist preservation. The Pinkham family's business was begun in 1875, but sold out to a commercial laboratory in 1968 when "faced with the reality of its shrinking market.." For the latter statement plus a promotional eulogy of the Pinkham effort see: Stage, S., *Female Complaints*, New York, 1979. The 19th C proliferation of spas, hydropathic cures, Turkish baths, many variants of herbalism, and patent and proprietary medicines is discussed by G. Williams in *The Age of Miracles*, Chicago, 1987.

[18] Chiropractic (from the Greek, "done by hand") was invented by Daniel Palmer, a Canadian magnetic healer, in 1895. The essence of Palmer's chiropractic as stated in B. J. Palmer's book, *History in the Making* (Davenport, Iowa, 1957, p. 43) was: "a reduction in the quantity-flow of mental impulse nerve force between Innate above and function below, between brain and body, was the cause of all dis-ease." Palmer was emotionally troubled, but at his 1906 trial he said: "I believe freedom also constitutes a patient having his choice in a doctor and to select the type of healing his intelligence finds best to regain his health. Because medicine has failed in these cases, do these poor souls have to spend the rest of their lives suffering?" Well stated, this explains much of the attraction of alternative therapies. Palmer's son, B. J. Palmer, to measure that "quantity-flow," invented the electroencephaloneuromentimpograph.

to control one's destiny rather than relegate it to a stranger. It is more satisfying to seek relief from illness using one's own knowledge and reason. What pride there is in an apparently successful outcome, to be the "master" of one's fate, especially if it is less expensive, more accessible, philosophically acceptable, and associated with less discomfort. The primitive medical empiricist had no choice but to use this approach, and while moderns do have a choice, no blame should be attached to it. The medical profession, however, should not recommend it, for its unfortunate consequences are seen daily in emergency rooms. Nevertheless, it will always remain a force to be reckoned with, for it is normal. It is also a source for the occasional observation that will prove accurate and useful. It should be viewed, within limits and when practiced by an individual rather than a conglomerate, as the loyal opposition working toward the same end. It should spur the profession to improve, not defend, itself. [19]

One way to improve itself was to polish the face of medicine. The Hippocratic writings contain several treatises of this sort, one being *Decorum*. Emulating these writings, the 19th C American physician was advised to dress appropriately, to exhibit proper demeanor, and to avoid undue familiarity, typical Hippocratic advice.[20] Another way was to improve the education of practitioners. In 1776, of perhaps 3500 practitioners in the United States only about 400 had received some sort of medical diploma. This was not unusual, for even in contemporary Great Britain the majority of practitioners obtained

---

[19] Roger Bean, Where are you?

Roger was arrested for providing, in his garage, inexpensive dental care to local citizens. The beneficiaries were said to be those who had limited incomes, principally the elderly. Roger was a denturist, not a dentist, and a denturist was not a recognized professional in his State of Florida. Nevertheless, he was much appreciated by his patients who came to him for dentures, paying him whatever they wished. It may or may not be relevant that he had previously been cited for drug violations. His garage was described as filthy.

In Florida dentures are the purview of the professional dentist. Given a choice most would select the dentist with the best dental outcome. But, despite his filthy garage, his lack of certification and oversight, absence of ancillary staff, want of professional guidelines or publications on preventive maintenance of teeth, no insurance coverage, no building and maintenance overhead, and aversion to advertising, Roger had plenty of work and was much liked by both patients and neighbors, who considered his arrest as unfair.

What would make people seek Roger out? The answer, of course, other than his just doing what his client wanted him to do, is primarily economic; he was cheap. He also simplified matters by not requiring or maintaining any paperwork regarding his operations. Roger is the perfect example of why people in post-Hippocratic Greece and Rome found little inconvenience in seeking out a local alternative medicine practitioner when true professionals were too expensive or in short supply. There will always be, to the frugal, the needy, and the niggardly, an attraction to the less expensive alternative, even in the face of overt evidence of an inferior product. This is human nature.

It is a waste of time to combat normality, far better to instruct. Roger, had he maintained a clean shop and standard sanitary safeguards, and if the facts are as those reported, should not have been arrested. He would have provided stiff competition for the dental profession, and the profession would be better off having to deal with Roger as a competitor rather than permit a State mandate that might outlaw Roger but, in return, would further regulate the profession. (Roger's story was distributed by *Fox News*, April 26, 2007.)

[20] See D. W. Cathell's *The Physician Himself and What He Should Add to the Strictly Scientific*, Baltimore, 1882.

their training through apprenticeships, usually to a surgeon-apothecary.[21] A third way to become more competitive was to knobble the competition, usually by legislation. Some nations found no difficulty at all in providing this service to a local profession, for that profession thereby came under obligation to government. But the desire of physicians to manage their own affairs led, in mid-19th C, to the development of national medical organizations in Canada, France, Britain, and America, organizations that on their own provided enlightened reforms and on their own promoted legislative protection against nonphysician providers. Dr. Baas singled out the United States: "In no country of the world, probably, has the principle of medical 'associations' been developed so widely and completely as in the United States. Besides the almost innumerable state and county medical societies...."[22] He was describing a cornucopia of koinons. Among these, the American Medical Association, founded in 1848, was intended from its very beginning to be a broad-based democratic organization to improve "the deplorable condition of medical education," one goal being the closing of schools of alternative medicine where, a contemporary observed, "the quacks abound as the locusts of Egypt." The status of medical schools had indeed been chaotic. The American Medical Association began as a "competitive rather than corporate" body, but it was to become very large, having many of the "attributes of a guild or labor union."[23] Although the American Medical Association served its membership well, in part because it was able, without outside assistance, to apply unified standards of quality to the profession, those competitive sects it tried to knobble have persisted up to the present day, just as the Methodists, Dogmatists, Empiricists and other sects competed in post-Hippocratic years. It was in the United States that medicine remained most aloof from state control, for neither the profession nor politicians desired government to assume healthcare responsibilities. In some countries, therefore, physicians in private practice were "self-employed petty capitalists" in a sometimes lucrative market that was "competitive and insecure."[24]

Prof. Roy Porter, in the preceding citation, p. 358, has given an appealing 19th C description of the overall picture:

> ". . . medical practice everywhere remained grounded on the ideal and reality of the private system, fee-for-service and market-driven. The personal relationship between physician and patient, perhaps sanctified by a framed copy of the Hippocratic Oath hanging above the physician's desk, confirmed cherished ideals of individual freedom, confidentiality and male honour. At its best, it was a system in which the doctor became a trusted family friend and, like the priest or pastor, a pillar of the community. Care, courtesy and compassion were valued even though the doctor's medications could do little...."

This nice description must not have applied to all regions, for who would not have preferred such physicians over alternative healers. If it had applied, far fewer tart comments about physicians would have emerged in poetry, picture, and prose of popular

---

[21] This and much other interesting information about early American and British medicine is related by Edward Shorter in his book, *Doctors and Their Patients; A Social History*, New Jersey, 1993, Chapter Two: The Traditional Doctor.

[22] Baas, J. H., *Outlines of the History of Medicine and the Medical Profession*, New York, 1889, H. E. Handerson, translator, p. 857.

[23] Paul Starr, P., *The Social Transformation of American Medicine*, New York, 1982, p. 92; \Means, J. H., *The American Association of Physicians*, New York, 1961, p. 29.

[24] Porter, R., *The Greatest Benefit to Mankind*, New York, 1997, Chapter 12.

American publications in the 19th C.[25] Therefore, this could not have been a typical practice. And yet even into the 21st C the description is an engaging one, and there is today no physician who has not heard many patients wish for the return of Dr. Porter's family doctor, who would, of course, be assisted by modern procedures and medicines.[26] Of the description by Porter, what particular is most reminiscent of Hippocratic times? It is the Oath and its relevance to the "personal relationship between physician and patient."

Underneath all the wrappings, however, the secret of success for this koinon of two was *compromise*. The less the authoritarian presence, whether from Church, Corporation, or Government, the greater is the necessity, and thereby the opportunity, to listen to each other, to work together, and when necessary to compromise. As unexpected as that subject may seem at this point, there is reason to invite another excursus.

Excursus on Compromise and Medical Practice

A compromise can be defined as "an agreement between two or more persons to settle matters in dispute between them."[27] It is implied that the cause of the dispute is held in common, has significant personal value to both parties, and its loss to one or the other will be considerable and perhaps intolerable. A compromise solution need not be a point midway between opposing views, nor must it require equal concessions from both sides. But at the end of the process each side surrenders something it values for something it values more.

The importance of compromise was understood by Heracleitus of Ephesus, a 6th C BC natural philosopher. He stated that "opposition is expedient, for from the fusion [of ideas] comes optimal combinations, and everything derives from rivalry." Among the virtuous oppositions he cites that of male and female and of bow and harp.[28] One aspect of compromise between competing expediencies is explanation and discussion, for what at first appears to be disagreement can turn out to be but a misunderstanding. The result may be an amicable agreement rather than contentious implementation.

In politics the opportunity to compromise is at the heart of democratic process. In psychology compromise can be internal and even pathologic, leading to the

---

[25] Witness Honore Daumier and his *Nemesis Medicale Illustree* (Paris, 1840), a panoply of amusing lithographs he contributed to many publications, all ridiculing the French medical system.

[26] A factor contributing to the high opinion of medical practicioners in the early days of our Republic was close identity with laiety. Medicine was poorly remunerative, and so it was often tacked on to the farming and various trades, crafts, and services that practitioners performed to earn a livelihood. Another estimable activity was participation in the Revolutionary War or other military service. The practitioner's office was usually Spartan in its accommodations, and most often was in his home.

[27] Black's Law Dictionary, 7th edition, 1999.

[28] This is a synthesis of three short statements attributed to Heracleitus by Aristotle (*Nicomachean Ethics*, VIII, 1, 6) as given in the *Loeb Classical Library, Hippocrates*, vol. IV, and translated by W. H. S. Jones: Heracleitus, Fragment 46, plus the examples in Fragments 43 and 45. There is also Fragment 8: "Opposition brings men together and out of discord comes the fairest harmony, and all things have their birth in strife."

"neuropsychoses of defense." And a person can compromise his principles, a daily seduction. Principles, especially moral ones, might not admit of compromise, sometimes not even of errors. Compromise can be between a principle and expediency, usually on moral or religious questions.

But in medical practice compromise is often between competing expediencies, and in this there is room for alternatives, allowance for error, and for adjusting to changing circumstances. For in medicine there is a common foe, disease, and the goal, its cure or control, is also held in common. Even "the personal value" of the goal for the physician and patient is the same: the patient's well-being. As this is generally understood, it explains why the physician-patient relationship has been to a great extent uncontroversial in the West and why compromise is seldom listed as a significant component in medical practice. The absence of authoritarian pressures guarantees its continuance. Although it is in great part subliminal, there are areas of compromise that frequently are necessary.

What good comes from compromise in the physician's office? Sometimes compromise may seem an unnecessary and perhaps even undesirable response in many situations and in medicine in particular. If a patient flatly refuses a recommended medical action, what more need be said? No patient should be forced into any action against his will. Freedom is personal choice. On the other hand, if a particular recommended medical plan is clearly effective, why argue? Alternative interpretations of a patient's data are routinely discussed in physicians' offices, and stubbornness is a very human trait. Nevertheless, in most instances a reasonable discussion of alternatives will lead to moderation of stance on the part of the patient and an improved display of options by the physician or a change in physicians.

Compromise does not apply equally to the "art," or physician-patient relationship, and to the "techne," or profession, of medicine. In the latter there is always a better way of doing something, and here the physician is in a position to anticipate the proximate superior result. The problem is that often no one knows just what that way is. If supported by sufficient evidence, professional judgment may not permit compromise because the degree and/or likelihood of harm to the patient makes any alternative action by the physician professionally unacceptable. There also are times when unequal influence is critically important, as in an emergency; equality can lead to unhealthy stalemate rather than compromise. But these tend to be extreme situations, every patient's situation is different, and another physician may have a different solution.

On a more ominous level, however, institutional authority, indeed any authority, can abrogate the need for compromise. Either the patient or the institution might have the luxury of demanding and thereby dictating management by the physician. The physician in such a circumstance might demand compliance. A guideline may specify actions to be taken, this being the promotion of a bureaucratic objective and the end of any compromise. Alternatives may thereby be obviated, but the result is more likely to be unsatisfactory, if not in this case then in the next, in part because the physician and patient will not be working in concert and because the patient's unique response to illness and therapy will have been insufficiently considered.

Until the day arrives when the best way of managing a particular disease is known with certainty, compromise will be needed. That day will not arrive soon, for biology is both complex and in flux as new problems and new solutions continually appear. And if it is prematurely assumed that certainty in any one area has arrived, there will be no further attempt at improvement for there will be no desire to waste one's time on improving what has already been declared to be optimal, whether it is or not. Again Heracleitus: "Everything flows," meaning all elements are in constant flux.[29] There is a constant need to reassess and readjust.

Almost inevitably, there are disparate views of a disease between the physician and the patient. The sources of difference include the following:

> 1. The physician's or the profession's limitations in knowledge or
> technology when facing an incompletely understood biological threat.
> 2. The physician's effort to educate and persuade the patient to do what is best to ameliorate an illness, an effort often confronted by the patient's certainty that he already knows the answer.
> 3. The patient's unrealistic expectation, be it cure, relief, or secondary gain.
> 4. The aptitudes of both the physician and patient, whether educational, physical, or intellectual.
> 5. The perceived value of the consultation, especially in estimating the contribution of natural course or divine intervention to the physician's efforts.
> 6. Peripheral diplomacy, confrontations, and assistance with or for family, friends, or beneficiaries.
> 7. What constitutes a successful conclusion.
> 8. Variation among patients in tolerance for discomfort, inconvenience, or other aversion.

The art of medicine is not found in merely being nice or wheedling. Indeed, the art of medicine (one of the three legs supporting the natural state of medicine), inasmuch as it comprises relationships, is in part the art of compromise. And the need for compromise arises mainly from the misery produced by biological threats for which there is inadequate understanding, imperfect relief, and from which none escape. As no disease can be assuaged with sufficient promptness or completeness, and no incurable disease can be cured, the inability of the physician to fulfill the hopes of the patient will forever be a potential source of contention between the patient and the best, most well-meaning, physician. This is evident in every physician's practice when, in a given case, every decision and action has been optimal but the limits of human knowledge have been exceeded or the nature of the disease under treatment is one of irreversible deterioration. It sometimes happens that the patient, or those close to the patient, because of disappointment, will broadcast the insensitivity or incompetence of the physician. No physician should be disturbed by this, for such is a natural human response to the tragedy of hope beyond attainment. In addition, societal or political expectations may be at variance with those of the patient and/or the physician. These differences may be economic, ethical, or statutory. Thus, what at first may seem an obvious and simple interaction between a physician and patient can be a contentious maze, and, although it is today a tribute besieged, it is a tribute to both physician and patient that the interaction seldom becomes a confrontation.

---

[29] "παντος ῥει."

The role of compromise in the evolution of medical practice as presented here has focused on the relationship between physician and patient, and its unheralded role in a free society has been indicated. Even reading the foregoing may seem a tedious exercise rather than a warning. But the natural state of medical practice can be considered a corollary of the natural state of social man in his interactions with others. And as these pages have shown, in most civilizations freedom has seldom been a characteristic of formal medical practice. The West has been the rare exception. This is because the physician-patient interaction is protected by another, and equally important, arena of medical compromise, the profession to which the physician belongs.

Which brings us to this conclusion: despite the seemingly unimportant role of compromise in the offices of today's physicians there are reasons to keep compromise as a guiding tenet. Yes, it promotes education and open discussion of competing expediencies and stimulates discovery of alternative solutions that may ease the patient's burden. But the reason to jealously guard this privileged dialogue is to prevent it being abrogated by uncompromising institutional concerns, *for the merits of compromise will be found no longer to be subliminal once the option of compromise no longer exists*. Willingness to compromise, to be open to contrary opinions, is the essence of a healthy democratic process; the shield of compromise is the koinon.

End of Excursus

With improved medical education, evidence of medical progress as presented in journals, and scientific inquiry that was open to all in the profession as expressed in "Letters to the Editor" or in questions raised during medical conferences, competitiveness improved as physicians did their job better. The stethoscope, the technique of percussion, instrumentation for internal examination, and, especially, the now vast network of physicians pooling their knowledge by medical publications and meetings, produced a precision in prognosis and prompted a respect for physicians' motives that no competing school or sect could match. The natural course of diseases now became better defined, distinctions were made between diseases that shared some common features, names were applied to newly characterized illnesses, and newly recognized diseases were promptly described in textbooks. And while Dr. Lewis Thomas, the prominent physician and writer, would lament the feeble therapies of the 1930s internist when compared to the surgeon, let not be forgotten those individuals without number whose deaths were prevented by the 19th C descriptions by the physicians Laveran, Manson, and Ross of the life cycles of *Plasmodia sp.* that led to control of malaria by destroying that infectious agent's arthropod host, the mosquito, and by the use of netting and insect repellents. This is but one example among hundreds of discoveries that, while not therapies, were not at all "feeble," just not flamboyant.[30]

The physician may not have been very effective in reversing the course of many

---

[30] Few will disagree that prevention of a disease is preferable to treatment. Yet drug therapies for human immunodeficiency virus infection (HIV) are daily topics in newspapers, as is the ingenuity, determination, and thoroughness of everyone involved in the research effort, all of which must be admired. And yet this disease is preventable immediately, completely, at no cost and without medication, a most modest and, for a third of a century, a completely unnewsworthy fact.

diseases, but he was better able to avoid worsening them. This was one way to counter alternative therapies. Drugs, whether useful or not, are all potentially toxic, and to know what will cause, aggravate, or disguise a problem, particularly when this knowledge can protect against extravagant claims and avert unwise delay, could not fail but to demonstrate the superior practice of the physician, if people would but listen.[31]

In a preceding chapter it was noted that Prof. Thompson acclaimed the 19th century as the Golden Age of Science, his witnesses including Faraday, Maxwell, the Curies, Kelvin, Roentgen, Edison, Darwin, Bruce, Ross, Einstein, Pasteur, and Ehrlich. None of these luminaries was a physician. And a 19th C physician, Emile Littre, editor and translator of the complete works of Hippocrates and the editor of the greatest of French dictionaries, felt "the real advancement of biological and medical science has nothing to do with theological dogma or metaphysical speculation, but simply depends upon collateral improvements in physical and chemical procedure." Apparently, Dr. Garrison, the historian of medicine who composed a synopsis on this topic, agreed.[32]

The reestablishment of the natural state of medical practice, however, did not require a revolution in medical science or any such "collateral improvement." The great technical advances of the 20th C are but a parallel experience in the history of medical practice and an intellectual short feature instead of the main show. And it is part of the dilemma of modern medicine to sort out the two, to avoid letting a technicolor, high density, flat screen with animated images draw attention away from the drama of the black-and-white classics that portrayed real life. Modern invention is here to stay, for a while, and a future Dr. McCoy may well have a pocket-sized PET scanner.[33] But what to do with the information obtained is the issue, just as was the diagnosis of pleural effusion by the Hippocratic physician who placed his ear against the patient's chest. For here, in essence if not in detail, is what was going through his head: What if the lung collapses when the effusion is drained? What if an intercostal artery is nicked? What if the effusion is an old one and causing little problem and should be left alone or is a new one and might drain itself or resorb given time? What if the patient is mentally incompetent, or competent but refuses all procedures that might cure the effusion? What if the cause of the effusion is an imminently lethal process that will not be favorably affected by removal of the effusion? What if the effusion decreases on its own, which it often does. What if? All of medicine is filled with "What ifs," no matter what the problem, no matter what the treatment, no matter what the setting. "What if" is never answered by gadgetry. A "negative" screening colonoscopy is no great pronouncement. "What if" is answered only

---

[31] For example, many tonics containing iron salts have been marketed over the counter for treating iron-deficiency anemia. But when taken without a clear understanding of the problem, the disease causing iron-deficiency anemia, perhaps a cancer of the colon with chronic inapparent blood loss in the stool, may go undiagnosed and worsen because the patient temporarily thinks himself improved because his anemia is improving and so will delay investigation of the cause. The chiropractor's spinal manipulation for back pain in an older individual who actually has bone destruction from multiple myeloma, whereby manipulation can lead to paralysis, is a perennial example given to medical students on the dangers of alternative therapies. At the time of this writing the disastrous inadequacy of a patient relying on garlic to treat his hypertension is confirmed daily in any large medical clinic. And on and on. On the other hand, certain procedures approved by the medical community, such as the previously ubiquitous tonsillectomy, have now been shown, by controlled studies, to be without merit in many cases.

[32] Garrison, F. H., *An Introduction to the History of Medicine*, Phila., 1921, 3rd edition, p. 338.

[33] PET: positron emission tomography. The Dr. McCoy referred to was in the popular television series, Star Trek.

by the physician. It is answered by being expert at prognosis. The Hippocratic physician, once he placed his ear against the patient's chest and diagnosed an effusion, would have posed, and likely answered, most of the "What if's" mentioned above. For the CT (computed tomography) scan, from the beginning to the end of this clinical scenario, is only one small part of the picture and most of the time adds nothing to management but greater certainty.[34] This is nothing to sneer at, but it is also but one of a hundred considerations in the mind of the physician. Yes, the CT scan can alter management, but by and large it just confirms the correctness of the original opinion. Gadgetry is but a tool, not an intellectual force. Circumstances may change, but the questions remain the same, and always shall.

In the 19th C the physician in the West again reclaimed the high ground. The Oath, improved abilities in prognosis, and a face-to-face medical practice affected only by local social pressures, was affirmed and buttressed by professional organizations that prided themselves on personal patient care, scientific objectivity, and adherence to the Hippocratic Oath. After two thousand years of being in an authoritarian shadow, the place held by Athenian physicians of the plague years was reestablished. And aspirin had yet to be discovered!

---

[34] In the surgical classic, *Cope's Early Diagnosis of the Acute Abdomen* (New York, 1987, 17th editor, revised by W. Silen, MD), there is this statement on p. 131: "Gentle palpation will often reveal a very hard mass slightly larger than a golf ball which cannot be mistaken for anything else once a few have been felt. Millions of dollars in diagnostic tests could be saved in this way." And yet there has probably not been a single case of acute cholecystitis in the past year in the United States that did not have both radiographic and sonographic, and perhaps even computed tomographic, or magnetic resonance, imaging studies to aid in *confirming* that diagnosis.

CHAPTER TWENTY-FIVE

OBSERVATIONS CONCERNING THE FUTURE OF MEDICINE

"Open your eyes to the fearful change which has been so noiselessly affected; and acknowledge BY STANDING STILL YOU BECOME A PARTY TO REVOLUTION." (sic)

Richard Hurrell Froude (1803-1836)[1]

Progress is not inevitable. In medicine the practitioner finds himself increasingly regulated, and it is ironic that the regulation stems from the profession's increasingly porous boundaries. Medicine's immigrants are becoming medicine's masters. The Hippocratic Oath is increasingly irrelevant, the work of the profession is ever more performed by those with inferior training, the professional organization is diluted by nonphysicians, medical practice is managed by nonphysicians, and, with the prize of medicine ever more fame and fortune, the attractions of a career in medicine are those of a business or a competition rather than a profession. The root of the problem lies not with those outside the profession who see advantage in a medical alliance. It lies, instead, with the profession that seeks them out. The koinon that guided the practice of medicine from superstition to science must redefine its limits and, reversing a forty-year trend, cease being bigger, and start getting better.

A. Progress is not Inevitable

Democritus (*ca.* 460-370 BC) reportedly said ". . . it is better to discover the cause of a single thing than to be the King of Persia."[2] With such ebullience in their making it is no surprise that good ideas emerge all the time, the modern success story for good ideas suggesting that prosperity will continue forever.[3] Yet individual genius is unlikely to invent much that is wholly new, for "organized invention" of modern industry has the momentum at present.[4] It has been said that Thomas Edison was the last, meaning final, great inventor, and he was born in 1847. New inventions for the most part occur by manipulating old discoveries and applying them to new problems, the photon, for

---

[1] Hurrell Froude was the elder brother of the famous English historian, James Anthony Froude. A cleric, Hurrell's statement is to be found in *Remarks on State interference in Matters Spiritual*, in *Remains of the Late Reverend Richard Hurrell Froude, M. A.*, vol. I of Part 2, Derby, 1839, p. 196. Although pertaining to "matters spiritual," Froude adds the comment, based on the principles of Hooker, that it "goes to any kind of State interference at all." Froude, part of the early 19th C Oxford Movement in England, was arguing a principle of 16th C Calvinism (p. 350).

[2] Vors. 68B 118. [*Fragmente der Vorsokratiker* – Diels] translation by the author.

[3] Dr. Iago Galdston wrote: "Unless some catastrophe overtakes our civilization, the continuous progress of medicine appears assured, and whatever may happen to the practice of medicine, whatever may be the economic destiny of the practitioners of medicine, will little affect the science [of medicine] proper." (Galdston, I., *Progress in Medicine*, New York, 1940, p. 326.) This is a great underestimation of the appeal and the danger of authoritarianism and is reminiscent of Plato's contention in the 4th C BC that medicine as a science had reached its zenith. See footnote below.

[4] W.B. Kaempffert, *Invention and Society*, Chicago, 1930. Kaempffert was pessimistic about the effects of "organized invention" by groups, for it would displace the novel idea of the individual with ideas from "insider" inventors whose organizations will make it difficult for a novel invention to be brought forward and properly recognized.

example, providing much grist for the invention mill. With the discovery of basic ingredients, there is available a vast field of application by virtue of mass action alone. Seen in this light, advances in medicine in the 20th C can be viewed, in the main, as elaborations on 19th C discoveries and inventions. Proof of the germ theory of infectious disease, the discovery of Roentgen rays, appreciation of the cell as the basic unit for understanding pathophysiology, the first understanding of immunity, all these and many more were 19th C developments. Even the discovery of modern antibiotics can be assigned to the 19th C, for Ehrlich was actively searching for them at the end of that century. Einstein had the beginnings of his theory of special relativity by 1896. It is a bit like the changes produced by the world of computers; today's capabilities are increasingly the consequence of gigabytes instead of ingenuity or common sense. There is, of course, nothing wrong with perfecting.

Modern progress, seen through the eyes of today's two or three generations, especially the youngest, appears predictable and permanent, the natural order of things. But it is these generations' descendants who will verify, or not, this assumption. One wonders how they will fare fifty years from now if alternative medical theories of the present day replace, on the hard-won platform erected by science over centuries, the child of the Enlightenment, or how they will judge today's focus on genetic minutiae to the detriment of practical preparedness for some imminent, obvious, or overwhelming biological calamity. It is perhaps presumed that man knows, or will soon know, all he needs to know to manage or prevent his illnesses, to regraft or regrow extremities, to modify genetically his progeny. But assurance of already attained perfection was Plato's opinion 2400 years ago, as well as opinions of thinkers in the 13th C.[5] And they were terribly wrong, both in overestimating the knowledge of their age and in underestimating the trajectory of the Western world. That such a trajectory can be internally misdirected has been proposed, for in 3rd C BC Greece the imminent triumph of a remarkably open society was willfully subverted by increasingly irrational institutions and behavior, a "fear of freedom," the "unconscious flight from the heavy burden of individual choice which an open society lays upon its members."[6] Although Aristotle viewed tyranny as an inevitable consequence of democracy, and Plato wrote that "Excess of liberty, whether in states or individuals, seems only to pass into excess of slavery,"[7] neither identified the mechanism of the march to tyranny as the "heavy burden of choice." And yet astrology, amulets, magic, preoccupation with spirits and occult forces replaced an earlier objectivity. Are today's examples of irrationality merely routine bedevilments that, playing on emotions, afflict all societies, or are they examples of an increasingly

---

[5] Plato valued knowledge to such an extent that he could argue that a craft such as medicine was not to be considered deficient or in error, any deficiencies and errors being instead the fault of the practitioner. See *Republic* I, 342 a,b. Some Hippocratics agreed: ἰητρικὴ δή μοι δοκέει ἤδη ἀνευρῆσθαι ὅλη, ἥτις οὕτως ἔχει,.... "Medicine in its present state is, it seems to me, by now completely discovered,..." (*Places in Man*, 46, translation of Paul Potter, *Loeb Classical Series*, *Hippocrates*, vol. VIII.) As for the Middle Ages, "The thirteenth century believed that it had realized a state of stable equilibrium, and because their extraordinary optimism led them to believe they had arrived at a state close to perfection." (Dewulf, M., *Philosophy and Civilization in the Middle Ages*, New Jersey, 1922, p. 267.)

[6] Dodds, E. R., *The Greeks and the Irrational*, Boston, 1957 (paperback edition), p. 252 and the final chapter, a brief but thoughtful review of possible causes for man's propensity to let individual freedom slip through his fingers.

[7] "Democracy terminates in tyranny." ἡ δεμοκρατία ἡ τελευταία τυραννισ ἐστίν. Aristotle, *Politica*, VIII, 10, translation of the author. Plato, *Republic*, VIII, 15, translation of B. Jowett.

systematic irrationality of an educated society turning primitive, as warned at the outset of this work (p. 33). Perhaps more relevant in this flight from freedom, will irrationality's ills emanate not from educated masses but from an elected but primitive central authority?[8]

If medical progress does grind to a halt the change will be subtle, for the benefits of scientific medicine and the natural state of medical practice, such as still exists, will not disappear at the same time. Society's benefit from medical inventions such as PET scanners and antibody-coated stents reflect, first and foremost, signal achievements of capitalism, not medical practice, and capitalism proceeds apart from the professions. Capitalism instead is the magnificent means of propulsion. By producing wealth, capitalism improves chances for the secure future that can be provided by sustained democratic governance.[9] It also is the amplifier of progress as it permits exploitation of invention and discovery by enlisting the assistance of experts outside the medical profession. But capitalism is incompatible with authoritarianism, and its potential benefits to society will be the first to succumb as its mechanisms of production are embraced by the State. Scientific medical practice then will slowly but inevitably follow.

It is appropriate here to recall the words of Flexner (p. 198*f*) concerning the bedside science of the clinician. This is an important arena for medical progress, an arena shared with the Hippocratics. It is one that costs nothing, is not affected by economic interests, and is not directed by funding priorities of proponents located in agencies of government. And it is an arena that has to a great degree become unexploited. There is probably not a single clinician in the United States who does not have interesting ideas directly relevant to the cure or management of malignant disease and of human immunodeficiency virus infection, ideas originating from personal clinical observations. Ninety-nine percent of the intelligent minds who have those ideas will never find anyone interested in listening to them, except, perhaps, for a friend or spouse or a local colleague. But there was a time when people did listen, when the average practicing clinician did put his thoughts on paper and had serious attention given to them by his colleagues. Important observations on physical examination, clinical course, therapy, and etiology awaited the careful clinician, and they still do.[10] Few, however, will be described in modern medical

---

[8] This has happened before. Erich Fromm (in *Escape from Freedom*, New York, 1941, chapter 1) wrote: "At first many found comfort in the thought that the victory of the authoritarian system was due to the madness of a few individuals, ... that men like Hitler had gained power over the vast apparatus of the state through nothing but cunning and trickery... In the years that have elapsed since, the fallacy of these arguments has become apparent. We have been compelled to recognize that millions in Germany were as eager to surrender their freedom as their fathers were to fight for it; that instead of wanting freedom, they sought ways of escape from it..." He quotes John Dewey: "The serious threat to our democracy .... is accordingly here – within ourselves and our institutions." (*Freedom and Culture*, New York, 1939.)

[9] Lipset, S. M., *Some Social Requisites of Democracy: Economic Deveopment and Political Legitimacy*, in *American Political Science Review*, p. 59, Mar., 1959.

[10] As an example, the Nobel Prize for Physiology or Medicine in 2005 was shared by Australians Barry Marshall and J. Robin Warren for their discovery of the role of *Helicobacter pylori* "in gastritis and peptic ulcer disease." See footnote, p. 410, for comments on this discovery and its earlier discovery by Dr. John Lykoudis (1910-1980). And decades ago the famed British weekly journal, the *Lancet*, had scores of Letters to the Editor submitted by clinicians everywhere describing their personal experiences with this or that topic, letters that contained educational, entertaining, and thought-provoking ideas on how to best diagnose or manage a broad range of illnesses. For example, the first issue of the 1967 *Lancet* had nine articles, all nine being of directly

journals, where points of view, political, social, theoretical, or technical, too often take precedence over clinical acumen.[11] Is this a sign of the change?

With this new millennium, therefore, it is appropriate to ask whether the medical profession is prepared to adapt to, or even survive, the unexpected. It is appropriate to look for evidence of vulnerability, for breaches, for misdirection. There are many potential sources for discontent, such as overspecialization, cost, and availability. But the five basic circumventions now to be described are greater threats.

B. Circumventing the ethical domain of the physician: the Hippocratic Oath

Dr. Ludwig Edelstein, famed medical historian, claimed that the Hippocratic Oath applied to only a small group of ancient Greek physicians because it was Pythagorean in nature, *i.e.*, it was sectarian and (presumably) only a few practitioners ascribed to this particular philosophical belief. Furthermore, the ancient Oath was seen to represent some philosophical ideal of a physician and impractical even at the time of its composition.[12] But Pythagoreanism as a regional or sectarian philosophy was perhaps as popular in ancient times as some religions are today.[13] It was probably still popular when the Oath was written. Therefore, the Oath, while represented to us as expressing "the ancient ideal of the physician," may well have been thought not only desirable, but realistic. Had not Christianity appeared, Pythagorus might now be quite fashionable. And yet the Oath would still be in place. In the eyes of those aware of its existence, the Oath was probably as admired when it was written as it is now. It would have been analogous to certain Christian oaths, perhaps hard to live up to, but admirable in the effort and vitalizing in the realization, regardless of its sectarian affiliation. Indeed, what arguments could be raised against it?

Whether Edelstein's opinion that the Oath had originally a very circumscribed effect on physicians is valid or not, the Oath is a venerable and universal statement on medical ethics. But the range of activities of today's physicians has extended so far beyond its original compass that for large numbers of practitioners the Oath is to varying degrees irrelevant, and many modified versions of the Oath have been proffered.

The Oath was written as a guide for clinicians at a time when the natural state of medical practice was close to existing, and it provides an ethical definition of the clinical

---

relevant to clinical care, and of thirty-one letters to the editor all but five were strictly clinical. This valuable clinical service for the general practitioner is now barely operative. See footnote, p. 370, for the equivalent contents of today's *New England Journal of Medicine*. Should someone inquire about the disappearing Internist, he should compare these two journals.

[11] See, for example, the article *Journalistic Malpractice* by Dr. Scott Gottlieb in the *Wall Street Journal*, May 29, 2007.

[12] Edelstein, L., *Ancient Medicine*, Baltimore, 1967, Pt. 1, *The Hippocratic Oath*, I. The Ethical Code, p. 9.

[13] See Iamblicus, *Life of Pythagoras*, translated by Thos. Taylor, in: *Iamblichus' Life of Pythagoras*, London, 1818. There is a modern edited paperback reprint published by Inner Traditions International, Ltd., Vermont, 1986. Iamblicus (*ca.* 245-325 AD) was one of the last of ancient writers that defended the pagan religion of the Greeks. He ascribes many Christian attributes to Pythagoras. In the 4th C BC there was a resurgence in the popularity of Pythagorus, although his message was somewhat altered.

physician in that particular medical environment. It does not describe the ethics of institutional healthcare programs, nor does it apply to practitioners in the pay of, and who have allegiance to, such programs. Thus, a threat to the ethical domain of the physician may arise when that medical environment is altered. Today the physician is, in many instances, under pressure to be a spokesman more for some institution than for his patient. This corporate environment did not exist in ancient Greece; the koinon existed for the purposes of the individual physician, not *vice versa*. It can only be expected that institutions, whether corporate or state, will at times infringe on an employee physician's ethical decision. Their intent is not founded in ill will, but the consequences are ominous.

Another threat arises when the physician's ethical code does not coincide with society's, or at least some segments of society. An ethic is acquired from the customs of a society and is, in the opinion of many, not to be judged as wrong or right. This is not a new idea. Ancient Greek sophists viewed goodness and justice as relative to the customs of each society. But it was soon realized that, within this interpretation, ethics could be a masquerade for interests of society's stronger members. Thus, it fell to Plato to argue for an objective and universal basis of judging behavior. But modern Western society is not Plato's city-state; it is instead diverse and cosmopolitan. The issue has become, therefore, not "custom of a society" but "customs of subgroups within a society." Excepting a socialist dictatorship, confrontations on the appropriateness of different patterns of behavior cannot be avoided, and, until a managed society finally hammers out the differences between people and between groups in its never ceasing march toward zero entropy, sectional morality must be diverted from medical practice; its intrusion into the physician-patient relationship must be prevented. For, if the medical profession becomes burdened with mandated moral responsibility, it should know in advance that, as the philosopher F. H. Bradley commented, "For practical purposes we need make no distinction between [moral] responsibility or accountability, and liability to punishment."[14]

Certain topics of morality will find both society and professional ethics always in agreement. For example, dishonest persons are not tolerated in the medical profession, for physicians will share society's distaste for dishonesty, and the dishonest could not be trusted to live up to the ethical requirements of the Oath. Beyond this, conflicts can arise when a divided society gives moral judgments the force of law, becoming a coercive force on physician behavior. In devisive issues, therefore, there are two options: (1) If the issue becomes law both physician and patient must follow the law; (2) If the issue is not regulated by law, the physician is an advocate for his patient, not a tool for a point of view. In either case the medical practitioner must be protected from demands for conformity by ethicist and moralist pressure groups.[15]

The Hippocratic Oath has remained intact for 2400 years. What Dr. Edelstein felt to have had limited application in early Greece is on office walls of physicians throughout the world. Over centuries there may have been squabbling about a few of its particulars, but the Hippocratic Oath has become the universal gold standard for a

---

[14] Bradley, F. H., *Ethical Studies*, Oxford, London, 1876, Essay I, *The vulgar notion of responsibility in connexion with the theories of free-will and necessity.*

[15] This is not a new thought. In the 2nd C AD Lucian wrote, in his satire involving a physician, *The Disinherited*, "Now physic, as nobody will dispute, is the most honourable and beneficial of all arts, and what is more equitable than that he who professes it should be allowed the most unbounded liberty to exercise it, or not to exercise it. So sacred an art .... can be subject to no command, to no control..." See: *Lucian of Samosata*, translation of William Tooke, London, 1820, vol. 2.

physician's conduct. There is little that is a more elegant confirmation of the similarity of the thinking between the modern age and the ancient Greeks. But new tenets are now being proposed and some original ones disavowed. Like the Constitution of the United States, there is pressure for reinterpretation and remodeling for convenience. Much of that pressure comes from outside the medical profession, from special interests. But the Oath was written by physicians for physicians.

The Oath, in the original Greek, contains only two hundred and fifty words as presented in the *Loeb Classical Library Hippocrates*, vol I. Prof. Jouanna states that the role of the Oath "was to preserve the interests and privileges of the family possessing medical knowledge," for it pertained to the "tribal" organization of the Asclepiadae of Cos and Cnidus.[16] Lines 16-32, however, bear on medical practice itself. Their meaning was, and is, universal, not tribal, and it is likely that by the time of their writing tribalism in Greece was for the most part a thing of the past.

While the Oath expressed a commitment to the profession, it was first and foremost a formal and unilateral commitment of the "compassionate medical scholar" to a sick patient. The Oath's summary words are "to help the sick," "never to injure," to "give place" to those best trained, "to abstain from wrongdoing," and "to not divulge" what is private and personal. Yet each of these five admonishments, translated below by the author, is threatened in today's world:

1. To help the sick:

> διαιτήμασί τε χρήσομαι ἐπ᾽ ὠφελείῃ καμνόντων κατὰ δυναμιν καὶ κρίσιν ἐμήν....   Lines 16-17
> "I will provide needed treatment for the benefit of the suffering according to my ability and judgment, ..."

The Hippocratics relied heavily on the natural healing processes of the body. Optimizing the patient's condition in order to promote healing was preferred to specific drug therapy, which in turn was preferred to surgery.[17] Modern medicine, of course, has a myriad of drugs and a myriad of surgical techniques. Its ability to help the sick is vast, and for the moment this capability is not threatened. At the same time, the elegant biological system it is meant to help is understood in many of its particulars to have an ability to heal with no help whatsoever. And although it is important to help others avoid sickness, the Oath admits of no role for physicians in treating the unsick, for investing the healthy in an aura of sickness, or for exploiting a synthetic repair mechanism in place of a successful natural one. The Introduction to this book has a more detailed explanation why the profession should distance itself from such practices.

2. Never to injure:

> ...ἐπὶ δηλήσει δὲ καὶ ἀδικίῃ εἴρξειν. οὐ δώσω δὲ οὐδὲ φάρμακον οὐδενὶ αἰτηθεὶς θανάσιμον, οὐδὲ ὑφηγήσομαι συμβουλίην τοιήνδε·
> Lines 17-20

---

[16] Jouanna, J. *Hippocrates*, translated by M. B. DeBevoise, Baltimore, 1999, p. 51.
[17] That which a drug does not cure, surgery can [might] cure; whatever surgery does not cure, cautery can [might] cure; but for those which cautery does not help, they must necessarily be termed "incurable." Hippocratic aphorism VII, 87, translation by the author.

". . . considering injury and injustice to be forbidden. And so I will not give deadly drugs even on being asked, nor will I give such advice."

Purposeful injury to a patient for personal gain is an apostasy and a criminal act to be punished accordingly. But today's problem arises when the means to help can sometimes injure. Some injuries result from individual proclivities for adverse drug reactions and allergic reactions. In other situations, the beneficial clinical effect of a drug is a consequence of an inherently injurious mechanism, as exploited, for example, in chemotherapy of malignant disease, and both good and bad effects predictably occur but they do so in a sometimes unpredictable way. The situation has grown more complex as previously unsuspected forms of injury, such as the late consequences of radiation exposure or the genetic injuries of thalidomide, have been recognized. One way to avoid the injury of treatment is to rely solely on the body's ability to heal itself. However, even natural defenses can be injurious, as in those diseases termed "autoimmune," and they often require treatment in their own right.

Risk/benefit assessment therefore enters into all therapeutic decisions. It is an important aspect in the physician-patient relationship, and one that invites no intrusion if the patient is competent to make his own decisions. It is true that from medicine's earliest days enticements have played a role in the management of some patients.[18] This is a natural response of the professional, who will usually know better than the patient the medical consequences, or risks, of action and inaction. The patient, in turn, can weigh the personal consequences. In occasional opposition are pressures from family and friends, should their opinions differ from those of the physician or the patient. Sometimes their counsels are wise, insightful, and helpful, at other times they reflect personal perspectives that may not benefit the patient. These aspects of the physician-patient relationship have not changed over the centuries and can be considered predictable human responses to inevitable medical quandaries.

But today there are institutional intrusions that represent societal and commercial interests, the former usually demanding conformity and the latter demanding economy. And so a closer look at risk/benefit must be taken, for any mechanism for diminishing risk attributable to a specific affliction comes with a price.

Excursus on Risk/Benefit

If purposeful action in diagnosis and treatment is undertaken, risk, in part and impersonally, is transferred from the disease to its management. Thus patient-physician communication is essential and can be complex, for the following reasons.

It is not rare for those who agree to a transfer of risk, meaning the acceptance of treatment, to have an unsuccessful outcome, a treatment failure, or a serious side effect, for example drug toxicity. Biology is far too complex to be completely predictable, and it is the rare treatment that approaches perfection.

Even successful treatment can have bad effects, such as secondary malignancies in patients who have undergone tissue or organ transplantation. Many decisions favoring a

---

[18] Sweetening mixed with medicines was used assist patients in taking medicines, as mentioned by Plutarch in *Moralia*, his work *On the Education of Children*, sect. 18.

good treatment would never have been made had the patient known in advance that some bad effect would occur at a later time. Enrolling patients in clinical trials are particularly susceptible to manipulation given our limited ability to accurately assess risk and benefit.

Then there is the morbidity or mortality associated with the act of determining whether a transfer of risk is even a consideration. Screening for disease falls into this category, and it applies especially to situations where the risk of the disease being screened for is low and the distribution of risk is uneven, which is usually the case. Therefore, the procedure used to ascertain the level of risk, for example a screening colonoscopy, is itself, for most people, a greater risk than doing nothing. But, of course, this is not known until the procedure is done and the results are known, and ways to explain aspects of risk have been devised, employing statistical manipulations such as the NNT ("number needed to treat").[19] Risk can be reasonably assessed by many people and informed decision made.

Next there is the nebulous situation in which there exists inadequate intellectual preparation to grapple with the abstractions of risk, even if capably described to the patient. This segment of a population is not small and presents obvious, sometimes insurmountable, problems in executing a risk reduction strategy. Nevertheless, it is one that presents itself on a case-by-case basis and it can often be managed given sufficient patience and the understanding and help of those looking out for the patient's interest.

But what is not manageable by any means in the transfer of risk is the dilemma whereby morbidity and mortality may result from a risk reduction strategy imposed by society on that part of the population which, had they not been inveigled or required to participate in the scheme, had no risk to begin with. A rare person who undergoes a colonoscopy may have had no lesion but may suffer a lethal perforation of the colon or renal failure from preparatory cleansing procedures. In this situation the price paid for discovering a zero-risk status has been a potentially mortal one.[20] Those that impose or popularize a risk transferring strategy should be able to justify, ethically, any negative consequences of their decision. The core issue is this: it is easy to make those decisions when a group mandate is involved, for the distribution of guilt resulting from a bad outcome is vague, even invisible. Individual accountability is avoided. All in the decision-making group

---

[19] The NNT, or "number needed to treat," refers to the number of persons who need to be treated in order that one person of the treated group will, on the average, benefit, as compared to an untreated group. It estimates the group effort needed to reduce the relative risk of a targetted problem. It is more useful in assessing economic benefits for a group than it is for individual decision-taking, but it is a number that at least can be comprehended. For example, the group of drugs used to regulate blood cholesterol levels, popularly known as "statins," requires up to two hundred persons be treated for several years to justify prevention of a heart attack in *one* person. A related calculation is the NNH, or "number needed to harm," the number of persons who, if treated, will, on the average, result in harm to one person.

[20] Of the variety of complications of colonoscopy, perforation of the colon occurred in approximately one out of every 500 procedures performed in persons over 65 years of age who were found to have no colon cancer (Gatto, N. M., *et al.*, *Risk of Perforation After Colonoscopy and Sigmoidoscopy: A Population-Based Study*, in *J. Nat. Cancer Inst.*, 95:230-236, 2003). A guideline promoting periodic screening colonoscopies where the perforation rate is one per thousand is, based on 1.5 million screening colonoscopies annually in the USA, knowingly assigning 1,500 colon cancer-free individuals to this dangerous complication, of whom up to 100 will die (perforation mortality rate approaches 10% depending on the health status of the patient).

will get the credit for lives saved, but none will get the blame for lives lost. The dilemma results from the imposition of injury on the healthy because of attempts to decrease the burden of a disease on society, on those destined, without its early discovery, to have it, placing it instead on some anonymous individual who would be found to have no such problem. It is an example of an age-old argument: harm to an occasional individual is justifiable because of a potential benefit to all, *i.e.*, the end justifies the means. Furthermore, that "occasional individual" still has his own burdens that fate has in store. It is indeed playing God when a committee advises or, especially, authorizes meddling in what should be a personal decision arrived at by the physician and patient. It has the additional disadvantage of permitting the physician to fall back on a committee recommendation as a justification for his decisions. This avoids difficult interpersonal decision-making and assumption of responsibility; less thought is required, less hesitation needed, and less office time is taken when committees have already done the work.

A corollary of the preceding is applicable to clinical research. Through tedious and harrowing empirical trial and error humans have sought relief from disease by use of local botanicals plucked or dug, and ingested *au crudité*, mashed, boiled, or mixed with some liquid. Empiricism remains a globally important experimental approach today, and it retains the same elements of the unpredictability and uncertainty it has always had, sometimes fraught with danger.[21] In a sense the brave subjects of this type of research are assuming those risks we might take if we were seeking an effective botanical on our own. In modern medicine, of course, the vast majority of the population assumes no risk in the seeking. Thus, by modern research methodology and "human studies committees" risk is removed from the general population and offered to volunteers. Those who volunteer for medical research studies accept this transfer of risk, for which the rest of us should be extremely grateful. Extreme caution, however, is urged when enrolling subjects in such projects, and the ethical justifications must be clear. They are not always so.

End of Excursus

---

3. "To give place" to those best trained:

> οὐ τεμέω δὲ οὐδὲ μὴν λιθιῶντας, ἐκχωρήσω δὲ ἐργάτῃσιν ἀνδράσιν πρήξιος τῆσδε. Lines 22-24
> "And I will not use a knife even on those suffering from stones, but will give place to craftsmen [experts] of this practice."

Debate has for centuries centered on the aversion to lithotomy as expressed in the Oath. But it is uncertain whether the "stones" referred to were gallstones, renal stones, or bladder stones, or whether a misspelling by some ancient scribe has obscured the intended sense of "castration."[22] It has been felt by some that the Oath excluded surgery from the work of the physician, relegating it to a presumably inferior but skilled technician. But

---

[21] See for example the consequences of administering a new and potentially useful medication to healthy volunteers (Suntharalingam, G, et. al., *Cytokine Storm in a Phase 1 Trial of the Anti-CD28 Monoclonal Antibody TGN1412*, in *N. Engl. J. Med.*, 355:1018-1028, 2006).

[22] Discussed by E. S. Kiapokas in *Analysis of the Hippocratic Oath*, Athens, 1986.

this is incongruous, for other surgical procedures were fully described and performed by Hippocratic practitioners.[23] Assuming the text is accurate, the sense seems clear to the clinician. First, lithotomy required critical technical skill, unlike a hemorrhoidectomy (although at times hemorrhoidal surgery can be complex and difficult), and second, the ability to perform a lithotomy improved with practice. Today's internist may perform lumbar punctures and aspirate pleural and peritoneal fluid, but he will not perform a percutaneous coronary angioplasty. The person who is most proficient should be the one to carry it out, and the more complex the procedure the more proficiency affects the outcome. This practice would seem consistent with the ancient Greek physician's use of able assistants, although that similarity pertained only when the physician himself had examined the patient and dictated the therapy.

In Hippocratic times an independently functioning equivalent of today's Nurse Practitioner or Physician's Assistant would have been either the physician's assistant or his competition, not his stand-in. But in recent years licensing of those only partially trained in medicine and then permitting them to operate with seeming autonomy by means of flow charts, guidelines, and telephone calls or Skype, assessing and treating patients not seen by a physician, has introduced into society, in deed if not in word, another type of physician, the inadequately trained one. It is true that a two-tiered medical system permitting inferior practitioners existed in early Greece. As Plato describes it, medical assistants were permitted to establish their practice on slaves but not on free citizens.[24] Perhaps the next time those living in rural areas are examined and treated by paramedical personnel in lieu of a physician, they should recall that ancient practice.

The Oath urges that the sick receive the services of the most skilled. Increased reliance on the less skilled is inconsistent with the Oath, even if it is more economical. Is

---

[23] These included thoracentesis, incision of abscesses (including those of the liver and the pelvis), removal of anal fistulae and hemorrhoids, and trepanation. Furthermore, specific instructions on preparatory technique and patient comfort are described in the Hippocratic work, *In the Surgery*. Celsus (25 BC - 50 AD) in Book VII, 26, decribes a perineal surgical technique for removal of lower urinary tract stones, citing Ammonius Lithotomos (3rd C BC) and his special instruments for the procedure, and praises Hippocrates for including both surgery and internal medicine as proper tasks for the physician.

[24] Here is the dialogue from Plato, *Laws* IV, p 720:

Ath. "And these 'doctors' (who may be free men or slaves) pick up the skill empirically, by watching and obeying their masters; they've no systematic knowledge such as the free doctors have learned for themselves and pass on to their pupils. You'd agree in putting 'doctors' into these two categories?"

Clin. "Of course."

Ath. "Now here's another thing you notice. A state's invalids include not only free men but slaves too, who are almost always treated by other slaves who either rush about on flying visits or wait to be consulted in their surgeries. This kind of doctor never gives any account of the particular illness of the individual slave, or is prepared to listed to one; he simply prescribes what he thinks best in the light of experience, as if he had precise knowledge, and with the self-confidence of a dictator. Then he dashes off on his way to the next slave-patient, and so takes off his master's shoulders some of the work of attending the sick. *The visits of the free doctor, by contrast, are mostly concerned with treating the illnesses of free men; his method is to construct an empirical case-history by consulting the invalid and his friends; in this way he himself learns something from the sick and at the same time he gives the individual patient all the instruction he can. He gives no prescription until he has somehow gained the invalid's consent; then, coaxing him into continued cooperation, he tries to complete his restoration to health.*" (Translation of T. J. Saunders, from *Plato, Complete Works*, editor, J. M. Cooper, Indianapolis, 1997. Italics added.)

it inconsistent with the natural state of medical practice or is it a worthwhile modern innovation? Insofar as it relegates the sick to receive less skilled attention, it is not the latter. And the time-honored Oath of Hippocrates, in its acknowledgment of the importance of skill, warns the profession not to be a party to it.

4. To abstain from wrongdoing:

> ἐς οἰκίας δὲ ὁκόσας ἂν ἐσίω, ἐσελεύσομαι ἐπ' ὠγελείῃ καμνόντων,
> ἐκτὸς ἐὼν πάσης ἀδικίης ἑκουσίης καὶ φθορίης, . . .
> Lines 24-26

> "And into whosoever house I may enter, I will enter it for the assistance of the sick, being above all purposeful wrong doing or harm, ..."

Occasional failure, inevitable in most human activities, especially complex ones, is unintentional, not a wrongdoing. But criminal behavior, the bane of all professions, is especially detrimental to medicine. The selection process for admission into the field of medicine must diligently exclude those who would engage in such behavior. In ancient Greece the ties of family or guild, in which the welfare of all members would be affected by the misdeeds of one, would naturally enforce consistent socially acceptable behavior. Apprentices were bound with similar ties of brotherhood, as mentioned in the Oath, which reflected on the Master's or the family's reputation. Ethical conduct was the purview of those most affected by its transgression, the public.

Today the selection process for medical school is in the hands of the medical profession, specifically the schools of medicine. Selection of future practitioners, therefore, is little changed in principle from the days of the profession's founding. But academic finesse cannot be permitted to outweigh ethical commitment in the selection process. As life would have it, personalities are shaped early on. By maturity one's nature has declared itself. And so it is that all medical school applicants are of an age that permits reasonable judgments on their ethical suitability, although by no means are those judgments perfect. A review of license infractions by American-trained physicians reveals most will be from personal abuse of drugs or alcohol, incompetence, and poor personal judgment rather than unethical medical practices directed at the patient.[25] The avoidance of wrongdoing as specified by the Oath resembles modern medical enforcement, but with one exception: the moral dilemma.

Excursus on Abortion and Euthanasia

Moral issues often have medical implications, and today's particularly contentious ones

---

[25] For example, when this footnote was written there were eighty-nine State Medical Board disciplinary actions among 34,342 licensed physicians in Ohio (pop. 11.500,000) during the year April 2005 to April 2006 (or, one per 386 physicians.) Of these, thirty-nine involved drugs or alcohol, including dispensing for family members, seven involved sexual misconduct, thirteen involved incompetence, including that resulting from medical disability, and nineteen were for fraud or felony, including issues of child support, poor medical records, registrations not reporting prior convictions, and carrying a gun onto an aircraft. See: State Medical Board of Ohio Disciplinary Actions, April 2005 – April 2006.

relevant to the Oath are abortion and euthanasia. As medicine is a social mirror it is uncertain how the individual practitioner must handle them, for Western practitioners mirror the moral variability of the greater society, and society is divided on whether the two issues are wrongdoings. If morality is based on religion, if abortion is inconsistent with morality, and if the state is of one religion, the solution is at hand. Present-day society is far different, and on this issue caring and thoughtful people have chosen sides.

It has been claimed that the Hippocratic Oath prohibits the physician from engaging in abortion, and some, viewing that prohibition as intolerable, have used this issue to diminish the reputation of the Oath and its ancient adherents and to justify the writing of alternative oaths. Here are the relevant words, as translated for the *Loeb Classical Library* series on Hippocrates by W. H. S. Jones in 1923:

> ὁμοίως δὲ οὐδὲ γυναικὶ πεσσὸν φθόριον δώσω. (Lines 20-21)
> "Similarly I will not give to a woman a pessary to cause an abortion."

In the days of Hippocrates was there a generic and moral injunction against abortion? Such would seem unlikely in a society that did not punish parents for practicing infanticide if they had an unwanted child, usually a female. Only under Emperor Constantine (280-337 AD) did the State come to the protection of that innocent. The Hippocratic injunction against abortion was most likely on another ethical basis, fear of harm to the mother. The feminine noun, φθορά, can, however, mean corruption, mischief, evil design, dishonor, even "seduction," in addition to "destruction."[26] In any case, although the Hippocratic statement on the subject may have been straightforward when first pronounced, its true meaning today is uncertain. In 400 BC what drug could have been a vaginal abortifacient? The answer is, none. Alternatively, given uncertainties of translation, perhaps the injunction was against contraception, surely a sensitive subject in a male-dominated society. But it is notable that in the classic early 20th C book on contraception by Marie Stopes, written before the development of modern birth control pharmaceuticals there is not a single chemical agent described that had as its mode of contraception some hormonal effect.[27] All depended on local spermatocidal activity or physical obstruction to prevent conception, this in spite of the endless accounts of herbal agents prescribed by practitioners of all sorts used as contraceptives over the ages. It is possible that the Hippocratic reference was to these methods of contraception, for their use might have resulted in a male heir not being produced. But while such an approach to preventing conception may have been "obstructive," it does not seem "destructive." Furthermore, many methods for contraception must have been common knowledge among women, requiring only a visit to a midwife or other woman familiar with the problem, and surely not to a physician. Were the woman desirous of keeping matters secret, no prescriptions would have been wanted or needed. Finally, could the sense of φθορά have been "mischief" or "seduction," and the purpose of pessary, perhaps soaked in a solution of sylphium, an extinct but apparently effective contraceptive botanical that

---

[26] Liddell and Scott, *A Greek-English Lexicon*. This is a standard work, first published in 1843, that has gone through nine editions.

[27] Stopes, M. C., *Contraception, Its Theory, History and Practice*, London, 1929. This is the "new and enlarged" edition, the first edition being in 1923. Several physicans appended their comments to the book's introduction, and they neither deny Stope's facts nor provide information on other forms of contraception.

was also touted as an aphrodisiac, have been the commercial equivalent of the modern sildenafil? Whatever its meaning, the Oath could have had nothing whatever to do with abortion, its use as an argument in any context being irrelevant in every sense to modern discussion of abortion, and the matter as regards Hippocratic medicine is hereby ended.

Having stated that, Oath or no Oath, the issue of abortion is with us. Today segments of western society are trying to impress legal sanctions on the medical practitioner for performing a procedure about which society has profound internal disagreement. Efforts by one segment of the population to invoke a technical filibuster using the medical profession as a straw man are surely an unfair mechanism for deciding the matter. There is presently no solution in sight for society's abortion dilemma. But for the medical profession there is. In the opening pages of this book were detailed those medical practices that were not to be considered relevant to the purposes herein, one reason being that the clinician is defined by his laboring for the sick. The example was given that some surgery for cosmetic purposes in healthy persons was not the domain of the clinician discussed herein and need not be offered the same protections the clinician should have. Many abortions are performed not for purposes of health but for convenience or fear. This is not the arena of the clinician, whose primary function is to help the sick, not abet the well, and pregnancy is not a disease. The medical profession has become entangled in a snare of society. It has no more right, as a profession, to intrude on social issues than social reformers have a right to intrude on medicine. The solution for the moment, therefore, is this: should a physician be requested by a "client" to arrange an abortion, the practitioner can then advise the "client" to seek assistance from some organization that provides the requested service, but he is not to be a spokesman for the medical profession nor the requested service, nor is the organization performing the service to be affiliated with the medical profession. It is up to society at some level to determine the legality of abortion, not the profession. If legal mandates are imposed on abortion, the abortionist, being outside the profession, must be subject to them, just as any citizen or business would be. By this means the regulation of this particular practice, except for agreed upon medical indications, would devolve solely onto society. It would immediately eliminate the need for professional debate on the issue. If society can recognize, legalize, and even authorize aromatherapy, naturopathy, homeopathy, and chiropractic, it can surely recognize and legalize a practice of a specialized nature such as abortion, one that actually works. And then any woman could decide to consult the office of an abortionist rather than a physician, just as she might consult an herbalist or an acupuncturist. Surely a woman in 5th C BC Greece would never have consulted a Hippocratic physician for an abortion. She would have consulted a midwife or knowledgable friend. And should any democratic society, through its elected officials, refuse to recognize the practice of an abortionist, that is the end of the matter. It is time to remove the physician from the phalanx of activists, time to cut the ties that have purposely been designed to enlist/enforce his collaboration for the purpose of strengthening arguments by appending his prestige. The physician can express his personal opinion via the same mechanisms as any other citizen.

An argument similar to the preceding can also be made for contraception. Apart from reasons of health that might require contraceptive medications by a physician, a "client" requesting the convenience of of contraception can apply to a nonphysician organization providing such a service. As of the date of this writing, emergency contraception is available over the counter to those who are seventeen years of age or older. Contraception for convenience should be removed from a clinical physician's daily tasks.

The preceding issue is comparable to euthanasia. Plato's "politic" Asclepius was, in *The Republic*, expected to not prolong the lives of those who could not be returned to a useful position in society:

> ". . . but bodies which disease had penetrated through and through he would not have attempted to cure by gradual processes of evacuation and infusion: he did not want to lengthen out good-for-nothing lives, or to have weak fathers begetting weaker sons; - if a man was not able to live in the ordinary way he had no business to cure him; for such a cure would have been of no use either to himself, or to the State."[28]

In such a State the aged or infirm would be viewed as sapping its strength, and euthanasia could therefore be viewed as morally justified for benefit of society, not for the afflicted person. Now this valuation of the individual bears directly on the role of the State in the provision of health care, but it is mentioned here for the purpose of discussing euthanasia. The place of euthanasia in society has been debated in the West since the days of ancient Greece and surely for thousands of years before. Plato and Aristotle disagreed on its role, the various arguments including avoidance of suffering, sanctity of life, divine injunction, and social usefulness. Today there is a general sense that the matter is a deeply personal one, its active pursuit by the State out of the question. But to whom should the individual willfully seeking the service turn? Not to the medical profession.

Again, the answer is to turn to an organization or individual that provides that service, one having no affiliation with the medical profession. A licensing procedure can be arranged that would assure the quality of the service, perhaps one that would be carried out under the aegis of a hospice. There are many circumstances in clinical practice that touch on the end of life. Questions relating to nutrition, surgical or pharmacological therapies, comfort, pain control, and anguish, for example, are daily issues for clinicians, and their management often bear on terminal illness. Clinicians and patients or their proxies can usually work out the preferred management. But for those who, for whatever reason, wish to deal with predictable rather than inevitable circumstance, a licensed euthanasiologist may be an alternative, but it must not be a physician.

To conclude, whatever the clinician's personal view on social problems might be, those problems are matters to be handled through public channels and the voting booth. The clinician's professional issues are not society's issues, and society's issues should not clutter medical journals. Thus, the purpose of this excursus is not to solve the problems surrounding the role of abortion or euthanasia in society. It is, instead, to disinvolve the medical profession. Physicians who, in the eyes of some, break moral rather than secular laws may be viewed as criminals. While society continues its great debate on the subject of abortion the medical profession should not choose sides and must oppose any efforts that make the profession a target for proponents and opponents. Individual physicians will have their personal opinions and express them through society's channels, and even when a societal consensus has been achieved the profession should remain aloof, for at issue there remains an ethical matter, namely, that physicians are to help the sick rather than to abet the well. The medical profession is not above society; it is part of it, and it

---

[28] Plato, *The Republic*, III, 407, d, translation of B. Jowett.

must be sensitive to the divisive issues of the day. The physician's opinion regarding abortion carries neither more nor less weight than a nonphysician's; it is absurd to think a physician should impress his own moral judgments on the laity (see p. 22). If physicians are to force a moral viewpoint on society because they consider themselves as uniquely privileged and qualified to do so, they exhibit the same irresponsible behavior as hypocrites of celluloid and tabloid who expound daily for personal advantage on moral issues far beyond what their intellects can bear.

End of excursus

---

5. To not divulge private matters:

> ἃ δ᾽ ἂν ἐν θεραπείῃ ἢ ἴδω ἢ ἀκούσω, ἢ καὶ ἄνευ θεραπείης κατὰ βίον ἀνθρώπων, ἃ μὴ χρή ποτε ἐκλαλεῖσθαι ἔξω, σιγήσομαι, ἄρρητα ἡγεύμενος ειναι τὰ τοιαῦτα. Lines 29-32

> In the course of patient care, and even outside it, that which I may see or hear concerning the circumstances of men which are not to be spoken abroad, I will keep silent, deeming those matters not to be divulged.

Universal agreement exists on the importance of keeping inviolable the communications between physician and patient. But as any hospital practitioner will attest, ready access to a patient's inpatient record is accorded to medical students, resident physicians, nursing staff, dieticians, administrative staff, numerous hospital committees, and social service staff, in addition to valid medical consultations. Often there are visits to a chart by researchers, legal authorities, paramedical personnel, external review committees, and on and on. Anyone recently hospitalized has no secrets from the general public. It is only a lack of public interest in the details that prevents the spread of that information back into one's individual social circle. If you have something you wish to keep secret, the hospital is increasingly the last place you should go. Despite the professed barriers to intrusion, protection of privacy in a modern hospital does not exist, and those barriers that enlist the services of government will but further their porousness. In centuries past one could with confidence keep no secrets from one's physician and one's confessor. No one should feel that way today as regards medicine.

Five tenets of the Hippocratic Oath have now been reviewed. Infractions abound. They originate not from the practitioner but from pressures exerted by those that surround him. As in early post-Hippocratic centuries, the consequences of organizational failure on the part of medicine are increasingly apparent. This time it is with medicine's permission rather than organizational insufficiency, its intrusions supported by collusion from within the medical profession itself, as the following circumstances will show.

C. Circumventing the Intellectual Domain of the Physician: Complementary and Alternative Medicine

Dr. Engelhardt, in *The Foundations of Bioethics*,[29] advances an extraordinary but increasingly appealing position, namely that physicians should prepare to embrace those who seek any and all forms of medical care. In anticipation of a growing list of alternative preventives, restoratives, treatments, and supervision that will inevitably result from the "loss of moral direction" that science has wrought, it is suggested that physicians prepare to practice within the "constraints of a secular pluralist morality" and to administer whatever makes a person feel right in his own, unique, moral universe. Another consideration is genetic engineering that could purposefully modify society's descendants.   Perhaps the new physician will have to not only heed "traditional" knowledge, but he will also make allowance for biological and social attributes of new life forms that, logically, could lead to a new species, beyond mankind.

Now the core knowledge of medicine is so vast that the addition of another area from the panoply that is alternative medicine to an already long list of medical things to remember, organize, understand, and apply is unreasonable. Englehardt seems to require that physicians be equipped like gods, so broadly mandated should be their knowledge and their charge. But enlarging the field of internal medicine is impossible, unless there be added another layer of subspecialists. Training of physicians now includes, on the one hand, recognition of the unfortunate consequences of unscientific medicinal practices, and, on the other, pressure to embrace or otherwise accommodate these same practices, a bizarre state of affairs, especially when legal liability is ever increasing for the physician in his own area of expertise.

The medical profession can hold its own with religious fundamentalism and alternative healers, not to mention charlatanism, for it has done so in the past. Social inconsistency is a perennial feature of a free, curious, and seeking society, and it is for the most part a sign of health, if not always a healthful path. It presents no threat. A homogeneous and submissive society is by far the greater threat. But the popularity of the various kinds of healers outside those of the modern medical profession can be used as a gauge of competitiveness, and any flourishing of the competition indicates a problem. Unless, of course, as Englehardt recommends, subjective medicine succeeds in infiltrating and, to varying degrees displaces, the scientific, in which case competition would be viewed as prejudicial and not to be permitted.

Complementary and alternative medicine do not include religious fundamentalism, a major social force throughout the world. How many times is heard, "You've done a good job, Doctor, but we all know it was the Lord who led to John's recovery." To which many physicians would wholeheartedly agree. And some religious sects view the use of many, even all, of the tools of medical science as irreverent gestures. But religious fundamentalism will not disappear. It has an eternal attraction, and for a reason. It is a part of man's intellectual equivalent to DNA, innate, struggling to provide inner direction, and, despite being manipulated to produce all-too-frequent intrusions upon man's technical progress, it is here to stay. Muons, pions, dark matter, and *Homo erectus* are irrelevant in this context, in part because thinking man knows that science in virtually all its aspects is but a descriptive process, a process that seeks to know and then proclaims "how" but not "why," one studded with curious and interesting theories seeking

---

[29] Engelhardt, H.T. *The Foundations of Bioethics*, Oxford, 1986 (1st edition).

an ultimate truth that is, in our hearts, known not to be attainable. Whatever the Grand Unified Theory may turn out to be, science will never answer the question of *why*. The force of religion will continue to influence man's progress as it always has, for its message is *why*. Godless States exist only where imposed; a democratic and truly free State will always be friendly to the religious.

D. Circumventing the Practice Domain of the Physician by the Inadequately Trained: Paramedicine[30]

Patient contact is increasingly relegated to nonphysicians, either because the local physician is overworked, unavailable, or because institutional economics mandate it. The fully trained physician is viewed more and more as a luxury rather than as essential. This is prompting many to leave their profession, even to the point of not recommending others to enter it. Many of these persons were trained several decades ago when their aspirations, their "calling," led them to accept lengthy schooling and an arduous apprenticeship as a small price to pay for a lifetime in an unambiguously useful, interesting, and honorable vocation. Now they are forced to face the reality that they are viewed as replaceable by technicians, expendable except for their signatures, liable because of their vulnerability, and questionable as to their motives.

Table 11: Competitors of the Medical Profession

Mechanism	Agent	Examples	
		Ancient	Modern
Populism	Politician	Mesopotamian medicine	Soviet medicine[31]
Amateurism	Quack	Roman medicine	Alternative medicine
Elitism	Aristocrat	Chinese medicine*	Treatment of the healthy
Mysticism	Cleric	Egyptian medicine	Religious cultism

*Classical Chinese medical practitioners, not the "itinerant doctors."

The Hippocratic physician had assistants who carried out his instructions,

---

[30] As defined in the Encyclopedia Britannica "paramedical" is: "healthcare workers who provide clinical services to patients under the supervision of a physician." It is not restricted to emergency response teams.

[31] Soviet medicine is the brainchild of the dictatorship of the proletariat, and epitomizes the consequences of collectivism. Physician density in the Soviet Union, per unit population, has, since the Revolution, always greatly exceeded that of the United States, being 429 vs. 225/100,000 in 1987. The profession of medicine has been utterly without power within the Soviet bureaucracy, the physician receiving a salary one-quarter less than the average *per capita* income. Populist medicine is, of course, medical care without cost, an overwhelming temptation for those wishing to avoid payment, and free medical care is the ultimate competitor and driver of "socialized medicine." Its true cost, however, is but too obvious. In late 20th C Russia was said to provide the worst health care in the world. Consult the *Foundation for Economic Education* and its newsletter of May, 2004, for an article by Anna Ebeling, *The Government Dream and the Soviet Reality*.

sometimes even staying in a patient's home to oversee their implementation. Some of the assistants were apprentices, some technicians, and perhaps some, or most, were slaves, for any other assistance would have been too expensive a service to provide. Today resident physicians, medical students, nurses, physiotherapists, home health aides, visiting nurses, and other specifically qualified personnel provide similar but superior service. Skilled within defined limits, they extend the utility of the physician in providing medical care, improving service and wonderfully increasing efficiency. Used in ancient Greece, they are natural corollaries of a properly run medical practice, and modern medicine has fully endorsed them.

But more and more it is the nurse practitioners and physician assistants and other medically affiliated practitioners who are practicing while the medical professional is preaching. The physician is removing himself, or being removed, from hands-on clinical responsibility, just another of history's long list of sophists or like the Mesopotamian *asipu*. Nonphysicians are being intercalated into the functioning body of the profession. By providing what some feel is the equivalent of physicians' services to patients, it might be expected that separate and freestanding organizations might consolidate around these services, just as Osteopathy became a distinct alternative to allopathic medicine over a century ago. Becoming competitive with, rather than joining with, physicians might well benefit by their autonomy. The competition would be healthy for the profession. Alternatively, additional training might permit many of these same paramedicine personnel to earn the title of "physician." In the experience of the author there have been some who would be warmly welcomed.

E. Circumventing the Professional Domain of the Physician by the Untrained: Eclectic Professionals

The Hippocratic physician was a professional, but he did not require a license to practice. His practice, unrestricted, depended on public perception of his effectiveness, ethical commitment, and perhaps the reputation of his apprenticeship. But this could only partially protect his medical practice and the general public from charlatans, who were also not licensed. The licensing of physicians in the West, first carried out in 1140 AD, was an important advance toward quality assurance. Now, however, nontraditional practitioners are also licensed. This official sanctioning of nontraditional and unproven practices by society's proxy, its government, has reversed the reason for physician licensing in the first place.

For the clinical physician has always been at one end of a continuum of all those who claim to be healers. The arbitrary cutoff in the West between the physician and nonphysician is not made by physicians but by society through its elected officials. Those who miss the cut off can still practice many aspects of medicine, can even term themselves "doctor," which term is, in the eyes of society, loosely synonymous with physician. They can advertise their expertise on a grand scale, can replace the rhetoric of the ancients with the photo-ops and subway posters of today, can be abreast of research data and select from that vast, complex, and even speculative knowledge anything they might wish to use for constructing their own theories of physiology that suit their own practices, products, or systems of logic. Still, this is all manageable.

But the new problem is that the medical profession is officially accommodating "affiliated" medical practitioners, thereby certifying to the public a huge, expensive, and risky or ineffective pattern of medical practice. Democratic government will increasingly authorize, in its perpetual effort to seek reelection by attempting to do everything for everybody, the investiture of unproven techniques and hypotheses. After centuries of being at the fringe of medicine, complementary and alternative medicine practitioners have not had to breach a wall; they are being pulled through the gates. The consequences of the profession's policy are (1) to give unfair advantage to untrained competitors, and (2) to imply a serious fault in traditional training that the nontraditional can repair, for otherwise, in the eyes of the general public, why would unscientific practitioners be championed?

The original purpose of licensing of physicians was to maintain quality in medical care delivery. But the licensing of quasi medical practitioners has been done to ensure their recognition so as to avoid the appearance of social inequity, for quality is not an issue when dealing with the ineffective.[32] This is not an improvement. It is a defect. Official recognition of these practices should be reversed. Then they would be permitted to take their traditional place on the stage and fairly compete on their own with the medical profession for public opinion rather than being listed on the profession's marquee.[33]

F. Circumscribing the Managerial Domain of the Physician: Subversion of the Koinon

A century ago in Western medicine the patient, consulting his doctor, may have had relatively limited choices in therapy, but the patient made the final decision. Now that option is increasingly under bureaucratic control. The patient, who used to come first, often is no longer so privileged. Prof. Samuel Bloom has summarized the bureaucratization of medicine.[34] From the viewpoint of the patient the provision of medical care varies according to social status, especially in the area of primary care; there is a loss of the interpersonal bond between physician and patient; and there are too many doctors involved, a "proliferation of providers." From the viewpoint of society this form of management is associated with high cost and inefficiency, dissatisfied patients, militant hostility to the healthcare establishment, legal challenges to the physician's autonomy, and an "intensified practice of defensive medicine." These sentiments were recorded a generation ago.[35] Their validity is even greater today. In Prof. Edward Shorter's book on a social history of medicine,[36] a statistic from the 1970s indicates the average consultation time for a family practitioner was six minutes in Great Britain and eleven minutes in the United States, but the former number is now being approached within some American

---

[32] By "quasi-" is meant "having some resemblance, usually by possession of certain attributes"; Merriam-Webster's Collegiate Dictionary, 10th edition.

[33] Perhaps there are some quasi-practitioners who do not realize that by allying themselves with the physician they are actually enlarging the catch that a government net will snare.

[34] Bloom, S.W. and Summey, P.: *Models of the Doctor-Patient Relationship: A History of the Social System Concept*, in E. B. Gallagher, editor, *The Doctor-Patient Relationship in the Changing Health Scene*. *Geographic Health Studies*, John E. Fogarty International Center for Advanced Study in the Health Sciences, New York, 1976.

[35] The National Institutes of Health, 1978, in a pamphlet entitled: *The Doctor-Patient Relationship in the Changing Health Scene.*

[36] Shorter, E., *Doctors and Their Patients*, New Brunswick, 1993, 2nd printing, paperback, p. 208.

health maintainence organizations.[37]

The effects of bureaucracy are especially obvious in the realm of the primary care physician, the general practitioner, formerly regarded as the acme of the professional pyramid. Now the general practitioner is at its base. The hands-on, involved physician has been displaced in public esteem by modern day Herophiluses and Erisastratuses, Dogmatists and Empiricists. The supplier of special medical services to the healthy seems more important to society than the frontline clinician, until that day arrives when one's own life-and-death decisions become unavoidable. The defendant on the witness stand is increasingly likely to be the physician who had to make a difficult but necessary decision in a moment of great stress, often under the direct gaze of potential litigants, rather than the health-promoting speakeasy that attempts to find disease where there usually is none, slickly congratulating the disease-free victims that they escaped that disease, or should one be found, immediately shifting all responsibility for its management elsewhere, usually, and fortunately, to someone who cares.[38]

In an earlier chapter the loss of the peripatetic physician was not lamented, but it was pointed out that he still practices today, a consequence of the interposition of institution between physician and patient. From this has come loss of continuity of care. The reasons are (1) Territorial: Loss of the role of the private physician when the patient is hospitalized or referred to a specialist who then co-opts care, for in the United States continuity of care was traditionally maintained by the primary physician even upon hospitalization of the patient; (2) Economical: Health maintenance organizations may have to increase efficiency by posting physicians for the convenience of the organization rather than for the benefit of the patient. This is a well recognized problem, for medical organizations require income to survive, and efficiency is a part of staying in business. But the loss of continuity of care is important and must be redressed. (3) Logistical: Emergency Room medicine or walk-in clinics as primary care providers have, by default, become in many areas the most convenient way to obtain the services of a physician. It is just easier most of the time to visit the Emergency Room than make an appointment to see a physician. This loss of the tradition of personal continuity of care by a physician by and large does not reflect the preference of physicians, and a return to this aspect of healthcare delivery of the past, within limits of feasibility, would greatly assist in strengthening the natural state of medical practice today.

Now the purpose of the final chapter in this book is not to affect the trend of socialization of medicine in Western society. Federal regulation of medicine is far too advanced to be rescinded. In a society that cries out for the security of entitlement that battle has been lost. In a change from the bitter and bloody 20th C revolutionary struggles, nationalized health care is, after open debate, despite its manifold defects, and in the full

---

[37] And here remember the words of Celsus: "From these things it may be inferred, that many people cannot be attended by one physician; and the man to be trusted is he, that knows his profession, and is not much absent from his patient. But they, that only practice from views of gain, because their profits rise in proportion to the number of patients, readily fall in with such rules..." (Celsus, *De Medicina*, Book III, Chapter 4, translation of J. Greive, Edinburgh, 1814.) By this Celsus is referring to the use of axioms to guide clinical decision rather than personal contact and clinical judgment, and that use of quidance rules allows the less competent physician to not only get by, but to inordinately prosper.

[38] For a sympathetic discussion of this issue see: Altschule, M. D. (ed.), *Essays on the Rise and Decline of Bedside Medicine*, Lansing, 1989, especially the introduction by Altschule.

light of day, being acclaimed by the majority. This book addresses instead only a minute part of the whole. But it is the physician's part, a part in which he alone is expert, along with 200,000 other clinicians in the United States. It is up to voters of a democratic society to determine if money from society's taxpayers will provide the means to dispense medicines and services such as nursing homes, transportation, and hospital care for all. But who will decide on the care itself? Data collection for those future decision-makers is well under way. Here is a clinical example from an article in the *New England Journal of Medicine* at the time this paragraph was first written (2004). It is typical in its conclusions in that it displays the orientation of those who will be making such decisions:

> "In addition, dexamethasone treatment reduced costs to the family and the health care system as compared with placebo. And although the cost savings per patient were relatively small, mild croup is so common that treatment of all these children with dexamethasone would yield substantial societal benefits."[39]

This book defends only the physician, who must remain apart from social legislation in order to maintain his own well-being and that of his patients. His protection is the koinon.

There are three levels at which medical organization, or koinon, is threatened, personal, local and regional:

Personal – The physician-patient relationship, or koinon of two, is threatened by legislation. So far this threat is limited, but legislation is interfering in areas such as end-of-life decisions, decisions formerly handled by those most intimately involved, not attorneys, legislators, and administrators. A most humane decision can, out of context and in the public eye, be made to appear horrendous, producing legislation that may affect not only that one situation but, impersonally, many thousands of others throughout the country and for many years to come. Certain life decisions have been, since the very first man, difficult and wrenching, for that is their nature. As they become placed in legal hands, those decisions can now be made with less inconvenience and with less feeling. Maybe it is easier this way. But it is ironic that the physician's clinical obligations under the Oath are being abrogated for the very reason they were written in the first place, abrogated by nonphysicians who also profess to serve the patient's interest. Interference is now common to the point of being unexceptional, even normal. The unsolicited third opinion no longer comes from the Church but from the Actuary, the Ethicist, the Attorney, the Senator. Now it may be observed that rewriting of an Oath is easy. But, as Dr. Dean-Jones has so elegantly put it, "Unlike medicine, writing does not require a knowledge of the opportune moment."[40] That moment, as well as the perception of that moment, is constantly shifting. It is the domain of the physician.

There also remains the potential, however much the topic may be minimized or evaded, to remove the role of the physician in end-of-life decision-making altogether. This has happened before, and it is relevant to reread Plato's statements on the subject found in Book III of *The Republic*.

---

[39] Bjornson, C. L., *et al.*, *Randomized Trial of Dexamethasone for Mild Croup*, in *N. Engl. J. Med.*, 351:1306-1313, 2004. For healthy contrast read the short but insightful and poignant article by Ellen More, PhD: *The Remains of the Profession, or What the Butler Knew*, in *Ann. Intern. Med.*, 134:255-259, 2001.

[40] Dean-Jones, L., *Literacy and the Charlatan in Ancient Greek Medicine*, in: *Written Texts and the Rise of Literate Culture in Ancient Greece*, Cambridge, 2002, H. Yunis, editor, chap. five, p. 103.

Another threat to the physician-patient relationship is the era of evidentiary medicine whereby physicians are pressured to base medical decisions on decision trees and decision analysis derived from studies performed on groups of people treated in a uniform way for a uniform condition.[41] As unrealistic as this is for the individual patient, it is not a new quandary. Here must be credited early 19th C French mathematicians and physicians, especially Prof. Simeon Poisson and Dr. F. Double, who, with their colleagues, questioned the extent to which statistical treatments of clinical phenomena should be trusted. Dr. Double (1777-1842) in particular argued that medical management based on statistics derived from data obtained from large groups would undercut the individualized assessment of a physician and thrust a major part of patient care into the hands of nonphyician scientists and statisticians.[42] This is exactly what is happening, for there is a major trend in modern medicine to base clinical management of patients as if they and their diseases conform to some uniform code, called a "guideline" as devised by a primordial medical constabulary.

While the physician will have undergone molding during an education that instills a degree of uniformity in medical knowledge and its application, the sick patient will always be approached as a singular individual. Two patients with pneumonia may be of the same age, gender, marital status, nationality, and a myriad of other details, but they will be treated as distinct by the physician, for, as any clinician will affirm, they are distinct. It is the gathering storm of present-day medicine that sees such distinctions give way to uniformity in approach, stratification, and standardization of therapy. This is not to deny that there is a "best" way to do something, and that there is a way that will benefit "most." But the physician-patient relationship is not about "most," for what is best for most may not be best for a given individual. Concern for the "most" is an institutional, perhaps even political, concern, but not a clinician's. In contrast to evidence-based medicine, a colleague has queried, "What about medicine-based evidence?," by that meaning the clinician's world rather than the statistician's. What is to be done when a plan for that unique patient does not comply with protocol? No, those who wish to be treated according to consensus guidelines derived from evidence-based medicine can be managed by paramedical or complementary and alternative medicine practitioners. For

---

[41] An anecdote of the author gives a friend's response many years ago when that friend was asked how he knew he was taking the study drug rather than placebo during an important national clinical trial: "Bill," he said, "do you think I'm a fool? I'm not going to take something that doesn't do a damn thing!" How he was certain in advance that he would not be taking the placebo will never be known, but it should strike a note of caution for all those who have unqualified faith in randomized clinical trials.

[42] Poisson, S-D., Double, F. J., *et al.*, *Rapports: Recherches de Statistique sur l'affection calculeuse, par M. Le docteur Civiale. Comptes Rendu Hebdomadaires des Seances de l'Academie des Sciences*, 1:171-172, 1835, as discussed in its modern context by J. R. Matthews in *Commentary: The Paris Academy of Science Report on Jean Civiale's…*, in *Internat. J. Epidemiology*, 30:1249-1250, 2001. This is not to be taken as a condemnation of the numerical methodology and quantitation preferred by Jean Civiale, a contemporary French physician. It is, instead, a warning about the abuse of, or unrealistic expectations from, statistical method. The advice of Morgagni is to be heeded: Neque enim numerande sunt, sed perpendendae, nec, nisi capitis diffectio accesserit, accipiendae. Morgagni, *De Sedibus et Causis Morborum*, Venice, 1761, 2 vols., Letter 51, art. 47, found in vol. 2, p. 294; "For they should not [merely] be counted up, but deliberated, and then only after dissection of the head has been provided" (translation by the author), meaning, in this example from his study of head wounds, merely counting cases of an abnormality is insufficient; they must also be individualy evaluated.

those who prefer individualized assessment and management by an expert who will know them as unique and who will, with their assistance, decide on a course, let them seek a physician. Twenty-four hundred years ago Aristotle recognized the complexities of medicine, the frequent inadequacy of fixed rules, and the need to judge matters on a case-by-case basis.[43] The physician must, of course, be aware of published medical studies based sound evidence, implementing hem or advising on their acceptance when appropriate. But only the individual physician can, in conjunction with the patient himself, determine what is best for the individual patient.

Local – The intellectual hub of medicine is found today in medical schools, and here it is the universities that pose a threat. The selection and education of physicians is for the most part in the hands of physicians. There are problems with the selection process, for many biases are involved, including the desire to forward the university's reputation. But the great emphasis on research rather than clinical care is particularly of concern. Teachers often are more researchers than clinicians.[44] One-on-one clinical teaching has become uncommon, relegated to farming out, for a few weeks, the occasional student to a harried clinic physician. Focus is less on the individual patient and more on research to save the world. It is a fact, however, that the true clinician's world revolves around one person and one person only, the patient of the moment. How instructive was Dr. Cronkite's editorial on chronic lymphocytic leukemia: the brilliance, the resources, the time, and the effort expended over forty years of research on this disease (plus many others, of course) and yet no improvement in survival.[45] This is often the case with research. But to be part of a successful outcome with even one sick patient, that is

---

[43] "but the agents themselves have to consider what is suited to the circumstances on each occasion, just as is the case with the art of medicine or of navigation." Aristotle, *Nicomachean Ethics*, II, ii, 4-5, translation of H. Rackham, *Loeb Classical Library*, 1990. This is not to disparage entirely the idea of guidelines, for they are valuable as memory aids and a way to avoid oversights. Indeed, *our textbooks are filled with guidelines* written by expert consultants who are solicited for chapters in their particular specialty. But guidelines vary from one expert to another, the ones furthest removed from the patient being federal guidelines whereas a medical association, group, or hospital can provide guidelines more closely tailored to the patient, the patient's circumstances, and facility capabilities. It is for this reason that physicians have Grand Rounds and other traditional public exchanges of clinical experience and opinion. It is claimed by some that guidelines will not restrict physician decision-making. See, for example, Reinertsen, J. L., *Zen and the Art of Physician Autonomy Maintenance*, in *Ann. Intern. Med.* 138:992-995, 2003. Experience has shown, however, that in the hands of government or an attorney that is often and patently not the case. Furthermore, guidelines not only must continually change as new knowledge accrues, but they must also reflect regional or organizational relevance. And the rate of change can be far too rapid for anything but a clinician's organization to manage. Otherwise it amounts to "cookbook medicine." See: Liang, M., *From America: Cookbook Medicine or Food for Thought: Practice Guidelines Development in the USA*, in *Ann. Rheum. Dis.*, 51:1257-1258, 1992.
[44] This trend can be traced to the early 20th C. Although Flexner praised the scientific potential of the bedside clinician, other leaders, such as Dr. William Welch of the Johns Hopkins University, urged that medical centers not rely on community clinicians. Instead he favored expanded laboratory research facilities and full-time paid staff to do research and to teach. See: Flexner, S. and Flexner, J.T., *Wm Henry Welch and the Heroic Age of American Medicine*, Baltimore, 1941.
[45] See: Reizenstein, P., and Cronkite, E. P., *Our Hematologic Heritage*, in *Leukemia Research*, 15:877-878, 1991, and Cronkite, E. P., *An Historical Account of Clinical Investigations on Chronic Lymphocytic Leukemia in the Medical Research Center, Brookhaven National Laboratory*, in *Blood Cells*, 12:285-295, 1987.

satisfaction, and it needs no editorial, indeed it shuns it.

Regional – The professional koinon, or large medical association, faces a threat in the uncritical inclusion of those who are not physicians, such as complementary and alternative medicine practitioners and representatives of government and other special interest groups. There is also a threat in permitting medical associations to be guided by nonclinicians, even nonphysicians.[46] The Hippocratic physicians guided and profited from their profession by engaging within a common council. But physicians are increasingly unable to withstand their traditional competitors because their organizations have joined forces with those competitors. It is the professional management of the medical associations that is leading this charge against itself. The purpose of a regional common council should not be to lobby, legislate, or enlarge the profession. Its purpose should be, instead, to improve the individual physician's performance through teaching and sharing of ideas, and to prevent fragmentation of the profession in the face of calamity by maintaining unity behind a common standard. It should minimize collaborations involving middlemen, one source of medicine's costliness.[47] Unfortunately the advanced nature of today's threats to the profession will require it to take political action to secure its autonomy, for circumscribing its influence as it exists today will offer an irresistible political target to those outside interests who would control it. But if action is not taken to return the field of medicine to medicine's practitioners the management positions of the medical associations will become civil service sinecures and some day any revitalizing changes will be viewed as a threat and perhaps even penalized.

Table 12:   Contemporary Threats to the Common Council (Koinon)

Level of Threat	Koinon Involved	Focus of Threat
Personal	Physician-Patient	Physician decisions
Local	Small Physician Organization	Physician training
Regional	Large Physician Organization	Physician identity

---

[46] "Are professions losing ground?," asks Michael Winter in *The Culture and Control of Expertise*, 1988. The answer is "yes" when considering increasing bureaucracy, complexity of organizations, and new technologies and occupations. Winter suggests there are now expanded opportunities for delivery of new professional services and for marketing, and this may avoid the "degradation of work" ethic by which computerized knowledge threatens professions. Medical knowledge alone, however, cannot replace the clinician, whose position should be secure unless he gives it away. See especially Winter's Chapter 3.

[47] The medical profession is not equatable to other businesses. Profit for profit's sake is the domain of the middleman. The middleman came to prominence when it was no longer possible for the physician to provide necessary services in his office, either because the machines became too costly to buy and maintain or because of regulatory agency requirements. The stethoscope, the electrocardiogram, the ultrasound machine, and even the x-ray unit need not, when within the individual practitioner's domain, be economic hindrances to care. But it is the cost of adhering to mandatory regulations and the expense of procedures and equipment outside the physician's office that so inflates medical costs, in addition to licensing and insurance fees.

G. Accountability

In some past time the physician-patient relationship was considered, in the words of Dr. Sigerist, "pure person-to-person," and "no person and no authority are to interfere," "as on a lonely island."[48] But that island has become crowded and "more and more... health and disease are not the private concern of the individual." Sigerist concluded that "the physician's profession is independent only in name." This analysis is not a good recommendation for attracting into the profession those individuals who would treat a patient as an individual. It is, instead, a call for those who would view their profession as an obligation to society and a venue for implementing policies of that society. Sickness, with the advent of Christianity, has undergone a metamorphosis from opprobrium to privilege, and "Society can ... demand that the individual be conscious constantly of his obligation to the general welfare of society." In turn the physician will advise the State on what services are needed, becoming Plato's *Asklepios politicos*. All appears to be, in the jargon of today, a "seamless social package." But it will be "seamless" only in that no exceptions will be permitted, for the nature of medicine's management will become ". . . the avowed and universal exception to the craft of healing from the action of Adam Smith's law of free competition, introducing legislative enactment and license into the public relations of medicine, thus constituting a virtual monopoly."[49]

The Hippocratic physician was a member of local society and his actions would have reflected the attitudes of that society. Prof. Jouanna even describes him as a "prisoner of judgment of the public."[50] He certainly was not antisocial or asocial, a fact that jumps out at any reader of the *Hippocratic Corpus*. And in this sense the Western physician has always been held hostage by his society, a point neither debatable nor worth debating. In the eyes of the Hippocratics, as for the American physician of but a few decades past, it was the patient who was the independent element. How critical this point is to our understanding of the problem at hand. Independence of the physician is justified only so long as there is independence of his patient. What Dr. Sigerist implied in his attack on individualism of the physician actually represented, in camouflage, his desire for a "seamless" entitlement package for patients without a choice, one in which medical decisions become decisions of society rather than the physician and patient. It is not so much that the physician loses his individuality as it is the patient who will be the involuntary recipient of society's decisions, for, in a democratic entitlement society, both society and society's leaders have already agreed on the inability of the individual to make his own decisions. In society as well as in nature, "there are consequences."

---

[48] Sigerist, H., *On the Sociology of Medicine* (edited by M. I. Roemer), New York, 1960

[49] *Practitioners letters to Lord Palmerston re: medical reform*, in *Edinburgh Med. J.*, Dec. 1857. The quotation comes from the final section "Free Competition in Medicine." An earlier statement is: "Make a clean sweep; remove every legislative enactment regarding the practice of medicine; leave it as free, as unprotected, as unlicensed, as baking or knife-grinding. Let our Colleges of Physicians and Surgeons, Faculties, and Worshipful Companies, make what terms they like for those who choose to enter them.... Give the principle its full swing, and, by so doing, be assured we would lose some of our worst quacks; but we would not lose our Alisons, our Symes, ... [and other great names]." In other words, let the professional organization, not government, act as its own "licensing agency."

[50] Jouanna, J. *Hippocrates*, translated by M. B. DeBevoise, Baltimore, 1999, chapter 5, for a description of the complex arena in which the Greek physician worked.

A clinician's wise decision may end with a bad outcome. Whether that decision actually was in error may never be known, but it will often be portrayed as wrong, especially in front of a jury. It was "wrong" despite being based on right reasoning as far as medical science could determine at the time, was not a deliberate error, and was done in the best interests of the patient. On the other hand, a clinically unwise institutional decision influenced by economic, social, and allocation policies may also end in a bad outcome. In that case the bad outcome would have been deliberate and the decision was not made on an individual's behalf; it was made on society's behalf, whether the institution making the decision was government or corporate. Ironically, this bad outcome will be viewed as acceptable, even though it was avoidable: "This is what we physicians are expected to do in a situation like this." Nevertheless, it was wrong, and wrong for a wrong reason, the wrong reason being the best interests of the society or institution rather than for the patient.

Sir James Spence underscores the covenant between the physician and patient that hinges on personal responsibility of the physician as the essence of medicine.[51] Many in society, however, view this differently; the group decision of the preceding paragraph may have been wrong, but it was wrong for the right reason: the best interests of the group. Those responsible for that wrong decision meant well, so how can they be culpable? But the clinician's decision is considered as wrong for the wrong reason inasmuch as he did not consider the welfare of the group and, therefore, he is culpable. How profoundly this threat stifles correct action. The practitioner is put in a position where he is safer implementing the group decision rather than the one he thinks is best, especially when there is an element of doubt, and doubt is the clinician's daily companion, that unseen force that propels him to study and study and to check, check, and check again. It is natural that in any collective action the individual will be cast below the group, and all this seems fine, until that day arrives when we, ourselves, become that individual. Then we, because of our self-deception, will have suddenly become the unenviable subjects of the greater good. But that unenviable practitioner now has his protection, for his accountability is no longer personal; it has been spread over society like jam on bread.

Accountability has implications for culpability. A bad outcome may trigger redress. Should the target be the group or the individual practitioner who follows the recommendation of the group? And who should determine whether a bad outcome resulted from malpractice? The lay public or the profession? Common sense answers both questions. The patient will have little chance for redress against the social establishment that caused the problem in the first place and from which it is essential that he retain his entitlements, and the physician will have little chance for redress against a jury seeking a scapegoat.

In the Garden of Eden no practitioner was needed, in the state of nature no practitioner was available, and in an imperfect world the natural state of medical practice is imperfect. Opinions, prejudices, and extent of knowledge are variables affecting both physician and patient, variables in a field of anxious action often tense with danger and pain. In ancient Greece, therefore, there were no laws expressly restricting the physician's domain. Plato espoused the eminent authority of the physician, as an expert, in patient management. Patients were not permitted to decline that advice.[52] Although Plato would

---

[51] Spence, J., *The Purpose and Practice of Medicine*, Oxford, 1960, p. 296.

[52] "We believe in them [doctors] whether they cure us with our consent or without it, …" Plato's *Statesman*, 293b, translation of C. J. Rowe, in *Plato; Complete Works*, Indianapolis, 1997, J. M. Cooper, editor. As per Plato, the source of the physician's authority is rather blatant; there is no one

have little or no autonomy assigned to patients, he did not circumscribe the physician's domain. He was, if nothing else, a champion of the expert. He would have restricted the independence of the patient, but not that of the physician, and in the event of a legal challenge with medical implications he would have the judges be physicians, not laiety.[53] Whereas other ancient societies threatened physicians with punitive measures should a bad outcome emerge, no such intimidation was made toward the Greek physician. This Greek concept had momentum, and Lucian of Samosata (125-180 AD) wrote: "But the medical profession should be left still more to their own discretion than other artists, in proportion to the greater nobility of their aims and usefulness of their work; this art should have a special right of choosing its objects; their sacred occupation, taught straight from Heaven, and pursued by the wisest men, should be secured against all compulsion, enslaved to no law, intimidated and penalized by no court, exposed to no votes or paternal threats or uninstructed passions."[54] In a word, no one presumed that a government or jury knew better than the physician about how to manage illness.

H. Medicine as a Career

It is a miracle that young men and women continue to choose medicine as a career. Remarkably, these acolytes agree to spend their lives amid other people's tribulations. And these are not the usual trials of life, the bad investment, the affront, the legal battle. They are profounder matters, another person's life or death, infirmity, human pathos. And the acolytes do so at the cost of accruing additional tribulations of their own. Plato frequently mentioned the physician, but he was no physician and could not be fully aware of the physician's cares and concerns, seemed not to realize that physicians and their families got sick and would be patients themselves and would die, that the profession of medicine provides its adherents no protection from the usual vicissitudes of life. In terms of risk/benefit it is indeed a miracle that anyone chooses it and does it well.

Dr. Edelstein argued that it was interest in the art of healing that attracted its practitioners and that provided the impetus for improvements and high standards of performance. And Plato concluded that in the ideal world the practitioner of an art would fulfill the aim of his art, income being an afterthought and not a motive.[55] Each profession would have its place to fulfill in society. And these sentiments are not far from the truth. Financial compensation alone should not attract any candidate to the profession, although the financial security that a decent salary will provide can be a secondary attractant. There

---

else who knows medicine better than the physician, so the matter is ended. Either this was just a point for argument's sake, or Plato had an extraordinarily optimistic opinion of contemporary medicine. This matter is discussed by G. Anagnastopoulos in: *Bioethics: Ancient Themes in Contemporary Issues*, Boston, 2002 (paperback edition), M. G. Kuczewski and R. Polansky, editors, p. 279*ff.*

[53] See Plato's *Nomoi* (Laws), 916 a-c.

[54] *The Works of Lucian of Samosata*, Oxford, 1905, 4 vols., translation of H. W. Fowler and F. G. Fowler, vol. 2, pp. 183-200. Admittedly, the cited words were spoken by a physician, and Lucian is known primarily as a satirist. But Prof. Christopher Robinson (*Lucian and His Influence in Europe*, Chapel Hill, 1979) considers this particular work, *The Disinherited*, to belong to his "ingenious" works, not the "comic" ones.

[55] Edelstein, L., *Ancient Medicine*, Baltimore, 1967, Pt. 3, The Professional Ethics of the Greek Physician, p. 319.

is a difference between medicine, and perhaps professions generally, and the world of capitalism. Money may reflect worth and perhaps even be viewed as a trophy, but the motivation for entering medicine is not money. Money may be an incentive for working in a particular environment, which means that higher income could attract some to work in difficult locations, a recompense for inconveniences. And money may be an incentive for longer hours or more difficult schedules or for becoming skilled in select procedures. And it may help level the playing field when it comes to physician availability. But it must not be allowed to entice persons to enter the field. And the reason is this: when the critical moment arrives, there is not enough money available to compensate a good clinician for his worth. The true clinician whose impetus for perfection is money will never exist.

There are many who sincerely wish to aid humanity and to heal the sick, many who profess a willingness to endure the inconveniences of a medical career. The popular regard for the physician and various financial and commercial attractions all contribute to the competition for this place in the sun. But medicine is not a place in the sun. Medicine is an arduous and stressful profession, one with many moments of great satisfaction, but it is not a particularly cheery one. Those wishing a career of cheeriness should enter vaudeville or perhaps politics. It would be nice if government were to make medicine a "cheerful" career. And it will certainly try. The collegiality associated with advisory boards, lobbying teams, disciplinary councils, and consensus panels provides the opportunity for fraternal coffee breaks, congratulatory dinners, and insider trading. But this is not the clinician's world. His is one of personal responsibility, personal accountability, and solo cups of coffee on the move. And so, for all those who would be a physician, decide which world you seek. If you choose the former you will be Dr. Sigerist's ideal physician, intent on transforming the world by furthering the general welfare of society, and you will often have the time and luxury to be cheery. Should you choose the latter you will be busy and burdened, but you will not be bored, and most of all you will be content.

I. Conclusion

Man the individual is, like other animals, reflexive and instinctive. Society, however, opens a new world of possibilities, for man can be optimally rational only in a group. It is in the hashing out of problems that the closest approximations to objective truth are found. Man's successes and failures, therefore, reflect his group. The Newtons and the Lockes would have been considered undesirables or irrational in many, indeed most, societies, and to a great extent England and Englishmen must be credited for their singular honors. Original and clever ideas, which all humans have, must be validated against other models to determine superiority. This can only be done in discussion in an open society, in an atmosphere that permits equitable give and take.

Dr. Kathleen Freeman concluded, from her studies of the Greek city-state, that "... the individual way of life in smaller units" was key to the phenomenon of a profusion of great thinkers arising from the city-state. This theory she felt was supported by their disappearance following the destruction of the city-state by Philip II of Macedonia (359-

336 BC).[56] With regard to medicine, the present work is in partial agreement, for evidence has been presented that geography, population, ethnicity, wealth, power, or even education cannot be credited with advancing medicine. But, in comparing Rome with transcendant Greece, she wrote: "The Romans were wonderful organizers, [but] an organization is not a place where people are encouraged to seek or to be free." What this work has attempted to show, in contrast, is that it is specifically the organization that is the *sine qua non* for progress, that the key to progress is not so much individualism, for that is ever nascent, as it is the ability of individuals to freely express their ideas and to freely associate with others doing the same. It is the nature of the organization that is the key, for it must be a koinon. And it is as a koinon that the threats to scientific medicine must be countered.

But an important feature of the koinon is size: it serves its purpose best when it is a forum for the individual. Greek city-states were relatively small by today's municipal size, and the number of voting citizens smaller still. Each voting citizen, therefore, having opinions about problems faced in common, could voice those opinions in open forum. As its value resides in individual expression, beyond a certain size it is impractical to permit any and all to express their opinions and to give those opinions adequate consideration. Politicization, therefore, is the natural consequence as blocs exploit legal venues, prominent persons, and rhetoric as they vie for control. A county or perhaps even a state medical association will qualify as a koinon, for each member can be heard, but a national association of physicians is a political animal, and it leaders often have political ambitions. Even further removed from a true koinon, of course, is a national health service, so far removed, in fact, that it is entirely a political tool. But the idea of the political economist, Arthur Young (1741-1820), that "there is but one all-powerful cause which instigates mankind, and that is government," hopefully has been utterly discredited by the preceding chapters.[57]

There are, however, a few problems that are best served by large groups, the most important being self-protection, for there truly is strength in numbers. But beyond a limited array of concerns, large organizations are a disservice, for they tend to be polarizing and, if they err, they do so on a calamitous scale. Plato specified in *Laws* the ideal size of a city-state, some 5040 voting citizens, but his calculation was the sum of people required to staff what he considered were the city-state's necessary committees, not a practical number that gave all individuals equal opportunity to voice their opinions. But several thousand may not exceed by much the maximum number supportable by a true koinon.[58]

---

[56] Freeman, K. *Greek City-States*, London, 1950; see her summary, p. 266. Elsewhere in that work Freeman decries Greek individualism in favor of a socialist compact, citing the destruction of Greece from unchecked self-interest.

[57] Arthur Young, a prominent English political writer, economist, and agriculturist, meant that government's ability to produce grand projects of great usefulness was the primary cause for progress, a concept prompted by the vastly improved conditions of the roads as he traveled from Spain into France. (See: Young, A., *Travels during the Years 1787, 1788, and 1789*, Bury St. Edmunds, 1792, p. 29.) While it is true that in matters of scale governments, by printing or appropriating mammon, can generate projects more massive than the wealthiest citizen could capitalize, but it is not logical that progress will inevitably follow. Such projects throughout history have primarily facilitated the extension of power and efficiency of the state. This is not the type of progress that is the focus of the present work.

[58] For an interesting discourse on city size and general agreement over the ages on its optimum size see: Sale, K., *Human Scale*, New York, 1982, chapter 5, "The Optimum City," pp.192-208.

As long as physicians' associations were comprised within the Greek city-state there was no pressure for them to be other than small and autonomous and no incentive for regional organization. But with the city-states fading from the assaults of Philip II and then the Romans, Hippocratic practitioners had no regional alliances from which to seek protection. The stability of such an alliance, whether of a governmental or commercial nature, might have proved to be the salvation of the profession. This book, by focusing on the individual and the small group, has circumvented a huge fact of the modern medical profession: there is a risk that physicians' groups or associations of insufficient size and political strength will permit the profession to be overwhelmed by political or commercial forces, in a way analogous to the overwhelming of Hippocratic medicine by the leviathan that was the Roman Empire.[59] A protection of the koinon is needed, and organizational size thus becomes a positive attribute. It is essential, therefore, that the protecting organization(s) representing the medical profession or segments of it be large enough not only to guarantee the credentials of its membership, but also to resist external regulation. On the other hand, it must not usurp responsibilities best left to the smaller koinon.

For Hippocratic medicine disappeared because it did not, or could not, do those things. The same may be occurring in Western medicine today. Viewed more and more as an employee and technician, more an expeditor than provider of medical care, the physician can seem an adversary rather than an ally if he disagrees with either an institutional guideline or an entitled patient's demands; he is himself becoming an entitlement, a serf. While physicians may attend national meetings of their profession, an expression of statutory allegiance, their functional allegiance is fragmented among ten thousand trifling bureaucratic structures.

Today's debate about the control of medical care, whether governmental or quasi governmental (such as health maintenance organizations), has unfortunately ensnared the physician and the medical koinon. To avoid taking the path followed by virtually all the failed medical professions of authoritarian societies in the past, it is necessary that clinical physicians remain free of this entanglement. It is often argued that American physicians, having received their training in institutions that have received varying degrees of financial support from the federal or state government, have an implied obligation to provide care such as society, within limits, may require of them. This is not a valid argument. The standard of clinical practice is understood by all to be the Hippocratic Oath; the Oath is recited in medical schools by many entering classes, and even those most detached from the medical field or its knowledge will still be aware of the Hippocratic Oath and its essential role in shaping medical practice. And nowhere in the Oath is there mention of society or society's medical needs. That discussion requires a separate arena. The Oath concerns only the individual clinical physician and patient. Public money, therefore, has been invested in medical education for the purpose of producing physicians that will abide by the Hippocratic Oath.

There is, furthermore, no mention in the Oath of a medical hierarchy within the profession itself, much less for medical leadership from the outside. The clinician's

---

[59] The issue here is basically a quantitative one, for both large and small groups become effective by passing through similar stages, namely those identified by Tuckman: the superficial acquaintances of formation, the turbulence ignited by discussion of serious issues, the subsequent acknowledgment of and trust in internal opposition, and finally the effective and efficient group use of resources (see: Tuckman, B., *Developmental sequence in small groups*, in: *Psychological Bulletin*, 63:384-399, 1965).

professional allegiance is solely to his patients and to his koinon. Although procedural issues require executive leadership in organizations, it is the individual member of the koinon, not some higher authority, who wields the power.

If the authoritarian shadow is permitted to continue its invasion of the profession, the accumulated knowledge stored in libraries and computers guarantee that knowledge will not, as in the past, become lost; it will merely become pointless. The individual patient will lose significance by micromanagement of the professions. At least in ancient Rome State regulation impinged only on providers of medical care, not on the recipients. Ethical solutions to issues of human mortality will be replaced by technical ones. As these trends persist and when a certain level of implementation has occurred, a degree of entropy will so completely characterize the field of medicine that it will cease to exist in the form recognized today. While it may retain some technical advances, in practice it will be impersonal, inefficient, and arbitrary. The Hippocratic Oath will be amended, not to make the Oath better but to make it more convenient for enforcement. And it will be majority representation by nonprofessionals that prioritizes medical education, treatment, and research. Selection of practitioners and rationing of diagnostic and treatment modalities will be legislative activities, and popular perceptions and special interest groups will promote society's research interests.[60] Perhaps over the next century the West will revisit the ways of ancient Egypt wherein medicine becomes totally the domain of State functionaries. It happened in the Soviet Union with the expected iniquitous results. It must not be forgotten that Hippocratic medicine vanished gradually, silently, and without a witness, yet in full view of society. In full view and in stealthy steps the same process is occurring today as societies surrender individual liberty in return for security imprudently thought to be provided by a powerful central government. If some calamitous global event occurs at a time when personal accountability is sufficiently effaced, there could be an even more rapid decline and fall of scientific medicine. At that point a dormant Hippocratic medicine will be awaiting the next global calamity that at its

---

[60] It is sobering to reflect on *Lysenkoism*, a phenomenon of the recent past. False hypotheses have always been, and will always be, part of man's search for the truth, a concomitant of the natural process of seeking causation. False hypotheses can be "a product of fanaticism" or merely the result of idle speculation, but the vast majority of false hypotheses result from honest error, usually an error of logic. There is, however, a natural process in an open society that permits false doctrines or hypotheses to be disproved or altered to accommodate new data, to be discarded or corrected bit by bit. In Soviet Russia, in contrast, T. D. Lysenko, disregarding "bourgeois" Western scientific evidence regarding DNA, postulated that the basis for hereditary was the cell itself, not a discrete subunit within the cell. He argued that cells could metabolically or otherwise adapt to environmental change and pass that adaptation to daughter cells, the "inheritance of acquired characteristics." He based his theory on virtually no scientifically validated evidence. But, under the crushing authoritarianism of a wishfully thinking dictatorship of the proletariat, his work, which began in 1929 and was praised by Kruschev well into the 1960s, prompted monuments, hymns, and portraits as *Lysenkoism* obtained, under the banner of Marxism, the status of a cult. This cult was exported "to other socialist states." Among its practical consequences were massive crop failures, the purging and deaths of top scientists, the quashing of careers, and a profound dampening of Soviet science. By restraining alternative ideas the State confers a monopoly that gives its preferred doctrine a life of its own. To succeed, a government susceptible to such reprehensible policies requires three things: centralization, censorship, and favoritism. It helps if the favored candidate is a fanatic, as was Lysenko, but a conspirator is also satisfactory. In medieval times the false doctrine thrived because of ignorance. Now it thrives because of politics. See: Medvedev, Z. A., *The Rise and Fall of T. D. Lysenko*, New York, 1969, translated by I. M. Lerner, and Soyfer, V.N., *Lysenko and the Tragedy of Soviet Science*, New Jersey, 1995, translated by L. and R. Gruliow.

passing will hopefully provide humanity another opportunity to escape self-imposed bondage.

Breaches in the organization and function of the medical profession have been reviewed. There are many. As a first step to reduce its vulnerability the following recommendations have been derived from a study of past successes and failures:

a. Adhere to the Hippocratic Oath.

b. Cease dependence on paramedicine by increasing the number of traditional clinical physicians and by training selected existing paramedicine practitioners to be physicians.

c. Become more competitive with alternative medicine; do not incorporate its procedures, do not join with it, and do not assail it.

d. Require all management positions in the profession to be filled by clinicians.

e. Identify only the individual clinician as accountable for his patient, group opinions having no legal force.

f. Avoid entangling alliances with commercial, governmental, and ethicist organizations, concentrating instead on the quality of clinical practice and communication among members.

g. Divest the profession of irrelevant and contentious specialties and subspecialties.

h. The independent medical koinon must be maintained at all costs, and maintained distinct from, and superior to, any larger medical organization(s) devised to protect it.

By these means survival of scientific Hippocratic medicine can be guaranteed in a democratic state and shored up against any future political chaos or authoritarian gambit until such time as essential freedoms can be reinstated. These recommendations do not reflect a sentimental return to the days of Hippocrates and the peripatetic physician; they are the means for retaining the fundamental values of the physician-patient relationship and the natural state of medical practice.

EPILOGUE TO PART I

"No systematic thought has made progress apart from some adequately general working hypothesis adapted to its special topic."

Alfred North Whitehead (1861-1947), referenced by
W. O. Aydelotte in *Quantitation in History*,
Reading, MA, 1971, p. 75

Part I, in seeking the natural state of medical practice, has presented contrasting interpretations of the course of medicine through the ages. On the one hand is the idea that mankind is inevitably, albeit gradually and erratically, improving its situation, that medicine since the first medicine-man has shown a continuum of improvement attributable to accumulated successes by which generations build on the work of earlier ones, and that this pattern, despite the occasional anomaly, will be sustained (Fig. 13, top). On the other hand is the idea that mankind has always recognized a certain basal level of empirical knowledge, its nature being relatively similar worldwide, and one that cannot be improved upon except in a free society. Absent protection from authoritarian forces, therefore, any advance can be erased and popular knowledge can return to the basal, and thereby primitive, level (Fig. 13, bottom). That the latter interpretation is reinforced by the course of medical science and the natural state of medical practice in the West following the age of Hippocrates should be obvious.[1]

This volume also has described the critical association of medical progress with individual and group freedom, an association to which the natural state of medical practice is indebted. Does it have a wider relevance? Whether a successful collaboration between group freedom and progress can be found in other arts and sciences is not addressed, although a recent Center for Hellenic Studies colloquium concluded that affluence and empire did not in themselves explain the greatness of the art, rhetoric, and other intellectual activities that was ancient Athens. In its publication of the proceedings of the colloquium there was this following summation: "As many essays in this volume suggest, it [Athenian dominance] was as much or more a consequence of specific conditions and

---

[1] It is on this point that the prominent sociologist, Dr. Nisbet, and the author part company (see footnote, p. 134, for a brief summary of Dr. Nisbet's position). While both are in agreement on the importance of the hostile interference with progress by authoritarian and over-weaning governance, Dr. Nisbet concludes that graded progress, even if slowed, will occur just as it has for thousands of years because the idea of "progress" is embedded in the Western mind. In the present work, however, evidence to the contrary has been introduced and posits a different mechanism for progress, namely, the free expression of innate human ability, an ability that is found in all people regardless of geography. Activation of this ability is greatly restricted in the authoritarian state, which explains both the inability of authoritarian governments to progress and the ability of authoritarian governments to inhibit progress. The European Dark Ages are a proof of this thesis. Thus, mankind's periods of progress have been sporadic, rare, and expungeable. To those who would argue that modernity and its lip-service to individual liberty is now globally embedded in too many cultures to be reversed, we need but look about us to see how quickly forgotten is the 20th C and its social engineering atrocities, authoritarian gambits on a scale affecting hundreds of millions of souls, some being fervent admirers, but most being forcibly fed, led, or dead. And forget not that the immutability of human nature as discussed in the Introduction persists, now being affixed to enormously destructive power available to petty authoritarians the world over.

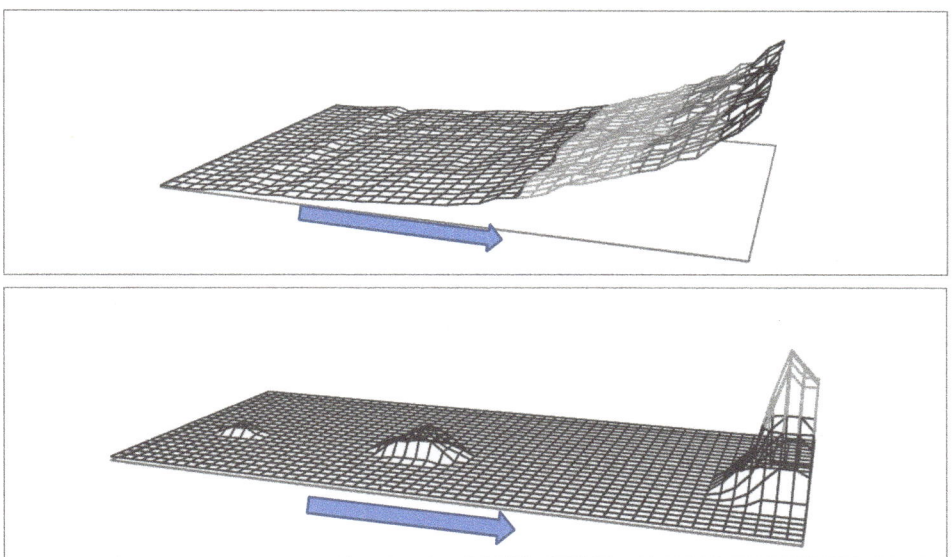

Fig. 13: Three-dimensional hypothetical and nonquantitative representations of medical progress over 5000 years. X axis (arrow) = time; Y axis = progress.

Top: Representation of the traditional view of human progress, in which advances, while global, sporadic, and either isolated or in clusters, are somehow cumulative, resulting in a gradual upward progress of mankind irrespective of social conditions. There are innumerable tiny peaks in an irregular global distribution, each representing some significant new discovery or invention that improves medical knowledge and contributes to medical progress of all mankind.

Bottom: Here the peaks are few, large, and focused, each peak representing documented periods of rational and increasingly scientific medical practice on a regional societal level, with the baseline representing steady state empirical knowledge that perpetually waxes and wanes as local discoveries are made and then are forgotten. The first small peak on the left coincides with the postulated appearance of rational medicine in Sumerian city-states and in predynastic Egypt, followed by the peak for Hellas of the Hippocratics and then the large peak on the right side of the graph associated with modern Western medicine. An increasing global population over the millennia invalidates any effort to semiquantitate the intensity and diffusion of medical discovery for the three periods.

policies created by the democracy."[2]

  Are these conclusions relevant to the present day? They are. The nature of social evolution as it relates to medicine would be a mere matter for academic debate were it not for the uncountable human tragedies that have followed on its errant development. The Dark Ages as presented herein represent one example of the consequences. John Stuart Mill noted that "the greater part of the world has, properly speaking, no history; because the despotism of Custom is complete," for "justice and right mean conformity to custom" that "no one ... thinks of resisting."[3] "Despotism" is the operative word here, but its agent

---

[2] *Democracy, Empire, and the Arts in Fifth-Century Athens*, Cambridge, 1998, D. Boedeker and K. A. Raaflaub, editors, chapter 15.

[3] Mill, J. S., *On Liberty*, chapter 3.

is rarely "custom." It is, instead, despotism in its colloquial sense that is able to manipulate "custom" to its own advantage, and it comes in many guises, whether an ideology, a ruthless and selfish faction, or specific individuals whose names have been seared into humanity's memory of 20th C despotism.

But medicine mirrors the status of society at large, especially the plebeian segment. The logic of the argument put forth in this work and its evidentiary support proposes that modern medicine was close at hand in Hippocratic times. Others have put forth explanations for the failure of a scientific revolution to occur either then or during the later Greco-Roman era. Their explanations have included (1) the reliance on deductive rather than inductive reasoning, on speculation rather than observation, (2) an inability to physically come to grips with the practical realities of experimental method, (3) the incapacity for comprehending that nature could be understood and manipulated ("dissected") apart from a natural philosophy of the cosmos as a whole, (4) restrictions inherent in a slaveholdingsociety, and (5) a quantitative deficiency of interested participants and an associated social "weakness" for science.[4] As this work has shown, however, it was due to none of these things. The cause is far simpler, basic, and relevant not just to Europe and the West but to global evolution of scientific process itself. The issue is individual and group freedom, and Hippocratic physicians simply were given insufficient time for fully developing broad-based scientific endeavors.[5] They were well on their way in medicine, and this might have been the catalyst for other disciplines. Given perhaps another century of unimpeded innovation, the equivalent of the many inventions and discoveries of 19th C clinical medicine should have been available and in everyday use before the time of Christ, inventions and discoveries likely to have stimulated similar progress in other scientific fields. Indeed, while perhaps fanciful, why not consider the possibility that a similar phenomenon could have occurred in ancient Sumer or predynastic Egypt? So adaptable, so marvelous, so creative and efficient is the human mind that, if comprehension is not clouded by emotion, facts unobscured by myth

---

[4] Cohen, H. F., *The Scientific Revolution: A Historiographical Inquiry,* Chicago, 1994. Chapter 4 contains a comprehensive review and critique of these and other recent scholarly opinions on the causes for the emergence of early modern science. In particular, the ancient Greek difficulty with combining "Ideas and Facts," discussed in relation to William Whewell's opinion as to why Greek science was not followed by a scientific revolution as occurred in the 17th C, is directly relevant to the present discussion, although addressed by formal logic.

[5] Let a generous one hundred years be assigned to the era of Hippocratic medicine during which its reputation was acquired: 500-400 BC. Now let Harvey's *De Motu Cordis* be dated from the time of his first lectures on the subject of the circulation (1616) and the state of medicine be described in England and Europe a century later (1716), only a few years after Dr. Samuel Johnson had his scrofula "cure" with the touch of Queen Anne on his neck. Theories and quackery were beginning to run rampant, and virtually all images of the physician, whether in oil or intaglio, were defamatory. Dr. Baas calls the vast array of medical frauds that provided care to the "masses" in Europe a "Corps of medical savages." (See his *Outlines of the History of Medicine*, New York, 1889, translated by H. E. Handerson, p. 771.) He also states that pharmacognosy did not significantly advance in the 18th C, and he includes an extensive passage on contemporary medical practice from a 1721 edition of *Artzney-Teuffel* by Ananais Horer, a classic publication that described the source of 1,500 medicinal botanicals for household use. Thus, even though *De Motu Cordis* was promptly acknowledged and accepted throughout the British Isles and Europe within thirty years (Weil, E., *The Echo of Harvey's De Motu Cordis* (1628) 1628-1657, in *J. Hist. Med. Allied Sci.*, 12:167-174, 1957), the mispractice of medicine remained undiminished for more than a century. From this one should be astonished by the progress of the Hippocratics over a similar period in the ancient world.

and falsehood, and salutary action not impeded by the bully, the ability of the human brain to deftly lift its entourage up from the fear and brutishness surrounding primitive circumstance will promptly lead to a life permitting healthful security and provide the occasion for introspection and wonder at the brief but glorious opportunity humans have been granted on earth. That has rarely happened, however, for a culprit, authoritarianism in its multifarious guises, has intervened as our social Satan. Not just the European Dark Ages, but also the wars, enslavements, and incalculable other injustices to all sentient beings can be traced to that same evil creation. Although human nature entails a social structure to restrain its brutish components, it is no answer to deny the expression of brutish behavior to most but relegate it to a few. And that is the context of the authoritarianism that has been under consideration herein. Twentieth century authoritarianism is now being revived and has resumed its march for control not only of geography but of the individual as well, this time perhaps on a global scale, and many an individual is now selfishly but gladly exchanging his freedoms for an idealistic security at the cost of chatteldom for his progeny. Should this process persevere the course of clinical medicine, already in disarray, will be profoundly transformed within a few generations, as has happened repeatedly throughout history. Perhaps salvation from its baneful effects will be realized by new and global means of communication, for no longer can the human mind be easily confined to an authoritarian cage, a doleful feature of the 20th C, as long as there are no infringements on our ability to responsibly communicate with one another.

It is the thesis of this book that the peaks indicated in Fig. 13 coincide as well with the intensity and diffusion of individual liberty of the citizenry.[6] Thus, a civilization that provides or permits individual freedom will register progress, but should that freedom disappear there will be, over time, a reversion to a primitive empirical status common to all authoritarian societies. A Greek word can be appropriated for the theory of human society that has resulted, by means of felicitous liberty, in the natural state of medical practice and medical progress. That word is "isagorial," from ἰσηγορία, meaning a society that demonstrates "equal opportunity to speak in public assembly" and, by modern extension, freedom of assembly.[7] An "isagorial" theory of human progress is appropriate because of its etymological derivation: ἴσος (isos, equality) and ἀγόρα (agora, popular assemblage). Its characteristics, as employed here, are:

---

[6] Part II of this volume, which includes an analysis of the social conditions contemporary with medical progress in ancient Sumer, Egypt, India and China, supports this thesis.

[7] ἰσηγορία was used by Herodotus in his *Histories* (Bk. 5.78) in comparing virtues of Persians and Greeks. Although he was reticent in his admiration for democracy, he could not avoid concluding the obvious, that freedom could be a great good, for it explained the military successes of the Greeks over vastly larger Persian forces. As for the word "isagorial," it is a neologism in it is not in the Liddell and Scott Lexicon. Instead there is ἰσηγορία. And ἰσογορία has seen academic use. But ἀγορεύω refers to speaking in public assembly. I have, therefore, used an "a" rather than the usual "e" or "o" because of the relative familiarity to readers of history of the ancient Greek "agora." A term for equality before the law is "isonomial."

1. It is the basis of *all* human apolitical progress up to the present time.[8]
2. It is sporadic, voluntary, inclusive, autochthonous, and independent of other social factors.
3. It is facilitated by and protected by democracy, but democracy is merely a permissive step for development of an isagorial society.
4. As a consequence of (3), it is not a political force and has no coercive function.
5. It is qualitatively proportional to the degree of individual liberty.
6. It is quantitatively proportional to the diffusion of individual liberty.
7. It is temporally proportional to the institutionalization of individual liberty.
8. It is most effectively expressed through its tolerance of voluntary and independent groups of free individuals with focused selfoldingest having equal opportunity to state their opinions without fear of retribution, groups identified herein by an ancient Greek word, the "koinon."

What is not at all clear is the course of medicine from this point forward. There are problems with today's profession as it drifts further from its natural state. Is it, as phrased in the Introduction, "on some unnatural course or merely an alternative pathway?" If it is on an unnatural course, will some minor corrective serve to return it to its traditional place, or are there signs that during this century an authoritarian blight will return mankind to the level of the subservient and the subjective and, by exploiting the medical profession as its accomplice, displace again the natural state of medical practice and prove the *isagorial theory of human progress* to be correct? But many brilliant experts of high political station are at work shaping our futures. Shall we not trust them and await events?

---

[8] A misinterpretation of the importance of the isagorial theory of human progress may result from the appearance of prosperity and growth of knowledge in an age of global authoritarianism. There are two reasons for this. (1) Many of the benefits of a free society are also desired by an authoritarian one, and the latter will purchase, copy, or steal fruits of the ingenuity emerging in a free society. (2) There are pockets of freedom in any large society, including strictly authoritarian ones, from which the occasional good idea can emerge. A combination of these factors can suggest forward progress of mankind independent of social structure. But the present work argues that the more authoritarian the society the less likely this will occur and the more likely that a trend, perhaps precipitous, to baseline empiricism will at some point reassert itself.

PART II: PREHISTORICAL ANALYSIS

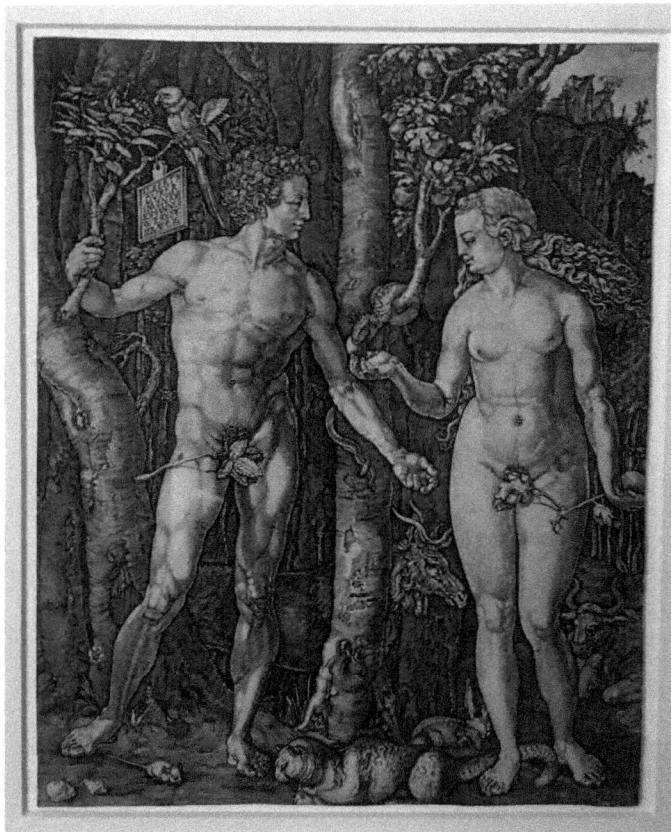

Fig. 14: This copy of the famous rendering by Albrecht Durer of the original sin opens this volume on a note suggesting a profound and universal significance to its topic, which is true. Can social egalitarianism be equated with eating an apple from the Tree of Knowledge of Good and Evil? The bite from the apple can be viewed, metaphorically or fundamentally, as an attempt to personally acquire the right to define good and evil. In doing it allows the strongest among us to define right and wrong in others, whereas natural law declares all humanity has in its collective conscience but one definition. It is argued here that the coerciveness of egalitarianism, by constraining human liberty, has stunted progress of mankind from its earliest days. In doing so, egalitarianism can be viewed as contrary to nature, as described by Dr. Murray Rothbard, and contrary to natural law, as defined by John Locke.[1] The temptation to have others do our bidding is not a violation if others can freely choose not to do so. But once coercive, the unhealthful consequences of the choice of egalitarianism, like the bite from the apple, can afflict untold generations of both its choosers and those innocents who had no choice in the matter. The focus of this book is the latter.

---

[1] References for the two works are: Rothbard, M. N., *Egalitarianism as a Revolt Against Nature*, Auburn (AL), 2000, 2nd edition, the opening essay, p. 1; John Locke's *Second Treatise on Government*, chapter 5, section 6: "The state of nature has a law of nature to govern it, which obliges every one: and reason, which is that law, teaches all mankind, who will but consult it, that being all equal and independent, no one ought to harm another in his life, health, liberty, or possessions." Also see *Essay* II, chapter xxviii, section 8; here he calls as Divine law what today is considered natural law. For a discussion of the *Book of Genesis* and its implications for natural law, see: Forte, D., *Eve without Adam: What Genesis Has to Tell America about Natural Law*, the Russell Kirk Memorial Lecture, from The Heritage Lectures, 1996.

CHAPTER TWENTY-SIX

EXEGESIS

"So adaptable, so marvelous, so creative and efficient is the human mind that, if comprehension is not clouded by emotion, facts unobscured by myth and falsehood, and salutary action not impeded by the bully, the ability of the human brain to deftly lift its entourage up from the fear and brutishness surrounding primitive circumstance will promptly lead to a life permitting healthful security and provide the occasion for introspection and wonder at the brief but glorious opportunity humans have been granted on earth."

> The author of the present work (from the Epilogue to Part I)

Given the present subject, its huge volume and its vast unknowns, this opening chapter for Part II offers such justification for its examination and interpretation of ancient civilizations as is seemly for a clinical physician with an eye to the dearth of effective medical care over the ages.

A. Justification for This Endeavor

Following such a prolix encomium on the human mind what can another book add? After thousands of years of practice it would seem that the human mind must already have things well under control, for today we in the West are generally quite comfortable, secure, and long-lived in comparison to the whole of human history. Alas, that is not the case. Part I of this volume began with a regional appraisal of historical medical practices around the globe, but it soon became apparent that only twice in human history has a natural state of medical practice been approximated and it was only during those two periods that sustained medical progress occurred, one being Hippocratic medicine during the age of Classical Greece (5th and 4th centuries BC) and the other being Western medicine since the late 18th C. The opportunity for the human mind to "lift its entourage" has, it seems, rarely occurred in the course of human history, and emotion, myth, falsehood, and the bully have proven able adversaries.

It was revealed in Part I that the collected knowledge obtained approximately 4,500 years ago during an embryonic stage of the specified civilizations included rational observations that over time became part of bureaucratic canon passed on as dogma from generation to generation with no significant additions and no significant challenge from new generations of official practitioners. Restating these observations, rational medical progress may have been under way in four disparate geographic regions much earlier in human social evolution than in Classical Greece. It was, however, commandeered by social forces with little interest in medical care other than as it might help maintain political hegemony. The "entourage," or body politic, appears not to have been "lifted."

Were the culprits that derailed early historic medical practices the same that derailed Hippocratic medicine, and are they a threat to modern Western medicine? Part I explained that, given the considerable medical insight obtained by Hippocratic physicians as indicated in recent translations of their clinical writings, the same interval of 2,000 years stood between Hippocratic medicine and modern Western medicine. That interval, from 300 BC to 1700 AD, was associated with a reversion of the entire Western culture to an extended period of profound medical ignorance, the years 500-1000 AD often being referred to as the European Dark Ages. It was shown that in the 18th C medical progress had to begin anew, starting from scratch.[2]

There is reason, therefore, to consider a larger view of the Dark Ages, namely, that most of humanity since its first appearance on this planet has lived in the Dark Ages, that here and there have been occasional dazzling glimpses of what the human mind was capable of doing, evanescent examples of genius and progress unfortunately doomed to disappear after a brief time in the sun. Hippocratic medicine was one of those examples. The others were the beginning of a rational clinical practice in ancient Mesopotamia (Sumer), predynastic or early Dynastic Egypt, the Indian subcontinent (Indus River Valley civilization), and predynastic China. Also in Part I, medical empiricism was shown to be the default system for medical practice. Once a progressing civilization fails, humanity must reinvent medical progress, once again beginning at the baseline level of empirical personal experience, a cycle repeated throughout the ages. In rediscovering medical progress we do not "stand on the shoulders of giants" of a previous age. This harmful piece of fiction has prompted undue reverence for the "great man" theory of progress whereby a civilization lionizes a few great personalities thought to make key decisions or discoveries that help set everything aright, whereas the true begetters and heroes of "setting everything aright" are, instead, the common man and woman of the brilliant species of hominid, *Homo sapiens*, who, if not suppressed or victimized, will automatically and without prompting drive civilization toward its zenith.[3]

But what factors led to development of rational medical practice in the first place? This may seem to modern readers a mere academic point of interest to archeologists, but the 20th C was flooded with examples of reversion to profound

---

[2] J. B. Bury, in his *The Idea of Progress: An Inquiry into Its Origin and Growth* (New York, 1932), makes clear his conclusion that the intellectual concept of "progress" is a recent human development that can be traced back only to the 17th C AD. This is in marked contrast to the present work, which views progress as being repeatedly attempted in all societies since mankind's origin, its absence from the prehistorical and historical record being a consequence of its inhibition rather than want of its initiation.

[3] The great importance of certain individuals in propelling progress was compared to governance and to economics by the eminent historian Herbert Butterfield (see: *The History of Science and the Study of History*, in *Harvard Library Bulletin*, 13:329-347, 1959). But his "individuals" (*e.g.*, Francis Bacon, Isaac Newton) are described as uniquely qualified for their role in the advancement of progress. Butterfield thereby minimizes the significance of both the social environment in which they worked and the innate intelligence of the human species. This is in contrast to the individualism posited in this work in which the underlying thesis is that since the first humans there have been innumerable Newtons. As for any demeaning comments about how we stand on the shoulders of giants, be assured that it is the historical interpretation of transmission of knowledge that is being demeaned, not the persons who made the discoveries. It is the fact that every advance must be rediscovered that is the issue. Another exception involves discoveries or inventions within the time-frame of a given civilization, for obviously if someone clever makes an important discovery and that discovery leads to other discoveries or inventions, it is appropriate to praise the original discoverer, for the original discovery is a "shoulder" on which others could build (or stand). It is akin to a meme, which is "an element of a culture or system of behavior that may be considered to be passed from one individual to another by nongenetic means, especially by imitation." Like genetic evolution, the more useful or interesting a discovery or invention is the more likely its transmission and mimetic effects will be extensive.

ignorance, including medical ignorance, of hundreds of millions of people manipulated through powerful State propaganda, physical exclusions or social and commercial activism. With modern communications of the digital age perhaps there will be no repeat of similar efforts to impress ignorance on millions, but with electronic marvels that can be manipulated with the flip of the switch, censorship is imposable on a vast scale. What will happen if modern medicine becomes, as has inevitably happened in the past, an authoritarian tool, a government bauble? It is reasonable, therefore, to understand how rational medicine began so that, should social calamity threaten, mechanisms of repair and prevention can be promptly instituted. Part II of this volume seeks the answer to that question. But in doing so it is swimming upstream against the studied opinions of great historians and sociologists of the past. Dr. Arnold Toynbee inferred, with an intellectual bias, a Western-oriented goal was the common goal for all civilizations, judging progress and self-determination to be a gauge of success and a failure to proceed in that direction the cause of their demise. In contrast, Dr. Henri Frankfort, from his Egyptian studies, concluded that each civilization could be understood only as a unique culture, its success gauged by internal constructs of its own culture rather than how it compared to other civilizations, a relativistic approach. Part II will elude both relativism and western tradition by focusing on the more fundamental nature of our species, more on a biological than a cultural basis for the passage of civilizations.[4]

The present work, therefore, will inquire into the authors, the social environment, and the fragile mechanisms that permitted and fostered the early medical classics in the first place. It is remarkable that scholars from four extensive regional civilizations have, over many centuries, assigned the authority for regional development of medical philosophy and medical practice to eras bordering on the prehistoric and technically designated the Late Neolithic and Bronze Ages, the dates in the range of 2500-2000 BC.[5] Those regions, their primary culture, their modern States, examples of their venerable medical writings, and dates of the oldest extant versions of those writings are reiterated here:

North Africa (Nile River culture) Egypt *Ebers* and *Smith* papyri   1550 BC
Near East (Mesopotamian culture) Iraq *Diagnostic and Therapeutic Manual* 1100 BC
South Asia (Indus River culture) India *Charaka* and *Susruta* Samhitas   100 BC
East Asia (Yellow River culture) China *Huang Ti Nei Ching Su Wen*   200 BC

This will then be followed by a comparison of that assessment with analyses from twelve pristine civilizations/proto-civilizations. All sixteen will also be viewed with an eye to pre-Hippocratic Greece and the city-state of Miletos.

B. Justification for the Use of Medicine as a Symbol of Progress

In Part I the history of medicine was examined for evidence of the natural state of medical practice, defined as "a clinically effective medical practice free from

---

[4] For a discussion of historical perspectives and criticism, see, for example: Frankfort, H., *The Birth of Civilization in the Near East*, London, 1951.
[5] Bronze Age dates are approximate and there is regional variation. Mesopotamian region: 2900-1200 BC; South Asia region: 3000-1200 BC; East Asia region: 2000-700 BC; North Africa region: 3100-1200 BC.

institutional influences or other forms of external coercion except for those social influences to which both physician and patient are equally exposed and susceptible." As clinical medicine was the fundamental issue it was appropriate that the author be a clinical physician licensed in the specialty of Internal Medicine, although the breadth of the topic at times strayed considerably from the field of medicine. Part II will seem even further afield, as it addresses evidence for the progress of societies generally, doing so by examining prehistoric and historic civilizations that have arisen in very different times and places. It is argued, however, that by using the profession of medicine as a yardstick, all societies can receive equitable assessment. Medical care, after all, is a universal marker of societal progress. Disease, with its infirmities, suffering, and mortal closures, is a primal, unrelenting, and pervasive motivational stimulus common to all mankind even when other motivational stimuli are inoperable. Although there is regional variation in type, cause, and treatment of illness, there is an overall similarity in the human condition as it pertains to health. Medical practices, therefore, are a generic marker of progress that can be applied to any human population, although writing can serve as well, albeit in a much more restricted way. The prominent Indian philosopher, Dr. Debiprasad Chattopadhyaya, has provided another reason for inquiring into medical practices as a mechanism for understanding the past: "In ancient India, the only discipline that promises to be fully secular and contains clear potentials of the modern understanding of natural science is medicine."[6] A further validation of the general significance of medical investigation was identified by Hippocrates himself in the work *Ancient Medicine*, XX: "I also hold that clear knowledge about natural science can be acquired from medicine and from no other source."[7]

It is also readily apparent that medicine is the easiest science to initiate and develop because so much of clinical medicine is based on direct observation of the patient. Observable fevers and rashes, simple commonsense techniques such as touching and direct auscultation (listening with the examiner's ear placed on the patient's chest or abdomen, and a rudimentary medical history are examples of the quick, simple, economical and painless procedures that can initiate scientific inquiry into causes and prevention of illnesses and effectiveness of treatment. And because of the ease of implementation and without the necessity of technical or procedural assistance from elsewhere the pool of contributors to a central "data base" for the sharing of information can be relatively small both in region and in the population being served. It is these four characteristics, namely universality, secularity, feasibility, and economy, that justify emphasizing medical practice as a generic indicator of progress in ancient societies.

C. Justification for Equating Ancient and Contemporary Human Intelligence and Motivation

As an opening generalization, all mankind, in all societies and cultures, historic and prehistoric, has had the benefit of an equivalent intellectual heritage, a feature that

---

[6] See: Chattopadhyaya, D., *Science and Society in Ancient India*, Bangalore, 1977, pp. 3, 4.
[7] Hippocrates' statement, here translated by A. H. S. Jones in the Loeb Classical Library series on *Hippocrates* (vol. 1), refers to "nature" and the "life sciences" rather than to an all-inclusive definition of the sciences. But the point is that the pursuit of knowledge must be observational (objective) rather than philosophical (subjective).

can be likened to or listed among those genetic traits necessary to be classified as *Homo sapiens sapiens* of the, presumably, same genetic strain that has peopled the globe in the last 30,000 years.[8] Charles Darwin viewed human intelligence as gradually improving over hundreds of thousands of years from man's hominid ancestors, which is consistent with his concept of morality and its variability among different ethnic and racial groups based on genetic distinctions. It must be admitted that if his conditions for genetic selection are accepted, there indeed might have been such a peculiar pattern of evolution of intelligence, although at what point intelligence would or will reach a stable level is unknown. But how the present group of *Homo sapiens* in aggregate would measure against the intellectual potential of preceding strains or species of migrant genus *Homo* is also unknown, although the cranial volume of present-day adult *H. sapiens* is smaller than some earlier species of genus *Homo*, including *H. neanderthalensis*. Another factor to be considered is what effect local environmental changes, perhaps some induced by activity of *H. sapiens* himself, might affect genetic transmission in the short term with consequent local alteration of specific neurological or intellectual capabilities. The role of intercurrent disease and the natural rate of mutation would, of course, play an additional part in survival and thereby might affect intellectual ability in some circumscribed populations. But if it can be accepted that, by and large, equivalent intellectual potential can be applied to any society, large or small, old or new, then ignoring the possibility that present-day humans are less intelligent than their distant forebears, it is fair to state that factors other than intellectual capacity have been the effectors of social change among groups of *H. sapiens* over recent millennia. Had this not been so, had intellect been the sole mediator of progress for human societies, once populations reached a critical size and density the superior intellect of humans should have triggered some internal self-propelling awareness of the desirability for optimal improvement in the status of their respective populations. The time to achieve a localized population of sufficient size for this awareness of improvability of the species may have required many centuries, but if local environmental stresses and external forces did not disrupt species-wide intellectual maturation, perhaps far-reaching modernization might have been accomplished long ago.[9]

---

[8] "Therefore it is meaningless from the biological point of view to attribute a general inferiority or superiority to this or to that race." This statement is from the American Association of Physical Anthropologists statement on biological aspects of race, proposition 6, published in the *American Journal of Physical Anthropology*, 101:569-570, 1996. An updated scholarly interpretation of new data published in 2012 is in agreement (as reviewed by Nisbet, R. E. et al., *Intelligence: New Findings and Theoretical Developments*, in *American Psychologist*, 67:130-159, 2012), although much new information on regional and environmental conditions, genetic interactions, and motivation is known to affect social success and IQ rating, as well as global evidence for very active genetic change in *Homo sapiens* from regional pressures.

[9] The merits of modernization, good or bad, are not the issue here, for the past is past. But in determining the best path for man's social progress going forward it is important to know what has restricted progress in the past. Also, "modernization" as used here is relative, meaning that the difficulties and dangers of existence have, as a consequence of intellect and motivation, been lessened when contrasted with preceding times. Similarly, the present-day issues relating to climate change reflect concern for the future. Civilizations of the past have often been profoundly affected by changes in climate, sometimes global, sometimes regional, as will be apparent in the pages to follow. But the equivalent intellectual status of all global populations indicates that, when mixed in with all the other potential forces that might induce genetic change in intellectual function, if there has been any species-wide change related to climate it has so far been undetectable.

Innate human factors other than intelligence that are relevant to individual and group survival and, ultimately, to societal change are curiosity and motivation. Curiosity is not an attribute of intellect or a species-specific phenomenon, and it is operative in all human groupings. It would not be readily susceptible to peripheral restrictions, and would, like genetic stability of the collective human intellect, be unlikely by itself to effect social change of a longitudinal nature. Which brings us to motivation, a more relevant phenomenon in the making of and benefiting from new observations.

Intelligence and motivation are linked in that objective measures of intelligence can fluctuate depending on motivation. In seeking an explanation for the delay in devolvement of scientific progress upon humanity, and if intelligence is a constant function, the answer may lie with a deficiency of some motivating factor. To be more specific, was a motivating factor lacking in early civilizations that led to delayed development of medical professionals and other evidence of progress? Factors that surely were motivational included sickness, trauma, difficult birthing, and early death, sufferings affecting all populations in all eras. Yes, sickness was a potent motivation, a propellant for progress and change, especially as the occasional long-lived individual would have been viewed as evidence of what was possible. Both intelligence and motivation were in play to a similar degree in prehistoric as well as historic times.

The simple scheme just presented must have existed in all early and primitive societies. But with so many motivational catalysts attached to sickness, there must have been strong inhibitory factors to explain why early civilizations that would have benefited from, and were intellectually capable of, medical progress remained without identifiable medical practices for so many centuries/millennia. Levels of motivation, or "hierarchy of needs," specified by the classic studies of Maslow are referred to here, for their relevance in many cultures has been examined.[10] Two factors, biological survival and safety, take precedence in Maslow's hierarchy of five levels of motivation, with the third level involving one's interaction with others, such as a family member or friend. These three factors represent "primitive" motivational requirements. The original Maslow scheme identifies two other factors as less primitive: the desire for esteem and the personal goal of self-realization. The relevance of this classification of levels of motivation to early culture can be questioned, but intuitively the "primitive" requirements seem reasonable, and they have been found generally applicable to a variety of modern cultures. Assuming the perceived universality of the "primitive" motivational factors as operative in ancient or primitive groups as well as modern, and that there is equivalent intellectual potential in ancient and modern man, could progress, as understood today, have resulted from attempts by early man to sustain himself despite an unforgiving environment?

A variety of local physical and biological impediments could intercept ancient attempts at progress. But mankind's attempts would have been perennial and at one time or another some must have led to an observation, discovery, or invention that would have prompted the motivational process to further improve the quality and length of human life, for everything we know of ancient times is consistent with fear, dread or fascination with death. In a small group the observation, discovery or invention of something of a vital nature could have been rapidly transmitted to others in the group or to nearby groups.

---

[10] See p. 286*ff* for more on Prof. Maslow and his book, *Motivation and Personality* (first ed., New York, 1954). Although there is scholarly criticism of the hierarchy of needs, most is directed at psychological fine-tuning of personality, whereas its value in the present work is as a referent for sequencing stages of early human social existence, or, as indicated by Prof. Maslow, the three "primitive" stages: survival, security, belonging.

Such a sequence in the right setting might have been the spark that would propel a further search for improvement, augmentation, and propagation of the original observation. But knowledge of a vital discovery will seldom be sustained to a point where it can permanently improve the lot of human society if it can be communicated to only a few family members or fellow tribesmen. A minimum level of population size, density and duration must be necessary, a focus of later discussion.

      Also important is a need for that observation, discovery or invention. If there is no perceived need for more water, there will be no progress in improving water supply. If there is plenty of game, there will be no need for domestication. In Eden, of course, there would have been no need for progress because everything was present that was necessary and useful, and nothing was present that was unpleasant or dangerous (with one exception!). In a sense, progress can be viewed as the path toward a secular Eden, for no other path will lead a society to a place where everything necessary, useful and pleasant is available. If, therefore, there were no perceived need for improvements, should there have been no foreseeable shortage of food or water, no external threats, no environmental hazards, there would have been little need for activating the "primitive" motivational factors conducive to survival and safety, and an early form of communal association would have little reason to change its social pattern, however simple, from generation to generation, perhaps for thousands of years.

      But primitive life was, whether in jungle or tundra, no Eden. Thus, to motivation must be ascribed a major role in societal evolution. Even if an Eden-like environment existed, surely human biological inevitabilities that include disease and death would have been a perpetual motivation to improve health and longevity. Motivation and intellect as universal human attributes are omnipresent equivalents and the engine of progress toward a secular Eden. *Ergo*, human "progress" comes with the blessing of Heaven.[11]

D. Justification for Selective Elevation of Mythology to the Status of Evidence

      In Part I it was concluded that only twice in the past 2,500 years has medical progress been systematically implemented: in the Hippocratic medicine of Ancient Greece and in the modern West. But even with certain societal constants that include (1) equivalence in intelligence and curiosity, (2) a levelling scale for assessing motivation applicable to a broad range of societies, (3) the "universal" yardstick of medicine for

---

[11] In the translation of Dr. Paul Sigmond (*St. Thomas on Politics and Ethics*, New York, 1988, p. 49): "… all the things to which man has a natural inclination are naturally apprehended by the reason as good and therefore as objects to be pursued, and their opposites as evils to be avoided." St. Thomas Aquinas made clear the role of free will, the appropriateness for the individual to seek happiness, and the equating of individual good with the common good, all this under the aegis of a natural inclination toward the good. To this end can be positively assigned the concept of human progress, as long as it can remain undiverted from the good. Insofar as untoward consequences can ensue along the path of progress, as long as all unambiguous attempts are made to avoid them, that path can be pursued. Disease, suffering, and premature death as causes of great unhappiness are "the good's" justifiable targets. St. Thomas indicated that no perfect happiness will be obtained in our earthly state, but he did not criticize the attempt to improve it. The role of natural law, a much-discussed topic and on which St. Thomas also expounded, will receive close inspection in later chapters of this work.

comparing progress among civilizations, and (4) modern archeological methods, can similar defendable conclusions regarding prehistoric societies be drawn?

A clearer picture of those earliest attempts at a medical profession is desirable, but data are few and the ancient texts have suffered alteration over many centuries. But myths and legends abound that relate feats of good and evil in the archaic inventories of all cultures and civilizations, stories of superhuman strength or wisdom or malevolence. Perhaps a source of valid information on prehistoric and early historic medicine can be found in folklore or teachings from oral tradition. The importance of myth and legend in telling the story of mankind has been enhanced in recent decades as archeological discovery has unearthed evidence supporting the veracity of significant portions of anecdotal prehistory. Heinrich Schliemann's Troy, the Great Flood of the Gilgamesh, and many biblical scenarios now being unearthed are examples of such narratives.

Given the ostensible conjunction of myth and legend with extant manuscripts, perhaps the historicity of medicine should be more closely considered with an eye to its mythical or legendary past. Medicine has had its share of seemingly unrealistic champions in the distant past. Four that are relevant to present discussion are: Huang Ti (the Yellow Emperor of prehistoric China, cosmic ruler, inventor of the wheel and writing, and composer of the *Huang Ti Nei Ching Su Wen*, often acknowledged as the foundation of Traditional Chinese Medicine; 2400 BC), Bharadwaja (Indian sage and architect of Ayurveda, to whom divine wisdom was imparted by means of the *Athava-veda*; prior to 2000 BC), Imhotep (semidivine Vizier, architect, high priest, astrologer, scribe, founder of medicine and purported author of the *Smith papyrus* in 3rd Dynasty Egypt; 2700-2600 BC), and Ninsun (goddess of medicine and mythical mother of Gilgamesh, 1st dynasty Sumerian king of Uruk (2900-2800 BC).

With justification to be offered in the following four chapters, literary instruments purportedly composed during the age of the legendary sages and masters will be teamed up with the status of society at or about the time of their purported authors. Rather than the fusion of early society and early works providing a level of veracity to the myths and legends, perhaps the reverse will result, *i.e.,* hints derived from myths and legends will be found to support the ancient origins of medical progress.

CHAPTER TWENTY-SEVEN

MILETOS AS THE ARCHETYPAL SOCIETY FOR THE FOUNDING
OF HIPPOCRATIC MEDICINE

The history of Miletos from its earliest days until its razing by the Persians in 494 BC is briefly
reviewed with a focus on its governance and commercial enterprise. Ancient Greek civilization is
second only to modern Western civilization in its embrace of progress and individual liberty.
Miletos is selected as a paradigm population for an attempt at understanding that success. Its
medical practitioners are assumed to have been the source of at least some of the earlier clinical
observations found in the Hippocratic Corpus, although it would be reasonable to assign a similar
course of political, commercial, and medical practice developments to other city-states in ancient
Ionia and the Dodecanese Islands. This chapter also introduces societal terms and concepts that will
frequently reemerge throughout Part II. Selected metrics and observations are summarized at the
chapter's conclusion against which sixteen other urbanized or proto-urbanized primary civilizations
will be compared in subsequent chapters.

A. Miletos and the Birthplace of Hippocratic Medicine

In Part I it was shown that the only approximation to a "natural state" of medical
practice other than 18th-19th C Western civilization occurred in ancient Greece. As we
are still living in the former, this chapter will review the era of Hippocratic medicine of
ancient Greece with focus on its origin.[1] The term "Hippocratic" is used to describe the
medical practice associated with the legendary practitioner with whom it has been
identified over the ages: Hippocrates (460-380 BC). In that tradition it must be
understood that the term does not include all medical practitioners, for no linguistic
distinction is provided in Classical Age or modern literature that separates those relatively
few in ancient Greece who practiced according to principles of Hippocrates from the great
majority and great variety of practitioners who did not. But the written record of
Hippocratic physicians, as reflected in the *Corpus Hippocraticum*, is sufficiently large
and detailed to provide irrefutable evidence of medical progress, whereas nothing of this
sort exists for other practitioners. Part I also describes the clinical achievements of
Hippocratic physicians, their social environment, and their disappearance. This will not
be repeated here. The point to be established, however, is that it was possible 2,500 years
ago to develop within a space of about two or three centuries a network of medical
practitioners capable of instituting a rational basis for making medical decisions, and that
this was done without benefit of technology and without being the recipient of prior
codified medical knowledge. Hippocratic medicine, therefore, can be considered the
universal *editio princeps* of medical practice against which other textual medical
traditions and their social environments can be compared.

The locus of origin of Hippocratic medicine has traditionally been identified as
the island of Cos, home of Hippocrates, just a few miles from the Ionian coast, now the

---

[1] The course and denouement of Hippocratic medicine is presentgreater ed in detail in Book 2 of
The Natural State of Medical Practice: An Isagorial Theory of Human Progress, Maitland (FL),
2019. Also mentioned in that volume, p. 218, is the uncertainty that surrounds the legend of
Hippocrates, although scholarly opinion presently favors the existence of the man.

western coast of Turkey. The ancient term that comprised the mainland sites of ancient Greek cities on that coast is Ionia, and Miletos was the most prominent city of Ionia in the 6th C BC. Miletos was sacked by the Persians in early 5th C BC, and little remains of that early city. For reasons given in Part I of this work there is reason to consider Hippocratic medicine as having its origin in an Ionic city such as Miletos rather than the small and relatively backward island of Cos. This analysis of city-state development, therefore, will use Miletos as the template for the civilization that would introduce Hippocratic medicine to the world. But it will not be the magnificent Miletos that was rebuilt in the 4th C BC; it will instead be the earlier Miletos as it emerged from prehistory only to be totally destroyed in 494 BC.

The ancient port city of Miletos has a complex and incompletely understood prehistory. Relevant to present purpose, a settlement on that location was associated with the Mycenaean empire and then the Carian culture in the 13th C BC, but in mid-12th C BC it was completely destroyed and the area remained deserted for one or two centuries.[2] Thus, from roughly 1050 to 650 BC, after it was settled anew by Ionian Greeks, it developed into a freestanding city-state with hegemony over roughly 700 square miles of territory, including the alluvial plain of the Meander River where it entered the Aegean Sea. Protected by a mountain range to the north and east, and with a fertile delta to support a flourishing agriculture, a self-sufficient Miletos became increasingly prosperous as an independent city run by an oligarchical government. It is relevant that by "oligarchical" is meant that city government, in its offices and deliberations, was in the hands of a wealthy socioeconomic group involved in commerce and trade, suggesting it was functionally a heterarchy, a management style much discussed in later chapters and defined on p. 13. It did not have, as a relatively new city, a powerful hereditary ruling class.[3] Turmoil erupted from time to time, and the importance of tradesmen and craftsmen is evident in that contention was not between rival nobility but between the wealthy and an increasingly wealthy middle class arising among the plebeians.[4] To counter this

---

[2] Excavations at Pylos of the Mycenaean palace and surrounding region have revealed a writing system called Linear B that is directly related to ancient Greek. An early form of the Greek word for medical practitioner (ἰατρός, iatros) was found in palace records, transliterated as *i-ja-te*, and a description of presumed medical instruments has been made by E. Protonotariou-Deilaki (Ανασκαφικαι Ερευναι εις Περισχήν Ναυπλιας, in Αρχαιλογικὸν Δελτίον 28:90-94, 1973), but neither claim can be considered definitive. Michael Ventris, who first translated Linear B, considered the translation of "physician" to be tentative, although this translation has subsequently not been questioned, and the "medical" instruments have also been considered by some to have been for cosmetic use. Stated comparisons of Pylos medical instruments with Classical era medical instruments must be in reference to those from Pompeii, 79 AD, or the Surgeon's House, Rimini, 2nd C AD, *i.e.*, 1500 years later. These details are mentioned here because it might be argued that Hippocratic medicine represented the natural progression of a nascent form of rational Mycenaean medical practice. To which it would be responded that evidence for this is frail and occurs at only one point in time. Nothing suggesting other than simple empirical treatments appear prior to the Hippocratic writings (*e.g.*, in Homeric epics, *ca.* 750 BC, or poetry of Hesiod, *ca.* 700 BC). It can be considered settled that there is no association of Hippocratic medicine to anything prior to the settlements of Ionia.
[3] See: Gorman, V., *Miletos, the Ornament of Ionia*, Ann Arbor, 2001, chapter 1. This excellent book is the source of much of the information on archaic Miletos used in the present work.
[4] It is from these two groups, or political parties, that the ἀειναῦται, or "perpetual sailors," were derived, their prominent leaders embarking on a ship to thrash out political differences, disembarking only when solutions had been decided. This preceded the tyranny of Thrasybulus,

menace as well as military threats from the nearby kingdom of Lydia, a highly regarded statesman, Thrasybulus, was chosen as tyrant to guide the city, which he successfully did between 650 to 600 BC, at the end of which time oligarchical control was reinstituted.[5]

But the period of special interest impinging on Hippocratic medicine is the century preceding the writings now attributed to Hippocrates, for it would have been during that century (600-500 BC) that clinical observations were made that would become the source of the wisdom imparted in early compositions of the *Corpus Hippocraticum*. In 560 BC the Kingdom of Lydia achieved hegemony over the Ionian city-states, at that time autonomous polities guided by commercial interests that were flourishing from maritime trade. Of those that bowed to the will of Croesus, the Lydian king, Miletos was granted special status and permitted to follow its commercial interests in return for supporting Croesus against the Persians. This was thwarted in 546 BC when the Persians defeated Croesus and assumed hegemony over the region, but again Miletos obtained special status. A tyrant, Histiaeus, was put in control of the city by the Persians. It does appear that, despite the "tyranny" of Histiaeus, the commercial and cultural well-being of Miletos was maintained. Both Croesus of Lydia and the Persians "did not impede in any way economic and cultural development."[6] It has also been stated that increased prosperity of Miletos coincided with the rule by Histiaeus, the Persian "vassal," and that the Persians in general interfered little in the internal affairs of their conquests. A contributing factor to Milesian prosperity may have been the assassination of Polycrates, tyrant of the neighboring island of Samos, for his previous blockades had restricted sea commerce in the area.[7] This would have helped soften the effects of any tribute and military support required of Miletos by the Persians. The favored status of Miletos persisted until about 500 BC when Histiaeus was replaced by his son, an event that ultimately would lead to a war with Persia in 494 BC during which Miletos was razed and its population dispersed or enslaved, thus terminating the history of that great city of Archaic Greece and leaving little tangible record of its existence. Years were to pass before Miletos again achieved prominence. Resettlement began in 478 BC, but by then Athens had become powerful and expanded its influence in areas previously under the aegis of Miletos. The city had to be repopulated, rebuilt, and social structures and networks reestablished. Although both Athens and the Persians maintained an association with the city it would remain a secondary regional force for two centuries. It is concluded, therefore, that it was during the earlier period of Persian hegemony over Ionia (*i.e.,* prior to 494 BC) that Hippocratic medicine first emerged. It is possible that Hippocratic

---

thus revealing the early 7th C BC prominence of commercial interests and the fruits of *heterarchy*, an organizational system much discussed later in this work.

[5] There was also this difference between the island of Cos and Miletos. Cos was Dorian, Miletos was Ionian. The Dorian culture venerated ancient customs to the point that the Spartans, who were Dorians, prevented contact with foreigners by having their cities inland rather than coastal, by restricting travel of their citizens, and closing their gates to foreigners. The Ionians, in contrast, welcomed novelty and interacted with foreign ideas, its morality repugnant to Dorians. The idea that the fount of medical knowledge of the Hippocratic era emanated from the small island that Dorian settlers appropriated from the aboriginal population of Cos is culturally and demographically highly unlikely. See: Muller, K. O., *History and Antiquities of the Doric Race*, two volumes, London, 1839, H. Tufnell and G. C. Lewis, translators, especially the first chapter of volume 2.

[6] See: Dandamaev, M. A., *A Political History of the Achaemenid Empire*, Leiden, 1989, translated by W. J. Vogelsang, p. 153 and p. 21. Also see: Meyer, E., *Geschichte des Altertum*, vol. 3, i, p. 57.

[7] See: Ure, P. N., *The Origin of Tyranny*, Cambridge, 1922, p. 270.

medicine prior to Hippocrates evolved in other Greek city-states, but if that were the case the basic argument put forth herein would likely be unchanged except for minor alterations in city-state metrics. The fact remains, however, that from all the other city-states that existed at the time of archaic Miletos there has appeared no information whatever on Hippocrates that would indicate an alternative site for the origin of Hippocratic medicine except for the well-known reference to "Hippocrates of Cos" in Plato (*Protagoras*, 311b) and in Soranus' *Life of Hippocrates* written 500 years later.

It is a reasonable assumption that a minor craft or profession such as a medical practice had little to fear from a change in early Milesian masters in the absence of widespread violence. At its peak the population of Miletos may have reached 65,000 and its urban size over 200 acres at the peninsular tip of an alluvial region of about 80 square miles. As a functionally autonomous city-state it lasted for 550 years. The importance of population size and density in supporting a small network of medical practitioners will be discussed in detail later, but a local population of about 10,000 is arbitrarily proposed as a necessary minimum. During the 8th C BC this number was surpassed in several population centers of Ionia, with Miletos being the largest.[8] There is no information on the health of its population prior to its destruction, and there is no archeological or literary information on its medical practitioners, although some famous personages prior to its destruction included Thales, Anaximander, Cadmus, Anaximenes, Aristides, Hecataeus, and Hesychius. These famous intellects (among many), the extraordinary Temple of Apollo at Didyma, and the thirteen-mile statue-lined road between Miletos and Didyma attest the greatness of Miletos prior to the Persian destruction. As for governance, the role of tyrants early and late in the 6th C BC having been discussed, there was in midcentury a mediation by Parians who were called to settle violent disputes between the wealthy and the artisanal class. The result has been likened to a "constitution," and in the short term it increased the power and municipal responsibility of a "middle class" composed of prominent landowners. The actual functioning of this arrangement is not evaluable, however, and it has been suggested that even with the proposed changes in governance that the highest offices remained within an established oligarchy.[9]

In the 70-80 medical treatises associated with the *Corpus Hippocraticum*, none mention Miletos, whereas Thessaly, the island of Thasos, Cyricus in northwest Anatolia, and Perinthus on the Sea of Marmara are specified as being the homes of some patients mentioned in those works, the latter three located near or on the route to the Black Sea where many Milesian colonies were established. Scholarly opinion holds that no Hippocratic works predate early 5th C BC and the destruction of Miletus. On the other hand, many clinical descriptions thought to have been written in the mid-5th C BC suggest their authors already had a background of knowledge that would have taken a group of physicians years to collect. It is that background of knowledge that may have come from Miletos as predecessors of Hippocratic physicians first began to form networks, organize, and collate and share their cumulative knowledge. Had a few Milesian practitioners escaped the Persian destruction a description of their practices might have been available,

---

[8] See: Morris, I., *The Growth of Greek Cities in the First Millennium BC*, 2005, p. 4 of this 29-page publication of *Princeton/Stanford Working Papers in Classics*. Prior to the 8th C BC it has been stated that there were no Grecian (Hellenic) cities, and that no settlements exceeded a 2,000 population. The city of Miletos can, therefore, be considered a city newly formed and without regional precedent.

[9] See: Dunham, A. G., *History of Miletus Down to the Anabasis of Alexander*, London, 1915, especially chapter 12, Constitutional History.

but medical practitioners were not highly valued in any ancient civilization, with the exception of those few who, for whatever reason, contributed to the welfare of the elite. And Athens had already denied its assistance to Miletos in the latter's plan for armed rebellion against the Persians. History, therefore, is left with no information on this point.

What is evident is that no other Ionian city-state, including Samos, Chios, and Ephesus, is likely to have been a fount of early medical knowledge. Furthermore, the home island of Hippocrates, Cos, is out of the question as a source of Hippocratic medicine, as is mainland Greece and its attendant islands. Given its wealth, importance, vast network of associations with other city-states, colonies, and empires, and being the home of famed pre-Socratic philosophers, for purposes of argument Miletos has been selected to represent the civilization that produced an archetypal medical practice, aspects of which have now persisted for 2,500 years. There is no practical alternative.

B. Social Structures of Miletos

In addition to the physical features of Miletos and the cities of other civilizations to be discussed in subsequent chapters, the freedoms and the limitations on individual and group enterprise that might have existed in ancient population centers is essential to an understanding of the concepts to be put forth in this volume, for its focus is the role of group freedom in the progress of any society. In Part I of this work Hippocratic medicine was uncoupled from traditional views that it represented or emerged from a medical school or a family of hereditary medical healers traceable to the legendary Asclepius. Instead it was placed within a network of medical practitioners formally communicating their clinical findings to a central source that, for a fee, communicated updated knowledge to its membership. It was likened to a "physician's cooperative," a group of persons with similar goals that was created voluntarily to improve the function and reputation of the "cooperative," in effect their profession. The commercial network of that group of Hippocratic physicians was also likened to a koinon (κοινόν) as used by Aristotle in a political sense (see p. 129 for further background of the koinon and related subjects). Essential to the success of a koinon was freedom from constraints by outside authority, equality in the rights of membership, a goal of self-interest, and the ability of members to speak freely without fear of reprisal. Implied in this, therefore, was the role of group liberty as the touchstone of progress. What information from Miletos, if any, bears on this point?

In all early or primitive societies the role of the family and its consanguineal and affinal social relationships has been dominant in social organization and power. Groups based on these connections, "kinships," are varied in content, size, structure, and purpose, but in early or primitive societies they consistently share one feature: egalitarianism, or, to more restrictively define the term for present purposes, a form of social egalitarianism. In this system there is a social structure within the kinship that assigns duties and obligations to all members depending on their status within the group. In an egalitarian society one obligation is the sharing of assets within the kinship, whether it be food, a product of work, or work itself. In modern times egalitarianism has come to include equal status and equal opportunity, but such philosophical details of equality would have been irrelevant to primitive and early kinships.[10]   It is also recognized that the degree of egalitarianism is inversely related to group size; the smaller the group, the more profound the role of the kinship on each member. Kinships were prominent features of ancient Greek society, and Dr. Kenneth Walters has stated: "Kinship cut across territorial concerns. Indeed, it may have been … a primary motive factor in the politics of the 6th century [BC]."[11] This would have included the city-state of Miletus.

But the hold of kinship on behavior weakened as cities formed and personal and family allegiances were shifting to economic and political associations according to personal preference. It was in ancient Greece that the political groundwork was laid that would formally support a greater degree of individual liberty and democratic process. The Greek city-states adopted it to varying degree, ranging from the elections by lot in Athens to the rigid authoritarianism of the Spartan State.   But one of the earliest manifestations of this revolutionary concept of democratic process occurred in Ionia, of which Miletos was the dominant city during the period of special interest for present discussion. Reference to democratic process is found on an early 6th C BC inscription from the island of Chios, approximately 90 miles northwest of Miletos.[12] The relative freedom enjoyed by merchants of Miletos allowed their maritime trade to proceed apace even though other aspects of social control in city-state life were administered by tyrants or oligarchies. There was, as a consequence, little interference in the mercantile networks that were the primary source of the city's prosperity.

This lack of State interference is consistent with recent scholarly analyses of a variety of urban areas: freestanding and self-sufficient networks of crafts, trades, and vocations provide stability to centralized populations despite disorder within hierarchical systems because their day-to-day work and associations are outside the range of leadership interests or control. Such networks and associations can determine the course of a polis irrespective of a coexisting hierarchy and are now thought to have been critical in maintaining an intact city or city-state in the face of hierarchical turmoil. The relative importance of these networks varies and can change over time, and therefore the term "heterarchy" has been applied to indicate that there is no one group having permanent direction over other groups. If there appear to be commercial networks in operation irrespective of the form of governance in the civilizations evaluated herein, (1) it will be assumed that medical practices could be counted among them, and (2) the primary governance of those civilizations will be listed as "heterarchy." It is a term now widely used in many scholarly discussions to explain functional successes in societies and other systems that were not adequately explained by hierarchy, the latter being a linear chain of command in which all but the highest level is sequentially nested in the next higher level. Heterarchy, as a term of management, clarifies much about social and economic dynamics

---

[10] This preliminary sketch oversimplifies the basis of kinship, which is an organizational latticework that is used to enforce an egalitarian ethic. See chapter 34.

[11] See: Walters, K. R., *Geography and Kinship as Political Infrastructures in Archaic Athens*, in *Florilegium*, 4:1-31, 1982.

[12] For the actual inscription see: Tod, M. N., *A Selection of Greek Historical Inscriptions*, Oxford, 1933, pp. 1-2. Dated by Tod to *ca.* 600-575 BC, the inscription is taken to indicate a popular council composed of representatives of subgroups that placed restrictions on its leadership and implied isonomia (equality before the law). As Tod states, "…the democratic tone of the Constitution is unmistakable." A perhaps earlier statement has been found at Dreros, an ancient Dorian Greek colony on Crete. Known as the Dreros Law and dated as Archaic, 650-600 BC, it imposed term limits and sanctions on the leadership of the colony.

of early societies and is often used in studies of ancient and primitive societies to explain their survival and growth despite little archeological evidence of a leadership or elite class to guide or entail labor from a population, especially in building monumental structures. Heterarchy and hierarchy commonly occur together, the former adding flexibility and valuable opinions that can help support or maintain a hierarchical system. But a heterarchy has its unique commercial or production services, sometimes even with its own separate settlements or neighborhoods, for the use of its labor force that are distinct from those of a political authority. The commercial ventures of Miletos, mentioned above, are evidence of heterarchy as inferred from historical comments on political events. Even earlier, during the 7th C BC colonization of coastal regions around the Black Sea by Miletos, many areas have been characterized as heterarchy. And the Greek Dark Age has been characterized as not "dark" but as a time of development of commercial interests that were considered heterarchy in an early stage of development.[13]

A final organizational feature to be sought in early or primitive cities is the existence of specialization. This is an indication of predictable surpluses in food supply that allow accumulation of products by storage that for reasons of commerce and stability can support trade and the luxury of technical specialization in other service and craft areas. "Specialization," therefore, is included in the list of features to be sought in the various civilizations to follow. Furthermore, the presence of specialization is part of the definition of "civilization" used herein (p. 13), and when present implies the capability, if not the probability, for a medical practitioner network. If specialization in a city can occur in the commercial stockpiling and trading of grain, ceramic production, and jewelry manufacture, it is possible that the prospering city will also have some citizens who would, if they could, join together to provide special services for a fee. There is at present absolutely no information about medical practitioners, Hippocratic or otherwise, in early Miletos. On the other hand, it is inconceivable than none existed.

To summarize this chapter, the location of the Ionian settlement of Miletos was unoccupied at its founding, and the evolution of Milesian governance, having no urban precedent and its economic development and provisioning of its population evolving locally, has been selected as an archetypal city-state governance in ancient Greece in which medical progress, as exemplified by Hippocratic medical practice, could have arisen. In that many of its initial settlers represented a forced emigration from the Greek mainland and shared some cultural behaviors and traditions, Miletos did not evolve from nomadic hunter-gatherers. But as a city it did not acquire prosperity by conquest, its future course depended on local decisions unguided by some distant center of power, and it was not a colony or satellite of an established civilization. These features indicating the development *in situ* of a permanent population center independent of outside authority is what sanctions Miletos as a prototype to which other large freestanding population centers, including prehistoric ones to be discussed later, will be compared, for they also will have developed independent of outside authority.

In the Table below it is not known if any of the nineteen listed characteristics and metrics were important to societal progress or, if relevant, whether quantitations

[13] See: Enverova, D. A., *The Transition from Bronze Age to Iron Age in the Aegean: A Heterarchical Approach*, Bilkent University Master's thesis, Ankara, 2012. Also see papers by Dr. Jan Driessen that propose an early Minoan system of economics based on commercial "houses," each with its dedicated workforce and administration probably directed along lines of kinship, a form of corporatism. Driessen, J., *A Prepalatial Matrilinear Society*, in *Back to the Beginning*, Oxford, 2012, I. Schoep, et al., editors, chapter 12.

represent minimum or maximum values. Other features of Milesian civilization may have been more relevant but are unavailable for assessment.

Summary Table for Miletos:

STAGE – Late Archaic

POPULATION, LOCAL – 65,000

POPULATION, TOTAL – unable to locate information; perhaps 100,000-200,000

PRIMARY AREA – 1 square mile (hegemony: 700 square miles, *ca.* half the size of Rhode Island)

URBAN DENSITY – 100 persons per acre

PRODUCTION – agriculture, ceramics, services and products relevant to commercial maritime trade

GOVERNANCE – aristocracy of wealth with intermittent tyranny, but primarily a commercial heterarchy that included colonies

EGALITARIAN ARCHEOLOGY[1] - no

PROMINENT EGALITARIAN KINSHIPS – not noted within the city boundary

WRITING – yes

DISTANT TRADE – yes; maritime colonies

SPECIALIZATION - yes

MONUMENTAL STRUCTURES – yes, temples and statues

DENOUEMENT – razed by Persians

MEDICAL PRACTICE – assumed

FORMATIVE PERIOD – 250 years

FLORUIT[2] – 300 years (starting with the time the first Ionian cities reached populations of 10,000)

CITY-STATE – yes

AVERAGE LIFE EXPECTANCY – n.a.[3]

---

[1] EGALITARIAN ARCHEOLOGY is defined on p. 13.

[2] FLORUIT refers to the period covering a society's mature prosperity, often a nebulous period.

[3] n.a. = not available.

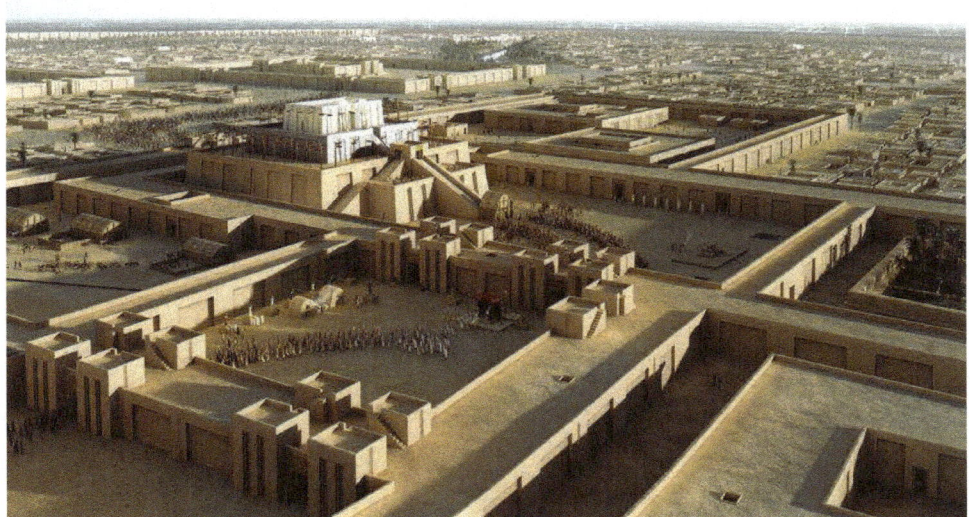

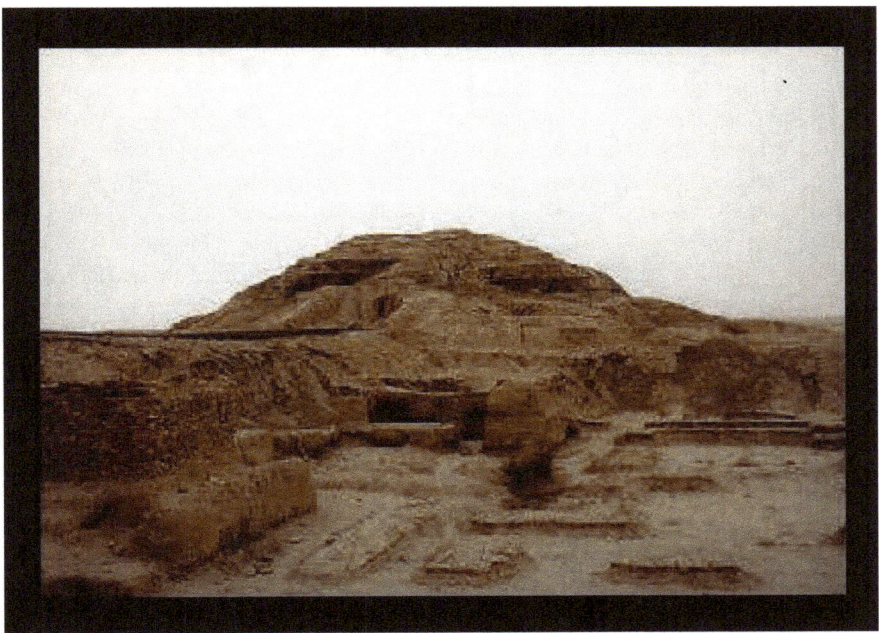

Fig. 15: (Top) Artistic reconstruction of the Eanna District of the city of Uruk *ca.* 3000 BC. This photograph is licensed under Creative Commons Attribution-NonCommercial-ShareAlike 4.0 International. (Bottom) Photograph, by Carmen Asensio and available in Wikimedia, of the Eanna temple of Uruk as seen earlier at the excavation site. Lying alongside a branch of the Euphrates River, Uruk was the largest city in the world at that time.

CHAPTER TWENTY-EIGHT

EARLY MESOPOTAMIAN CIVILIZATION

Sumer is the first of four great primary civilizations to be compared to Miletos, all four having been the source of ancient medical classics. The prehistory of Sumer and the founding and rise of its largest city-state of Uruk are presented, and the agricultural and commercial prosperity of that city before conquest by Akkadians (2350 BC) is proposed as the social milieu in which a network of medical practitioners acquired the ancient wisdom of clinical medicine that would find its way into later Babylonian medical writings. Writings and myth suggest that the independent *azu* ("physician") was recognized as a commendable member of society probably as early as 3200 BC, although a mature cuneiform probably was unavailable to record his observations until 2900 BC. As scholarly literature has a number of fine articles revealing the clinical acuity of some Sumerian clinicians, only one example is reviewed in detail in this chapter. The rise of an autonomous city-state at a time of (1) weakening of egalitarian kinship ties, (2) commercial prosperity, and (3) prior to authoritarian centralization of power is proposed as containing the window of opportunity for the formation of a medical network capable of initiating medical progress. A companion to medical progress, another product of commercial prosperity, is writing.

A. Early Sumer and the City-State of Uruk

Like Miletos, all four of the great riverine civilizations discussed in this and the subsequent three chapters (the Uruk and Jemdet Nasr cultures of predynastic Sumer abutting the Euphrates River, the Naqada culture of predynastic Egypt along the lower and middle Nile River, the Shandong culture of predynastic China along the Yellow River, and the Harappan culture in the Indus River Valley) developed in alluvial plains. Their association with the large river valleys and deltas can be ascribed to a hospitable agricultural environment capable of supporting a large population. This, rather than any innate superiority of the inhabitants, explains the prominence of the four large riverine civilizations in world history. The intention now is (1) to identify characteristics of the earliest days of each of the four great civilizations that developed medical practices so that they can be compared to early Miletos and to a group of prehistoric primary civilizations/proto-civilizations to be discussed later, and (2) to assess socioeconomic evidence that the classical medical writings associated with those four great civilizations could be traced back to their originating (primary) civilizations. A degree of repetition of chapters 2-5 is unavoidable.

Human settlement with primitive agriculture surrounding the upper Tigris and Euphrates rivers was occurring as early as 9,000 BC. A progressive southerly expansion and maturation of the northern cultures is proposed as an early phase of what is now called the Ubaid culture (6500-3800 BC) in the area that would become known as Sumer. This culture with its numerous small communities evolved a system of urbanization, temple building, and irrigation. Its settlements were without walls, and projects were undertaken that required organized communal effort. It has also been proposed that over time a hierarchical form of governance developed with a temple-associated system of centralized redistribution of food, although social stratification was minimal. This pattern was continued into the Uruk Period (4000-3100 BC) that supplanted the Ubaid, social stratification surging as the Uruk Period came to a close. Despite this, the Late Uruk

Period (3400-3100 BC), the formative phase of Sumer, saw the early evolution of larger villages and early developmental stages of city-states, the development of writing, and the expansion of trade into distant regions. This important cultural expansion proceeded apace in some regions for the next 200 years, now called the Jemdet Nasr period (3100-2900 BC), during which city-state populations exceeded 10,000.

An important social change during the Late Uruk and subsequent periods was the change from traditional small group kinship intrafamilial ties to ties with the more successful families. In the process of changing affiliation the egalitarianism of traditional kinship structure was gradually replaced by a less domineering inter-kinship association, one more personal than that provided by a traditional hierarchy of power defined by class.[1] The affiliation of a kinship was now with another kinship, one that was more successful and might prove a profitable companion and provide leadership in commercial ventures. Both the traditional and the new "nested" kinship alliances were probably patriarchal, but the latter infringed much less in one's personal life. Evidence of this is the cosmopolitan composition of neighborhoods. These shifts were taking place in the late 4th millennium and ultimately would lead to dynastic Uruk, its significance being discussed in chapter 2 as the proposed time a nascent network of medical practitioners would begin to compile their medical knowledge for future colleagues.

The role of natural disasters, especially flooding (including the great flood mentioned in *Genesis*), during this period of Mesopotamian civilization is heatedly debated, and so all that can be inferred is that flooding of some degree was not a rare occurrence in the region and how any flooding that did occur affected regional society is uncertain. In either event, in the subsequent Sumerian early dynastic period (onset: 2900 BC) the city-states grew in size, proliferated, and remained autonomous for centuries until united under a single Akkadian ruler *ca.* 2350 BC. The history of this period (2900-2350 BC) is poorly attested, but intercity rivalry was important. Some have argued that city-states during the early dynastic period may have resembled monastic centers in medieval Europe whereby the monastery often served as a commercial and distribution center as well as a religious center for the surrounding region.[2]

The largest Sumerian city during the period under consideration, and one of the earliest, was Uruk, for which the Uruk Period is named. In the Jemdet Nasr phase (the final stage of the Uruk Period) the city was at its peak, with a population of about 50,000 in 2900 BC. It may be the same city as the biblical Erech. Earlier construction had produced some stone buildings, a ziggurat, elaborate temples, baths, courtyards, and monumental structures with cone mosaics, and Uruk was, by 2900 BC, a walled city with hegemony over much of Sumer. The large size of the city has been explained by an extensive system of irrigation and the agriculture of domesticated grains that provided large food surpluses. Initially a market town of moderate size, the agricultural success of early Uruk and the region was the basis for most of its early economic development, and

---

[1] See: Ur, J., *Households and the Emergence of Cities in Ancient Mesopotamia*, in *Cambridge Archaeological Journal*, 26:2, 2014.

[2] As an example, Cistercian monks at Fountains Abbey in England in the 13th C had about 15,000 sheep on their granges (land holdings) and provided the economic surge that changed Yorkshire and surrounding areas from their previously described "desolate" state to a thriving countryside dotted with fields, villages, and marketplaces. See: Internet Homepage of Petyt, A., and her monologue on *Medieval Monasteries in Yorkshire* (2001), at Learning Centers at Ancestry.com; ("The contribution of the Cistercian Order to the economic development of the North was little less than revolutionary.")

the initial urbanization was in response to that excess production. So effective was agriculture that trade and commerce over great distance was initially established for that surplus, subsequently followed by mass production of pottery, figurines, finished jewelry, textiles, and weapons. To produce these commodities, specialized crafts and vocations appeared. Although arising from and surrounded by small agricultural communities, Uruk had, by 2900 BC, a system of small colonies, a developed military, and slaves obtained from peripheral conquests. The first nonmythical king also emerged as a ruler during the 1st Dynasty (2900-2800 BC) of Uruk. That king is now thought to have been the legendary Gilgamesh, hero of the *Epic of Gilgamesh*, commonly recognized because of its inclusion of a description of a calamitous flood. As such, the *Epic* is now considered by many a source of information on the social status of Uruk at that time. A stratified society, thirty-foot walls surrounding the city, and its militarization indicate it had become involved in destructive wars.

Despite its militarization, however, the statement is made in the *Epic of Gilgamesh* that King Gilgamesh consulted with an "assembly of men" from the city when considering war with the city-state of Kish, the approximate date of this being *ca.* 2800 BC. The nature of the assembly is not specified, but it is made clear that support from within the community was required for such a strategic decision. Dr. Samuel Kramer proposed there was a bicameral representation of citizens, the lower house composed of plebeians.[3] Even as king and presumably as the head of a large military force, unilateral action ordered by Gilgamesh himself was not possible. A purely hierarchical system of governance, therefore, is not supported.

Egalitarian governance was also unlikely, for, during the Jemdet Nasr period (3100-2900 BC) that preceded the 1st Uruk dynasty, tablets with administrative accounts of a commercial or distributive nature indicate careful tallying of products by a central authority. The vast storage of grain and the attraction of commercial ventures added population to the enlarging city-states and document the commercial consequences of agricultural achievement. This required leadership that, in the absence of evidence of a hereditary or political ruler, could only have been achieved by either commercial ventures (perhaps a heterarchy) or approval by the target population as a whole working through its leadership (a form of corporatism, as defined on p. 13).[4] In either event, the *Epic of Gilgamesh* interpretations would suggest that even into the 1st Uruk dynasty the functioning of city-state daily life was still primarily in the hands of mercantile interests rather than a dynastic kingship.

There is a similarity between the metrics of Uruk and Miletos. The smaller agricultural settlements adjacent to Uruk provided surplus agricultural products to the city in return for goods and services and for storage and perhaps redistribution in times of need or to provide a settlement specializing in one particular product with essentials produced by another settlement. It is unknown if the distribution of goods and services by the temple and religious offices of Uruk should be viewed as an egalitarian process or a commercial one, but given the vast size of grain storage the latter is most likely, although,

---

[3] See: Kramer, S. N., *The Sumerians: Their History, Culture, and Character*, Chicago, 1963, p. 99.
[4] "Heterarchy" and "corporatism" are defined on p. 13. There is also a recently described mechanism of social relations that springs from group interactions in which the groups have roughly equivalent prominence in the early stage of urbanization. It called a "settlement hierarchy" and it is proposed as the natural way intergroup adjustments take place as an enlarging population center that has had no prior experience with a leadership hierarchy becomes more complex and must deal with new goods and services needed by the evolving society.

with input from the people regarding storage and distribution, a system based on corporatism as mentioned in the preceding paragraph is possible.[5] There was a formal ruling dynasty in Uruk by 2900 BC, but the importance of the temple in daily life of citizens was great in its early years. It may, therefore, have provided a stabilizing social network that operated independent of a titular king, gradually being replaced as commercial interests assumed day-to-day functioning of city life. As for sharing of provisions and other essentials, it is one thing for a society to be egalitarian when there is little to distribute, as in small hunter-gatherer groups. The distribution is by personal effort and the survival of a small group is likely to be affected by the disability of one or a few members. But if redistribution is overseen by contributors, a voluntary agreement on equitable distribution is needed. This is more likely within a commercial network, although if the population involved sought its own arrangements for storage and distribution of commodities, the functional system might then have been a form of corporatism.

Among the specializations there should have been medical practitioners serving the central and peripheral populations during the period discussed here. When the temples had become fully secularized under Ur-Nammu (*ca.* 2100 BC), the fee for the "physician" (*azu*) is mentioned in the *Laws of Ur-Nammu*. Before this time, therefore, the *azu* must have been independent and perhaps free to form a network with other medical practitioners. Life expectancy at this time in Uruk is not certain, but in the contemporary Bronze Age Sumerian city-state of Kish the age at death averaged 30 years for men and 28 years for women.[6]

B. Uruk and the Early Sumerian Medical Writings

The three famous works attributed to the civilization of Sumer include: (1) a tablet of fifteen medical prescriptions from the final phase (Ur III) of Sumerian dynastic rule *ca.* 2150 BC, (2) the *Therapeutic Handbook*, also written about 2100 BC, and (3) the *Medical Treatise on Prognosis and Diagnosis*, an extensive work on general medicine discussed in chapter 2, that exists only in a 11th C BC copy. That copy, however, is thought to have been derived in part from a composition of the Old Babylonian period (19th-16th C BC). Furthermore, some of the text is linguistically attributed to the Ur III period, indicating that at least part of its content was much earlier Sumerian origin.[7]

---

[5] There may be some equivalence with the early Minoan economy, which began to flourish about 2500 BC. See: Driessen, J., *A Prepalatial Matrilinear Society*, in *Back to the Beginning*, Oxford, 2012, I. Schoep, et al., editors, chapter 12.

[6] See: Rathbun, T. A., *A Study of the Physical Characteristics of the Ancient Inhabitants of Kish, Iraq*, Coconut Grove, 1975, p. 187.

[7] *The Medical Treatise on Prognosis and Diagnosis* was compiled in the 11th C BC by the scholar Esagil-kin-apli, a nonphysician. It contains Sumerian text as well as later additions, and the trend of the additions and alterations became progressively mystical over time. There is even controversy as to whether the diagnostic component, which reflects observational skill, was to be used as a guide for exorcism or for medical therapy. As the *Treatise* was directed at the *asipu*, the exorcist, it is proposed that primordial physicians, the Sumerian *azu*, was the source of the clinical observations, but that it was the *asipu*, the Akkadian exorcist who entered the medical scene in the late 3rd millennium, who became dominant over time, reflecting an unfortunate degradation of the medical practitioner that was effectively perpetuated by Esagil-kin-apli and his "innovative" interpretations of the texts in the 11th C BC. A convenient review of this complex sequence is available: McGrath,

Given the affinity of post-Sumerian cultures for Sumerian intellectual property, in conjunction with their limited ability to develop their own (the Amorite empire of the 20th to 16th C BC was considered primitive in the eyes of the conquered and had no written language of its own), it is possible that most of the contents of the *Medical Treatise on Prognosis and Diagnosis* was of Sumerian origin. Many cuneiform medical texts, when transcribed, distinguish Sumerian terms from Akkadian ones. This indicates that their contents could be Akkadian but that certain technical terms in Sumerian were retained, just as Latin and Greek roots underlie many technical terms in modern medical texts. Furthermore, it is scholarly opinion that documents with retained Sumerian terms tend to be from Sumerian originals.

An important consideration is social stability during these several centuries. When Sargon the Akkadian won the battle of Uruk (*ca.* 2300 BC) the walls of the city were destroyed and much of the population fled to other Sumerian cities. Sargon proceeded to form an empire by military conquest. A previously symbiotic association between Sumerian and Akkadian peoples was disrupted as the Akkadian language was imposed in some areas. Wars near and distant were waged as the Akkadian Empire expanded, and at times of weakness chaotic conditions occurred in some Sumerian cities. After only 180 years of dominion, Akkadian rule was overthrown by the Gutians, considered at that time also a barbarous people. Again there was considerable destruction, principally of Akkadian society, and the Gutian presence was borne for almost 50 years. Then followed the period of Ur III (or third dynasty, 2112-2004 BC), which saw a resurgence of Sumerian hegemony by the king, Ur-Nammu, over a region that included several city-states. Under his leadership important communal projects were carried out, and at this time the law code of Ur-Nammu was written.[8] It included several laws directed at medical practitioners, the purpose being to limit the size of payment for various surgical procedures. The son of Ur-Nammu carried on the legacy of his father by instituting a calendar, maintaining civic archives, and developing a standing army. Sumerian writing and literary form were maintained despite the preceding two centuries of disruptive rule.

As the Akkadian reign lasted 180 years, the Gutian reign for 50 years, and the Ur III period lasted about 100 years, periods that began and ended with military conflict and during which the temples, fundamental in and unique to the existence of each city-state, were placed under central secular management, it is difficult to imagine how a group of medical practitioners could have not only formed a network for the purpose of improving their services to the public, but also would have compiled and authored their collective knowledge. Furthermore, the city of Uruk must have been badly damaged in the process of conquest, both in structure and population, and it is conceivable that, like ancient Miletos under the Persians, the destruction was sufficient to wipe out evidence of a preexisting medical profession.[9]

There are, however, much earlier mentions of Sumerian medical practitioners in letters and documents. The *azu* appears to have been a private citizen. There is evidence of a professional medical practice already existing in 2350 BC in Ebla, a hegemonic kingdom that was in communication with Sumerian city-states 550 miles distant. The finding of a room in a palace in ancient Ebla that was apparently reserved for herbs with medicinal value and in which their more active components could be extracted by boiling

W., *The Diagnostic Series SA>GIG: Ancient Innovations and Adaptations*, a Master of Arts thesis from the Department of Near and Middle East Civilizations, University of Toronto, 2016.

[8] See p. 44*f* for more on the *Law Code of Ur-Nammu*.

[9] See: Hamblin, W. J., *Warfare in the Ancient Near East to 1600 BC*, London, 2006, chapter 3.

or perhaps even distillation in making salves and other medicaments is evidence that at least as early as 2400 BC there was enough information on their use to suggest professional management of medicinal therapeutics made from herbs.[10] Furthermore, the listing of contents thought to be for a medical practitioner's kit in Ebla would have been appropriate for a professional rather than a local empiricist, and a short pharmaceutical tablet devoid of mysticism that mentions the *azu* has also been uncovered.[11]

Thus, the events and items in the preceding paragraphs predate the Ur III period and support the contention that the wisdom found in the Sumerian pharmaceutical tablet, the *Therapeutic Manual*, and the *Medical Treatise on Prognosis and Diagnosis* were collected by Sumerian medical practitioners prior to the destructive era initiated by the Akkadians, *i.e.*, prior to 2350 BC. Perhaps Uruk was the home of that nascent medical profession and, like Miletos, its evidence of a professional medical group or network being destroyed during the city's conquest. There is increasing scholarly agreement that the mother of Gilgamesh, an early king of the 1st Dynasty of Uruk, dated to *ca.* 2800 BC, was, in the mythological telling, Ninsun (also Ninisin or Gula), a goddess who included among her attributes the gift of healing, both medically and by incantation. In one description of Ninsun found in other writings she holds a scalpel and is identified as an *azu*, a physician. For the lowly *azu* to be associated with a deity by 2800 BC there must have been social recognition of effective medical practitioners for at least two or three preceding centuries. The (so far) earliest mention of the *azu* in cuneiform was also dated to this same period by Dr. Leonard Wooley.[12] Although dating of the fragments and the amendations to the *Epic of Gilgamesh* is an inexact science, there is some similarity between this "legendary" association of a superhuman king with medicine and (1) the polymath Vizier Imhotep of the Egyptian 3rd Dynasty (2650-2575 BC; see p. 55*f*), and (2) the Yellow Emperor of ancient China (*ca.* 2400 BC) and his superhuman feats that included the composition of the famed Chinese medical classic, *Huang Ti Nei Ching Su Wen* (see p. 74).

A peripheral reason to consider the late 4th or early 3rd millennium as the source for the knowledge in the *Medical Treatise on Prognosis and Diagnosis* is that there clearly was contact and intellectual exchange between Sumer and Protodynastic Egypt (Naqada III, 3300-3100 BC).[13] The question has been raised as to whether medical wisdom from Sumer entered the intellectual realm of predynastic Egypt, centuries later reappearing in the Ebers and/or Smith papyri to be discussed in the next chapter. To have done so would suggest that Sumerian medical wisdom was already being acquired by medical practitioners during the Uruk III and Jemdet Nasr periods in Sumer, although this is not to say that the specific writings referred to above had their origin at that time.

---

[10] See: Wachter-Sarkady, C., *Consuming Plants. Archaeobotanical Samples from Royal Palace G and Building P4, in Ebla and Its Landscape*, Abingdon, 2013, Matthiae, P. and Marchetti, N, editors, chapter 23.

[11] See: Fronzaroli, P., *A Pharmaceutical Text at Ebla (TM.75.G.1623)*, in *Zeitsch. F. Assyriologie*, 88:225-239, 1998.

[12] Cited by: Kramer, S. N., *The Sumerians: Their History, Culture, and Character*, Chicago, 1963, p. 99. The physician's name was Lulu, presumably a prominent figure.

[13] See: Rice, M., *Egypt's Making: The Origin of Ancient Egypt 5000-2000 BC*, London, 2003, 2nd edition, chapter 2.

C. Clinical Assessment of Sumerian Medical Writings

The Sumerian pharmaceutical text, devoid of mysticism, offers a fleeting glimpse into medicine's scientific past. It has been explicated by a prominent pharmacologist and thereby has revealed a convincing measure of technical knowledge and scientific process.[14] The *Therapeutic Manual* also has been translated into English with an astute clinician's help and is now known to contain much that is empirical and rational. But it is the *Medical Treatise on Prognosis and Diagnosis* that is the primary source of the clinical knowledge that has elicited admiration for the quality of Sumerian medicine.

It has been proposed that medical knowledge displayed in the *Medical Treatise on Diagnosis and Prognosis* was obtained through a gradual accretion of knowledge over centuries, from the Old Babylonian Period (1830-1531 BC) down to the 11th CBC, an ever enlarging book of knowledge of tediously acquired observations somehow maintained by a central authority that collated it despite intervening years of war, famine, and natural catastrophe.[15] This seems unlikely, for Near Eastern civilizations all had their own paths of conquest, and military ventures were common. A physician's organization that might preserve clinical wisdom of its members would have had a difficult existence given the incessant social disruptions. It is far more likely that the clinical foundation for the *Medical Treatise of Diagnosis and Prognosis* was a local Sumerian effort and was obtained at a specific time and over a fairly brief span, perhaps several generations, *i.e.*, 50-100 years. It may, of course, have been subsequently disassembled and then reassembled.

---

[14] Webb, J. L., *The Oldest Medical Document*, Medical Library Association, 1956.

[15] This is the expert opinion of Prof. JoAnn Scurlock, the prominent historian and cuneiformist. See: Scurlock, J. A., and Andersen, B., *Diagnoses in Assyrian and Babylonian Medicine: Ancient Sources, Translations, and Modern Medical Analysis*, Urbana, 2005, p. 6. She contends the 11th C BC *Medical Treatise on Prognosis and Diagnosis*, being lengthy, did have an earlier origin, perhaps Old Babylonian, but was changed in "format and wording" and amended over the centuries with new observations continually added by generations of physicians. She provides examples that are considered uniquely Akkadian rather than Sumerian and considers the recipient professional of the medical knowledge in the *Medical Treatise* to be the *asipu* rather than the *azu*. It may be, however, that just as Romans were to the ancient Greeks, the Akkadians were but excellent students. Furthermore, the conservative nature of the writing is shown by the finding of cuneiform copies as late as the 2nd C BC that retain recognizable features of the Diagnostic Series parts of the *Medical Treatise*, indicating that aspects of the original composition remained functional after 1500-2000 years. Dr. Robert Biggs commented that the wording of some Neo-Assyrian medical texts were exact copies of texts a thousand year older (see: Biggs, R. D., *Medicine, Surgery, and Public Health in Ancient Mesopotamia*, in *Civilization in the Ancient Near East*, J. M. Sasson, editor, New York, 1995). While undoubtedly new information was added at times, some of which might have been valid improvements, overall the course of the *Medical Treatise* was probably similar to that of the Ebers and Smith papyri in ancient Egypt: the 11th C BC version of the *Medical Treatise*, like the two 16th C BC Egyptian papyri, reflect sequential canonical versions of original writings made over a thousand years earlier. As for the *asipu* and *azu*, the present work champions quite different clinical roles for the two practitioners, the former being essentially an exorcist, the latter the true clinician.

Excursus on *The Medical Treatise on Prognosis and Diagnosis*

It is not a purpose of this excursus, or indeed of the entire volume, to judge the accuracy of an ancient medical work by modern scientific knowledge. It is instead to determine the accuracy of the observations expressed in ancient medical writings as estimated by clinical techniques available to practitioners of any age and to identify those observations that must have resulted from repeated observation, *i.e.,* had what can be called scientific confirmation. If it so happens that a specific disease or disease process is identifiable, the value of that identification lies not in the correctness of the diagnosis but in inferences that can be drawn about the accuracy and relevance of the original clinical observations. For there is to be found the starting point for medical progress, one that is available to every age and every society. At that starting point and once an accurate observation has been made, inductive reasoning can be applied and the validity of the reasoning confirmed or not based on further observation. Once both variety and quantity of observations have been adequately acquired it becomes possible to opine on mechanisms and associations. From these ideas spring the recognition of syndromes and the consequences of treatment. Progress is under way. But the starting point lies always with an accurate initial clinical observation and the motivation to do something with that information.

Unfortunately, progress can be stopped at any point, be it by war, famine, directive, or loss of opportunity. If we wait for the stage whereby syndromes, named diseases, and optimal treatment have been identified we may be able to define how medical progress endured or ended, but we will have missed the opportunity of determining how it began. And the present focus is on its beginning. Although observations obtained from taking a medical history and performing a physical examination on a patient tend not to be complex, there are qualitative aspects of the procedures. Pulse-taking at various points of the body can be made complex as it was in ancient China, but the basic observation is a simple one. In contrast, the Hippocratic physician who 2,400 years ago identified the clinical evidence of pupillary muscle paralysis as a significant finding in a patient now known, with a high degree of certainty, to have had diphtheria made a much more keen observation (see p. 209).

Just when the earliest steps in clinical medicine occurred in prehistoric times is impossible to say, for accurate oral tradition can travel through many human generations. But for such a prominent civilization as ancient Mesopotamia, generational characteristics, grouped into archeological phases, can provide a scholarly chronological backdrop against which early medicine appeared. Furthermore, those archeological phases are dated, which permits inferences about stability of the civilization. It takes only a few generations of medical practitioners to acquire a base of knowledge from which not only prognosis, but also effectiveness of treatments, can be extracted, and the "generations" of practitioners need not be familial. It is sufficient that they be in convenient periodic contact with each other to exchange experiences and ideas and to transmit the updated material to the next generation. Social stability for a century might be a reasonable minimum for a network of knowledgeable clinicians to form, acquire, and then transmit their combined observations in the form of a treatise. Clinical acumen of medical professionals is rapidly acquired in a stable social setting, but if average life expectancy, expressed as age at death, is about thirty-five years this places an additional limitation on the individual practitioner's medical experience, especially as medical practitioners were not of an elite class and would have shared the universal workload of daily living, may have been subject to being impressed for military ventures, and would have contributed to the effort required for communal projects. Thus, the requirements for this are an adequate number of practitioners covering a sufficient population for their combined experience to permit reasonably accurate generalizations and clinical predictions, and sufficient time in the day to carry this out, just as do other crafts and trades.

As for a critique of the *Medical Treatise on Diagnosis and Prognosis* itself, a definitive and convincing translation and commentary has been published by Drs. Scurlock and Andersen.[16] Clinical insight for the translation was the work of a knowledgeable clinician, an Internist with a subspecialty of Infectious Disease, and it therefore is unnecessary to repeat here the abundance of empirical-rational elements that are found throughout the text, with the following exception.

A recent publication by one of the authors includes an additional description of what might be drainage of an empyema of the chest.[17] That translation, however, concludes that an incision is to be made at the level of the fourth rib from the top, although an earlier translation had specified the enumeration was to be from the bottom. As there are twelve ribs the fourth rib from the bottom would also be the ninth rib from the top. Anteriorly, of course, the fourth rib overlies the heart, and the side of the empyema is not specified. But prior to the ready availability of ultrasound examination the usual site for needle insertion has been the eighth intercostal space (between the eighth and ninth rib) in the posterior axillary line, a level that would in most situations be performed safely on either side of the chest. Thus, unless examination of the chest wall by the ancient practitioner showed localized external evidence of internal inflammation as the spot to incise, just above the third rib (*i.e.,* below the fourth rib) *counting from the bottom* posteriorly would likely be the best place for an incision. If this were the thinking of the ancient practitioners who performed the procedure it would indeed be an amazing feat, for it must have been based on prior experience and anatomical knowledge of unexpected degree. The alternative, incising below the fourth rib from the top, would probably have been disastrous, inducing a pneumothorax or lacerating a large blood vessel, perhaps the aorta, or at the least unproductive, because gravity causes free fluid to layer in the lower chest

---

[16] Scurlock, J., and Andersen, B. R., *Diagnoses in Assyrian and Babylonian Medicine*, Chicago, 2005, p. 181.

[17] Scurlock, J., *Sourcebook for Ancient Mesopotamian Medicine*, Atlanta, 2014, pp. 484-486. This is from the *Babylonisch-assyrische Medizin* version of the text (BAM 39), and it and the preceding footnote provide both transcription and translation of the pertinent sections. But as reviewed by Kinnier Wilson (*Diseases of Babylon: An Examination of Selected Texts*, in *J. Royal Soc. Med.,* 89:135-140, 1996), the incision was above the third rib from the bottom, *i.e.,* in the eighth intercostal space if counted from the top (there are twelve ribs). It was assumed, however, that the purpose, as pointed out by Dr. Scurlock, was to drain a liver abscess, whereas the associated pulmonary sounds and the apparent placement of a lead tube for drainage indicate the clinical problem was a pleural infection, a collection of pus called an empyema. In modern procedures care would be taken to avoid the blood vessels on the underside of the bottom of each rib. This extensive explication of management of empyema is provided because of the extraordinary implications attendant to the Scurlock translation.

when the patient is upright. In either instance this is a notable example of medical progress.

End of excursus

D. Conclusion

There is abundant evidence of clinical competence in early Mesopotamian texts that could only have been acquired by a professional group over time, perhaps three or four generations in one productive century. It would have required a preceding century or two for the first individual practitioners to appear and establish the notion that specialists in medical care were superior to the care provided by friends or family. The only question is to what early era they belong, for it may have been as early as the Late Uruk Period (3400-3100 BC). On the other hand, it would have been unlikely after 2400 BC, when city-states in Sumer began to lose their autonomy. For purposes of comparison of Sumer with other civilizations, Uruk at its peak (during the Jemdet Nasr phase, 3100-2900 BC) has been chosen as the archetypal Mesopotamian city-state where a nascent medical profession might have existed, for Uruk was the largest regional population center for the longest period and, as a religious center for much of Mesopotamia, it was relatively stable up to the time of its destruction. Miletos had some two or three centuries after its population reached 10,000 to develop a network of medical practitioners, which would be consistent with independent practitioners in Uruk appearing at roughly 3100 BC. The clinical compilations may have occurred over the next two centuries.

The principle clinical writings of early Mesopotamian medicine of which excerpts are, directly or indirectly, extant, have now been reviewed in the context of prevailing culture and changes in ruling dynasties. Several points can be made about the nature of these texts. (1) Neither the earliest tablets, the *Therapeutic Manual*, dated to Ur III (*ca.* 2100 BC), nor a pharmacologic tablet containing fifteen medical prescriptions as presently published, has any supernatural connotations. (2) More complex in origin is the *Medical Treatise on Diagnosis and Prognosis*. From the Old Babylonian period (*ca.* 1600 BC) there are cuneiform tablets of an extensive work containing diagnostic and prognostic methods that were later compiled and substantially edited in the 11th C BC. The latter text includes much that is clinically perceptive, but it is also brimming with mysticism. (3) There is scholarly evidence that much of the *Therapeutic Manual* of Ur III and the *Medical Treatise on Diagnosis and Prognosis* share common features, the two texts seemingly part of a single work, or perhaps two works designed to complement each other. If this is so, then the original *Medical Treatise on Diagnosis and Prognosis* itself probably existed as early as the *Therapeutic Manual*. (4) The differences between the earlier and the 11th C BC edition of the *Medical Treatise of Diagnosis and Prognosis* need, however, to be explained. It is tempting to infer that the mystical component is entirely an attempt at emendation of an originally rational Sumerian work, much as the earliest Ayurvedic tracts were greatly altered centuries later to accommodate Brahminic religious practices in India. Similarly, the earliest clinical medical tracts of ancient China were greatly altered centuries later to accommodate both acupuncture in the 1st C BC and the philosophy of Yin and Yang that was first espoused in the 3rd C BC. These points are discussed in later chapters.

It is proposed that the initial collection of medical wisdom occurred in the predynastic period or 1st Uruk dynasty sometime between 3200-2700 BC, probably closer to the former date. The actual writing down of such a compilation might have occurred perhaps one or two centuries later. A weakening of egalitarian kinship ties and the lure of prosperity occurring in a rapidly growing population yet to be impeded by a coercive centralized bureaucratic governance would have been the optimal time for a group of medical practitioners to combine their knowledge and collate it. From this temporary repository of freedom their knowledge would become the mainstay of rational medical wisdom that would find its way into later Babylonian and Assyrian medical treatises after being dramatically altered in the 11th C BC by the learned scribe, Esagil-kin-apli (for more information on the role of this scribe see p. 49, footnote).

Summary Table for Uruk:

STAGE – Bronze Age
POPULATION, LOCAL – 50,000 (2900 BC)
POPULATION, TOTAL – 1,000,000 (hegemony, not domination)
PRIMARY AREA – 2.3 square miles
URBAN DENSITY – 33 persons per acre
PRODUCTION – initially food surplus from irrigation, with subsequent commercial trading ventures producing a burgeoning economy and population growth.
GOVERNANCE – practical everyday governance during the period of interest was initially one of corporatism which then evolved into a commerce-based heterarchy, with subsequent centralization, secularization of temples, and strengthening of kingly authority.
EGALITARIAN ARCHEOLOGY - no
PROMINENT EGALITARIAN KINSHIPS – no, nested
WRITING – yes
DISTANT TRADE – yes
SPECIALIZATION – yes
MONUMENTAL STRUCTURES – yes, temples
DENOUEMENT – declined after annexation by the Akkadian Empire (2350 BC)
MEDICINE – yes, the *azu*
FORMATIVE PERIOD – 900 years
FLORUIT – 700 years (the Jemdet Nasr and early dynastic periods: 3100 to 2400 BC)
CITY-STATE – yes
MEAN LIFE EXPECTANCY – 31 years (Kish)

CHAPTER TWENTY-NINE

HIERAKONPOLIS AND THE EARLY NILE RIVER VALLEY CIVILIZATION

This chapter places the original compositions that would be transcribed *ca.* 1550 BC and subsequently known as the Ebers and Smith medical papyri to the Protodynastic or Early Dynastic periods of Egyptian history. Apart from distinctive linguistic differences, reasons for this are presented, the principal one being the status of society adjacent to the unification of Egypt under the Pharaohs (3085 BC), a period noted for flourishing commercial manufacture, population growth, and prosperity. As the largest urban area along the Nile at this time, the city-state of Hierakonpolis is selected as the most likely site for the acquisition and collation of medical wisdom that is present in the two famous medical papyri. A clinical appraisal of some of their contents confirms their objective nature and supports the notion of a collaborative effort of a group of medical practitioners in the collecting and recording of their findings. Both writing and medical progress occur independently but contemporaneously as a consequence of prosperity and vigorous commercial activity, as they did in ancient Sumer. The dissimilarity between Sumerian cuneiform and Egyptian hieroglyphic/hieratic clinical descriptions does not support the notion that Egyptian medicine was an importation from the Mesopotamian civilization.

A. Dating Ancient Egyptian Medical Writings

The history of ancient Egyptian medicine is largely based on two papyrus manuscripts, the *Papyrus Ebers* representing internal medicine and the *Smith Papyrus* representing surgery. The date for their production is approximately 1550 BC, although it is scholarly opinion that they are copies of works composed many centuries earlier. One estimate suggests a date as early as 3400 BC for *Papyrus Ebers* and 3000 BC for the *Smith Papyrus*, although some authorities feel the latter preceded *Papyrus Ebers*. Archeological study supports the following approximation of societal shifts in ancient Egypt surrounding dates of the presumed original composition of the two works:

6000 BC – beginning of rapid immigration back into Egypt of a people who had previously moved to the Near East because of hostile environmental changes.
3800-3085 BC – the Naqada culture
3085-2686 BC – Early Dynastic Period (1st and 2nd Dynasties) initiated by unification of Upper and Lower Egypt

Narrowing down the proposed dates of the original medical compositions, or at least the period in which the clinical observations were made, it is argued herein that the social conditions of the later Naqada culture or early dynastic period were the most appropriate times for a nascent medical profession. Naqada culture has been divided into three periods, then evolving, with chronological uncertainties, into the 1st Dynasty:

Naqada I – 3800-3500 BC
Naqada II – 3500-3300 BC (a few villages began urbanization, with populations as high as 5000)
Naqada III (Protodynastic) – 3300-3085 BC (lasted *ca.* 215 years)
1st Dynasty – 3085-2890 BC (lasted *ca.* 195 years)

From these sequences, which to nonspecialists seem reasonably consistent, attention can focus on the social period and its characteristics, more than the dates themselves, most likely to have been associated with, and conducive to, the wisdom found in the two papyri.

As background, ancient Egypt is for the most part considered to have been throughout its prehistory and early history a rural and relatively peaceful region. As late as the Old Kingdom (2686-2181 BC) the estimated total population of Egypt was no more than about one million contained within a cultivatable agricultural region of only 15,000 square miles, little larger than the state of Maryland (the present population of Maryland is about six million). There is little evidence that early population centers had defensive construction. Consistent with this, it is generally held that there were no autonomous archaic Egyptian city-states, suggesting that in their earliest times the various population centers were so diminutive and culturally similar that they readily grouped together in provinces rather than contesting territory. Perhaps the necessity of communal efforts to control the flow of the Nile river was at the heart of this apparently benign early relation.

But beginning with the Naqada period, perhaps as a response to a growing population, scattered small villages began to coalesce and cluster around centrally located larger settlements. It has been proposed that these represented chiefdoms. Implied in this term is that the underlying society was partitioned along the lines of egalitarian kinships, as defined on p. 13. It was at this time that distant trade and commercial development are first noted. Society became more complex as the central locations began to amass excess agricultural production, perhaps to sustain the general population through difficult times.[1] This has been termed a redistributive economy, a management method whereby that which was available or abundant in one community could be made available to others that were deficient. Population continued to increase and to become more concentrated, now sometimes within walls, as small communities disappeared and the central administrative settlements merged to become divisions of larger organizational strategies that had in their turn more powerful central bureaucracies. It is thought that the population increase of the centers was primarily from immigration from peripheral settlements rather than proliferation. Evidence of conflict now became common as the Naqada II period approached. Nevertheless, a hieroglyphic/hieratic writing was developed in response to commercial development, a remarkable degree of specialization in crafts and trades appeared, fermented beverages were mass-produced, remarkable art forms were created, elite cemeteries were established, and a multitiered stratified society emerged, presumably essential to accomplishing large-scale tasks that were beginning to appear.[2] A few population centers now developed what might be termed true cities, one being Hierakonpolis, to be discussed below. It might be asked if these large administrative units would be considered city-states, to which most scholars would answer in the negative. But, as this early coalescence does not seem to have been a matter of conquest, for present

---

[1] A relatively new perspective is that of Dr. Ian Hodder, who, from his studies of the ancient community of Catalhoyuk (see p. 563), thinks some prehistoric settlements were not the consequence of herding, agriculture, and resulting sedentism. They were, instead, religious or ritual centers that attracted regional nomadic groups, those centers then becoming agricultural to support the increasing number of workers and visitors; i.e., their decision to institute agricultural techniques was the result, not the cause, of settlements. Regardless of origin, it is among stable settled societies that a nascent medical profession would later develop.

[2] Much of the information in this paragraph is adapted from: *Before the Pyramids*, Chicago, 2011, E. Teeter, editor, especially chapter three by Renee Friedman and chapter four by Branislov Andelkovic.

purposes they will be considered to have evolved in response to commercial ventures and needs, thereby autonomously developing into city-states as defined on p. 13. Ultimately there evolved at the end of the Naqada culture, and often out of conflict, a unified Egypt. Throughout this period the delta region remained agricultural and organizationally slower in evolution. A concurrent phenomenon, as concluded from examination of royal cemeteries of the Naqada III (Protodynastic) period, was "stark social differences" within the population, a forecast of the profound authoritarian governance that would follow. In support of this dismal outlook is the (limited) archeological evidence that support a mean life span of peasants of 30 years, whereas the upper class more often reached ages of 50-60. Childhood mortality is estimated at about 50% of those under five years.[3]

B. Hierakonpolis

Egyptian legend places the origin of medicine and the first named physician, Imhotep, in the 3rd Dynasty (2686-2613 BC).[4] For present purposes, however, the late Naqada city of Hierakonpolis will be used as the most likely locale for those early medical professionals who could have compiled the medical experience provided in the Ebers and Smith papyri. As the dominant city of Protodynastic and early Dynastic Egypt, Hierakonpolis was located in Upper Egypt beyond the Wadi Hammamat, the principle and shortest trade route between the Nile and coastal trading communities that bordered the Red Sea. Its location permitted ready access to gold mining further east. At its peak Hierakonpolis is thought to have been the home of about 10,000 people, but it held bureaucratic sway throughout the south of Upper Egypt and into neighboring Nubia. A rough estimate of the population in that region is 30 percent of the total Egyptian population of perhaps 350,000, or in the range of 100,000. Hieroglyphic/hieratic writing is first found there, probably a necessary invention in response to the development of commercial interests which included mass production of ceramics, importation of wood, precious metals, and significant interactions with Mesopotamian cities, especially Uruk.[5] Jewelry, trade in ivory, and other ventures as noted led to development of specialization of crafts. Hierakonpolis was the administrative center for the region and burial site of Narmer, probably the first Pharaoh of a united Egypt (3085 BC). In Egypt of the Protodynastic period, Dr. Juan Castillos, a noted authority on predynastic Egypt, has concluded an important social characteristic of the period was that "Kinship ties [were]

---

[3] A recent study of a non-elite cemetery at Hierakonpolis concluded that the age at death of those who reached 15 years of age was, during the late Naqada period, 30.6 years for men and 35.1 years for women. See: http://scholarworks.uark.edu/edt/565. Batey, E. K., *Population Dynamics in Predynastic Upper Egypt: Paleodemography of Cemetery HK43 at Hierakonpolis*, a Ph.D. thesis, Univ. of Arkansas (Fayetteville), 2012.

[4] The irrelevance of Imhotep to the history of medicine is discussed on p.73*f*. Nevertheless, the legendary/mythological attribution of the profession of medicine to a recognized 3rd Dynasty notable supports the idea that the event of a medical profession, if not the inventor, was not only wrought by this early date, *ca.* 2700 BC, but had developed to the point of being admired.

[5] See: Meza, A., *Ancient Egypt before Writing*: From Markings to Hieroglyphs, XLibris Corp., 2012. This book contains an extensive account of evidence supporting both a close commercial effort between predynastic Egypt and Mesopotamia and a significant Mesopotamian influence on Egyptian culture.

played down and largely replaced by other types of allegiance to semi-divine king ruling over a large territory."[6]

The archeological structure of Hierakonpolis is said to encompass in close proximity both the ancient city and an even more ancient, and larger, settlement area. Its development over centuries as described in the preceding paragraph has received more scholarly attention than other areas and has provided many of the findings that define the transition over time of predynastic Egypt. But with unification of Egypt *ca.* 3085 BC and a change of in the course of the local Nile, its significance decreased as the center of power moved to the as yet undiscovered city of Thinis. Thereafter, Hierakonpolis became primarily a religious center.

Earlier in the Protodynastic era the towns and small cities must have had their own medical practitioners, for practical management of abscesses, dental disease, and trauma demands attention in any era, and the person who learns how to manage them would be appreciated by the local community. Although they might have been appreciated, they may not have been paid, for they would have been merely common folk. But with prosperity things could change. And after transition to dynastic rule, a unified Egypt during the 1st and 2nd dynasties has been characterized as a time when specialization occurred among plebeians, and there was a period of "great creativity and inventiveness."[7] Certainly one of those specializations could have represented medical practitioners, commoners able to devote more of their time to medical care. These are the people who would have provided the clinical wisdom present in the Ebers and Smith papyri.

Religious practices in ancient Egypt included a variety of deities, the deity varying from city to city.[8] Shamanism is not a recognized feature of the mystical life of ancient Egypt. Nevertheless, it has been pointed out that pharaohs, like shamans, were viewed as mediators between the people and the afterlife, an interesting analogy that may be correct. Shamanism is a very individualistic enterprise and has even been characterized as entrepreneurial, and yet it has been associated with egalitarian societies. Perhaps one reason for the shaman's success in egalitarian societies everywhere may reside in the unique and unrestrained practitioner and his or her relative freedom from social controls. The people might view with awe such freedom of action that they forbade each other. Even the elite and the chief might fear the shaman. In this sense the shaman may have satisfied an egalitarian group's unstated desire for a power broker that could override an intrinsically fractious community or leader. In contrast, the priesthood, which would tend to smooth out differences between people and to maintain a ritualistic and predictable similarity within the larger group, was the friend of the leader. In any event it was the shaman who often held the individuality card under which the people were socially managed. The shaman and strong leader might vie for a monopoly on their positions, but the great power of a shamanistic pharaoh lay in his or her combination of the two.

In the days prior to the development of the pantheon of Egyptian deities and prior to the formal Egyptian priesthood of the Old Kingdom (4th Dynasty, a period of great pyramid building), individual medical practitioners would have had little or no official recognition. As members of a small and poorly remunerative society they would have received no special attention or remembrance. The point to be made is that this may have

---

[6] Castillos, J. J., *The Development and Nature of Inequality in Early Egypt*, in *British Museum Studies in Ancient Egypt and Sudan*, 13:73-81, 2009.

[7] See: Trigger, B., *et al., Ancient Egypt: A Social History*, Cambridge, 1983, p. 66.

[8] See: David, R., *Religion and Magic in Ancient Egypt*, London, 2002, chapter 2.

been the time, *i.e.,* during late Protodynastic or Early Dynastic periods, when empiric observations and decisions could be made by plebeian practitioners to form a collegial network, for by the time of Imhotep and the 3rd Dynasty the shamanistic façade of authoritarian pharaonic rule was becoming indelible.[9]

C. Clinical assessment of *Papyrus Ebers* and the *Smith Papyrus*

To better appreciate the significance of the work of ancient Egyptian practitioners a limited review of the texts of *Papyrus Ebers* and the *Smith Papyrus* in modern context will reveal the careful observations that underlie their clinical descriptions. A lengthy exposition is unnecessary as decades of focused attention have led to their popularity in the modern mind, but some mention will be made of modern analyses. It is important that these works be seen as the result of a concerted group effort.

Excursus on *Papyrus Ebers* and the *Smith Papyrus*

The two most important of the ten ancient Egyptian papyri that contain valid clinical information are the Ebers and the Smith papyri. Of the remaining eight papyri, much of their medical content can be traced to the Ebers papyrus and therefore of little help in determining the origin of its knowledge. But who collected and collated the original wisdom, and what was its nature? The medical knowledge in the Ebers and Smith papyri has been repeatedly assessed over the past century, and some claim ancient Egyptian medicine to be the foundation of Western medicine. Is that knowledge so unique, sufficiently rational and scientific, and widespread over time to justify that claim?

---

[9] Despite suggestions that in ancient shamanism is found the origin of religious feelings and the easing of physical stresses via hypnotic "altered states of consciousness" that might give a sick patient some survival advantage, classic histories of medicine, including those of Baas (*Outlines of the History of Medicine*, 1889), Nutton (*Ancient Medicine*, London, 2004), and Edelstein (*Ancient Medicine*, Baltimore, 1967), do not even mention the term "shamanism," confirming its insignificance in the history of medicine. A prominent physician, Dr. William Corlett, in his book *The Medicine Man of the American Indian and His Cultural Background* (Springfield, 1935), while providing a beautifully sympathetic (unjustifiably so, and racially demeaning as well) picture of the North American shaman, contains absolutely nothing of medical value, the few attempts at "treatment" often being grotesque. Also see: McClenon, J., *Shamanic Healing, Human Evolution and the Origin of Religion*, in *J. Scientific Study of Religion*, 36:345-354, 1997. This is in part based on a misrepresentation of the shaman's role, however, for the goal of the shaman was to control events. The fear and awe some tribal societies had for their shaman was but a shadow of the prodigious power surrounding the pharaohs. As the intermediary between the people and the gods, unlimited power was granted to pharaohs in all aspects of Egyptian life. While this was not implemented via drug-induced trance, other altered states of consciousness, or psychotic behavior, the mystical role of the shaman provided the same veneer of mystique surrounding and protecting the pharaoh. This shamanistic role of the pharaoh was not in competition with or shared with medical practitioners, but in exercising his powers over the people medical practitioners would have been swept up with all other components in society and used to the benefit of the ruling class. Thus, while the priest, like the shaman, had no reason to display other than benign neglect toward medical practitioners, the pharaoh's wide-ranging power in ancient Egypt made priests of his practitioners.

The complete hieratic texts of the Ebers and Smith papyri have been edited with commentary several times in the past by scholars but not by clinical physicians. The texts upon which commentary apropos ancient Chinese and Indian classics of medicine are based are readable to a limited extent without special training. In contrast, scholarly interpretation of hieroglyphic and hieratic texts, like cuneiform from Mesopotamia, requires familiarity with a form of writing that is the domain of few people. Fortunately, there has been interest by some physicians in assessing the role of their profession in the early papyri, both in literal translations and idiomatic expressions. Their specialized knowledge, often with the help of linguistic scholars, has provided meaningful interpretations of otherwise incomprehensible translations. It is for this reason that this Excursus will review some modern physicians' perspectives of ancient wisdom as presented in the Ebers and Smith papyri.

The *Smith Papyrus* and Neurosurgery:[10]

The text of this papyrus contains 48 descriptions of injuries to the head, arms, chest, and spine. One new perspective is an interpretation of the Smith papyrus that posits it comprises case studies that were not from actual patients, instead being idealized patients used to point out instructive clinical features to its readers. The authors of this theory point out that the clinical acuity present in descriptions of orthopedic injury in the manuscript is remarkable given the early state of the written language of the time. These opinions are supported by a review of the examination signs described in the text, *i.e.,* physical examination findings rather than a medical history provided by the patient, although it is apparent in many of the descriptions that the patient would have been in no condition to provide any information whatsoever. Those physical findings include:

a. Nuchal rigidity, an involuntary (reflexive) rigidity of the neck that resists flexion, results from blood in the cerebrospinal fluid or inflammation of the meninges as seen in meningitis. It is here differentiated from simple pain in the neck from local trauma in which, even though painful, the neck can be rotated and flexed (usually not a wise thing to do!).

b. A forerunner of the Lasegue straight leg-raising test is described in a lumbar spine injury.

c. Description differentiating a vertebral compression fracture from a "burst" fracture, the latter being a vertebral compression fracture with neurological deficits.

d. Knowledge that neurological complications from a cord injury depend on the level of the injury, a concept that implies an anatomical continuum of central nervous system control of peripheral nerve function.

e. Knowledge of anatomical changes resulting from axial trauma to the spinal cord, something unlikely to have been known without information obtained from dissection.

f. Knowledge that vertebral injury could cause peripheral sensory and motor deficits. As open bone-against-bone injuries, commonly encountered in armed conflict, produced no such deficits elsewhere, it is implied that the spinal cord,

---

[10] See: van Middendorp, J. J., Sanchez, G. M., and Burridge, A. L., *The Edwin Smith papyrus: a clinical reappraisal of the oldest known document on spinal injuries*, in *Eur. Spine J.*, 19:1815-1823, 2010.

rather than the vertebral bones, was involved in neurological function. But only in two cases were spinal cord deficits described, which implies that if cord damage, as opposed to vertebral damage, was evident the case was hopeless and there was no reason to teach that type of information to others if nothing could be done.

These six points of clinical deduction were made from six of the forty-eight cases described in the Smith Papyrus. That the person(s) who first made them was a keen and logical observer is without question, and that the selection of the cases as demonstrating six distinctive injuries was based on prior experience with similar injuries is also beyond doubt. Medical colleagues involved in translations such as this are to be commended for permitting modern readers to appreciate the subtleties of clinical examination that were apparent to those ancient practitioners but unapparent in most translations that followed.

The Smith Papyrus and wound management:

The following is based on Dr. Majno's interpretation of Case 47 from the Smith Papyrus.[11]

a. The patient had a wounded shoulder and a sequence is described for its management. Although washing the wound is not described, perhaps that had already been performed, for the next recommendation was to suture the wound. This is interesting, for in the recent past a "dirty" wound, one received in an unsanitary environment or by an unsanitary device, has, after superficial cleaning, often been allowed to heal without suturing, a slow process called "healing by secondary intention." This requires careful nursing attention, but the fear is that a focus of infection might be enclosed within the wound if it is sutured. But it has been stated that in every war surgeons quickly relearn that prompt cleansing and suturing even "dirty" wounds is often quite satisfactory, and so apparently thought the practitioner who wrote about Case 47; sew up the wound, apply a grease and honey mixture, and it may well heal satisfactorily.

b. On repeat examination if the sutures are loose, tighten them and apply more salve, and here the practitioner says that, as the swelling is decreasing, the procedure he is recommending can be applied anywhere on the body, not just the shoulder.

c. If, on the next examination the wound is inflamed and the patient has a fever, the practitioner does not bind (close) the wound, for enclosed infections are, for the most part, much more dangerous that draining ones. Thus, the general approach to this patient has been sound.

d. Another interesting aspect of this Case is the definition of "inflamed," for the ancient practitioner had no term for the redness, swelling, pain, and heat associated with infection, but Dr. Majno has convincingly described the hieroglyphic signs meaning "heat" in context. With this the implied terms of local heat (from inflammation) and generalized heat (fever) seem appropriate translations.

The Ebers Papyrus and "cutting:"

---

[11] See: Majno, G., *The Healing Hand*, Cambridge (MA), 1975, p.97-99.

Although the Ebers Papyrus is primarily a pre-Iron Age therapeutic composition and contains almost 800 recipes, it has snippets of clinical work that help to assign it to an empirical-rational document. One is the use of "knives" for making incisions. Several are mentioned, and Dr. Majno has convincingly pointed out that one form of knife was made from papyrus reeds, and those who have suffered a "paper cut" will recall the strength of thin and seemingly fragile pages of paper. But beyond this, Dr. Majno mentions three types of swellings conducive to incision:

a. Paragraph 871 probably describes an abscess and is to be incised and drained, with care being taken to avoid cutting any nearby blood vessels.

b. Paragraph 872 suggests a vascular tumor (swelling) that can be excised if the knife is hot, which implies that the anticipated bleeding will require a hot knife. Proteins coagulate at about 60 degrees C (140 degrees F), so a knife made from papyrus reed could have been heated to boiling 100 degrees C (212 degrees F) and perhaps helped minimize bleeding or oozing from an incision. [12]

c. Paragraph 876 describes a swelling where a physical blow had occurred. If bleeding occurred a level of heating approaching cautery was necessary, and a "fire-drill" was used, presumably a slender piece of wood heated by friction.

d. Dr. Majno also notes that the wounds in the Smith Papyrus were generally not infected, at least initially, whereas in the Ebers Papyrus the lesions probably were all infected. As such, there often would have been local collections of pus that required incision and drainage if they did not drain themselves.

e. In Paragraph 522 a section on assisting healing of a wound restates the importance of maintaining drainage until the wound has healed, but it also mentions the use of "spoiled" bread to assist if the purulent drainage is excessive. [13] Perhaps this was to help dry the wound, but moldy bread has at times been suggested as a source of salutary antibiotic activity.

f. Finally, some swellings could be removed cleanly whereas others required care so that retained material would not cause a recurrence of the swelling. In other words, it was important to allow an infected wound to completely drain, or the infection would flare up again.

All these points confirm a practical empirical approach to management of visible lesions of various types, including a probable umbilical hernia and the removal of a Guinea worm. [14] That instructions would not only be given on handling such patients but that they would be recorded is proof sufficient for the existence of collaborating medical professionals in that distant age.

---

[12] Bamboo knives were common in ancient southeast Asia.

[13] The potential for some penicillin-like activity from moldy food has received attention for topical use (see p. 379*f*). The Egyptians also used honey and copper salts on wounds, also significant sources of antibiotic activity. There is also evidence that herbal "wines" were available in the late Naqada period, which suggests that alcohol extraction might have been used to obtain more active principals from botanicals. (McGovern, P. E., Mirzoian, A., and Hall, G. R., *Ancient Egyptian Herbal Wines*, in *Proc. Nat. Acad. Sci.,* 106:7361-7366.)

[14] See: Strouhal, E., Vachala, B., and Vymazalova, H., *The Medicine of the Ancient Egyptians*, New York, 2014, especially chapter 3, *Ancient Egyptian Surgery*, which updates thinking on this section of *Papyrus Ebers*.

Papyrus Ebers and the vascular system:

In paragraphs 854 and 856 are found descriptions of a distribution system extending throughout the body. At the center of the system was the heart. Pulsations of the heart were recognized and could be felt at different sites around the body. Confusion arises in this interpretation because the ancient Egyptian practitioner(s) who inferred this distribution system could not, as did not the early Hippocratic physicians centuries later, differentiate between cord-like (tendons, nerves) and tube-like structures (blood vessels) that were found throughout the body. Assuming this to be the case the term "pulse/vessel" will be used here to include (1) palpable pulsations and (2) cord- or tube-like structures that were known to exist but were not palpable and therefore not susceptible to pulse taking. A comprehensive review of anatomical descriptions in the Papyrus Ebers is provided by Dr. John Nunn, an accomplished physician. A slight modification of the opinions expressed in that work is provided here: [15]

a. There were three pulses/vessels in each arm: the radial pulse at the wrist, the brachial pulse at the elbow, and the axillary pulse in the axilla.

b. There were three pulses in each leg: the femoral pulse at the groin, the popliteal pulse in back of the knee, and the dorsalis pedis pulse on the dorsum of the foot. As the popliteal pulse is not so obvious the third pulse could have been the posterior tibial pulse on the medial aspect of the ankle.

c. There were four pulses of the temple: the superficial temporal arterial pulse is noticeable in two places, immediately in front of the ear and on the forehead lateral to the eye. As this would be bilateral the total would be four.

d. There are two pulses for the nose that carry blood and two that carry mucus: the dorsal nasal artery is bilateral and felt on the bridge of the nose near the inner angle of the eye. It is possible that the other pair was thought to be internal and the cause of the common nosebleed. The responsible area is now called Kiesselbach's plexus, wherein lies an anastomosis of five small arteries that would not have been identifiable. That plexus is bilateral, one on each side of the nasal septum. If the two thought to be carrying blood represented the latter, the palpable ones (the dorsal nasal arteries) near the bridge of the nose may have been those postulated to carry mucus.

e. The two pulses referable to the bladder are thought to have been ureters, the tube-like structures that carry urine from the kidneys to the bladder.

f. The two pulses to the testes are thought to have been the bilateral spermatic cords. (These are fully palpable but do not pulsate.)

g. The four pulses to the liver: the bile duct, hepatic artery, portal vein and hepatic vein. These would have been identified easily in the butchering of animals or in mummification of humans at the time the liver was removed. As the incision was not long and usually on the left side, the four tube-like structures would have been identifiable on the removed wedges of liver. Although not routinely performed until the dynastic period, organ removal was occasionally practiced as early as 4,000 BC.

---

[15] See: Nunn, J. F., *Ancient Egyptian Medicine*, Norman (OK), 2005, p. 48.

h. There are four pulses for the spleen and lungs: the spleen has two vessels, the splenic artery and vein; the lung has the trachea which splits into two mainstem bronchi, one to each lung.

i. There are two pulses for each ear: the external ear canal and the Eustachian tube.

Although the association of pulse with vessels other than arteries indicates gross ignorance of the physiology involved, the mere palpation of peripheral pulses in some of the sites noted above indicate an element of assiduity in observation and examination that would not have been undertaken, and certainly not recorded, by a layman. Again, this is evidence of an early professional at work, but not merely one professional. It was the work of a group of professional practitioners who maintained a collegial network.

In conclusion, those ancient Egyptian writings that have come down to us may not have laid out a scheme of physiology, anatomy, and physical examination that would lead to modern medical discovery, but it was a solid commencement by persons who were capable of improving their original work. That their observations would never be built upon by others was not a fault of theirs.

End of excursus

D. Conclusion

The location of the compilers of the wisdom of the Ebers and Smith papyri was likely to have been Heirakonpolis, for it had the largest concentration of people. But there is no reason that a network of practitioners could not have existed in proximal peripheral settlements, periodically exchanging ideas and observations. Remarkably, however, there is no contemporary documentation of any medical practitioner or medical instrumentation so far discovered from either the Protodynastic or the Early Dynastic periods.

Nevertheless, the argument is proposed here that would place the original compositions of the Ebers and Smith papyri (or the fragments from which the later copies would be made) after the Naqada II period and before the 3rd Dynasty of a unified Egypt, *i.e.,* between 3300 and 2700 BC. Population centers before this time would have been small and scattered, and after 2700 the uniting of Upper and Lower Egypt by the 3rd Dynasty pharaoh, Djoser, initiated monumental projects that included fortifications, pyramids as burial monuments with sacrifice of humans and animal, military conquests into the Sinai that indicate profound control over most of the Egyptian population by an elite class and military. Pharaonic priest physicians soon followed. Consistent with the argument is the statement by Manetho, the 3rd C BC Egyptian historian, who wrote that the 1st Dynasty's second pharaoh, Athothis (ruled *ca.* 3050-3000 BC), was a "physician" and that he wrote an anatomical text.[16] While it seems unlikely that a pharaoh would have

---

[16] Manetho's text: "Athothis his son, [he ruled] 57 years, he built the palace in Memphis; anatomical books were brought forth, for he was a medical practitioner." This is found on p. 28 of the Loeb Classical Library text of Book 1 of Manetho's *History of Egypt*. Manetho, a 3rd C BC Egyptian priest, is not known with certainty to have been an authentic figure. But this leads to an intriguing suggestion by Prof. Calvin Schwabe in his fascinating book, *Cattle, Priests, and Progress in Medicine* (Minneapolis, 1978, p. 71), in which he reasonably posits that Athothis, being a healer,

done such a thing, the placing of a medical work early in the 1ˢᵗ Dynasty is (1) consistent with the reasoning put forth in this section regarding Hierakonpolis, and (2) chronologically believable because of the mention of the 1ˢᵗ Dynasty fourth pharaoh, Den (ruled 3000 to 2960 BC), in paragraph 856a of the *Papyrus Ebers*. It also suggests that the information in Athothis' book on anatomy must have been acquired during at least the preceding century or two to have been considered so important. Thus, the timing of the professional collation of medical wisdom of the Ebers and Smith papyri, based circumstantially on social environment and legend, is likely to have been between 3300 and 2700 BC, with a probability it was close to the earlier date, *i.e.,* Protodynastic.

As for population metrics, the local concentration of the population at Hierakonpolis at its peak was considerable smaller than the Greek city-state of Miletos, although it is likely that the size of the regional population interacting at Hierakonpolis was not too different, perhaps 100,000. Its population density also was considerably smaller but the area of hegemony was larger. Protodynastic Egypt was undergoing a period of growth and centralization, with development of extensive distant trade, surplus production of food, and foci of groups involved in production of a variety of products, including luxury items of individualistic design, that seemed unrelated to any central authority and were often organized outside the central city. As a functional urban center it must have been the trade network that provided the necessary cohesion for a stable city. Indeed, Protodynastic Egypt has been identified with "industrial scale mass production."[17] Of the different possibilities, a heterarchical system of commercial, and thereby social, governance (perhaps a "settlement hierarchy," see p. 13) existed, also similar to Miletos.

Moving away from egalitarian kinship villages and into population centers, the new citizens of the city, now prospering, could have supported small groups of medical practitioners that remained in contact over time and communicated their medical observations to one another. A recent analysis of Egyptian state formation by Dr. Alice Stevenson includes the following statement: "… intractable and permanent inequality was established at the end of the Predynastic…"[18] This may have reflected an elite class of wealth, a consequence of successful commercial ventures. But to many plebeians this must have meant opportunity. Writing was available to a limited population, namely those benefiting from its use in commerce, thereby also contributing to establishment of an elite class. But it should be borne in mind that not only the earliest Egyptian medical writings but also those of Sumer emerged concurrently with the invention of writing not because writing was necessary for their intellectual composition but because clinical knowledge

---

must also have been a veterinarian, thereby gaining knowledge from comparative anatomy that explains in part the contemporary and subsequent misinterpretations of human anatomy. Were the present volume not an abridgement more time would be spent on the important but unsung role played by animal healing and dissection in the earliest history of medicine as described by Dr. Schwabe, a veterinarian. And its contemporary importance is underscored by the Dean's advice to the author's entering medical school class at the Ohio State University many years ago: "When you begin your practice in a town the first person you should meet is the local veterinarian." That person would know the endemic medical environment and its health risks to humans as well as other animals.

[17] See: Hikade, T., *Urban Development at Hierakonpolis and the Stone Industry of Square 10 N5W,* in *Egypt at Its Origins*, Dudley (MA), 2004, S. Hendrickx, et al., editors.

[18] See: Stevenson, A., *The Egyptian Predynastic and State Formation,* in *J. Archaeol. Res.*, 24:421-468, 2016, the final paragraph. The basis for other statements in this and the preceding paragraph can also be found in this excellent scholarly review of the subject.

already compiled in preceding centuries may have just been awaiting the opportunity for a more durable perpetuation.

Thus, while the complexities of Egyptian development overall suggest early trends to centralized bureaucratic control in the region, more generally there was prosperity and a variation of enterprise. A meaningful manuscript collation of medical experience previously obtained in the Protodynastic could now appear within a network of medical practitioners.

Summary Table for Hierakonpolis:

STAGE – Protodynastic (Neolithic)
POPULATION, LOCAL – 10,000
POPULATION, TOTAL – 105,000
PRIMARY AREA – 0.5 square miles (300 acres)
URBAN DENSITY – 31 persons per acre
PRODUCTION – ceramics, jewelry, ivory, beer
GOVERNANCE – fading of kinship social organization as population increasingly joined local elites in urbanization and became involved in commerce (heterarchy), later developing bureaucracies and then rigidly hierarchical pharaonic dynasties
EGALITARIAN ARCHEOLOGY – no (some elite burials)
PROMINENT EGALITARIAN KINSHIPS - no
WRITING – yes
DISTANT TRADE – yes
SPECIALIZATION – yes
MONUMENTAL STRUCTURES – no; large walls or forts and the first (step) pyramids appear in the second dynasty or later
DENOUEMENT – change in course of the Nile River, and then subsumed by dynastic Egypt as a religious center
MEDICAL PRACTICE – presumed, but no artifacts
FORMATIVE PERIOD – 1200 years (Naqada culture)
FLORUIT – 400 years (beginning of Protodynastic [3300 BC] to end of Dynasty I [2900 BC])
CITY-STATE – yes (by the definition given on p. 13)
AVERAGE LIFE EXPECTANCY – 30 years

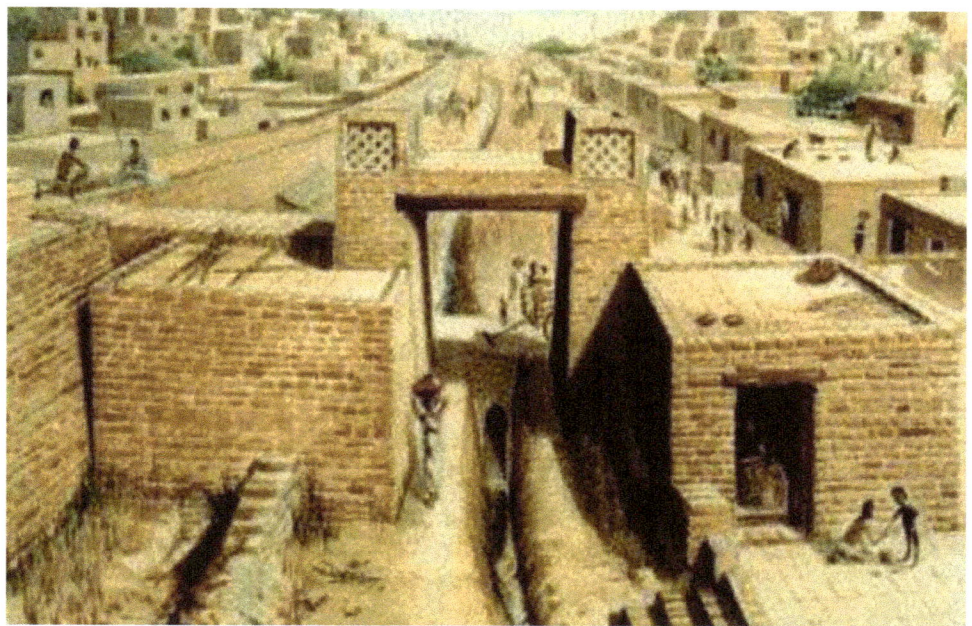

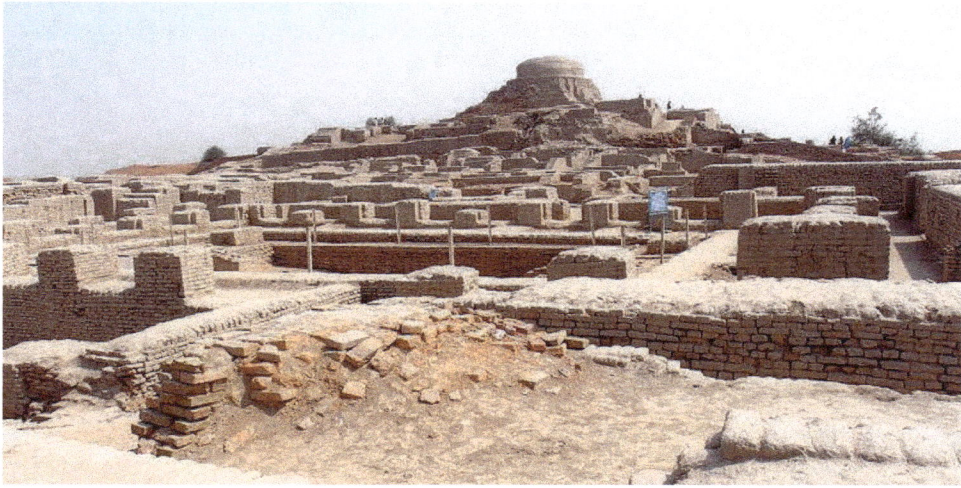

Fig. 16: Top: An artist's depiction of the gateway to the city of Harappa, a companion city to Mohenjo-daro in the Indus River Valley civilization, showing a facet of the drainage system as it may have existed about 2500 BC, the earliest urban waste management system known. The photograph, unattributed, can be seen on the Crystalinks website. Bottom: Photograph by Saqib Qayyum of the excavation site of Mohenjo-daro located in the present-day Sindh province of Pakistan, is available through Creative Commons Attribute-Share Alike 3.0 unported. Prominent in the distance is a domed Buddhist stupa, a much more recent construction.

CHAPTER THIRTY

MOHENJO-DARO AND THE EARLY INDUS RIVER VALLEY CIVILIZATION

Recent archeology has revealed the remarkable remnants of an Indus River Valley civilization that may parallel in scope the Mesopotamian civilization. In contrast to Uruk, the minimal evidence of fortifications and social stratification provide traditional support for an egalitarian social organization in the region for much of its history. Over time it evolved extensive trade based on agriculture, pottery, sculpture, jewelry, timber, textiles, and ivory, quite different from that of Mesopotamia which was primarily based on exportation of agricultural products in return for metals, wood, and other items. The Indus River Valley civilization had access to the Arabian Sea, to central Asia, east through the sub-Himalayan belt across the Indian subcontinent, and to the tropical south. New findings indicate the local culture, rather than an Indo-Aryan immigration, was the likely source of at least a portion of the Vedas that have guided Indian culture ever since. The principal relevance to medicine has been the *Atharva Veda*, the foundation of Ayurvedic medicine. There is controversial evidence of a written, non-cuneiform, language for the Indus River Valley civilization, as yet undeciphered. The *Charaka Samhita* and the *Sushruta Samhita*, roughly 2,000 years old, are the classic expressions of Ayurvedic medicine, and they contain a wealth of clinical material unfortunately rewritten over the ages to support a theocratic elite class. But the original objective observations in the two works probably derive from the period when the Indus River Valley civilization was commercially flourishing (2600-2000 BC), suggesting the presence during that period of a network of medical practitioners.

A. Overview of the Indus River Valley Civilization

In contrast to the Mesopotamian civilization that evolved relatively quickly in a newly formed geographical region, an alluvial plain and delta north of the Red Sea, the Indus River Valley civilization is now considered to have encompassed an unbroken cultural prehistory extending back to at least 8,000 BC. For present purposes, however, interest is focused on the era and the locale that produced the Vedas, a group of four expansive spiritual-philosophical hymns that (1) were later integrated into Hinduism, and (2) were the prehistoric source of traditional Indian medicine, Ayurveda, first primitively expressed in the tract designated the *Atharva Veda*.

The early Indus River civilization was coeval with Sumer in Mesopotamia and Protodynastic and Early Dynastic Egypt along the Nile River. Its distance from Uruk would have been about 1,800 miles, almost twice as far as Hierakonpolis in Egypt was from Uruk. Even in its earliest cities there is evidence of a progressive culture as manifested by its constructions, city planning, standardization of weights, and widely available in-house plumbing that included toilets. It seems appropriate to consider its waste disposal system and water supply as true evidence of progress, for fired bricks that can last for centuries were devised for construction of wells and drains, and the onset of their use can be dated to *ca.* 2600 BC. Prof. Jonathon Kenoyer stated, "For the first time, we find widespread evidence of formally tiered settlement hierarchies complete with specialized craft settlements ... ."[1]   There may have been a type of writing, as yet undeciphered, that was present prior to 3000 BC and which changed little over subsequent centuries, although the exact nature of the symbols remains undetermined.   The population of the Indus River Valley civilization at its peak has been estimated as high as five million.

When the Indus River Valley civilization is divided into phases the Vedas are often assigned to the Late Harappan era (Harappa was a major city of the Indus River Valley civilization), dated 1900-1300 BC, but an analysis of new data by Dr. Subash Kak offers 2000 BC as the latest possible date for the earliest formulations, or "samhitas," of the Vedas and possibly much earlier.[2, 3]   The dates are important, for during its existence the large Indus River Valley civilization changed dramatically, moving from egalitarian villages to an archeologically egalitarian city-state culture with no city centers, temples, monumental structures, or royal tombs, then through an urbanizing culture with evidence of hierarchical organization to a period of decline as presumed environmental changes prompted a migration of many of the population to the east.[4]

The earliest cities appeared in the pre-Harappan phase of the civilization, *ca.* 3300 BC, with at least one city, Rehman Dhari, having a population of perhaps 10,000. But it was in the Harappan II phase (2800-2600 BC) that the civilization rapidly grew, and a major city was ancient Mohenjo-daro on the Indus River. It was settled in the early 3rd millennium BC and over several centuries is thought to have grown to a population of 40,000. Because of limited evidence of defensive protection, it has been proposed as a major administrative center for the surrounding region. Covering almost a thousand acres, it had, by 2300 BC, a central "citadel" on which was a large public "Great" bath, wells, a priest residence, and a marketplace. Its advanced system of urban planning with streets laid according to a grid, a remarkable system of sewage drainage including flush toilets in most houses, local wells, bathhouses with heated water, courtyards, and some two-story houses. The egalitarian face of the city has been inferred from the similarity in dwellings and their contents, whether in the city itself or in the peripheral settlements, in the widespread access to water, sewage drainage, and in the absence of palatial structures. There is little evidence for social stratification or a ruling class, but it has been suggested that such a well-devised urbanization must have had elected officials. Indeed, the similarities among several of the Indus River Valley cities have been interpreted by some as supporting a central State-level authority for the region.

---

[1] See: Coningham, R., and Young, R., *The Archaeology of South Asia: From the Indus to Asoka, c. 6500 BCE-200 CE*, Cambridge, 2015, p. 172.

[2] See: Kak, S., *On the Chronological Framework for Indian Culture*, in *Indian Council of Philosophical Research*, pp. 1-24, 2000, for a convenient updating of the history of ancient India based on recent archeological and literary research. The author notes that the *Rig Veda* may have been composed before 3,000 BC if, as it states, the Sarasvati river emptied into the sea at that time.

[3] There is great controversy not just over dates but regarding the nature of the Indus River civilization itself. Questions include: (1) was there an influx of Indo-Aryans from the Western Siberian Plain carrying with them the foundational concepts that would, over the next thousand years, determine the initiation and nature of Hinduism, or (2) was there instead an emigration of the same concepts out of the Indus River valley and into western Asia and the Middle East. All this bears on the dating of the Vedas. For a summary of evidence see *The Indo-Aryan Controversy*, Abington, 2005, E. F. Bryant and L. L. Patton, editors, especially chapter 11 by Michael Witzel.

[4] Schug, G. R., et al., *Infection, Disease and Biosocial Processes at the End of the Indus Civilization*, 2013, PLoS One.2013; 8(12):e84814.

Importantly, Mohenjo-daro had an Upper and a Lower section, the latter being large and divided into "spatially discrete" neighborhoods based at least in part on commercial enterprise and perhaps kinship/ethnicity. Within each neighborhood there was a focus of larger dwellings for a small segment of the population, perhaps for those directing the commercial venture or a prominent family within a kinship-based neighborhood. Of note, a few prominent structures in each neighborhood bore resemblance to what are considered large public structures of the Upper section. This commonality of architecture is thought to have linked the various neighborhoods together, in doing so bridging the natural resistance that occurs between traditional kinship allegiances and those forces of centralization necessary to maintain a cohesive urban center.[5] The planning necessary for the mature city of Mohenjo-daro suggests that, whatever its humble origin, it developed in such a way as to suit a population needed for commercial ventures. Neither an egalitarian nor an authoritarian governing structure is supported by the newest evidence. It is appropriate, therefore, to consider its social organization during the centuries of prosperity one of heterarchy, or perhaps corporatism, despite archeological indicators typically associated with egalitarianism. Economically it was a corporate city and its organization was an expression of convenience, efficiency, and an attempt to satisfy its citizenry. Perhaps it can be likened to the corporate development of the Endicott-Johnson shoe manufacturing company in New York State in the early 20th century. George F. Johnson, the chief executive of this prominent business, initiated the *Square Deal* for company employees that involved profit sharing, healthcare, and home financing. City planning was involved. In a sense, it was a joint venture between company management and its employees, one term applied to it being "welfare capitalism."[6] It was highly successful in every way. If a similar arrangement evolved in Mohenjo-daro and if the citizen employees were involved in shaping the urban environment, this would qualify for the term "corporatism" and differentiating it from either an authoritarian hierarchy or a heterarchy.

Another city, ultimately a city-state, was Harappa, for which the Harappan culture has been named. It had its origin about 3800 BC. A thousand years later it had the beginnings of craft specialization, *i.e.,* about 2800 BC. It was after this time that urbanization occurred, so that by 2600 BC it could be classified as a city-state for its hegemony stretched, like Mohenjo-daro, over many nearby small villages. It also flourished in the Late Mature Indus River Valley civilization phase (2200-2000 BC). At this time there was important trade with Mesopotamia and other distant regions. But studies of skeletal remains reveal, despite the suggestion of minimal social stratification, evidence of disease and violence against some of the community, as identified in remains of non-elite cemeteries but not in elite ones. Both Harappa and Mohenjo-daro went into a precipitous decline *ca.* 2000 BC.

The major factor behind the growth of population centers in the Indus River Valley was commercial development, for extensive trade existed across the sub-Himalayan region of northern India, the southern tropical region of the Indian subcontinent with its spices and exotic animals, and central Asia with its ores and precious stones. Casting of metals, practical mathematics (standard weights and scales, use of a binary decimal system), perhaps an early form of writing, mass production of ceramic

---

[5] See: Mosher, M. S., *The Architecture of Mohenjo-Daro as Evidence for the Organization of Indus Civilization Urban Neighborhoods*, Univ. of Toronto, Ph.D. thesis, 2017.
[6] See: Zahavi, G., *Workers, Managers, and Welfare Capitalism: The Shoemakers and Tanners of Endicott Johnson, 1890-1950*, Urbana, 1988.

goods and textiles, seals such as occurred in Mesopotamia, and trade with Mesopotamia also provide documentation of its economic life. There also was river access to the Arabian Sea. A broad-based cultivation of crops with irrigation and the domestication of animals also developed, this probably being secondary to commercial development and trade in order to accommodate the increasing population. Although city populations might number in the tens of thousands, the region was flush with surrounding small settlements that interacted with commercial efforts in the cities and provided their sustenance. It is for this reason that Mohenjo-daro and Harappa are identified herein as city-states, for interaction with the peripheral settlements was not one of domination but of coordination, presumably through commercial networks, and for this reason overall governance of the region will be designated as a heterarchy of commercial ventures.

The limited information on the Indus River civilization makes identification of the social context for any medical compilations uncertain, but it is clear that, for the peripheral and agricultural arm of society, kinships were intact, their role in agricultural surpluses centering around water sources, with consensual kin-based management of water resources.[7] This type of management would have been assigned to leaders or patriarchs from the various kinships, and while they might assign a kinship to fulfill a specific role or task in water management the internal social structure of the kinship would remain unchanged, its egalitarian aspects retained.

Within the cities themselves, however, it is not easy to imagine a role for traditional small kinships given the many options and opportunities. Typically, this is the time when a nuclear family is able to assert its independence from the clan. Traditional ties of kinship are considered to have been especially strong prior to an urbanizing India, and there is evidence that in prehistoric times land ownership that often accompanied a kinship helped maintain its influence. It has even been proposed that the neighborhoods found within the boundary of Mohenjo-daro represent kinship holdings, in which case they may have been a real source of power.[8] But over time the kinships of the more powerful that initially represented commercial interests would establish themselves in the city-state and become "oriented to the stabilization of new power structures," whereas plebeian kinships that represented the majority of the population would have had a decrease in influence.[9] Thus, because of urbanization both a loss of influence and a weakened hold over individual members diminished the kinship.

It must be remembered, of course, that the role of early or primitive egalitarian kinships is not merely a matter of redistribution of assets; egalitarian kinships represent assigned status and obligations to fellow members. As Dr. Jared Diamond has stated it, the egalitarian component in these small societies may require redistribution of resources but it does not mean equal status. Rather, egalitarian leadership is informal and there is no formal stratification or monopoly on leadership, information, or decision-making.[10] And should several kinships within a settlement jointly agree to initiate or participate in

---

[7] See: Miller, H. M.-L., *Surplus in the Indus Civilization: Agricultural Choices, Social Relations, Political Effects*, in *Surplus: The Politics of Production and the Strategies of Everyday Life*, Boulder, 2015, C. T. Morehart and K. De Lucia, editors, chapter 4.

[8] See: Ratnaga, S., *Townsman and Tribesman at Mohenjo-Daro* in *Annales Histoire Sciences Sociales*, 59:39-71, 2004.

[9] See: Basant, P. K., *Urbanization and Society in Early India*, in *A Social History of Early India*, p. 81, Delhi, 2009, B. D. Chattopadhyaya, editor, volume 2 of *History of Science, Philosophy and Culture in Indian Civilization*, D. P. Chattopadhyaya, editor.

[10] Diamond, J., *Guns, Germs, and Steel*, New York, 1999, a paperback, chapter 14, p. 269.

a commercial venture, that outcome could lead to a form of corporatism in which the kinships would not represent just employees but could actually contribute to the nature of that venture. In contrast, should there be an agreement to have a central storage for the kinships' grain for redistribution as needed, that would be an example of collectivism. Of the two scenarios, corporatism and trade would invite prosperity and collectivism would provide security. Equally of the two scenarios, corporatism would foster growth, whereas collectivism would contain it, for without commerce there would have been no inherent reason to enlarge. A growing city may be thought a desirable goal in modern times, but with primitive urbanization there would have been nothing of the sort. When considering the sources of power or influence in a developing city-state, collectivism is unimportant. This is not meant to reflect its desirability, but it is a reflection of its actual status. Simply put, a city-state could never exist without a successful commercial base unless coercion were involved. Just as early writing and mathematics were developed as tools for commerce, early cities also developed in response to commercial needs. Thus, the commonsense conclusion must be that alliances within plebeian kinships gave way to alliances with commercial ventures as Indus River Valley city-states prospered. This attracted others who wished to share in prosperity rather than remain within traditional village kinship boundaries of obligations, customs, and status. The shift apparently was voluntary. It is, therefore, within the city of the city-state, not the surrounding settlements, that a network of medical practitioners might have initially evolved, the city a place of opportunity, the peripheral settlements a niche for stability and tradition.[11]

The decline of the Indus River Valley civilization is usually dated *ca.* 2000 BC, but the decline was slow and asymmetrical over centuries. Separately, for over a thousand years tribal kingdoms with clear class distinctions developed throughout the subcontinent. None became dominant until dynastic empires developed, the Mauryan Dynasty being the one that unified the region in the 4th C BC. Thus, the Indus River Valley civilization did not decline because of incorporation within a powerful empire. But it was during this Late Harappan period that it is proposed the Vedas assumed their prominence throughout India and, in later centuries, that Hinduism and the caste system were promulgated.

B. The Vedas

The Vedas, four extensive hymns that provide the early scriptural base of Hinduism (The Rig Veda [hymns and their mystical exegesis], the Artharva Veda [procedures for everyday life], the Yajurveda [prose worship rituals], and the Samaveda [holy songs]), have been considered of divine origin and presented to humankind through the words of inspired ancient sages. From them the Vedic age has been thus named, its chronology being fixed between the end of the Indus River Valley civilization (*ca.* 1500 BC) and 600 BC. In the past they were thought to have been introduced into India by an influx of Indo-Aryan populations from the Western Siberian Plain, people who entered

---

[11] In: Mosher, M. S., *The Architecture of Mohenjo-Daro as Evidence for the Organization of Indus Civilization Urban Neighborhoods*, Univ. of Toronto, Ph.D. thesis, 2017, the following statement is found: "… lie at the heart of the motives by which people initially abandoned local autonomy for a more restrictive and asymmetrical social order." It is one conclusion of this volume that, when it comes to judging motives, the reverse is more accurate. People were taking advantage of early urbanization for relief from the restrictive social order of egalitarianism, in the process preferring to accept the unknowns of city life in hope of a better one.

northern sections of the country west of the Himalayas, their religion being superimposed on local religious practices as they displaced or integrated and then superseded the large population living in the Indus River Valley. But modern scholarship, based on new archeological evidence, has been shifting to a dramatically different interpretation, namely that events and findings previously attributed to foreigners can now be considered, at least in part, indigenous, especially those in the region of the Indus River Valley.[12] This, however, has led to controversy with regard to the origin of the Vedas, their actual presence previously being considered an Indo-Aryan linguistic marker. The issue will not be resolved here.

If the Vedas did not arrive from regions northwest of the subcontinent, the regional location for the proposed sages that saw the production of the Vedas may have ranged broadly across northern India, roughly covering the territory of the Indus River civilization and further east over the Indo-Gangetic alluvial plain, stretching sea to sea across northern India. Houses that have been declared to be Harappan in construction in the west have been found as far east as Uttar Pradesh.

At some point, however, mention of datable events in the Vedas permit this frequently mystical work to become at one with reality in the context of identifiable societies. It is here proposed that it was primarily in the Indus River region during the "mature" Harappan era (2600-2000 BC) that a prospering and urbanizing people formally integrated local concepts into the Vedas, for that region had by far the greatest population, highest population density, prosperity, dominant culture, and, central to present discussion, a proposed network of medical practitioners, an argument clarified below. It must be remembered that present discussion is about the Vedas and medicine, that the ancient treatises that entered the Charaka and Sushruta Samhitas are assumed to have derived from a group of medical practitioners, and that this would have required a practitioner network residing in a city, not in scattered rural villages. Thus, the *Atharva Veda*, which is the oldest Veda but one, has the most extensive reference to medicine and evidence of a rational approach to medicine. It must originated in a city or had medical elements incorporated into its text by city dwellers.[13]

It is notable that some Dravidian terms are found among the *Rig Veda* Sanskrit, and a Dravidian language was used in parts of the ancient Indus River Valley.[14] This suggests that the original material was amended in the Indus River Valley. Furthermore, while much scholarship places Veda composition between 1500-500 BC (the Vedic age), it has been pointed out that mention of courses of rivers (especially the Sarasvati river, which ceased to flow about 1900 BC) and events (astronomical mentions, the Bharata war, and genealogies) in the earliest Vedic compositions permit a much earlier date for

---

[12] Some findings previously considered to have been introduced by foreign invaders can be explained by Indus River civilization trade with other cultures/civilizations that included Mesopotamia and Egypt. These include cylindrical engraved seals for commercial and ritual use.

[13] It has been pointed out that the word "caraka" has been considered the origin of Charaka in the Charaka Samhita, and that it has been translated as wandering mendicant, suggesting peripatetic practitioners were the source of the samhita's clinical material. This may be analogous to early Greek practitioners who traveled from city to city. While all this may be true as far as it goes, there would have been no Charaka Samhita unless there were a coordinated collation of data from many practitioners, and this could have occurred only in a populous area where practitioners had convenient contact with one another, most likely after shifting from wandering medicants to a settled existence.

[14] See: Parpola, A., *The Roots of Hinduism: The Early Aryans and the Indus Civilization*, Oxford, 2015.

their origin, at least for the *Rig Veda*, the first and foremost of the Vedas. Thus, Dr. Subhash Kak is able to propose that the early Vedic literature was composed prior to 2000 BC (footnote reference, p. 505). This information is important for it permits, in turn, an earlier date for the composition of the *Atharva Veda* and thereby the collection of the scientific clinical observations upon which is based Ayurvedic medicine. If there were a climatic or other catastrophe that led to the slow disintegration of the Indus River Valley civilization *ca.* 2000 BC, which seems likely, the associated social disruption would make the intellectual production of the Vedas less likely after that upheaval than during the preceding prosperous Harrapan era. The prehistoric origin of the Vedas may never be accurately determined, but for present discussion the Kak estimate will be used with the understanding that the chronology, but not the sequence, of these early events may err by half a millennium or more. Extant manuscripts of fragments of the Vedas are chronologically unhelpful, the oldest being Nepalese manuscripts dated to the 11th C AD.

This confusing section can be summarized as follows. Like Uruk in Sumer and Hierakonpolis in Egypt, Mohenjo-daro arose among humble villages to become a major commercial and trading center. In the process, its central populations traded a kinship-structured rural life for an urbanized society in which personal and family allegiances were now switching to stable and prospering commercial ventures. Living in neighborhoods, even clans or entire tribes may have agreed *en masse* to join in a commercial venture, suggesting a form of corporatism in which the workers helped determine the course that commerce and urban development would take.[15] It is proposed that during this period, *ca.* 2600-2000 BC, networks of medical practitioners arose and objective and empirical observations of a medical and biological nature were made. The unprecedented objective perspective of illness and nature pursued philosophically in the *Atharva Veda* had to come from somewhere. While not wishing to detract from the role of venerable sages, a practical conclusion is that it originated in the freethinking medical practitioners of the Indus River civilization, practitioners who could not have previously existed in small villages and whose disciples would fade away with the civilization itself, but leaving a trail of medical wisdom that somehow survived to be included in revered medical classics of India.

C. The Vedas and the Medical Samhitas [collections]; Their Origin

The philosophical and empirical foundations of modern Ayurveda and therefore the basis for the two classic works of Indian medicine, the *Charaka Samhita* and the *Sushruta Samhita*, are found in the Vedas.

Of the four Vedas the most medically oriented is the *Atharva Veda*, considered the earliest but one of the Vedas. But the problem with postulating that work as the source of the good clinical information to be found later in the two medical samhitas is that most English translations of the Vedas do not support such a claim. Virtually all mention of disease is presented in simplistic, although poetical, descriptive terms of external clinical findings within a mystical context. One exception to this interpretation of the work comes

---

[15] This would be a most remarkable phenomenon and suggest a level of fraternity existed throughout the civilization unlike any other. Curiously, the author has a 16th C drawing entitled "Cain building the city of Henochia," showing Cain and many laborers at work constructing a *de novo* city that must have been predesigned. Some liken the Biblical city of Henochia to the ancient Mesopotamian city of Eridu.

from Dr. Chattopadhyaya, a prominent Indian philosopher who has demoted the mythological content of the Vedas by pointing out the scientific, and in his view, areligious nature of the early Vedas.[16] He supports this with his reading and interpretation of both the *Atharva Veda* and the *Charaka Samhita*, thereby highlighting the underlying scientific and clinical astuteness of those works and the philosophical association between the two not previously inferable from other translations. He also is convinced that the wisdom from the *Atharva Veda*, a collection of 730 hymns, is the product of many authors. Finally, although specific clinical descriptions of diagnosable diseases cannot be found in that Veda, it is clear to him that its evidence for objectivity and for nature's physical laws has been transmitted into the *Charaka Samhita*, which would explain both the nonmagical aspects of that text and provide the factual aspect for Ayurveda as it evolved into a clinical discipline.[17] His argument is convincing, if for no other reason than his translations provide solid support for his conclusions, something that cannot be easily inferred from other translations.

Traditionally the source of Ayurveda has been attributed to the Vedic sage, Bharadvaja, and placed in the Vedic era. Compared to the other three Vedas the *Atharva Veda* has been criticized in its appeal for objectivity to the point of being considered by some religious authorities to not be a Veda. Dr. Chattopadhyaya has described it as an entreaty for an objective and even democratic approach to knowledge and to medical practice, to which he attributes the disdain of that Veda by the Brahmin caste of Hinduism. The principles of Ayurveda, as attributed to Bharadvaja, are: (1) a belief in causality, (2) acknowledgement of a disease as an entity rather than a status, and (3) acceptance that curability (of curable diseases) can reside in the actions of a physician. These principles, plus the clinical observations found in the two medical samhitas, underlie their great significance and reputation despite, as Dr. Chattopadhyaya states (*ibid.*, p. 425), "the heap of intellectual debris eventually dumped on them." Much of the discussion of the *Charaka Samhita* and the *Sushruta Samhita* that follows will find its support in the translations and references in the work of Dr. Chattopadhyaya and in the well-known translation of the *Charaka Samhita* by P. V. Sharma, famous Ayurvedic physician and scholar of Sanskrit and Hindi.[18]

A first consideration is whether a work itself is worth the effort of discussion, and to that point is the authenticity of translation. It was demonstrated in Part I that at times ancient works were translated by persons with a level of technical knowledge that was inferior to the original authors. For fictional and entertainment works this is not of great concern, but for technical professions it is imperative that technical terms be accurately translated, for if accuracy is lacking much of a work's imbued knowledge will not be apparent and even seem absurd. It is for this reason that Hippocratic treatises as translated by the author are accompanied by a wordlist and commentary that provide a degree of specificity to terminology that other translations have lacked.[19]

---

[16] The prevailing opinion, however, is that the Vedas represented religious scripture in their own right, a primitive form of religious devotion and instruction that was later subsumed and altered to become the foundation for Hinduism.

[17] Dr. Chattopadhyaya's excellent book, *Science and Society in Ancient India* (Bangalore, 1977), is to a great extent an explication of this topic.

[18] Sharma, P. V., *Caraka-Samhita*, published in 2014 (4th edition), Varanasi, 2 volumes.

[19] Adams, W. H., *The Natural State of Medical Practice: Hippocratic Evidence*, Maitland (FL), 2019.

The same problem with technical accuracy applies to the Charaka Samhita. The wording and implied meaning of the translation by Dr. Avinash Kaviratna in 1896 today make little sense to modern readers. And this is because scientific knowledge has made early translations functionally archaic. The translation of Prof. P. V. Sharma, updated in 2014, is much more understandable, and even when seeming obtuse the logic behind his discourse comes through. Optimal translations of Hippocratic works are often found in short journal publications on specific medical problems authored by specialists in those fields.[20] For present discussion, however, the Sharma translation will be used, with full knowledge that much of the wisdom underlying the text will be missed. What will not be missed, however, is its evidence that practitioners long ago were careful and insightful observers and that the subsequent course of medicine on the subcontinent would have been vastly advanced had they been permitted to build on initial successes. The transmitted wisdom reached its first stage in its mention in the *Rig Veda*.

The *Rig Veda*

The first and most revered Veda is the *Rig Veda*. In chapter 10, verse 97 is stated: "Oh bright herbs, you are like mothers. In your presence I promise to offer to the physician cows, horses, clothes and even myself ... ."[21] Another entire hymn is devoted entirely to a healing herb. Elsewhere it is stated that "the wise physician is one around whom the herbs gather... . He wages war on sickness of all forms."[22] Dr. Chattopadhyaya has commented that the text of the *Rig Veda* is "totally unaware of the hierarchical society." This plus other statements do not suggest an inferior status of physicians, proof that the Vedas predated their (the Vedas) accommodation into Hinduism, for with that association physicians became relegated to a relatively lowly status. But the key point is that physicians are identified as worthy community specialists. Thus, the foremost Veda sets the stage with a medical profession already evolved.

The *Atharva Veda*

The next stage is found in the *Atharva Veda*, the Veda most concerned with the profession of medicine. It has received the greatest criticism from religious teachers for its attention to care of the body at the expense of caring for the soul. Not surprisingly it contains lines that provide philosophical support for the physician's work. At that early stage, however, it relies on magic and incantations to rid a patient of demons. Even when botanicals are discussed, and only a few are mentioned, they are approached as if they are themselves

---

[20] An example is: Kokate, K. K., and Kulkarni, N. G., *Endometriosis in Ayurvedic Perspective*, in *J. Homeop. and Ayurv. Med.*, 2:142-3, 2013. While not fully consistent with modern allopathic medicine, the clarification of "yonivyapat" as a clinical description of endometriosis (but not of its pathological features) and the explanation of terms given to its different clinical presentations makes the original Charaka description much more understandable, logical, and, given its archaic nature, remarkable.

[21] Chattopadhyaya, D., *Science and Society in Ancient India*, Bangalore, 1977, p. 235.

[22] This, like the previous reference, is a translation by Dr. Chattopadhyaya of *Rig Veda* X, 97, 4 and 6, a section of the *Rig Veda* clearly laudatory of the physician and praising his ability to use botanicals to return people to health.

amulets. Nevertheless, the use of certain botanicals must raise the question of "Why these and not those?" The effective use of these living amulets must have instilled some sense of dependency on the botanical itself. Furthermore, the village women would have known local lore about the value of certain plants passed down to them from generations preceding the Vedas. The distinction between magical use and empirical use is cloudy in this context. And that distinction may have been what prompted Brahminic writers to attack the content of this Veda in carefully chosen ways, one being the forbidding of gathering "roots" for treating disease and the statement that "he who practises [sic] for the multitude is pronounced impure." Democratic process was not in the plan for Hinduism's priests.

Despite the opposition to an empirical-rational approach to managing sickness, those who provided the clinical basis for classics of medicine that would include the Charaka Samhita, the Sushruta Samhita, and others somehow managed to retain earlier, and forge newer, wisdom.

The *Charaka Samhita*

With similarities to the Cnidian (symptom-oriented rather than patient-oriented medicine of the ancient Greek colony of Cnidos) and Egyptian approach to medical diagnosis, the Charaka Samhita primarily uses specific symptoms as a basis for understanding and dealing with a medical problem. In its theoretical construction, an aberrancy or imbalance in factors that maintain health produces various symptoms, and treatments are needed to realign them. For example, vomiting can be caused by neurologic disease, vestibular disease, gastric irritation, bowel obstruction, and as a side effect of drugs and toxins, yet it is approached as a specific aberrancy, a singular disease in itself. If a person has vomiting, fever, diarrhea, and a skin rash, each symptom or sign is thought to have a specific and different explanation. Thus, the treatments are designed to counteract the various causes of the various signs and symptoms of a disease rather than pursuing a primary treatment that, by treating a single diagnosis, will control the basic cause of the disease and leave symptomatic treatments as a separate goal. There is an inadequate effort to develop the concept of a "syndrome" that would group signs and symptoms and permit true identification of causation. If this were done and if the basic disease process is thereby controlled, ancillary symptomatic therapies in most instances would not be necessary for long. This is not to say that there is no attempt at a unifying model of disease. In Book 2, chapter, 3, it is proposed that something enters the "mouth of the uterus" that causes a "tumor" or mass to develop. But the development of the concept stops there. For this reason, Book 5, "Signs of Life and Death," is here explicated first because causation of signs and symptoms are less diffuse. The unabridged edition of *The Natural State of Medical Practice: An Isagorial Theory of Human Progress*, chapter 4, can be consulted for a discussion of other Books of the *Charaka Samhita*.

From Book 5:
Chap. 1 - Two significant observations: (a) the phenomenon whereby the lower part of the body becomes more livid as the upper (higher) part becomes more pallid shortly after death (*livor mortis*) as gravity causes blood to settle downward promptly after blood circulation ceases, and (b) the deep purple that can be seen in cyanosis

associated with some deaths, especially on the lips, as indicated by the cited color of the black plum (jamun) found in India.

Chap. 2 – The smell of a patient's breath associated with lethal diseases is described using the metaphor of "flower." This physical examination finding could include *fetor hepaticus* in liver cirrhosis due to thiols, a fruity smell present in diabetic ketoacidosis due to ketones, and *uremic fetor* due to ammonia present in advanced uremia. Such a relatively subtle physical finding is not likely to make an impression on anyone except a person who is specifically looking for evidence to objectively characterize or diagnose disease.

Chap. 3 – The response to touch at approaching death includes discussion of palpating the pulse, observing the respirations (deep respirations indicating severe metabolic acidosis, shallow indicating neural unresponsiveness to oxygen lack or carbon dioxide excess), observing lack of response to a painful stimulus (tested by pulling of a hair), the presence of sweating despite the body being cool, and stiffness of the body.

Chap. 4 – Loss of senses were noted, with unresponsiveness to sound, a general diminishing of senses, the patient hearing no "heart sound" on plugging the ears (a remarkable, if irrelevant, observation), sudden darkness of vision, and delusions that commonly occur with approaching death.

Chap. 5 – Poor prognostic signs were described, including opisthotonos (tetanus was always lethal), the attraction of flies to land on the body (a clinical dictum in the past that indicated imminent death), onset of delirium (a common acute finding in severe systemic disease such as sepsis), vivid end-of-life dreams and visions (not hallucinations), and certain skin rashes.

Chap. 6 – Physical abnormalities often superimposed on the cachectic patient included constipation plus thirst, anasarca, "viscous" urine (high specific gravity usually indicating recent poor fluid intake), and the combination of fever and diarrhea (not uncommon in terminal infectious disorders).

Chap. 7 – This chapter discusses color and "luster," usually relating to approaching death: a patient who faints every time he is lifted upright (orthostatic hypotension), cachexia with excessive urine or stool, losing weight while eating satisfactorily, shallow respirations with twitching (the latter probably indicating myoclonus, a common sign *in extremis*), advanced cachexia, and mania. (Note that there is frequent repetition of events, phrases, descriptions among chapters.)

Chap. 11 – In sections 25 and 26 is found the statement that when a patient refuses both treatment and the physician's assistance, he has "moved under the control of God of death" and is not to be treated.

Chap. 12 – There is mention here that a powdery substance sometimes appears on the head as death approaches. This might mean terminal uremia, except that uremic "frost" is white, whereas the powder described in the Charaka Samhita looks like powdery cow dung. Medicinal cow dung is presently purchasable as formulated into a substance that is purported to have anti-infective qualities.

At the conclusion of Book 5 it is stated that the patient can be advised of his impending demise if he requests it, but the physician should not do so if it is thought it might cause earlier death or if it would cause affliction to others. It also states that some of the signs and symptoms mentioned do not mean inevitable death, and that there may be moderating effects if certain omens or portents are observed. But it is clear that close observation of a great many end-of-life circumstances was required to provide the confident and mostly correct interpretation of signs and symptoms presented in these chapters. It was not arrived at by random anecdotal experience, and it was not derived from a great list of observations over centuries that had been added to, one by one, by generations of practitioners who felt obligated to add their jot of information to a greater pile. It certainly did not come from one man or sage. It could have only come from professional procedures laid out by some person or group, its final form representing their considered opinion. A similar conclusion was reached by Dr. Chattopadhyaya.[23]

In addition to specific reference to signs and symptoms that indicate the *Charaka Samhita* to be the dedicated work of true clinicians, the philosophical orientation of those ancient physicians is highlighted by Dr. Chattopradhyaya. He translates verse 36 of Book 3, chapter 3 as: "Now, of all types of evidences, the most dependable ones are those that are directly observed by the eyes. Here are some of our views based on the observation of thousands of instances" (see p. 81 of preceding citation, for its author indicates this is a "loose translation"). He finds numerous statements throughout the work that "placed the ancient doctors among the pioneers of the materialist outlook in Indian history." Spiritual connotation is "scrapped." Prior to development of class and professional hierarchies he considers ancient doctors "the scientists par excellence of the age," pointing out at the same time that "pioneers of science are to be judged not by the actual success of implementing their programme but by the success of their formulation of the programme." Dr. Chattopadhyaya's work is especially valuable for he is able to provide a living translation that detects, rather than ignores, the objectivity and the respect for physical laws that are not obvious to those unfamiliar with the language. The original formulation of their "programme" is thereby rendered visible and preserved for the ages.

Tracts in both the Charaka and Susruta Samhitas advise the physician to be personally familiar with medicinal herbs, to know how they are to be grown and harvested. This work with the soil, as well as the physical touching and manipulation of patients and their wounds and sores, is what made the profession of medicine a very menial, even detestable, endeavor to the upper classes for centuries. Manu, the giver of laws, prohibited high-caste Hindus from accepting any food from doctors because that food "is like pus and blood." The attention directed at the body at the expense of the soul was the source of the criticism by the upper classes, a criticism Dr. Chattopadhyaya says is joined by Plato. This is a bit unexpected, for Dr. Chattopadhyaya, a philosophical devotee of communism, would have been expected to admire Plato because of many aspects of Plato's ideal city. In conclusion, the stamp of greatness can be applied to the original wisdom of the *Charaka Samhita*, if not to those who subsequently edited and manipulated it to their own ends.

D. Conclusion

The metrics of the Mohenjo-daro civilization were similar to Miletos, but the absence of monumental structures and lack of evidence for social stratification suggest an egalitarian civilization. The absence of large municipal works also might be consistent with an overall egalitarian social management of the city, for physical coercion in building monumental structures was not needed. The two most viable options are (1) an early form of corporatism with workers/members as a group involved in aspects of management of a specific commercial interest (the city was divided into neighborhoods, and there were

---

[23] See: Chattopadhyaya, D. P., *Science and Society in Ancient India* (Bangalore, 1977), p. 28.

some large assembly spaces in the city center), or (2) a heterarchy of commercial and trading interests in which a significant part of social control was not just over those affiliated with specific types of production but was also included within the entire network of commercial ventures, a corporate structure. This would not have interfered with peripheral settlements and their egalitarian kinship traditions. For those within the new commercial neighborhoods, however, their association within either a heterarchy or commercial corporatism would have weakened any kinship allegiance. As a part of the apolitical settlement hierarchy that developed as the city's early population enlarged, specialties useful to commercial and private interests must have developed, including medical practitioners.

Based only on circumstantial social evidence, it is tentatively proposed that the objective medical wisdom to be found in later Ayurvedic tracts was first collected in its cities such as Mohenjo-daro. It is also likely that, as proposed by Dr. Kak, it was at this time, if not the place, that formal collation of the Vedas took place. The *Atharva Veda*, therefore, may in the future be found to attribute its perspective of objective science to the stimulus of the work of networks of medical practitioners, in a sense a Baconian preview of work to follow. This proposed scenario accommodates aspects of the philosophical orientation of the Vedas as primarily a creation of the subcontinent.

Summary Table of Mohenjo-daro (similar for the city-state of Harappa)

STAGE – Bronze Age
POPULATION, LOCAL – 40,000
POPULATION, TOTAL – unknown, but total Indus River region population was *ca.* 5,000,000 divided among about 70 cities = 71,000 per city and its environs
PRIMARY AREA – 1.6 square miles
URBAN DENSITY – 56 persons per acre
PRODUCTION – pottery, agriculture, jewelry, textiles, ivory, extensive distant trade
GOVERNANCE – municipal coordination from agreements among trading and commercial operations (a heterarchy) or from corporatism within neighborhoods
EGALITARIAN ARCHEOLOGY - yes
PROMINENT EGALITARIAN KINSHIPS – in peripheral villages for control of resources and coordination of agriculture
WRITING – uncertain, but possibly an early form with only a few hundred symbols, so far undeciphered
DISTANT TRADE – yes
SPECIALIZATION – yes
MONUMENTAL STRUCTURES - no
DENOUEMENT – possibly environmental changes, but uncertain
MEDICAL PRACTICE – so far no evidence
FORMATIVE PERIOD – 800 years
FLORUIT – 500 years (2500-2000 BC)
CITY-STATE – yes
AVERAGE LIFE EXPECTANCY – 35 years[24] (for the better off)

---

[24] Based on statement that "almost half" of the population from the R-37 cemetery reached their "mid-thirties." See: McIntosh, J., *The Ancient Indus Valley: New Perspectives*, Santa Barbara, 2008, p. 253. It seems that neonatal and early childhood deaths were not included in the estimate, and that the buried population may have been more affluent that the general population.

CHAPTER THIRTY-ONE

LIANGCHENGZHEN AND THE EARLY YELLOW RIVER VALLEY
CIVILIZATION

Legend holds that it was in the time of the Yellow Emperor (*ca.* 2400 BC) that the Chinese medical classic, the *Huang Ti Nei Ching Su Wen*, a dialogue between the Yellow Emperor and his ministers, was composed. The location was Shandong Province in what is now northern China. An example of a contemporary Shandong city-state is Liangchengzhen, a prominent coastal commercial center flourishing at that time. Although no medical presence has so far been uncovered from archeological sites, it is proposed that the medical observations in the *Huang Ti Nei Ching Su Wen* were first made in such an urban environment. As the clinical contents of the composition, such as have been handed down to us, reveal much that is objective and insightful, it is suggested that at the time of its writing, or prior to it, there was a small network of medical practitioners who shared their medical expertise that ultimately made its way into the received text. Over the centuries substantial new content was amended. But underneath the "new age" additions and the heavy editing in the 8th C AD by Wang Bing, the practical, and sometimes acute, observations made by those ancient practitioners can be detected. These, the true authors of the authentic portions of the *Huang Ti Nei Ching Su Wen*, will remain unknown, but we can opine about the social world in which they worked.

A. Longshan Civilization and the Yellow Emperor

In the early history of medicine in China the famous *Huang Ti Nei Ching Su Wen* (one translation being the *Inner Canon of the Yellow Emperor*, the title of the standard English language translation by Dr. Ilza Veith; see footnote, p. 77, for reference) eclipses in prominence all other ancient manuscripts as a guide to clinical practice, a position it still holds today in Traditional Chinese Medicine.[1] Although modern Western analysis of its content finds most to be irrelevant or fanciful, three elements confirm its significance: (1) it has no mystical component, (2) it is patient-oriented in that its focus is the individual patient and each patient is considered unique, and (3) it contains fragments of clinical description that clearly represent attempts at accurate clinical assessment, evidence that practitioners who wrote them had experience with other patients having similar problems. The modern version of the *Huang Ti Nei Ching Su Wen* provides no important insight to modern practitioners, but it is necessary to determine how its practical features were derived, for they contrast markedly with the rest of the work.[2]

As the recent scholarly estimate for the earliest date for composition of the *Huang Ti Nei Ching Su Wen* is the 1st C BC rather than 2400 BC, what could have been the source of its fragmented wisdom? Was it merely a compilation of observations by contemporary practitioners of the Eastern Zhou (770-256 BC), Qin (221-206 BC) or the

---

[1] The companion work to the *Huang Ti Nei Ching Su Wen* is the *Huang Ti Nei Ching Ling Shu,* an acupuncture treatise. As acupuncture was first mentioned in 1st C BC Chinese documents, it does not, as a relatively recent addition to Traditional Chinese Medicine, directly bear on the present discussion.

[2] *The Huang Ti Nei Ching Su Wen* contains some acupuncture and much theory derived from the 3rd C BC concept of Yin and Yang, again both probably late additions to a set of pre-existing clinical observations.

Han Dynasty (206 BC – 220 AD), or did that work represent the residuum of dispersed clinical fragments of a school of medical thought that had existed in much earlier, perhaps even prehistoric, times? Legend and myth suggest the latter, for authorship of the *Huang Ti Nei Ching Su Wen* has been attributed to the Yellow Emperor (reigned *ca.* 2400 BC) of the Longshan Culture (2900-1900 BC and 2600-2000 BC are proposed dates), declared the formative era of a distinctive Chinese culture. The Yellow Emperor is considered the source of numerous examples of beneficence to mankind, a functional parallel to that ascribed by ancient Greeks to Prometheus, the mythical Titan overthrown by the Olympian god, Zeus, for stealing fire and giving it to mankind. An important difference is that the Yellow Emperor is claimed to have united, by carrot and by stick, much of the Central Plain of China. Like Prometheus, however, many consider the Yellow Emperor to be myth rather than legend. What is the place of Longshan Culture in Chinese history?

There seems to be general agreement that the proximal Neolithic culture preceding the Longshan, the Yangshao (*ca.* 5,000 to 2,500 BC), was an early agricultural culture associated with somewhat mobile populations periodically seeking more bountiful harvests and returning to sites they previously had occupied. Their distinctive pottery was not made with a potter's wheel, and descriptions of their "round wattle-and-daub huts, each with reed roof and plaster floor and an oven in the center" closely mirror Bronze Age huts of Flag Fen in Cambridgeshire, England, the latter being proposed as seasonal dwellings for a more distant but dispersed population in approximately 1500 BC.[3] The Yangshao people had neither central government nor a temple culture and lived in villages covering perhaps 10-50 acres with estimated populations averaging about 300.[4] There is no evidence of martial effort, the small peaceful villages often being surrounded by a ditch considered insufficient to protect against human invasion. The later years of Yangshao Culture saw deterioration and a degenerative decline in quality of workmanship traceable in its pottery. This presumably egalitarian society was then replaced by the Longshan people.

Whether the early Longshan people were indigenous or had migrated from the north down the coast to settle in the lower Yellow River valley is debated. It was during this age, one characterized by a rapidly growing population, greater competition for available resources, and strong defensive and offensive military postures, that the Yellow Emperor is thought to have unified the Chinese people, preparing them for the postulated Xia dynasty of a confederation of states (2100-1600 BC) and the Shang dynasty (1600-1046 BC) that followed. Population estimates of Neolithic China are sparse and mere guesses based on things like village size and characteristics of dwellings, but pursuant to present discussion, the average size of a sample of Longshan villages is calculated to have been 43,000 square meters (about ten acres) for an average population of 640. This contrasts with the average village population of the antecedent Daxi and Dawenkou cultures estimated to be in the range of 300 or less, but with notable larger exceptions.[5]

The Yellow Emperor is one of several sages and demigods of Chinese prehistory traditionally placed in the Longshan Culture, a late Neolithic culture notable for its

---

[3] Sullivan, M., *The Arts of China*, 4th edition, Berkeley, p. 5.

[4] See: Maisels, C. K., *Early Civilizations of the Old World*, London, 2001, p. 271; Wang, J., *Population Pressure and Growth of Chinese Primitive Agriculture*, in *Agricultural Archaeology*, 3:58-73, 1997.

[5] Extracted from: Min, L., *Settling on the Ruins of Xia: Archaeology of Social Memory in Early China*, in *Social Theory in Archaeology and Ancient History*, Cambridge, 2016, G. Emberling, editor, chapter 13.

distinctive pottery and development of the pottery wheel, rammed earth walls, advances in agriculture and domestication and herding of animals, and an early silk industry. Jade, metal tools, and rice as the dominant grain appeared. Some suggest an early form of writing was developed, although supposed inscriptions on bone have yet to be translated.[6] Dr. Li Min has described ancient Longshan communities: "The flow of raw material, finished goods, and knowledge among them [the Longshan communities] created a well-integrated Longshan world. The political experimentation in the late third-millennium BCE proto-urban centers, the formation of large religious and political networks, and the expansion of technologies and knowledge in animal, plants, metallurgy, and religious communication mark the Longshan period as a time of unprecedented social and cultural transformation in early China."

The early rapid expansion of the Longshan population led to numerous small agricultural communities rather than a few large ones, those that were large tending to be located in more isolated regions, the many smaller ones (with areas of roughly 5-20 acres) distributed throughout the flat Central Plain, the region now considered the heartland of Chinese culture. Clusters of small communities then began to surround a central larger one. Over time many communities became fortified, with population estimates for the larger central sites ranging from 15,000-50,000 protected behind imposing walls. To the earlier advances now came the practices of ancestor worship and divination.

B. The City-State of Liangchengzhen and Its Demography

The observation has been made that of the total area that might be considered the Longshan eastern region, where the Yellow River empties into the China Sea and identified as Shandong, was the region least involved in militarization and which displayed the least disparity in wealth. Perhaps pertinent is the local geography, for the Shandong area was relatively isolated and thereby protected from proximal cultures by extensive marshes, only later opening to other areas when climate change led to drying of wetlands. The clustering of settlements in conjunction with an apparent social integration, rather than segregation, of a communal (commercial?) hierarchy has been taken as evidence of a functional network for crafts and trades that provided regional social cohesion distinct from any vertical hierarchy that may have existed or was imposed. Indeed, the development of this pattern, termed a settlement hierarchy, has been proposed by scholars as an attractant for movement of smaller settlements and individuals toward an urban environment.

The Longshan civilization is considered to be the opening phase of a united Chinese polity and culture from which is derived its subsequent intellectual heritage.[7] An

---

[6] Dematte, P., *Longshan-Era Urbanism: The Role of Cities in Predynastic China*, in *Asian Perspectives*, 38:119-153, 1999.

[7] See: Dematte, P., *Longshan-Era Urbanism: The Role of Cities in Predynastic China*, in *Asian Perspectives*, 38:119-153, 1999. Relevant to this discussion is the concept of "city-state," and M. E. Lewis, among others, has cautioned that Chinese city-states must not be considered similar to Greek city-states, for the former were always governed by a strict hierarchy and the concept of equality among its citizenry was never contemplated in city-state operation. But this interpretation of data may not apply to predynastic China, a period prior to the formation of a culturally unified collection of larger city-states with a strong sense of cultural identity and class hierarchy that could contain disharmonious activity. Dr. Dematte even uses the term "koine" in describing the earlier

important and typical Longshan city, some might say a "city-state," is Liangchengzhen, located in Shandong province.[8] It developed in a sparsely populated area *ca.* 2600 BC, and by 2200 BC covered *ca.* 700 acres (slightly more than a square mile). Liangchengzhen was centrally located within a cluster of communities that diminished in size according to distance from the center, an organization indicating commercial/economic integration of a region covering perhaps 200 square miles, somewhat less than the size of New York City. Travel by foot to most of its peripheral settlements probably could be made in a day or two. In the absence of information on its population and using 200 square meters as an average size devoted to a city household in studies elsewhere, the city population may have included 14,000 households, and a recent analysis based on regional sustenance suggests the regional population was *ca.* 70,000. Based on archeological findings it is thought that the city was the central distribution point for the region's communities, and both utilitarian and prestige goods were produced there, presumably to be commercially exchanged for commodities obtained from outlying villages.

　　Between the early and middle phases of the Longshan civilization the population of Liangchengzhen increased probably because of movement of villagers from peripheral settlements into Liangchengzhen itself. With this in mind the recent report of marked local variation in components of clay used for ceramics in urbanized Longshan regions implies an absence of centralized control of production, but it leaves in place the need for a social apparatus in marketing of the product. This pattern, found elsewhere in the Yellow River region (as well as in other Neolithic and Bronze Age civilizations around the world), suggests a commercial heterarchy existed, perhaps functioning in parallel with a self-organizing hierarchy as urbanization proceeded, and would remain evident centuries later in the Shang Dynasty.[9] As in many other city-states the surrounding communities functioned as suburban neighborhoods and provided specialized products and services to the other communities by using the organizational resources of the central city revolving around commercial products, thus also suggesting heterarchical organization. Importantly, Liangchengzhen was located within a few miles of the Yellow Sea and thereby it was also a commercial center for trade with distant populations. Given its size, population, duration of occupation and importance there would have been local

---

pattern, and κοινή is the term used by Aristotle for confederations of city-states and for "mutual advantage." This change in organization would have occurred in the Longshan era, probably during its earliest stage, although the Shandong region, with a large area being relatively isolated geographically, might have avoided this transition until a later date. The Shang cities have been classified as territorial, by which is meant they were larger and with a strong hierarchy, whereas late Neolithic cities were "city-states." For a discussion of this point see: Trigger, B. G., *Understanding Early Civilizations: A Comparative Study*, Cambridge, UK, 2003, p. 92*ff.*

[8] See: Yates, R. D. S., *The City-State in Ancient China*, in *The Archeology of City-States: Cross-Cultural Approaches*, Nichols, D. L. and Charlton, T. H. (eds.), Washington, D. C., 1997, p. 77. Dr. Bruce Trigger (see above footnote) has an opposing view regarding city-state status.

[9] See: McIntosh, R. J., *Ancient Middle Niger: Urbanism and the Self-Organizing Landscape*, Cambridge, 2005, the section in Chapter 6 discussing Dr. Kwang-chih Chang, the eminent archeologist and Sinologist, the urban development in northern China, and the coexistence of heterarchy and hierarchy in ancient China.

medical practitioners providing basic medical care to both the central city and surrounding communities, but there is at present no information on this point.[10]

It is thought that in its earliest stages Longshan culture may have been egalitarian in that evidence of hierarchy in dwellings and burials is minimal. Liangchengzhen is thought to have less evidence for social stratification than most other sites. But as time passed social stratification appeared contemporaneously with an increasing population, movement of people from peripheral settlements to cities, shamanism, and a more intensive farming with reuse of land. Dr. Li Liu identified social rank in burial sites and stated "kinship-based Longshan communities were internally and externally stratified."[11] On the other hand, Liangchengzhen was not one of the studied populations cited, and some of the recognized hierarchy may merely have involved the settlement hierarchy that can naturally occur as a centralizing population increases in size.[12] Probably relevant is the opinion that the size of the polis increased in the Middle phase of Liangchengzhen development (2400-2200 BC), and that this was associated with a decrease in size of peripheral settlements, suggesting something was triggering urban immigration. That "something" most likely was commercial activity. At this time archeological study indicates the city was a four-tiered settlement hierarchy.[13] A wide panoply of goods and services would have evolved within the polis to support commercial ventures, and this should have included medical practitioners. All this supports the conclusion that a commercial heterarchy was guiding the development of the city. Furthermore, a search for dietary evidence of an elite population has provided no more than suggestive evidence of its existence. As for overall social control, the study of ceramic production technique in Liangchengzhen mentioned above concluded that the production and distribution of ceramics was managed through "flexible, self-organizing systems" and a multiplicity of production sites with no evidence of centralized control, even for high quality products, and this organization was found at several other Longshan sites up through the middle of the Longshan period.[14] This also suggests there were other functioning commercial

---

[10] For a recent updating of archeological findings in the Yellow River area see: Son Bo, *The Longshan Culture of Shandong*, in *A Companion to Chinese Archeology*, Chichester (UK), 2013, A. P. Underhill, editor, chapter 21.

[11] See: Liu, L., *Mortuary Ritual and Social Hierarchy in the Longshan Culture*, in *Early China*, 21:1-46, 1996.

[12] The association between nuclear population size, its natural pattern of organization, necessary agricultural support and the number of services available has been one way to look at urban growth. In this scheme medical practice could be considered one of the services likely to appear as a centralized population reaches a certain size. The otherwise generally close relation of population size with variety of services suggests the form of governance and social structure should be relatively unimportant in determining when medical practitioners will appear to serve the population, its size being the major determinant. But a service based on providing wood for fires within a city is quite different from provision of a service with which a culture has had no prior experience. For present purposes population size is considered one possible determinant for a network of medical practitioners, but only inasmuch as it represents opportunity, not causation. Nevertheless, this would be an interesting area of study. See: Ortman, S. G., et al., *The Pre-History of Urban Scaling*, PLoS ONE 9(2): e87902, 2014.

[13] For a recent review of the status of Liangchengzhen see: Lanehart, R. E., *Patterns of Consumption: Ceramic Residue Analysis at Liangchengzhen, Shandong, China*, 2015, Graduate Theses and Dissertations, Graduate School at Scholar Commons, especially chapter 2.

[14] See: Druc, I., et al., *A Preliminary Assessment of the Organization of Ceramic Production at Liangchengzhen, Rizhao, Shandong: Perspectives from Petrography*, in *J. Archaeol. Sci: Reports*, https://doi.org/10.1016/j.jasrep.2017.12.050.

heterarchies. Finally, in contrast to the flagrantly hierarchical contemporary city of Liangzhu to be discussed later, the burial sites in the Shandong region that includes Liangchengzhen have provided no clear evidence that would suggest a hereditary elite class.[15] The point to be made is that for a significant part of its predynastic existence Liangchengzhen appears to have been a marketing center utilized by various commercial enterprises and traders and unencumbered by a meddling political hierarchy. In this environment the strong kinship alliances that existed weakened as a kinship-based community evolved into a commerce-based city, at least in its formative years.

It is not argued that a notable feature of Chinese history is the formidable role of kinship in state formation. In its prehistory kinships were, as everywhere, the basic structure of society. To this was added ancestor worship, a manifestation of the importance of lineage within a kin group and "a reflection and extension of kinship behavior." This was essential to State, religious, and political associations beginning with the first Chinese dynasty. Characteristically, therefore, the focus of ancient Chinese society was on kinship rather than the individual, that a person's worthiness was not based on individual accomplishment but on the adherence to, and support of, his or her function within the larger kinship group, whether at the family or State level, a social obligation with a religious orientation, an extensive ritual and a goal of living up to the expectations of one's predecessors. With such sweeping social saturation involving kinship, a weakening of kinship ties usually occurring during urbanization would not be expected. This does not require that kinship lose it meaning, and kinship-based burial sites and other common features can continue to be observed. But it is likely that the assigned status, duties, and obligations of kinship would have to make room for the anti-egalitarian and self-serving nature of the nuclear family.[16]

It was during this period, roughly 2500-2300 BC (the middle Longshan period), that the Yellow Emperor is reputed to have lived, the grand descriptions of his accomplishments presumably accounting for or in response to the dramatic proliferation of the population and culture at that juncture.[17] Relevant to present discussion this culture

---

[15] See: Barnes, G. L., *Archaeology of East Asia*, Oxford, 2015, especially chapter 7, Emergence and Decline of Late Neolithic Societies (3300-1900 BC).

[16] Discussions of the nuclear family often focus on its egalitarianism and the destructive changes in it brought on by the modern world. But gender, age, and physical size guarantee limited success in enforcing equality beyond being helpful. Also, definitions of the nuclear family tend to be specific, whereas in prehistoric settings definitions are not available: grandparents were rare, one parent often deceased, and the "nuclear" family could be non-affinal, nonconjugal, or "nonnuclear" (the latter by circumstance rather than by choice). In nomadic bands the nuclear family might change according to circumstance, the mother in charge of her children as communal property. Despite this, individual prehistoric dwelling sizes commonly accommodated perhaps four or five persons, estimates of a prehistoric city's population is sometimes based on an estimate of five persons per dwelling, and anthropological descriptions of prehistoric communities often use the term "nuclear family." So the point to be made is that the family by whatever name has always existed because its focus is children and their propagation, and the adjective "nuclear" comprises the children and those immediately responsible for their well-being. Finally, the idea that the egalitarian entitlements of tribal members would voluntarily supersede the needs of a "nuclear" family's children is inconceivable. The "crop" of new members born into a prehistoric society was essential to its survival, and to permit want in one's children so that another family's children could benefit would have been a source of conflict. Thus, the linking of nuclear family with egalitarianism, whether intra- or extrafamilial, is immaterial to present discussion.

[17] In the past it was popular opinion that the Han Chinese as an ethnic group could trace their origins to the Yellow Emperor, and a recent article provides genetic analysis as support for a Central Plain

would be expected to include his acquisition and dispersion of medical wisdom. About 1900 BC the city and its dependencies were gradually subsumed by the social changes that would lead to the 1st Chinese dynasty.

But what medical wisdom was there? Evidence of trepanation in the Dawenkou Culture that preceded the Longshan Culture has been discovered, the skull indicating long-term survival of the recipient of the procedure.[18] Other Neolithic findings include evidence of tooth extraction that is postulated to have been a social custom, and a comparison of burial sites of hunter-gatherer *vs.* agricultural eras in the Yellow River region, *ca.* 6000 *vs.* 3000 BC, reveal skeletal remains in the latter to be smaller, with more evidence of osteoporosis, degenerative joint disease and anemia (criteria for these conclusions unstated), but skeletal ages were older, suggesting the agriculturalists were less healthy but somehow longer-lived. Beyond this type of fragmentary information there is no information on the health status of the region under discussion, and nothing on available medical care.

Thus was the social circumstance surrounding the age of the legendary Yellow Emperor, and it was this time of territorial contests among autonomous city-states that has been proposed as the time he came to head a confederation of them. Today a monument located in Shou Qiu, Shandong Province, is said to mark his birthplace, about 150 miles inland from Liangchengzhen. Confucius came from the same region.

Liangchengzhen and many other Longshan settlements declined, some disappearing, *ca.* 2000 BC, their place taken by a developing Bronze Age territorial state with centralized commercial and social controls. Most prominent was Erlitou, a large city with palatial buildings and a walled section behind which the elite lived. Ceramics now revealed a uniform pattern of production. Central control was now in place. It is postulated that this new arrival in the region represents the legendary first dynasty of China, the Xia.[19]

C. The *Huang Ti Nei Ching Su Wen* and Social Circumstances surrounding Its Origin

The Yellow Emperor's Classic of Internal Medicine,[20] or *Huang Ti Nei Ching Su Wen*, is first mentioned in the *Hanshu* (the *Book of Han*, written in 111 AD, and is a history of the early Han Dynasty, 206 BC to 23 AD). It is one-half of a work entitled

---

origin for the Northern Han Chinese, although epidemiological specifics, particularly the randomness of the ancient samples studied at the Hengbei site, is unstated. And there is today a grand mausoleum dedicated to the Yellow Emperor located in Shaanxi Province that claims to exhibit his footprint. This site is about 600 miles west of Liangchengzhen. See: Zhao, Y-B., et al., *Ancient DNA Reveals That the Genetic Structure of the Northern Han Chinese Was Shaped Prior to 3,000 Years Ago*; PLoS ONE 10(5): e0125676. doi: 10.1371/journal,pone. 0125676. Published May 4, 2015.

[18] See review: Han, K. and Chen, X., *The Archaeological Evidence of Trepanation in Early China*, in *Indo-Pacific Prehistory Association Bulletin* 27, pp. 22-27, 2007.

[19] See: Liu, L., *On the Chronology of the Three Dynasties*, a Special Report found on *The Ancient East Asia Website*; Liu, L., *Urbanization in China: Erlitou and Its Hinterland*, in *Urbanism in the Preindustrial World*, Tuscaloosa, 2006, G. R. Storey, editor, p. 161.

[20] This is the title of the book by Dr. Ilza Veith that is considered a key work informing Westerners about ancient Asian medicine. See: Veith, I., *The Yellow Emperor's Classic of Internal Medicine*, Baltimore, 1949. Veith's translations used herein are placed in quotation marks. Her work included only 32 of the 81 chapters of the *Huang Ti Nei Ching Su Wen*.

Huang Ti Nei Ching, the other half being the *Huang Ti Nei Ching Ling Shu*. As the latter is said to refer only to acupuncture, and as acupuncture cannot be identified as a therapy prior to the 1ˢᵗ C BC, it is not discussed here. The *Huang Ti Nei Ching Su Wen*, in contrast, was stated in the *Hanshu* to contain medical wisdom from ancient times. As such it is important to add a confirmatory note that the Han dynasty has never been cited as the source of the wisdom in the *Huang Ti Nei Ching Su Wen*, merely its composition/collation, thus confirming the existence of a reputable medical profession at some point prior to 206 BC, the onset of Han rule.

There are differing accounts of the authorship and editing of the *Huang Ti Nei Ching Su Wen*, but the principal editing, which all concur has provided the most authentic version, is that by Wang Bing in the 8ᵗʰ C AD. Wang was a minor functionary of the Tang dynasty and there is no evidence that he was a physician. He nevertheless revised the work, heavily annotated it, and added to its content (just as more than one-third of the ancient Ayurvedic work, the *Charaka Samhita*, was written by Drdhabala, a nonphysician, in the 9ᵗʰ C AD, and major editing of the *Medical Treatise of Prognosis and Diagnosis* in ancient Mesopotamia was undertaken by another nonphysician, Esagil-kin-apli, in the 11ᵗʰ C BC), and in doing so made it more consistent with contemporary theories of physiology that authenticated acupuncture, moxibustion, and their relation to the cosmos. Notably, there is much in the *Huang Ti Nei Ching Su Wen* that involves acupuncture, both its theory and its actual performance. It is therefore certain that those sections mentioning acupuncture are not the ancient part of the *Huang Ti Nei Ching Su Wen* referred to in the *Hanshu* bibliographical entry, for the earliest mention of acupuncture and the earliest evidence for its practice is during the 1ˢᵗ C BC, not long before the *Hanshu* was written. While it is clear that many hands were involved in acquiring the clinical wisdom that lies within that classic work, far fewer were involved in enfolding that wisdom into a philosophical unity consistent with respect for authority demanded by China's bureaucracies. That unity, that "onto-cosmological whole" with its profound effects on anatomical and physiological theory, beclouds the deeper truths in the *Huang Ti Nei Ching Su Wen*. For an explication of many chapters, see the unabridged version of this work.[21]

The *Huang Ti Nei Ching Su Wen* contains numerous extracts of good clinical information, many of which would not have been made had not the original observer been knowledgeable about a personal medical history, physical examination, and pathophysiology. It can be further inferred that the practitioner had seen several patients with a specific disorder and that he had enough respect for the accuracy of his observations and their relevance to the care of the sick to write his findings and interpretations down, for he would not have done so had he not wished to broadcast his findings to other practitioners.

The range of medical information in the *Huang Ti Nei Ching Su Wen*, while superficial, is broad, as is the variety of medical problems that are described. Comments on management of diseases, while often bizarre to Western physicians, are presented in an authoritative way that suggests the authors had a breadth of experience. Note that the plural of "author" is used here, for it is unlikely that the range of valid clinical descriptions in the *Huang Ti Nei Ching Su Wen* was collected within the practice of a single person. How does this bear on the origin of a nascent medical profession in ancient China?

---

[21] See: Adams, W. H., *The Natural State of Medical Practice: An Isagorial Theory of Human Progress*, Maitland (FL), 2019, chapter 5.

That a physician's history and physical exam underlay many of the clinical descriptions is apparent both in their factual nature and in the sensitive and perceptive metaphorical imagery of physical signs recognizable by today's clinicians. It can be concluded that at least some medical care in the original writing of the *Huang Ti Nei Ching Su Wen* was not perfunctory. Although it is conceivable that only one person was its author, that person must have been privy to the experience of a large number of practitioners.[22] What social setting would have tolerated or supported that group effort?

It is probable that there were no local medical practitioners in the small peripheral settlements, for inhabitants had to support themselves through agriculture or crafts. There needed to be some attraction within large population centers for those who would provide full-time medical care. Thus, the knowledge found in the *Huang Ti Nei Ching Su Wen* must have been derived from a large population center. If a city of 50,000 persons included 100 practitioners, such a number could have provided over time a handful of interested practitioners willing to work together to collect the type of objective clinical information that would have been included in the "original" *Huang Ti Nei Ching Su Wen.*[23]

From demographic considerations it can be postulated that organized medical knowledge was unlikely prior to the Longshan era, but with the evolution of autonomous city-states, an opportunity existed for individual entrepreneurial medical practitioners to organize collegially. Being of a common mind, these practitioners could, over time, have collaborated in an organized network for collecting and sharing medical experiences, their names unknown but their heritage encompassed by and ascribed to the legendary Yellow Emperor.

It can also be postulated that the original *Huang Ti Nei Ching Su Wen* was unlikely to have been composed after the Longshan era:

a. The post-Longshan period is vaguely defined, and some postulate it was the time of the Xia dynasty. If so, that interval may have been commanded by the central bureaucracy of Bronze Age Erlitou culture that would merge into the Shang dynasty. But the uncertainties of this period of four hundred years resists for the moment any conclusions about the formation of a territorial state. Scholarly opinion, however, cites a deterioration of Longshan culture and its replacement with the Yueshi culture, one of lesser technical achievement; no large cities are identified.[24] If features of social organization of the region are so nebulous as to be undescribed and if an apparent

---

[22] A similar conclusion based on similar but much more specific and accurate clinical examples is described in *The Natural State of Medical Practice: An Isagorial Theory of Human Progress,* Maitland (FL), 2019, Book II, chapter 6, where evidence is provided showing that the works of Hippocrates represented not one man's brilliance but were instead the combined wisdom of many clinicians affiliated with a regional network.

[23] For example, the ancient regional center of Liangchenzhen in Shandong was at the center of a cluster of perhaps thirty small villages and the grouping may have represented a political unit. In the preceding Dawenkou culture there was no clustering of villages and therefore a population of size/density insufficient for the study required to support the descriptions of the *Huang Ti Nei Ching Su Wen,* whereas the population of Liangchenzhen and its outlying villages may have been sufficient. See: Shelach-Lavi, G., in *The Archeology of Ancient China: From Prehistory to the Han Dynasty,* Cambridge, 2015, p. 130, and Liu, L., *The Chinese Neolithic: Trajectories to Early States,* Cambridge, 2004, p. 199.

[24] See: Liu, L., *The Archaeology of China: From the the Late Paleolithic to the Early Bronze Age,* Cambridge, 2012, p. 275.

deterioration of culture occurred over the four centuries, it is difficult to imagine a network of medical practitioners emerging during this time.

b. The later successor to the Longshan Culture, the Shang dynasty (1600-1046 BC), was a hierarchical society with highly regarded military and political classes, and it has been classified as a territorial state. There is nothing of a medical nature in the vast trove of inscriptions found on animal scapulae collected from Shang dynasty sites that suggest any association with medical practice. Instead, most scapular inscriptions that bear on illness are oracular and seek the cause and prognosis of symptoms in responses from ancestral spirits as part of a strongly shamanistic culture. The complexity of the written language progressed over time and it has been postulated that it may have reached 3,000 characters by the end of the Shang dynasty.[25] With writing well developed, had a mass of medical knowledge been acquired by Shang practitioners some of it would surely have been preserved in writing and at least the existence of a medical practice or medical composition would have been mentioned in a few of the inscriptions among the tens of thousands of scapular inscriptions so far translated. A separate scholarly review of ancient Chinese medicine concludes that the Shang dynasty was saturated with ancestral worship, oracular diagnosis and prognosis, and mystical wu-shamans that dealt with spirits and demons.[26] Shamanism is absent from the *Huang Ti Nei Ching Su Wen*.

c. The subsequent Zhou Dynasty (1046-256 BC) also has no record of medical accomplishment. The *Rites of Zhou*, composed in the 3rd C BC, is usually mentioned in discussions of ancient Chinese physicians, for it specifies, in effect, a medical department of 22 physicians, including physicians for animals, within a clearly defined hierarchy. This indicates that even at such an early date State physicians were there to serve the leaders and elite class, leaving the local practitioners unnamed and unrecognized. This is not surprising given the rigid hierarchical and feudal system imposed by a Zhou family monarchical system that, considering itself morally justified by divine right, was perpetually at war. During the Zhou dynasty writing improved and medicine was recognized as a vocation. But medicine's primary function was to rid a sick person of demons or to prevent sickness by warding off demons. So pervasive was the demonological concept that all medical illness was considered to be the consequence of a single disease, namely the nasty work of a demon who could manipulate its manifestations so as to range from arthritis to famine. There is nothing in the historical record of the Zhou Dynasty that suggests any association with *Huang Ti Nei Ching Su Wen*, even though the later years of that Dynasty saw the age of many of the great philosophers and thinkers, including Confucius, and produced profound books and treatises on many subjects, including the principle text of Daoism and the *I Ching* (Book of Changes). With such august intellectual company, why would no profound medical work have emerged at this time. Scholars have identified peripheral commentary and anecdotes of a medical nature among a number of compositions done during or after the Zhou dynasty, but none were written by physicians or for physicians and thus shed no light on clinical practice of the time.[27] It is nevertheless irrefutable that at least a small medical profession existed

---

[25] The number of characters in modern monolingual Chinese dictionaries can exceed 50,000.

[26] See: Unshuld, P., *Medicine in China: A History of Ideas*, Berkeley, 1985, especially chapter 1 (Shang) and chapter 2 (Zhou).

[27] See: Gwei-Djen, L., and Needham, J., *Records of Diseases in Ancient China*, in *Am. J. Chinese Med.*, 4:3-16, 1976. Perhaps most relevant for present purposes are the anecdotal descriptions of a medical nature found in the *Tso Chuan* that recount events in mid-Zhou, but they are social descriptions rather than medical ones.

and was held in good repute during latter years of the Zhou Dynasty, shortly before the earliest mention of the *Huang Ti Nei Ching Su Wen* but many centuries after the Yellow Emperor.

    d. Following the Zhou was the short-lived Qin Dynasty (221-206 BC) when all of China was unified under one master. This supremely authoritarian regime was responsible for some monumental undertakings and for significantly diminishing the population of the region as it attempted to stamp out any menace to the centralized state. There was a period of purging of intellectuals and a ridding of literary works that were not consonant with official policy. Perhaps treatises on medicine from earlier dynasties were burned or otherwise lost during this destructive era.

    It can be concluded that: (1) the erudition in the *Huang Ti Nei Ching Su Wen* is unlikely to have been collected prior to the Longshan culture, if for no other reason than there were insufficient concentrations of population to support medical specialization, (2) the Shang, Zhou or Qin dynasties posterior to the Longshan culture provide no historical evidence of the medical wisdom found in the *Huang Ti Nei Ching Su Wen* even though writing had been invented, and (3) when mentioned in the *Hanshu* of Han dynasty it was already considered ancient. Thus, its origin, or part of it, can, with a certain looseness of logic, be assigned to its traditional place, the Longshan era of the Yellow Emperor. Even in Han dynasty documents which reference the ancient nature of the *Huang Ti Nei Ching Su Wen*, a similar status has been ascribed to another famous Chinese work, the *Shen Nong*, a pharmaceutical and agricultural treatise also written in the late Han Dynasty but stated to be a summary of knowledge obtained prior to that dynasty. Shen Nong, the purported author, has been described as related to the Yellow Emperor. Just how early wisdom was passed down over two thousand years to be rediscovered during the Han dynasty is a mystery. Epic tales have been passed down using poetical mnemonics, and there is rhyming in the *Huang Ti Nei Ching* (so stated in the *Memory of the History of the World*, a UNESCO publication), although whether this was in the original is unknown.[28] The overall level of scholarship, integration, and cohesiveness of the work suggests an originally coordinated assemblage of knowledge.

D. Conclusion

    It is proposed that two of the most famous productions of medical literature in Chinese history may well be of prehistoric origin as popular tradition and opinion suggest, perhaps the product of a brief interlude in the early political evolution prior to dynastic China that was characterized by the rise of autonomous city-states prompted by

---

[28] There has been a legend in the oral history of a Native American group (the Heiltsuk Nation) on the west coast of Canada that mentions a coastal area that was a climatic sanctuary for its predecessors during the last glaciation. The *Smithsonian Magazine* (Smithsonian.com, April 5, 2017) has reported archeological confirmation on Triquet island. This suggests that the oral history of this extraordinary population has maintained an element of accuracy for as long as 14,000 years. It has also been pointed out that oral tradition has perpetuated down to the present-day herbal remedies found in ancient Egyptian papyri, a 3,000-4,000-year passage, among individuals with no access to those papyri.

commercialization and population increase.[29] Cities of the Longshan civilization such as Liangchengzhen remained relatively autonomous and operated in a heterarchical environment for several centuries. They were unique in that they, being earlier, retained autonomy even during the formation of confederations, whereas all others, which can be principally ascribed to the late Longshan Culture and the Xia, Shang and Zhou dynasties, were regional population centers and territorial states of a cultural system that at all levels incorporated a rigid hierarchical authority and would become tributaries to centralized government.[30] The metrics for Liangchengzhen were similar to those of Miletos, and, like Miletos, it was close to the sea. Protected by its environment for centuries, also like Miletos, its artisanal production could develop regional networks without coercion of a hereditary or political hierarchy.

Summary Table of Liangchengzhen:

STAGE – late Neolithic
POPULATION, LOCAL – 50,000 (Liangchengzhen city)
POPULATION, TOTAL – 70,000, based on estimates of agricultural sustainability
PRIMARY AREA – 1 square mile (hegemony: 200 square miles)
URBAN DENSITY – 78 persons per acre
PRODUCTION – lithic tools, jade, mass production of ceramics, aquaculture, jewelry from imported turquoise and jade, rice, trade center function for the region, maritime trade
GOVERNANCE – a settlement hierarchy supporting a trading heterarchy of a commercially prosperous elite; commercial interests linked the central urban area with peripheral settlements inland and distant regions by coastal trade
EGALITARIAN ARCHEOLOGY - no
PROMINENT EGALITARIAN KINSHIPS – a later development among elite classes
WRITING – ?
DISTANT TRADE – yes
SPECIALIZATION – yes
MONUMENTAL STRUCTURE - no
DENOUEMENT – uncertain, but replaced by Bronze Age settlements and cities
MEDICAL PRACTICE – none identified to date
FORMATIVE PERIOD – 500 years (Longshan; 3000-2500 BC)
FLORUIT – 500 years (2500-2000 BC)
CITY-STATE – yes
AVERAGE LIFE EXPECTANCY – n.a.

---

[29] There were many city-states in ancient China, but within dynastic China cities ranged greatly in size and were without exception tributaries to central authority, *i.e.*, components of a territorial state, rather than being autonomous.
[30] For a scholarly review of Chinese city-states see: Yates, R. D. S., *The City-State in Ancient China*, in *The Archeology of City-States: Cross-Cultural Approaches*, Nichols, D. L. and Charlton, T. H. (eds.), Washington, D. C., 1997, chapter 5, pp. 71-90. It is pertinent that the author sees a common thread centered about ritual that would permit merging of local, but always hierarchical, societies into larger ones. This would permit some degree of non-destructive autonomy for the individual city-state aggregation of villages, but the degree of autonomy permitted to citizenry is open to debate, for classes of citizens included those of lower status who provided manpower for military ventures and for construction of the huge rammed-earth walls of later Longshan and Shang dynasty centers of power.

CHAPTER THIRTY-TWO

REVIEW AND SUMMARY OF THE FOUR GREAT CIVILIZATIONS
AND MILETOS

A distinction is made between so-called "great" civilizations and primary civilizations, the former being a sequence of civilizations that depreciate over time but their apparent longevity is viewed as a manifestation of "greatness," whereas the latter can lay the groundwork for subsequent prosperity and progress. Urban examples from the four primary civilizations of the "great" civilizations, all city-states previously discussed, are then compared to the ancient Greek civilization city-state of Miletos, along with their chronological relation to the great medical classics associated with them. Then the results of all five civilizations are combined and metrics averaged, followed by a discussion of cities and urbanization.

A. The "Great" Civilizations

A summary of the early status of the four great civilizations at the time they developed specialization in trades and crafts, including a nascent medical profession, will now be compared with the Ionian city of Miletos. But first it is necessary to define "civilization" and "great civilization." Included among the many orthodox definitions of "civilization" is a population with self-sufficiency in agriculture, a government, trade, cities, a form of written communication, and an established religion. Modern definitions of "civilization" include "a high level of cultural and technological development" and "a culture characteristic of a particular time or place," but the former is too restrictive and the latter too vague for present purposes.[1] For this volume, inasmuch as it analyzes the earliest stages of urbanization, the definition presented on p. 14 is sufficient in that it specifically identifies two interrelated characteristics inevitably underlying the formation of all civilizations: a surplus production of food and the presence of specialization. This simple definition can be applied to prehistoric and historic population centers of any culture.

There is no consensus as to what constitutes a "great" civilization. Geographical size, duration, and relevance to the modern age are often implied. But do any civilizations merit the praise usually reserved for something truly great? Modern popular history agrees they do: "Today's civilizations owe an immense debt to the powerful empires and mighty cities of antiquity."[2] But it is one of the lessons conveyed in Part I of this work that, on the contrary, "the powerful empires and mighty cities of antiquity" have been devastating to the mass of humanity and contribute to the cause of mankind's Sisyphean attempts at progress. Despite the hubris of modernity by which we seem to justify the atrocities of ages past as merely the inevitable path to our present greatness, we owe to those mighty empires and cities little but thousands of years of ignorance, want, and wars. Even the origin of cities is suspect, for, as this volume will show, early urbanization was not sought because it was so good but because the egalitarian kinship life of the band or

---

[1] Webster's New Collegiate Dictionary, 1979.
[2] See: *Ancient.eu* for the *Ancient History Encyclopedia*, "Ancient Civilizations."

tribe was so bad. People were leaving something rather than going to something, escaping rather than arriving.

As a first step in understanding "great civilization," a succession of minor civilizations may incorrectly suggest a single long-lived civilization. Unless this is realized, any analysis of the origin of progress can be misattributed to the whole rather than the essential part. To avoid this mistake, the term "primary civilization" will be the focus in this book, *i.e.,* a civilization that has not been "shaped by substantial dependence upon or control by other, more complex societies."[3] Using this as a guide the selection of the early cities of Uruk, Mohenjo-daro, Hierakonpolis, and Liangchenshen discussed in the previous four chapters qualify as major settlements of "primary" civilizations. It is relevant to note that the four primary civilizations were not particularly long-lived, ranging approximately 600-800 years for their evolution from tiny settlement to prominent city-state, whereas the full extent of the four regional civilizations that succeeded them is often viewed as spanning the entire settlement period of their respective regions, from the earliest times even up to the present day, a conflation that equates civilization with geography. Reckoning from the earliest date of cultural identification of the four regions, the span of the Chinese civilization has been stated to be 4,000 years (to the present), the Egyptian civilization 3,000 years (ending with the conquests of Alexander the Great), the Mesopotamian civilization 3,300 years (ending with conquest by the Romans), and the Indus River civilization 2,000 years (from early-Harappan to the post-Harappan phases). Except for the latter, much of their physical existence and perceived greatness was a reflection of military conquest. For purposes of the present work militarization counts for little, and assuredly not for "greatness," as a measure of quality.

How did each of the four primary civilizations end? Uruk was superseded by Akkadians who promptly established an empire and a "secondary civilization" that included most of the Sumerian cities; Hierakonpolis was promptly subsumed by Dynastic Egypt and transformed into a religious center; and Liangchengzhen, perhaps diminished by climate change, was subsumed *ca.* 1600 BC by either the territorial state of Erlitou or the Shang Dynasty, a familial dynasty that established hegemony over the Longshan culture and is considered by some as the first Chinese dynasty. The Indus River Valley civilization is different in that an imposed yet cohesive governance over the entire riverine region is not known to have existed if the theory of an Indo-Aryan influx is in error. The course of local conflicts and rulers in that region is only beginning to be understood. In general, however, the procession of three of the four "great" civilizations can be viewed as a succession of secondary civilizations, at least in their early phases, rather than a singular expression of a logical continuum of cultural maturation. Indeed, perhaps all human prehistory and history is being viewed through the wrong end of the telescope in a subconscious attempt to justify events that have led us to where we are today. Looking through the telescope from the proper end may permit our better judgment to come to bear on causation of specific events and losses rather than just victories, to chapters rather than (in the modern mind) a completed manuscript. In the final analysis, the reason that the great civilizations came to be considered "great" is not that they became better but because they became bigger, either in size, population, or duration. And they became bigger because they were crueler. They became bigger rather than better, they acquired rather than invented, they socially deteriorated rather than progressed, and, relevant to

---

[3] See: Trigger, B. G., *Understanding Early Civilizations,* Cambridge (UK), 2003, p. 19.

present discussion, they copied rather than conceived. Nevertheless, in this process the great civilizations managed to retain elements of successes of their forebears, *i.e.,* their primary civilizations, and thus fragments of earlier medical progress have been somehow dragged even into the modern age. Just why that happened is of course a story already told in Part I.

But why is this important for present discussion? If the interpretation expressed in the preceding paragraph is accepted, at least for sake of argument, a comparison of lesser civilizations to the "great" ones becomes less like comparing "apples and oranges," for the "great" ones were merely the physical progeny (but not the posterity) of primary ones. It also simplifies analysis. For example, the 11th C BC extensive 4th Babylonian dynasty editing of the *Medical Treatise on Diagnosis and Prognosis* is no longer a variable to be considered in assessing the qualities of Sumerian medicine. What is being evaluated is its quality at the time the clinical material was obtained, at the latest 2350 BC, rather than what was added, if anything, between 2350 BC and 1100 BC. The focus is no longer Mesopotamian medicine; it is Sumerian medicine.

B. The Significance of City-States and an Introduction to Heterarchy

It was explained in Part I that all four "great" civilizations subsequently incorporated the good practices of early medical practitioners in such a way as to enhance central power over the general population. It is also apparent that they impressed into duty the good reputation of those early practitioners. For many centuries, credit for the early medical wisdom described in classical writings has been popularly ascribed to the secondary civilizations that followed, to the point of actually being used to define the remarkable intellectual prowess and humanity of authoritarian empires. Sumerian medicine is now usually presented as Babylonian or Mesopotamian medicine; Egyptian medicine has been declared the foundation of Western medicine; the principles of Ayuvedic medicine are taught as being the work of inspired Hindu Sages, with Hinduism being the dominant religion of India; and Traditional Chinese Medicine is ancient wisdom accumulated by the work of its unique Chinese Sages and tirelessly carried on by a formal coterie of physicians recognized by the Chinese State. Credit is being given where credit is not due. It should go instead to those early practitioners of the primary civilizations. The successful use of rhetoric to improve the image of one society (the secondary civilization) at the expense of another (the primary civilization) is to be ignored as evidence of progress. A large and powerful militaristic State that parasitizes other States for its survival is impotent in effecting true progress. It is not surprising, therefore, that the earliest evidence of medical progress is traceable to a phase of human social development preceding the authoritarian territorial State. This section of the present chapter is intended to invoke a sense of patent protection for those early practitioners.

Archeological and literary studies of the cultures of the four primary civilizations have suggested that at an early stage of urbanization a nascent form of an effective medical practice existed. In each instance its presence and quality have been expressed or implied in ancient medical documents. In each instance there is reasonable circumstantial evidence that traces the origin of some of that medical knowledge to Neolithic or Bronze Age medical practitioners. In each instance there is a chronological association of that accretion of medical knowledge with practitioners affiliated in some way with early city-states as defined herein. In tabular form the associations, roughly approximated, are:

Primary civilization	Documents	Earliest extant version	Phase of society
Uruk Culture Jemdet Nasr	*Medical Treatise on Diagnosis and Prognosis*	11th C BC	Predynastic (3100 BC)
Naqada Culture	Ebers and Smith papyri	16th C BC	Protodynastic/1st Dynasty (3100 BC)
Harappan Culture	*Charaka samhita*	8th C AD	Predynastic (2200 BC)
Longshan Culture	*Huang Ti Nei Ching*	9th C AD	Predynastic (2500 BC)

Progress to improve the lot of society's members is not intended just for an elite class of an urban population. It should instead comprise the total population, including dependent settlements and domiciles in its proximity. To this end, some view the structure and functioning of cities throughout history, and now prehistory, as fairly similar even when those cities have been completely independent in their development. An important mechanism in this process has been described by Dr. Monica Smith as "the use of networks to increase information transfer," which means that networks developed within populations in which networking members were often at a distance from one another.[4] On this point Dr. Smith has concluded that a hierarchical system with an elite class is inherently limited in its power to change the course and momentum of urban development unless it is able to enlist the cooperation of citizenry. This is because the multitude of networks of groups operating on different levels throughout the urban population will propel development in a way that more closely serves the whole of the citizenry rather than a closeted hierarchy. Indeed, the ability of a city to flourish at all is a function primarily of such networks that foster cooperation in economic activities (*ibid.*, p. 24-27).

A term for the system that guides an organization or community by autonomous networks, each having its own sphere of influence/power and unable to avoid interacting with other networks because of proximity, is "heterarchy," the antonym of "hierarchy." A heterarchy has no central hierarchical system to organize society; there are instead many foci of authority, autonomous and fluctuating in influence. It would not be surprising, therefore, that the first glimpses of the existence of professional medical organization would be found in some early independent city-states in the absence of an elite class. In ancient Mesopotamian cities a picture of its inhabitants going about their daily tasks can be easily imagined from archeological remains of neighborhoods, private

---

[4] Smith, M. L., in *The Social Construction of Ancient Cities*, Washington, D. C., 2010 (paperback), M. L. Smith, editor, Introduction, p. 7. This recent book is of special interest in that it highlights the dynamic nature of cities and their effects on proximal communities.

houses, a variety of workshops, bakeries, mills, taverns, commercial shops, and barbershops. Unless specifically targeted by elites, the day-to-day functioning of most of a city-state's enterprises would have been more affected by the weather than by bureaucratic dictates, in part because if commercial ventures were to cease for any reason there would be no "city." In this environment the idea of medical practitioners could be recognized by citizens as a useful service. This was elaborated in Part I when discussing the koinon, a small democratic group of like-minded persons proposed to have been organized by Hippocratic physicians for the networking of their medical practitioners to improve their functioning and effectiveness. The transformation of the local or itinerant medical practitioner into a member of a network of practitioners is the consequence of not only population size and density (as will be discussed later) but also of a shift in professional paradigm, *i.e.,* from the limited knowledge of the individual to the arithmetic increase in knowledge that results from collaboration within the group. This group would develop spontaneously because of need rather than by direction, and it would remain independent as long as the social setting was amenable. As the archaic medical practitioners in all four of the primary civilizations previously described were not shamans, instead being merely local persons who drained abscesses, pulled teeth, set fractures, and bandaged wounds, such unpleasant tasks would unquestionably have been carried out by those of lower class, whereas the shaman was of the elite. But in a heterarchy the plebeians were both the source and the recipients of an embryonic form of professional medical care.

Features that support a distinction of city-states from other polities, collectively the "territorial" states, have been summarized by Dr. Bruce Trigger: territorial states are often larger, but because leadership elite and their retainers concentrate in the urbanized areas the central population is smaller. They also typically have monumental architecture and other large projects made possible because of greater excesses of products, especially foodstuffs, that can support a large labor force that is under their control. Distribution of command and control, especially as pertains to the economy, remains in the hands of relatively few people, and centralization of power, by redistributing the population according to changing circumstance, permits focus on efficiency, a factor that increases the wealth of the upper class at the expense of the farming class.[5]

City-states, in contrast to territorial states, generally have a centralized city surrounded by many smaller communities. Sometimes these communities provide a particular service or commodity needed by the general population, in return for which they might receive commodities produced in another village. The central city tends to contain the bulk of the population, including those with specialized trades and services and many of those involved in agriculture who would leave the city daily to tend their lands. The city's central location makes it accessible to those living in the surrounding villages. In the early stage of development there was an opportunity for a broader representation in governance when outlying citizens could walk to the central city in one day, and it has been pointed out that in southern Mesopotamia the city-states were

---

[5] See: Trigger, B. G, *Understanding Early Civilizations*, Cambridge (UK), 2003, pp. 110-113 and 266-270. Another intriguing difference between city-states and territorial states was suggested in which the latter, because of absolute controls on production, produced artistic products that conformed to a specific ideal that was not disposed to change over time. The art that was produced for the elite class, therefore, was of higher quality than for lower classes and tended to become rigidly distinctive, but in city-states the nascent individualistic enterprise fashioned a greater variety of product based on the common experience.

separated by about twenty miles and often visible to each other, an observation supporting the practicality of the suggestion that even the peripheral population could represent a political force. Finally, with the central city in a city-state representing more a marketplace and central storage facility than an elite enclave for ruling the territorial state, there is broader exposure of the general population to a greater variety of goods and services. Regional clusters of city-states can share cultural characteristics but are usually autonomous and distinctive.

Although there is differing opinion about the validity of differentiation, or even the need for differentiation, of city-states from territorial states in explaining the development of subsequent great empires, this is not relevant to present purposes. Whether city-states were a prerequisite for, an alternative pathway to, or a regression from, a territorial state does not alter the social consequences of an autonomously organized coalescence of small groups within a central locus for fostering unity, security, and stability. It is proposed, therefore, that it was in the archaic city-state that an opportunity presented itself for development of a form of medical care that surpassed in effectiveness the primitive empirical care that had been available from a family member or neighbor in other archaic forms of social organization. The function of the local adept at wound care, tooth extraction, and draining of abscesses could, by networking with similar healthcare practitioners, now be expanded to include prediction and management of illnesses hitherto a mystery; the adept was now a primordial practitioner. His status, however, was to change when city-states became integrated into a more powerful hierarchical political structure. In Egypt the prominent medical presence became an arm of the State and the State religion; in China it was an additional branch of an elite class with allegiance to, and at the service of, the State; in Mesopotamia it was the victim of State-promoted mystics and was destined to disappear; in India it came under the hegemony of an authoritarian religious sect and subsequently demeaned by its incorporation into religious canon.

But the evolution in medical care permitted by the city-state structure, while it would be expected to have occurred at a time when a form of writing was available to expand horizontal and vertical transmission of knowledge, may have been accumulating in the minds of some prehistoric practitioners who would then have passed on their wisdom to their progeny or interested persons by example or by recitation. Despite limited transmission, at least it provided protection against its loss. For example, some knowledge in the *Huang Ti Nei Ching Su Wen*, if composed in the early Longshan era, may have been transmitted orally for perhaps five or six centuries before writing was developing during the Shang Dynasty and into the Zhou Dynasty. Similarly, Ayurveda, as practiced according to the Charaka and Sushruta samhitas, might have been passed orally through generations for perhaps twice that, a thousand years.

To summarize, an early form of empirical/rational medicine occurred in all five civilizations described so far, in two of which a mature form of writing did not exist. A list can be proposed of characteristics and metrics associated with such evidence of progress as existed in a major city selected from each of the five. They include the structure of an autonomous city-state arising from an agricultural base, then becoming a commercially prosperous heterarchy with a spontaneously formed governance of convenience (a settlement hierarchy) existing during the transition from egalitarian to the inevitable authoritarian governance.

C. Overview of the Four Primary Civilizations

The common measure of progress can be acquired by evaluating a society's state of medical practice, for medical need is a universal need, and strength of the motivational stimulus for better medical care is expected to be equivalent in all societies, large and small. A problem for small societies may merely be a numerical limitation in talent about which there is little that they can do. Miletos may have been of sufficient size to see the birth of medical professionals. As concluded from the preceding four chapters, the other primary "successful" civilizations had the beginnings of a nascent medical profession. What was the touchstone that permitted that early step? Integration of the data from the "successful" primary civilizations follows:[6]

1. Assessment of the four primary civilizations:
   a. Central and peripheral populations:
      The Sumerian, Indus River, and Yellow River populations were large, with core populations in the range of 50,000 persons living within an area of approximately 1-2 square miles. Populations in the large surrounding territory from which were drawn those who supported or interacted with the central populations numbered in the hundreds of thousands. The Egyptian populations, however, were smaller by 80% because of the limited narrow strips of fertile land bordering the Nile available for agriculture. As all four primary civilizations survived long enough to have medical professions capable of medical progress, the minimum total, or "integrated,"[7] population required for a network of medical practitioners based on their combined experience can be as low as the Egyptian population in and under the hegemony of Hierakonpolis (*ca.* 100,000). Other factors, of course, would modify that result, such as geographical features or a higher population density of the central population.
   b. Production and specialization for vendable benefit:
      All four areas evolved from small agricultural communities that unified in efforts to increase food production, the primary effort in all instances being water management and irrigation. With the resulting food surplus, market towns initiated internal and distant trade that extended to other commercial ventures. Production of utilitarian and luxury items benefited from population increase and the emergence of specialization in crafts and trades. The large alluvial plain setting permitted expansion of food production to support a growing urban population.
   c. Intellectual advances:
      Writing, like mathematics, made necessary by commercial interests, developed in both Sumer and Egypt. It originally functioned as a tool of commerce, only later as a tool of intellect. With some scholarly opinion to the contrary, an

---

[6] The definition of a "successful" primary civilization as used in this work refers to the ability, either demonstrated or circumstantially implied, to develop a network of medical practitioners. The justification for identifying the five civilizations as "successful" is based on the medical treatises associated with each of them. The logic of "successful" is based on the assumption that if evidence of a medical practice is found, so will other specializations, and specialization is required for progress.

[7] By "integrated" is meant the interaction between a population center, or nuclear population, and peripheral populations that cooperate commercially to sustain each other.

untranslated "script" has been found in the Indus region, and commercial and identity seals were produced with inscribed characters. No treatises have been uncovered. Early inscribed figures suggesting Chinese characters have been found on oracle bones from the late Longshan culture, although nothing has been identified that would permit communication of ideas or instruction. At present, therefore, only two of the four primary civilizations (not including Miletos) can be considered as supporting literacy. Nevertheless, the need for a permanent record in writing was making its appearance in the other two primary civilizations. Although literacy is a nonessential convenience in the early evolution of medical progress, it is co-respondent with medicine as a marker of societal progress.

d.   Evidence of a medical practice:
This is well-established for Sumer and it probably existed in Egypt at this early stage, although this is an inference derived from later medical papyri. The earliest specific mention of the *swnw*, considered the term for "physician," is from the 3rd Dynasty (*ca.* 2700-2600 BC), by which time these "physicians" had been firmly impressed into government service; *i.e.,* they must have already existed for centuries. Nothing on this point is known from the Indus and Yellow River primary civilizations. Although presumably there were medical practitioners, the evidence is far more indirect than for early Egyptian medicine, being based on legend, status of society, and medical knowledge from manuscripts that is of uncertain, but surely archaic, origin. The clinical material transmitted down to later medical classics from the Indus and Yellow River regions, however one may view its origin, must have been the product of astute practitioners at some point in regional prehistory. Here is a summary listing proposed for the collation of medical wisdom found in the regional classics of medicine:

	Mesopotamia *Medical Treatise and Therapeutic Manual*	Egypt *Papyrus Ebers*	China *Huang Ti Nei Ching Su Wen*	India *Charaka Samhita*
Proposed origin	3100 BC	3100 BC	2400 BC	2000 BC
Disassembled	yes*	yes*	yes*	yes*
Manuscript, extant	1050 BC	1550 BC	8th C AD	9th C AD
Extensive redaction	yes (11th C BC)	yes (previous)	yes (8th C AD)	yes (9th C AD)
Extraneous conepts	yes (mysticism)	yes (mysticism)	yes (theory)	yes (religion)

*Scholarly assessment suggests multiple authorship, perhaps an assemblage of fragments.

e.   Political status and governance:
All four cities considered archetypal for their primary civilization were to varying degrees autonomous city-states as defined on p. 13. Three of the four were, at least in their formative years, classified as "Protodynastic:" Uruk as Uruk IV/Jemdet Nasr prior to Early Dynastic period in Mesopotamia, Hierakonpolis as Naqada III/Protodynastic prior to the Early Dynastic Period in Egypt, and Liangchengzhen as Longshan culture prior to the 1st (Shang or Xia?) Chinese dynasty. Mohenjo-daro was but one city-state of an extensive Indus

River civilization with many city-states that apparently had no political unification. All four had, at least during their protodynastic existence, archeological evidence of egalitarian systems of social management, and consistent with this is the absence of monumental structures in three (Indus River, Nile River, and Yellow River). Burial sites have revealed limited evidence of elite populations. In Mesopotamia it has been proposed that a theocratic structure with central temples for collection of produce and crafts existed in many city-states that provided a redistribution of items to contributing settlements as needed. Nevertheless, in all four civilizations the prominence of commerce and distant trade suggests that as prosperity and population increased, internal order was maintained at least in part by such management as was integrated within the commercial ventures themselves. The archeological evidence of egalitarianism can be otherwise interpreted as the absence of an elite class, which is quite a different thing. Urbanization occurred at a time of no central bureaucracy or other preexisting hierarchical structure and had to be worked out internally as prosperity and population grew. Physical coercion was apparently unnecessary.[8] The strategic governance that sustained these commercial patterns, given the size of the involved population and lack of evidence of physical coercion, could hardly have been egalitarian. Most likely there existed a heterarchical system of commercial enterprises or commercial consortiums of a corporatism nature that were not centrally regulated. A hierarchical control may have been present within the commercial operations themselves, but the larger force at work was that of a heterarchy, with coordinated commercial enterprises guiding urban prosperity and growth.

f. Duration and denouement of the civilization:
Of the four primary civilizations the end of Sumer is clearly defined with the bureaucratic takeover of the city-states *ca.* 2350 BC by the Akkadian empire. Mohenjo-daro began its decline around 2000 BC along with many other Indus River Valley cities. The Yellow River city of Liangchengzhen deteriorated as the population emigrated *ca.* 2000 BC. Perhaps this was because of changing climate, although Liangchengzhen was ultimately integrated into a territorial state. Hierakonpolis ceased being a bureaucratic and commercial center *ca.* 2900 BC as the Nile changed its local course and Egypt was unified within a dynastic empire with its capitol elsewhere. Thus, the dynamic endpoints of prominent cities from each primary civilization under discussion are reasonably pinpointed despite uncertainty of their cause. As for total duration as prominent centers of primary civilizations with the structure of a city-state, it is similar among the four, approximately 1000 years.

g. Quality of life:
An estimate of life expectancy is a valuable statistic because wisdom of older members obtained from experience would be expected to facilitate progress in a society. From limited information in published reports estimates, especially

---

[8] In Uruk this statement is true only for free citizens. Slaves/debtors were at the service of the more powerful groups or families. But the existence of slavery in early Hierakonpolis, Mohenjo-daro, and Liangchengzhen is not documented as a significant fact of society, so the contribution of slavery to their initial commercial success, if any, was not great. The same holds for Miletos, for there was no identifiable slavery in Ionia prior to the 6th C BC and when it did appear it was quantitatively a very small part of the work force.

those that use age at death for estimating life expectancy, are: Hierakonpolis – average life expectancy of 28 years for working populations; Uruk (data of Kish), 31 years; and Mohenjo-daro 35 years, but this may be biased toward the more well-to-do. Liangchengzhen is unreported.[9] These values are consistent with most estimates for other Neolithic and Bronze Age civilizations. Such data should ideally reflect the status of plebeians rather than the elite, for reasons to be discussed. One conclusion is that the quality of life for the greater population was not good.

h. Duration of flourishing phase (FLORUIT):
Another possible contributor to progress and perhaps a more accurate and easier one to estimate than duration of the period from formation of a civilization to its denouement, is duration of a flourishing economy. Using this measure, the average duration for the four was about 500 years. The time from village to city-state was also about 500 years, but this is, because of uncertainties, virtually a meaningless number.

2. Assessment of the four primary civilizations as compared with Miletos:

Table 13 compares individual metrics of the four "successful" primary civilizations alongside the prime example of a successful city-state, Miletos. Miletos is obviously not a civilization unto itself, its early development being representative of the greater Hellenic culture rather than a derivative. Its founding, however, was autonomous and its subsequent course, historically relatively well documented even though archeological information on its early years is poor, mirrors the other four city-states surprisingly well.

The mean size of the local population of the four primary civilizations plus Miletos is 43,000 with a standard error of the mean of about 9,000, indicating, assuming a Gaussian distribution of data, the range comprising 95% of similar populations would be 25,000 – 61,000.[10] For "total population" the mean is 111,000 with a standard error that includes 95% of similar populations being 51,000 – 171,000. This calculation does not use the Uruk datum because (a) it is far in excess of the others, and (b) the focus of interest is the minimum rather than the maximum size of population necessary for progress. For a city-state's primary location the mean area is 1.3 sq. mi., with a standard error to comprise 95% of similar populations being 0.7 – 1.9 sq. mi. Other important conclusions are:

a. The time from small but recognizable settlement to a population capable of initiating specialization (set when possible at an urban population approaching 10,000), was 250 years for Miletos, whereas the mean for the

---

[9] The value of 28 years for Hierakonpolis is derived from: Podzorski, P. V., *Their Bones Shall Not Perish*, New Malden, 1990, a study of pre-dynastic skeletal remains from Naga Ed-Der, Egypt. It represents age at death of a non-elite population that had reached 15 years of age, meaning deaths in infancy and childhood are not included in the calculation.

[10] The assumption of a Gaussian distribution is without scientific foundation in this instance, its justification not being the distribution of the actual population but instead being the consequence of the myriad of external factors that would come to bear on that population, so many and so varied in each case that the end result would have been an equalizing effect just as the averaging of a multiplication by a series of random numbers might have an equalizing effect.

other four was 850 years with the range of standard error as above being 530 – 1,100 years. This reflects the preexisting culture that may have

Table 13: Comparison of Metrics of Prominent City in Each of the Five "Successful" Primary Civilizations.

	Miletos	Uruk	Hierakonpolis	Mohenjo-daro	Liangchengzhou
POP., LOCAL	65,000	50,000	10,000	40,000	50,000
POP., TOTAL	200,000	1,000,000	105,000	70,000	70,000
PRIMARY AREA	1 sq. mi.	2.3 sq. mi.	0.5 sq. mi.	1.6 sq. mi.	1.0 sq. mi.
POP. DENSITY	100/acre	33/acre	31/acre	40/acre	78/acre
HEGEMONY	700 sq. mi.	3000 sq. mi.	500 sq. mi.[6]	1000 sq. mi.[2]	200 sq. mi.
GOVERNANCE	heterarchy	heterarchy	heterarchy corporatism	heterarchy	heterarchy corporatism
WRITING	yes	yes	yes	?	?
DISTANT TRADE	yes	yes	yes	yes	yes
MONUMENTS	yes	yes	no	no	no
SPECIALIZATION	yes	yes	yes	yes	yes
DENOUEMENT	destroyed	subsumed	transformed	abandoned	subsumed
MEDICAL PROF.	yes, ἰατρός	yes, azu	yes, swnw[4]	?	?
FORMATIVE	250 yrs.[3]	900 yrs.	1200 yrs.	700 yrs.	500 yrs.
FLORUIT[7]	300 yrs.	550 yrs.	400 yrs.	600 yrs.	500 yrs.
CITY-STATE	yes	yes	yes	yes	yes
LIFE EXPECT.	n.a.[5]	31 yrs.	28 yrs.	35 yrs.[1]	n.a.

[1] Based on cemetery R37, the population judged "better off." [2] Crude estimate based 1-2 days travel from city, radius = 20 mi. [3] Estimated as the time needed to achieve (1) excess agricultural production, (2) specialization in manufacture, and (3) a local population of 5,000-10,000. [4] The term for "physician" is derived from extant papyri, especially the Papyrus Ebers, and the otherwise earliest inscription is from the 3rd Dynasty (2670-2617 BC) as applied to Hesy-ra. [5] n.a. = no proposed or estimated data available. [6] Crude estimate of 50 miles in length along the Nile plus 5 miles in width on each side of the river. [7] FLORUIT estimates the years of relatively stable prosperity, and it is during this period that it is proposed that specialization could occur, including the medical observations were made that found their way into the medical classics associated with the four "successful" civilizations. The duration of Floruit is upper limit.

facilitated the path for the founders of Miletos, one already advanced in comparison with the *de novo* evolution of the other four civilizations from small agricultural settlements.

b. For duration of established prosperity (Floruit) the mean is 470 years with a standard error as above of 360-575 years. Miletos was 300 years and for the other four it was 510 years with a standard error as above of 430-600 years. The duration for Miletos was prematurely shortened by its total destruction in 494 BC. The total time for both the formative and prospering periods for Miletos was 550 years, whereas the mean for the other four was 1,330 years, with the standard error as above being 1100 - 1600 years. The total socially integrated population that can be expected to support the initiation, *de novo*, of a network of medical practitioners may be at least 50,000, and that includes an urban statistically derived component of at least

25,000, these numbers being at the low end of the standard error, although if only Hierakonpolis is used (which it will be) the latter figure can be lowered to 10,000.

c. The geographic area that can accommodate the density component of the demography, a probably irrelevant statistic given archeological uncertainties, is nevertheless interesting because mean and standard error of urban population density of the five civilization was 56 persons per acre (95% confidence limits: 29-84), perhaps more consistent than one might expect.

d. The total integrated population can vary hugely, although if a minimum value exists it might be that population found in the area around the nuclear population within one day's travel, perhaps a radius of ten miles, approximately 300 square miles.

It is of interest to relate the five "successful" civilizations to the development of modern Western civilization. In Part I the date by which Western medicine matured to become a proper profession was estimated to be about 1750 AD. If 1300 AD is picked as an average date for a Europe emerging from the Medieval period (cities with populations greater than 10,000 were then appearing), then 450 years was the time needed for Western civilization to produce a medical profession, similar to (b) above, assuming the nascent profession was manifest near the end of Floruit. The Floruit for Miletos was short because of its destruction, but its medical professionals were already at work. The estimate for Western civilization is altered if it is considered a product of the preexisting Roman civilization. On the other hand, if the Dark Ages are considered an impedance to development (which is true) and the onset of Floruit is given to be the Reformation, the value of almost 250 years (1517 to 1750 AD) is not so different from Miletos.

The speed of evolution of progress within a civilization may not depend heavily on the upper limit of population size, for the circum-Aegean population in the 5th C BC was *ca.* one million, whereas 13th C AD Europe had a population of *ca.* eighty million. Details are needed, however, because medieval Europe contained numerous locales where progress might have been initiated based on the minimum requirements postulated from Table 13, p. 539, namely self-sufficient city-states encompassing a total population of 10,000 or more. Nevertheless, in 1087 England had only 18 towns with populations above 2,000, and by 1377 the population of London was 23,000, with all others containing far fewer than 10,000. The population of medieval France, which had 25% of the entire European population, numbered 17,000,000 in 14th C prior to the plague epidemics, but had only ten cities larger than 10,000, and Paris, by far the largest city in Europe with an estimated 80,000 population, would not have been much larger than ancient Miletos.

However fanciful the above statistical inferences may be based on quality of the data, they can now be compared to twelve lesser primary civilizations that are well-known to scholars of anthropology, archeology, and related fields. The reason for this comparison is the contention made in Part I that human ingenuity is ubiquitous and perpetual. The question of "Why did we not reach this point much sooner?" posed on page 23 may be answered.

CHAPTER THIRTY-THREE

SETTLEMENT, DEVELOPMENT AND DISAPPEARANCE OF
TWELVE OTHER ALLUVIAL PLAIN CIVILIZATIONS

After locating and defining a "lesser" civilization there is an explanation for the inclusion of the twelve civilizations in this chapter, including a discussion of the significance of alluvial environments, geography, reasons for nonselection, and issues related to identifying form of governance. A precis of the twelve lesser civilizations is then given, along with a list of metrics and other characteristics for each. A summary of those characteristics relevant to present purpose and an overview of the group of twelve with names of prominent population centers concludes the chapter.

A. Definition and selected characteristics of twelve lesser civilizations

The common features of early civilizations necessary to be included in this chapter are (1) archeological recognition, (2) some knowledge of both origin and denouement of the civilization, (3) no association with a dominant culture (*i.e.*, must be a primary civilization), (4) presence of sizeable settlements, (5) association with an alluvial plain, and (6), as with all civilizations as defined on page 13, evidence of agricultural surplus and specialization of labor of some segments of the population. They are termed lesser civilizations merely because they would have remained unknown but for the fine efforts of modern scholars.

They were selected from among hundreds of civilizations/cultures now recognized around the world that have received scholarly study. There were certain selection preferences in mind in addition to those mentioned above: evidence of durability, inhumation practices that permit estimation of life expectancy and social organization, evidence over time of specialization of tasks and improved lifestyle, self-sufficiency, and absence of evidence that the culture developed or was sustained by conquest rather than agriculture or commerce. For example, alluvial plain environments tend to be more amenable to agricultural development and a settled lifestyle, but isolated settlements of a few hundred persons would represent a population of insufficient size to support specialization, a short-lived settlement would be unable to sustain generational passage of knowledge and, in the absence of writing, it could not accumulate wisdom. A civilization that grew by conquest rather than productivity might limit its specialization to offensive ends and thereby be merely a parasitic culture, its growth and improvements not being a manifestation of intrinsic maturation. Finally, a settlement that was a fringe extension of a larger centralized culture would probably retain aspects of authoritarian population control used by the parent culture. On the other hand, contact with other cultures and evidence of distant trade and imported products is not a basis for exclusion because it is becoming clear that late Neolithic and Bronze Age cultures were so numerous in most regions that almost all had contact with or knowledge of proximate, and often distant, cultures. Some degree of awareness of novel ideas practiced or entertained elsewhere was in most situations unavoidable.

The twelve lesser civilizations were also selected in part to provide a broad geographical coverage, and when added to the five successful primary civilizations the distribution of the total of seventeen is as follows:

North America ---- Cahokia, Anasazi, Poverty Point
South America ---- Marajoara, Norte Chico
Africa ---------------Egypt (North Africa), Djenne-Djenno (sub-Sahara)
East Asia ----------- Liangchengzhen, Liangzhu
South/Central Asia -- Mojendro Daro (Indus River), Sintashta
Europe ------------- Terramare, Miletos
Middle East -------- Sumeria, Shahr-i Sokhta
Eastern Europe ---- Cucuteni-Trypillia, Catalhoyuk

Another consideration was chronology, for a range of values was desirable, although some concentration on ages approximating the dates of five successful primary civilization was also favored.

Examples of cultures not selected because the above requirements were not met included, but were not limited to, the following:

a. In the Mekong alluvial region there was an extensive complex of settlements connected by waterways permitting both local communication and access to the sea and distant commercial targets. But the earliest large settlements described so far (Funan, 1st C AD) are considered by some scholars to be Indian in name and culture, implying that their formation was subsequent to early Indian script and therefore an extension of a preexisting Indian civilization (*e.g.*, Mauryan).

b. A different situation arose in the region of the upper Nile River with the Kerma culture. Distinct from dynastic Egypt further downstream, it emerged from a herding society that in the 4th millennium BC settled near the Nile in response to climate change. From 2500 to 1500 BC it was a flourishing kingdom, at times rivaling Egypt in power. It had no written language, however, and the archeological remnants are so far very limited. Little information is available except for what is mentioned in Egyptian texts. There is no information on medicine. Skeletal remains suggest inequality of hard labor, but the major remains appear to represent retainer sacrifice, and thus not relevant to the age and social status of the population at large.[1] With so little information at hand about some of the key parameters being followed in the present work and because of the proximity of and interactions with the Nile River civilization downstream it was not included as a lesser civilization.

c. The Australian aborigines might seem an ideal group for evaluation, especially as they have been the object of two centuries of much social and scholarly attention. But there have been, despite uncontested access to an entire continent for 50,000 years, no settlements. This may seem remarkable, but considering that permanent settlements elsewhere did not evolve until the Late Glacial Period receded 11,000 years ago, and even then evolving hesitantly, perhaps the Australian experience is not so unusual. Its uniqueness is discussed further in chapter 34 in the context of the role of motivation in social change. But as there

---

[1] See: van Djyk, J., *Retainer Sacrifice in Egypt and in Nubia*, chapter 7 in *The Strange World of Human Sacrifice. – Studies in the History and Anthropology of Religion*, vol. 1:135-155, Leuven, 2007, J. N. Bremmer, editor.

were no permanent settlements the Australian aborigines are not relevant to present analysis.

Form of governance was not a consideration in selection of a lesser civilization. But upon deliberation it was thought, despite limited data, to be a most important category, and standard definitions were needed for a consistent analysis of early development. Most were a mixture of types, but the principle categories used are: hierarchical, egalitarian, heterarchical, and corporatism. Their definitions are found on pp. 13-14, and what is considered the primary governance providing guidance and cohesion for the community at large has been selected for the Summary Table given for each lesser civilization. It will be seen that there is a pattern to social evolution over time. For convenience, an anticipation of that pattern is herewith previewed.

The scheme often begins with egalitarian agricultural domiciles and settlements, small and sparse, each organized by family tradition. Agricultural success then breeds surpluses which can be either stored centrally or traded in a conveniently evolving market town, essentially an agricultural cooperative, for tools, essentials unavailable locally, and luxury items. The market town enlarges and becomes more important as trade increases, now featuring trade in both agricultural surpluses and those needs available through specialized production by a workforce within the central polis (urbanized citizens). Catalytic components for this process include a harsh physical environment or a threatening external social environment. Those few individuals involved in directing and coordinating their own specie of trade become more important and prosperous than other members of society because they are essential in that (1) they cannot be easily replaced by novices (whereas small farmers and manual laborers abound), and (2) they also work to make certain that they are not replaced. The relatively few commercial leaders become more powerful, but their influence is limited for the most part to their areas of production. Specialization in production is assigned for convenience and efficiency to specific neighborhoods within the emerging polis, and interdependency between peripheral settlements and polis become essential. The enlarging polis is segmentally managed by commercial interests that interact to organize essential needs for the population. The next phase is a gradual takeover of the entire mercantile city-state system for political purposes, sometimes being an issue of physical defense of the polis and its property, sometimes being personal aggrandizement, and sometimes being the installation of a traditional leader, perhaps a hereditary one, to prevent social disruption. Over time what initially was a hierarchy of convenience or a naturally developed settlement hierarchy becomes overtly authoritarian and thereby a hierarchy of inconvenience to development and innovation.[2]

During the course of these changes a profound social change takes place as the group loyalty of kinship is traded for personal choice within a sodality. And it is at this stage, *i.e.,* heterarchy, that the relatively unhampered and unregulated small groups arise to provide support services for commercial ventures and their labor force. But with further growth and prosperity the politics of power appear that lead to a political hierarchy. Interests, opportunities, and threats replace the commercial sodalities with political ones.

---

[2] This is not a new idea. Lao-Tzu (6th C BC) is said to have commented:
    The more restrictive the laws,
    The poorer the people.
(Chapter 57 of the *Tao Teh King*, translated by Dr. Isabella Mears, Glasgow, 1916.)

It is within the pattern of social evolution just described that a small group might emerge as a network of medical practitioners. There is one important difference, however, between medical practice and the other services. As an example, a person who sees that wood is necessary for the polis (a term defined here as the urban area of a city-state) or for a commercial operation can decide to not only collect wood for his family fire but also to initiate a small commercial venture on his own by collecting extra wood and selling it. A medical practice at the early stage of civilization under discussion, however, would have had no precedent and would surely take more time to be initiated and developed. Furthermore, the location of the practitioner network must lie within a polis rather than among the peripheral settlements, although intimate exchange of knowledge and networking between the two could take place.

One particular social pattern will receive special attention: the kinship. Although egalitarian kinship affiliations are universal, the importance attached to kinship in the present work is in part based on its dominance among the plebeian class, the source of medical practitioners. Laboring units are usually found in the peripheral settlements and in the urban neighborhoods housing kin groups engaged in particular aspects of production. In both situations, kinship obligations and commercial operational requirements would probably conflict and dominate personal decisions, with the kinship affiliation thereby weakening. It is the moderating of egalitarian ties that would ultimately facilitate the formation of a medical practitioner network.

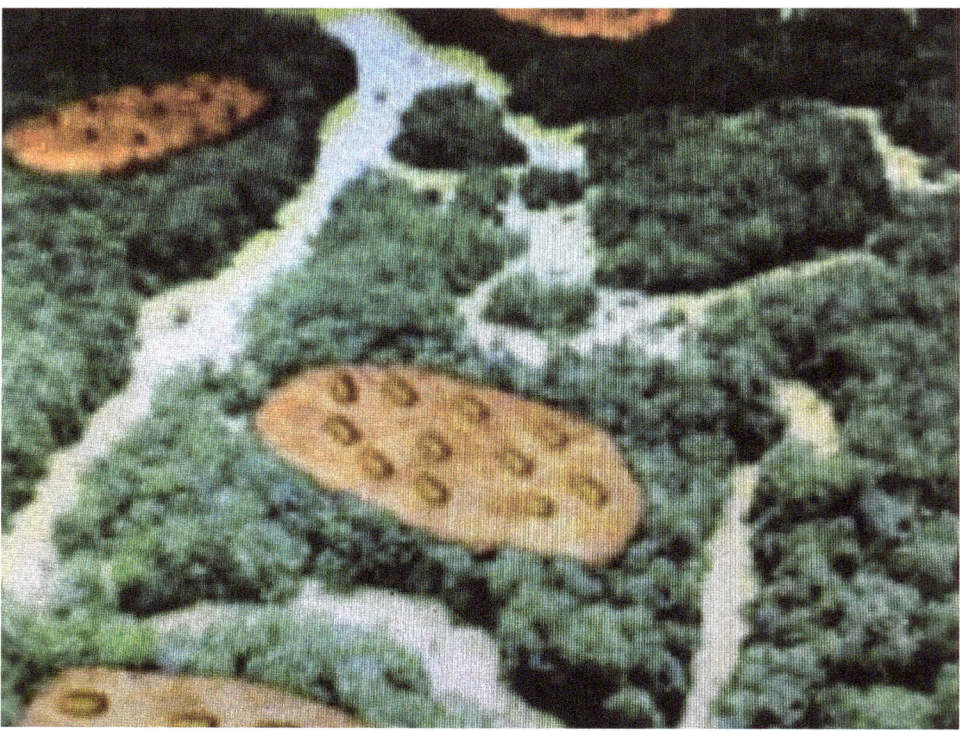

Fig. 17: Artistic rendering of inhabited mounds, clusters of which made up the population centers of the Marajoara civilization located at the mouth of the Amazon River. One, Os Camutins, comprised forty mounds containing a population of about 10,000, suggesting an average population per mound of about 250, consistent with a modest sized kinship grouping such as a clan.

B. Precis of Twelve Lesser Civilizations

1. The Amazon River Basin civilization of Marajoara

Pre-Columbian America continues to amaze as its early civilizations/cultures are being rediscovered.[3] One region now receiving attention is the vast (2.7 million square miles) Amazon River Basin. The veracity of reports by the first European explorers of flourishing settlements along rivers and in plains drained by the Amazon river is being confirmed. This new information is opening a broad area for research into historic and prehistoric America, for it is postulated that the large area under consideration once was home to an estimated eight million people and that what has been considered to be pristine rainforest is now being viewed as having been pocketed with inhabited and partially man-made open regions or savannahs in ancient times, the present rainforest in some areas being to a significant extent secondary growth, some of which originated with botanicals domesticated in those early settlements. Raised bed agriculture was used. But with the arrival of Europeans and the introduction of diseases never previously encountered in the region, it is now thought that there was great attrition among the populations of villages and cities, although this conclusion is open to debate.

In some areas, particularly those in proximity to rivers, unbroken settlements extending for miles had been reported by early European explorers, and cities with populations in the tens of thousands may have existed in late pre-Columbian times. Roads between settlements linked cultures, and linguistic families covered broad areas. Some settlements may have been multiethnic. One of the more prominent ancient civilizations in Amazonia was the Marajoara, located on the large alluvial island of Marajo and its seasonal floodplain near the entrance into the Atlantic Ocean of the Amazon River.[4]

Marajo is a sizeable island, and the area assigned to the Marajoara civilization covers about 7,000 square miles, somewhat larger than the State of Connecticut. With inhabitation dating from the early 1st millennium BC the island population would grow over the next thousand or so years to perhaps 100,000 during its prominent period, from 800-1300 AD. As there were no igneous rocks in the region, hard stones were imported, and utilitarian ceramics were an early product. Stability of the culture was provided as follows: over centuries numerous hillocks developed as the inhabitants enlarged existing elevations by adding construction and debris, and in this way the mounds, already sizeable, became sufficiently large and high to permit communities a safe haven from flooding by the Amazon River.

Many of the resulting mounds contained large habitations, often with several hearths that indicated several families or an extended kinship shared the longhouses, mound sizes ranging from a few acres to over 100 acres. The two large population centers, Marajoara

[3] For reviews see: Roosevelt, A. C., *The Rise and Fall of the Amazon Chiefdoms,* in *L'Homme,* 23:255-*283,* and Clement, C. R., et al., *The Domestication of Amazonia before European Conquest,* in *Proceedings of the Royal Society B, Biological Sciences,* 282; 2015. http://dx.doi.org/10.1098/rspb.2015.0813.

[4] Roosevelt, A. C., *Maritime, Highland, Forest Dynamic,* in *The Cambridge History of the Native Peoples of the Americas,* vol. III, part 1, Salomon, F., and Schwartz, S. B., eds., Cambridge, 1999, pp. 264-348.

and Os Camutins, included up to forty mounds, each center with total populations perhaps as high as 10,000. The larger centers tended to be surrounded by a group of smaller ones, and it is this feature that justifies the appellation of "city-state" to the most densely populated areas, although no central structure other than a cluster of mounds could have been the source of "city" management. It is proposed that canals and causeways permitted convenient travel and communication, but the nature of the island delta at the mouth of the Amazon has not permitted such structures to survive.

Many mounds are in the proximity of former ponds, and it is proposed that the ponds filled during periods of flooding by the Amazon River, thus providing a supply of readily available fish, turtles, and other marine food sources that took the place of traditional agricultural techniques. In addition, a complex of canals and channels accessible by canoes permitted wide-ranging penetration of the large island for purposes of foraging. There was little formal agriculture, but dams were devised to retain water in flooded areas after flooding receded. The only tools produced relevant to farming were axes, and, with the poor soil, limited area on the populated mounds, and periodic flooding, agriculture was principally represented by grain from local growths of spreading grasses rather than root crops, except for cassava. Edible palm fruits and palm oils were staples. There is the opinion, based on skeletal remains well-preserved in urns, that the general health of the population was probably better than found in other areas. The average human population density for the island would have been about ten per square mile. Primitive horticultural societies, including recent ones in the Amazon Basin, generally average "at least 1 – 10 people per square mile."[5]

The several largest mound clusters are surrounded by many smaller ones, and the variation in findings among the mounds indicates specialization of some proportion of the population. A major speciality of Marajoara, and principal item of trade, was production of much-prized ceramics, including dishes, figurines, urns, ceremonial ware, and a great variety of ceramic vessels for everyday use. In return, a variety of stone was imported, inasmuch as nothing of this sort was available on the Marajoara delta. Trade may have extended as far as Central America.

Local populations of 1000-2000 persons were common, although the largest were as high as 10,000. Some assume a form of hierarchical social system existed, one suggestion being a chiefdom, but the means, or even its necessity, by which the population was coordinated is as yet unknown.[6] There was no written language, but some idea of the status of inhabitants can be inferred from skeletal remains (mostly male) deposited in funerary urns that often were placed within the mound area. Female figurines dominate the artistic forms, and some have suggested authority was particularly vested in women. Although it has been proposed that there was an elite population, the distinction between elite and non-elite was modest and may have reflected leadership of commercial ventures rather than a hereditary or political elite. It is uncertain if shamanism was important, the evidence based only on certain female figurines. No evidence of a formal medical

---

[5] See: O'Neil, D., *Horticulture*, in a tutorial by the Behavioral Sciences Department, Palomar College, San Marcos, CA, www2.palomar.edu.

[6] For a review of current scholarly opinion of how Marajoara society was organized see: Moore, J. D., *A Prehistory of South America*, Boulder (CO), 2014, chapter 8.

practice has been uncovered, and osteological data on age at death of the inhabitants have not been presented.

Temples and ceremonial structures have not been found, and there were no offensive or defensive weapons or evidence of violence. The relatively large central and extended populations suggest a centralized egalitarian form of social management for the region was unlikely. Traditional egalitarian relations within a kinship structure probably existed on inhabited mounds, and families apparently were matrilocal. If this is accurate, it suggests that the social environment impressed on the population residing in a geographical environment of mounds would have favored persistence of egalitarian kinships and a disinclination to allegiance with sodalities arising from Marajoara's commercial ventures.

Some metrics of the Marajoara civilization are similar to Miletos, but the size of each of the two population centers on Marajo Island is much less than Miletos city although the overall population over which Miletos had hegemony was about the same and the region of hegemony was double that of Miletos. Lack of archeological evidence of a high-level governing elite suggests that coordination of commercial ventures was managed locally by those involved in production networks. Thus, the network of mound clusters might be likened to production nodes that would vary in importance depending on population and competitiveness. This would temper social interactions between communities, mounds, and mound clusters. An alternative social organization is likely within kinship units residing on their respective mounds in longhouses. Forced separation of subunits of the population, a consequence of seasonal dispersion of settlements by waters of the Amazon, may have deterred social integration even in the large centers, resulting in small self-sufficient kinships that could be likened to delayed gratification hunter-gatherer groups with internal egalitarian social controls and duties.[7] Medical networking is conceivable, for the larger centers and peripheral settlements had sufficient populations to support a number of medical practitioners. But environmental restrictions may have limited any attempt at a medical network within the larger civilization. On the other hand, the remarkable duration of the civilization, well over a thousand years, might be regarded as time enough for its development. The variable Floruit appears to be irrelevant to the development a network of medical practitioners, at least in Marajoara. The absence of evidence of a medical practice despite a stable, peaceful, and relatively prosperous civilization over five centuries suggests one would never have developed.

Summary Table for Marajoara

SOCIETY – pre-Columbian
POPULATIONS, LOCAL – 1,000-10,000
POPULATION, TOTAL – 100,000

---

[7] There has been new appreciation of the social complexity of hunter-gatherer groups with the recent recognition of two types, one type exhibiting "immediate-return" behavior in which ready partnering is used to acquire the day's necessities and to make the day's decisions, and the other exhibiting "delayed-return" behavior in which storage of essentials and limited husbandry permit crystallized personal relationships. The latter more readily accepts features associated with agriculture and sedentarism, whereas the former, because of its stricter egalitarian nature, is resistant to change.

PRIMARY AREA – *ca.* 50 clusters of inhabited mounds unequally distributed along streams throughout 1,500 square miles, most well within a few miles of another site; for the Os Camutins residential and ceremonial site, *ca.* 0.2 sq. mi.

URBAN DENSITY – 78 persons per acre (Os Camutins)

PRODUCTION – fish, ceramics, stonework

GOVERNANCE – heterarchy for commercial ventures, egalitarian at home

EGALITARIAN ARCHEOLOGY – yes, except for some burials

PROMINENT KINSHIPS – yes, in villages (small mound clusters)

WRITING – no

DISTANT TRADE – yes

SPECIALIZATION – yes, in family units

MONUMENTAL STRUCTURES – none recognizable

DENOUEMENT – deterioration of culture over time, then abandoned, cause unknown

MEDICAL PRACTICE – ?

FORMATIVE PERIOD – 1200 years (first inhabited mounds)

FLORUIT – 500 years (900-1400 AD)

CITY-STATE – yes (Marajo, Os Camutins)

AVERAGE LIFE EXPECTANCY – no published information

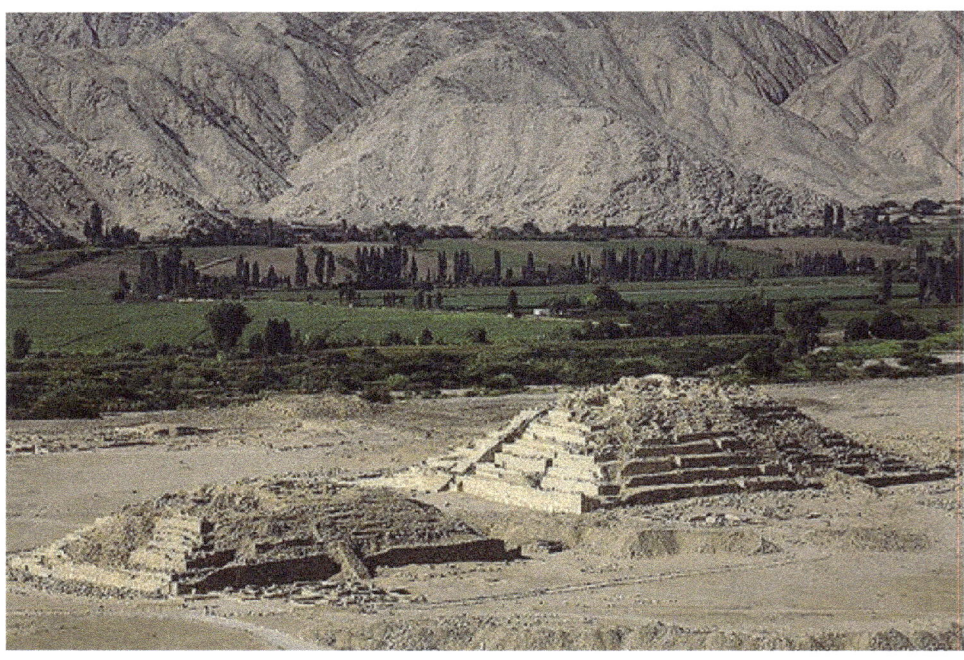

Fig. 18: Archeological remains of Caral Supe, the major temple complex of the 3rd millennium BC Norte Chico civilization in present-day coastal Peru. Although the central population of Caral Supe was only 3,000, that of satellite villages in neighboring river valleys was about 20,000. This photograph is to be found on the World Heritage Site through UNESCO.

2. Norte Chico civilization of coastal Peru (Huaca Prieta preceded, Caral Supe subsequently emerged)

In the North Chico region of Peru is found the ancient city of Caral Supe, about ten miles inland from the Pacific Ocean and a major center of a civilization that flourished on an alluvial desert terrace of the Supe river valley and nearby valleys *ca.* 2600-2000 BC, although initial settlement may have been as early as 3500 BC.[8] The population in the Supe river valley is estimated to have been as much as 20,000 within an area of 35 square miles, with an estimated 3,000 residing in Caral Supe itself, a central area of about 200 acres postulated to include habitation for an elite subpopulation and an uninhabited locus for large communal gatherings. But most settlements paralleled the nearby several rivers that emptied into the Pacific Ocean, and the overall settled region extended over 700 square miles, with commerce in fishing pursued in coastal settlements and agricultural commerce with inland communities. The network of rivers in the region was vital as it made an extensive irrigation system possible. Numbering about twenty, the affiliated communities initiated irrigation of the generally arid region for sustenance of the population of the valleys and beyond. There was variety in their domesticated crops, which included corn. Food was cooked by roasting, as this was a preceramic culture. Cotton was an important commercial product, one use being fishing nets. Techniques of textile manufacture were evolving. The nearby maritime and agricultural settlement of Aspero, which antedated Caral Supe and was not as large, was located near the coast and also had ceremonial buildings and platforms, but it is now evident that monumental structures were located in many locations.

Small in central and total population but with regional settlements over an area similar to that of Miletos, Norte Chico civilization was stable for many centuries with growing prosperity and with a suggestion of central guidance over some aspects of daily life as they pertained to monumental constructions. The Norte Chico region, like the Miletos region, was on or near the seacoast, but in contrast to the Aegean Sea there would have been little or no maritime commerce. The growth in size and area of the human settlements was fluid over time, with the greater monuments occurring later in the prehistory of the region.

Evidence is accumulating that distant trade was a major contributor to the survival and prospering of the region. Cotton fishing nets and other items made Norte Chico have been identified in other coastal areas. An agricultural surplus was available for exchange with goods imported from further inland, including jungle populations. Thus, the agricultural foundation of the Norte Chico region permitted the formation of communities that produced in turn a prospering regional commercial center. With little evidence to suggest a formal arrangement existed among the communities it is assumed they functioned autonomously in their commercial ventures. As such, this is consistent with a heterarchy. If so, cooperation among the communities may have been mediated by patriarchs or an assigned leader. Another possibility is that the population of each community determined the nature of its commercial operation, thereby representing an early form of corporatism. But, as with Marajoara, within family units there was little to

---

[8] See: Haas, J., et al., *Power and the Emergence of Complex Polities in the Peruvian Preceramic*, in *Archeological Papers of the American Anthropological Association*, 14:37-52, 2004.

shift allegiances away from the place of traditional egalitarian kinship for, being in separated communities, integration within a larger commercial structure was not an issue.

The monumental structures of Caral Supe and of Aspero are thought to have required significant central organization and a large labor force, but there is no evidence whatever of coercion or a militaristic component, either offensive or defensive. One explanation for their construction is that the surrounding settlements actually functioned as a "confederation of communities" and that the communities, autonomous, were competitive with each other in supporting the religious cult that was common to all the communities and located at Caral Supe.[9] They contributed a labor force to the beautification and magnificence of their shrine, much as ancient Greeks competed in their opulent offerings to shrines at Delphi and elsewhere. As a consequence, visitors and traders from distant regions brought desirable products and prominence to Norte Chico, surely another reason for local communities to support their local monumental edifices.[10]

Musical instrumentation has been recovered in Norte Chico, but pictorial art is virtually absent, with only a few painted figurines being found so far. Some think a quipu system was used for tabulation, but there was no system of writing. The nature of governance is unknown and there is presently no evidence supporting a theocratic system of redistribution of resources as is postulated to have occurred in early Sumerian city-states. Burial sites have provided no evidence for class stratification and no evidence of violence or warfare. The prehistory of this region, however, is still incomplete, and perhaps Caral Supe with its monumental pyramids was built as a regional center for religious ceremony or other common use purpose. If the total population of the region of 20,000 is correct, most of the peripheral settlements must have had populations of under 1,000.

Initially it was assumed that a central hierarchy was necessary for the organization and effort required to build monumental structures. But the elite may have fulfilled only religious or mystical needs of the region, and, while that class may have been responsible for organization, design, and upkeep of the monumental structures, the peripheral communities functioned autonomously. Although there is evidence of production of sumptuous items in the temple area (just as there was a building assigned to production of copper ornamentation at the temple area of Cahokia; see p. 555), there were no storage sites designed for distribution of provisions to peripheral settlements.

Nothing has yet been found in the North Chico region that suggests there was a system of either medical practitioners or shamans, although the absence of a written record and of artistic renderings restricts the options available for identifying them. No skeletal remains have been reported that might reveal evidence of surgical treatment. Although trepanation has been reported in other American cultures at an early date it has not been detected in Caral Supe burials. One explanation for this that fits the previous paragraph's

---

[9] See: Korol, D., *Gobekli Tepe and Norte Chico: Structural Monumentalism and Protocivilization Manifestations in Pre-Pottery Societies*, (2015) ENG. English translation of the work is available on the Internet.

[10] A similar dispersion of population and a central temple area is seen at Cahokia in North America (discussed on p. 555). At famous Gobekli Tepe in Anatolia the 12,000-year-old temple area was not surrounded by settlements, but it must have been visited frequently by hunter-gatherer bands in order to exist at all.

speculations may be that the total permanent population was fragmented, a "confederation," rather than being under the control of a central polity. An explanation for the absence of medical practitioners is not obvious, but population size and density of the individual settlements was relatively small, perhaps ranging from a few hundreds to a thousand or so. There was no high-density central population. Like Marajoara, while six centuries of prosperity, peace, stability, and modest growth might seem sufficient for a small network of medical practitioners to appear, perhaps egalitarian customs with their necessary assignment of duties, responsibilities, and status to individuals at a local level and the need for donated services for monuments and shrines were sufficient to hinder formation of a medical network. Like Marajoara, environment (river *vs.* aridity) necessitated a partitioning or separation of the settlements, a natural inhibitor to network formation and to a supervisory elite. Kinship affiliations therefore prevailed. The Caral Supe-centered civilization flourished until *ca.* 2000 BC at which time it went into decline, the reasons not clear. There now is evidence that a physical catastrophe centering around earthquakes and flooding may have occurred.[11]

Summary Table for Norte Chico civilization

SOCIETY - pre-ceramic, Late Archaic
POPULATION, LOCAL – 3,000 (Caral Supe)
POPULATION, TOTAL – 20,000 (30 settlements no larger than a few hundred to 2,000)
PRIMARY AREA – 200 acres (hegemony, 35 square miles, but the total area including sparsely settled river valleys was 700 square miles)
URBAN DENSITY – 20 persons per acre (Caral Supe)
PRODUCTION – cotton textiles, netting, seafood and agricultural products, jewelry
GOVERNANCE – confederation of communities (considered as kinships), each with its own commercial orientation; consistent with either a heterarchy or perhaps a form of corporatism. Social organization was community-based and must have been one of traditional egalitarian kinships, either clusters of small kinship units such as extended families or small clans. Elites probably provided supervision of monumental sites.
EGALITARIAN ARCHEOLOGY – "no" based on monumental structures, but "yes" on inhumations, no militarization or evidence of coercion; as pyridamal mounds were associated with many villages, "yes" is the overall conclusion.
PROMINENT KINSHIPS – yes (in the villages)
WRITING – no
DISTANT TRADE – yes
SPECIALIZATION – yes
MONUMENTAL STRUCTURES - yes
DENOUEMENT – declined, earthquake?
MEDICAL PRACTICE – ?
FORMATIVE PERIOD – 600 years (from first monuments)
FLORUIT – 600 years
CITY-STATE – no, except perhaps late as the Caral Supe "religious" center became the focus of ritual for the confederation of communities
AVERAGE LIFE EXPECTANCY – n.a.

---

[11] See: Sandweiss, D. H., *et al.*, *Environmental Change and Economic Development in Coastal Peru between 5,800 and 3,600 Years Ago*, in *Proc. Nat. Acad. Sci.*, 106:1359-1363, 2009.

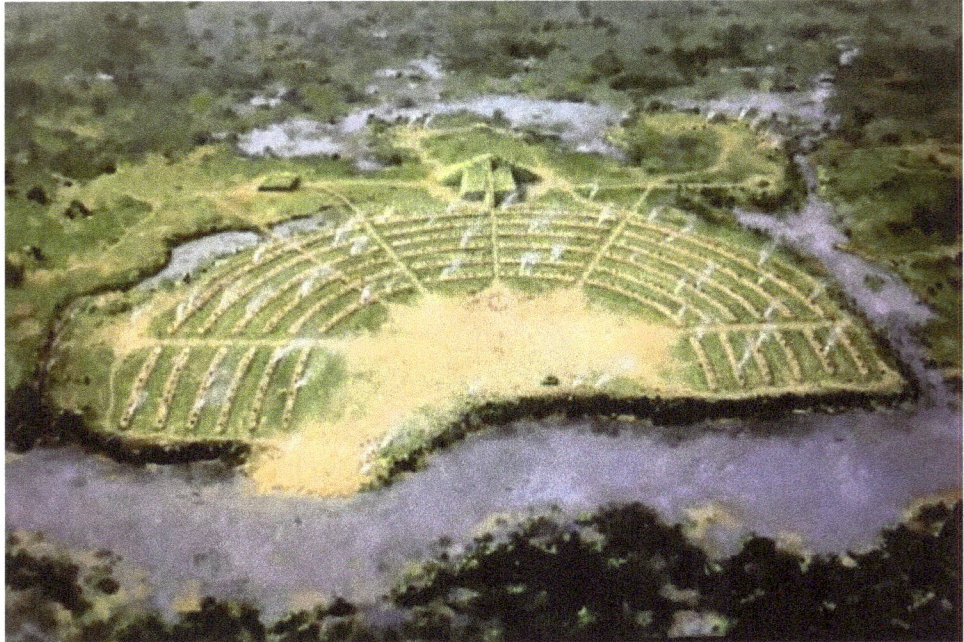

Fig. 19: Located in northeast Louisiana not far from the Mississippi River is the central site of an early Mississippian mound building civilization referred to as Poverty Point, a modern name for the area. Although its prominence comes from a unique and large mound complex, culturally and commercially related small settlements extended out several miles. This is a Martin Page image courtesy of Louisiana State Parks, and it is available on the Internet.

3. Mississippi alluvial, Poverty Point:

The alluvial plain of the lower Mississippi river encompasses about 7,000 square miles and contains the focal point of the Poverty Point civilization, a long-lived early mound building tribal culture that first appeared *ca.* 2200 BC, although the earliest mound building in America can be dated to *ca.* 4000 BC. It flourished from about 1700 to 1000 BC. Its settlements bordered the Mississippi river for perhaps a hundred miles, but a thirty-seven-acre plaza at Poverty Point in present-day northern Louisiana is thought to be a central gathering place for ceremonial practices. It is estimated that the remarkable symmetrical ridges constructed around the site were carefully laid out and required a massive construction effort, although the mounds and central plaza were constructed over centuries. It is likely that the tops of the mounds were occupied by residences for perhaps several thousand people. Although simple stone and clay pottery, tools, and effigies that include human figurines have been found, it appears that many tons of flint, iron ore for weights for fishing nets, and a great variety of other minerals, including copper, were imported from hundreds of miles away for the purpose of producing finished products, and polished stone beads and art forms (effigy beads and pendants) have been uncovered. Study of a cache of unfinished stone beads from fifty miles east of the river documents the use of a lathe in their production, which must have been employed by a specialist in the craft. This indicates that Poverty Point was a major center for commercial production, and examples of that trade have been found hundreds of miles away.

Perhaps Poverty Point should be viewed as similar to Norte Chico civilization in that it was composed of autonomous small settlements along the Mississippi River and its branches that provided a commercial trading center for the southeastern North American continent in addition to its own production of goods for trade. It had no competition. Poverty Point itself may have been a pilgrimage site with some permanent residents to maintain and organize the mound area. But despite the attention to Poverty Point itself it was the clustering of local autonomous villages containing a variety of ethnic groupings that provided the stimulus for commercial ventures. [12]

Within twenty-five miles of Poverty Point are found many smaller settlements, and it is thought that they represented an integrated part of the civilization and its commercial activities by producing or providing specialized goods and services related to the center's commercial activities, although the method for coordinating production is unknown. An interesting hypothesis suggests that the great mounds were able to be built because the person(s) or tribe controlling the area would give parcels of land to those who wished to join the community on the condition that they would construct their section of mound as directed. Thus, it might have been self-interest rather than coercion that made the monumental effort possible. But an alternative explanation posits a materially egalitarian society guided by a "knowledge elite" that was powerful and influential enough to acquire voluntary manpower for monumental construction.[13] Otherwise how can one explain commercial production in a society that had no local natural resources for export? Were some of their imports actually gifts from distant peoples? Could the "knowledge elite" have been shamans? The nature of some of the stone carving and decoration is likely of a religious or ritual nature. As there are no burial sites described at this point, nothing can be attributed to this proposal with certainty. The possibility of shamanism is unproven, but Poverty Point products must have had a significance beyond simple barter.

This civilization is extraordinary in that it was hunter-gatherer and had no agricultural base, a factor that would have limited the size of its central population and favored commercial integration of nearby small settlements to support the commercial efforts associated with Poverty Point civilization. It was a trading center established over many centuries, as were its mound constructions, but ultimately it led to a flourishing commercial period for its affiliated communities lasting, some think, as long as 1000 years. With no evidence of coercion, the mechanism whereby its monumental structures were completed and commercial production was coordinated is speculative. Those settlements closer to the center were involved in commerce, whereas those more distant are thought to often have been unrelated socially or politically. Still, those settlements that lined many miles of the Mississippi river were probably linked via waterways and are considered components of the Poverty Point civilization. They varied in size from

[12] The source of much of the preceding information is: Gibson, J. L., *Poverty Point: A Terminal Archaic Culture of the Lower Mississippi Valley*, second edition, 1996, *Anthropological Study Series, Louisiana Archaeological Survey and Antiquities Commission*.
[13] See: Kelly, L., *Knowledge and Power in Prehistoric Societies*, Cambridge, 2015. Dr. Kelly lists ten characteristics consistent with an elite group within an apparently egalitarian society that directs use of its resources and has its source of influence embedded in oral tradition.

several family units to scores of dwellings and are also considered to have been permanent rather than seasonal. As for local political organization, all that can be said is that, because of the massive effort involved in the earthenworks of Poverty Point and environs, some form of important central organization must have existed. Its nature and whether there was a hierarchical social scheme is unknown, but there must have been an underlying sense of identity, tribal or communal, that permitted the civilization to persist as it did. Consideration should also be given to the concept of heterarchy whereby groups of persons involved in various commercial ventures, such as production of stoneware and metalwork, importation of raw material, and trading networks, were each located in the various autonomous communities. The activities of daily living required for a nonagricultural society, however, may have taken up the time of most community members.

There is as yet no evidence of any medical practice, although there is little archeological evidence left with which to reconstruct village life, for modern farming has destroyed most of the sites where residences would have been constructed. Remnants of a presumably egalitarian kinship-based society may have hindered development of a medical practitioner network, even though the total population, the proximal settlements, and stability of the site might have supported such a network.

Although more like a "proto-civilization." the reason Poverty Point is included here is (1) the long period in which it was peacefully sustained and the long-distance trade that was its source of stability, (2) its unique status as a trading center with connections to distant cultures, (3) extensive settlements near and far with clear evidence of their association with Poverty Point as a pivotal ritual center, and (4) the associated settlements, where most commercial activity must have taken place, would have been occupied by a plebeian population, and if medical practitioners were to arise, it would be from that population, but there is no evidence of it.

Summary Table for Poverty Point

SOCIETY – Late Archaic
POPULATIONS, LOCAL – 3,000-5,000
POPULATION, TOTAL – certainly many thousands along the Mississippi River for up to one hundred miles
PRIMARY AREA – 1.4 square miles (hegemony, 100 square mile; on the shores of the Mississippi River)
URBAN DENSITY – 3 persons per acre
PRODUCTION – stonecraft, tools, figurines, ceramics, and some copper work
GOVERNANCE – heterarchical arrangements supporting commercial networks, but with the autonomous communities retaining traditional egalitarian kinship patterns
EGALITARIAN ARCHEOLOGY – with monumental construction, local villages that appear not to have been under coercion, and a central elite population that has not been identified, the answer for the moment is "yes"
PROMINENT KINSHIPS - yes
WRITING – no
DISTANT TRADE – yes
SPECIALIZATION – yes

MONUMENTAL STRUCTURES - yes
DENOUEMENT – slowly declined over several centuries
MEDICAL PRACTICE – ?
FORMATIVE PERIOD – 500 years
FLORUIT – 700 years
CITY-STATE – no; probably a confederation of kinships with a common ritual center
AVERAGE LIFE EXPECTANCY – n.a.

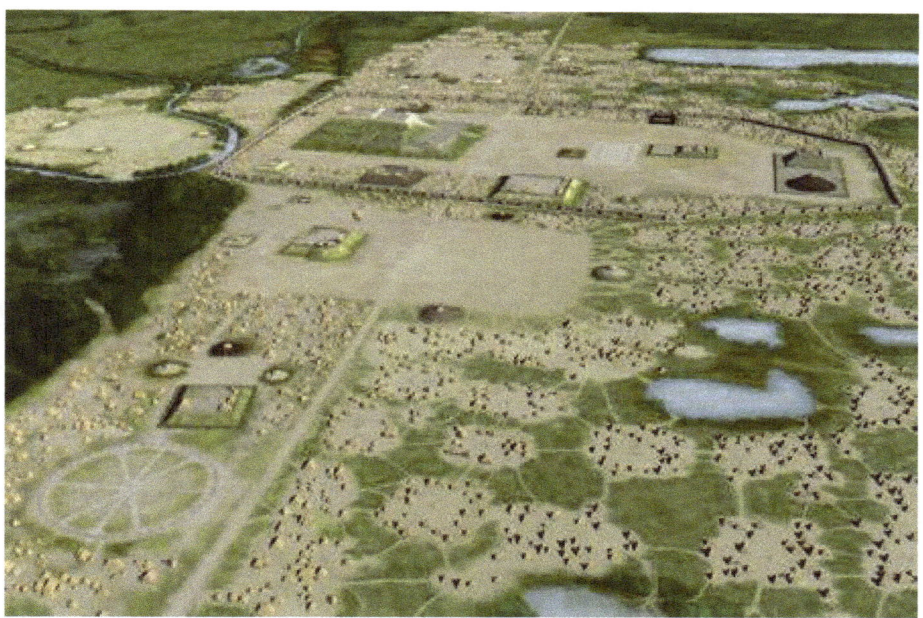

Fig. 20: Cahokia, center of a late Mississippian mound building civilization, was located in present-day southern Illinois, flourishing from 900-1300 AD. With a central population perhaps exceeding 20,000 at its peak, it was a commercial center connecting the Great Lakes region and the southeastern United States. This artist's rendering of Cahokia, done by Hieronymous Rowe, is provided here courtesy of Wikimedia and licensed under Creative Commons Attribute-Share Alike 4.0 International.

4. Cahokia, part of the Mississippian culture

Modern paleohydrological research now indicates that major flooding events occurred in the region of the central Mississippi River in approximately the 6th C and the 14th C AD.[14] It was during the interval between those events in the floodplain of the Mississippi River that the Cahokian civilization developed, flourished, and then declined. It was also during

---

[14] See: Munoz, S. E., *et al.*, *Cahokia's Emergence and Decline Coincided with Shifts in Flood Frequency on the Mississippi River*, in *Proc. Natl. Acad Sci.*, 112:6319-6324, 2015.

that interval that forest clearing and the evolution to sedentism and an agricultural lifestyle took place. The Cahokian civilization, which was sustained for about 800 years, is considered a manifestation of the greater Mississippian civilization, a mound building civilization that, like Cahokia, was composed of "urban" centers surrounded by smaller settlements that extended from the Great Lakes to the Gulf of Mexico. Cahokia was the largest and oldest of its settlements. Many of the Mississippian settlements were chiefdoms, and social classes did exist.[15]

From scattered small agricultural settlements the Cahokian population grew and developed intensive farming practices and fostered trade that would extend from Mexico to the Great Lakes and throughout the southeast of North America. Copper was acquired from which artistic pieces would be traded as well as used locally for ceremonial purposes. Production of tools from imported lithic raw material, copper products, jewelry and ornamentation, pottery, and agricultural surplus, especially corn, made Cahokia, located conveniently near the Mississippi River south of the Great Lakes, the trading center connecting for the southeast with the rest of the North American continent, an urbanized commercial center that functioned like a giant mall for the more immediate surrounding region.[16]

It is likely that it also became a focus of religious ritual, for over several centuries, beginning about 900 AD, more than 120 mounds were raised within a 6 square mile area. In its center was the Monk Mound, a dirt pyramid of great dimension used as a ceremonial platform, and a fifty-acre open area. In the periphery were smaller settlements and mounds. Presumably the agricultural and commercial successes of Cahokia preceded its religious significance, but the prehistory of monumental mound building in North America dates to 3000 BC and earlier. The permanent population of Cahokia may have exceeded 20,000 during its phase of rapid growth, the 11th and 12th centuries, and evidence suggests a large migration into Cahokia of people from distant regions with no ethnic ties to local inhabitants. The enormous human effort expended in building the giant mounds and platforms required organized community effort. This was likely a voluntary effort, perhaps with transient or semi-permanent groups contributing to the production of their own particular mounds. The reason for this is unknown, and indeed the reason that Cahokia developed at all is a mystery. But if religious ritual were sufficiently unique and important, this could explain its attraction for distant groups. The finding of ceremonial pipes with shamanistic features would suggest shamans might have provided charismatic guidance important to controlling or manipulating the population.[17] The pipes were found, however, in peripheral sites rather than near a central location. It

---

[15] See: Hudson, C., *The Southeastern Indians*, Lincoln (NE), 1995. This and other scholarly works stress the rigid and often ruthless nature of the authoritarian chiefdoms of the Mississippian culture. Cahokia, however, seems an unlikely example of this form of social order. The true nature of its social organization will probably be discerned as archeological study progresses. The consistent importance of commerce in initiating urbanization is one of the underlying themes of this volume of *The Natural State of Medical Practice*, and a "chief" of a large population would have functioned more as a ruler than as a Chief Executive Officer. Although a "chief" might commandeer a commercial enterprise he would not have initiated one.

[16] See: Bolfing, C., *The Paradigm of the Periphery in Native North America*, an Honors Thesis submitted to Texas State University, San Marcos TX, 2010, especially chapter 3, Cahokia.

[17] See: Emerson, T. E., *Materializing Cahokia Shamans*, in *Southeastern Archeology*, 22:135-154, 2003.

also has been pointed out that as populations transition from hunter-gatherer to an agricultural way of life the traditional shaman is replaced by more communal and ritualistic behaviors, *i.e.,* a priest-figure. Perhaps the pipes were a remnant of earlier organizational efforts of a band or tribal unit, whereas the center of Cahokia with its massive mounds and burials reflected a change toward public ceremony and ritual rather than individualistic displays of a mystical nature. A second finding is a copper workshop, the only one known in North America, near the great Monk Mound. It is now thought that the principal use of the copper was for ceremonial items related to officiating that occurred on the great mound. Interestingly, heating to high temperature and annealing were used in Cahokian metallurgy. A third point presently being proposed is an astronomical basis for the location and alignment of many structures, suggesting that the concept of a cosmos was part of religious conception. But probably the most important factor directing the course of Cahokia was its kinship arrangements as highlighted by Dr. James Brown. With the finding of "diverse origins in ceramic producing social groups," the latticework upon which society was formed can now be postulated to be a hierarchy not of a few individuals but of relations between kinships.[18] There was no central coordinating authority. The variation in food storage facilities, most located peripherally, indicates leadership was dispersed. Immigrant groups, formerly autonomous, joined with and intermarried with local kinship groups so that there were "kin-ordered modes of production," the distribution in responsibility and importance varying with the power status of the kinships.[19] This led to an inequality among Cahokian residents, for the surplus of labor provided by the immigrants meant that their bargaining power was lessened. But interactions were between or among kin-based groups, not a coercive central authority.

Putting this all together, perhaps the attraction of Cahokia was something of a cult-like nature, or perhaps Cahokia was a site for religious pilgrimage. There may even have been a processional route for visitors to follow.[20] But otherwise, the economic cohesion that maintained this vigorous and sizeable population was a stable class-oriented society based on kinship groups, large and small, weak and powerful, although it is curious that according to Dr. Craig Lockard "nobility" were required to marry into the plebeian class.[21] Relations in and between groups would have been formally structured with assigned duties. There are similarities here with the "nested kinships" postulated for early Sumer (p. 481). Further afield were small farming hamlets, based on corporate kin-groups, and even these had evidence of "village-level specialization" for production of commercially useful items. While small egalitarian settlements and agriculture were commonly found in regions extending out from the Mississippi River, Cahokia was the exception, its motivation being a commercially derived hierarchy, probably guided in ritual by a separate elite class, although the peak period of prosperity and size, *ca.* 1200 AD, has also been attributed to an elite group commandeering the mechanism of religious ritual. Although the importance of this is debated, the theory does fit the archeological evidence

---

[18] See: *Brown, J. A., and Kelly, J. E., Surplus Labor, Ceremonial Feasting, and Social Inequality at Cahokia: A Study in Social Process*, in *Surplus: The Politics of Production and the Strategies of Everyday Life*, Denver, 2015, C. T. Morehart and K. De Lucia, editors, pp. 221-244.

[19] See: Wolf, E., *Europe and the People without History*, Berkeley, 1982, pp.88-99.

[20] See: Pauketat, T. R., et. al., *The Emerald Acropolis: Elevating the Moon and Water in the Rise of Cahokia*, in *Antiquity*, 91:207-222, 2017.

[21] See: Lockard, C., *Societies, Networks, and Transitions*, Boston, 2008, vol. 1 (of 2), p. 346.

that this hierarchical phase of Cahokia social life in which the peripheral population shifted from sprawling settlements to the ritual center was sandwiched between much more extensive periods of egalitarianism within kinship groups.

The apparently clear-cut era of prosperity of the Cahokia civilization was attended with several stable and prosperous centuries. With agricultural surpluses, especially corn, and subsequent involvement in commerce that prospered from Cahokia's convenient location along the Mississippi River between the Great Lakes region and the southeastern North American continent, it became secondarily a great center of ceremony and ritual. Cahokia can be considered a civilization with a commercial base in corporatism but at the same time firmly within a social hierarchy built on kinships. There also may have been a tolerated elite deemed necessary for ritualistic practices and guidance of monumental construction. It is unknown if that separate elite class had more than nominal influence over the daily life or prosperity of Cahokia. No one has yet proposed that some of the large mounds may have been the work of specific ethnic or tribal groups, similar to the monuments of Norte Chico. While there was some hierarchical governance based on kinships, there is so far nothing to dispel the idea that Cahokia was essentially the product of a confederation of autonomous groups with frequent visits from more remote neighbors. The surrounding egalitarian agricultural communities were incorporated into the hierarchical kinship system that developed. But it has been pointed out that the consequence of this social change was not permanent, and when difficulties finally threatened Cahokia the individual kinship units ultimately disavowed the new system and voluntarily departed in order to return to their simpler egalitarian ways. Having marched a short distance along the path to "progress," they turned back to the stability of ever unchanging tradition.

Dispersal of the surrounding settlements may have terminated the Cahokia civilization. But as Cahokia declined in the 13th C, geological evidence supports the notion of increasingly devastating floods. Its disappearance in the 14th C does not appear to have involved conflict or epidemic disease. But the lives of the people of Cahokia were probably difficult at all stages. In the absence of data from burials of inhabitants of the Cahokia region, the life expectancy of contemporary groups adjacent to the Mississippian culture was sixteen years in those who reached the age of fifteen.[22] The findings in a burial site of evidence of a singular large-scale human sacrifice remains unexplained. As there was no written record their lifestyle remains hypothetical, and nothing of a medical nature has been uncovered that describes the nature of day-to-day medical care. Metrics of Cahokia could have supported a network of medical practitioners, for the four-century duration of its prosperous and peaceful period and the size of its population at the zenith approximates the lower range of similar values for the five successful primary civilizations. But the overriding fact of this civilization is that it not only arose amidst a confederation of egalitarian kinship communities and remained so throughout much of its existence as a hierarchy of kinships, but it also ended with a resumption of egalitarian existence as its composite social units dispersed in response to environmental changes. As the "common man" who would be the first medical practitioner in Cahokia was never freed from the demands of kinship to make the attempt, Cahokia can enter no candidate

---

[22] This calculation is derived from data from the Steed-Kisker archeological site to the west of Cahokia. See: Obrien, P. J., *Cultural Resources Survey of Smithville Lake, Missouri*, volume 1, *Archeology*, Kansas State University, 1977, pp. 113-127.

for the honor. A comparison of Late Woodland Cahokia with the Late Archaic culture of Poverty Point suggests that after three thousand years there was no change for the better, although things did get bigger. Although there is a vague similarity with the predynastic Egyptian culture and its subsequent pharaonic dynastic monumental structures in that there is a sequence of mound building civilizations in the Mississippi region (Poverty Point, 1400 BC; Adena culture, 500 BC; Hopewell culture, 100 BC; and Mississippian culture manifested in Cahokia, 700 AD) that produced ever larger monumental mounds, no link among the four has been found. In contrast to most of the twelve lesser primary civilizations, it is now reasonable to attribute the decline of Cahokia to calamitous environmental change.

Summary Table for Cahokia civilization

SOCIETY – Late Woodland
POPULATION, LOCAL – 20,000
POPULATION, TOTAL – ?; fluctuated with coming and going of kinship groups, probably tribes
PRIMARY AREA – 6 square miles (hegemony: may not be relevant in this context)
URBAN DENSITY – 5 persons per acre
PRODUCTION – agriculture (corn), copper metallurgy, hand tools, jewelry, ornamentals,
GOVERNANCE – locally and peripherally egalitarian kinship communities or small chiefdoms (and chiefdoms are based structurally on kinship), but functionally a commercial enterprise with production based on hierarchical kinship relations beginning in the 12th C. As groups came and left apparently voluntarily this can be viewed as an example of corporatism, for kin-group decisions provided direction rather than a central ruling elite. With a plebeian structure built of kinships, Cahokia, most unusually, withstood a formal centralization of power. Egalitarianism remained a potent force.
EGALITARIAN ARCHEOLOGY – no (extensive central monuments)
PROMINENCE OF KINSHIPS – yes
WRITING – no
DISTANT TRADE – yes
SPECIALIZATION – yes
MONUMENTAL STRUCTURES - yes
DENOUEMENT – flooding
MEDICAL PRACTICE – ?
FORMATIVE PERIOD – 400 years
FLORUIT – 400 years (900-1300 AD)
CITY-STATE – yes
AVERAGE LIFE EXPECTANCY – 31 years if there were survival of infancy and childhood (data from adjacent site)

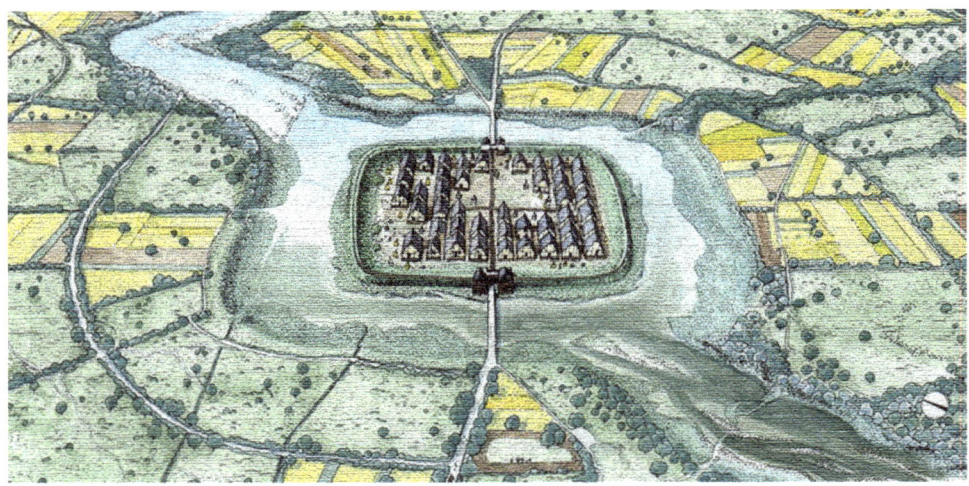

Fig. 21: Artist rendering of a village of the Bronze Age Terramare culture that developed in the region of the Po river in Italy. About seventy villages are known and are characterized by similarities in construction. The total population, estimated at 150,000, suggests an average village size of 2,000, of which some were clustered to give a higher regional concentration. Production of bronze tools and weapons was a major commercial effort. This photograph of an artist's rendering of a Terramare village can be found at EXARC.net in the context of the Terramara Park of Montale and is published under a Creative Commons Attribution-NonCommercial 3.0 license.

5. The Po River Valley civilization of Terramare

The Po river, which begins in the western Alps and empties into the Adriatic Sea south of Venice, drains a valley that covers about 18,000 square miles. In its central region the Po valley was home to the Terramare civilization, a Middle/Late Bronze Age (1650-1150 BC) people initially scattered in small hunter/agricultural settlements. It is viewed as a unified culture of networked villages based on (1) architectural style of their dwellings, quadrangular settlements with houses on pilings surrounded by redirected river channels for protection and water source, and (2) the rapidity with which it appeared in the region, suggesting immigration over a century of people with a common heritage. One theory is that the population migrated down from trans-Alpine pile dwelling communities. Once established it was an agricultural culture with fields and herds, horses, ploughs, and carts. Over time the small clan-sized settlements with an average population of about 130 coalesced into large communities that could cover up to fifty acres and contain perhaps 2000 people, but in general each settlement was within 1-4 miles of its neighbors, and clusters of settlements might contain as many as 6,000 persons.[23] It is estimated that at its peak the Terramare population reached 150,000. Overall population density for the region at its peak is about 40-50 individuals per square mile.

The Terramare civilization, with its seventy villages of identical construction, appears to have been socially well-integrated, and no primary administrative center or central source

---

[23] Cardarelli, A., *The Collapse of the Terramare Culture and Growth of New Economic and Social System during the late Bronze Age in Italy*, in *Scienze dell'Antichita* (15), 2009.

of power has been identified. Given the commercial venues and self-sufficiency in agriculture for sustenance, it is likely that interpersonal covenants were devised to optimize production, the result being a commercial network distributed throughout a cluster of settlements. There may have been several such networks, each specializing in a particular aspect of the commercial product or procedure. But for day-to-day functioning, maintenance of canals and roads, and protection of villages, there is little to suggest anything other than an egalitarian kinship social order. As time passed there was a movement of the populations of small settlements to a few larger ones. Despite lacking a central authority for social management, the close-knit community network had some metrics similar to Miletos and might have developed a network of medical practitioners at some point, although no evidence for this has been identified.

Metalworking in bronze was an important focus of the region, as was commerce that extended as far as the Baltic. It shared with Etruria common features in its ceramics but maintained its otherwise unique culture. Amber was imported and made into ornamentation. Figurines were produced. Cremations and burial practices were unpretentious, with few goods accompanying the deceased. While the development of the early settlements may be viewed as a *de novo* event introduced by an immigrant population, European populations at that time were generally enlarging and migrating to new regions. It is likely that metallurgical knowledge had been acquired prior to the Terramare settlements, although defined networks of metallurgical manufacture were most developed toward the end of the Terramare civilization.[24] But the origin of the people remains undetermined at this time.

Despite its growth and prosperity and evidence that some citizens/families were wealthier than others, the Terramare civilization at no point appears to have developed an elite class of citizens that maintained control over the others. There was evidence, however, of a class of citizens that might be denoted as "warrior," a merit of distinction that could be extended to family members, but the villages were in close contact and any defensive effort would have been directed at outsiders, not at other Terramare settlements. Social organization was based on family units, and perhaps some were primarily involved in commercial ventures and others in defense. In any case, it is thought that close social integration of the communities was made necessary by the effort required to maintain waterways. For these reasons a reasonably nonauthoritarian society was retained despite its growth in population and wealth over five centuries. Interestingly, Dr. Cardarelli considers this civilization as "isonomic," equality in civil or political rights before the law. Based on limited data, the life expectancy at the age of fifteen was at least twenty-five years, significantly higher than most other civilizations described in this volume.[25]

---

[24] See: Hardin, A. F., *The Mycenaeans and Europe*, London, 1984, in which he refers to this network as a "koine" on p. 11, an interesting and relevant analysis.

[25] Derived from the data of Canci, A., et al., *La Necropoli della media e recente Eta del bronzo di Olmo di Nogara (Verona)*, in *Preistoria e Protostoria del Veneto*, Florence, 2015, a conference paper, pp. 327-340. In calculating mean age at death the age used for all those estimated to be 50 or greater was 50, meaning that the final value was certainly greater than 40 years but by how much was not calculable. More relevant is the proportion of persons over 50 years of age: 13% for men and 28% for women. The validity of the data in terms of random sampling is, of course, unknown. The investigators, however, do not report that the inhumations suggest an elite subgroup within the general population.

It is interesting that a network that functioned to optimize production and distribution of bronze products has been termed by a scholarly source as a "koine," considered (p. 129) as a voluntary and democratic group of equals. In other words, this cohesive group of villages functioned as a heterarchy, its commercial ventures being primarily production of bronze tools and weapons. Within each village, however, there remained an egalitarian system directed by leadership within a kinship, especially as some processes in tool-making required no special skills, which means all able-bodied family members could be employed in the process.[26] It was a kinship-vested process rather than one directed by a hierarchy.

Near the end of this culture it is proposed that changes in river level, drought, and overuse of the land precipitated a departure of the population, although the timing of the event approximates the end of the Mycenaean empire in the nearby Greek Peloponnese, and thereby may have shared the same fate.

The lack of evidence for medical professionals may have been a consequence of kinship-oriented egalitarianism that persisted throughout most of the Terramare civilization. There also may have been an insufficient population density until its later years. Also, the physical separation of villages may have limited the chances of a network of medical practitioners, although the separation between villages was only one or a few miles.

Summary Table for Terramare:

SOCIETY – Middle Bronze Age to Final Bronze Age
POPULATION, LOCAL – 2,000 (clusters up to 6,000)
POPULATION, TOTAL – 150,000 (200 settlements)
PRIMARY AREA – 50 acres for a later sizeable settlement (hegemony of the culture, 3,000 square miles)
URBAN DENSITY – 16 persons per acre
PRODUCTION – agriculture, herding, metalwork, ceramics
GOVERNANCE – egalitarian within communities comprising established kinship neighborhoods, heterarchy for metallurgy and cohesion of the overall civilization
EGALITARIAN ARCHEOLOGY - yes
PROMINENT KINSHIPS - yes
WRITING – no
DISTANT TRADE – yes (Aegean, Verona, Baltic)
SPECIALIZATION – yes (ore and amber imported)
MONUMENTAL STRUCTURES - no
DENOUEMENT – abandoned, cause unknown
MEDICAL PRACTICE – ?
FORMATIVE PERIOD – unknown prior to immigration
FLORUIT – 300 years (1450 -1150 BC)
CITY-STATE – yes, in terminal stage as larger settlements developed, sometimes with peripheral small subsidiary hamlets
AVERAGE LIFE EXPECTANCY – 40 years (minimum estimate)

---

[26] See: Barbieri, M., and Cavazzuti, C., *Stone Moulds from Terramare (Northern Italy): Analytical Approach and Experimental Production* , in *Experimental Archaeology*, issue 2014/1.

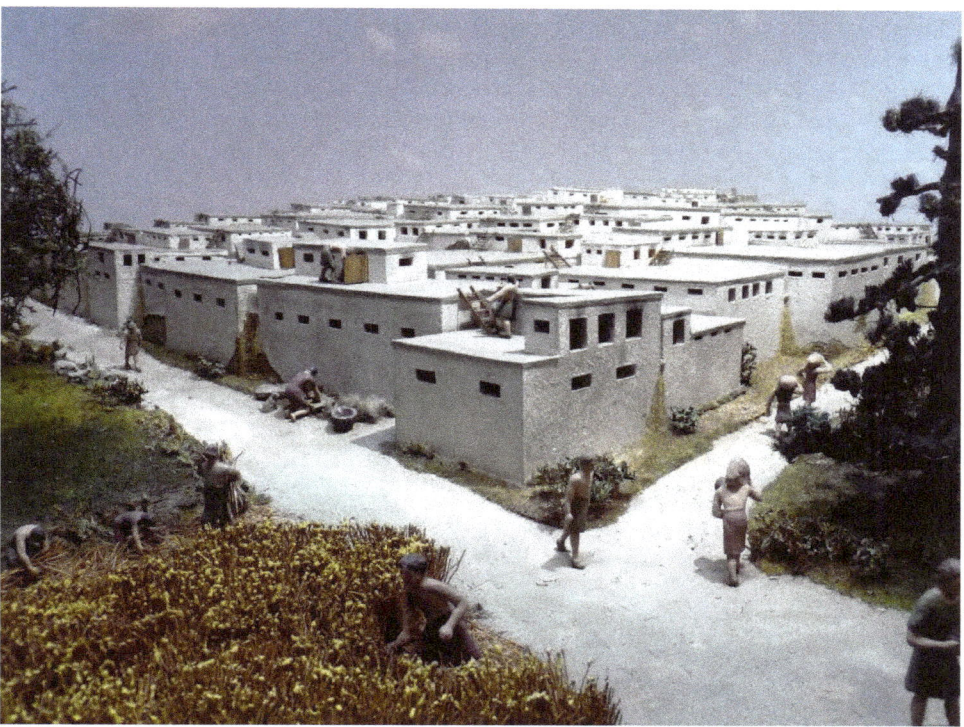

Fig. 22: The famous Neolithic "proto-city" of Catalhoyuk, located in modern-day south-central Turkey, flourished for a millennium about 7000 BC. There is little evidence of a commercial base, nor are there public buildings or evidence of warfare. The population, estimated as high as 10,000, is thought to have been partitioned into neighborhoods probably based on kinship. This photograph of the artistic reconstruction by Wolfgang Sauber of Catalhoyuk from the *Museum of Prehistory and Early History in Thuringia* through Creative Commons 4.0 International.

6.   Catalhoyuk

On the ancient alluvial plain of a former river channel in southern present-day Turkey is found the remnants of the Neolithic and early Bronze Age city of Catalhoyuk. The site was populated by 7000 BC and lasted for about 1400 years. Pictures of its unique development of 1,500 densely packed dwellings without streets and entered from their roofs are widely familiar. Every dwelling was of similar design and had a room for habitation and small ancillary rooms, some with plastered walls, often with wall paintings. Inhumation occurred within the settlement itself, but despite many human figurines no site for religious practices has been found.[27] More surprisingly for a town of this size, no public buildings have been discovered.

No evidence of social hierarchy has been identified, as suggested by the remarkable similarity of construction and contents of dwellings, this being supported by only limited

---

[27] See an overview by: Farid, S., *Catalhoyuk Comes Home*, in *Archeology International*, 13:36-43, 2011.

evidence of specialization based on proximity of dwellings containing similarly produced goods. The interesting idea of Catalhoyuk being formed by two large kinships in such a way as to promote intermarriage has been proposed as an explanation for the large population at the site, which might have reached 10,000 at its peak. The culture was sustained primarily by hunting, although early domestication of animals and agriculture was under way before the area was abandoned. Agriculture was of little importance for most of its existence, and food surplus was an unlikely basis for its settlement and long duration. At the time it was inhabited, the region around Catalhoyuk was swampy and probably flooded annually. Over time agriculture was initiated, but the location of the fields was a mile or more from the settlement, placed there because of the drier land. An important reason for agriculture may have been to provide forage for domesticated animals. Pottery, obsidian mirrors, fishhooks, and a great variety of tools of local production have been found, and there appears to have been some trade with Mediterranean and other peoples, including importation of colored stones that were then made into high quality tools and jewelry. Ceramic products were locally made, and it is suggested that there were ownership seals on some of them indicating private ownership.[28] Pictorial art was produced, and animal figurines are abundant. There is no evidence of militarism, offensive or defensive.

An extensive study of burial bones from the settlement suggests the average life expectancy was about 32 years. This rather low value was from a population that included a few individuals of age 60-70, so the mean age at death of the others would have been somewhat lower than 32 years. There is no evidence of human violence, but there was a significant presence in the community of chronically severe anemia (undiagnosed as to cause) as demonstrated by "porotic hyperostosis" and evidence from skeletal analysis of a high level of physical effort. The extraordinary statement has been made that the description of Catalhoyuk just presented applies to the settlement and its people for over twelve hundred years.

At this point no medical practitioners have been identified, although in early days of investigation it was suggested that there were some dwellings that could have been used as "hospitals." This Neolithic town comprised a homogeneous domestic society that lived in virtually identical circumstances for fifty generations before abandoning the settlement and leaving no evidence of a hierarchical or overtly coercive mechanism of social control. Such a description is so remarkable that the reason for social cohesion would seem to be immediately obvious, but it is not. The uniqueness of the Catalhoyuk community has been attributed to a surprisingly well-adjusted communistic society. A selected quotation from the earliest archeologist who explored this ancient settlement said: "...: they concentrated instead on ... the continuity of life ... and the ways of achieving it."[29] Indeed, the social system that permitted survival, without evidence of a hierarchical organization, of so many people living side-by-side in such a small area is so remarkable that there must have been a potent social force, perhaps religious or moral, that forbade or obviated confrontation and violence. Recent evidence may explain these findings. There are groups of attached dwellings that are distinctively walled off from neighboring

---

[28] For an extraordinary jump of faith but nevertheless an interesting one see: Brosius, B., *From Cayonu to Catalhoyuk: Emergence and Development of an Egalitarian Society*, originally in German (Vergessene Welt), in *Inprekorr*, 400/401, 24-29, 2005.

[29] Mellaart, J., *et al.*, *The Goddess of Anatolia*, Milan, 1918, in volume 2, p.11.

groups even though physically contiguous. It has been proposed that these clusters were inhabited by kinships and that Catalhoyuk can be considered an "agglomeration of neighborhood communities" rather than a early urban community.[30] Were this the case, social organization and control may have been internally managed, *i.e.,* within each kinship, with a cohort of kinship leaders mutually making decisions related to overall management of settlement needs. Any coercion would have emanated from within the individual kinships rather than a central elite.

For present purposes, however, Catalhoyuk is unlike Miletos in a number of ways, including its Neolithic origins, small size, absence of surrounding settlements, and no initial agricultural base. But what it does have is a flourishing era (1200 years) to be envied by great empires, surely time for social specialization to occur and a medical practitioners' network to form. The evidence for a short life expectancy (32 years) having survived childhood might be considered an important feature that could abort development of a number of trades and professions, but that life expectancy is not much different from other civilizations over the millennia (remember that the plebeian in ancient Egypt averaged about 28 years at the time of death). Surrounded by high infant and childhood mortality followed by a laborious existence and early death from disease and injury, generation after generation should have spurred such a stable population to attempt control of predictable health problems that repeatedly presented themselves. With the few elderly persons indicating to their neighbors that an older age was possible and yet with age at death averaging 32 years or less in the absence of warfare, it would have been expected, from a culture that, from initial settlement to abandonment, lasted almost 2,000 years, that from such a large population several persons would spontaneously, or by a selection process, take on the responsibility for providing medical care for portions of the community at large.

But the nature of governance is consistent with an egalitarian society, not surprising given the limited farming and the reliance on hunter-gatherer sources for sustenance. With no food surplus the initial investment in commercial ventures was futile. And it is the nature of an egalitarian society that everyone contribute to the communal effort at sustenance, survival, and security so that everyone could benefit thereby. This requires assignment of the necessary duties and tasks to individuals throughout the community. Egalitarianism is a characteristic of most small kinships, and one's position, including age, within the kinship is associated with certain obligations and responsibilities. It is possible that leaders of the various kinships (Catalhoyuk "neighborhoods") in the settlement considered the Catalhoyuk community to be a "super-kinship," with obligations and responsibilities assigned to each kinship. Thus, totally immersed in obligations and responsibilities, there was no room for maneuvering for a better status and no hope of the same. Successful completion of assigned tasks prevailed over any other course of action, thus inhibiting the conception and initiation of novel ideas and formation of networks of production. It is also in primitive egalitarian societies that shamanism dwells, and certain recurrent designs in Catalhoyuk have been interpreted as manifestations of shamanistic practices, perhaps another inhibitor of attempts at empirical-rational medical interpretation of sickness, not by antagonism to medical care but by usurping a large

---

[30] See: During, B. S., *The Anatomy of a Prehistoric Community*, in *From Prehistoric Villages to Cities: Settlement Aggregation and Community Transformation*, New York, 2013, J. Birch, editor, chapter 2.

proportion of community effort or resources. Egalitarian societies tend to be small groups where no member is a stranger. The population of Catalhoyuk is remarkably large for a strictly egalitarian society. In addition to its divisions into smaller neighborhoods, two possible explanations are: (1) a shamanistic form of social control, or (2) an external environment so dangerous that the existence of the usually small hunter-gatherer group was impossible. Neither possibility would be friendly to an empirical/rational professional medical network. Whether the proximity of the imposing Mount Hasan volcano, which erupted during the early formation of Catalhoyuk, affected the people's perception of the supernatural is unknown.

Key to progress, however, is commercial success. Agricultural surplus was unlikely except during the final stages of Catalhoyuk, and commercial prosperity must have been minimal given the settlement's early position in urban development, limited evidence of trade with the Mediterranean region, and lack of specialization (no particular area of the site or family unit appears to have been tasked with producing a unique manufacture). Unless new discoveries provide a basis for a different social organization, the concept of Floruit as applied to most of the twelve lesser primary civilizations must be greatly constricted in this instance, for by no measure can Catalhoyuk be said to have had a flourishing period. From beginning to end it lumbered along as a purely egalitarian success story, with success as defined by Elbert Hubbard (see p. 640).

But what of those bones that registered evidence of hard work? Hard physical work, as defined today, is sometimes considered a healthy lifestyle, and where one's job does not provide the opportunity for hard physical work popular exercise clubs and gymnasiums can make up the balance. But if that hard work were dangerous, then the short life expectancy of primitive societies becomes more understandable. And the hazards of daily life may not have been merely physically arduous and dangerous work. Attrition from toxic comestibles or specific nutritional deficiencies may have been considerable at times. Remember that Catalhoyuk is so early an attempt at urbanization that the foundation of folklore that has always been so valuable to primitive societies was in its infancy as well. Indeed, the search for medicinal herbs is often touted as an admirable effort by our ancestors, but just the obtaining of a clan's daily bread must have taken a great toll in human life during those early years. Even the decision to settle in one location and initiate farming was probably undertaken as much to avoid toxic botanicals by planting what was known to be safe as it was to have a dependable store of foodstuffs.

After a long and culturally conservative existence the Catalhoyuk community resettled nearby for a few centuries and then abandoned the location, perhaps because the adjacent river and regional streams and swamps began to disappear, although the specific cause remains unknown.

Summary Table for Catalhoyuk:

SOCIETY - Neolithic
POPULATION, LOCAL – 8,000
POPULATION, TOTAL – 8,000
PRIMARY AREA – 100 acres
URBAN DENSITY – 83 persons per acre

PRODUCTION – specialized stones, jewelry, obsidian
GOVERNANCE – confederation of egalitarian kinships
EGALITARIAN ARCHEOLOGY - yes
PROMINENT KINSHIPS – yes; neighborhoods
WRITING – no
DISTANT TRADE – yes, but little (Mediterranean, Jericho)
SPECIALIZATION – yes, but little
MONUMENTAL STRUCTURE - no
DENOUEMENT – abandoned
MEDICAL PRACTICE – ?
FORMATIVE PERIOD – 500 years
FLORUIT – 1,300 years
CITY-STATE - no
AVERAGE LIFE EXPECTANCY – 32 years[31]

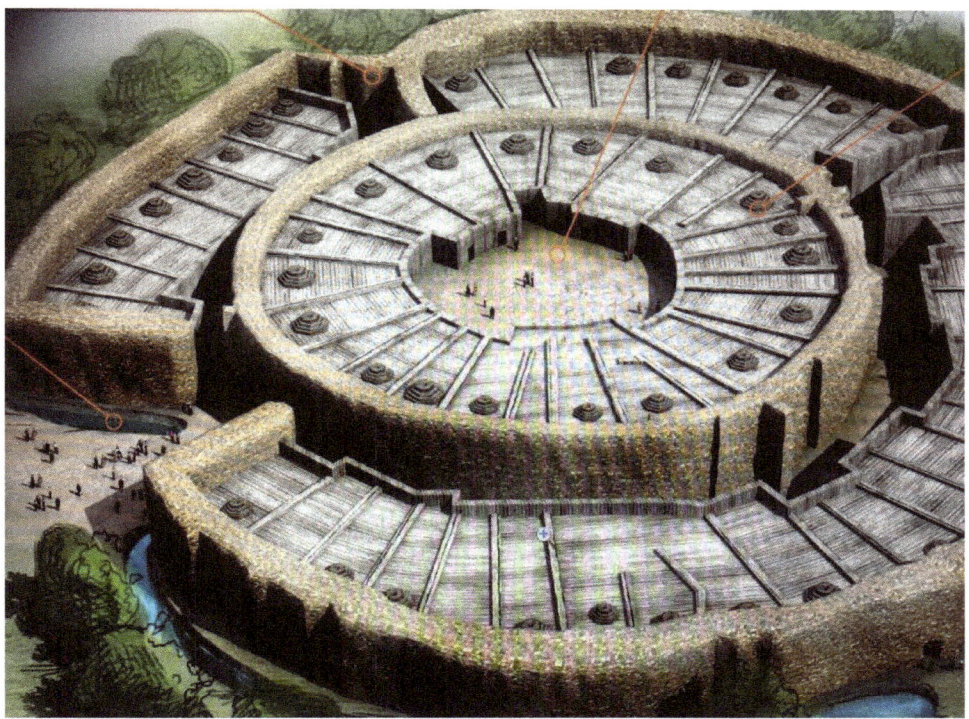

Fig. 23: The walled city of Arkaim, one of twenty Bronze Age settlements comprising the Sintashta civilization on the eastern side of the Urals. Although not arranged as a city-state with surrounding complementary villages, each "city" had about 2,000 inhabitants. The commercial activity of each centered on metallurgical productions, but there was no coordinated manufacture. Dwellings appear to have been partitioned to accommodate kinships. This artistic rendering is made available under the Creative Commons CC0 1.0 Universal Public Domain Dedication.

---

[31] See: Bodley, J. H., *Cultural Anthropology: Tribes, States, and the Global System,* Lanham (MD), 2011, Table 5.8.

7. Western Siberian Plain: Sintashta Civilization

Extensive Late Neolithic and Bronze Age settlements are being discovered worldwide, opening new vistas for understanding archaic human social settlements and their progression to modern nationhood. Expanding knowledge has revealed a far more technically and intellectually complex series of civilizations and cultures in diverse geographic locations around the globe than previously suspected. Indeed, given the authoritarian crudeness, atrocities, and impoverishment of vast populations in many modern states, it is not unreasonable to surmise that the present political state of affairs represents not the latest modern and improved manifestation of human progress, instead being a regressive or atavistic inversion of progress from those early settlements that, had they been seized upon and managed differently or had they not been railroaded by authoritarian bullies in ancient times, might long ago have led to a peaceful and prosperous longevity. This, of course, is one of the important reasons that archeological research is carried out, for if archeology did not have a goal in furthering human understanding about its past as a way of improving its future it would be little more than a hobby.

One active archeological region of interest that has emerged in the last twenty years is the largest lowland and flood plain in the world, the Western Siberian Plain covering about a million square miles. Much of it is uninhabitable and covered by permafrost, but beginning on the eastern slopes of the Ural Mountains and extending eastward this Cenozoic alluvium was the site of the Sintashta civilization (2100-1800 BC), so-named from the originally excavated city. Another of its settlements is Arkaim, a five-acre home to an estimated 2000 people who lived in variably sized houses arranged in circles around a central square. It was solidly walled and surrounded by irrigated fields. Bones recovered in the area are from horses, cattle, and other domesticated animals. That its overall construction and orientation suggests an analogy with Stonehenge is considered by most to be fanciful. Strikingly, furnaces for metalworking were found in most of the houses. There were exterior wooden walkways. Details of its social makeup are unavailable, and it was evacuated by its population before there was evidence of destruction. It has been suggested it was the administrative center for the region, and the planning of the settlement indicates a coordinated effort with central planning.[32] But there is no local cluster of smaller villages to suggest either Arkaim or Sintashta was the center of a city-state. Furthermore, the ubiquity of evidence for metallurgy throughout the settlement and in many other regional settlements is evidence that metallurgical manipulation of copper and bronze was an important activity of the population over a large region, although perhaps not on a large scale. There was an unusually strong defensive design to the settlements indicating a militaristic society, but it also included difficult entryways into the village, perhaps to prevent outsiders' access to the villagers' method of extracting ores from local sources for production of bronze and weapons made from bronze. The metallurgical techniques involved may have been intended to be kept secret, but the idea of a warrior class and a culture engaged in frequent warring is been

---

[32] See: Shnirelman, V. A., *Archeology and ethnic politics: the discovery of Arkaim*, in *Museum International*, 50:33-39, 1998.

strongly supported.[33] Half of adult inhumations contain weapons thought to indicate an extensive warrior caste, and so it would seem that warfare was a constant companion of the Sintashta settlements. But it has been also noted that almost all "weapon" types were utilizable for hunting, and osteological evidence of trauma of warfare is lacking. As these further discoveries show, the warfare scenario now seems much less likely.[34] Warfare also has been noted to directly correlate with population density, and as a concurring argument the permanent population of the Sintashta region was low outside the settlements.

The Sintashta people had been preceded by a prominent culture, the Yamnaya, which has been credited with expanding the Indo-European language and genetic heritage to a wide area. But, relevant to present interests, it was a seminomadic herding culture. Although there was a daughter intermediary culture between it and Sintashta, it may be that Sintashta was a settled subgroup of a larger ethnic population that remained seminomadic. Perhaps these other nomadic people were dependent upon the many metalworking settlements in the Sintashta region to provide them with implements of war and hunting, including chariots. It is otherwise difficult to explain the prompt emergence in the region of Arkaim and other settlements, for farming was not one of their features, and successful agriculture is the usual cause of the surplus sustenance that leads to a focal population increase. But it has been suggested that a preceding aridity of the region restricted herding and that seminomadic populations would sometimes form permanent settlements near more plentiful sources of water, their fortifications being necessary in order to maintain exclusive use of the area. This was not a matter of fertility for agricultural development; the issue was grazing territory for their herds.

It also appears that there was unequal access to ores and other items throughout the Sintashta region, that the various settlements were not involved in the actual mining of metals and their ores, and that trading occurred between settlements. The network thus established may have provided the leadership needed for Sintashta settlements, a veritable "Ruhr Valley" of industrial centers, with some scholarly opinion favoring an egalitarian form of social control in Arkaim. The idea that Sintashta settlements were seasonally occupied to take advantage of geological resources for smelting is presently considered unlikely. At least some settlements were not only capable of self-sufficiency in maintaining a long-term survival, but also were intent on producing iron products primarily for their own use rather than being part of a network set up by some distant power exploiting local resources for the purpose of supporting nomadic warrior groups. Gravesites have yielded items clearly consistent with an extensive trade network with distant peoples, and receipt of tons of copper products sent from the region is documented in the Mesopotamian city of Ur. Arkaim and its congeners functioned as small industrial towns. Regarding life expectancy, the statement has been made that very few were of advanced age.

---

[33] See: Epimakhov, A. V., *Settlements and Cemeteries of the Bronze Age of the Urals: the Potential for Reconstructing Early Social Dynamics*, in *Social Complexity in Prehistoric Eurasia*, Hanks, B. K., and Linduff, K. M., eds. Cambridge, 2009, chapter 5.

[34] See: Johnson, J. A., *Community Matters? Investigating Social Complexity through Centralization and Differentiation in Bronze Age Pastoral Societies of the Southern Urals, Russian Federation, 2100 – 900 BC*, Doctoral dissertation, University of Pittsburgh, 2014.

Arkaim is in the midst of about twenty similar communities all located within an area of about 20,000 square miles and all are situated adjacent to rivers. It bears similarity to the original Sintashta archeological site in the same region, the two usually being linked together in Bronze Age descriptions. All twenty communities suggest some similarity in construction design. Furthermore, settlements were separated from each other by 20-40 miles, suggesting a large area was required to sustain each settlement. One obvious explanation is that the metallurgical enterprise required much wood to maintain the furnaces required for smelting.[35] An indication that the strong walls surrounding Arkaim were defensive protection of the population is reflected in the invention of the wheeled chariot in the Sintashta region at this time. Much has been made of the Arkaim region as a locus of early Indo-Aryan culture, but no written language has been found, nor has evidence relevant to medicine been uncovered. Kurgans and other gravesites have revealed war chariots suggesting a military cast and supporting the idea a hierarchical society, but there is no other evidence that this was the case. There is agreement that the population in each site seemed archeologically egalitarian, and some settlements reveal a domiciliary pattern consistent with neighborhoods, suggesting grouping by kinship. Several hundred inhumations have been recovered that include all ages, and the overall similarity in ornamentation, ceramics, and "weapons" in five burial sites do not support a traditional hierarchy for social control (see Johnson citation on preceding page). It is likely that the capacity for producing bronze implements and weapons was primarily for personal or communal use, the weapons and the stockade-like construction of the walls being for defensive purposes only.

Yet some form of leadership was necessary to coordinate trade and production. An interesting theory suggests the Sintashta proto-civilization is but one manifestation of a greater regional organization, in effect a territorial State, that integrated metallurgy, mining, and agricultural sustenance. This suggests the culture might be likened to some sort of prehistoric benign Gulag and therefore was "not built on the principle of kinship."[36] State management would necessarily have been coercive, of which there is no evidence in the Sintashta settlements. More convincing is the conclusion of Dr. Ludmila Koryakova, who, based on the closeness of the dwellings, their comfortableness, and the homogeneity of households and their involvement in production, considers their governance a form of corporatism, one in which special interests (in this case the citizenry *in toto*) made communal decisions regarding commercial production and municipal operation, an extraordinary phenomenon.[37] Corporatism needs not be authoritarian, and indeed it can blunt the authoritarian hand. Insofar as it might be considered democratic, it can be tyrannical if all involved kinships are committed to specific duties to maintain a commercial enterprise. It would then be functioning as a super-kinship and harbor all the advantages and disadvantages of egalitarian control. This is one feature that distinguishes it from a heterarchy, for in the latter there are numerous distinct commercial ventures that would vie for the available labor force, thereby offering choices for the community at

---

[35] See: Shaparov, D., *Middle to Late Bronze Age Transition in the Southern Urals (Russia): A Settlement Pattern Perspective*, Saarbrucken, 2011, for an extensive and detailed account of regional settlements and metallurgy that include Sintashta, especially chapter 5.

[36] See: Alekseevna, O. E., and Aleksandrovich, P. V., *Early State of the Bronze Age: Arkaim – Kargaly Case Study*, in *International Journal of Humanities and Cultural Studies*, 3:121-128, 2016.

[37] Koryakova, L., and Epimakhov, A., *The Urals and Western Siberia in the Bronze and Iron Ages*, Cambridge, 2014, p. 181.

large, whereas the corporatism of Sintashta, if indeed it existed, would have been monolithic. An alternative mechanism of social control that would not rely on kinship might be a sodality involving the entire community, but in an otherwise sparsely populated region the possibility of iron production by a community of like-minded but otherwise unrelated individuals and families seems remote.

There must have been a wide-ranging trading network that included all Sintashta settlements and which provided a stabilizing influence on community life. Both the size of the population and the settlement are tiny compared to the five successful civilizations, and, given the small population, 300-400 years may have been insufficient for a medical profession to develop. If Sintashta society required the full strength of its members to maintain, sustain, and defend their outposts in an iron ore-rich geography there would have been little chance for an empirical-rational medical practitioner to develop a network of clinicians. Such persons might have been especially useful, for metallurgy and production of copper and iron products would have introduced unique health hazards into this society.

As the predecessor of the Sintashta civilization, the Yamnaya culture was characterized by nomadic chiefdoms, societal stratification, herding, and mobile settlements, it would not be surprising if aspects of authoritarian governance existed within Sintashta settlements. But study of inhumations does not support this notion. An egalitarian social scheme existed, at least when it comes to personal wealth. Can Sintashta be compared to Sparta? It may have had, like Sparta, a warrior caste and was at least superficially egalitarian. Its size was too small, however, and there is no evidence of conquests or a slave or serf workforce. Like Sparta, the appearance and practice of equality in what might have been a warrior society could have masked the authoritarian nature of egalitarianism.[38] But the equal distribution of wealth suggests another mechanism of social control, corporatism (see p. 13 for definition). The homogeneity of household production of commercial products may have been the basis for special interest groups, which in this case several large kinships would comprise the community as a whole, directing governance in which decision-making would represent majority opinion or patriarchal or kinship leadership.

Interestingly, some have proposed that this site was not continuously inhabited during its 300-400-year existence, but was used intermittently according to season, for there was herding. The disappearance of the Sintashta civilization has been blamed on climate change, but meteorological studies indicate the environment preceding and during the Sintashta civilization was stable and conducive to agriculture. A better explanation has been put forth by Dr. Denis Shaparov in which the unique and closeted production of bronze by Sintashta settlements was, in a sense, put out of business by the finding of extensive deposits of ores in other areas and the spread of metallurgical technology to populations that migrated into the region, forming permanent settlements with an agricultural base.[39] As a consequence, the Sintashta populations may have emigrated to these less rigorous social environments.

---

[38] See: Hanks, B. K., and Linduff, K. M., *Social Complexity in Prehistoric Eurasia*, Cambridge, 2009, especially chapters 4 (p. 47, by D. W. Anthony) and 9 (p. 146, by B. K. Hanks) for discussions of the role of warfare and metallurgy on the social fabric of Sintashta civilization.

[39] See: Sharapov, D., *Middle Bronze Age-Late Bronze Age Transitions in the Southern Urals (Russia)*. This is available at ScholarWorks@Georgia State University, 5-15-2011.

Summary Table for Sintashta/Arkaim

SOCIETY – Middle/Late Bronze Age
POPULATIONS, LOCAL – 1,000
POPULATION, TOTAL – 20,000
PRIMARY AREA – 5 acres (hegemony: 20,000 square miles for 20 settlements)
URBAN DENSITY – 200 persons per acre (perhaps 400 per acre in Arkaim)
PRODUCTION – copper, bronze, bronze implements and weapons
GOVERNANCE – egalitarian, perhaps a form of corporatism or super-kinship
EGALITARIAN ARCHEOLOGY - yes
PROMINENT KINSHIPS – kinships present but social significance uncertain
WRITING – no
DISTANT TRADE – yes (central Asia and the Near East)
SPECIALIZATION – yes
MONUMENTAL STRUCTURES - no
DENOUEMENT – abandoned (to escape egalitarian kinship for larger sodalities?)
MEDICAL PRACTICE – ?
FORMATIVE PERIOD - ?
FLORUIT – 400 years
CITY-STATE – no
AVERAGE LIFE EXPECTANCY – "very few elderly;" 28 years[40]

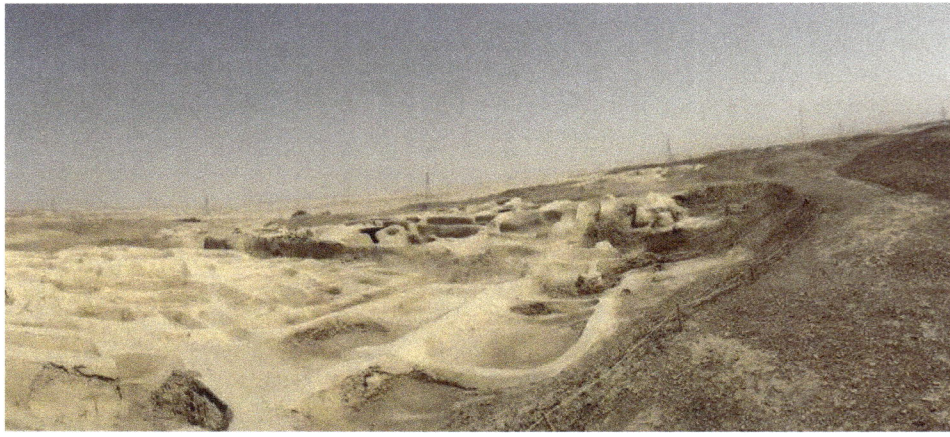

Fig. 24: Ruins of the eastern residential area of the city of Shahr-i Sokhta that developed in the region of the Helmand river (in present-day Sistan Provice of Iran) during the mid-3rd millennium BC. It was a commercially active region situated between Mesopotamia and the Indus River Valley and yet is considered to represent a distinct culture. Its peak population may have reached 20,000. This is photograph is found under the Creative Commons Attribution-Share Alike 4.0 license.

---

[40] See: Baumer, C., *The History of Central Asia: The Age of the Steppe Warriors*, New York, 2012, translated by Miranda Bennett, p. 146.

8. Shahr-i Sokhta

The Sistan Basin, a region the size of Connecticut (*ca.* 6,000 sq. mi.) located in the south of modern Afghanistan at its juncture with southeast Iran and Pakistan, was the site of numerous Bronze Age settlements. Its geology, which provides an inflow of water via several rivers (primarily the Helmand river) that drain nearby mountain ranges but have no outflow, permitted year-round access to water for much of the time but great susceptibility to intermittent periods of drought. Despite its reputation for aridity it was the site of an important Central Asian civilization that developed slightly later than those of Mesopotamia to the west and the Indus river valley to the east. It is reported that 900 Bronze Age sites have been located in the Basin. The largest city to be identified is Shahr-i Sokhta, a commercial center with a population as high as 20,000 with a central area covering 350 acres (over half a square mile) that flourished for much of the 3rd millennium, peak prosperity being *ca.* 2600-2400 BC. It developed from a small town of about twenty acres on the alluvial plain (delta) of the Helmand river, arising amidst a myriad of dispersed small settlements only a few acres in size that would surround the enlarging city and thus support its designation as a city-state. Because of its proximity to raw materials, including mines for various ores, and being geographically amenable to east-west commercial traffic, its increasing population in the mid-third millennium was supported agriculturally by efforts at irrigation based on the incoming and subsurface water of the Sistan Basin. Work with flint, textiles, lapis lazuli, turquoise, and chlorite, production of pottery from numerous kilns established in the central city and peripheral settlements, smelting of copper, and transport of ores provided the region with numerous distinct commercial ventures. Each unique trade would have had its own regional location within the city-state, defined supporting population, and system of production and distribution. It is not clear that kinships were a significant basis for social organization, and Dr. Philip Kohl has proposed that, because of the fluid social structure throughout Central Asia and the Middle East at that time, "it is likely that only the "elites" formed tightly integrated, politically uniform kinship groups."[41]

It is with some hesitancy that this civilization has been included among the "lesser civilizations" described in this chapter, the reason being the proximity of two of the five large "successful" civilizations (Mesopotamian and Indus River valleys). But Shahr-i Sokhta is the unexpected product of the intrinsic population of a region subject to geological uncertainty and yet grew to become a strategically located major center of commerce. The nature of the original settlement is unknown, but the region does not lend itself to agricultural prosperity. In contrast to the other primary civilizations described in this chapter, the origin of Sharh-i Sokhta is likely to have begun as a small trading settlement rather than a small market town. At the present time there is little evidence of hierarchical control of the population except for minor gravesite evidence that appeared in the waning years of the city. It can therefore be archeologically classified as egalitarian. Like the Indus River Valley civilization there is no evidence for a militaristic society (the early Uruk dynasties of Sumer had an army), its success being the consequence of commerce rather than conquest. Given the many distinct kinds of production and trade and the specific activities attached thereto being located in their specific sections of the city and surrounding settlements, it is reasonable to suggest that the management of the

---

[41] See: Kohl, P. L., *The Bronze Age Civilization of Central Asia: Recent Soviet Discoveries*, Armonk, NY, 1981, the Introduction by Dr. Kohl.

region was partitioned among the various parties involved in each commercial activity. As such it resembles a heterarchy, a group of networks each with its own area of social hegemony, that presumably worked together to further the best interests for local commercial networks. In some respects the functioning of Shahr-i Sokhta resembles Djenne-Djenno (see following section), although it is likely that the successes of the former were very much tied to the fortunes of Mesopotamian and, especially, Indus river valley civilizations. Thus, the fading of the Indus river valley civilization and the end of dynastic Sumer coincided with the rapid decline of Shahr-i Sokhta because the commercial basis for a cohesive polity was gone.

Archeological finds confirm its contact with distant civilizations, and over several centuries a close commercial association evolved with Mesopotamian city-states. Nevertheless, its cultural similarities with several other nearby smaller urbanized sites have been sufficient to propose the region to be peopled by the Helmand culture. Scholarly opinion holds that the intrinsic culture of this region was clearly distinct from that of the Indus river civilization and was also unrelated to Mesopotamian civilization, with the exception that evidence from a tablet considered to be written in Proto-Elamite suggests some features of Shahr-i Sokhta may have evolved within the cultural sphere of Susa, a city under the hegemony of Uruk approximately 400 miles further west. Despite this finding there is yet no evidence that writing was adopted or invented. The city was not a colony of a distant polity, its people were native to the region, and it grew in size because of commercial prosperity rather than conquest. There is, however, evidence of a variety of cultures from distant regions consistent with the presence of traders passing through the region, a feature reminiscent of Cahokia.

The population itself lived in modest dwellings, for the most part single rooms but sometimes with an internal courtyard. The relatively limited evidence of storage containers of grain and other food in the dwellings has been taken as evidence for a central authority having commandeered from the citizens essentials for sustenance and redistribution as required. This, however, is total conjecture, as central storage facilities have not been identified. Time and further excavation should provide more accurate information on daily life of the population.

Evidence of city planning became apparent only after the city had reached its most prosperous state. Thus, the occurrence of sections of the city involved in a specific commercial production spontaneously appeared, presumably in response to convenience for production. At the present time there has been no report of evidence of an elite population, from either the nature of the dwellings or the presence of an elite section of the city. It has been assumed that there must have been central control of the city-state of Shahr-i Sokhta, but in most archeological sites with known hierarchical power structure the focus of that power has been readily discernible, including the presence of monumental structures. It is not apparent here, and even the two larger buildings so far identified at the site may have merely been variations of local dwellings rather than centralizing features. One thing is clear: urbanization of Shahr-i Sokhta was a purely commercial invention, and its leadership came from traders and producers of goods. Evolution of the city, therefore, was one of convenience for commercial purposes. Without good evidence of central governance it must be considered a relatively pure form of heterarchy. This is consistent with the analysis of some Near and Middle East societies by Dr. Yuri Berezkin who noted that the development of surprisingly large centralized acephalous populations could occur, sometimes with evidence of private ownership and "the corresponding weakness, both of corporate ownership rights and of kin-based institutions in general ... ."[42]

A remarkable source of information that has only been partially exploited is its sixty-acre grave site. Located outside the city and protected in part by the tendency of the superficial layers of soil to form a thick crust of salts, hundreds of inhumations have been examined out of what has been estimated to be 19,000.[43] A variety of techniques of inhumation were employed, something to be expected in that burials in this location occurred over many centuries (2800-2100 BC), and a characteristic of many of them is the presence of some aspect of the interred's occupation, either tools or the products themselves. Up to the present time a section or a burial technique of the grave site that might suggest an elite class has not been reported. Dress did not differ significantly between male and female, and evidence of ownership (from seals) was found on both sexes. Except for one knife, no evidence of a militaristic population has been found, consistent with the absence of any surrounding fortifications. From osteological study it is estimated that little more than one in twenty of the population reached forty years or more of age, and antemortem tooth loss is considered very high. There has been no scholarly comment thus far on evidence for a medical profession, but two grave site findings raise the possibility. One was a much publicized orbital prosthesis found in the eye socket of a woman, surely a cosmetic device but one with surprising detail. The other, a recent finding, is a triangular trephination defect in the cranium of a 13-year-old girl with hydrocephalus that has clear evidence of healing, indicating significant post-surgical survival.[44] Whether a medical person performed the procedure is unknown.

It is intriguing that the extremely limited medical evidence available coexists with extremely limited evidence of a form of writing. Had the city continued to survive and prosper might it have become a "successful" civilization in which a group of medical practitioners could join to collate their findings for the assistance of future colleagues just as happened in Sumer? Alternatively, as there was commerce between Shahr-i Sokhta and Sumerian city-states with known medical practitioners, why would not the idea be copied? Perhaps there was little trade with Sumer, 600-800 miles further west than Susa. Likewise, writing was invented for commerce. Even though the writing found near the city has been attributed to Susa, located on the fringe of Mesopotamia, the origin of Proto-Elamite writing is unknown, although it is cuneiform in nature. Given the prominence of Shahr-i Sokhta in commerce it might be asked if it is possible that Proto-Elamite writing could have originated there. Shahr-i Sokhta is much closer to the Indus River valley (400 miles) than the Mesopotamian region (1,200 miles). As unlikely as that is (a great

[42] See: Berezkin, Y. E., *Apa Tanis and the Ancient Near East: An Alternative Model of Complex Society*, Uppsala Univ., Arkeolgi och antic historia<htt;://www.arkeologi.uu.

[43] See: Piperno, M., and Tosi, M., *The Graveyard of Shahr-i Sokhta Iran*, in *Archeology Magazine*, 28:186-197, 1975, and Piperno, M., and Salvatori, S., *Recent Results and New Perspectives from the Research at the Graveyard of Shahr-i Sokhta, Sistan, Iran*, in *Instituto Univ. Orient.*, 43:173-191, 1983. These and other scholarly publications by the coauthors are the basis for much of the information in this section.

[44] See: Moghadasi, A. N., *First Skull Surgery in Iran: The Burned City and a 4800-Year-Old Skull*, in *Iranian J. Publ. Health*, 43:249-251, 2014.

majority of the writings come from Susa), further excavations should clear up the matter as well as providing additional evidence relevant to the medical practice.

The rapid decline of the city in 2300 BC and abandonment in 2100 BC has been attributed to climate change with worsening droughts. But the more likely explanation is the unification of the region of Sumer under the Akkadians, a simultaneous dwindling of the Indus River Valley civilization, or increasing trade competition that included sea transport. The loss of valuable markets and its consequent diminishing role in regional trade probably led to emigration. Without a commercial base there was no longer any benefit to being a city dweller.

Summary Table for Shahr-i Sokhta:

AGE – Middle Bronze Age
POPULATION, LOCAL – perhaps as high as 20,000
POPULATION, TOTAL – n. a.
PRIMARY AREA – 350 acres (hegemony: based on one day's journey (10 mi.), *ca.* 300 sq. mi.)
URBAN DENSITY – 62 persons per acre
PRODUCTION – ceramics, textiles, turquois, copper, bronze, lapis lazuli, implements
GOVERNANCE – commercial heterarchy
EGALITARIAN ARCHEOLOGY - yes
PROMINENT KINSHIP - unlikely
WRITING – primitive ?
DISTANT TRADE – yes (central Asia, Mesopotamia, Indus River Valley, and the Near East)
SPECIALIZATION – yes
MONUMENTAL STRUCTURES - no
DENOUEMENT – abandoned 1900 BC, commercial failure
MEDICAL PRACTICE – possible
FORMATIVE PERIOD – 600 years (*ca.* 3100-2500 BC)
FLORUIT – 600 years (2500-1900 BC)
CITY-STATE – yes
AVERAGE LIFE EXPECTANCY – uncommon to exceed 40 years of age (4 out of 86

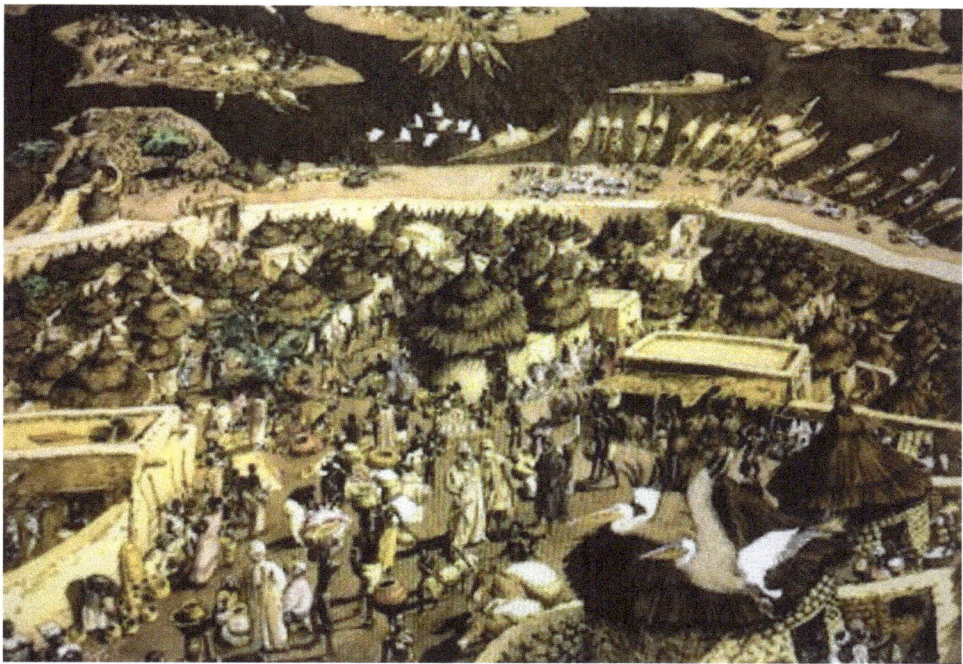

Fig. 25: Artist's rendering of bustling commercial activity centered in the ancient city of Djenne-Djenno, located in present-day southern Mali. With its central and peripheral population estimated at 50,000 and most inhabitants living on large riverine mounds that supported kinship groups, each engaged in its particular commercial venture, the absence of a controlling hierarchy was particularly notable. It flourished from 450-1050 AD. Photograph presently found on the *Making of Cities* website, makingofcities.org,

9. Djenne-Djenno

A more recently discovered alluvial settlement has been described in the Niger River Valley in the sub-Saharan section of the African country of Mali. Djenne-Djenno was settled by nomadic groups in the 3rd C BC as the previously swampland was drying. Over time the population retained herds of cattle, sheep, and goats and developed an agricultural base that was to include rice, the latter being a staple surplus that initiated the growth of the settlement. The settlement increased to cover about 25 acres, its dwellings constructed of mud bricks. Predictable flooding permitted rice production, and the population flourished both in self-sufficiency and in north-south trading from its agricultural base. Small satellite settlements developed nearby, perhaps by immigrants into the area, some becoming the locus of specialized production such as pottery. Habitation was primarily situated on mounds that were man-made and on which there is layer after layer of evidence of habitation over time. Ultimately the mounded settlements numbered about 40 within a 20-square mile area, and at its zenith the population of the Djenne-Djenno area may have reached 50,000. Although the social reasons for initiating this pattern of mound-based settlement are uncertain, periodic flooding probably necessitated a mechanism for escaping rising flood waters. What is certain is that on each of these mounds the inhabitants adopted or introduced specializations in pottery, masonry, and other crafts and skills, efforts assisted by ready transfer of product, goods, and services to and from the polities within reach of the growing riverine "urban" center.[45] The variety of products and adjoined ethnic groups made Djenne-Djenno an attractive trading center. One activity was iron smelting, and to do this iron ore had to be imported. As time passed, metallurgical processes were moved out to the peripheral clusters of dwellings, perhaps because necessary fuel was more accessible. Unusual imported items found in the settlement indicate that distant trade networks were already functioning and specializing at an early date, perhaps, as suggested from other archeological investigations in the region, even in the Late Neolithic. The resulting Djenne-Djenno iron manufactures and artistic productions are now highly prized. Whatever the mechanism underlying the Djenne-Djenno prosperity and duration (1,150 years, of which its most productive period extended over 600 years: 450-1050 AD), it appears to have been due to the concatenation of opportune resources, geography (river transport), manufactures, and sources of sustenance, especially a surplus production of rice.

Archeological evidence does not suggest a ruling hierarchy during either the early development or the maturation of the culture that developed, implying that supply and demand of goods and services were contracted at a local level or what has been termed "horizontal power relations" suggesting power was located in "overlapping agencies."[46] This is consistent with the concept of heterarchy, a system of shifting community influences based on commercial rather than political interests which it can either replace or ignore. The absence of "chiefly power" elites is consistent with the absence of temple or monumental structures that would have suggested authoritarian central management. The principal investigators of the archeological site report no evidence of Mediterranean influence before the arrival of Islamic peoples in the 12th C.

Like Catalhoyuk (see p. 563), Djenne-Djenno survived in the same location for over a thousand years without evidence of a central governance. Likewise, Djenne-Djenno is regarded by many as an egalitarian civilization, with early founding families having implied authority to guide the city's rituals and development but without much power. Frugal gravesites, no monumental structures, and absence of elite housing and regalia confirm that social organization was egalitarian kinship at the clan level. It has been stated that "the social function of any feature of a system is its relation to the structure and it continuance and stability, not its relation to the biological needs of individuals."[47] The longevity of the Djenne-Djenno system suggests it had a very successful system indeed. Given the population size, suburban settlements for specialists, river access for distant trade, and duration of the settlement, a medical profession should have developed there, but there is no evidence for it. Why is this so?

---

[45] LaViolette, A., *Ethno-Archaeology in Jenne, Mali*, Oxford, 2000.

[46] See: McIntosh, R. J., and McIntosh, S. K., *Early Urban Configurations on the Middle Niger*, in *The Social Construction of Ancient Cities*, Washington, D. C., 2010, Smith, M. L., ed., chapter 5. Most of the information related here about Djenne-Djenno is the result of extensive archeological investigations by the authors as described in that chapter. The theory of urbanization suggested by their investigations is given in a singular phrase: "heterarchy rather than hierarchy," a topic covered in detail in chapter 13 of the present work.

[47] See: Radcliffe-Brown, A. R., in the Introduction to *African Systems of Kinship and Marriage*, Abingdon, 2015, A. R. Radcliffe-Brown and D. Forde, editors, in the Introduction, p. 82, the 1st edition published in 1950.

Perhaps the reason no evidence of medical practice has been found is the persistence of egalitarian social organization attached to each residential/vocational mound. In kinships there are obligations and duties of each member. Medical practitioners emerge from the plebeian class rather than from the wealthier population, and the egalitarian nature of kinship groups may have restricted any tendency of its members to involve themselves in extra-kinship responsibilities. And if residential mounds and periodic flooding meant a degree of isolation of the attendant districts similar to that of the Marajoara civilization (p. 545), the enforced separation of segments of the population may also have made a network of medical practitioners less likely.

In any event, the population was settled, stable, and had agricultural abundance. There is empirical evidence of shamanism. The overall development of the city-state is consistent with many others: first a small herding, then agricultural, settlement among many that then grew in response to the need for a market town to manage storage and trade of surplus food, a process which, if the town is geographically conveniently located, attracts commercial ventures. The result in Djenne-Djenno was population growth and development of distant trade. Usually a central management would then emerge as a politically hierarchical form of governance superseded both the horizontal governance of commerce and the egalitarian governance of peripheral kinship communities. This, however, never occurred in Djenne-Djenno. The regional cultures of the middle Niger River suggest a similar pattern of urban expression elsewhere, and from this there is consideration given to a mysticoreligious concept that may have added a degree of cohesiveness among these seemingly disparate clusters of specialized autonomous settlements that had a certain homogeneity in pattern. In the absence of elite regalia, separate elite burials, monumental structures, and walled enclosure, group to group business interactions are thought to have been important in maintaining cooperative arrangements, and thus there is the inference that spirits and shamanism common to the area may have added support to that link. Such a theory remains unproven.

The inherent stability provided by this multifaceted support system, one that can be interpreted as a step toward urbanization, was, if foreseen by its early inhabitants, a brilliant production. Such prescience, however, may not have favored a longer life for its citizens. There is extremely limited information on this point from the archeological investigations of Djenne-Djenno, but of eleven adult burials adequate for assessment from the late phase of its existence, six were no more than twenty-five years of age and only one survived to age forty-five years.[48] The average of the maximum estimated ages for the eleven was thirty-one years. Few skeletal specimens have been found satisfactory for analysis, in part because cremation was common.

The timing of the decline of ancient Djenne-Djenno is consistent with the entry of the Islamic influence into the region and nearby urban development, to which the citizenry of Djenne-Djenno may have emigrated as environmental pressures developed and, as some propose for Sintashta and Arkaim, if the personal obligations of their traditional egalitarian kinships were found to be less burdensome in the new city.

---

[48] McIntosh, S. K., and McIntosh, R. J., *Prehistoric Investigations in the Region of Jenne, Mali*, Oxford, 1980, 2 volumes, p. 188 of volume 1.

Summary Table for Djenne-Djenno

PERIOD – Historical African
POPULATION, LOCAL – 50,000
POPULATION, TOTAL – 50,000
PRIMARY AREA – 100 acres (hegemony, 20 square miles)
URBAN DENSITY – 500 persons per acre
PRODUCTION – iron and iron products, rice
GOVERNANCE – vocational networking of mound-based egalitarian kinship communities for specialized production and trade (a commercial heterarchy)
PROMINENT KINSHIP - yes
WRITING – no
DISTANT TRADE – yes (trans-Saharan)
SPECIALIZATION – yes
MONUMENTAL STRUCTURES - no
DENOUEMENT – abandoned
MEDICAL PRACTICE – ?
FORMATIVE PERIOD – 750 years
FLORUIT – 600 years
CITY-STATE – no, as there is no evidence of central governance
LIFE EXPECTANCY – 31 years (derived from statistically insignificant data)

10. The Liangzhu Civilization

Emerging in the Yangtze River Delta and spanning 3400-2250 BC, a late Neolithic culture with a central city of considerable size and complexity has been termed Liangzhu. It was preceded by the Songze culture (3800-3300 BC) of which there is limited information other than that obtained from its pottery and gravesites, from which it has been concluded that authoritarian military dominance was in place in the region. The Liangzhu urban center with its suburban periphery covered almost two square miles, including a central walled area of about 100 acres and two other outer walls that would have been major construction efforts. The culture was Neolithic and agricultural, with rice production a major economic resource, although a silkworm-based industry was developing. The layout of both the urban and suburban areas is thought by some to have been planned in advance, as there is little evidence of earlier settlement in the area. The number of the peripheral settlements is presently set at 400.

The abrupt migration of settlers into an area adjacent to the lower Yangtze River brought with it an early jade industry. Ceramic pottery, slate sickles, stone adzes, varieties of whetstones, art work, and evidence that diamond was used to finish their tools complement the culture's famous work done with jade. So detailed was some of their engraving that it has been suggested that some form of magnifying lens was used. As Liangzhu's importance increased, there was increasingly specialized craftsmanship with workshops dedicated to different phases of production of finished jade products. Constructed near the Yangtze River, water was dammed and diverted for flood control and watercraft communication. Dockage and piers were built. Expansion of the population, upwards of 30,000 in the central Liangzhu site alone, and its new settlements was southward. At its peak the population of the entire civilization may have been in the "hundreds of thousands."[49] Lower classes had dwellings raised on pilings and connected by wooden walkways, whereas the upper classes resided on more substantially constructed mounds. Regional archeological investigation has identified approximately 150 small settlements adjacent to a network of rivers and streams surrounding Liangzhu and presumably subject to the central city. In contrast to the usual agricultural settlement pattern, the central Liangzhu site has been characterized more as a "city" than a redistribution point for agricultural products.[50] Waterways permitted efficient transport of goods and services to and from central distribution points. There is evidence of a local observatory for astronomical study.

It is thought that the Liangzhu had a well-established hierarchical governance, with an elite class easily identified from the wealth surrounding its inhumations. This was apparent during its earliest stage, for burial sites, rather than being large and similar as in most egalitarian societies, were now smaller and focused, with evidence that an elite class/families preferred interment of their own. The basis for disparity in wealth appears related to jade production in the period from 3000-2600 BC. The empowered class ultimately lived within the walled central area of the city, its construction dated to the late stage of development of the site. Some suggest that earlier there were a number of smaller chiefdoms, autonomous kinship groups evolving into commercial elite rather than a single centralized authority, for the noted variations in burial wealth are scattered around the region rather than concentrated in on location. Others think the clustered settlements around Liangzhu were not autonomous and were under direct control of a central ruling class.[51] Perhaps both views are correct, with peripheral "bosses" or foremen overseeing certain small settlements assigned by the central authority to provide a particular specialization in commercial production. Evidence of a stratified social arrangement has been identified for the Songze culture that preceded the Liangzhu, and a thousand years was time enough for a hereditary concentration of power to develop. Some authorities have made the generalization that cultures of the Central Plain region along the Yellow River, which would include the Longshan culture (see p. 518), were more "collectively oriented" and cultures from the Yangtze River Delta were more "ruler-centered."[52] There also was a slave population and mortuary evidence of human sacrifice in the latter.

This extraordinary civilization inherited its hierarchical governance from its preceding culture, but then developed technical and artistic vocations at an early era contemporary

---

[49] See: Major, J. S., and Cook, C. A., *Ancient China: A History*, Abingdon, 2017, especially chapter 33, The Neolithic Era and the Jade Age.

[50] See: Qin, L., *The Liangzhu Culture*, in *A Companion to Chinese Archaeology*, Oxford, 2013, A. Underhill, editor, chapter 28. Nevertheless, the sequence suggesting that Liangzhu as a manufacturing center emerged without evolving from a market town is so disengaged from the usual that it must be questioned. It is proposed instead that rice production with its surpluses coupled with the town's coastal geography may have resulted in a commercial market place and therefore to be a more likely location chosen for further commercial development, in part because market access and a labor force would already have been in existence.

[51] Much of this information comes from the preceding reference and: *The Formation of Chinese Civilization: An Archaeological Perspective*, Beijing, 2005, Sarah Allan, editor.

[52] Fang, H., Feinman, G. M., and Nicholas, L. M., *Imperial Expansion, Public Investment, and the Long Path of History: China's Initial Political Unification and Its Aftermath*, in *Proceedings of the National Academy of Science*, 112:9224-9229, 2015.

with Sumer in Mesopotamia. The culture was indigenous. Scholars have suggested hierarchical guidance was present from the city's earliest years in the planning and implementation of extensive dams, waterways, and monumental constructions. Given scholarly focus on the evidence for hierarchical control, it is difficult to fit into Liangzhu's development any role for commercial networks of a heterarchical nature for production or trade distinct from a ruling elite. The absence of writing appears to have had a limiting effect on its development when compared to early Mesopotamian and Nile River civilizations, although it must be acknowledged that it is unexpected that such a prosperous mercantile polity would have no form of permanent recording of commercial interactions. There has been the recent discovery in the Liangzhu area of etched artifacts that some think represent a primitive form of writing, but further study is under way. The size of its central population and many other features were shared by Miletos, but the area of influence was much greater. Given its duration as a city-state, it seems there should have been professional medical practitioners, although there is no evidence of this.

The metric similarities between Liangzhu and the Shandong Longshan city of Liangchengzhen are quite striking, and in the latter there also has been found no evidence of medical practitioners. The latter, however, is thought to have had little evidence of a social hierarchy in its earlier states, whereas Liangzhu exhibited from an early stage distinct class division. Liangchengzhen, approximately 700 miles north of Liangzhu, was chosen as the likely source of the medical classic, *Huang Ti Nei Ching Su Wen*, because it was a prominent city characteristic of the age and in the locale of the fabled Yellow Emperor, whereas the Liangzhu culture has no such cultural heritage. Disappearance of Liangzhu occurred abruptly around 2250 BC and is so far unexplained, but it was not destroyed by military violence, and indeed there has been no evidence so far suggesting the culture was militaristic in any way.

Summary Table for Liangzhu

PERIOD – Late Neolithic
POPULATION, LOCAL – 30,000
POPULATION, TOTAL – "hundreds of thousands"
PRIMARY AREA – 4 square miles (hegemony, 40,000 square miles)
URBAN DENSITY – 12 persons per acre
PRODUCTION – jade, rice, tools, ceramics
GOVERNANCE – political hierarchy, probably based on kinship
EGALITARIAN ARCHEOLOGY - no
PROMINENT KINSHIPS – elite kinships, settlement kinships
WRITING – no
DISTANT TRADE – yes
SPECIALIZATION – yes
MONUMENTAL STRUCTURES – large city walls
DENOUEMENT – unknown, but abrupt and nonviolent
MEDICAL PRACTICE – ?
FORMATIVE PERIOD – 500 years
FLORUIT – 750 years (3000 BC to 2250 BC)
CITY-STATE – yes (400 smaller settlements)
AVERAGE LIFE EXPECTANCY – n. a.

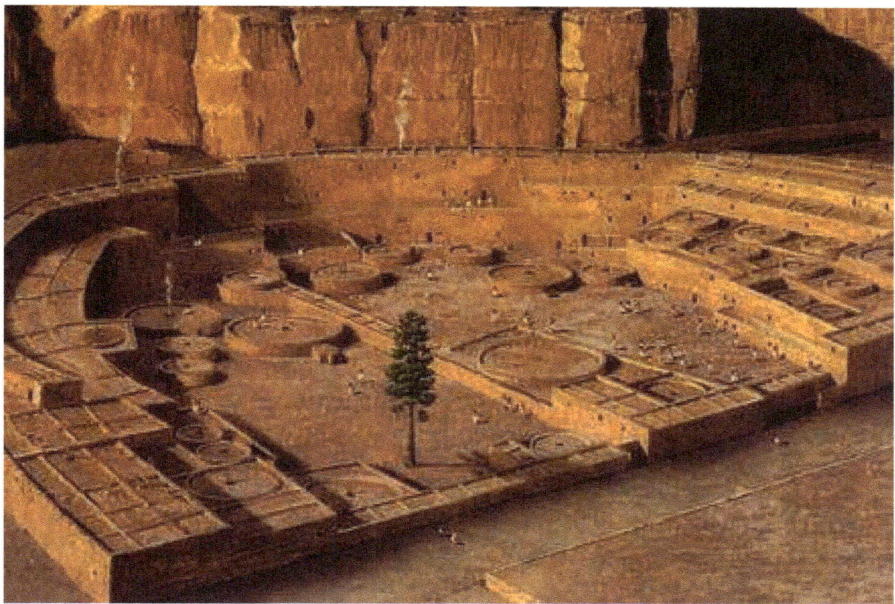

Fig. 26: Artistic depiction of Pueblo Bonito in Chaco Canyon as it may have appeared in the 12th AD. It was a "great house" constructed at enormous effort by the post-Archaic Woodland Anasazi civilization. As initiator of the Pueblo culture, this civilization was dispersed over perhaps 50,000 square miles in the Four Corners region of the American Southwest, but its dominant centralized population lived in the Chaco Canyon region, home to 5-10,000 people, although there were many smaller centers with "great houses." There was commercial interaction with Central America and the Mississippi cultures. Although matriarchal governance is suggested, the role of coercive leadership in Anasazi development is not yet defined. This photograph is a digital construction of NASA/Ideum and is in the public domain.

11. The Anasazi Civilization

Presently dated to the 1st C BC, the Anasazi civilization appeared when a hunter-gatherer society in the North American West added farming to its means of subsistence. Its culture would persist for 1400 years and its oscillations would provide archeologists with a superfluity of observations on the demography and lifestyle of an ingenious and determined people. The progress of Anasazi society over the centuries, therefore, has been well-studied, but this thumbnail sketch will concentrate on its periods designated Pueblo I (750-900 AD), Pueblo II (900-1150 AD), and Pueblo III (1150-1350 AD).

Corn and squash were introduced from Mexico and remained staples throughout Anasazi prehistory, corn being especially important as it was capable of long storage, a major determinant of its value in early cultures. Basket weaving, ceramic production, and a jewelry industry subsequently developed. But it was lifestyle and dwellings that have received most attention. Initially there were scattered small farming communities of up to 100-200 persons living in pit-houses, but over time clusters of farmsteads began to surround larger village centers with large pueblo structures built of local material, stone or mud, that were used for community activities, meetings, and ceremonies. This was the Pueblo I stage. Then smaller pueblo buildings were adjoined over time to form multiunit structures several stories high, usually surrounding a central plaza. "Great houses" were built in towns throughout the region (over 200 have been identified). It is estimated that "great houses" in Chaco Canyon, the center of Anasazi civilization, included in their construction some 200,000 logs hauled from fifty miles away. This is thought to have been completed by 900 AD (Pueblo I, early Pueblo II). The social organization for this effort and for the Anasazi Culture as a whole is unknown. For most of their existence the great houses were not residential dwellings for most of the people, who lived in small individual dwellings on the hillsides adjacent to the area containing the central plaza. Placement of the larger and well-organized communities is thought to have been guided by defensive considerations, as was the frequent use of ladders to enter the dwelling units. This suggests a serious threat of attack. The largest pueblo contained 800 rooms, many being used for food storage. Some of the settlements became quite large, and it has been estimated that the population of the Chaco Canyon site may have reached 30,000, and that the total number of homesteads scattered over the region reached 20,000.[53] Thus, there were dozens of large pueblos and a vast surrounding area containing hundreds of small settlements, and, although quantitation can be misleading, there were associated Anasazi settlements scattered over tens of thousands of square miles in what is now the "Four Corners" region of southwestern United States, the elevation generally 5-6,000 feet. These settlements participated in a network for trading, for traditional cultural events, and presumably for meetings of local councils.

It is thought that the Chaco Canyon site was the primary focus for the entire region. It is not known if organizational decisions from the Chaco Canyon site amounted to governance, but evidence of specialization in production in peripheral settlements has not been reported, suggesting their value to the civilization was primarily agricultural. A complex of roads, estimated at 400 miles, and the great effort involved in erecting the large pueblo buildings imply that some form of central authority coordinated such complex efforts. Archeological findings have included remains of colorful macaws that could only have come from tropical Mexico, thus adding to the data indicating distant trade with populations in Mexico, the Pacific Coast, and even the Mississippi region. Intricate jewelry was produced by the Anasazi, including much from turquoise, that would have been exported. Some Anasazi sites had well-developed dams and irrigation systems that supported agriculture in what would become an arid environment. Food surpluses were thereby produced and traded for ceramics and other items.

In all but its last stage most of the population lived in small individual dwellings set apart from the population centers in the larger settlements and Great Houses, and it appears that the latter over time grew to house an elite class. Life was difficult for the common man if the findings at a peripheral settlement located on Black Mesa is any indication. A study of a "household group" of a farming community dating from 1000-1150 AD (Pueblo II) has been presented. Over 200 skeletons have been recovered that span the period from 800 to 1150 AD. Of those that were able to be studied, 10% were infants and 50% were adults. "Life expectancy" was estimated at 25 years and was associated with slow childhood growth, shorter adults (by about 4 centimeters less than elites), childhood mortality triple that of the elites, evidence of heavy labor, a diet short on meat, and a

---

[53] Important Anasazi sites include Montezuma Valley (a broad valley that may have contained as many as 30,000 people), Cedar Mesa, Mesa Verde, and Canyon de Chelly, each area containing dozens of small villages.

prevalence of evidence of anemia set at 87%.[54]   In contrast, the population centers were prosperous and growing, and the concentration of power and wealth, the elaborate burials of a few of its inhabitants, and skeletal evidence of a less rigorous lifestyle within the relatively few large communities support the notion of hereditary leadership of great influence. This has recently gained support from the finding that, of a cluster of 14 burials in Chaco Canyon's largest pueblo spanning 800-1130 AD, the period of Chaco Canyon's dominance, remarkable generational similarities in DNA indicated not only hereditary passage of wealth over that entire period, *i.e.*, a dynasty, but one that was matrilineal and perhaps matriarchal.[55]   Just when this presumed shift from clan council to a hereditary nobility is uncertain, but it probably occurred at an early stage (Pueblo I).

The Anasazi developed no written language.   Although "religious" ritual has been considered a very important force in the culture, its role in moral guidance and deference to authority is unknown.   In some quarters there is presumption of, but no scholarly discussion of, shamanism, and the practice may have not existed at all.   There is no evidence of any form of medical practice.   By about 1200 AD, the Anasazi population, which had begun to evacuate its peripheral small settlements and move to population centers, was rapidly declining, probably by emigration southward, subsequently disappearing as a regional culture.   The reasons for the decline are debated but it followed on the most prosperous Anasazi period.   Climatic issues, overcultivation, and mismanagement by an elite class are mentioned as possibilities.

But there is an interesting cultural sequence attached to Anasazi civilization when viewed over the 1,400 years of its existence.   There is scholarly agreement that during the earlier centuries common customs and rituals held together regional tribes, and egalitarianism within the various kinships was the means of social control.   But once a sedentism evolved and surplus food and commercial trade could be sources of wealth it became possible for a subpopulation to prosper and to acquire power.   This may have occurred, and over about 200 years there developed a prominent elite class, with the lowest class being subject to poverty and arduous toil.   An alternative scenario is that over time the populations outgrew the capacity of local systems of agriculture and water sources in areas that were to become arid, the consequence being that an increasing number of farming families were in marginal areas, leading to poverty and malnutrition in peripheral farms and communities.   In either event, soon after reaching its zenith the Anasazi civilization deteriorated, its emigrants joining new groups or reestablishing tribal ties elsewhere such as those who are now called the "Pueblo people."   There also was a reversion to egalitarianism, one so rigid that in more recent centuries it has been documented that

---

[54] See: Martin, D., *et al.. Black Mesa Anasazi Health: Reconstructing Life from Patterns of Death and Disease*, Carbondale (IL), 1991, chapter 2.

[55] See: Kennett, D., *et al.*, *Archaeogenomic Evidence Reveals Prehistoric Matrilinear Dynasty*, in *Nature Communications*, Feb. 21, 2017. There was a parallel arrangement in Nepal in the not so distant past. Management of the nation at that time was in the hands of hereditary prime ministers from the Rana family. One of their largest palaces in Kathmandu had 1,700 rooms and 7 courtyards. From their palaces the Ranas controlled a region of 55,000 square miles, not too different in size from that of the Four Corners area over which the Anasazi exerted hegemony. It is tempting to suggest that the 650-room Pueblo Bonito that contained the 14 burials mentioned above was, in effect, the abode and the palatial center of a powerful family that ruled the widespread Anasazi nation. What is missing, of course, is evidence of a mechanism for physical coercion or cooperation from a dominant power.

"nonconformists were driven out."[56]   For present purpose note that (1) the period of greatest prosperity and influence occurred at a time authoritarian governance was in place, and (2) local events and the means of social control during the interval between the earlier egalitarian period and the development of an elite class have not yet been defined. Nevertheless, it has been proposed that the temporary experience of the Anasazi with inequality and prosperity made them eager to regain their egalitarian ways.   But let another scenario be proposed: after centuries of stable social organization based on egalitarian kinship, greater attention was paid to water resources, and dams, irrigation canals, and reservoirs permitted expansion of agriculture to the point that commercial benefit could be obtained by the Four Corners people.   This benefitted the population as a whole and had been undertaken by the population as a whole, and it was not done with an eye to becoming prosperous.   It was instead done to survive during the drought of 850-900 AD.   Great houses were begun, and their construction was of a defensive nature, again a matter of survival.   It is suggested, therefore, that it was during this difficult period that the ingenuity of the Anasazi not only managed to survive, but to thrive.   That success is what may have brought early tribal leadership together to consider regional organization under a ruling family.   Community successes may then have been commandeered by some means, and an authoritarian era imposed.   At this point one must take note of a series of papers by Dr. D. L. Martin who has described a very nonegalitarian pattern of violence and desecration of bodies in the American Southwest during this period, including some focus on the Chaco Canyon region.[57]   By filling in gaps in the osteoarcheological record and offering a variety of explanations for violent behavior it is clear that the Anasazi culture was permeated with this aberrant social conduct and its consequences throughout Pueblo I, II, and III periods.   This reinforces the conclusion of this section, that the preexisting egalitarian Anasazi culture was promptly transformed into an authoritarian hierarchical society.

In final analysis, the time available for development of a professional medical network for the Anasazi civilization was about 400 years, as the earlier years were hampered by climate vicissitudes and the necessity of constructing defensive housing.   Furthermore, the short life-expectancy of the non-elite would profoundly impair the founding of a medical profession, for the elite class would not have undertaken medical care as an occupation.   Medical care, in contrast to shamanism, was no source of power, but for the Anasazi there is little to no evidence of either.   But did the Anasazi socially evolve to the point where specialization and commercial prosperity would have provided the circumstances needed to foster a network of medical practitioners?   It certainly had commercial success in trading and agriculture, that success resulting, at least part of the time, in surplus produce.   But evidence in support of heterarchy or corporatism is not present, and the widespread role of violence as a solution to social problems makes it clear that a coercive hierarchical system of social organization was in play.   A medical network would have been inconceivable given the constant threats of violence, both internal and external.   Corporatism could explain why an elite matrilineal hierarchy could be noncoercive, for the plebeians could voluntarily enroll in projects that had communal benefit in mind.   But later the archeological evidence of frequent violence favors

[56] Stuart, D., E., *Anasazi America: Seventeen Centuries on the Road from Center Place*, Albuquerque, 2014, p. 208.
[57] See: Martin, D. L., *Hard Times in Dry Lands: Making Meaning of Violence in the Ancient Southwest*, in *J. Anthropol. Res.*, 72:1-23, 2016s.

development of a ruthless elite class or external threat as the culture became prosperous. Thus, the time between the initial egalitarian kinship (patriarchal?) governance and the subsequent central authoritarian governance was too disruptive and short to permit the development of noncommercial entities such as a medical practice. This could also explain why the general community, rather than coalescing in neighborhoods or hamlets based on kinship, tended to disperse in individual family units surrounding ritual centers. Their allegiance was no longer to their kinship but to the central elite leaders either for safety from marauders or for fear of disturbing their ruling class. It would also explain why the people so quickly reverted to egalitarian kinships as the culture disintegrated. They had found something even worse than egalitarianism.

Summary Table for the Anasazi

PERIOD – post-archaic Woodland
POPULATION, LOCAL – 5,000 (Chaco Canyon; highest estimate: 30,000)
POPULATION, TOTAL – 100,000 in small settlements were dispersed over a very wide area[58]
PRIMARY AREA – 30 square miles (hegemony, 50,000 square miles)
URBAN DENSITY – 270 persons per acre (at Pueblo Bonito)
PRODUCTION – turquoise, jewelry, pottery
GOVERNANCE – egalitarian kinships initially, later merging into hereditary coercive authoritarianism
EGALITARIAN ARCHEOLOGY – yes, initially
PROMINENT KINSHIPS – yes, early, with bands/tribes joining in common effort; later elite kinships control
WRITING – no
DISTANT TRADE – yes (Mexico, Pacific coast)
SPECIALIZATION – yes, but limited
MONUMENTAL STRUCTURES – yes
DENOUEMENT – abandonment
MEDICAL PRACTICE – ?
FORMATIVE PERIOD – 700 years
FLORUIT – 400 years (Pueblo II and III periods; 900-1300 AD)
CITY-STATE – yes, with roads to network with distant settlements
AVERAGE LIFE EXPECTANCY – 25 years for plebeians (limited data), but this included early childhood deaths.

---

[58] See: Lockard, C., *Societies, Networks, and Transitions*, Boston, 2008, vol. 1 (of 2), p. 346.

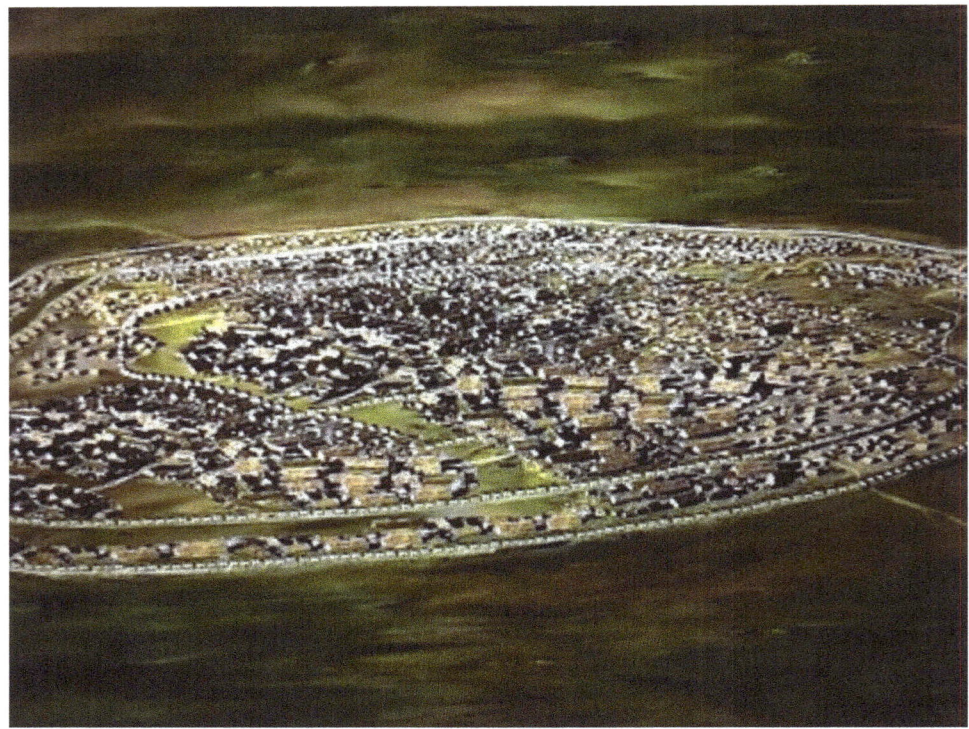

Fig. 27: The 4th millennium BC "proto-city" of Maidanets is schematized here, although its social dynamics are uncertain. Located in modern-day western Ukraine and northeastern Romania and with a possible population of 30,000 but with few peripheral communities and no evidence of organized commercial activity, the basis for the large population centers of the Cucuteni-Trypillia civilization remains to be determined. The hegemony of the Cucuteni-Trypillia civilization has been estimated at 140,000 square miles, almost the size of the State of California, but there is no evidence of any centralized governance. This photograph is made available via license of Creative Commons Attribution-Share Alike 4.0 International.

12. The Cucuteni-Trypillia civilization; Maidanets

In eastern Europe archeological findings over the last 30-40 years have raised many questions regarding traditional theories on the origin of European civilization. The earliest culture that supports this reassessment is the Cucuteni-Trypillia civilization (5000 – 3000 BC), and it grew and prospered in the region now occupied by Moldova, southern Ukraine, and northern Romania. Its settlements tended to be small, perhaps a dozen households, but local crops and domesticated animals, plus hunting, were sufficient to maintain a local population as large as 500. It is estimated that such settlements lasted no more than one hundred years before being abandoned or purposely burned. The same sites were in general not reinhabited for another two centuries. But ultimately the civilization spawned scores of large population centers. One of the largest was the settlement of Maidanets, and it will be used as an archetypal settlement of the Cucuteni-Trypillia civilization.

Differing dates are given for the duration of this civilization that borders the western Black Sea, and an approximation is 2,000 years. Large population centers were evolving by 4300 BC, and the flourishing period for this civilization can be considered to have lasted at least 1,000 years. There is general scholarly agreement that over this entire period the Cucuteni-Trypillia civilization was relatively stable. At least some of the large centers appear to have developed quickly and with a plan in mind for the layout for houses and corridors. Weapons were few and it can therefore be concluded that threats from surrounding cultures or intercity rivalry were also few, as least for much of its duration. The initially small population was engaged primarily in hunting, fishing, and limited agriculture, but over the centuries the population increased, as did settlements, the latter number estimated at 3,000 at its peak. Agriculture and domestication of animals supported more people, and soon the civilization contained many large towns and cities. Maidanets' population has been estimated as high as 30,000 in an area of one square mile. Like city-states elsewhere the large population centers, generally termed "megasites" rather than cities, developed some form of association with or hegemony over many small satellite settlements. The nature of that interaction is unclear, however, for there is no evidence of central urban management, no central stores, no delineation of property or monumental structures, no evidence of tribute and no obvious commercial enterprises that required interaction between the polis and the peripheral settlements. Although some work with copper occurred late in its course, Cucuteni-Trypillia civilization is considered Neolithic.

It is remarkable, given the size of the population centers, that there is little evidence of a hierarchical political system or of an elite class until the final stages of the civilization. Dwellings and the planned design of various communities were of a similar nature, although each of the cities had its unique features, and this pattern was unvarying for most of its span. Much has been made of (1) the apparently planned destruction by fire of many of the dwellings in a 70-80-year cycle, and (2) the vast number of figurines, the majority being female representations. But for present purposes the issue is not why the population did what it did, but why so many did it. For example, many dwellings were burned according to a particular pattern, but they were primarily from the central city rather than peripheral settlements. The unity in the social scheme over much of the Cucuteni-Trypillia region seems unlikely to have been a spontaneous response of citizens. Perhaps there was a relatively rigid adherence to some common social factor that required or coerced communal agreement and thus aided planning.[59] Alternatively, as subgroups of "megasite" dwellers were intermittent residents, perhaps newly admitted subgroups destroyed dwellings of prior inhabitants in the neighborhood they intended to occupy. Nevertheless, the overall opinion of scholars is that from beginning to end this was an egalitarian society, and this supports the idea of egalitarianism as a potent mechanism for population control. Unlike Catalhoyuk, where individual dwellings were physically contiguous, "megasites" such as Maidanets had their dwellings for the most part separated by sufficient space for each household to provide for its essential daily needs and chores without encumbering others. This finding, plus the large open areas and nearby but separate settlements have led to the classification of these cities as "low density urban

---

[59] See: Chapman, J., and Gaydarska, B., *Low-density Agrarian Cities: A Principle of the Past and the Present*, in *Trypillia Mega-Sites and European Prehistory: 4100-3400 BCE*, Abingdon, 2016, J. Muller, K. Rassmann, and M. Videiko, editors, chapter 17, pp. 289-300. The entire volume contain valuable updated information and perspective on this interesting civilization.

sites." and others include Cahokia, the Anasazi communities, some Longshan sites in China, and population centers in Amazonia, all being discussed in the present work. There is interest in present-day low density urban sites, but the significance of this settlement pattern in prehistoric times is uncertain. It does suggest the possibility that by maintaining family self-sufficiency, it had the effect of placing physical and economic limits on any effort that might be made to develop a central political authority. At the same time, the autonomy of small family units and their modest physical separation would have retained the egalitarian ethos of the underlying society, *i.e.,* a counterbalance to heterarchy, and would have limited any tendency to form specialized groups. This is consistent with the findings: there is virtually no evidence of specialized production of any kind. It is probable that this low-density urbanization with its autonomy of individual units was specifically sought by families as preferable to the relatively isolated small settlements during threatening times. How else can be explained the absence of dense urban housing usually brought about either by commercial ventures that preferred a close-knit labor force or by the necessity for a common defense.

This settlement pattern also is consistent with other findings: there was very little trade with distant sources, and even that occurred only late in the course of this civilization. It becomes difficult, therefore, to assign any particular form of governance to such large polities, for an egalitarian society that tends to redistribution is not consistent with autonomous family units that prefer to fend for themselves.[60] Nuclear families are not considered egalitarian, and, if there is a choice, as a unit a family would want what is best for itself, not for its neighbors. For this reason, the nuclear family rather than kinship will agree to accept corporatism: it realizes that it can be better off as part of a commercial group, *i.e.,* corporatism, than a kinship group. Indeed, the reference just cited states in its Abstract that "It is during periods when extended families operate more independently of band political structures that the opportunity for unequal access to resources and wealth emerges." But unequal access to wealth associated with commercial ventures in early urbanization is inconsistent with the Cucuteni-Trypillia civilization for neither the central polity nor the peripheral settlements show significant variations in wealth to distribute or acquire. The egalitarian inhumations of this civilization probably also reflect absence of wealth throughout its population, for a community that has no commercial activity of significance has little individual wealth. New discoveries suggest two relevant factors affecting the size and social makeup of the "cities." One is that large numbers of dwellings were burned at times, thus meaning that the overall population at any one time was significantly less than proposed earlier. The second is evidence of housing clusters

---

[60] In prehistoric Canada the rise and decline of Native American settlements has been attributed to the movement of family units into dense villages and back into autonomous domiciles in response to perceived threats to survival of the small units from climate change or other external pressures. When things were stable the autonomous unit was preferred, apparently because the egalitarian ethos that pervaded the dense settlements was in itself viewed as a threat. There was a reversible exchange of autonomy with security. See: Harris, L., (2013) *Heterarchy, Egalitarianism, and the Archaelology of Complex Hunter-Gatherers: Reinterpretation of Social and Political Dynamics in the Aggregated Villages of the Mid-Fraser Region, Bristish Columbia (2000-800 B. P.),* a paper read at the 78th annual meeting of the Society for American Archaeology.

that suggest neighborhoods, and the size of each neighborhood might be consistent with the requirements of a kinship group.[61]

The extensive and long-lived Cucuteni-Trypillia civilization is in some ways similar to the long-lived Catalhoyuk civilization in that a thousand years passed with little social change. It likewise developed neither a significant commercial agricultural base nor commercial trade. Being profoundly egalitarian as judged by archeological evidence, this may merely have reflected the absence of a means to acquire wealth. By extending its borders primarily westward it accommodated an increasing population without conquest. And yet it was profoundly different from Catalhoyuk in that the individual families retained great autonomy, a most inegalitarian characteristic and in marked contrast with the strict and dense domiciliary pattern of Catalhoyuk. Perhaps the population was quite satisfied with its circumstances and had little motivation to change, the little change that occurred being associated with knowledge acquired from neighboring cultures. After all, its agriculture, herds, and natural resources for hunting sufficed for its population as long as it could match an increasing population with an enlarging geographical footprint. But it did not develop any features essential for progress to the point that the members of the culture had a significantly improved life. Indeed, one wonders what the attraction was that initially led them to this clustering of family units in the large settlements in the absence of commercial development, for this civilization seems to have been devoid of both a commercial heterarchy and an elite hierarchy. What did they have to gain? One possibility is mobility. Extended families and larger kinships could move in and out of the large population centers in response to changing conditions, perhaps environmental or hostile threat. The possibility of corporatism seems unlikely as a form of governance as there was no elite group to combine "corporate" ideas with action and no large-scale commercial projects to benefit from a corporatism approach. In the absence of a source of prosperity through surplus, storage, and trade, the expected role for specialized services did not exist. *Ipso facto*, it would be unexpected for a medical practitioner network to have emerged despite such extended stability. Whatever the final determination may be, the static existence of this civilization over two millennia would be more startling but for the well-studied Egyptian civilization that also saw two millennia pass without progress. If one puts aside monumental structures and craftmanship, the Cucuteni-Trypillia civilization, just like ancient Egypt, got bigger but not better, even though one was an authoritarian hierarchy and the other was subdivided among egalitarian kinships. The affiliation of kinship units, rather than weakening within a larger urban venture as is usually the case, remained strong and its people "... still lost in kinship ties... ."[62]

The neighborhood arrangements in the Cucuteni-Trypillia civilization megasites, if proven, bear some resemblance to mound dwellers of Marajoara, Poverty Point, Terramare, and Djenne-Djenno except that the Cucuteni-Trypillia populations had no environmental features that would segregate kinship units; it was done by choice.[63]

---

[61] For a discussion of recent thinking on "ground up" neighborhoods in this region see: Chapman, J., *The Standard Model, the Maximalists and the Minimalists: New Interpretations of Trypillia Mega-Sites*, in *J. of World Prehistory*, 30:221-237, 2017.

[62] See: Chapman, J, and Gaydarska, B., in chapter 17 (pp. 289-300), in *Trypillia Mega-Sites and European Prehistory: 4100-3400 BC*, Abingdon, 2016.

[63] See: Chapman, J., et al., *The Second Phase of the Trypillia Mega-site Methodological Revolution: A New Research Agenda*, in *Eur. J. Archaeology*, 17:369-406, 2014.

The life expectancy of the populations of the Cucuteni-Trypillia region is unknown, for no cemeteries and virtually no inhumations have yet been discovered. Presumably it was similar to most other prehistoric populations, 30 – 40 years. As Cucuteni-Trypillia populations span the shift from a hunter-gatherer society to sedentism between 5000 BC and 3000 BC, report of a 6000 BC population declared to be the first farmers in Europe had an estimated average age at death of 31 years for men and 29.9 years for women.[64]

Summary Table for Cucuteni-Trypillia civilization, Maidanets

SOCIETAL STAGE - Neolithic
POPULATION, LOCAL – 30,000 (recent estimates less than 10,000)
POPULATION, TOTAL – ?
PRIMARY AREA – 660 acres (hegemony: 400 square miles, but the entire civilization extended over more than 100,000 square miles)
URBAN DENSITY – 31 persons per acre
PRODUCTION – subsistence until late period
GOVERNANCE – a large cluster of neighborhoods, each an egalitarian kinship
EGALITARIAN ARCHEOLOGY - yes
PROMINENT KINSHIPS – yes, the basis for neighborhoods in the megasites
WRITING – no (although there is the controversial regional Vinca script)
DISTANT TRADE – late period, and then with neighboring cultures.
SPECIALIZATION – only in late period
MONUMENTAL STRUCTURES – no, but some large buildings are compatible with the function of community center
DENOUEMENT – ?
MEDICAL PRACTICE – no evidence
FORMATIVE PERIOD – 900 years
FLORUIT – 1000 years (4300-3300 BC, although perhaps "expanding" is a better term than "flourishing" for there was little commercial activity)
CITY-STATE – no; voluntary agglomeration of kinships
AVERAGE LIFE EXPECTANCY – n.a.

C. Overview of the Twelve Primary Lesser Civilizations

Relevant to the definition of "city-state" on p. 13, two of the lesser civilizations (Catalhoyuk and Sintashta) had no peripheral settlements, two (Norte Chico and Poverty Point) had central polities primarily for ceremonial use, one (Cucuteni-Trypillia) had no significant commerce, and one (Terramare) developed peripheral settlements as a late phenomenon, leaving only six of the twelve lesser civilizations with a semblance of an autonomous city-state. Furthermore, the civilizations evolved in quite different eras:

---

[64] These data are from a 6000 BC early Neolithic settlement in northern Greece, Nea Nikomedeia, perhaps 500-600 miles south of Moldova. See: *European History: A Survey*, Buffalo, 2002, S. Milisauskas, editor, pp. 184-185. A more general source for comparison is: Boldsen, J. L., and Paine, R. R., *The Evolution of Human Longevity from the Mesolithic to the Middle Ages: An Analysis Based prion Skeletal Data*,

three were Neolithic, two were Bronze Age, one each was pre-ceramic, Late Woodland, and Late Archaic (all American), and three (Marajoara, Anasazi and Djenne-Djenno) merged into the modern era. Other characteristics include the following:

a.   Production and specialization for vendable benefit:

All the lesser primary civilizations achieved self-sufficiency and were able to produce surplus food or provide commercial products, but the degree of success varied. Catalhoyuk and Cucuteni-Trypillia had very little, and Marajoara, a large island at the mouth of the Amazon River, had, by virtue of geography, limited resources and limited access to distant cultures. Poverty Point, near the Mississippi River, had distant trade in stonecraft, but trade was not transported by river, for its location was near the mouth of the Mississippi river as it forms a delta that carries into the Gulf of Mexico. The variety and luxuriousness of its product was thereby limited.   Nevertheless, as these four civilizations had archeological evidence of distant trade, they will be assessed as marginally specialized in that they had something to trade in return.

b.   Political status and governance:

Most of the twelve seemed bereft of a central hierarchical political structure, or at least their sustenance and artifacts do not suggest such a thing. Of those with an elite hierarchy, only Liangzhou was clearly and rigidly so, the Anasazi evolving later an authoritarian elite.   Shahr-i Sokhta was purely heterarchical but with commercial neighborhoods presumably kinship-based. Sintashta suggests an organization of kinships consistent with corporatism, and Catalhoyuk is now considered a collection of neighborhoods despite its dense population. The latter three plus the remaining seven centralized populations can be viewed as confederations of kinships. Even Terramare, where there probably were kinship neighborhoods, might represent a coordinated effort of a kinship confederation, although the idea of a formal alliance of kinships developing within each settlement area would seem unlikely. The role of confederations of kinships as the mechanism whereby egalitarianism is maintained and enforced is part of the big story of this book.

c.   Archeological egalitarianism:

Egalitarianism as defined by archeological finds was present in seven of the twelve lesser civilizations.   None, with the unlikely exception of Sintashta civilization, provide evidence of aggressiveness as a mechanism for prosperity, although Liangzhou had defensive structures and violent aggression characterized the late Anasazi civilization, although its source is uncertain.

d.   Duration and denouement:

The duration of each lesser civilization is given in two parts: the time for a prospering civilization to appear and the time that it flourished. This was done because it would have been during the centuries the civilizations flourished, rather than during their formative years or their decline, that progress would have been manifested in a network of medical practitioners. The shortest duration of the flourishing period (Floruit), 300 years, occurred with the Terramare civilization, the three longest in Catalhoyuk (1,200 years) and Cucuteni-Trypillia and Poverty Point (1,000 years each). The causes of their terminations are often speculative, with climate change frequently being a possible mechanism. As best can be determined, none were overtaken by conquest. Flooding is quite likely for Cahokia. But it can be concluded that conscious decision was behind the vacating of all twelve sites, as there is no evidence of terminal conflict.

e.   Contact with other cultures:

All twelve had some evidence of trade relationships extending beyond local, some for obtaining raw materials, others being markets for finished products or crops. This was very limited in some, *e.g.* Catalhoyuk and Cucuteni-Trypillia, but for the present all are considered to have had contact with outside cultures and thereby some idea that heterogeneity of lifestyle existed among foreign populations.

    f.   Quality of life:

An indirect measure of this variable is life expectancy, inasmuch as it might reflect community health. For purposes of this book, the interest in life expectancy resides primarily in the number of older persons in the community at any given time. Generational wisdom becomes a more significant contribution to community living and planning than it is in nomadic societies because the older, and therefore more likely infirm, population can be assigned sedentary tasks, thereby contributing to society rather than being a burden to a mobile band. Some idea of the rigor of existence can be gained in those few instances where life expectancy data are available. If life expectancy calculations include infant and childhood mortality, the resulting figure would more accurately reflect community health, but calculating life expectancy of those who survived to the age of 15-20 years gives a better idea of the number of older individuals in a community population and thereby its susceptibility to progress. Although the data vary in quality, the average age at death was consistently in the low thirties (Terramare being a modest exception). The variable of greatest interest for present purposes is age at death, a value that can be only modestly estimated in adults from skeletal remains.

CHAPTER THIRTY-FOUR

THEORETICAL CONSIDERATIONS FOR SOCIETAL PROGRESS
AS DERIVED FROM THE FIVE SUCCESSFUL PRIMARY
CIVILIZATIONS (CHAPTERS 27-31); A COMPARISON WITH
TWELVE UNSUCCESSFUL CIVILIZATIONS

Early decisions about the preferred lifestyle of small kinships, especially hunter-gatherer bands, were based on rational considerations and personal preferences rather than a preset propensity to settle in villages as soon as the warmer climate of the Late Neolithic made it possible. Those decisions ultimately were the determinant for or against urbanization. If "against," it could result in 50,000 years of nomadism as occurred with Australian aborigines. If "for," subsequent commercial enterprise and discovery could lead to market towns and then to urbanization, from which subsequent generations might people a vast civilization. Some variables derived from the analysis of the five "successful" primary civilizations in which early forms of scientific medical practice appeared are reviewed for their relevance in evolving a civilization capable of progress.

A. Rejection *vs.* Selection

Summaries of twelve lesser civilizations having been reviewed, a most unexpected observation is that in none of the twelve is there evidence of medical practitioners. Yet many of their metrics resembled to a modest degree those of the autonomous Greek city-state, Miletos, and the four primary civilizations with historical evidence of a true medical profession appearing in their early stages of cultural and commercial development. As it has been proposed at the outset of this work that (1) progress in medicine could have occurred fairly quickly because the intelligence of ancient humans was equivalent to ours and could have supported scientific complexity, (2) morbidity and mortality in daily life would have been a perennial motivating force in all ages to avoid or assuage illness or injury, and (3) many important clinical observations are cheap, quick, obvious, and require no technology, why did the capacity for early progress fail to produce any evidence of a medical practice? The absence of medical practitioners as a unanimous finding in the twelve lesser primary civilizations is so striking it suggests that some explanation has been overlooked or that our reasoning has been faulty or based on false assumptions. It is especially remarkable given the stability and durability of some of the civilizations. How are nuanced developments in thousand-year-old ancient societies to be judged when such gross anomalies defy understanding?

The most obvious explanation is that the cause of this apparent aberrancy will someday be uncovered by further archeological exploration. But could a clue be found in study of the indigenous population of Australia?

Excursus on Australian Aborigines

The extraordinary history and prehistory of Australian aborigines has received much scholarly attention for many years, especially the complexity of its kinship associations.

But a striking observation has been the absence of permanent settlements that might be called a village at any time during the 50,000 years of aboriginal habitation of the Australian continent.[1] At first glance, this suggests there was no motivation to form permanent settlements, indicating an existence relatively free from deprivation and danger, or that the alternative, agricultural settlement, was too difficult, dangerous, or repulsive. Indeed, the present opinion is that much of the Australian landmass has been poorly amenable to agricultural development, in part because of its aridity. There are acceptable regions, however, in the east and west, such as the Liverpool Plains region in the southeastern state of New South Wales, an alluvial plain that is an important agricultural region today. Here can be found very early aboriginal "occupation sites," art, and petroglyphs, but no aboriginal settlements have been identified. While aridity has been an important feature of large parts of Australia in recent millennia, it was not always so. When the first aboriginal population arrived, the region is thought to have been lush. Archaic settlements usually have been in the proximity of rivers, and there are many river systems in Australia, in addition to which the option for establishing fishing communities along the extensive ocean coastline would have been as available in Australia as in any other part of the world.

In one of the more curious intellectual exchanges of today, the subject of intelligence, as measured by testing, is sometimes invoked to explain differences in the development of entire cultures. The Australian aborigines have received attention in this regard, and it is postulated that below a certain point on a standard intelligence quotient scale, a point not reached by the aborigines, the ability to recognize methods of adaptation becomes inefficient, thereby explaining their lack of communities; it simply did not occur to them to change. There is an interaction between intelligence and motivation, however, and if limitations on motivation exist there may be repercussions in assessing intelligence.

Earlier it was pointed out that motivation to change is required for progress, and, if there is insufficient motivation to change, a society can remain frozen in time, and this appears to have happened with the aboriginal people of Australia. As an alternative explanation, however, there may have been motivation to *not* change. It was noted by a French explorer of the upper Mississippi region that among indigenous people of North America a nomadic existence often was the preferred existence; settling down in one place and growing crops was demeaned. What could be better than moving about as one pleases? There may have been other factors, of course, such as those related to sanitation, that made it preferable to move from place to place rather than to devise waste disposal systems that to them may have seemed repellant.[2] Or perhaps some early attempts at settlement living had been met with epidemic disease of either human or animal origin, the fear of which made permanent settlements not an option. Staying in one place for an extended period, therefore, may to them have seemed primitive, dangerous or evidence of disability. But one thing certain is that resistance to change need not be blamed on

---

[1] The one or two exceptions are on the seacoast and may have been the production of stranded seafarers from some unknown region.

[2] There is the anecdote by John Hersey in his book, *A Single Pebble*, when, during a period when he was employed as a worker on a boat that carried freight on the Yangtze River, he pulled a thin square of white cloth from his hip pocket, blew his nose, and replaced the cloth in his pocket, a procedure that drew rude comments and displays of disgust from his Chinese co-workers who preferred to vigorously expel nasal mucus on the ground and be rid of it.

insufficient collective intellect of a society. The primitive society's communal intellect had knowledge of factors of which we are unaware that militated against sedentism and an agricultural subsistence, and, if recent evidence of limited agriculture and domestication by Australian aborigines is confirmed, this would indicate the concept of sedentism was not unknown. Absent nutritional deficiencies, regional genetic maladaptations, and considering environmental and social priorities and threats, the primitive society's intellect merely was otherwise occupied.

Nomadism has been the norm for most of mankind's time on earth, and sedentism may in some ways be an aberrancy. Nomadic societies are notably egalitarian, although this has not prevented devastating behavior toward one another. It is a popular notion that aboriginal Australians were nonviolent relative to other societies, but this is not supported by evidence in skeletal remains indicating organized conflict and physical trauma, particularly head trauma among women. Some restraint on individualism is an unavoidable necessity in any form of communal living. And it has been proposed that this restraint on individualism has permitted social progress to occur, the destructiveness of the individual being prevented at the level of the average member of a society. Disruptive behavior would be evident to all and promptly controlled. Were this the case, however, egalitarian nomadic groups effective in suppressing individualism should have been the first with evidence of progress, including some form of progressive medical care. Instead, as with the Australian aborigines, they have been the last.

There was a global move toward human settlement with the end of the Late Glacial Period (10,000 BC). Prior to that human settlements were more like encampments. Australia was affected as well by that climatic phenomenon, although the climate of the Late Glacial Period was not as severe as occurred in the Northern Hemisphere. Elsewhere a settled existence and a turn toward an agricultural subsistence sometimes evolved. But this change was not forced upon early populations, and it took thousands of years before the Neolithic Revolution and its turn to agricultural settlements gingerly began, so gradual in fact that it can be considered reticent. Glaciation at its peak covered only a small proportion of the global land mass, and although accompanied with extensive drying and desert formation, habitable regions would have been abundant for the tiny global human population of that era. There is also evidence that a human population increase began long before the regression of the glaciers. Finally, the Holocene glacial retreat began 19,000 years ago, but the first permanent human settlements date from about 11,000 years ago. And another five or six thousand years had to pass before the Neolithic "revolution," the switch from hunter-gatherer to agriculture, took place and the Bronze Age population proliferation occurred. And even when sedentism was adopted, large areas such as northern Europe and the British Isles were populated not by villages and towns but by individual or tiny clusters of houses. In other words, if environmental and social dangers were not great, village and town life or other dense population centers were not sought.

Post-glacial climate change apparently was not viewed by Australian aborigines as a reason for altering their traditional lifestyle. Perhaps the reason was not that they rejected sedentism in favor of nomadism, even though that option was always present. Nor was the reason the demeaning "it just did not occur to them to change." Perhaps the reason lay in the coercive power of egalitarian kinship in restraining any inclination to change. Kinship was of overwhelming importance. It defined land boundaries, ceremonies, traditions, membership and place in society, and even individual representations of the popularly known "Dreamtime," the cosmic worldview shared by the many clans. To be part of and to uphold one's part in that worldview required obeying its tenets and and its enforcer, the kinship. Thus, both ethnical and ethical identity of the individual served to bind him or her to the clan rather than merely marking his or her place in it. In leaving the kinship one left more than a community support structure.

The nature of the Australian aboriginal egalitarian kinship-based society and its oral tradition has been well-studied, and despite a suggestion of limited farming it is considered a hunter-gatherer culture divided into small bands and clans. But clan interactions and strict regulation of membership, marriage, ritual and age/gender-defined responsibilities and duties made for a rigid social system. Although considered egalitarian in that leadership was neither hereditary nor politically determined and family units shared sustenance, with no social classes the authority for enforcement of egalitarian intolerance was engrained into the band or clan structure by a kinship that provided the mechanism for its enforcement.

Attributing such a display of the power of the kinship in prehistory is not to be viewed as unusual. When some brave souls in other global locations did decide to leave their nomadic egalitarian cage, it was not because of attractions elsewhere. It is proposed here that this was done to escape an unsatisfactory social environment at home, an escape from egalitarianism and a theme to be repeated in this book. They were not going to; they were leaving from. From wherever humans first appeared on earth, they did not, like bacteria, form an ever-enlarging colony; they instead dispersed at every opportunity, ultimately to every corner of the globe. But for the Australian aborigines, once arrived, sea level changes allowed them to disperse no further. Perhaps external dangers or an arid climate kept them from dispersing in family units; maybe safety resided in bands. This may have increased the hold of kinship on restricting personal choice: to remove oneself from the security of a band may have been considered a dangerous choice, danger coming from either the environment or marauding bands. There was no place to which they could escape. Without commerce no urbanization could occur to which they could apply.

Of pain and debility, mankind's perpetual motivation for self-improvement, nothing appears to have been developed in Australian aboriginal society that suggests the presence of medical practitioners. Even shamanism is barely in evidence except in its modern reincarnations. Local empirical treatments, including some herbs and mud casts for fractures, in most instances would probably have been provided by a knowledgeable family member or friend. The local person who pulled teeth or set bones was probably viewed merely as a useful technician, not one who heals with knowledge. But based on present knowledge, that medicine as a specialized skill "just did not occur to them" cannot be used as a criticism, for it also did not occur to any other nomadic population or to any of the twelve lesser civilizations described in the preceding chapter. Medicine as a specialization would not appear until urbanization was under way, a major point being made in this book. Had Australia and its aboriginal population remained undiscovered, another 50,000 years would likely have passed without a change in its nomadism and without improvements in medical care, health or life expectancy.

A nearby example that duplicates much of the foregoing occurred in Tasmania. When the land bridge between the Australian continent and Tasmania was lost because of the rise in sea level of the post-glacial era, the aboriginal population of the island was isolated from other human contact for 10,000 years until visited by European settlers.[3] This population has been considered the least technically advanced of all prehistoric societies, one investigator concluding that there were only thirteen tools (*e.g.*, spherical pebbles for throwing, digging sticks, throwing sticks, wooden spears) used in procuring food that would separate their culture from chimpanzees, a separation considered "narrow." Whether prehistoric Tasmanians could even start a fire remains a debatable point.[4] With no social classes, the only organizational structure of the nomadic hunter-gatherer Tasmanian society was the clan, usually numbering from 20-50 persons, although territorial delimitation was assigned to a group of clans that were assumed to belong to a larger common kinship. The difficult life of ancient Tasmanians has been reviewed by the eminent anthropologist, Dr. Robert Edgerton.[5] It is awkward to assign the term "egalitarian" to a society such as the aboriginal Tasmanians, for evidence indicates a gross inequality among the population, especially the harsh existence of women and the frequent violent raids for women and for food, despite an environment that, unlike the Australian continent, is considered to have had abundance. But egalitarian kinships are rarely egalitarian in the sense of being a group in which all members are treated as equals. It is understood that age- and gender-based inequalities are inevitably present in egalitarian groups, elders being favored and women subject in varying degree to domestic abuse and violence, and that violence in general is commonplace.[6] Clans are egalitarian in that, to serve the greater good, there is a redistribution of labor, redistribution of essentials, and no social class. But with no mechanism to restrain bullies or those vying for influence, personal differences can be more readily resolved by force than by reason. Although anything produced or captured is supposedly for the welfare of the group, perhaps Tasmanian men ate more nutritious food and labored less than the women because the men felt they had to be fit and ready to defend the clan. Such details are unknown. But in an environment that might have been a little Garden of Eden for a socially acculturated population, the rules of the clan turned Tasmania into a Hell, especially for the women.[7] For 10,000 years there was not a single sign of betterment for society, and it is even thought that the ancient Tasmanians lost some of the more advanced

---

[3] An important source of information in this section is: Roth, H. L., *The Aborigines of Tasmania*, Hobart, a *ca.* 1970 reprint of the second (1899) edition.

[4] For a recent review of this topic as it relates to the capacity to improve lifestyle see: Haidle, M. N., *Lessons from Tasmania – Cultural Performance Versus Cultural Capacity*, in *The Nature of Culture: Based on an Interdisciplinary Symposium "The Nature of Culture,"* Tubingen, 2016, Haidle, M. N., Conard, N. J., and Bolus, M., editors, pp. 7-17.

[5] See: Edgerton, R., *Sick Societies*, New York, 1992. Dr. Edgerton considered the poor and often brutish conditions of primitive society a generic manifestation of maladaption to circumstances, but the cause of maladaption was not identified. To attempt that identification one must first distinguish among the defects of egalitarianism: the absence of hierarchical controls that restrain violence, the destructive effect of redistribution on motivation, and the presence of nonviolent coercion that restrains individualism. Dr. Edgerton was focused more on the first. More on this matter is found in the next chapter of this volume.

[6] Some perspectives on egalitarianism in this section are discussed in *Oxford Studies in Political Philosophy*, Oxford, 2017, volume 3, David Sobel *et al.*, editors.

[7] Even reports of 18th C French explorers, while describing an intrinsic courtesy and interest by Tasmanians in their interaction with the explorers, mention the difficult tasks assigned to women while the men were not so tasked. And pertinent to life expectancy, when they met a group of about 60 Tasmanians, an estimate of individual age ranged from infants to roughly thirty-year-olds, but for one fifty-year-old man.

practices they brought with them from their continental Australian forebears. They had, in fact, regressed.

And that brings up the point of this excursus and a point highlighted in this volume regarding all early and primitive societies: egalitarian kinship as a potent force resistant to change. The problem is not the degree of violence inflicted by some members on others, for there was little choice but to work within the existing system. The problem is not the nastiness of life in an egalitarian prison. If a man or a male-directed subgroup decided to leave the security of the band it would either not survive, merely join another band, or become a band unto itself. The greatest problem for the egalitarian band is egalitarianism itself, not its susceptibility to turmoil. Although turmoil and a short life expectancy bedevil the egalitarian society, the most profound inhibition to progress was the necessity for every member to work for the common good, under coercion when necessary. Working to improve one's personal lot in life or to make oneself less miserable than others in the kinship was not possible. Without hope of improvement and with escape from the clan an unacceptable alternative, it is a wonder that this situation did not persist forever. One might even view the Australian and Tasmanian aboriginal experiences as evidence that it could. The isolation of Australis has provided a test case whereby we can see the importance of social construction on the brilliant species of *Homo sapiens*, that species capable, on the one hand, of remaining unswervingly attached, without change, to its nomadic bands and clans for many of years, come what may, and on the other hand, separating from the bands and clans and sending man to the moon, splitting the atom, and devising instantaneous communication around the entire planet, all this being accomplished within three centuries. Now please see Figure 28.

This excursus is not meant to explain why Australian aborigines remained nomadic. It is, instead, to explain that they had a choice, although that choice was unacceptable. But it underscores the astonishing potential of *Homo sapiens* and the consequences of departure from the band on the capacity to think and act as an individual or personal interest. To do this those egalitarian bonds need first to be broken.

End of excursus

It is suggested that the absence of evidence of early medical organization in the twelve lesser primary civilizations, if subsequent study confirms that to be true, was, as is the case of the culture of nomadic egalitarian groups, the consequence of choice, the choice being to remain within the security of the kinship or to risk destruction outside it. It was a selection that had the effect of rejecting change. Members thought they were merely accepting a sensible system of social control and mutual assistance. The stultifying effect of egalitarian kinship was not recognized because there had never been an alternative. This will be discussed at greater length below in the context of efficient use of resources and the role of food surplus and commercial ventures in assisting the birth of progress. But for the moment it is sufficient to propose that primitive societies remained primitive for many centuries, even for thousands of years, not because of any inadequacy of intellect but because of a social prison that they purposely constructed and in which they unknowingly incarcerated themselves, a prison in which they themselves were the jailors, and often nasty ones at that.

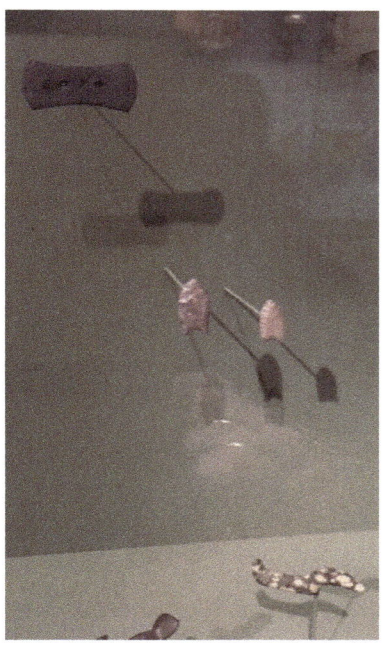 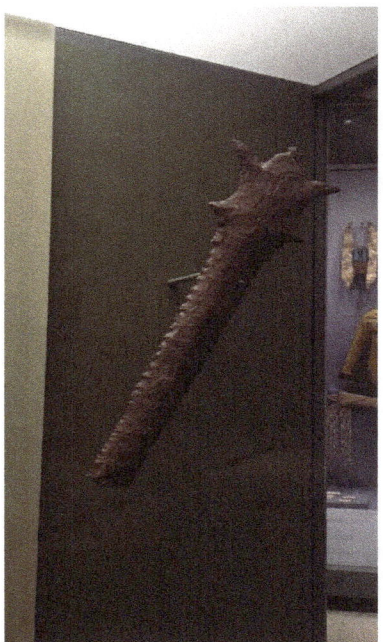

Fig. 28: From the Museum of the American Indian in New York City: (Left) Two Clovis projectile points from Washington county, New York, dated to about 10,000 BC. Made from knapped flint, it is proposed that the technology spread across North America in but two or three centuries. (Right) A scepter of the Mississippian culture found in Le Flore county, Oklahoma, made from knapped flint about 1200 AD. In a little more than 11,000 years technological advances permitted things to get bigger but not better. Photographs by the author.

B. Longevity (Life Expectancy)

A demographic factor relevant to progress is the age of a population. By this is not meant maximum life span, which is defined as the number of years a person is able, likely or not, to reach. Presently that age is thought to be about 120 years, the limit to which the physiology of the human body is not expected to exceed. In a sense any death occurring at an earlier age is premature. It is generally agreed that this measure has been unchanging for humans over recent millennia. More relevant to the status of a society, however, is the life expectancy for each individual born into it. As a demographic, a number of variables enters the calculation of the average life expectancy of a society, an important one being infant and childhood mortality. These young deaths are consistently high in primitive, ancient, and poorly governed societies, and if the calculation of the average age at death for a community includes deaths in infancy and childhood, the mean life expectancy of the total population, skewed by inclusion of that early peak in premature deaths, will differ greatly from the average duration of life of those that survive to adulthood.[8]

---

[8] The mathematical "mean," or "average," is the value obtained by dividing the sum of a data set by the number of data in the set, not the mode (the most frequent value in a data set) or median (the

As the variables in demographic analyses are many and often difficult to quantitate, this has given rise to complex statistical methods by which estimates of life expectancy are derived.[9] Because of limited data for present discussion, a recent summary of life expectancy according to archeological era has been published as derived from a paper by Doctors MacLennan and Sellers that discusses age at death of ancient populations:[10]

Era	Life Expectancy (yrs.)
Paleolithic	40 or more
20,000-6,000 BC	under 40
Neolithic	25-28
Bronze Age	24
Iron Age	?40
Classical Age	66-72
Dark Ages	36

If these figures in any way approximate the true nature of life expectancy in ancient societies, it should be no surprise that only rare foci of organized medical knowledge are found prior to the Classical Age in Greece, being the four primary civilizations discussed in chapters 28-31 of this work. Perhaps only in major alluvial regions could a civilization's population become large enough to have sufficient older members, and therefore experience, in close contact with each other to make organized medical thought possible. The numbers in the above list, however, are extracted from an article that does not present the mass of raw data from archeological excavations. They are, instead, very limited samples containing few data points that are provided by the authors as examples of their respective ages, rather than the mass of data points sometimes obtained from large inhumation sites. But even with such data there is no way of knowing how closely the inhumed represent the total population of a community, nor can statistics be adjusted to account for unpredictables such as epidemic disease or warfare.[11, 12] Inconsistencies are

---

middle term in a data set). For a better understanding of the complexity of the subject of life expectancy, see: Hacker, J. D., *New Estimates of Census Coverage in the United States, 1850-1930*, in *Social Science History*, 37:71-101, 2013. And to further complicate the issue, the modal age at death is now being proposed as a superior gauge for comparing health outcomes in modern nations with relatively high populations of elderly.

[9] See: Hoppa, R. D., and Vaupel, J. W. (editors), *Paleodemography: Age Distributions from Skeletal Samples*, Cambridge, 2002.

[10] See: MacLennan, W. J., and Sellers, W. I., *Ageing through the Ages*, in *Proc. Royal College of Physicians*, 29:71-75, 1999.

[11] Those injured or killed in battle often can be identified by archeological study, but the lethal consequences of war to noncombatants are unable to be differentiated from the pathologies of other times except in their quantity. How much is unappreciated of the full consequences of warfare. A true accounting of the tragic history of the common man, the detritus of families, the deaths of infants, helpless children and the infirm, starvation, slavery, all left in the shadow of great events, remains, and will probably always remain, unknown and, sadly, unacknowledged. This, of course, is one impetus for the present work.

[12] See: Boldsen, J. L. and Paine, R. R., *The Evolution of Human Longevity from the Mesolithic to the Middle Ages: --An Analysis Based on Skeletal Data*, in *Exceptional Longevity: From Prehistory to the Present*, Odense, 1995 (updated in 2000 by V. Castanova), Jeune, B. and Vaupel, J. W., editors, pp. 25-36. It is notable that females had a significant decline in survival during this period. As for males, assuming a mortality of 50% in infancy and early childhood, of ten male newborns,

common. In prehistoric cultures discussed in the preceding chapter, for example, limited data are provided for the Terramare Bronze Age culture in Italy, where the average age at death of men and women in one site was at least 40 years, somewhat longer than that listed above for the Bronze Age, as were some Old Kingdom Egyptian (2650-2150 BC) burials: 36 years. But a critical review using specific criteria and ancient European sites supports the conclusion that, from approximately 7,000 BC to the classical age (500 BC) the chance of a 20-year-old man surviving beyond 32.5 years was fairly stable at 40%. [13]

Most osteoarcheological studies have as a goal a clearer understanding of the health status of a population. The classic paper by Angel, based mainly on skeletal studies of ancient Europeans, included not only assessment of life expectancy, but also data on stature and pelvic inlet depth, both reflecting aspects of health status. In addition to suggesting that paleolithic man was in general healthier and lived longer than agrarian man, there was a very modest increase in life expectancy in Hellenistic times that succeeded the age of Classical Greece, the age of Hippocrates. [14] The issue at hand,

---

five might live to age 20 years, of which two might live past the age of 32.5 years, of which one, with luck, might live to 49 years or more. It has been pointed out, therefore, that with statistics like these few prehistoric children knew their grandparents. The situation was actually worse, for recent statistical demographic analysis of Classical antiquity, which included references to cemetery stele and the like and therefore more wide-ranging than the ages of the rich and famous, has pointed out the frequency of fatherlessness (with motherlessness not far behind). On average, about half of those reaching 20 years of age had lost their father. See: Scheidel, W., *The Demographic Background, in Growing Up Fatherless in Antiquity*, Cambridge, 2009, S. R. Hubner and D. M. Ratzan, editors, pp. 31-39. And excavations of almost 700 skeletons from the prosperous Greek colony of Metaponto located in the south of Italy indicate that in the 7th-2nd C BC life expectancy at birth was in the 20s and age at death having reached 15 years of age was 40 years, far short of the estimate for the Classical Age given on the preceding page (see: Henneberg, R. J., and Henneberg, M, *The Diet of the Metapontine Population as Reconstructed from the Physical Remains*, in *Living Off the Chora: Diet and Nutrition at Metaponto*, A. Prieto and J. C. Carter, editors, Austin, 2003, pp. 29-36). In Neolithic Orkney Islands, data from hundreds of burials show the additional life expectancy of 15-year-old boys to be 13 years (average age at death: 28 years) and pubescent girls to be only 9 years (average age at death: 22 years) and only four out of ten were over 12 years of age. (See the remarkable book of J. W. Hedges, *Tomb of the Eagles*, New York, 1987, for the extraordinary story of the ancient Orkney Islands, especially the section on Tribal Orkney I.)

[13] Life expectancy if one reached the age of 20 years in the United States, as detailed in the 1852 census, was 40 years, the average age at death being, therefore, 60 years (average of men and women combined) in Massachusetts, and for "colored" men and women in New England it was 36 years and 40 years, respectively, the average age reached being 58, whereas the same statistic for the ancient European sites based on 40% of twenty-year-olds reaching 32.5 years would be in the range of 30 years, barely one-half the U. S. 1852 data.

[14] The average age at death of prominent Greek personages has been estimated at *ca.* 70 years. The Gerousia in Sparta required its members be over sixty years of age, and many prominent Greeks are known to have been seventy years of age or older (Sophocles lived to age ninety). In contrast, the early study of J. L. Angel (*The Length of Life in Ancient Greece*, in *Am. J. Gerontology*, 18:18-24, 1947) found the average age at death to be about 40 years, and an extensive study of workers in Imperial Rome indicates an average age at death of about 30 years (see *Bones: Orthopedic Pathologies in Roman Imperial Age*, New York, 2015, Piccioli, A., *et al.*, editors). And of 880 late Holocene inhumations in Indian Knoll in Kentucky (estimated at 3,000-2,000 BC) only one skeleton was judged to be that of an individual over fifty years of age. In predynastic Egypt (Naqada) only one skeleton out of 266 examined was felt to be over sixty years of age, and in *ca.* 1500 BC there was a similar age distribution. There are many who believe Classical Greece life expectancy was significantly longer than that of prehistoric civilizations based on statistics such as this, but hard

however, is to determine to what age a sufficient number of adults of a population need to survive in order to provide a productive workforce that can sustain both family and culture and provide an institutional memory to instruct and guide its younger members. And to do this the dominant role lies with the life expectancy of the plebeian population.

Thus, the demographic requirements for present purposes are relatively few. They are: (1) only the ages of adult skeletal remains (*e.g.*, over fifteen years of age) need be used for calculation, (2) evidence that plebeians in the population comprise most inhumations, an obvious elite status being grounds for exclusion as being less likely to represent life expectancy of the population as a whole, and (3) size of the population being studied, as well as its variations in density, values usually obtained from study of dwellings and estimating the number of individuals who may have lived therein. The weakness of this approach, as always in statistics, is in the sampling, for calculations are almost always derived from a miniscule and nonrandom sample, and in the state of preservation of specimens.

It has been proposed from data reviewed in Part I that the time necessary for an urbanized society to develop a reasonable grasp of clinical medicine basics, meaning recognition of syndromes, the body's responses to acute injury, a concept of infectivity, contagion and its prevention, basic principles of physiology, and judging the effectiveness of therapies, is in the range of a few hundred years. Might life expectancy of the population affect this value?

Taking as an example the Djenne-Djenno civilization (see p. 577) which flourished for about 600 years, there is no evidence of medical practitioners. This is unexpected because a coeval pan-Mediterranean civilization (the Eastern Roman, or Byzantine, Empire flourished from 330-1453 AD) that included Egypt was 2,000-3,000 miles from this major trading center that had a population at its peak of perhaps 50,000. Yet there is no evidence of contact by Djenne-Djenno with either civilization prior to the arrival of Islamic influence in the 11th C AD, a time that coincided with the city's deterioration. Up to this point the civilization was thriving, self-sufficient, and enlarging. In view of the evidence for a general prosperity in Djenne-Djenno over many centuries and the lack of evidence for a coercive political hierarchy, what features affecting life expectancy might have restrained development of an early medical profession?

a. Deficiency of experienced members:
Just how close the cited average of 31 years of age at death comes to the true value for adult plebeians in Djenne-Djenno is unknown, but it is consistent with all the other ancient sites from which data are better. There would have been few adults old enough to have acquired firsthand medical knowledge worthy of passing on to younger members and fewer still that an older knowledgeable person could consider collegial peers.

b. Egalitarian kinships:
Throughout Djenne-Djenno egalitarian kinships would have assigned roles, duties, and obligations to their members, and an environmentally partitioned civilization like Djenne-

---

data on the point are few. The variables necessary to calculate life expectancy in various ages are many, so all that can be said is that the larger the population the more likely it is there will be a larger number of individuals whose life experiences could be useful to survival. The presence of many prominent persons who might be expected to live longer on average than plebeians may in fact reflect an increase in life expectancy of the general population, but for Classical Greece it remains an assumption. In the absence of writing, oral transmission of experience is especially valuable if there is to be any hope of progress, for otherwise new and useful observations vanish in a generation or two.

Djenno with its residential mounds would have maintained traditional kinship duties and obligations within households while at the same time working within boundaries set for commercial production. In other words, even if a person should live to forty or fifty years, the status assigned by kinship would have had priority over other activities, and the chance of developing a peer group focused on any innovative venture must have been slim.

    c.   Social class:

Although Djenne-Djenno had no obvious ruling class, some of the population had superior status. In a hierarchical society it often happens that the life expectancy of the elite classes tends to be significantly greater than that of the plebeians. In the presence of an elite population that is spared some of the toil and danger and is the recipient of a proportionately greater share of the society's productivity, it follows that a hierarchical society will have more older members than an egalitarian one. But it is thereby obvious that neither form of governance, egalitarian nor elitist, is likely to favor development of a network of medical practitioners: the egalitarian society will have no individuals it wishes to spare, or those that are available will have few years as a mature adult in which to acquire sufficient practical wisdom worth exchanging with others, whereas the elite, although longer-lived, will have no interest in doing a plebeian's work.[15]

    d.   Prosperity:

When people are safe and the food supply is better this brings another benefit: a larger population. A more secure food supply and a settled lifestyle that characterized the switch to an agricultural and then a commercial society might improve fecundity and lower neonatal and early childhood mortality. Another valuable consequence would be an increase in the general population and thereby in the absolute number of more mature and experienced. That proportion may not increase, but with a growing population in a defined space there would be a greater density of elderly. Interactions among the more knowledgeable segment of the community (*i.e.,* the older population) would be more likely and more information would be shared, if for no other reason than being a manifestation of the increased social interaction that is a concomitant of urbanization. The greater density of those longer-lived individuals would be expected to improve linear passage of acquired wisdom so that each succeeding generation would be better able to avoid dangers and to benefit from the historical experience of elders.

    e.   Sedentism:

With the change to an agricultural and sedentary way of life the elderly might be useful at home doing many of the more monotonous tasks related to daily living, this resulting in more elderly but experienced members. But prior to sedentism the outlook for those few who became elderly was not good. As the injured, infirm and aged became a hindrance to the group and physically contributed little to its survival, they would not receive group benefits. Although this did not always happen, the great variety of ways by which hunter-gatherer groups shed responsibility for the elderly has frequently been catalogued, and geronticide is a recognized solution in many areas.[16] In not so ancient times, for example, some Pacific atoll populations would release such persons on a separate but otherwise uninhabited island apart from the rest of the population. Village

---

[15] In ancient Greece apprentices starting at an early age learned medicine from existing practicing physicians, but the new primary civilizations described herein would have no prior experience with "physicians."

[16] See: Brogden, M., *Geronticide: Killing the Elderly*, London, 2001. There is no one section of the book that can be highlighted as a summary, for documentation of a subject, more comprehensively termed "death-hastening" and seldom popularly discussed, is extensive.

young people would then be assigned to periodically visit that island to replenish its food supply, but otherwise there was no assistance provided. Although geronticide may have eased physical burdens on a small band or tribe, knowledge was lost because of it. By casting away the elderly infirm, options for action would be limited by the inexperience of the myopic young, a further hindrance to progress. The few burials of elderly found in prehistoric times may sometimes reflect the practice of isolating or leaving behind those who were burdens to society; *i.e.*, they may have received no burial, merely being left behind with a parcel of food. This was no Garden of Eden.

Excursus on Eden

"And the Lord God planted a garden eastward in Eden; and there he put the man whom he had formed."

Genesis 2: 8

Modern lifestyles in the West and in culturally similar countries, regions, and cities around the globe have produced a level of convenience, security, a prosperity for so many people over recent generations that, despite the billions who share little of that abundance, it may seem, especially to the younger population, that prosperity has always been with us, was deserved and inevitable, the natural state of things, and will, with the digital age upon us, remain so. A future without limitations or cares, a secular Eden on a global scale, is eagerly anticipated and is impelling ideological political thought, although overt and pending hazards periodically dampen enthusiasm.

One marker that supports faith in such a future is life expectancy. Biblical statements declare 120 years to be the expected duration of life for humans, and over the past two centuries it has risen from 35-40 years to almost 80 years in many countries.[17] There have always been exceptional persons, exceptional in health or exceptional in luck, who far outlive the average for their societies, but to have so many live for so long and so well is a remarkable fact of modern times. This has never previously happened. Perhaps this *is* the path to a secular Eden. Pertinent to that path and to the purpose of this book is human progress, and life expectancy can be viewed as a measure of human progress.

But first is the issue of priority. Should the increase in life expectancy of modern times be attributed to progress, or is progress merely an inevitable consequence of an enlarging population of older, and thereby wiser, members? The wisdom of the patriarch, the sage, old wise men and women, church elders, oral histories, and biblical declarations (Job 12:12 – "Is not wisdom found among the aged? Does not long life bring understanding?") has reportedly been objectively confirmed.[18] Is a society where children usually do not know their grandparents inherently disadvantaged? If so, then most societies since the first man and woman have been so disabled, and this might explain the slow evolution, perhaps tens of thousands of years, of progress among humankind. And it is true that

---

[17] See: *Genesis* 6.3. But the conclusion about life span is not without its critics.
[18] See: Li, Y., et al., *Compensating Cognitive Capabilities, Economic Decisions, and Aging*, in *Psychology and Aging*, 28:595-613, 2013.

there are two periods that are usually considered to have significantly longer life expectancies: modern times (proven) and the Classical Age of Greece and Rome (unproven). As the present volume proposes, these two eras are credited with great success in advancing human progress, and if a larger mature and experienced population can be shown to inevitably explain the periods of progress, then this, the present volume, has been a waste of time. The issue is readily resolved for modern times, for life expectancy and population should increase prior to evidence of progress if progress is their inevitable consequence rather than a cause. A recent analysis confirms a significant increase in European populations by 1850, first evident in western Europe and then in eastern Europe.[19] Using a significantly increased life expectancy as it relates chronologically to new health practices, Europe at baseline (1770s) did not have a significant increase until 1900, and this includes a significant decrease in infant mortality.[20] As medical progress and movement toward the natural state of medical practice as proven in this volume, began in 18th C Europe, these data confirm that progress in Europe, and subsequently in the global populations, preceded population growth and increased life expectancy.[21]

There is some scholarly debate about life expectancy regarding the merits of a Paleolithic hunter-gatherer diet over a Neolithic agriculturalist diet, with evidence that the former resulted in longer-lived and healthier humans. Both the hunter-gatherers and the agriculturalists, however, still had a life expectancy shorter than gorillas and orangutans. This seems odd in that the human brain is given great credit for mankind's 19th C "survival of the fittest" narrative to the point where he has obtained mastery over virtually every facet of the planet, whether animal, vegetable, or mineral. Such dominance has been declared or is implied as proof of a genetic *tour de force*, survival in the best Darwinian sense, that has produced the rise in posture, stature, and nature from four-legged forebears illustrated so frequently in cartoons, by some sort of triumphant yet inevitable consequence of the blind chance of a hypothetical Big Bang, producing gradually more upright, taller, and brighter human specimens, each little development of each of the big and little bones of the shoulder and spine and feet, each millimeter in height, each point of the Intelligence Quotient, coming into play slowly by molecular selections of infinitely small gradations in survivability generation after generation for millions of years, perhaps with infrequent leaps and bounds by "punctuated equilibrium," to improve mankind's chance of survival in life-and-death competition with other earthly life-forms and myriads of environmental threats that would finally lead to an increase in life expectancy countless thousands of years in the future, specifically our 19th and 20th centuries. What a masterstroke of luck that our ancient forebears accommodated such an extraordinary sequence of events for us, and what a misfortune that they knew not what was occurring.

---

[19] See: Max Roser (2018), "*Life Expectancy*." Published online at OurWorldInData.org. Retrieved from: 'https://ourworldindata.org/life-expectancy' [Online Resource]

[20] See: Riley, J. C., *Estimates of Regional and Global Life Expectancy 1800-2001*, in *Population and Development Review*, 31:537-543, 2005, and Haines, M. R., *The Population of Europe: The Demographic Transition and After*, in *The Encyclopedia of European Social History*, Encyclopedia.com, 10 December 2018.

[21] Complexities of demography are great, however, and just how much benefit can be ascribed to medical progress and to other factors is a matter for debate, but not here.

How did this all begin in the first place? What set the continuum in motion that stealthily led, over fifteen million years, from the two-foot tall, four-legged, forty-pound *Proconsul africanus* to *Homo sapiens*? If the human species has exhibited, society-wide, a level of intelligence that has been both unchanging for millennia and universally similar, how is it that a "survival of the fittest" theory can explain the following: that as early as there is objective evidence, primarily from osteology and going back to Paleolithic times, human life expectancy is routinely found to be in the range of 30-35 years, a finding that changes little until modern times.[22] In a related observation, the infant mortality rate of gorillas in the wild (*i.e.*, mortality in the first three years of life, including stillbirths) varies considerably although 25% may be a reasonable approximation. But a recent textbook states that Paleolithic humans (9000 BC) had only a 50% chance of survival to age 15, and study of a Bronze Age inhumed population in 500 BC Italy revealed that from 33-50% of the interred were under 5 years of age.[23] Such an abbreviated life expectancy and early childhood mortality in a biological body that is thought to permit living to an age well over 100 years does not seem to be a positive indicator of superior survivability, especially as gorillas, chimpanzees, and orangutans have a life expectancy of 35-50 years in the wild and 50->60 years in captivity.[24] And yet at Indian Knoll, a permanent

---

[22] See: Angel, L., *Health as a Crucial Factor in the Changes from Hunting to Developed Farming in the Eastern Mediterranean*, in *Paleopathology at the Origins of Agriculture*, Orlando, 1984, M. N. Cohen and G. J. Armelagos, editors, pp. 51-73. This informative paper has been updated in many ways, but the definitions of life expectancy are so varied, vague, or unstated, that it is difficult to group findings from different papers into one statistical base. The listing of approximate longevities (in years) of ancient populations provided by Angel can be used as a starting place for a general statement such as is discussed here: Late Paleolithic (30,000-9,000 BC) – 35.4 (males) and 30.0 (females); Mesolithic (9,000-7,000 BC) – 33.5 (males) and 31.3 (females); Early Neolithic (7,000-5,000 BC) – 33.6 (males) and 29.8 (females); Late Neolithic (5,000-3,000 BC) – 33.1 (males) and 29.8 (females); Early Bronze Age (3,000-2,000 BC) – 33.6 (males) and 29.4 (females); Middle Bronze Age (2,000 BC and for varying periods afterwards) – 36.5 (males) and 31.4 (females); and Early Iron Age (1,150-650 BC) – 39.0 (males) and 30.9 (females). (Note that dating of major divisions of the Stone Age vary.) Taking a more specific study for comparison, a well-defined population from a Late Neolithic tomb in Spain dated to 3,700 BC had an average age at death for 38 individual skeletal remains as follows: 17 were "subadult" (under 20 years of age) and 21 were "adult" (over 20 years of age). The mean age of the latter group (male and female grouped) was 30.5 years (determined from the average of the individual age ranges reported, minus 7 adults in whom an age range was unable to be determined. Violence was not the cause of death, and they "exhibited a moderate number of pathologies." See: Alt, K. W., et al., (2016) *A Community in Life and Death: The Late Neolithic Megalithic Tomb at Alto de Reinoso* (Burgos, Spain), PLoS ONE 11(1): e0146176. Doi: 10. 1371/journal.pone.0146176.

[23] See: Stockwell, E. G., and Groat, H. T., *World Population: An Introduction to Demography*, New York, 1984, and Tafuri, M., *et al.*, *Diet, Mobility and Resident Patterns in Bronze Age Southern Italy,* in (unable to identify), pp. 45-56, 2003.

[24] The Center for Great Apes reports the following life expectancy (in years) for gorillas – 40-50 (wild), 50-60 (captive). Type of gorilla not stated. The National Geographic Institute reports 45 years for chimpanzees (wild), type not stated. Other estimates include orangutans as 35-45 years (wild, with maximum observed being 53 for a female and 58 for a male) and baboons as 30-45. Some local reports give significantly shorter survivals than these estimates, but the difference is generally in the range of only 5-10 years. And a study of chimpanzees in the Mahale Mountains (Tanzania) indicate female fecundity greatest between ages 20-35 years. (Nishida, T., et al., *Demography, female life history, and reproductive profiles among the chipanzees of Mahale*, in *Am. J. Primatol.*, 59:99-121, 2003.) In Dr. Dian Fossey's book, *Gorillas in the Mist* (Boston 1983),

prehistoric habitation site in Kentucky that flourished between 3000 and 2000 BC, a recent reanalysis of data has concluded that, of an interred population over centuries of 880, only one was deemed over fifty years of age.[25] The Neolithic hunter-gatherer of the Jomon people of Japan had an average age at death of 36 years if those individuals managed to survive to age 15 years; more recent hunter-gatherers of the Japanese Neolithic who survived to age 15 years had an average age at death of 44 years.[26] Very premature death at every age category seems to have been unavoidable until the last two centuries. A reasonable conclusion is that survivability of our early ancestors, or even their first appearance, is not the consequence of a preceding period in which gradual expression of a superior fitness was operative generation after generation. If so, those ancient humans might early on have approached that 100-year life expectancy as a consequence of their superior attributes and survivability, primarily the complexity of their brain, that their ancestors lacked. Instead, the complex brain of *Homo sapiens* seems to have provided no survivability benefit at all. Evidence even suggests that the life expectancy of early Upper Paleolithic man (considered "modern" man) was no greater than that of roughly contemporary Neanderthals.[27] It almost seems as if humans had not been biologically evolving to inhabit a "survival of the fittest" world, instead just being plopped down in the midst of a dangerous world after emerging from some other state in which their evolution was guided by quite another process, one in which survival was not predicated on confrontation of danger and chaos, one that was perhaps even Eden-like. If evolution of the complexity of the human brain was not a matter of natural selection, one might wonder why it did so happen.

An unanswered question, of course, is, to what use is the elderly population to survival? If the more complex brain resulted from a selective force for propagation of the human species rather than longevity, there might be a Darwinian explanation for its development. That, however, would require evidence for increased fecundity or some other mechanism for increasing the number of births and their survival into childbearing years.[28] If there is

---

appendix C, 9 gorillas on whom autopsies were performed that did not die from poachers included one that was between 50-55 and the other between 55-60 years of age.

[25] See: Johnston, F. E., and Snow, C. E., *The Reassessment of the Age and Sex of the Indian Knoll Skeletal Population: Demographic and Methodological Aspects*, in *Am. J. Phys. Anthropol.*, 19:237-244, 1961. Subsequent reassessments have been made regarding techniques, both osteological and statistical, of this unusual population that displayed much evidence of violence, but the rarity of an "elderly" adult in this ancient Native American population, mostly from ca. 3000-2000 BC, is obvious. In the United States in 2016, almost 30% of 300,000,000 people were 55 years of age or older, whereas among the approximately eight hundred Archaic period (8000 – 1000 BC) skeletal remains of Indian Knoll only one was classified as over fifty. The 30% in 2016 can be compared to 0.1% at Indian Knoll, a 300-fold difference or, as usually presented in current popular media, a 30,000% increase.

[26] See: Kaplan, H., et al., *A Theory of Human Life History. Evolution: Diet, Intelligence, and Longevity*, in *Evolutionary Anthropology*, pp. 156-186.

[27] See: Bocquet-Appel, J., and Degioanni, A., *Neanderthal Demographic Estimates*, in *Current Anthropology*, 54:S202-S213, 2013.

[28] One area that would have contributed more to species survival than a bigger brain might have been an increase in fecundity, something impossible to quantitate over the ages, in part because risks attendant to bearing children is blamed for the generally shorter life expectancy of women in prehistoric times, especially for the primigravida. This is one reason why fecundity is not more important in the survival of the human species: its mechanism for success decreases the fecund.

no correlation between the two (*i.e.*, brain size/complexity is found to be unrelated propagation), then to what is the modern brain an adaptation? Why did development not follow some other course and inhabit the cranium of a long-lived and peaceable genus such as *Chelonoidis nigra*, the Galapagos tortoise that can live as long as 170 years.

To this end, the finely tuned biological system that each us is contains so many variables that are susceptible to genetic alteration may have been meant for some other state. What that state might have been has always been the grand question. It is in regard to this that it is appropriate to consider Darwin's conclusion on the construction of the human eye in its complexity and fine integration of functions that permit normal sight.[29] His statement was that it seemed absurd to think that such a complex biological system as the human eye could have been the result of a series of selective genetic mutations whereby each genetic change permitted one member of a species to survive where others could not, that survival benefit being the consequence of improved vision or merely by chance. Nevertheless, he considered his theory of evolution, first expounded in 1859, to be so excellent that he believed it was the truth, despite its element of seeming absurdity. One wonders what Darwin would have to say about this were he to return today and see the true complexity of the eye and vision as far as modern science has been able to ascertain it. That complexity is so incredibly vast and multifaceted, from the simple optics of refraction to the intracellular production of innumerable species of proteins that make up the eye's tissues and fluids, that modern knowledge cannot be mentioned in the same breath with the simple concepts of the mid-19th C of Darwin. And even now we know our knowledge of the entire process of vision to still be at an elementary stage. Were Darwin here today and aware of all that has transpired in modern understanding, perhaps he would revert to his original position.

And think again about mankind's increase in life expectancy that has occurred only over the past 200 years. There is no evidence of a gradual increase in life expectancy over hundreds of millennia to match the gradual or intermittent march posited in cartoons for early hominid to upright man. Prior to the 19th C life expectancy was in the range of 35 years for the average person, even since the beginning of mankind itself, give or take a few years as suggested by the modest increase geographically and chronologically localized to the Hellenistic period (323-31 BC) (Table 14, p. 611).[30] It was little different

---

[29] See: Darwin, C. A., *On the Origin of Species By Means of Natural Selection*, New York, 1860, p. 167: "To suppose that the eye, with all its inimitable contrivances for adjusting the focus to different distances, for admitting different amounts of light, and for correction of the spherical and chromatic aberration, could have been formed by natural selection, seems, I freely confess, absurd in the highest possible degree." Modern biology has integrated Darwinism within the larger scope of genetics that many feel dispels absurdity, but the point is best debated elsewhere rather than here.

[30] Life expectancy in the Greco-Roman world is uncertain even though accurate ages of some of the elderly are known. Socrates, Sophocles, Plato, Seneca and Archimedes lived to age 71, 90, 77, 93, and 75 years, respectively, but they reflect the lifestyle of the rich or famous rather than the average worker or mother. Another major unknown is infant and childhood mortality. Phlegon of Tralles in the 2nd C AD wrote *On Long-Lived Persons* in which he claims to have identified seventy individuals in one area of Italy who lived to be older, some much older, than one hundred years, and Pliny also comments on centenarians in 1st C AD Italy, but see T. G. Parkin, *Old Age in the Roman World* (Baltimore, 2003), especially chapter 6, pp. 173-189, for a discrediting of such claims. The Greco-Roman world was vast and varied, and a meaningful single estimate of life expectancy applicable to either Greek or Roman "culture" in that period of history is unavailable.

from the average of 35 years during the European Dark Ages. It is not hyperbole, indeed, it is a fact, to point out that mankind has, since its very commencement, been living in a perpetual Dark Age except for the last three centuries. With the exemption of the controlling elites of human society who might live longer than the plebeians, mankind from the beginning has provided little evidence for improved survival because of an ongoing genetic selection favoring some mythical "fitness." Fitness for what? Despite his vaunted brain mankind's life expectancy did not exceed that of the gorilla until 200 years ago.[31] Events suggest instead that man first appeared on this planet quite unprepared for the survival of his species.[32] Despite his capacity for brilliance, life has been for most humans very much as Hobbes noted, short and brutish, but not so much from man's unsociable disposition, instead being due to an inability to cope.

Table 14: Mean Stature in Feet and Median Life Span in Years of Humans in Prehistory and History[33]

	Mean Stature (ft.)		Median Life Expectancy (yrs.)	
	M	F	M	F
Paleolithic	5.81	5.47	35.4	30.0
Mesolithic	5.66	5.24	33.5	31.3
Early Neolithic	5.57	5.10	33.6	29.8
Late Neolithic	5.29	5.06	33.1	29.2
Bronze/Iron Ages	5.46	5.06	37.2	31.1
Hellenistic	5.64	5.13	41.9	38.0
Medieval	5.56	5.15	37.7	31.1
Baroque	5.65	5.18	33.9	28.5
19th C	5.58	5.17	40.0	38.4
Late 20th C (USA)	5.72	5.36	71.0	78.5

Increased age, of course, cannot be viewed as evidence for natural selection ("survival of the fittest") because at some point increased age and its inevitable infirmities impose a burden to society rather than a benefit, and age-related decreases in fertility obviate any genetic mechanism for fecundity that might otherwise apply, although it might be a

[31] Wich, S. A., et al., *Life History of Wild Sumatran Orangutans (Pongo abeleii)*, in *J. Hum. Evol.*, 47:385-398, 2004, reports wild orangutans reaching the age of 58 for males and 53 for females, and for gorillas the "life span" usually given as 35-40 years in the wild and 40-60 in zoos. Hakeem, A., et al., in *Handbook of the Psychology of Aging*, 4th ed., Birren, J. D. and Schaie, K. W., eds., San Diego, 1996, 79, states, however, that "Long-term observational data suggest that the maximum life spans for zoo-living and wild primates may be about the same." (Life span is not the same as life expectancy.) The life expectancy of the same species contemporary with ancient civilizations discussed in this book is unknown, but when available data are compared to that of humans listed on p. 602, the point is made: parallel branches on the hominid ancestor tree support the conclusion that life expectancy of humans relative to other hominids is no better and may well be inferior.

[32] Unprepared, unless his preparation was not meant primarily for propagation of his species. But if not for that, then for what? An intriguing question.

[33] This Table is modified from that used by: Wells, S., in *Pandora's Seed: The Unforeseen Cost of Civilization*, New York, 2010, p. 23. Measurements of stature could reflect nutritional status or childhood disease.

marker for other features that are beneficial. It has long been known that the brain of modern man is smaller than some of his proposed forebears and related species such as *Homo neanderthalensis*. Maybe the idea that the size of man's brain has produced his modern mastery of the world has actually been associated with a decrease in brain size rather than an increase.

But, if man's brain and his fecundity were truly associated with a bettering of his status in life, why, given our great expectations and predictions, has his progress been so middling that in the 18th C Alexander Pope acknowledged him "Created half to rise and half to fall; Great Lord of all things, yet a prey to all;... the glory, jest, and riddle of the world."[34] Whatever has propelled humankind to its apogee has not been its prehistory and early history, of this we can be sure. And whatever humankind was capable of doing 10,000 years ago, it is no more capable of doing now. But a few hundred years ago something happened, some other circumstance intervened that, after millennia of mankind's milling about in self-imposed incarceration, opened the cage, progress was unchained, with the betterment of the mass of mankind finally improving and doing so at a previously unimaginable rate.

In conclusion, what explains this phenomenon, this sudden appearance of longevity? With human history packed with successes in all sorts of ventures, whether building of empires, climbing mountains, winning great battles, building massive monuments, or growing the largest pumpkin, why is it only now that life expectancy clearly exceeds that of man's fellow hominid, the orangutan? As it turns out, there *is* a path to a secular Eden, a path that is now evident. That path, born of the Reformation (see p. 349) and bred by parliamentary process, is characterized by three features: recognition of the importance of the individual, liberty of conscience, and freedom of self-determination. Their mechanism of operation and its importance in human collaboration will be discussed in later chapters, but for time on earth, for appreciating the pleasantness that life can offer, for the personal interactions with others that provide meaning and fulfillment, a long life, perhaps even one of Biblical proportions, might be desired and attainable, unless humanity reverts to its unpleasant default state. But why has it taken so long for mankind to realize this path, and will it be permitted to continue the journey? That is a question to be answered, in part, in this volume.[35]

End of Excursus

C. Population Size and Density

Large city size is apparently irrelevant to mechanisms that induce progress in a society, for there have been hundreds of large cities in prehistory and early history, and

---

[34] From Pope's second epistle of *An Essay on Man* (1734).

[35] It is curious to note, with regard to Eden, that the calculations of F. A. Hassan (*On Mechanisms of Population Growth during the Neolithic*, in *Current Anthropology*, 14:535-542, 1973) show that, beginning with a single fertile couple and a population growth rate of 0.1 percent per year, the total world population at the time of Hassan's article would have been reached in 20,000 years. And in preparation for the chapters to come it may be useful to revisit the frontispiece of Part II of this volume and its commentary.

prior to the modern West virtually none have been the source of institutionalized progress and none have been the reason for its initiation. Cities may become larger and more elaborate, and monuments, colorful markets, and a fascinating polyethnicity may indicate accommodation, but they do not mean progress. There may repeatedly be small foci of progress in the midst of city bustle, but they become lost in the crowd. A large city, even if rigidly authoritarian, would not be expected to impede individual medical practitioners, but if those practitioners became organized or a source of wealth authoritarian strictures might appear, as historically occurred with the *Code of Ur-Nammu* in Sumer or that of the code of Hammurabi in Babylonia, both discussed on p. 45*f.*

For evolving small cities, however, population kinetics as size increases can have positive consequences. Previously parochial kinships and personal interests now can interact with others and foster new ways of thinking and doing things. The concept of "settlement hierarchy" has been used to explain the tendency of a population to naturally structure itself, with an increasing population leading spontaneously to more complex hierarchical organization as the community adjusts to changing needs. The many special interest groups who organize will share their unique perspectives or impress their influence on local issues and so contribute to overall development of the community. It is at this point, when the bond of knish ip has weakened, that a medical practice network is likely to appear, and it will appear in the plebeian population.

The demographic point at which egalitarian process and kinship regulation are affected by size has received scholarly attention. It is observed that, given time limitations on discourse, the larger the egalitarian population the more arguments and disagreements occur and the greater the difficulty in reaching a consensus and in maintaining group cohesion. For egalitarian bands as an example, the Dunbar number has been proposed as a population size beyond which social cohesion weakens.[36] That number, presently estimated at 150, will vary according to a number of factors, but the concept is of value here not because of the number but because the elements of truth embedded in it provide a reasonable explanation for the initiation of hierarchical controls in societies as population size increases. Importantly, it is the loss of power previously distributed throughout the egalitarian community that is compromised as an organizational hierarchy evolves. Because egalitarianism denies a fundamental right that humans be "agents of their choices," individualism emerges from the weakening of its grasp.

An analogous situation exists with kinship. It has been observed that, "Increases in the rate of population growth increase the size of kin groups but decrease their inequality and vice versa."[37] This occurs as the kin group, or some of its more politically forceful members, seeks ways to maintain cohesion in response to the enlarging population. Again, the point is that kinship regimentation, *i.e.*, the assigned status of its members, weakens beyond a certain group size.[38] Thus both egalitarianism and kinship

---

[36] See: Dunbar, R. I. M., *Neocortex Size as a Constraint on Group Size in Primates*, in *J. of Human Evolution*, 22:469-493, 1992.

[37] See: Hammel, E. A., *Kinship-based Politics and the Optimal Size of Kin Groups*, in *Proc. Nat. Acad. Sci.*, 102:11951-11956, 2005. A model of this consequence of rate of population growth has been proposed.

[38] This should not be confused with the "kinships" of brotherhood with a specific goal, *e.g.*, a brotherhood of railroad workers. It has been pointed out that in large cities new kinships abound as humans congregate around a common cause or ethnicity. This type of kinship is one of friendship and mutual assistance prompted by a common need rather than the term's use herein as a way of life from birth to death that finds its origin in the relationship between members of the same family.

authority diminish as urbanization evolves, and traditional controls are replaced by new options and alliances. Contributing to this process, at least in evolution of medical services, is the presence of more experienced persons in the population, an increase reachable by either increased longevity of the population or increased population density.

The importance of demography in effecting progress should now be clear. Even without any improvement in life expectancy, the mere increase in a focal population size may suffice to concentrate the basic skills and knowledge for progress in specialized fields. The five successful civilizations of chapters 27-31 with at least circumstantial evidence of a medical practice network were neither villages nor sprawling metropolises at the time their medical networks began. This excludes that ubiquitous mystic, the shaman, and it does not include the empiric medicine of a family member or friend nor the closeted medical knowledge of midwifery that might be held in common by a group of women in a community, all of which can be found in small societies. This, by the way, is not to diminish the inestimable role of midwifery in the course of human events. That groups of women who looked after their own at a critical juncture in life did not become a formal group of medical practitioners was no fault of theirs. It may still be discovered that early groups of male medical practitioners who are behind the classical medical writings presently under discussion got their inspiration for forming their medical groups and networks from observing the unobtrusive dedication of self-proclaimed midwives as they communicated with one another. And if ever there is a question raised about the humaneness of *Homo sapiens* in view of its sordid history one merely need point to the selfless midwives who, anonymously, without pomp and without remuneration, have helped or attempted to help minimize the trauma and distress attendant to childbirth throughout the ages.

Interest for the moment, however, is focused on small polities and the minimal size required to initiate and sustain progress, and now an attempt at understanding can at least be surmised. The populations of the five primary civilizations identified in chapters 27-31 as having done so averaged about 40,000 in their nuclear populations. There would be a better chance of a subgroup of practitioners meeting up and organizing if there were 200 in the area of a square mile rather than 10. On the other hand, if ten years were the average practice duration (because of a short life expectancy), the opportunity for collegial accumulation of knowledge would be much lessened. But, in general, it can be hypothesized that, based on experience (the five "successful" civilizations) and theoretical considerations, a central population in the tens of thousands is sufficient for a nascent medical profession and for sustained progress generally.

The population density for the five "successful" civilizations was 56 persons per acre (95% confidence interval: 29-84). But little has been mentioned heretofore about population density because it is even more phantasmagorical than some of the other parameters in the prehistory data. In Table 15 (pp. 622-623) the population density is derived by dividing the largest believable population at the time of interest (*i.e.*, Floruit) by the dimensions reported from archeological studies, and both numbers are highly variable because of poor quality data. The final number does not reflect published scientific estimates for each site because they are seldom available or, if available, are given with significant qualifications that preclude a reasonable generalization.

D. Duration

Once a primitive settlement was established and had expanded into a city-state it took on average about 400-500 years to develop a nascent medical profession in the five successful civilizations, one that could provide a collegial mechanism for progress in medicine. Dogged by their short lives, the early city-state inhabitants had previously relied on a family member or friend for advice on health matters, herbal remedies deemed effective, and botanicals to be avoided. At this point may have appeared the earliest empirical practitioner who would make some cogent observations and perhaps institute generational passage of his knowledge. If there were serial passage of knowledge, perhaps a century would pass as new knowledge accumulated among his descendants. A familial and generational practice of practitioners was born. At different locales throughout the enlarging city-state this could have been repeated to varying degrees until the time came when one of the practitioners would hail another and ask if he had seen people with an unusual rash and fever such as had recently sought his help. The two might then have discussed the possibility of meeting with several other practitioners with whom they were familiar. When the meeting transpired the several practitioners may then have decided it would be useful to all if there were future meetings, thus essentially founding a primitive medical society. After another few generations passed the now "members" may have determined that their experience was decidedly better than that of other types of practitioners. It would behoove them to organize their pooled wisdom, for it would help guarantee that their superior type of practice would invite prosperity, and, now comprising a rather bulky amount of information, they might want to pass on their knowledge to future practitioners. At first this would have been oral transmission, but as the civilization continued to flourish and commerce become more complex, early forms of writing appeared. This practical invention could then have been acquired by the practitioners, the ultimate result being the original form of the classics of medicine attributed to the five successful civilizations.

The fictitious scenario of the preceding paragraph is but one way of speculating on medicine's earliest days, although some of its particulars conveniently fit with factual observations of the medical profession's history. These include: (1) the role of certain families being identified as the source of medical practitioners, such as the purported Asclepiad families of ancient Greece, (2) the pooling of knowledge from a number of practitioners that explains the evidence of a broad experience in dealing with the sick that is a feature of the classic medical writings under discussion, (3) the generous and probably self-serving association of the source of the information in those medical classics with prominent, now legendary, individuals in the distant prehistoric past (such as the Greek god, Apollo, the Yellow Emperor, the sage Bharadvaja, Asclepius, and Imhotep), and (4) the astuteness of some of the observations in the classical writings that indicate scientific confirmation by sequential practitioners.

Admittedly the forced assembly of this jigsaw puzzle into a narrative covering a few centuries is unscientific, but it was pointed out in Part I that medical knowledge is cheap, obvious, and quickly and easily obtained. Thus, once under way it would not take many people or much time for medical practitioners and their knowledge to flourish just as the local society was flourishing. A wide window of time is not required for the transformation to take root. Once a *de novo* city-state had reached a stable prosperity (*i.e.*, Floruit), a few centuries should have sufficed for a nascent medical profession.

Obviously, this does not apply to newly developing cities of an empire with preexisting specialization and communication.

E. Prosperity

Who would undertake the responsibility of providing medical care on his own other than what might be requested by family or friends? It is unlikely, given the struggle for existence, that a member of a primitive nonegalitarian community who acquired some medical expertise would otherwise offer his services without some form of compensation. A member of an egalitarian community would not even conceive the idea. It is also unlikely that a community that required total communal involvement to merely exist could produce such a person. The importance of a settled and flourishing community now becomes apparent. With a commercial base in agriculture or in the production of something desirable, whether a tool or decorative bauble, the benefit to a community is two-fold: (1) it can provide wealth and stability extending over generations, and (2) some form of personal benefit could now become available to those who provide useful specialized services. A person who acquired excess grain could trade some of it for assistance, including asking for help from a person recognized as knowing a therapy that might help in overcoming an infirmity. It is necessary, therefore, that a community be not only of sufficient size, but also sufficiently prosperous, to entice the occasional member of the community to initiate a service previously unknown outside the family circle. If this picture is approximately correct, it is unlikely that any medical care could ever have emerged from bands or tribes other than that suggested by word of mouth and implemented by a family member. Their populations were small and their egalitarianism, while it may have ensured that what little was known of medical care was available to all, its quality would never improve. It is the commencement of profitable heterarchical structures within the greater society that would open the door for improvements in daily life and in services obtained by barter.

A possible issue of a minor nature related to prosperity of a polity as it evolves professions is the life expectancy of the plebeian population in general and medical practitioners in particular. A useful development would have been a longer life span for the individual practitioner. He could then acquire more knowledge, experience, and expertise and instruct more novices. One thing that would improve his life chances would have been a bettering of his personal station in the community, for he then might join the more elite population in sharing the benefits of a less arduous and less dangerous lifestyle and thereby live longer. Thus, prosperity might provide two possible benefits to the medical practitioner: (1) it introduces a profit motive that provides the fuel for entrepreneurship and (2) it might contribute to a longer life in some of the community, including medical practitioners, who can now provide for their personal needs without hazarding the daily dangers confronting the majority of the plebeian population. The last statement has, of course, not been validated, and given the exposure of medical practitioners to all manner of infection, local and contagious, there may have been, on average, no increase in life expectancy.[39] Finally, if the practitioner indeed personally

---

[39] A recent study of medical professionals concluded, "Our results are in line with the many nineteenth-century studies showing that medical professionals, compared to other 'civilized classes', had a somewhat lower average duration of life." See: Van Poppel, F, *et al.*, *The Life*

benefited from a better station in life, the ultimate beneficence would accrue to the general population as medical practitioners improved their skills and knowledge that would be available in times of necessity. That such a distinction could conceivably be significant in promoting intellectual progress may seem absurd, but the mean age at death for males over many centuries in pre-Classical Greece as measured by Dr. Angel was 38.6 years, whereas for Classical Greece it was 42.6 years.[40] This was enough for Dr. Angel to state "It is clear that a small but definite increase in length of life accompanied the rise of civilization in ancient Greece." Furthermore, the mean length of life of 83 "men of renown" in Classical Greece was found to be 71 years.[41] Social mobility of prospering plebeians leading to an improved lifestyle and life expectancy suggests an increasing length of life, even a modest increase, at least be considered among those factors underlying the initiation of a medical profession. Credit for this must go to the prosperity of early urbanization when it extended to the plebeian class.[42]

F. Demographic Conclusions

Despite insufficient data to scientifically prove the point, it is proposed that a concatenation of several demographic conditions need to be satisfied before an adequate nucleus of potential talent is available that would permit the initiation and maintenance of an occupational specialty.

A further variable is that the community remain politically stable for an extended period, perhaps three centuries or thereabout. If several prosperous centuries pass without evidence of medical practitioners, it is likely none will ever appear. The civilizations of Catalhoyuk, Poverty Point, and Cucuteni-Trypillia all "thrived" for at least a millennium and left no evidence of medical practitioners. Their way of life precluded that possibility.

Another requirement is anticipation of personal benefit, usually prosperity, and that prosperity may result from an element of "fee for service," in which case the medical practitioner, acquiring some form of wealth, might be able to avoid some of the dangers associated with daily living and become longer-lived and more effective in his work. Prosperity would not be limited to a specialization, and therefore this requirement is essentially the development of a middle class.

An increase in "knowledge years" could be obtained by starting education early (*i.e.,* making the profession familial). But the shift from familial professions to freestanding professional groups as occurred in Hippocratic Greece is best explained by an increase in the wealth among some of the non-elite population as commerce flourished.

Assuming, therefore, no prior experience with, or knowledge of, such a thing as a clinical medical practice, demographic requirements for initiation of a progressive

Expectancy of Medical Professionals in the Netherlands, Sixteenth to Twentieth Centuries, in *Population,* 71:619-640, 2016.

[40] See: Angel, J. L., *Length of Life in Ancient Greece,* in *J. Gerontol.,* 2:18-24, 1947.

[41] See: Batrinos, M. L., *The Length of Life and Eugeria in Classical Greece,* in *Hormones (Athens),* 7:82-83, 2008.

[42] But this burden of the common man has persisted into modern times. A careful study published in 1885 found the "rich" class in Budapest had an average age at death of 52 years, whereas for the "middle" and the "poor" the values were 46 and 41 years, respectively (von Korosi, Josef, *Ueber den einfluss des Wohlhabenheit und der Wohnverhaltnisse auf Sterblickkeit und Todesursachen mit besonderer Berucktsichtigen des Auftretens der Infectiosen Krankheiten,* Stuttgart).

medical practice, as derived from study of the five ancient "successful" civilizations might include:

1. A collegial network of at least several medical practitioners
2. Several centuries of social stability
3. Prosperity, as evidenced by trade and specialization, sufficient to support medical practitioners working for profit
4. A total population in the tens of thousands, perhaps as low as 10-20,000.

G. Preceding and Succeeding Civilizations

Of the five successful primary civilizations described in chapters 27-31, four had long delays between original settlement and evolution to a phase that permitted development of medical professions. If the FORMATIVE and the FLORUIT periods are totaled, the average duration of the four is 1,340 years (standard deviation: 256), whereas the average for the same periods for six of the longest-lived lesser civilizations is 1,640 years (standard deviation:191), a difference that is marginally not significant (p = 0.06) and the difference does not favor the longer duration. This is relevant to the lesser civilizations of chapter 8 because it does not suggest that total duration of a civilization is a significant factor in initiating progress or in initiating a medical network. The reason for lack of progress lies elsewhere.

Consider the course of medical practice in a primary civilization specified as successful. Roughly 1,600 years (4400 to 2800 BC) separate the early Naqada settlements in Egypt from the proposed time of the original composition from which was copied the Ebers papyrus. For most of that time empirical recycling of limited knowledge was taking place, generation after generation passing limited wisdom on to the succeeding one, its limited value further limited by short life expectancy. New clinical observations and new attempts at remedies surely were made throughout that period, most to be forgotten because there was no network of practitioners for remembering. There was no central locus in which to record that knowledge as it became available, and there was probably no one else in the community capable of doing so. And this is the important point: the idea that there is somehow a gradual communal accretion of medical knowledge over centuries that accumulates to the point it can be considered the organized wisdom of a superior civilization is false. The accumulation of knowledge comes in bursts if the time is right.[43] But if there is no one to record or otherwise develop and report a new finding at the time, it is likely to be forever lost.

But if there is an organization that preserves the event, whether in writing or in a common memory, the event can live on for centuries. The dramatic flowering of

---

[43] It may be helpful to review Fig. 13 in the Epilogue to Part I of this work. There is a faint increase in knowledge above background empiricism attributed to nascent medical practice in Sumer and ancient Egypt (to which the present volume would now add India (Indus River Valley) and China (Liangchengzhen)), a larger increase associated with ancient Greece (Hippocratic medicine), and a vast flowering of Western medical knowledge over the last two centuries. Also compare these flourishing periods with the life expectancy of the Hellenistic and 19th C periods as presented in Table 14. If there was an increase locally during the Late Neolithic Period it is undetectable. It is proposed that the periods of longer life expectancy concomitant with the flourishing of medical knowledge indicate a general flourishing of salutary aspects of lifestyle other than medicine, the outbursts of medical knowledge merely reflecting community-wide enterprise.

Renaissance art, produced by gifted individuals who are always plentiful in any society, was possible not because a flood of geniuses happened to be born in Renaissance Florence and environs in the 15th and 16th centuries, and not because they were lucky enough to have been selected by their patrons, but because they were provided a degree of individual freedom to pursue their art that included the freedom of networking with colleagues also protected by patrons to inform each other of new works and ideas about that art.[44]

Thus, if the original medical composition of the Ebers papyrus that was copied in 1550 BC is dated to 3000 BC, the data on which it was based was not amassed over the preceding millennium; it was instead collected within a few generations of its writing. It occurred during a brief window of opportunity that was preceded by a long period of linear transmission of medical lore, most of which was lost and the rest of little consequence because it was of poor quality, unverifiable, and succeeded by a Pharaonic Egypt that impressed upcoming generations of medical practitioners into government service.

Applying the same assessment to Sumer, the principle content of the *Medical Treatise of Diagnosis and Prognosis* and the *Therapeutic Manual* has been assumed to represent medical thought in Sumer prior to its appropriation by the Akkadians in 2350 BC. The millennium or two preceding the collection of the wisdom underlying the cited medical texts was not one of gradually accumulated knowledge to be assigned to an entire civilization. Nor is it to be assigned to the succeeding age of Sargon when all Sumer and other city-states were merged into one man's empire. Instead, the wisdom that would be found in the medical classics was collected over a few generations, most likely during the Late Uruk or Jemdet Nasr period, *i.e.*, sometime between 3200 and 2900 BC, a period of rising prosperity.

For China, similar estimates, although less reliable, can be made by referring to its prehistoric culture as outlined in chapter 31. The size of settlements of the Dawenkou culture that preceded the Longshan civilization were small, no more than a few hundred persons, and incremental increases in medical knowledge prior to the rise of Longshan culture cities is inconceivable. There is scholarly opinion, however, that the Dawenkou period (4100-2600 BC) represented a formative step in developing the Longshan culture, and the Longshan culture is considered by many to be the principal begetter of Han China, the era of early unification and the Yellow Emperor. The earliest acquisition of medical knowledge has traditional and legendary ties with Longshan culture. Furthermore, the Iron Age Yueshi culture that replaced the Shandong Longshan culture has been clearly associated with a pronounced cultural decline. Thus, both demographically and intellectually the earliest collection of medical wisdom is unlikely to predate 2600 BC Longshan culture, and for reasons mentioned previously unlikely to postdate 2200 BC, the onset of decline of the Longshan culture. It is proposed that these four centuries are the window of time during which a few generations of medical practitioners began to work together as a nascent profession. Legend would be more specific and place its origins before and up to the time of the Yellow Emperor, *i.e.,* 2600-2400 BC. It would have been a time of commercial prosperity and growth in Liangchengzhen before political classes and elite kinships became powerful.

---

[44] They may not have been free as individuals, but, beginning with medieval guilds, venues for artists in training, for exhibiting and selling their works of art, and by virtue of these organizations to exchange ideas. The importance of guilds and patronage is discussed in vol. 1 of this work and recently received scholarly attention in: *Encyclopedia of Social Networks*, Los Angeles, 2011, G. A. Barnett, editor (see *Artists Communities*, p. 57*ff.*).

Parallel changes in the Indus River civilization exist but are unfortunately even more vague. The Early Harappan period (3300-2600 BC) was for the most part a time of villages that progressed to city-states during the Mature Harappan period. Given the sequence of social changes, an argument can be posed that a window of time for the original collection of medical wisdom transmitted through the classical clinical medicine texts in India could well have been a sequence of generations sometime during the years of the Mature Harappan culture (2600-1900 BC) of the Indus River civilization. The Vedas are often dated prior to 2000 BC, and many agree that a primitive and an as yet undeciphered Indus River script was in use at that time. It was during this period of growing population and commercial prosperity in Mohenjo-daro (or an equivalent size city-state), *ca.* 2600-2300 BC, that medical insights would have been gained and reputation established within the city that would later be interpreted and incorporated into the Atharva Veda.

In summary, it is proposed that the origin of all the classic medical writings of antiquity did not gradually emerge over the ages from this or that great civilization in this or that region now identified with modern nations. Their origins instead are to be found in ancient city-states that had few or no ties with preceding or subsequent civilizations. Their origins are not related to a race, ethnic group, or beloved national identity. They are, instead, somehow related to a system of governance, in all instances the product of a relatively autonomous and generally prosperous commercial city-state. This, of course, is consistent with the situation that existed in ancient Greece and the city-state of Miletos. In a word, they were related to governance that supported or ignored rather than interfered with commercial ventures, thereby promoting population growth, stability, prosperity, a middle class, and options for specialization of services. A window of opportunity appeared as early cities spontaneously attempted to establish order in their polity through a process now called "settlement hierarchy." At this time social complexity increased as newly created special interest groups burst into being to support the growing city. This should not be surprising, for, as expressed in *Why Liberty*: "Spontaneous order: it is common for people to assume that all order must be the product of an ordering mind, but the most important kinds of order in society are not the results of conscious planning or design, but emerge from the voluntary interaction and mutual adjustments of plans of free persons acting on the basis of their rights."[45]

H. The Five Successful and the Twelve Lesser Civilizations Compared

All seventeen civilizations discussed in this volume have now been characterized by nineteen criteria. The features common to all twelve of the lesser civilizations and to the five "successful" civilization, are demographic, commercial, chronological, and social structure at both the municipal (central) and village (peripheral) components. Table 15, pp. 622-623, includes features of Table 13, p. 539, so that sixteen characteristics of all seventeen "civilizations" are displayed and can conveniently be compared. Consult the author's unabridged version of *The Natural State of Medical Practice: Escape from Egalitarianism* for a more extensive discussion of differences between the five successful and the twelve unsuccessful civilizations/proto-civilizations.

---

[45] See: Palmer, T. G., *The History and Structure of Libertarian Thought*, in *Why Liberty?*, Ottawa (Illinois), 2013, edited by Tom G. Palmer, p. 32.

The following statistical analysis, an abridgment of Appendix A of *The Natural State of Medical Practice: Escape from Egalitarianism*, based as it is on acknowledged but presently unavoidable uncertainties, is subject to arbitrary definitions, approximations, and interpretations. Arguably, therefore, much of the data might be considered unworthy of statistical analysis. This is one reason for the simple statistical tests applied; complex tests are unmerited. As a result, all statistical conclusions come *caveat emptor*. "Successful" refers to those five civilizations, each represented by an archetypal city of their age, that are presumed to have had networks of medical practitioners whose knowledge is, in part, found in ancient medical classics. "Unsuccessful" refers to the twelve lesser civilizations arbitrarily chosen for reasons cited herein, but from whom no known medical presence emerged. That distinction is used only in this Appendix. The term "lesser," used elsewhere in this volume, was retained because it reflects the "null hypothesis" status of those civilizations before it was known that they had no medical presence. As this volume approaches its conclusion, we now know. Numbers and some "p" values have been rounded to 2 places for convenience. Tests used were the two-tailed Z-test (Z) for comparing two population proportions and the two-tailed Student's t-test for differences between two independent samples (S). All values are drawn from Table 15 (pp. 622-623).

a. Size of central population
Difference (S):   Significant, $p < 0.01$
Conclusion: Central populations were significantly larger, on average, in the successful civilizations. And if a Z-test is used to assess the proportion of successful vs. unsuccessful civilizations using both size (> or < than 20,000) and presence or absence of heterarchy, the level of significance is unchanged.

b. Size of central population of those identified as city-states
Difference (S):   Not significant, $p = 0.1$
Conclusion: There was no statistically significant difference in size of representative polities between the five successful and those six unsuccessful civilizations identified as city-states: Marajoara, Anasazi (Chaco Canyon), Cahokia, Sharh-i Sokhta, Djenne-Djenno and Liangzhu. The following conclusion can be drawn: it is possible but unlikely that the success of the five successful city-state civilizations can be solely attributed to the size of their urban centers.

c. Population density, excluding suspect values
Difference (S):   Not significant, $p = .8$
Conclusion: Population density shows no association with successful civilizations. Inadequate data exclude the Anasazi, Poverty Point and Cahokia civilizations from the calculations (Pueblo Bonito of Anasazi being too small, Poverty Point not being urbanized, Cahokia because of extensive central ritual areas), although all the estimates are crude and of suspect validity.

Table 15: Parameters for Comparative Analysis of the 17 Civilizations Discussed in Text.

	MILETOS[1]	URUK	HIERAKON-POLIS	MOHENJO-DARO	LIANG-CHENG-ZHEN	MARA-JOARA	NORTE CHICO	CUC-TRY
OPULATION F OLIS, AXIMUM	65,000	50,000	10,000	40,000	50.000	10,000	3,000 CARAL SUPE	20,0
OPULATION EGEMONY	200,000	1,000,000	105,000	70,000	70,000	100,000	20,000	?
RIMARY AREA	1 SQ. MI.	2.3 SQ. MI.	0.5 SQ. MI.	1.6 SQ. MI.	1 SQ. MI.	0.2 SQ. MI. OSCAMUTINS	0.3 SQ.MI. CARAL SUPE	1 SQ.
OVERNANCE AY-TO-DAY	HETER-ARCHY	CORPOR-ATISM, HETER-ARCHY	HETER-ARCHY	HETER-ARCHY, CORPOR-ATISM	HETER-ARCHY, CORPOR-ATISM	HETER-ARCHY	HETER-ARCHY, CORPOR-ATISM	KIN HIE ARC
ROMINENT GALITARIAN INSHIPS[3]	NO	NO	NO	YES, BUT NOT IN POLIS	NO EVIDENCE SO FAR	YES,[2] ON INHABITED MOUNDS	YES,[2] IN VILLAGES	YES NEI HOC
RITING	YES	YES	YES	PROBABLE	POSSIBLE	NO	NO	NO
ONUMENTS	YES	YES	NO	NO	NO	NO	YES	NO
ENOUEMENT	RAZED	SUB-SUMED	SUBSUMED	DECLINED	SUBSUMED	DECLINED	NOT KNOWN	NOT KNC
EDICINE	YES	YES	YES	?	?		NO	NO
ORMATIVE ERIOD	250 YEARS	900 YEARS	1200 YEARS	700 YEARS	500 YEARS	1,200 YEARS	900 YEARS	900 YEA
LORUIT	300 YEARS	550 YEARS	400 YEARS	600 YEARS	500 YEARS	500 YEARS (900-1400 AD)	800 YEARS	1,00 YEA
ITY-STATE	YES	YES	YES	YES	YES	YES	NO	NO(
EAN AGE AT EATH OR LIFE XPECTANCY	N.A.[4]	31 YEARS	28 YEARS - COMMONERS	35 YEARS - BETTER OFF	N.A.	N.A.	N.A.	N.A
ERIOD	LATE ARCHAIC	LATE NEO-LITHIC, BRONZE	LATE NEOLITHIC	BRONZE AGE	LATE NEOLITHIC	PRE-COLUMBIAN	PRE-CERAMIC	NEC ENE
RCHEOLOGIC L GALITARIAN`	NO	NO	NO (ELITE BURIALS)	YES	YES	YES	YES	YES
OPULATION ENSITY	100/ACRE	33/ACRE	31/ACRE	39/ACRE	78/ACRE	78/ACRE	20/ACRE	45/A

[1] The first five columns contain features of the "successful" primary civilizations and the remainder are the lesser ones. Because of fluctuating characteristics over time, archeological uncertainties, approximations in dates, and disparities in data as presented by different scholars, the dates and statuses in this Table must be considered crude estimates as interpreted by the author from an extensive review of scholarly literature.

[2] Persistent kinship control of individual life affected mostly those who had no large geographically contiguous central population or whose central population was a temple or ritual elite.

[3] Includes extended families, clans, tribes, chiefdoms.

[4] Data unavailable.

	POVERTY POINT	CAHOKIA	TERRA-MARE	CATAL-HOYUK	SIN-TASHTA	SHAHR-I-SOKHTA	DJENNE-DJENNO	LIANG-ZHU
	1000-3000	20,000	6,000	8,000	1,000	20,000	50,000	30,000
NY	? - MANY VILLAGES	? 40,000	150,000	8,000	20,000 20 TOWNS	?	50,000	200,000
	1.4 SQ. MI.	6 SQ. MI.	0.1 SQ. MI. (LARGE)	0.15 SQ. MI.	5 ACRES	0.5 SQ. MI.	0.15 SQ. MI.	4 SQ. MI.
Y	HETERARCHY	CORPOR-ATISM	CORPOR-ATISM	KINSHIP HIERARCHY	CORPOR-ATISM	HETERARCHY CORPOR-ATISM	HETER-ARCHY	KINSHIP HIERARCHY
	YES,[2] IN VILLAGES	YES, NESTING KINSHIPS	YES,[2] IN NEIGH-BORHOODS	YES, NEIGH-BORHOODS	YES, NEIGH-BORHOODS	KINSHIP NEIGHBOR-HOODS	YES,[2] ON INHABITED MOUNDS	YES, ELITE KINSHIPS
	NO	NO	NO	NO	NO	POSSIBLE	NO	NO
	YES	YES	NO	NO	NO	NO	NO	NO
	DECLINED	FLOODING	VACATED	VACATED	VACATED	DECLINED	VACATED	?
	NO	NO	NO	NO	NO	POSSIBLE	NO	NO
	500 YEARS	400 YEARS	?	500 YEARS	?	600 YEARS	750 YEARS	500 YEARS
	1,000 YEARS	400 YEARS	300 YEARS (1450 TO 1150 BC)	1,200 YEARS	400 YEARS	600 YEARS	600 YEARS	750 YEARS
	NO	YES	YES, LATE	NO	NO	YES	YES	YES
E	N.A.	31 YEARS, IF SURVIVE INFANCY	40 YEARS, MINIMUM ESTIMATE	32 YEARS	"FEW" ELDERLY, 28 YEARS	FEW OVER FORTY YEARS	31 YEARS, POOR DATA	N.A.
	LATE ARCHAIC	LATE WOODLAND	BRONZE AGE	NEO-LITHIC	BRONZE AGE	MIDDLE BRONZE AGE	HISTORIC AFRICAN	LATE NEOLITHIC
	NO (MONUMENT)	NO (TEMPLES)	YES	YES	YES	YES	YES	NO
	3/ACRE	5/ACRE	40/ACRE	80/ACRE	200/ACRE	62/ACRE	50/ACRE	12/ACRE

    d.   Presence of city-state status

Difference (Z):   Significant, p = 0.01

Conclusion: There was a significant correlation between city-state status, as defined herein, and a successful civilization status, *i.e.,* being a city-state improved the chances of a civilization becoming successful. In fairness, however, the present definition of "city-state" is very broad. The excluded civilizations were Cucuteni-Trypillia and Catalhoyuk (no commercial interaction with surrounding communities), Sintashta and Terramare (no networks of interdependent peripheral villages), and Poverty Point, Norte Chico and Djenne-Djenno (no evidence of central coordination of commercial operations with peripheral communities).

    e.   Presence of monumental structures (commonly attributed to hierarchical authoritarian governance)

Difference (Z):   Not significant, p = 0.8

Conclusion: There is no significance difference in the erection of monumental structures between successful and unsuccessful civilizations (includes massive functional constructions, shrines, and temples).

    f.   Presence of writing

Difference (Z):   Significant, $p = {} < 0.01$

Conclusion: There is a significant association between the successful civilizations and proven evidence of writing, a significance that persists ($p = .02$) even if Sharh-i Sokhta in the "unsuccessful" grouping is credited with a form of writing. But if it is confirmed that the "inscriptions" found on oracle bones from the Longshan era and on seals in Mojendo-daro constitute early writing the association will be even more significant.

    g.   Medical practice and egalitarian kinship in nuclear populations

Significance (Z):   Significant, $p = {} < .01$

Conclusion: There is no statistically significant association of a formal medical practice with prominent plebeian egalitarian kinships. "Not egalitarian" describes Miletos, Uruk, Hierakonpolis, Mohenjo-daro, and Liangchengzhen. The latter two are classified as "not egalitarian" based on more circumstantial grounds, but even if they are excluded from the calculation the p value remains $< .01$.

    h.   Archeological egalitarianism

Significance (Z):   Not significant; p = 0.49

Conclusion: Traditional archeological findings associated with the designation of "egalitarian" (from inhumations, dwellings, absence of monumental structures, no inner walls for elites) do not significantly differ between the successful and unsuccessful civilizations described in this work.

    i.   Egalitarian kinship (*i.e.,* strong kinship presence in the centralized population)

Significance (Z):   Significant; $p < 0.01$

Conclusion: There is a strongly positive correlation between prominent egalitarian social groupings and the unsuccessful civilizations. This refers to centralized populations rather than peripheral settlements where kinship ties would be expected to persist. The exceptions in the unsuccessful group are the Sintashta civilization (status uncertain; could be solely corporatism) and Poverty Point (role of the central population regarding peripheral villages is uncertain, although all the riverside villages in the region would have their own egalitarian kinship management). Liangzhu has been included even though the egalitarian aspect of egalitarian kinship may have decreased as a dominant kinship claimed political control. Shahr-i Sokhta was included because the city neighborhoods may have been kinship enclaves.

j.   Association of egalitarian kinship with writing
Significance (Z):   Significant; $p < .01$
Conclusion: The invention of writing is statistically unassociated with egalitarian kinships. Mohenjo-daro and Liangchengzhen are not included among the nonegalitarian civilizations because of the circumstantial nature of the existence of writing.

k.   Importance of heterarchy
Significance (Z):   Marginally significant; $p = 0.05$
Conclusion: Heterarchy, in this case meaning municipal guidance mediated primarily through commercial interests, is likely to be a significant contributor to the success of a civilization. Reworded, the absence of heterarchy is significantly associated with unsuccessful civilizations (level of significance is unchanged). But when applied just to larger civilizations (10,000 or more) the level of significance ($p = 0.06$) is not improved. By disassociating heterarchy from size, this suggests heterarchy is at best a permissive rather than a contributing variable to "success."

l.   Importance of the duration of the FORMATIVE PERIOD
Significance (S):   Not significant; $p = 0.31$
Conclusion: The length of the FORMATIVE PERIOD (from early established settlement to a flourishing polity with population growth) is unlikely to be related to development of a successful civilization.

m.   Importance of the duration of the FLORUIT PERIOD
Significance (S):   Not significant, $p = 0.18$
Conclusion: It is unlikely that a longer duration of a civilization's flourishing period (growing or sustained prospering of a central population) will contribute to the success of a civilization if it has not happened within the first few centuries.

n.   Writing and population size
Significance (S):   Significant; $p = 0.05$
Conclusion: Writing, in this small sample, is marginally associated with a larger population. "Successful" in this context indicates the presence of writing. Mohenjo-daro and Liangchengzhen are excluded because of circumstantial nature of their "writing."

o. Writing and FLORUIT

Significance (S): Not significant; p = 0.18

Conclusion: Writing, in this small sample, is not significantly associated with duration of a prospering and growing polity.

p. Writing and egalitarianism

Significance (Z): Significant; p < .01

Conclusion: In this calculation neither Mohenjo-daro nor Liangchengzhen is included as having a form of writing, although Dr. Paola DeMatte considers the Longshan culture of China to have had "incipient forms of writing." The p-value indicates a significant association between nonegalitarian societies and the development of writing.

q. Prominent commercial activity

Significance (Z) Not significant; p = 0.33

Conclusion: Commercial activity as a prominent social feature was not significantly different between successful and unsuccessful civilizations. Excluded from the "unsuccessful" category were Cucuteni-Trypillia and Catalhoyuk, neither of which had evidence of commercially significant external trade. It is concluded that commerce alone is insufficient stimulus for a civilization to progress.

r. Writing and a network of medical practitioners, the latter being considered "successful"

Significance (Z) Significant; p < 0.01

Conclusion: Writing is strongly associated with "progress" as identified in this work by evidence of a network of medical practitioners, excluding two (Mohenjo-daro and Liangchengzhen), both with limited evidence of writing.

s. Writing and commerce

Significance (Z) Not significant; p = 0.48

Conclusion: Writing was found only in civilizations/proto-civilizations with a commercial base, but, with only two having no such base, the quality of any statistical result is poor. Nevertheless, there is no significant difference. The association of medical practice with commerce would give the same statistical result.

The following is a list of the more relevant conclusions that can be drawn from the cursory statistical analysis of data presented above:

1. Central populations were significantly larger in five successful city-state civilizations, but not significantly larger than the six unsuccessful city-state civilizations.
2. Population density showed no significant association with a successful civilization.
3. There was significant association between city-state status and a successful civilization.
4. Archeological egalitarianism was similar in successful and unsuccessful civilizations.
5. There was a strong association between a prominent egalitarian kinship presence and the absence of a medical network (*i.e.*, the "unsuccessful" civilizations).
6. Heterarchy was marginally associated with the successful civilizations.

7. The lengths of both the FORMATIVE and the FLORUIT periods were unassociated with a successful civilization.

8. Commerce/distant trade: similarly present in successful and unsuccessful civilizations.

9. Writing and medical practitioners were each unassociated with egalitarian kinships.

10. Writing was not significantly associated with FLORUIT duration.

As a final comment, many attributes of the lesser, or "unsuccessful," primary civilizations are shared by the successful primary civilizations. Important is the fact that many of these factors might have been thought to be significant, but now have been determined not to be. In other words, by excluding things like total population, durability of the civilization, and extensive trade as factors determining the ultimate social fate of the twelve lesser civilizations/proto-civilizations, the negative association between "egalitarian kinship" and progress gains logical strength, if not statistical power.

CHAPTER THIRTY-FIVE

EGALITARIANISM

Egalitarianism is closely examined because its effects are greatest in that segment of ancient populations from which medical practitioners arose, the plebeian (commoner) class. Definitions of egalitarianism are discussed, with social egalitarianism as a practical answer to social organization in early/primitive societies. With permanent settlements, selected archeological characteristics have been the means by which scholars recognize egalitarian communities. As the mechanism by which an egalitarian social organization was usually selected, Maslow's system of motivational hierarchy is discussed. The primal levels of the hierarchy, survival and safety, are personal motivations and considered irrelevant to egalitarianism. But now the "need to belong" motivation comes into play as each member attempts to adapt to or modify the behavior of others to accommodate his or her own behavioral preferences. Differences of opinion are presented so as to attract others to a particular opinion, and at some point the more forcefully impelled or popularly held opinion restricts opposing ones. Thus, a seemingly democratic result can, in the hands of the majority of the society, shut down completely all alternatives. Motivation can be stifled. But egalitarianism decreases as trade promotes urbanization, prosperity, and population growth. Urbanization, a consequence of commercial ventures, weakens kinship allegiances and provides a window of opportunity for individuals and families to break free.

A. What is Egalitarianism?

It is necessary at the outset to define egalitarianism as it might be considered to have existed in early or primitive societies. Egalitarianism, being a popular and adversarial issue in modern times, has led to categories of egalitarianism that are unlikely to have existed in premodern societies. As an example, "luck egalitarianism" is based on the premise that it is wrong for some people to have less than others because of misfortune not of their own making. Society is therefore obligated to correct this by redistribution of goods and resources. Isonomia is the basis for "legal egalitarianism," where equality before the law is the issue. Other categories of egalitarianism include gender, racial, and economic. But it is hard to imagine that premodern societies would have identified race, gender, economic status, class distinctions, or codified laws as discussable issues when deciding distribution of effort or products of that effort. Those societies were small and their principal adversaries were the physical environment and their own ignorance. The morality of their redistribution of effort and products of that effort was not an issue, or if it was it was overshadowed by the necessities of daily life. For these reasons the definition of egalitarianism will be minimalist, indicating the focus is on its implementation more than explanation and on its consequences more than validation.

Archeological studies of prehistoric populations frequently identify a community with a common lifestyle expressed in similar dwellings, appurtenances, luxury goods, and burial practices lacking affluence as being egalitarian in that there appears to have been no privileged class, family, or person. The term is also applied to most primitive hunter-gatherer societies who possess little of a private nature. It is often assumed these egalitarian venues indicate a society's desire for equality among its members, an equality that includes access to food, to comforts, and to a voice in group decisions. The efforts of men and women in procuring daily necessities are also considered equally shared, although childbearing and physical size and strength guarantee gender inequality in tasks. Group decisions are made by common consent. It is furthermore often assumed that egalitarianism in a society has been chosen by its members because it seemed to be a good way to live together in harmony.

Egalitarianism is especially important to the origin of medical practice for its effects are most pronounced on plebeians, and it is from the plebeian class that medical practitioners arise. It is for this reason, unfair as it seems, that monarchies, priesthoods, and other elite groups are mentioned but little in Part II except as objects of criticism. It would be otherwise if the elite political classes were the source of societal progress, but they instead supply the abusers of that segment of society which is the source of progress, bent on keeping their privileged status by preventing the plebeian in seeking his.

It may, of course, be inappropriate to designate any ancient primitive society as "egalitarian." The ethical implications of the term in modern minds implies a purposeful selection from a collection of different philosophical lifestyle choices. This obviously did not happen, for prehistoric populations had no political history from which to make a choice. In fact, the similarity in choice of population management used by most primitive societies, a choice regarded as "egalitarian," was probably followed by them in part because it was their human nature as families to do so, guided by practical considerations of survival and security. The grouping in clans and tribes also was probably a further response to the latter two concerns. One sociological sequence in complexity specifies an initial phase in which "egalitarian" bands or tribes are based on kinship reciprocity with equal access to resources, a second phase that includes only the system of redistribution of egalitarianism now managed without threat of force by hereditary elites (chiefdoms), and the ultimate phase, a stratified society with "unequal access to basic resources" supported by threat of force and exploitation. Placed in juxtaposition with the proposed alternatives, a harmonious and stabilizing egalitarianism seems quite a tempting lifestyle.

A reason for the modern popularity of egalitarianism is its presumed pacific nature. Evidence against this assumption, however, is plentiful (see excursus on Australian aborigines, p. 595). But even if egalitarianism were inherently pacific, if a warlike society appeared on the scene, the peaceful society will be quickly eliminated.[1] The Society of Friends and other pacific groups and sects can be admired in the West and have the benefits ascribed to being "conscientious objectors" because they are protected by Western democracies, their pacific nature unthreatened. But should authoritarian political forces continue to centralize power within democracies around the globe, those groups will quickly disappear once they have been declared expendable.

There also has been much scholarly investigation into lifestyles of primitive bands and tribes, both extant and historic, and support for the notion of caring and altruistic societies capable of surviving on their own is lacking. Whether it be longevity, harmonious rapport, care for the elderly and infirm, or pacific interaction with outsiders, anecdotes inconsistent with a congenial and caring egalitarian society abound to the point of being cliche.[2] The importance of geronticide as a solution to those whose age or

---

[1] It is not denied that a well-run hierarchical state can tolerate and protect egalitarian groups as well as oppositional views. In the United States the Quakers and other pacific groups and sects are protected and admired, but in most other historical settings their separate identity and existence would have been short-lived.

[2] Classic works such as that of Sir James Frazer (*The Golden Bough: A Study in Comparative Religion*, ultimately in twelve volumes, 1906-1915) and of Joseph Campbell (*The Masks of God*,

infirmity are deemed deleterious to the band or tribe is an example of egalitarian thinking that finds its equivalent in discussions of modern medical practice. One must, therefore, doubt whether egalitarianism as fairness or a moral concept ever entered the mind of either ancient or contemporary primitive people whose survival was focused on a coordinated and physically capable membership to withstand the threats of an unforgiving environment. It must have been more important that as many as possible of a group's membership be prepared for the next day's sally with Nature, and if a lucky catch by one member permitted a personal feast while other members went hungry, there could be unpleasant repercussions. Others propose egalitarian social practices originated not from innate tendencies of generosity or fairness but from the fact that bands could not travel with surplus food, and so it was distributed to all as needed rather than wasting it. In other words, a practical reason for sharing, an amoral rather than moral basis for what superficially might be termed egalitarianism, may better explain its pervasiveness. If this is correct, then modern definitions of egalitarianism are irrelevant, for they carry the baggage of philosophy and morality that probably did not exist for primitives.

It is, therefore, not possible to accurately define the egalitarianism practiced by ancient societies, although it has been thoroughly parsed for modern primitive ones. Perhaps archeological evidence has been misinterpreted and presumed egalitarian ancient societies were not so. Certain cities as well as nomadic bands called egalitarian are so utterly distinct that their forms of egalitarianism must also be distinctive. It has been pointed out, therefore, that direct evidence of egalitarianism in large ancient societies is nonexistent, mostly being an assumption based on negative evidence, *i.e.*, archeological studies revealing no evidence of a nonegalitarian society. But what is called egalitarian may mask powerful but unexpressed internal forces regulating community behavior by means of secret knowledge such as shamanism. Dr. Keith Otterbein maintained that even among hunter-gatherers there was no such thing as egalitarianism, that threat and mental or physical coercion was present and was guided by a hierarchy of power even though there was no named headman.[3] For present purposes the following characteristics, in whole or in part and in line with current scholarly opinion, will be used to objectively identify a prehistoric society as "archeologically egalitarian:"

1. No differential wealth present in burials, within dwellings or in architecture
2. No monumental structures
3. No distinctive longer-lived population
4. No separate habitation district based on class
5. Absence of militarization and of defensive barriers

As an unqualified "egalitarianism" in present context is meaningless because so many qualifiers have been attached to the word, for present purposes the term as applied to early societies will be qualified and either stated or implied as "social egalitarian." This melds into an egalitarian ethos the position, duties, and responsibilities a member has to other members in his society regardless of his personal preferences, for redistribution comes with a price. It is a reminder that egalitarianism is always coercive, and therefore but another expression of authoritarianism. Even though egalitarianism is now commonly

---

four volumes, 1959-1968) include plentiful anecdotes of often bizarre or grotesque practices from ancient and primitive societies. And see p. 605*f* for end of life care of elderly in primitive societies.
[3] See: Otterbein, K., *How War Began*, College Station (TX), 2004, especially p. 77, the section on The Myth of the Egalitarian Band.

used in describing economic redistribution, it includes within its tenets enforcement in the production of products that are to be distributed.

B. The Source of Primitive Egalitarianism

What might have been the pragmatic cause of ancient lifestyles now declared to be egalitarian? Was it merely a matter of familiarity with a social pattern followed by parents and grandparents to which there was no experience with an alternative? Perhaps it was a result of understanding the vagaries of human nature, that some persons could disrupt a tenuous lifestyle to the detriment of the group as a whole by actions that exceeded a communal norm, or perhaps it was a matter of like and dislike of personalities that considered themselves superior to the rest of their society, an inherent psychological antipathy to hubris.[4] An interesting recent theory proposes that nomadic hunter-gatherer bands began with a hierarchical structure. This seems logical in that families are not naturally egalitarian, and consanguineal kinship provides the basic structure for most hunter-gatherer bands. But the level of intolerance in small bands for unequal access to food or other resources is such that there develops a "counter-dominant mentality" that renders the troupe egalitarian, or, if there is a leader, reverse dominance allows the troupe to dominate the leader so as to render the troupe coercively egalitarian.[5] Or was it a matter of communal efficiency intended to combat daily vicissitudes of primitive life by minimizing need and waste and avoiding excesses? A "scattered and unpredictable" sustenance as the origin of coercive egalitarianism has been proposed because it is the "leveling mechanism" of success and failure, something bordering on "luck egalitarianism" that prevents undue accumulation of power in any one person. In this scenario, egalitarianism, while temporarily essential to survival, will be shed to some degree when predictable sustenance becomes available.[6] In other words, egalitarianism could be good in situations that threaten survival. But what if egalitarianism itself is inescapable?

A tendency for humans to form groups is important to progress, for by forming groups there is more interface of ideas and a greater ability to act on them. Indeed, the essence of Part I series was the critical role of the small group of autonomous individuals pursuing a common goal of self-interest, the "koinon," in promoting progress within a society. Why, then, did hunter-gatherer groups not promptly come upon novel ways to improve their lives, instead persisting in a way of life that was unceasingly arduous and dangerous, sometimes for thousands of years?

It may be relevant that there appears to be an optimal group size for decision-making. For example, some suggest six to eight people is optimal, for beyond that number the frequency of social interactions increases exponentially and the time permitted each member to present his or her thoughts decreases. Egalitarian bands on average have fewer than fifty members. Thus, the band might be considered more amenable to good ideas

---

[4] See: Zaluski, W., *The Psychological Bases of Primitive Egalitarianism: Reflections on Human Political Nature*, in *The Emergence of Normative Orders*, Krakow, 2016, J. Stelmach et al., editors, pp. 83-106.
[5] See: Boehm, C., *Egalitarian Behavior and Reverse Dominance Hierarchy*, in *Current Anthropology*, 34:227-254, 1993.
[6] See: Cashdan, E. A., *Egalitarianism Among Hunters and Gatherers*, in *American Anthropologist*, 82:116-120, 1980.

than the tribe or clan that operate more on the level of subgroup interactions rather than individual ones, with quite different consequences. There is, however, no evidence of this, as neither band nor clan is, over time, associated with any improvement in the primitive state. Thus, the size of an egalitarian society seems unrelated to this outcome. Another factor for consideration is disruptive behavior. Within hunter-gatherer groups antisocial behavior by an individual might be met with force, either physical or by public ostracism. But as population size increases, overt social pathology is less effectively recognized and managed. The larger the group the more likely it has the potential for this disruption embedded within it. While it is unknown how many early/primitive societies, ranging in size from bands to tribes and clans, were brought to an end by internal dissention, the issue again is improvement in their primitive state. And again, increasing size of population is not an obvious determinant for improvement, for if larger size favored progress the world would have been populated with cities far earlier than has happened.[7] Thus, the persistence of an egalitarian social structure and the tardy devolvement of urbanization cannot be attributed to a surfeit of good ideas. The absence of change within egalitarian groups is, instead, associated with the *absence* of good ideas. The answer seems obvious: something about egalitarianism itself is inimical to the interface of ideas. The proliferation and persistence of small egalitarian groups is not a consequence of intelligence or of wise decision-making.

In volume 1 of the unabridged version of this work it is stated: "This opportunity [to compromise] is diminished further by a finite earthly existence during which cumulative experience is seen through a myopic lens: each generation feels justified, even compelled, to reinvent the wheel and considers itself especially favored by new ideas to forego the old ones." Given the short life expectancy of ancient/primitive populations and their narrow institutional memory in populations where children rarely knew a grandparent and frequently did not know their biological parents it is a safe assumption that egalitarianism was not carried forward generation after generation because of custom. Instead, it is likely that the same social organization was utilized century after century based on contemporary circumstances. What was the overweening circumstance?

As the most basic level of motivating factors listed by Maslow in his "hierarchy of needs" is a threat to survival, perhaps ancient egalitarianism finds its roots there.[8] The

---

[7] If the disruption is not sociopathic but instead is just a matter of justifiably contentious issues or rivalry between peers for leadership, the band can split, each contender taking with him his allies. This is probably the reason for the innumerable small hamlets and individual domiciles scattered throughout some prehistoric, primarily Bronze Age, regions of the world discussed in section C of this chapter. It may have seemed wiser to exist in a small group with single leadership than a larger group in which desire for leadership prompted grounds for contention and discord that could affect all members of the group.

[8] In 1943 Maslow (*A Theory of Human Motivation*, in *Psychological Review*, 50:370-396) put forth his hierarchy of needs as the basis for personal and societal motivation. Some of his ideas and observations were obtained from studies of "primitive" modern societies. His five-tiered hierarchy listed physiological survival as the most basic motivational force, followed by security, belonging, esteem, and self-realization, in that order, and the more basic need(s) had to be satisfied before moving on a less basic ones. Endless parsing of his scheme has followed over the years, but most criticism has been directed at the upper, less basic, tiers (see, for example, Kenrick, D. T., et al., *Renovating the Pyramid of Needs: Contemporary Extensions Built Upon Ancient Foundations*, in *Perspectives on Psychological Science*, 5:292-314, 2010). As the present subject matter concerns prehistoric man, the Maslow hierarchy will be used as a basic reference on motivational factors for the ancient societies discussed herein. Walter Rostow (*The Five States of Economic Growth*,

communal enforcement of sharing, if the small society overcame "scattered and unpredictable" threats to survival and were healthier because of that sharing, would be conducive to survival. And the second most powerful basic motivational factor is security, and personal security might have been promoted by belonging to a larger group, a band or tribe.[9] Thus might be explained the apparent affinity in primitive society for egalitarianism and then tribal membership; the need for survival was fulfilled by egalitarian behavior and the need for security by tribal affiliation. But this is an error.

It is here argued that the need for survival and security was fulfilled not by purposeful egalitarian behavior; it was fulfilled by common sense. It is inappropriate to infer a planned political motivation to such basic behavior in which choice is no issue. There was no intention to prevent or erase inequality *per se*; the need was to meet threats to survival.[10] Maslow's most basic elements of his hierarchy of needs were survival and security. They are personal motivating factors and therefore are identical attributes in all individuals; if survival as an independent individual or family unit was unlikely, then egalitarianism was, in a sense, not a matter of choice.

It is the next level that is problematic. Matters now become complicated in that each member of a society becomes subject to the organizational structure of the society inasmuch as he or she has voluntarily exchanged some degree of individual liberty for group security. And it is here that the third, and yet "primitive," level of motivating factors from Maslow's hierarchy of needs comes into play, and that is the desire to belong, to be one of a group. The issue is no longer survival and safety, these having already been transcended in that the larger society can now maintain its existence. It is at the third level of motivation where the intellectual basis and modulator of ancient egalitarianism can be found.

The desire to belong invokes issues not found in the desire to survive and to be secure. The nature of interactions with others varies from the productive and pleasant to the destructive and hateful. In a society the latter must be controlled to protect the other members of that society. The means employed is egalitarianism. Its essence is to control.

Egalitarianism is related to the desire to belong, to belong to a group, but implicit in this is that the group be socially acceptable to the individual joining it or deciding to remain in it. There is considerable modern discussion of the merits and demerits of such a scheme in large modern societies, but they may not be relevant to ancient, and perhaps primitive, small societies where, for example, one disrupter out of fifty members is controllable, whereas one million out of fifty million in a modern society is controlled with great difficulty. A large population thereby ensures that coercion will be needed from a central authority, the State, but a small population such as a band or tribe can function as a committee of the whole in pressuring an individual to act in accordance with customary behavior even when it is against that individual's personal interests, or else

---

Cambridge (UK), 1960) also provided a nuanced theory of societal evolution, but the focus of the present work is more basic: a free society contrasted with an authoritarian one.

[9] An inconsistency in this statement is that personal security would be expected to include one's health, and yet not one of the twelve lesser civilizations examined in chapter 8 left evidence of a medical presence even though the average age at death was in the low to mid-30s.

[10] The factor of personal attachment is not addressed here, but this has nothing to do with egalitarian behavior.

depart.[11] Some degree of coercion seems reasonable and at times unavoidable, given the range of personalities in any human society, in order that society be not critically disrupted. And is it not but realistic that a person be agreeable to some personal limitations if those limitations improve the status of the society that might redound to his or her personal benefit? But it may not be a wise trade-off. This is not an issue that a primitive or ancient band or tribe is likely to have addressed, for there would have been no knowledge of consequences of the coerciveness of egalitarianism over the long run, no knowledge of other forms of social organization, and no concept of progress as a means of permanent improvement of society. Egalitarian coercion was an immediate solution to an immediate problem in the same way that parenteral coercion is to raising young children. It is only in light of knowledge accumulated over time that we can now look back and judge the consequences of that early form of egalitarianism. One thing is certain. The basis for the adoption of egalitarianism by each generation of ancient or primitive "egalitarian" societies was not prior knowledge of it or its consequences except for that form of egalitarianism within which existing members came of age. In the dangerous world of the Neolithic, were a form of governance to be found unsatisfactory, none would have survived to implant that information into local lore that could be transmitted orally from generation to generation.

Under all the layers of interactions that make up human society, the primary cause for social egalitarianism was, and is, to control the disrupter, the person not like you. In the small group the disruptor is an individual; in large groups the disruptor is the small group. In a nation the disruptor is the large group, the party or movement. And it is the tragedy of egalitarianism that the coercion that restrains the disruptor includes in its pattern of restraint the innovator, the sentinel, and the protester as well as those who would do harm. And there is always the possibility that the disruptor may be right. It follows that efforts to suppress the disruptor will suppress innovation and options for social change. There are other arguments against egalitarian systems, including the philosophy that taking something from someone and giving it to someone else is immoral, an issue for later discussion. But the perspective here is different: it is not one of ethics or of material gain or loss; it is one of restriction of choice.

Egalitarian systems were rendered acceptable to members of bands and clans not because they were good systems but because the only option was leaving the security of the group. But, if they did leave, their new social structure was preferably small. If the environment was relatively safe for an individual or family, living in individual units or hamlets was preferred, as was done during much of the Bronze Age (*ca.* 3200-600 BC) across Europe and the British Isles. This was possible because the immediate environment permitted the family or extended family a degree of safety with arable land and animal domestication sufficient for survival. There were no large population centers such as were occasionally found in the Neolithic era. The early settlements in that period can, like the Bronze Age individual settlements in much of Europe, be attributed to development of agriculture. But unlike Bronze Age Europe, Neolithic towns and early cities developed because of social forces requiring monumental construction (*e.g.*, Durrington Wall adjacent to Stonehenge) or a need for security, whereas much of Bronze Age Europe did not feel a necessity to urbanize for security or markets. A market site

---

[11] One example of this is "reverse dominance" as described on p. 631. In small societies where there is, by necessity, a leader, the total society membership can dominate that leader, something that is suggestive of presidential governance in a democracy.

might, by mutual consent, be freestanding at a crossroads or in a small village, but with nothing likely to occur that would require a more populous center for commerce.

The fact that small egalitarian groups were mankind's representation on earth for thousands of years was not a product of a small total global population, for human population doubling time could have given rise to cities in the Paleolithic had there been no environmental disruptions. If people really wanted the company of their own species close at hand, there would have been cooperation in many facets of life to make the transition to cities possible and rapid. But there were disruptions, and the most important disruption was purposeful: the method meant to control disruption was itself disrupting.

C. Egalitarianism, Settled Existence, and Commerce

What leads hunter-gatherer societies to assume a settled agricultural or herding society when the opportunity presents itself? In certain primitive egalitarian societies it has been proposed that hunter-gatherer groups that rely on an "immediate return" lifestyle employ a system of assertive, meaning "coercive," social control that requires the sharing of work and rewards among its members.[12] In such a system there is no accumulation of affluence, no hoard of assets of one's own. With such a system of sharing there is no place for personal gain because the planning needed for a "delayed return" on expended effort that is part of an agricultural lifestyle is so different from "immediate return" hunter-gatherer thinking and implementation.

A variety of theories have been presented to explain the shift from a nomadic to a settled existence. In many of the theories the motivating factors have been environmental change or inadequate sustenance available by foraging. Alternatively, this shift may not have been a nomadic group response to external forces, instead merely being an innate preference for a closer association with other encountered groups, a preference prevented until global meteorological changes permitted it. In the balance, foraging wins out over sociability, for it has been noted that nomadism is typically associated with regions having longer growing seasons, thus supporting the foraging theory. There also are numerous theories regarding group formation, but for present purposes socially "needy" theories will be avoided and Maslow's levels of primitive motivation will again be consulted. Maslow's second most profound motivating factor affecting one's choices is safety and security. Should a small nomadic group combine with another the greater will be group strength for protection and for capturing large game. Perhaps this explains why Australian aborigines did not develop settlements; they felt sufficiently secure in small groups, and large game was unavailable for most of their prehistory. It was not a matter of avoiding large hostile populations; they had no experience with such. That human settlement has been viewed as a global phenomenon, enough so that, despite differences in local circumstance, an age of human development has been named for it: the *Neolithic Revolution*. The term suggests that most humans had been looking for the opportunity not only to settle rather than to roam, but to settle in the proximity of others.

But that avoids the issue of those who did not join the rush to polity. As pointed out in the excursus on Australian aborigines (p. 595), humanity's switch to agriculture was reticent and sometimes never occurred. Quantitation of that change would be welcome, but in its absence it is proposed herein that it was not the attractiveness of a

---

[12] Woodburn, J., *Egalitarian Societies*, in *Man* (N.S.) 17:431-451, 1981.

sedentary existence that caused the change. People were not switching to village life primarily to abide among other people. They were just tired of abiding among their own people and the coercive egalitarian kinships that controlled every aspect of daily life. Furthermore, many preferred not to exchange one onerous system of control, the egalitarian kinship, for another system of control and health threats that might result from living in a larger communal setting. Many therefore chose a third path.

In the Neolithic period and into the Bronze Age, from British Isles to northern and eastern Europe to the original Austronesian population of Taiwan and to many other areas around the globe, human settlements over extensive regions were composed of only one or a few dwellings. The previously hunter-gatherer peoples began to form settlements. But hamlets were tiny and no large towns or cities existed. Each cluster would have been surrounded by sufficient natural resources and enough land for agricultural sustenance of at most a few family units. This pattern might exist for many centuries, and sometimes, like the Jomon culture of Japan, for millennia, without any development other than what might be termed local market towns. Even the occasional natural resource that might be useful for trading was inadequate for stimulating communal commercial exploitation. The extensive (100 acre) flint mining complex at Grime's Graves, located in a farming region in the east of England, was worked for centuries in the Late Neolithic and Bronze ages without an associated commercially active town developing nearby. Flag Fen, a Bronze Age settlement also in eastern England, required extensive human effort in construction of causeways, weirs, and ritual sites, but only few dwellings built on pilings and scattered roundhouses in a fishing area suggest a settlement. The Neolithic site of Durrington Wall several miles from Stonehenge was a settlement of as many as 3,000 persons, but it was occupied primarily for needs of monumental constructions. In the Neolithic Hongshan culture of northeast China (4000-2900 BC) inhabited districts (estimated populations, *ca.* 1,000) are clearly distinquished and some evidence of inequality of prosperity are present, but the population density of a large surveyed area was approximately one household per square kilometer, estimated from the district with the highest overall density.[13] The Bronze Age Bell Beaker culture and early Unetice culture (2300-1600 BC) of Eastern Europe (now the Czech Republic, Poland, Germany and further east), despite a few larger settlements, had the "vast majority" of its settlements being "several houses" in a hamlet.[14] This Bronze Age pattern throughout Europe with settlements seldom larger than fifty persons would give way only when population increase led to a need for security and the building of Iron Age hillforts. And in China, with its great emphasis on kinships and clans, the famous *Treatise on Food and Money*, composed in the 1st C AD as part of the *Han Shu*, noted that in preceding centuries families preferred rural life. As winter approached farmers and their families were ordered to leave their farms and live cooped up in close quarter in the cities, a disheartening proposition ("I sigh to my wife and children"), whereas in the spring families happily ("glad as can be") looked forward to exchanging the crowded city for the detached life of the farm.[15] And even in apparently inhospitable circumstances there is a

---

[13] See: Peteron, C. E., et al., *Hongshan Chiefly Communities in Neolithic Northeastern China*, in *Proc. Nat. Acad. Sci.*, 107:5756-5761, 2010.

[14] See: Makarowicz, P., *The Construction of Social Structure: Bell Beakers and Trzciniec Complex in North-Eastern Part of Central Europe*, in *Przcglad Archeologiczny*, 51:123-158, 2003.

[15] From: *The Book of Poetry* in *The Treatise on Food and Money*, part of the *Book of Han*. The English translation is by Nancy Lee Swann: *Food and Money in Ancient China*, Princeton, 1950.

desire to lead a socially detached life, for the Fayu of Papua, Indonesia, lived in nomadic single family units in a swampy area, only meeting biannually with other Fayu families.[16]

That many such scattered populations over large regions did not naturally coalesce into towns and thence to city-states unless there was a pressing need such as security suggests they were in no hurry to get too close to their neighbors. Even in the Early Bronze Age northern Mesopotamia previously large urban sites gave way to regions of much smaller settlements with extensive networks of paths, rather than remain large urban sites with primarily radial roadways.[17] One might even wonder if humans have instilled in their psyche a preference for a degree of distance from one's neighbors. This could teleologically explain the rapid spread of *Homo sapiens* around the globe shortly after its appearance on Earth. Just as trees branch out permitting leaves better exposure to light, perhaps a basic urge of humans is to branch out to maintain personal liberty. An increase in probability of survival of a society would logically be expected from an increase in fecundity, but as a further guarantee that humans would succeed in establishing their genus and species it would make sense to instill in them a preference for avoiding others of their kind, thus enforcing their spread in small groups inexorably over all the Earth to seek optimal residence and only then to propagate a colony. After all, the strongest factors regulating population growth for most organisms, large or small, are (1) density, in which rate of growth is roughly inversely proportional to population density, and (2) dispersion, in which there is a tendency of an animal species to disperse in one of several patterns that are species specific. In the Orkney Islands north of Scotland the total human population about 3000 BC may have reached 6,000, but its dispersion of family units tended to be peripheral on each island with some distance between each settlement. In ancient Japan, the Jomon hunter-gatherer culture of 3000 BC had a total population estimated at 260,000,[18] yet the largest and probably permanent settlement, Sannai Maruyama, held no more than 500 people, with most of the culture living in clusters of five or six pit-houses, each of which housed about five individuals. Throughout the entire area of the British Isles, 120,000 square miles, and for thousands of years up to the end of the Bronze Age, only two or three settlements have been described that can be considered small villages, a pattern found throughout northern and southeastern Europe for the same periods. An apparent exception, Durrington Walls, mentioned on the preceding page, dates to *ca.* 2500 BC, was unoccupied after a few centuries, and was not intended to be a permanent commercially self-supporting community. To counter the argument that settlements remained small because technological immaturity could not support large ones, in other areas of England larger farmed lands have not been consistently associated with larger settlements.[19] As the level of personal interaction in such an autonomous dispersion of tiny populations in homesteads and hamlets, some of which were only inhabited intermittently, must have made any higher level of social order unnecessary, it would be inappropriate to designate

---

[16] See: Diamond, J., *Guns, Germs, and Steel*, New York, 1999, a paperback, chapter 14, p. 265.

[17] See: Ur, J., *Emergent Landscapes of Movement in Early Bronze Age Northern Mesopotamia*, in *Landscapes of Movement: Trails, Paths, and Roads in Anthropological Perspective*, 2009, Snead, J. E., Erickson, C. L., and Darling, J. A., editors, chapter 9.

[18] See Koyama, S., *Prehistoric Japanese Populations: A Subsistence-Demographic Approach*, Senri Ethnological Studies, 4:187-198, 1992.

[19] For much information in this paragraph see: Rathbone, S., *A Consideration of Villages in Neolithic and Bronze Age Britain and Ireland*, in *Proceedings of the Prehistoric Society*, 79:39-60, 2013.

scattered family units as egalitarian. Indeed, egalitarianism for all intents and purposes did not exist in the Late Neolithic and Bronze Ages in the British Isles and northern Europe. Beyond this, it is presently considered that the nuclear family is a great hindrance to egalitarianism, and thus disruption of the nuclear family by enforced separation of its members is a common procedure in communistic societies just as it was in ancient Sparta. There was in many regions, therefore, no egalitarianism from which to escape.

It is thought that the tiny settlements alluded to above were based on kinship and comprised the nuclear or extended family, from which one might also conclude that it was not the kinship structure of the group that people sought to leave, instead being the intellectual limitations and coerciveness of egalitarianism so integral to nomadic hunter-gatherer life. With the greater assurance of proximal sustenance, the option of growing a surplus of a commodity, and the ability to store some commodities the coercive and redistributive components of egalitarianism were evaded but the leadership component of the family, the kinship, small though it was, was retained. There was little desire to crowd. The distinction between kinship and egalitarianism is discussed in the next chapter.

This makes one wonder about the perverse influences that compelled people to join together in the large Late Neolithic and Bronze Age centers of Sumer, ancient China, ancient Egypt, and elsewhere. An important one was the threat of hostile groups, but a new attraction appeared that explained compact populations centered in towns and cities: commerce. Associated with this demographic change, the larger populations that developed from commercial ventures had a division of labor. Decision-making within commercial production and trading networks remained with those actively involved in them rather than with the associated community at large. A higher level of organization was still unnecessary. Whether in producing ceramics, growing millet or rice, exploiting a local resource such as flint or jade, or producing luxury items, as commerce developed it attracted a larger local population. In a "trickle-down" arrangement, agriculture and herding necessarily increased to support the enlarging population bent on commerce. If local geography and environment were sufficient to support population growth, from clusters of small settlements there was a coalescence of some into a central polity and some entered satellite communities that interacted with that polity, the interdependency representing a city-state, at least as defined on p. 13. Inequality in personal possessions appeared, and personal interests became varied and specialized. In this process the peripheral settlements may have maintained elements of an egalitarian kinship structure, but otherwise this traditional social structure, especially its egalitarianism, was diminished. Why did the "great" cities of ancient times appear where they did rather than in Europe, the British Isles, and elsewhere? It was not because of a special gifted local population or a gifted local leader. True, enemies and natural disasters were often the cause for "circling the wagons" for the common defense. But for the voluntary part of urbanization played by mankind one need look no further than the natural human preference to be autonomous and unencumbered by demands of others that interfered with personal choice. If a reasonably safe existence for a freestanding family unit was impossible, either because of environmental threats or marauders, larger egalitarian kinship groups such as the band and the tribe were available for protection. But that protection came with a price: egalitarian conformity within the community. Commercialism with its prosperity and specialization also offered security in numbers, but, importantly, it helped people avoid egalitarian conformity.

Thus, the appeal of prosperity offered by urbanization plus the release of the individual from egalitarian bonds prompted a move to commercial centers, a move acceptable only if a sense of security was not lost. The larger populations seemed to provide that, for now irrigation, walls, large-scale agriculture and specialization became available. For the small surrounding settlements the only additional issues to be managed were those necessary for maintaining their part in commercial operations. Traditional egalitarianism might locally persist. The central polity, however, now the focus of commercial ventures, devised its own social structure as a spontaneously designed hierarchy and specialization of services responded to a prospering and enlarging urban population. The hierarchy, the consequence of commercial success, was presumably a collaboration among commercial leaders and the labor force, for this early hierarchy, termed by scholars a "settlement hierarchy," was not yet hereditary or political. It arose as a way to peacefully coordinate the varieties of communal effort. As for decisions relating to the overall course of the city-state, the presence of several commercial networks would have functioned as a heterarchy or a form of corporatism that included the labor force and would maintain social organization with or without the inevitable evolution of a political hierarchy.

The importance of commercialism cannot be overstated. Without commercial ventures people living within a coercive egalitarian system in an unsafe region had no where to go. The many dusty tells and other heaps of ancient rubble show that once commercial stimulus declined the population also declined as people resumed their traditional kinship-focused ways and moved on.

Catalhoyuk had a large central population but remained profoundly egalitarian, but it is exceptional in that there was little to suggest any commercial activity. Its agricultural sector ensured self-sufficiency but not surplus. It is considered a "proto-city" because it had no leadership; it was but a large town. This is not a criticism, for it probably reflected the lack of safety of the regional environment in that early age (7000 BC). There was no commercial activity to speak of that might decline for there would have been limited trading opportunities. Thus, for Catalhoyuk there was no way to escape the egalitarian kinship trap. There is no other way to explain a completely static society the size of Catalhoyuk that existed for over a thousand years, great effort being spent on planned renewal of dwellings but no evidence of improvement or progress.[20] Even in those instances, for example the Cucuteni-Trypillia civilization, where large central populations did arise but commercial operations did not exist to an important degree, the "urban" area was inhabited only in time of need, with its families and kinships coming and going according to their individual circumstance. But in areas where food resources were abundant and commerce was established, cities emerged, and it becomes more understandable why the five successful civilizations analyzed in this book formed large cities that later evolved over many centuries to become territorial states with regional identities: they were in very large and fertile alluvial plains.

Yes, this was the time, within the developing city, for transformation, for individualism, for the transferring of allegiances from the coercive egalitarianism of kinships to new social organizations that were less personally intrusive. This would lead to liberal interaction of ideas and progress. But it would not last long.

---

[20] From recent excavations at Catalhoyuk some scholars feel there is evidence of armed conflict, that the structure of the dwellings was selected to check invasion, and that flint tips of weapons and other features indicate armed attacks were not rare, although it is not stated by whom. That there might have been marauding bands or roaming bears is not debated, but the overall sense of the previous discussion is unaltered.

D. More on the Nature and Consequence of Egalitarianism

In an egalitarian (immediate-return) society unwritten rules include the core issues of sharing and no accumulation beyond one's daily need. In less egalitarian (delayed-return) societies some aspects of the immediate return society are also found, but an individual who finds himself more prosperous than his kin will soon be invaded by distant family members who have the right to their share of his good fortune, thus hindering any attempt at self-improvement. This is a common finding in village life in many areas of the world today. Individualism would not be an admirable trait unless one member of the community were superior to all the others in a specific achievement clearly useful to the kinship or community at large. But in immediate-return societies even this can be socially reproachable.

The issue here, however, is the initiation of a novel idea. In describing the immediate-return and delayed-return primitive societies Dr. Woodburn (see footnote, p. 635) observed that "non-competitive, egalitarian hunter-gatherers limit the development of agriculture because rules of sharing restrict the investment and savings necessary for agriculture." The same would have applied to medical care. The individual who realized the potential of concentrating effort at diagnosing, treating and preventing illness might, on his own, have attempted empirical and rational pursuit of medical knowledge. But that was not his decision to make. The decision was made by his kinship and its tradition, within which there may have been no other person with an interest in the matter when weighed against day-to-day problems. While there was surely freedom in some egalitarian societies to move about, even to leave one's group and join with another egalitarian group, it was the freedom of a cellblock, with freedom to move around or between prison cells. The early 20th century writer, Elbert Hubbard, defined a prison as: "An example of a Socialist's Paradise, where equality prevails, everything is supplied, and competition is eliminated."[21] In small egalitarian kinships bent on survival and security there may have been no practical choice, but in larger egalitarian societies there was no permission. Methods to restrain expression of individual superiority by primitive egalitarian societies have been presented by Dr. Boehm, and one mechanism for opposing inequality is the previously mentioned "reverse dominance" in which the community at large opposes individuality that suggests superiority by mocking or shunning the suspect individual.[22] If this prevailed in ancient egalitarian societies, which were usually small, as it does for modern primitive ones, the final judgment on individual undertakings would have been society itself. Dr. Boehm points out that "such societies are deliberately shaped by their members." And therein lies the heart of egalitarianism in the early/primitive society: an intentional coerciveness percolating throughout a society that assures all its members will be no more than average. In doing so it ignores a fundamental truth: in one way or another, or at one time or another, *every* person is above average. Although there may indeed be some transient survival value to minimalizing the "Alpha" personality and thereby permitting open group discussion of pressing issues in primitive "egalitarian" societies, the damping effect of egalitarianism and its singular focus on immediate survival, guarantees that that survival, while perhaps benefiting the persistence of clan structure, will never improve the quality of life of individuals in the clan nor their clan

---

[21] From: Hubbard, E., *The Roycroft Dictionary*, Aurora (New York), 1914.
[22] Boehm, C., *Egalitarian Behavior and Reverse Dominance Hierarchy*, in *Current Anthropology*, 34:227-254, 1993.

descendants.[23] This, the coercive face of egalitarianism, when added to the negating effect of redistribution of effort and assets on personal motivation, ensure that the sameness of lifestyle will endure for those clan descendants. If to this there is added a system of enforcement, the kinship, that "sameness" may persist thousands of years.

A person in a kinship may be required to fulfill certain duties, but if his opportunity for survival benefits from this arrangement, the issue is a matter of personal choice; losing his kinship status could be fatal (outside the kinship). This is an obligated trade-off, and a way out of kinship was present but not taken. There is also the possibility that leaving a kinship might not be desired because of devotion to the kinship itself, a personal feeling that one does not mind the limitations imposed by the kinship because of a personal attachment to its members. Only when the leadership of the band, or the band membership itself, imposes limitations that are sufficiently onerous might one then wish to leave the group. The kinship then becomes viewed as a prison: it is too dangerous to leave and too burdensome to stay. At a certain point the risk of leaving the kinship may become acceptable and the individual can depart. For those who leave the egalitarian kinship, there are two options: (1) if the environment is relatively safe, establish the nuclear family on a small plot of land sufficient for self-preservation, or (2) if the environment is not friendly, join a larger, non-kinship, group involved in commercial activity, the initial phase of urbanization.

It is the variety of ideas spawned by innumerable perspectives, not just those of a docile herd, that provides the apparatus for a better life for all humanity, including the "common man and woman." The amalgamation of ideas from an enormous variety of sources is today doing what it was meant to do, one clear measure of success being a remarkable increase in healthful longevity around the world. And the reason this has not previously happened is that overwhelming forces have successfully denied the innate morality of individuality, impressing a docile and obedient sameness to the mass of mankind (excepting, of course, those who fight to be in charge and thereby reap the benefits of the labor of others). Given the conclusions of Part I, the many facets of modern western life we now enjoy, including medical care, scientific invention, sources of energy, and commerce, have been merely transient novelties in the prehistory and history of mankind and unable to escape the grip of the egalitarian cage to benefit everyone. The grand question is whether the present attempt, so wonderfully institutionalized by America's Founding Fathers, will this time succeed. For one part of the answer, the grand question must begin to focus on natural law.

E. Egalitarianism and Transgression of Natural Law

Adam was to be a farmer, not a hunter-gatherer, and his progeny started settlements. The first family favored sedentism over nomadic or horticultural lifestyles. But prosperity was not to be their lot and the farming was ordained to be difficult. Adam, Eve and family were expected to exist in a social system unrestrained in their daily choices by any secular authority for no such authority existed. Using the metaphor of the previous section, they were the first small branches of the human tree. But they already had

---

[23] See: Boehm, C., *Hierarchy in the Forest*, Cambridge (MA), 2001, for Dr. Boehm's extensive work on primitive humanity and his evidence supporting the essential role of egalitarianism in promoting human social evolution, a view that contrasts markedly with that of the present volume.

instilled in their intellects not only the self-indulgence that led to their downfall but also the moral guidance to help them to live together and survive. The descriptive name of such a society or group, one that was settled but not urbanized is "rural agrarian,"[24] but more important is the moral guidance, or "natural law." Although the latter is discussed in detail in the following chapter, here the competition between natural law and egalitarianism is briefly considered. Natural law for the moment will be approximately defined as the Golden Rule, a manifestation of our conscience, a self-awareness of moral goodness or blameworthiness in our actions and intentions. It is often argued that natural law underlies all systems of justice and governance, but at issue here is the coerciveness of egalitarianism. Can egalitarianism be consistent with the message offered by the Golden Rule? And the Golden Rule is "Do unto others as you would have them do unto you." Another version is "Do not do unto others what you would not want done to you." One implication is that one should not take from another what is not freely given. And yet it is in egalitarianism that allocation of effort and redistribution of resources requires the taking, under threat, the industry and products of those most productive in a society. Could it be that egalitarianism has hidden among its tenets a transgression of natural law? And if the answer is "Yes," perhaps this explains in part the stagnation of Catalhoyuk, the militarism of Sparta, and the absence of progress in all lesser primary civilizations of chapter 33.

F. Sparta and Imposition of the Egalitarian State

Widely regarded in the past as an admirable example of an egalitarian state, Sparta was not always so. Present scholarly opinion supports the notion that Dorian ancestors migrated into the northeast of the Peloponnesian peninsula during the years now identified as the Dark Age of ancient Greece, a time that spans the decline of the Mycenaean empire (1200 BC) to the commencement of Archaic Greece (750 BC). A nearby early center of Dorian prominence was Argos, and from 800 to 500 BC this city flourished as a prosperous center for bronze metallurgy, pottery, agriculture, horses, silver coinage, and an artistic culture. Argos and Sparta were enemies for centuries. Sparta likewise developed into a powerful city-state, and, despite its frequent wars, by the 7th C BC its culture likewise flourished in music, poetry, bronze sculpture, ivory carving, pottery, and figurines. Later in that century the legendary Lycurgus is said to have devised a "constitution" that was meant to produce "internal political equilibrium," but in doing so provided a mechanism whereby Sparta became a stable but egalitarian and militaristic state. Two initial steps included land redistribution and the withdrawal from the populace of gold and silver to prevent individuals from acquiring wealth.

Apparently in response to concerns about not only about its enemies but also its serfs and dependencies, Sparta's citizenry became in effect a standing army. That the social result was selectively egalitarian has been fully explored by scholars, but sufficient communistic activities and avoidance of displays of opulence were retained that reinforced Sparta admirers' view of its egalitarianism even though a sizeable and powerful elite class existed. The inequities of the Spartan system regarding land tenure, the relation between citizens and their serfs, and movable wealth have been well

---

[24] The sequence is: Hunter-gatherer, Rural agrarian, Urban, Commercial, Industrial, Post-industrial.

described.[25] The subsequent decline in Sparta's power and influence has been attributed to the social inequities thus produced, although a major factor was a marked decline in its population of citizens, due in part to casualties of war. Argos also had a change in governance and acquired a tyrant, Pheidon II, at about the same time as the Spartan "constitution" was instituted. Pheidon is remembered primarily for his expansionist policies, but the city itself continued to prosper and, to a limited extent, allied itself at times with Athens. In contrast, by the 6th C BC Sparta had instituted social controls that led to loss of crafts and a "reduction of non-military wants to the barest minimum."[26] By the 4th C BC Sparta was in political and social decline, but Argos built monumental structures such as the largest theater in ancient Greece, an odeum, a large agora, and became the host of what were formerly the Nemean Games.

Sparta, as can be seen, changed its nature prior to its decline. In its initial Dorian character it was part of just another expansionist population, and when settled in the Peloponnese it initially assumed the general character of many other Greek city-states in its commerce and culture and it flourished. Its "constitution," however, as voluntarily accepted by the citizens of Sparta, led ultimately to an isolated, militaristic, illiterate, and, for a great many of its citizens, a superficially egalitarian but divided class society that would persist as Sparta became less and less significant. Egalitarianism proved to be no defense against political authoritarianism, instead becoming its ready partner.

In Part I Sparta was compared to contemporary Athens and other Greek city-states with regard to developing a medical profession. There should have been true physicians in Sparta, given the importance of medical care for its citizen army and nearby examples of Hippocratic medical practice in other city-states, but the only Spartan medical personnel mentioned by historians are those individuals, nonphysicians, who retrieved the wounded in battle. Furthermore, before the time of Hippocrates, citizens of Sparta had restrictions placed on their autonomy. To maintain military readiness they were not permitted to do the physical work unrelated to that readiness. Those tasks were assigned to noncitizens and serfs. This was no setting conducive to group networking by citizens concerned about providing for the community's medical needs. All thinking was guided by military priorities, communal oversight, and spying. Whereas elsewhere in early classical Greece the "elite" class did not avoid manual labor as a way to personal wealth, the egalitarian "elite" of Sparta remained aloof, letting slaves and serfs manage the practical matters of the polis. Whereas Hippocratic physicians practicing in different cities around the eastern Mediterranean formed a professional network that produced a volume of medical wisdom that would be admired for centuries, the egalitarian citizens of Sparta were forbidden even to travel to a nearby town without permission.

Such single-mindedness of purpose stunted the growth of whatever knowledge and culture might have sprouted from Spartan ingenuity. And this brings into focus the role of coercive egalitarianism in suppressing progress. Here the problem is not only with "egalite'." For the greater society the problem is the limited number of issues upon which a community will focus. It is the consequence of doing nothing rather than something, the disavowal of change, that is such a damper on progress. The number of issues is necessarily small because of the need for consensus, or at least the concurrence of the larger or more powerful portion of the polity. Those issues that may seem important to one individual, and in fact may be important to all, can be ignored by the community at

---

[25] See: Hodkinson, S., *Property and Wealth in Classical Sparta*, London, 2000.
[26] The source of much information and the quotation in this paragraph are found in: Cartledge, P., *Sparta and Lakonia*, London, 1979, especially chapters 8 and 9.

large because of an enforced preoccupation with a consensus-limited set of issues. It is not a matter of dislike of originality or novelty; it is a matter of assigning priorities, and the ever curious mind of the individual is therefore disregarded by communal demand. But the egalitarian community is not anti-intellectual; it is pro-survival. It is not anti-individual; it is pro-community. It is not anti-progress; it is pro-stability. Egalitarianism as an amoral issue is not a matter of redistribution to make all equal; it is redistribution to assure that all in the community are equally prepared to do their part in the next battle. It is not, or should not be, a matter of jealousy or envy; it is a matter of efficient organization to guarantee survival. And if spiritual forces are considered an ally, they too would take precedence over the individual, not because of deep faith in something but because egalitarians would accept an ally from any source. In all these matters egalitarianism that pervades a community is not an intended evil but as a democratic form of authoritarianism in which most of the community resent the unpredictability of individualism and demand unanimity of action in the name of survival of the way things are perceived to be; ingenuity has become an enemy.

Finally, egalitarianism is not instituted as a matter of morality that might be traceable to natural law. Instead, by ignoring the natural inclination of humans to individual liberty it is disobeying natural law and thereby narrowing the path to progress. While egalitarianism as a moral political force is a relatively new idea, its use in this way today is but a ploy, for its purpose is the same: a rejection of change and a way to control others. The control over others in an effort to suppress the uncommon man is not urged on by ill will. It is inspired by the fear of what might happen if there is no control or if control is, or might be, put in the hands of others who are viewed as objectionable. Its modern popularity, as stated by Erich Fromm in relation to the 20th C democracies' tendency to embrace dictatorship, is based in part on idea that, when there is a loss of supervisory authority in a person's life and yet there is no freedom to pursue personalized goals, people will chose the populist authoritarian.[27] He also noted that the ultimate freedom "…the ideal – if only man's nature could rise to it – is communism." What was not mentioned by Dr. Fromm is that communism, a form of social egalitarianism, was, at the time of his writing, pursuing its tragic course.

And what about unexpected threats? It might be a present or future human conflict, a preparation for a natural disaster, or other imminent threat. Egalitarianism would not, however, be prepared for the unexpected. Indeed, the tunnel vision engendered by social control of the individual is a guarantee of susceptibility to the unpredictable, as well as an incoherent response to a threat once realized. Perhaps "abandoned" would not be cited after so many early civilizations listed in Table 15, pp. 622-623, had incompetence bred by egalitarianism not been in play. As for Sparta, although credited with a survival of one thousand years, its time in the sun was barely two hundred years.[28] And so the consequence of Sparta's ascetic rebirth as egalitarian was use of social coercion rather than leadership hierarchy to restrain any individual desire to stray from the normative, and: "… by accentuating social inequalities and the sense of distance between individuals, they aroused envy, produced discord within the group,

---

[27] See: Fromm, Erich, *Escape from Freedom*, New York, 1941 (1st American edition, the original, in German, having been published the same year). For a rebuttal to Dr. Fromm's characterization of the mass of mankind with regard to its fear of freedom, at least when it comes to America, see p. 680 of this volume.

[28] From the time Chilon of Sparta (fl. *ca.* 570 BC) to the battle of Leuktra in 371 BC.

threatened its equilibrium and cohesion, and divided the city within itself."[29] To its external threats Sparta unwittingly added an internal one.

Another element of intellectual restriction has been newly defined, and for convenience it has been categorized as "groupthink." Egalitarianism limits options available to a society by restricting novelty, whereas groupthink, in which a subgroup puts forth its opinion as the superior one and manages to inculcate that opinion throughout a society, also limits options of society, but it causes a further problem: in that the subgroup opinion is the opinion of likeminded people, there is the likelihood that the opinion will be unrealistic or less favorable because the subgroup would not have had an open discussion that could have disclosed faults in its favored opinion. Egalitarianism restricts choice and groupthink can prioritize the wrong choice, a bad combination.[30]

The final common denominator of the various ways that egalitarianism imposes restrictions on society is not one of equalization. It does not equalize; it "stamps out diversity."[31] In a primitive stage of existence, therefore, having shut off avenues of escape from a primitive state, a society afflicted with egalitarianism will remain primitive forever, until some inevitable calamity leads to its demise. In the meantime, life in such a society will remain "solitary, poor, nasty, brutish, and short." Whether it be Catalhoyuk or pharaonic Egypt, whether it be egalitarianism of the small group or tyranny of the large, the consequences will be the same, with three important observations: (1) Sometimes the authoritarian can be right and a tyrant's actions efficient, and this can lead to willful lack of appreciation of the dangers in political authoritarianism. (2) There may be no place to which to escape. "There is ample evidence that even primitive tribesmen themselves are not fond of their primitivism and take the earliest opportunity to escape from it;" wrote Dr. Rothbard (as cited above, p. 270). And thus they do try in our age, but in Catalhoyuk that option was absent. (3) In the overtly political authoritarian society, coercive power will be in the hands of a relatively small group, and those individuals will live relatively well, whereas in social egalitarianism none will do well. That is why the citizens of Catalhoyuk remained chained and unchanged for a millennium with a life expectancy of about 30 years, whereas in ancient Egypt the magnificent art and massive monuments of the pharaonic elite with an average life expectancy of 40-50 years looked down upon the simple masses who, over 2,000-3,000 years, also had an average life expectancy of about 30 years. Prominent individuals were memorialized in ancient Egypt and some idea of daily life and misery faced by its people are available to modern scholars. For Catalhoyuk, however, it was but a stroke of luck that the archeological site was discovered, for otherwise Catalhoyuk would have remained an unknown, and in a sense tragic, lesson in the history of mankind.

G. Egalitarianism and Spontaneous Order

"Spontaneous order" is another consideration that might bear on group behavior and function. It has been likened to the "invisible hand" of Adam Smith that is associated

---

[29] Jean-Pierre Vernant: *The Origins of Greek Thought*, p. 64, Ithaca, 1996, 4th printing of Cornell Paperback.

[30] See: Whyte, G., *Recasting Janis's Groupthink Model: The Key Role of Collective Efficacy in Decision Fiascoes*, in *Organizational Behavior and Human Decision Processes*, 73:142-162, 1998.

[31] See: Rothbard, M. N., *Egalitarianism as a Revolt against Nature*, Auburn, 2000, 2nd edition, p. 277 in the essay entitled Freedom, Inequality, Primitivism and the Division of Labor.

with the effectiveness of free market economics, and it is in this capacity that it is a present-day issue in modern economic theories. Spontaneous order also bears some resemblance to natural law.

> Definition of "spontaneous order:" Order which emerges as a result of the voluntary activities of individuals but is neither a product of the execution of human design nor a creation of government.

Spontaneous order represents the unintended but good and proper consequence that results from a certain similarity of action of members of a population in response to a stimulus. The innate tendency that leads to this effect is present in all rational individuals. The idea is not new. Lao-Tsu (6th C BC), in the 57th chapter of *Tao Te Ching*, stated:

> Therefore the sage says:
> I take no action and people are reformed.
> I enjoy peace and people become honest.
> I do nothing and the people become rich.
> I have no desires and people return to the good and simple life.

Kant (1724-1804) would have the liberty of interplay of ideas, good or bad, in the long run resulting in a good result. He would say it is the back-and-forth nature of arguments more than the quality of the ideas expressed in those arguments that is the key to success, because an initially successful but defective argument may lead to a bad result, but continued interplay and more arguments will automatically and over time lead to a good result, "spontaneous order."[32] With Kant there is no mysticism or Divine intervention involved. The success of the freedom to argue and disagree in contributing to progress in this context could be framed mathematically. Presumably what appears to be a chaotic mix of opinion will have the possibility of good and bad outcomes. The bad ones will ultimately wither because they do not work, whereas the good ones will be more likely to work. Thus, the bad will slowly be eliminated, especially as people become more enlightened about the critical nature of individual liberty in promoting progress and about the bad consequences of certain categories of decisions. All this sounds Pollyannaish, and human history suggests that "over time" can be unconscionably long. Other scholars, however, would argue that it is the innate moral sense, or conscience, present in all humans that leads to spontaneous order, and, if abnormal limitations are not imposed, spontaneous order will become apparent because the unopposed moral sense will, in a population over time, lead to the proper result, *i.e.,* it will be consonant with natural law. The critical point here, however, is that, in both approaches, liberty of expression of conscience for all members of society is necessary for progress.

Egalitarian society, therefore, affects spontaneous order in a negative way. In egalitarian society the intolerance of its reign of nonsovereignty can be absolute in the demotion of innovative thought by inhibiting normal interactions, and thus spontaneous order will have no opportunity to emerge. Furthermore, people have different aptitudes, skills, and interests, characteristics that make a person an individual rather than a worker

---

[32] The value of crossing of swords of opinion as an expression of "unsocial sociability" is clearly explained by Dr. G. H. Smith in Part 12 of his series *Ayn Rand and the History of Philosophy*, "*Immanuel Kant on Spontaneous Order*," 2016, http://www.libertariansim.org/columns/immanuel-kant-spontaneous-order. In Kant's philosophy humankind's inherent antagonism to others who disagree is the basis for human progress.

ant. These native talents, if not inhibited, may permit that individual to provide a unique service, and by that progress, whether in lifestyle improvement, longevity or prosperity. It can open to the rest of the community the good news of his talents. This the coercion of egalitarian society prevents.

H. Egalitarianism and Kinship

Throughout this work the term "egalitarian kinship" is commonly applied to early and primitive groups. This differentiates it from "kinship," a term now applied indiscriminately to many groups of all sizes, including larger ones that form around a common cause or ethnicity. Egalitarian kinship has no formal definition and it is therefore defined herein as:

> Egalitarian kinship - a consanguineal and affinal group in which assigned status implements opinions and traditions of an egalitarian society.

This definition implies that the prevention of diversity and the equalization of effort and the results of that effort are a product of the egalitarian group, with the kinship, by inserting a hierarchy, being useful in implementation and enforcement.

The pervasive nature of kinship has always influenced attempts to escape coercive egalitarianism. Familial bonds are strong and may override a personal desire for greater freedom of action. Egalitarianism is a characteristic of small kinships, but the larger the kinship institution the less egalitarian is its hold on behavior. Although usually viewed as a compassionate and sensible response to external threats and an admirable interpersonal social bond that helps ensure social stability and continuance, its basic nature was clearly identified by the eminent Scottish jurist, Henry Sumner Maine (1822-1888) when he defined kinship's legal position as depending on a person's "status" whereas Western jurisprudence has replaced "status" in favor of the "contract." [33] The consequence has been to shift the focus of legal implications of a personal action from one's place in society to the individual himself. By means of contractual understanding one can now make personal choices for personal benefit rather than holding a social position assigned to him by an unyielding social tradition, its enforcement in small societies being, in effect, one's neighbors. It has been noted that kinships standardize social life in a highly prefigured way, and, by regulating the behavior of different categories of kin, "leave little leeway for spontaneity or individual differences." [34] In band societies kinships are usually bilateral in that both spouses contribute to the social pattern, and that pattern is inevitably coercively egalitarian, one of family dependency rather than individual obligation. Everyone in such kinships has a role, but not of one's choosing.

---

[33] See chapter 5 of Sir Henry's famed *Ancient Law*, London, 1861.

[34] The modern relevance of the change "from status to contract" has been recently analyzed by M. S. Weiner in his book *The Rule of the Clan* (New York, 2013), which supports its significance with modern examples. At the same time, even bands express their egalitarianism in different ways, including the way children are raised, so that it is acknowledged herewith that the generalizations that are the source of criticism of egalitarianism in this volume may not apply to all small groups. But this is not a study of sociology. It is a review of the changes in civilizations/cultures over the ages, from which the importance of the effect of egalitarianism has emerged.

But Dr. Nisbet notes that "centralization and bureaucratization of power" is a potent influence against kinship in that persons will identify less with their own kinships and will be more open and tolerant with other individuals.[35] In larger groups it is more difficult to maintain the kinship pattern. Thus, the social organization of "corporatism" has been applied to several of the lesser civilizations in chapter 8. This may be confusing inasmuch as there are many forms of corporatism, including liberal, fascist, progressive and absolutist. Relevant in present context, however, is kinship corporatism. In the Sintashta civilization dwellings were nestled close together and each household had evidence of contributing to the overall production of metal products. This has recently been described as a corporate arrangement, in which the entire population was entailed, voluntarily it is assumed, in the manufacturing process.[36] With little evidence of a social hierarchy other than that adult males may have been warriors when needed in addition to being metallurgists, it might be thought that the villagers represented several kinship groups, each with inherent leadership structure, specific social positions, and an understanding of traditional rights and duties to each other. And this sounds fine until it is realized that the goal of kinship, as mentioned above, is stability and continuance of the kinship, not the needs of the individual. And it is here that corporatism comes into play, for a corporate social structure can replace the intricate kinship system by appealing to the nuclear family to join with other nuclear families within the larger social environment of a corporate social structure in an organization designed specifically to benefit all its members in that the members control the course of the organization rather than a chief of a tribe, elder of a band, or strongman. Furthermore, its leadership could be held accountable for decisions made. It has been pointed out, after reviewing the evolution of corporations through medieval Europe, that most people belonged to some form of corporation as the centuries went by, and with the economic security of belonging individuals could make personal decisions with less interference from kinships. Dr. Avner Greif has underscored the benefits: "Corporations and nuclear families embody and reinforce a culture of self-government, cooperation among non-kin, the legitimacy of majority rule, respect for minority rights, the accountability of leaders, and individualism."[37] This may seem irrelevant to ancient societies, but it is to be remembered that the European Dark Ages saw a return to profoundly primitive societies devoid of advances of the Classical Era. Viewed in this light the Sintashta experience might represent an early attempt at a form of "corporate kinship," an intermediate step away from traditional kinship, a transegalitarian attempt to escape from the injustice of egalitarianism, and toward a degree of personal responsibility, individual choice, and benefits attached thereto.[38] It will probably never be known if this is relevant to the present task, for neither the size nor duration of Sintashta civilization were likely to support the development of a network of medical practitioners, the present gauge of progress.

---

[35] See: Nisbet, R., *Prejudices: A Philosophical Dictionary*, Cambridge (MA), 1982, p. 52, in his discussion of social deterioration attributable to capitalism.

[36] See: Koryakova, L., and Epimakhov, A., *The Urals and Western Siberia in the Bronze and Iron Ages*, Cambridge, 2014, p.181.

[37] See: Greif, A., *Institutions and the Path to Economic Modernity: Lessons from Medieval Trade*, Cambridge, 2006, especially chapters 8, 9, and 12 which deal with family structure, institutions, and growth.

[38] See: Hayden, B., *The Dynamics of Wealth and Poverty in the Transegalitarian Societies of Southeast Asia*, in *Antiquity*, 75:571-581, 2001.

With the exception of Liangzhu, which early on turned its kinship base into a ruling class and politically stratified the society, and Sharh-i Sokhta, which was a straightforward commercial heterarchy that adapted kinships into a corporatism structure, all the other lesser civilizations discussed in chapter 8 involved kinships and were, or can be assumed to have been, subject to powerful social forces from them. Kinships are considered a "cultural universal." Nevertheless, there are different types of kinships, often quite versatile depending on local circumstance, and biological affiliations could be ignored in the acquisition of members. In ancient Greece, Rome and India specific religious affiliations could serve as the basis for kinship.[39] The size of kinships varies from the nuclear family to the hereditary phratries of ancient Greece, the latter encompassing thousands of "brothers" within a proposed, sometimes fictional, ancestral lineage, usually attached to a geographical location. Given the various guises and sizes that comprise kinships it is not surprising that their adaptability has brought the kinships great credit as a social model of stability and longevity and as such have become models for guilds, corporations, and religious institutions. There are restrictions in kinships, however, especially in primitive ones, that place significant obligations upon members, including their place in society, *i.e.,* their "status" as referred to by Dr. Maine. For this reason, and based on evidence, Dr. Nisbet noted a "partial decline of the kinship community can be a significant force in the eruption of the golden ages in the history of the mind," indicating that kinship "affects liberation of the individual spirit and the expansion of individual imagination."[40] The egalitarian kinship status of all seventeen civilizations is recapitulated here, beginning with the five associated with medical practitioners:

a. It was the reform of Cleisthenes, who in 508 BC abolished phratries (a form of kinship) in Athens, thereby opening further the door to democracy, increasing individual mobility, and leading to the remarkable phenomenon of Classical Greece. This was a formal acknowledgement of the victory of democracy over tribalism in ancient Greece, a process that had been under way for a century throughout the Greek city-states. Indeed, the earlier selection of the tyrant, Thrasybulus of Miletos (*ca.* 600 BC), has been viewed as a primitive form of democratic process.

b. Prof. Jason Ur, in studying the role of households in "urban origins," noted that while the Ubaid period of Mesopotamia was "characterized by kinship organization," it is generally held that with the appearance of cities during the succeeding Uruk phase there was a "disappearance of kinship as a structuring principle...." Dr. Ur proposes another explanation that retains the essentials of kinship through "nesting" of households. This interesting idea removes the nuclear family away from the larger extended family, band, and tribe kinship groups and toward a particular household that has, for whatever reason, attained prominence. This alliance, when multiplied, leads to a chief or titular head, *e.g.,* a king, emerging from the prominent household, but one with which the subservient households, not being conquered, can interact as with other households but at the same time benefiting from the new hierarchical arrangement. This freeing up of the

[39] See: Fustel de Coulanges, N. D., *The Ancient City*, Garden City (paperback), n.d. (first published in 1864), as translated by Willard Small, bk. 2, ch. 5.
[40] Nisbet, R., citation on preceding page, p. 115. He also (p. 126) states that "Feudalism is an extension and adaptation of the kinship tie with a protective affiliation..."

nuclear family to make decisions in its own best interests is similar to the evolution of corporatism. The key point to be made is that such an allegiance leaves behind the coercive egalitarianism of the original kinship and, rather than replacing it with bureaucratic authoritarianism, it introduces the voluntary interaction of nested households, or at least that is the conclusion *vis-à-vis* Uruk.[41] Overall, Dr. Marc Van de Mieroop concludes it is unlikely that familial kinship ties carried over in cities even though persisting in peripheral communities. Documents from Uruk indicate that within the city only rarely were neighbors found to be related. Thus, it was the nuclear family that regained some of its autonomy in the city, whereas the extended family or clan remained active in the smaller settlements outside the city.[42]

c. In Egypt, the common man in early settlements might have been fully immersed in kinship obligations, although as populations increased it was the nuclear family that predominated, even to the point that there were no status names for those more distantly related. But as Dr. Juan Castillos pointed out, any kinship association weakened as local individuals began to realign themselves with more attractive prospects for their future, namely, commercial and bureaucratic ventures, and the kinship tie, limited as it was, was broken.[43] It is noteworthy that the three civilizations just cited, late Archaic Greece, predynastic Sumer, and Protodynastic Egypt, were the source of medical classics postulated to have been compiled or composed during the transition from a coercive egalitarian kinship to central political governance.

d. Even for Liangchengzhen, the city-state representing the age of the Yellow Emperor, Dr. Rheta Lanehart has recently discovered that ceramic production was not under centralized management but was instead made with local, chemically distinct, substances and techniques by dispersed settlements, families or neighborhoods.[44] While this might be interpreted as an indication of a flurry of activity from small kinships, the fact that it was a local commercial effort within the larger population center identifies it as an entrepreneurial effort of the nuclear family or small extended family that permitted a degree of individual choice uncharacteristic of traditional kinships; they were curtailing aspects of egalitarian kinships for a better life.

e. The shift away from egalitarian kinship for cities in the Indus River Valley civilization is less uncertain. An urban habitation pattern consistent with extended families is proposed as an explanation of the observed neighborhoods. Corporatism might explain the remarkable design and features of the city, for it suggests its residents had a role, directly or indirectly, in its formation. Corporatism, by enlisting the recommendations of its plebeian organization, would shift allegiance from kinship to a mutual

[41] Ur, J., *Households and the Emergence of Cities in Ancient Mesopotamia*, in *Cambridge Archaeological Journal*, 26:2, 2014.
[42] See: Van de Mieroop, M., *The Ancient Mesopotamian City*, Oxford, 1997, pp 103-110.
[43] See: Castillos, J. J., *The Development and Nature of Inequality in Early Egypt*, in *British Museum Studies in Ancient Egypt and Sudan*, 13:73-81, 2009.
[44] Lanehart, R. E., *Patterns of Consumption: Ceramic Residue Analysis at Liangchengzhen, Shandong, China*, 2015, Graduate Theses and Dissertations, Graduate School at Scholar Commons, especially chapter 2.

interest, commercial ventures and support structures such as housing. Generic architectural designs in the neighborhoods that mimicked those of central leadership designs suggest their purpose was an enticement to plebeians to reorient their sympathies to their new urban institutions and away from traditional egalitarian kinship.

Within the twelve lesser civilizations described in chapter 8, there was a notable persistence of smaller kinship configurations despite enlarging central populations:

a. Marajoara – The kinship arrangement of this egalitarian Amazonian civilization was sculpted by the environment in that traditional housing in settlements was on segregated mounds. Also, the work done on many of the mounds was characteristic of each particular settlement, in this way assuring there would be an additional limit on the opportunity for external pressure to alter the traditional social pattern of a mound's small kinship group.

b. Norte Chico – The scattered small settlements along the four rivers emptying into the Pacific, considered egalitarian, contributed to the commercial and ritualistic features of this civilization. With each community having a population in the hundreds, the basic social organization was probably a kinship clan, each community with its own internal controls and an agreed-upon association with an organizational hierarchy that existed for purposes of ritual. Commercial ventures did not require a large population living in close quarters, thus requiring no separate authoritarian structure for maintaining social order over the confederation of clans.

c. Poverty Point – The scattered settlements surrounding the remarkable residential mounds and stretching along the Mississippi River and its tributaries were likewise separated by environmental barriers from any coercive central authority and would have maintained tradition kinship relations.

d. Cahokia – Despite being the "mall" for the central and southeast North American continent, the individual egalitarian settlements surrounding and supporting a professional hierarchy of ritual specialists retained traditional kinship social structures as evidenced by their ethnic diversity and their coming and going as kinship groups. The permanent peripheral settlements may have owed some allegiance to a central authority, but if this were a voluntary choice the kinship scenario should have remained in effect.

e. Terramare – The physical separation of villages within a network of riverine channels may have limited the opportunity for central control in this apparently egalitarian civilization. Within the village, each populated by perhaps a thousand persons, there would have been local leadership, for each village was a complete production unit in itself, consistent with the idea that metallurgical production was spread via kinships. Commercially each settlement would have functioned as a node in a civilization-wide heterarchical network, but there was no higher level of organizational power to counter or weaken the underlying traditional kinship systems.

f. Catalhoyuk – This egalitarian community had, based on recent assessments, neighborhoods. To this can be added the proposal that stability for the entire settlement is to be found in the side-by-side association of two distinct kinships in such a way as to permit intermarriage. The "neighborhoods" were small clusters of attached dwellings, each cluster separated by architecturally distinct walls from the otherwise contiguous settlement. There is little reason to consider anything else than kinship organization with all its social stability as the explanation for the longevity of this remarkable civilization.

g. Sintashta – As noted above, recent assessment of the Sintashta settlement social system suggests this civilization was built around corporatism. Its dwellings were comfortable but physically close and consistent with a homogeneous social pattern. With no evidence of chiefdom, this would therefore represent a voluntary commitment of kinship groups to the purposes of a common commercial venture. While commercial success resided in the cluster of kinships that agreed to function as a single commercial organization with characteristics of corporatism, social cohesion was found in "jural elements in social relations" provided by the individual kinships.

h. Shahr-i Sokhta – The commercial center that arose from small settlements in the Sistan basin primarily centered on trading, but it was a heterarchy of commercial operations. Presumably life of the common citizen was tied to one of the commercial trading ventures, and with no need for a military, no defensive considerations and a ready supply of food there should have been few limitations from the city itself on activities of its citizens, in other words, no central organizational authority. Its seemingly discreet neighborhoods were probably based on distinct commercial and trade interests in alliance with kinships.

i. Djenne-Djenno – Segregated settlement mounds, each settlement a separate production unit of a heterarchical commercial center, were also kinship units within this remarkable egalitarian civilization. Other than some presumed traditional guidance and recommendations from the established earlier families at the site, no centralized power existed. Social cohesion resided in the kinship.

j. Liangzhu – It would seem, given its early dates, that kinship relations must have been essential to the cohesion and success of this commercial city. It is likely that the marked social stratification found its basis in commercial ventures. A kinship prominent in organizing a commercial venture became elite, thus leading to stratified class distinction, with traditional kinships persisting and the lower class kinships subservient to the dominant kinship.

k. Anasazi – Undoubtedly kinship associations were essential as tribes made up the social composition of this commerce-based civilization. Central storage and the ability to acquire the labor of many members for projects orient`ed toward the public good suggest a form of corporatism, and, as there is no evidence of coercive central governance, a reasonable conclusion is that traditional egalitarian kinships provided the social cohesion necessary for public works. There is the additional factor of geographical separation among the many smaller settlements over a large region, a feature that would favor continuance of local egalitarianism.

l. Cucuteni-Trypillia – This civilization of egalitarian "cities" and small settlements with no commercial base has been recently analyzed regarding settlement patterns within the cities. It was concluded that one explanation for the unique layout of the large population centers was the localization of each kinship or band to a linear cluster of dwellings.

I. Egalitarian Kinships

From Table 16 it might be concluded that the pervasiveness of kinship-based organization in evolving civilizations is by itself a powerful nullifying force in pursuing progress. But kinship is a social constant worldwide and underlies the structure and function of myriads of organizations, large and small, and its presence can be minimal or profound. Dr. Nisbet has pointed out the following: kinships do not prevent intellectual achievement, and, indeed, rather than struggling against traditional kinships the Founding Fathers of the United States Constitution "incorporated rather than dismissed" the concept. Kinship is not necessarily related to egalitarianism, for he noted that kinship has a strong tradition in authoritarian societies, and it does provide a latticework for social interaction that averts chaos. He states instead that: "Egalitarianism represents the leveling of all those 'inns and resting places' of the human spirit which are found in social hierarchy, tradition, kinship and institutionalized religion." [45] And this brings us to the relevance of Tables 15 and 16 and to the attaching of the term "egalitarian" to "kinship." These two terms are not causally linked and their definitions are distinct. Placed together they usually refer to small primitive groups such as a band or tribe. With larger kinships, however, chiefdoms develop from skillful manipulation of positions within the kinship that enable a dominant figure to enforce traditional egalitarian mechanisms. In contrast to positions of leadership within a successful commercial enterprise, the assigned status of those within the kinship is arbitrary and unrelated to ability. But the decisions and redistributive power of the larger kinship no longer rests with the shifting and tractable social interactions within the community but with the permanent power to assign roles and to dispense favors by the chief. Formalized coercion is now available to manipulate the individual for the benefit of the kinship and its leaders. In short, whereas egalitarianism resists change, leadership within a larger kinship provides the mechanism for enforcement of the egalitarian ethic. As population increases, coercion changes from a more passive horizontal implementation to a more rigid and vertical authoritarian and one. This is implied in the combined terminology "egalitarian kinship" of Tables 15 and 16. It does not suggest a diminishing of functional egalitarianism.

J. Conclusion

When considering the five successful primary civilizations there seems to exist a window of opportunity between the successful founding of a primary civilization and the apparently inevitable takeover of governance and population control by a centralized political and authoritarian, usually male dominated, hierarchy. Dr. Rita Wright has captured that moment in a statement about Uruk: "This urbanism occurred in the absence

---

[45] See: Nisbet, R., *Prejudices: A Philosophical Dictionary*, Cambridge (MA), 1982, p. 18, in his discussion of authoritarianism and p. 125 for egalitarianism.

Table 16: Characteristics of Social Organization for the Twelve Primary Lesser and the Five Primary "Successful" Civilizations* during Early Urbanization.

Lesser Civilizations	Archeological Egalitarian	Egalitarian Kinship**	Commercial Heterarchy***	Authoritarian Hierarchy	Primitive Corporatism
Marajoara	-	+	+		
Norte Chico	-	+	+		
Poverty Point	+	+	+		
Cahokia	+	+	+		
Terramare	+	+	+		
Catalhoyuk	+	+	-		
Sintashta	+	-		+	
Shahr-i Sokhta	+	+	+		+
Djenne Djenno	+	+	+		
Liangzhu	-	+	-	+	
Anasazi	+	+	-	+ (late)	+
Cucuteni-Trypillia	+	+	-		

Successful Civilizations****

Greece (Miletos)	-	-	+		
Sumer (Uruk)	-	-	+		
Egypt (Hierakonpolis)	+	-	+		
India (Mohenjo-daro)	+	-	+		
China (Liangchengzhen)	-	-	+		

* Social status of the five "successful" primary civilizations at the proposed time the original compilation and/or composition of their classic medical writings took place. Most of the seventeen civilizations had more than one mechanism in play.
** Low-level kinships (bands, clans and tribes).
*** Heterarchy, often concurrent with hierarchical characteristics.
**** Successful in that a nascent medical profession developed.

of a strong centralizing state and was able to thrive for at least a brief moment under the control of decentralized local groups."[46] During the unfolding of this process the hold of egalitarian kinship was weakened by commercialism, traditional duties and responsibilities diminished, and individual action could be taken. It is during this fragile period, flanked by a weakened egalitarian kinship and a coercive authoritarian State, that there can be a freeing up of minds and bodies to explore new ideas and processes. Dr. Trigger states: "In early civilizations, …, class displaced kinship and ethnicity as the main organizing principle of society."[47] According to this sequence kinship affiliations were exchanged for social classes, suggesting little room for individual or group freedom in either camp; the average man merely jumped from the frying pan into the fire. But this

[46] See: Wright, R., *Prehistory of Urbanism*, in *Encyclopedia of Urban Cultures: Cities and Cultures around the World*, Danbury (CT), 2002.
[47] Trigger, B., *Understanding Early Civilizations*, Cambridge, 2003, p. 47.

profound shift in allegiance was not effected immediately. The interval between the two positions might have been years or decades.

Egalitarianism has been discussed by Dr. John Kekes as an ideology, one of many "isms" upon which social order has been theoretically constructed.[48] Although Dr. Kekes reveals the irony, the illogical nature, and the human misery that has followed on attempts to impress egalitarianism on populations in recent history, he has also pointed out that the ideological methodology used to promote such a social change is an even more fundamental social defect than egalitarianism itself. This is because ideologues, by stifling alternative thinking, prevent realistic dialogue and openness in relation to other social constructs that might prove practical, if only in part. As a consequence of the work of Dr. Kekes and others in Western society, previously held sympathetic views of egalitarianism are now giving way to a better understanding of its modern authoritarian threat and its tragic historical documentation.

Somewhat different, however, is the context of egalitarianism in the present work. In early and primitive societies alternative "isms" were nonexistent. Ideology and the ideologue were, therefore, not the issue, for there were no competitive alternatives except for group schism or isolation from one's band or tribe. Likewise, the concept of personal liberty would not have existed, and therefore could not have been infringed in those ancient times because survival of the individual superseded personal fulfillment. And so it is the intrinsically authoritarian nature of egalitarianism itself, rather than its ideological enforcement by marginalization of social alternatives that, at an early and vulnerable state of human social evolution, is at issue in this work. It has been shown in this volume that, despite the apparent absence of social coercion by ideologues, personal ambitions were still held in check in early societies. Notwithstanding their relatively small size and thereby the necessarily close personal interactions within those societies, the egalitarian threat was omnipresent, whether in physical strength of a headman or in compulsion or expulsion by the kinship itself, the latter recognizable today in the tyranny of the majority, a concern of democracy that requires constant attention.

One might even view egalitarianism as an example of tyranny of the majority. The course of an egalitarian society may change according to circumstance and with the blessings of the society as a whole, thus giving the appearance of free and equal "egalitarian" competition of ideas. But enforced uniformity, by its infringement on human liberty, is logically immoral, a point touched on in the next chapter.[49] It is only when the element of kinship enforcement relaxed that an element of individual and group autonomy could occur, and this happened only when a less coercive, albeit temporary, option opened: commercial prosperity and early urbanization. This option was not chosen for its attractiveness. It was chosen because it was a way to escape egalitarianism.

---

[48] Dr. John Kekes, Emeritus Professor of Philosophy, State University of New York, Albany, has exposed, for many years and through many books, the troublesome issues and illogical thinking associated with egalitarianism. See especially his *The Art of Politics: The New Betrayal of America and How to Resist It*, New York, 2008.

[49] And yet, justification by claim of morality often underlies the egalitarian's coercion, a modern-day social menace as seen in many African secret societies such as the Poro in West Africa. Here morality, with its basis in kinship, is relative to power. Thus, the "egalitarian ethos" has "condemned its followers to flatlining stagnation" by "not allowing for individualism, private initiative or personal success." See: Ellis, S., *The Mask of Anarchy*, New York, 2001 (paperback), especially chapter 6, and Butcher, T., *Chasing the Devil*, New York, 2011 (paperback), p. 272.

CHAPTER THIRTY-SIX

NATURAL LAW

Definition of Natural Law: A body of unchanging moral principles regarded as a basis for all human conduct.

Oxford English Dictionary

Following a definition of natural law that includes its applicability to all mankind, it is axiomatic that it must apply equally to both early and modern man, including ancient hunter-gatherers. As far as it is a "law," it exists to guide the community of man. Because of the varying definitions of natural law, the term as used here is equated with the *moral sense* as described by Dr. James Q. Wilson. Evidence supporting the existence and general applicability of natural law in historical and modern societies is reviewed. Its relevance to early human societies is then discussed in relation to specific areas in which moral valuation is displayed. The consequences of actions in accordance with, or inconsistent with, natural law as they affect the development of early man's social organizations are then discussed. The conclusion is that coercive egalitarianism and egalitarian kinships include within their strategies such practices as are inconsistent with natural law, thereby inhibiting proper societal evolution and the realization of progress. Sadly, the felonies of a few have devolved great misery upon the many.

A. A Review of the Concept of Natural Law

If there were an innate natural guide that provides mankind with a means for discerning right from wrong, a moral compass that is universal and timeless, it should have applied to the first humans and must have attended the association of individual humans into small, then larger, groups as they moved in ancient times from a nomadic to a settled existence. As a uniform code of just and fair conduct it should have been available to assist group cohesion and protection, the making of decisions, the management of crises and the use of local resources. If the intellect of mankind has not deteriorated over the last ten thousand years, then neither has that internal guide, our conscience. Had it been a part of every member in a community it should have helped keep the community communal, assisting in its survival and realization of a better life for its individual members.

Described above in the subjunctive and in view of the generally pathetic course of mankind's social organizations in providing a better life it may be easy to dismiss the concept of innate moral guidance as fanciful or merely an appendiceal religious conviction. But nothing could be further from the truth. The innate moral guidance under consideration has been proposed, corroborated and studied for thousands of years. Its traditional name, "natural law," commonly presented by scholars as first applied by the Stoics in the phrase νομός κοινός, will be used herein.[1]

---

[1] Interpretation of the Stoic phrase is usually given as "natural law," although linguistically its meaning is closer to "common law" or, less likely, "law as commonly understood." But in reviewing the various ancient Greek statements regarding natural law, it is the statements made in context, more than traditional lexical definitions, that make clear it is an innate moral sense of Divine origin that is meant.

As an opening statement, the purpose of natural law, as far as human reason can discern, is to help the human community survive and thrive. It is not a guide to personal fulfillment; its role is to help human society overcome obstacles to survival and security. It is directed at the group. And while it is commonly discussed in terms of human interactions within a large society, it should be operative in small groups as well. In this volume it applies both to the urbanization of large populations and to the entrepreneurial function of the small group, the "koinon."

One might suppose that language development within early communities had to be sufficiently advanced to transmit philosophical concepts among their members for natural law to come into play. But the components of the moral compass ascribed to a "natural law" are few and simple even though a huge bibliography representing untold hours of study and thought on natural law has accumulated over the ages. For example, there has been a distinction made between "natural law" and "natural rights," with extensive explication and scholarly dialogue attached thereto. Modern references to natural law vary widely, from what quaintly can be termed the wise regulations of Mother Nature to the desire to conflate the basic mathematical structure of the universe with its functioning, including the purpose and future of humankind.[2] In recent literature an equivalent concept has been called "the moral sense."[3] But the definition of natural law at the beginning of this chapter, short and simple, is useful because it identifies natural law as being a matter of principles, thereby bypassing legal arguments about the popular Western identification of the topic as "law" in common usage.

It is essential that the definition of natural law be understood to mean that certain moral principles are innate in every human being, regardless of time, place, or social setting. It implies that natural law need not be taught; it is already in play in every person, although its expression might be buttressed in an individual raised in an environment consonant with natural law. Because of varied social environments and because expression of natural law must inevitably come via a human agent, characteristics of the times, places, and social settings can be dragged along with that expression, sometimes masking the profound principle involved, sometimes cloaking it within secondary gains of the society or the individual invoking it, and sometimes being explicitly denied because of deemed necessary "human" priorities. The moral principle in question has been characterized as not self-evident. But they are self-evident in human actions because there is no alternative explanation for first principles underlying man's moral foundation. On the other hand, most persons have never thought much on the matter, and therefore natural law may be indirectly self-evident via its effects even though it goes unrecognized by individuals unaware of the expressed concept but active in its application. While not codified, the commonality of natural law expression throughout the family of man and its independence from genetics and human dialogue underscores its fundamental nature and thereby its chronological precedence and primacy over human law, which hereafter will be termed "positive" law consistent with current scholarly use.[4] The source of natural

---

[2] See: Heisenberg, W. K., *Das Naturgesetz und die Struktur der Materie/Natural Law and the Structure of Matter*, Stuttgart, 1967.

[3] See: Wilson, J. Q., *The Moral Sense*, New York, 1993. Wilson uses sympathy, fairness, self-control and duty as chapter headings and addresses them as characteristics of the moral sense.

[4] Darwin (*The Descent of Man, and Selection in Relation to Sex*, London, 1874, 2nd edition, chapters 4 and 5) commented on the importance of morality as a feature distinguishing man from other animals, and that the basic tenet – "the prime principle of man's moral constitution" – is, in effect, the Golden Rule. Furthermore, this social instinct was acquired (*i.e.*, not innate) "for the good of

law is not a matter for discussion here. Dr. James Q. Wilson generously included natural selection as a potential mechanism for its generation (as cited above, p. 23), although just how natural law happened to have found a place on the list of characteristics usually considered to be naturally selected by an unforgiving state of nature is not pursued in depth. C. S. Lewis cleared up the matter for many by pointing out that natural law is not an instinct, for an instinct is a propensity to act in a specific way, whereas natural law is a guide for what to do, a guide for choices, and it therefore helps us decide the right choice between two instincts.

A profound philosophical basis for natural law is expressed in the writings of Immanuel Kant, the German philosopher. As for its foundation, he stated, "Autonomy is therefore the ground of the dignity of human nature and of every rational nature." The natural end of man's actions is his happiness, a goal that requires autonomy, and it is only from a position of autonomy that morality is expressible. Furthermore, as a "principle of reason" independent of circumstances, a morality encasing good will is an expression of a universal law that each individual, on reflection, could conclude by himself. By confusing legislated laws with the moral law, to the extent that the former is inconsistent with the latter, the supposed positive benefits of the former can return negative results on the proposer and all others. What prescient words! Kant avoids identifying the source of moral law beyond the individual, but it has a reason for existing in every human in that reasoning humans exist; it is inherent in all.[5] From this perspective Kant is providing intellectual and logical support for what mirrors the Golden Rule and our conscience. Indeed, his concept of the Categorical Imperative is in part considered a restatement of the Golden Rule: "Act only in accordance with that maxim through which you can at the same time will that it become a universal law."[6] To the extent that he requires autonomy for expression of morality he is at one with advocates of political freedom such as John Locke and other icons standing behind the Framers of the Constitution of the United States.

The intertwining of natural law with positive law in recent years is confusing. Dr. A. Dicey (1835-1922), the famed English jurist whose three principles for the supremacy of the ordinary law of the land over all citizens made no reference to the role of an innate sense of right or wrong in deriving the laws of the land, is nevertheless often stated to base his references to personal freedoms on natural law.[7] One reason for the

---

the community." He was puzzled by the proliferation of "absurd" rules of conduct and religious beliefs in the face of "self-regarding virtues" that "now appear to us so natural as to be thought innate...." He also felt that persons whose actions were inconsistent with virtue had a greater mortality rate than the virtuous, and that there was, as a consequence, a gradual but favorable movement in social integration of mankind over time, like the changes in behavior of domesticated animals. Furthermore, he considered virtuous traits transmissible via heredity: "If bad tendencies are transmitted, it is probable that good ones are likewise transmitted." Natural law in its present context, however, is present in every individual, and its variability in expression bears not on the presence of the "law" (it is always present) but on the awareness and receptivity of the "law" by the individual personality.

[5] The quotation from Kant is found in *The Moral Law*, a translation and analysis of Kant's work on morality by H. J. Paton, London, 1964, 2nd edition, p. 103.

[6] See: Kant, I., *Groundwork of the Metaphysics of Morals*, Cambridge, 1997, as translated by Dr. Mary Gregor.

[7] See: Dicey, A. V., *Introduction to the Study of Law of the Constitution*, New York, 1915 (8th ed., initial version published in 1885). He identifies three principles: all citizens are subject to "ordinary"

confusion is in not realizing that natural law, or moral guidance, is an attribute of an individual, not an organization. The freedom of the individual is not granted him or permitted him by some organization. Nor is it based on what his predecessors have determined by trial and error over centuries is best for that organization and therefore for him. Nor is it part of some social contract under which his freedom is inherently linked with everyone else's in some sort of organizational give and take. Nor is it part of some cosmic idea of how we think things should be run. Rather, his freedom is based on the innate understanding of other individuals around him that he is not to be kept from doing what he wants to do, just as he is not to interfere with them. Natural law is a moral orientation, not a legal document. But if an individual purposely invades the territory of another, whether by preventing an action, taking away a possession, injuring, misrepresenting, or deceiving in the absence of a provoking invasion of his own territory, there has then been a disregard of his moral guidance, and that is wrong. In its most general expression it is the Golden Rule, variations of which have been found in virtually all cultures, one of the scholarly proofs of the existence of natural law.[8]

It can be argued that, while ignoring natural law carries no penalty for the individual unless there is a positive law of society that is consistent with moral guidance, there is a price extracted from the community, and that price, the consequence of ignoring moral guidance, may be the failure of the community to thrive or survive once sufficient indictments have accrued. The failure is not so much in the nature of a penalty as it is merely the consequence of choosing the bad option. Natural law, or moral sense, or the Golden Rule, provides guidance, through the actions of its members, to a community on how its members should get along with others. It is not an individual's key to the Kingdom or a pathway to Heaven.[9] It follows that when controverted, a price might be extracted from the community by the turn of events. And that is the reason, it is proposed here, that nineteen "great" civilizations of mankind identified by Toynbee have disappeared (the remaining four, including Western civilization, presently in the balance).

B. Spontaneous Order and Natural Law

General principles of natural law can influence community perspective on a broad front and lead to a general concordance of opinion. For example, the principle of noninterference with another's actions (assuming no harm was intended or predictable) might provide "moral" guidance that would diminish intrusions into each individual's attempt to improve his or her prospects during the early stages of urbanization. The "settlement hierarchy" is an organizational model relevant to urbanization that predicts

---

law rather than arbitrary, ordinary courts must apply the ordinary law, and fundamental rights are "rooted in the natural law" rather than abstract constitutional concepts.

[8] Scholarly descriptions of a maturational path to morality (Kohlberg's stages of moral development) have received much attention in recent decades, and there has been some attempt to compare those stages with morality as acquired by primitive societies. This is not, however, an appropriate analogy, either on principle (adults, primitive or no, are not children) or with regard to natural law (which is innate and complete from its onset, is unlearned, and is not imprinted, although it can become more obvious in a social environment that does not suppress its expression).

[9] The individual, however, is inevitably involved. Natural law provides for the good of the individual in that the individual is the beneficiary of group action, and natural law is a guide for the group.

hierarchical evolution as a consequence of population increase.[10]   The greater the population, the greater are the levels of hierarchy needed to provide a level of efficiency and support for the growing population to prosper. This type of hierarchy is not imposed on the community; it is devised by the growing community as needed, functioning more as a mechanism for coordination and instructing rather than commanding. And as population increases commensurate with prosperity, existing supports for the community can increase or enlarge, and new supports for the community can be acquired. At some point, an individual may find that his ability to effectively treat some medical issues in the community can be used as a source of income. Population continues to increase, other individuals take up the provision of health care as a source of income, and soon a commercial network of medical services can be identified.

All this did not happen because it was ordered by a central bureaucracy. It was made possible because the community became more prosperous and freely exchanged ideas. But note that the changes developed from the bottom up, not from the top down. This is because those who affected change did so because of self-interest, not because they were commanded to do so. And that is the point to be made about a settlement hierarchy. The concept of settlement hierarchy is deceptively simple: a ranking of population centers by size. But of great importance is that development of the self-regulating hierarchy is in the hands of the people themselves, not a political, hereditary, or occupying power that dominates society and dictates development. The latter will happen soon enough, but before authoritarian interference takes charge there is a period in development where there is little infringement on normal human interactions that permit coordination, cooperation, disagreement and dissent to the benefit of all. It, like a free market, is an example of spontaneous order as discussed on p. 646f. It occurs as a nucleus of people, each working to improve life for themselves and their families (whether or not they act as individuals or as constituents of a commercial venture), seize upon a variety of individual mechanisms for that improvement, but the common outcome of the effort is progress toward an improved condition for all, a feature unintended at the onset. No one said, "Come everyone, we can make a great city if we work together." Instead, the sentiment was, "We will be free of the bullying from the tribe if you and I and the children move to the settlement and help John sell firewood to the folks making those nice ceramic pots." The stimulus was self-interest.

Earlier the susceptibility of spontaneous order to disruption was discussed in relation to egalitarianism. As has been proposed in this volume, progress was thereby unable to be initiated. But the settlement hierarchy can provide a window of opportunity for improvement in the human condition. It is a point in time sensitive to a variety of human ideas and ambitions that, if left alone, will see a potpourri of individuals work out their differences by compromise rather than command. Bargaining and bickering, individuals can seek and find opportunity. This latch pin to progress has been lifted, and spontaneous order, as corollary of natural law, has been permitted to work.

If an issue with a moral aspect arises in a free people and a vote is taken to initiate action the myriad of votes cast would ideally represent the group's decision within a moral

---

[10] For a recent review of early urbanization see:

Sandeford, D. S., 2018, *Organizational Complexity and Demographic Scale in Primary States*, in *R. Soc open sci.* 5:171137.http://dx.doi.org/10.1098/rsos.171137. The text also includes an overview of specific primary "states," and there will be some demographic data at variance with that included in this volume (*e.g.*, Sandeford reports Hierakonpolis with a greater population), but that is the nature of scientific inquiry when data are limited.

framework of natural law that, regardless of their personal motives, would in general be the good rather than the bad decision. Insofar as spontaneous order also will be displayed in the actions of a free people, the conflation of spontaneous order and natural law seems logical, for individual liberty is an indispensable feature of both. People must be free in order to ensure that their assent on social direction reflects their unfettered opinions and discussions on any moral issues attached thereto, the key word being "unfettered." Spontaneous order can be viewed not as complementary to but as a subsidiary of natural law.[11]

Pertinent to present discussion, spontaneous order should not be an issue in a heterarchy, for the options of members of a heterarchy are primarily technical details relevant to commercial ventures and relevant to relatively few people, whereas spontaneous order is the result of a universal prompt to avoid immoral action. In a heterarchy the questions to be solved include appropriate management, nature of competition, and logistics.

Spontaneous order is also not an issue for the specialized group such as the koinon, for the focus of the koinon also is narrow and technical, factors open to discussion are well-defined, and the group size is usually small.

But there is a troubling implication of spontaneous order as a manifestation of controverting natural law that has prompted present discussion. Inasmuch as the consequences of spontaneous order are dependent on a society's openness to natural law, a society that is, for whatever reason, not open to it will receive no benefit from it. And when nonbeneficial consequences inevitably appear all members of the society will suffer, whether or not some members would have acted in a way consistent with natural law. One is reminded of the many tragic vicissitudes that befell Biblical populations or cities that must have included among their numbers many individuals who would have chosen a course of action consistent with natural law but were caught up in the consequences of an incorrect alternative selected by authoritarian leaders. The wrath brought down on the heads of innocents was the consequence of their being unable to put forth their arguments for correct action.[12] In this sense, their sad endings were, like the denial of progress, a result of egalitarian communal action (or of communal inaction in not replacing defective leadership). The untoward results also may be viewed as built into human misresponse in such a way that humans, through their errors in judgment, inflict their own punishment. The population or its leaders brought those consequences upon themselves because its form of governance, whether egalitarian or authoritarian, ignored or suppressed opinions of those through which spontaneous order could have been expressed. One can understand, even if not agree with, the ancient claim of the superiority of democracy with equality before the law over hierarchical authoritarian governance, and with the claim, first implemented by the Founding Fathers, that democracy alone is insufficient for the protection of minorities, and therefore protections were provided so that all opinions would have the opportunity for free and open discussion. Without exercising these options, humanity will remain at the whim of authoritarians and will continue to be the recipient of tragic consequences because of their own poor choices or poor choices of the authoritarian leadership. It is through the

---

[11] This is not just a personal judgment. See: Skoble, A., *Natural Law and Spontaneous Order in the Work of Gary Chartier*, in *Philosophy Faculty Publications*, Paper 49, Bridgewater (CT), 2014.

[12] This is identified in Ecclesiastes, 8:14: "… that there are just men to whom it happens according to the work of the wicked; again, there are wicked men to whom it happens according to the work of the righteous." (King James translation.)

workings of spontaneous order that one can more easily understand that humanity is endowed with natural law in order that societies, rather than individuals, be enabled. It is, however, obvious that if a society benefits from natural law and spontaneous order benefits will redound to the individual member as well.

C. Natural Law in Major Civilizations

Much has been written about natural law in recent centuries, with the great impetus coming from the profound analysis of St. Thomas Aquinas (1225-1274 AD), but reference to innate moral guidance that transcends the laws of man is an ancient concept, which one would expect were it a feature of the human mind everywhere and in all times. Historically, Classical antiquity in the West included Sophocles describing its importance and its origin in Antigone's reply to Creon, ruler of Thebes: "Nor did I think that your decrees were of such force, that a mortal could override the unwritten and unfailing statutes given us by the gods. For their life is not of today or yesterday, but for all time, and no man knows when they were first put forth."[13]

Aristotle applies natural law to the political arena, stating that political justice is part legal and part natural: "...; by general laws I mean those based upon nature. In fact, there is a general idea of just and unjust in accordance with nature, as all men in a manner divine, even if there is neither communication nor agreement between them."[14] He then proceeds to offer the analogy of Antigone, just mentioned above, so that there is no question as to the point he was making. And Cicero made numerous references to natural law that are frequently cited and which formed an important part of Roman law, subsequently to be passed on to Western constitutions. This innate moral guide, he said, was born with us: *non scripta, sed nata lex*, and was not a product of the State for it existed before States were established.[15] Furthermore, in *De Officiis* (3.69) it is made clear that moral law supersedes civil law, whether the latter is just or unjust: "The civil law is not necessarily also the universal law, but the universal law ought to be also the civil law."[16] With regard to slavery, Dr. Muller reminds us that Ulpian (170-223 AD), Tryphonimus and Cicero considered freedom as included under *jus naturale*.[17]

---

[13] From Sophocles play, *Antigone* (Ant., 476), first performed in 441 BC, translation of Richard Jebb. For a relevant and encompassing review of Greek references to natural law see: Le Bel, M., *Natural Law in the Greek Period,* in Natural Law Proceedings, 1949.

[14] Aristotle's *Rhetoric*, 1373b2; translation of J. B. Freese.

[15] In *Pro Milone* (4.10) Cicero stated the following about law in the context of self-defense: *non scripta, sed nata lex* ("This, therefore, is a law, O judges, not written, but born with us, - which we have not learnt or received by tradition, or read, ... imbibed from nature herself,...", translation of C. D. Yonge). It is a statement on morality in that Cicero was arguing that it is not immoral to forcibly defend oneself from "plots," "robbers," and the like.

[16] "Quod civile, no idem continuo entium, quod autem gentium, idem civile esse debet." Translation in text by Walter Miller in the Loeb Classical Library, volume XXI, Cicero, *De officii*, 1.10.31. In *De Officiis*, 3.26 and 3.27, a discussion of the difference between what is right and what is expedient, he notes it is a law of nature not to harm another human. In 3.70, 71 he decries fraudulence and cites civil law as based on a "natural feeling for the right," therefore suggesting an example of the appropriate conjunction of natural law with civil law, a form of positive law (although the force of the argument is lessened in the section mentioning vending of slaves).

[17] See: Muller, H. J., *Freedom in the Ancient World*, New York, 1961, p. 265.

St. Thomas defined at length the concept of natural law as a manifestation of God's omnipresence in his earthly creation, and this has generated much scholarly discussion ever since. Natural law is not Eternal law, the latter representing God's plan for the Universe and perhaps being closer to Heisenberg's concept of "natural law" (see p. 657 for footnote reference), and it has been suggested that the Mosaic laws were prompted by the insufficient attention given by the favored of God to His internal directives (*i.e.,* natural law). But natural law is the moral compass each individual possesses, and it can be followed or willfully bypassed, its guidance ignored in the face of a complex or chaotic society or undue self-interest. It has been frequently suggested that natural law varies from region to region, from society to society, because each society has it unique history and needs. But natural law does not vary according to region or society. It is found in every individual, and it has been present since the first man and woman. There is a natural inclination to follow natural law. It has made group living successful over the ages and may have been absolutely necessary for survival of our species. Had humans not been the fortunate recipient of natural law, they may have remained, in the mind of the evolutionists, but king of the jungle in a real struggle against gorillas, lions, and cobras for survival. St. Thomas included the following as internal expressions of natural law guidance:[18]

1. We know good is to be done, evil to be avoided.
2. We know our actions should be guided by reason.
3. We know we should not harm others.
4. We know we should not kill others.
5. We know we should not commit adultery.
6. We know we should not take from others.

In the writings of St. Thomas circumstances exist whereby these moral prerogatives have been modified, and this has been the source of differences in interpretation of the concept of natural law.

Within the Judeo-Christian ethos of Western civilization natural law can be discerned *ca.* 1300 BC, the time of Moses. Had Hebrew society abided by natural law just what the consequences would have been over time are unknown, for early Hebrew society was soon transformed by kingship, an undemocratic transition that blunts individual responsibility and choice of each member of the community. The interval between these two events was about two or three centuries. Great troubles followed. Much later the Romano-Jewish historian, Josephus, viewed life itself, insofar as it was desired, as a law of nature, and therefore to take a life was evil.

Regressing further in time, early writings from the four "successful" primary civilizations studied in this work have been interpreted as historical evidence of a universal judicial process consistent with a realization of innate moral guidance, or natural law, although the fit is far from perfect. In ancient Egypt this was manifested through Ma'at, the universal power that regulated physical and moral matters. Although the physical laws were not elucidated by ancient Egyptians, the moral law was clear and was meant to be followed by every individual, including the pharaohs. It was not written down

---

[18] This list is extracted from: *St. Thomas Aquinas on Politics and Ethics*, New York, 1988 (paperback), translated and edited by Paul E. Sigmund, pp. 48-50. St. Thomas' comments on natural law and its varying interpretation according to circumstance makes clear understanding difficult for many of its readers.

but delivered by the pharaoh or judge who was subject to that innate moral sense and thus guided by Ma'at. Prof. Brague considered this "close to the notion of natural law."[19]

In ancient Sumer expression of an innate natural law is minimally documented. In the *Code of Ur-Nammu*, dated *ca.* 2100 BC, the king of much of southern Mesopotamia listed a number of laws (fifty-seven are known), but relevant to natural law is the prologue. Ur-Nammu indicates that his laws, which were to benefit all the people, were in accord with the god of justice, Utu (the sun-god). This implies a divine origin for the nature of his code of laws, although Ur-Nammu took credit for their pronouncement. An earlier legal writing under an earlier king, Urukagina (24th C BC), is considered a "reform" document rather than a law code, and Urukagina wrote that his kingship was divinely bestowed, but it is unknown if he considered the justice he proclaimed also divinely bestowed.

In predynastic China, contemporaneously with the preceding, similar considerations were expressed in the Huang Lao philosophy. Whereas Confucius (551-479 BC) considered the innate expression of justice to be found in the "discretionary judgment of exemplary persons" rather than being a "universal ethical principle," the Taoist movement attributed to Lao Tzu (604-521 BC) as incorporated into the Huang Lao philosophy states that ultimate justice is found in the rule of law rather than the rule of man, meaning "...natural law grounded in a foundational natural order."[20] Interestingly, the origin of this philosophy, as indicated by recent excavations, is in some manuscripts attributed in part to the Yellow Emperor, Huang Ti, the mythical sage of *ca.* 2500 BC who is referenced with regard to medical writings discussed on p. 74*f.* Even C. S. Lewis has used the word "Tao" (The Way) as a way of expressing natural law in terms of beneficence, duties, justice, honesty, mercy, and magnanimity.[21] Another prominent philosophical religious movement in ancient China was founded by Mo Ti (5th C BC), and its stand that political justice was up to the "Will of God" to judge laws, penalties, and government itself found disfavor with Confucian governments. One might wonder what course Far Eastern Asian culture might have taken had Confucianism not been adopted as its cultural paradigm.

The Indus River Valley is the region associated with the origin of the Vedas, the foundational compositions of Hinduism dated to *ca.* 2000 BC. In the centuries that followed the Vedas Hinduism emerged, and the Laws of Manu were composed, at the earliest, about 500 BC. But with the earliest texts written about 100 BC the most that can be said about the origin of Hinduism is that it is derived from "ancient" precursors. Some of the Dharma writings provide the closest approximation to universal natural law in that there is recognition of what is proper conduct and what is good for society:

---

[19] Brague, R. *The Law of God: The Philosophical History of an Idea*, Chicago, 2008, English translation by L. G. Cochrane, pp. 16-17, first published in Paris, 2005.

[20] This interpretation is based on the relatively recent discovery of the *Huang-Lao Boshu*. See: Shih, H., *The Natural Law in Chinese Tradition*, in *Natural Law Institute Proceedings*, pp. 119-153, 1953, and Peerenboom, R. P., *Law and Morality in Ancient China*, Albany, 1993, the first chapter. Essentially, non-assertion and non-interference were proposed as attributes of good governance. "I do nothing, and the people will be transformed of themselves." (From p. 127 of the first citation.)

[21] Lewis, C. S., *The Abolition of Man*, especially chapter 2 and the Appendix. And in chapter 25 of Teh King (translated by Dr. Isabella Mears, Glasgow, 1916): "Man finds his law in the Earth. The Earth finds its law in Heaven, Heaven finds its law in Tao, the Tao finds its law in the affirmation of itself." As for the Tao itself, It "was a Being already perfect before the existence of Heaven and Earth."

"Hindu thought counts *Dharma* as the true Sovereign of the State, as the Rule of Law. The king is the executive called the Danda to uphold and enforce the decree of *Dharma* as the spiritual sovereign. Thus the king or temporal sovereign, is not the source of Law in the Hindu State. The sources of Law are above and beyond him. They are not his creation. He has only to see to their observance."[22]

It is pointed out that *Dharman* is mentioned sixty-three times in the oldest Veda, the Rig-Veda. And it is the term *dharma*, which includes meanings of law, order, and justice, that is most often considered, in its parts, roughly synonymous with natural law. Sometimes written "Rta," Dr. A. Parpola describes it as the "active positive force of truth" that pervades the universe and controls all behavior of gods and men.[23] In doing so it coordinates "everything," which can be interpreted that it is also responsible for "spontaneous order," which has been discussed. But the specificity of the *Dharma sastra* and the range of human guidance it provides has come down to us through the sages and scholars of Hinduism, and the principals of natural law thus evolved have come to encompass lifestyle and civil law, somewhat similar to the way that natural law in the eyes of some refers to the workings of the universe. For example, the rigid class system that evolved in Hinduism prevents any universal relevance to much of the classic writings, as working for the overall good of every individual in society is inconsistent with a society that has been inherently and incredibly inequitable. Hinduism, being a synthesis of Indian religious and philosophical thought, emerged historically no earlier than 500 BC. But what is relevant here is that much of its content comes from prehistoric oral tradition of the Vedas perhaps as much as 2,000 years earlier. It is reasonable to conclude that innate moral guidance (natural law) is embedded in the Vedas, the precursors of formal Hinduism, at that early date, even though a succinct statement of natural law has been overgrown by extensions of its interpretation into activities of daily religious life.[24] Indeed, the very act of composition of the Vedas can be considered the best proof of an awareness of natural law at the time of the early Indus River civilization.

From the above synopsis, the admixture of parochial and universal interests attached to prehistorical origins of historical writings, not to mention insufficiencies in translated definitions, make it awkward to seek out clear-cut features of natural law that would apply to all four successful primary civilizations discussed in this volume. But it can be said, and sufficiently demonstrated, that all of them had considered an innate and overweening moral code as a guide to social behavior that overrides or guides the positive laws devised by mankind, and for this to happen a higher order of existence must have ordained that code which, in the West, is called natural law. It is the confusion produced by man's attempts to apply his specific interpretation of such "law" to the law of the land that has caused great difficulty in understanding or defining natural law. But that moral guidance of natural law supersedes the positive laws of mankind was undisputed among the four civilizations is the point to be made, rather than an analysis of differences in its application.

---

[22] Mookerji, R. K., *Chandragupta Maurya and His Times*, 4th ed., New Delhi, 1966, p. 49. (First published in 1945.)

[23] See: Parpola, A., *The Roots of Hinduism: The Early Aryans and the Indus Civilization*, Oxford, 2015.

[24] See: Sundaram, M. S., *The Natural Law in the Hindu Tradition*, in *Nat. L. Inst. Proc.*, 1951, pp. 69-88. Also see p. 511 of the present work and Dr. D. Chattopadhaya's view that the original rational intention in medicine of the Atharva Veda was an entreaty for an objective and even democratic approach to knowledge and to medical practice.

In the eyes of many, natural law is eternal, irreducible, unchanging, and irreplaceable. In that it precedes and supersedes human law, its moral principles are not the result of consensus, instead being etched into the human conscience from the very beginning. Given this general assessment of the topic of natural law and the physical/literary evidence supporting the existence of natural law in some format in all five of the successful primary civilizations discussed in this section, it is concluded that the presence of moral guidance is indeed a universal human attribute, that the ability to distinguish between what is right and what is wrong is a part of every human conscience, and its presence and consequences therefore can be postulated in early and prehistoric societies to be discussed below.[25]

D. Natural law in recent history

For an example of the conflation of natural law with positive law it is convenient to review the biography of Dr. Friedrich Hoffmann, the great German physician and philosopher of medical ethics at a time when medicine was about to escape the thralls of medieval authority. A contemporary of Dr. Hermann Boerhaave (1668-1738), the physician who put medicine back on track as a scientific clinical profession and thereby promoting the return of a natural state of medical practice, Dr. Hoffman (1660-1742) wrote an influential work on medical practice, his *Medicus Politicus*, published in 1738, in which he promoted the concept of natural law as part of the justification for his philosophy of ethics. But in his effort to align his ethical philosophy with natural law he permitted his personal biases, including his religious opinions, to influence the final product. As a consequence, he intended that physicians be the public face of his idea of morality to the point that he thought physicians themselves should be natural law philosophers. So important was their work to be that part of his method was to prepare physicians for public office, and in fact a number of his students did just that.[26] This is entirely consistent with the cosmic role of the physician put forth by Dr. Rudolph Virchow (1821-1902) a century later, as discussed on p. 22. It is this sort of confusion that is sowed when personal opinions intrude on the moral orientation of natural law; we cannot help but bring our own perspectives to bear on its expression so that we might improve others and impress on them our superior personal insights.[27]

---

[25] For an interesting and unexpectedly broad review of natural law with many historical examples see: Dymond, J., *Essays on the Principles of Morality*, New York, 1836, pp. 60-66, first published in London, 1829.

[26] See: Baril, T. E., *Philosophical Analysis of the Concept of the Politic Physician in Friedrich Hoffmann's Medicus Politicus*, University of Texas, 2008, a PhD dissertation.

[27] Darwin did not deny the importance of conscience and morality in forming human communities, and, consistent with natural law, he considered a significant part of human conscience as innate, a genetic trait with an expression that was variably expressed, even in different ethnic or racial groups. But, like intelligence, he viewed it as a "gradual advance" from man's hominid ancestors, and there are some who have postulated that there has been continued improvement in morality in historic man up to the present, presumably by the same mechanism (*North British Review*, July 1869, p. 531; also Lecky (*History of Morals*, vol. 1, p. 143). Darwin names that mechanism "social instinct." It is clear from his commentary, however, that his idea of the source of morality is distinct from the definition herein. See: Darwin, C., *The Descent of Man*, Chicago, *ca.* 1874, Pt. 1, chapter 4, "Moral Sense."

The eminent 17th C jurist, Hugo Grotius, based much of his work on natural law, although despite extensive writings it is not always clear what he means. The reason is that he uses natural law as an argument for relatively specific 17th C problems, and a clear "general" definition of the term is not easily extracted. But in his opinion natural law was a trait implanted in all of mankind, not just Christians, and was implied in man's ability to reason. He did not indicate that natural law was of Divine origin, but, as he was prominent in contemporary Christian theological issues, his writings, being of international relevance at the time, may have been an attempt to avoid stirring up partisanship based on culture.[28] Montesquieu (1689-1755) expressed a premonition of natural law when he not only wrote that primitive man, before he made any laws whatever, would have had a sense of justice, but that, like laws of physics, a law of justice predated the existence "of intelligent beings" (*des Etres intelligens*). This gentle suggestion of a natural law pertaining to justice being equated with, but distinct from, laws of physics, is further validated by his description of its invariability: "To say there is nothing of just or unjust, but what is commanded or forbidden by positive law, is the same as saying that, before the describing of a circle, all the radii were not equal."[29]

But the orientation of natural law, *i.e.,* its moral guidance, is not subject to personal interpretation, and its purpose is to provide a latticework on which to build man's positive laws. There is no contradiction here, for if a particular positive law is consistent with our innate moral guidance the resulting structure is more likely to stand the tests of time, whereas a positive law that is inconsistent with our moral nature is likely at some point to invite disavowal and to fail. Such a description, of course, is too simplistic, for improper positive laws abound in most societies, yet many seem to thrive. This is deceptive, however, for survival today does not mean survival in ten years or a century from now. The history of the world so far is the history of fallen civilizations, and our own history is now being written. Inconsistencies between natural law and authoritarian directives, as discussed in this chapter, can be blamed for failed policies that repeatedly return civilizations to a primitive state, for there seems to be some powerful yet undefinable force declaring those civilizations were on the wrong path rather than merely an alternative pathway and that their misbegotten ventures must be brought to an end. The great hope, of course, is that someday there will be sufficient congruence between natural law and positive law that previous inconsistencies, some by their nature deemed malevolent and some for the moment deemed necessary, will become obsolete, and that all of mankind's disagreements will then be minor ones.

This brief section, however, has not been inserted to opine on mankind's future. Its purpose here is to propose one reason for the decline of civilizations, and not only the

---

[28] See his famous work, *De Iure Belli ac Pacis* (the Rights of war and peace), first published in 1625.

[29] Montesquieu, *The Spirit of Laws,* I, i, translation of Thomas Nugent. The first publication of work, in French, was in 1748. Nugent's translation of that first edition was published in 1750. But to imply that a sense of justice, and therefore a sense of right and wrong, was imbued in the Creation suggests an acknowledgement of the Creator, whereas Montesquieu's commitment to religion has been questioned. Interestingly, in Book I, chapter 2, Montesquieu discusses laws of nature as they apply to primitive man, of which he lists four. The first, based on fear, deals with survival, the second with security/safety (includes nutrition), the third with social interaction (direct, interpersonal), and the fourth with a desire to live within a society. Except for the fourth, the list reflects the first three levels of motivation proposed by Maslow (see footnote, p. 286), his fourth being the motivation for esteem of others, which, of course, can only occur within a society. This list of Montesquieu's, however, is not a formulation of natural law but a response to laws of nature.

nineteen great ones identified by Toynbee, but also a myriad of minor ones, including all twelve that were described in chapter 33. But one cannot help but consider that *The Natural State of Medical Practice* described in this volume is a verification, however burdened its analysis with human error and ignorance, of not only the existence of, but the critical role of adhering, through democratic governance, to natural law and thereby contributing to, if not actually causing, the global intellectual dominance of Western thought and beneficence, as well as being the sole arbiter and architect of human progress.[30]

---

[30] See also: Wilson, J. Q., *The Moral Sense*, New York, 1993. In this excellent book evidence is collected to show that humans have an innate moral sense. He does not mention natural law in his book, but the objective evidence accessible to mankind for both is similar. Dr. Wilson does not specifically state that the origins of the moral sense and of natural law are different, and separately he has indicated he hoped they were the same (see interview at Acton Institute in *Religion and Liberty*, Vol. 9, No. 4, *The Free Society Requires a Moral Sense, Social Capital*). But in doing so he has avoided a formal listing of "absolute" natural laws sometimes given by others in descriptions of natural law, preferring more generic mechanisms of moral guidance: sympathy, fairness, self-control, and duty, each of the four being a title of a chapter in his book. This is a convenient way to look at the issue, for specific laws suggested by scholars can be interpreted in various, often confusing, ways, not always good or helpful, that support of their preferred dogma or positive laws, *i.e.*, laws propagated by man. And who would want to make a law against sympathy? Wilson also stated that in the West there has been an increase in scope of the moral sense. It is flourishing as a concept, and its precepts for moral guidance in the West are considered relevant in more and more circumstances, including international ones. A major area is in laws governing the use of the seas. All this is not a result of the teaching of natural law or moral sense to modern generations. This cannot be done and is irrelevant. It means, instead, that the universality and reality of natural law is beginning to emerge through millennia of layers of human (positive) law. And with an appreciation that intrinsic moral guidance, spontaneous order, and natural law are perspectives of the same innate counseling all humans possess, the potential role they can play in shepherding human events becomes even more powerful. At the same time, an understanding of the history of and the potential role of human agencies in preventing their effects becoming manifest have also become more obvious. This is a debate that requires further discussion, but the present work supports the critical role of liberty in permitting natural law to be felt and followed.

But it is not natural law *ipso facto* that leads to progress, for, as discussed earlier, progress is primarily a consequence of group liberty, and the focused nature of small group interests is less likely to benefit from natural law guidance than those interests that are distributed throughout the general population. On the other hand, when human reason has proposed positive laws consistent with natural law it will naturally follow that individual and group liberty and thereby progress are more likely to become manifest. The period of greatest liberty in the development of a civilization is the same period in which progress in medical knowledge has emerged, doing so coincident with the flourishing of medical practice best exemplified historically in the ancient Greece of Hippocrates. All of this can be seen to be integrated into a philosophical unity that can explain not only the repetitive cycling of civilizations but also the thousands of years of delay in evolution of, at long last, a civilization capable of immense progress in all areas affecting mankind. And that progress has occurred over a very short time, but several centuries, and with no assistance from any other agency, nor sword nor prayer, except the one that counts most: natural law. Beginning with religious freedom in the 16th C, its propagation in the 17th C, proceeding to parliamentary governance of the 18th C, and thence to the consequent widespread shower of knowledge and commercial prosperity of the 19th C, the West has been the fortunate recipient of the consequences of obedience to natural law, and it has done so despite the great wounds to our civilization imposed by desperate attempts of a long list of prominent villains and fanatics who have ignored moral guidance and imposed their blinded visions on hapless millions.

E. Natural Law in Early Society

Innate guidance on human interactions should have made its effects apparent in those prehistoric attempts at communal living at a time before social complexity and population size began to camouflage the internal conscience residing in all persons. This has been pointed out by James A. Donald, who stresses that early society knew natural law because it had to know it for survival.[31] It is because many other factors, including man-made laws, impinge today on natural law that make its effects so difficult to assess that its very existence is questioned by many. Although Donald argues that natural law is more a method than a list of laws, for purposes of discussion of its relevance in primitive society some reasonably implied attributes have been summarized as follows:[32]

1. protection of life
2. keep promises
3. do not wrong another
4. trust
5. individual liberty
6. protection of property

From the subjects on this list it is clear, for example, that protection of life in its various forms, primarily human life, is a fact of life in ancient civilizations as well as modern, anthropological detail that jumps out at us from burial practices, monumental ritual structures, religious and mythical artistic renderings of females relevant to birth, death, and transfigurations, and matrilineal societies. The primacy and veneration of life and birth before all things is unassailable. Issues of infanticide, geronticide, human sacrifice, and wars of conquest are the warped superimpositions on mankind of the positive laws of man. It is indeed the awesome magnitude of this evil that in turn inflicts on the powerless the conclusion that those few in charge who ordain what would otherwise be evil must be supported by some unearthly power. People view an execution for its profundity, not its fun. To think that people in any age would view human sacrifice as a good thing is incorrect. It is considered merely a better thing than the reason for the sacrifice in the first place, which must have been very bad indeed. Human sacrifice is, therefore, an entirely human production, a particularly grotesque formulation of positive law.

Item 2 on the list can be similarly treated. The inviolability of certain social interactions is universal, such as the trading routes and message sticks used over centuries by Australian aborigines under time-honored rules of safe passage. The keeping of promises is topical in that its political relevance is being debated even today, but its relevance to the formation of early societies must have been as fundamental then as now. The importance of keeping of a promise would have applied to all members of ancient and primitive societies, and this reciprocity is commonly displayed in barter and exchange and other commercial trading. It can be implied in gift-giving, courtesies and reputations.

Items 3 and 4 are issues of doing wrong to another and of trust, and are related items and are not discussed here.

But disregard for the last two items on the list of the inferred moral guides would have been in conflict between natural law and communal survival. They involve

---

[31] See: Donald, J. A., *Natural Law and Natural Rights*, from the James's Liberty file collection index, licensed under the Creative Commons Attribution-Share Alike 3.0 License, n.d.

[32] Johnston, J. F., Jr., *Natural Law and the Rule of Law*, 2003, The Philadelphia Society.

individual liberty and personal property. Just as moral sense can be veiled or superseded by a desire for something that may be amoral or immoral, the natural desire of an individual to follow a benign personal inclination or to own something of personal value may not have been considered acceptable behavior by other members of an egalitarian society. Egalitarianism and its coveted security founded in homogeneity of thought and action would have been a way to minimize conflict or to control distribution within the community, and behavior to the contrary would have resulted in efforts to stop it. By redistribution of material needs, greed would not have a chance to progress to robbery and conflict even though greed may have been an unspoken part-and-parcel of the decision for redistribution in the first place. This might be considered a fair trade-off: on one hand greed was confined by social coercion, but on the other hand greed was acknowledged. But what might have been the consequences of primitive egalitarianism in the overriding the two inferred moral principles of natural law?

Individualism may have been considered antisocial or irrational behavior in egalitarian societies where every member was expected to contribute to communal goals. But there is a natural desire of the individual to think, travel, explore, and attempt based on personal inclinations, *i.e.,* to be at liberty to act on one's own behalf, whether out of curiosity, interest, or self-interest. As this is constrained in egalitarian society, there must have been continuous tension between anyone expressing novel interests and the rest of the community. The cry of the egalitarian to this day is for a predictable homogeneity of society, to make everyone else as good as we are, although this wish for homogeneity often is made to masquerade as a humanitarian desire for economic equality.[33] But this ccomes with a price. Now the confusion of what is "good" according to our conscience is to not interfere with the actions of others, and this is supported by early mankind's tendency to disperse in small independent groups. This conflicts with the "opinion of what is good" for our convenience, this is supported by the illusion of fairness.[34] The resulting loss of innovative ideas ensures a static society and prevents progress. Catalhoyuk is an example of this. Over a thousand years, approximately the time from the Battle of Hastings to the present day, roughly fifty generations of its people followed the same unwritten social directives. One consequence was that few reached the age of 45 years. There is no way to judge whether they were a happy people, but if they were it was because they knew not what they were missing. Egalitarian society, by disarming the moral consciences of its members in its infringement of individual liberty, is inadequate in defense, unprepared for the unexpected, incapable of progress, and, while perhaps not overtly intemperate, chronically disgruntled.

---

[33] The opposite end of this social spectrum is the free society, where individual freedom is prized and censorship abhorred. Lack of homogeneity results in a social analogue of Brownian motion that contrasts sharply with enforced homogeneity of egalitarianism. As a static society contrasts with an enterprising one, it is the former that is the more organized, unified, and easily commanded, whereas the latter, when healthy, is of such varied interests that it is more difficult to organize, impossible to reach unanimity, and, because of intrinsic differences, fractious. To outsiders it will seem disorganized and lacking a communal sensibility and common goal. This can quickly change, however, when a point is reached where its freedoms are threatened.

[34] The "activities of others" is not an invitation to libertines. But it needs repeating that individual liberty under natural law does not include the liberty to do wrong. This distinction and its philosophical support and political implications are lucidly discussed by Dr. Hadley Arkes in *A Natural Law Manifesto,* available on the website of the *James Wilson Institute on Natural Rights and the American Founding.*

The protection of property is an equally complex and important issue in that acquiring property, whether land, an invention, a special tool, or a secret cache of something desirable would have been contentious in strictly egalitarian societies. In them, attempts at ownership, if successful, are presently thought to have introduced a propensity for permanent settlements.[35] Thus, by obstructing ownership, nomadic populations were guaranteed a future of nomadism and forever denied any possibility of progress within their societies.

Natural law, in summary, provides a moral guide for every individual in a society and, as a consequence, a judicial way of life, a protection, and a guide for society itself. Self-interest is very much served if all in a society are permitted to respond to their own moral compass, for it is the same moral compass in all. It is, therefore, not only a stabilizing influence on society's individual membership but one that quietly works, through human reason, to the benefit of everyone, not just the few in charge or the few who make or interpret the laws. In a sense it allows society to function as a koinon: by permitting all in a society to freely give their opinions in open forum discussion, the final decision will have had the benefit of many minds concentrating on the problem at hand. And democracy can permit natural law/moral guidance to emerge because in a democracy each individual should have a protected freedom of expression. In this sense natural law can never find adequate expression under egalitarian and authoritarian governance, for in the latter the individual must speak for the leader, and in egalitarianism the individual cannot speak.

Natural law will, however, lose its influence if enough members do not observe it or are prevented from observing it. Among the variables that can destabilize a society a difficult one is the refractory member, and it has been suggested that as many as one in twenty-five persons in modern society can be considered a sociopath, *i.e.,* a person with an unclear distinction between right and wrong.[36] These individuals, who will be more likely to consider the end to justify the means, have bedeviled all societies over the ages, especially when in positions of leadership. They can be managed at an early stage by social pressures if they can be identified, but as populations increase such individuals become lost in the crowd and can proceed to mischievous ends by attracting similar

---

[35] Woodburn, J., *Egalitarian Societies,* in *Man* (N.S.) 17:431-451, 1981.

[36] Let the population of a small ancient settlement comprise 100 persons, of whom there are 10 infants, 20 children, 30 subadults, and 40 adults. Of the 40 adults, half would be men. Of the twenty men 5% (*i.e.,* one) might be a sociopath/psychopath or functional equivalent. (A recent book by a Harvard psychologist estimates 1 in 25 Americans is sociopathic.) That person would easily be controlled or ostracized by the others in the settlement. And if there were 1000 people in a village, each of whom knew most of the others, and 10 were sociopaths and worked in concert, they would be dangerous, but the other 390 adults would know of them, recognize them, and could probably contain them. But if there were a small city of 10,000 and miscreants numbered 100, there would be a big problem. They could be unrecognizable within the larger population and able to foment fear and attract others to join with them to control part or all of the community. But as a civilization expands, it appears that the opportunity for authoritarian personalities to control events in a population arises. If sociopathic behavior were merely the lower end of a Gaussian curve of normal human behavior rather than an aberrancy, then their authoritarian risk to a society would be inherent in all societies, a risk of danger that will increase proportionally as the population increases unless there is a form of governance that does not restrict individual liberty for the great majority but is able to prevent antisocial behavior in the few. That risk should be susceptible to calculation and thereby quantifiable.

persons into their cause and become sufficiently powerful to the point of destabilizing society. It has been truly said that "the bigger the pack, the meaner the dog."

In conclusion, natural law is not a scientific construct, and its origin can be debated. But if it is a uniquely human quality then its origin must be traced back to mankind's creation. Darwinian natural selection based on genetics, particularly genetics relevant to neurological function and thus affected by millions of nucleotides, seems an unlikely explanation for any survival advantage. Any relevant genetic changes from selective pressure would necessarily have gradually evolved, step by step, over many thousands of years. As a way of explaining behavioral characteristics and the human conscience this seems unreasonable, especially as, based on life expectancy, any claim of survival advantage is disingenuous. It is not surprising, therefore, that natural law is considered an argument in support of creationism. And insofar as egalitarianism undermines the moral conscience (natural law), egalitarianism itself can be considered logically immoral. If this is the case, the perpetuation of human misery within its purvue can be blamed on that immorality. The epithet of "immoral" has often been cast at promoters of egalitarianism. But note the timing in the evolution of society of this particular type of immorality. It begets two distinct forms of expression. In an established society, egalitarianism undermines individualism and is used as a tool to control the common man, whereas in early/primitive society communal coercion prevents his development.

How did natural law impact human civilization at the earliest stages of society? In recent history natural law has been invoked in the formation of laws of the United States guaranteeing individual liberty. This aspect of natural law, if active in a primitive society, should have prompted efforts to improve that society by permitting progress in that individuals in that society could search out what was personally best. Everyone could could then benefit from one individual's effort or discovery, the benefits being much greater and more enduring than occasionally sharing a good meal. But this did not happen until egalitarian kinship was abandoned, with the consequences now to be discussed.

CHAPTER THIRTY-SEVEN

HETERARCHY AND THE KOINON

The role of writing in promoting progress is reviewed and it is concluded that inscribed symbols first develop as a tool for commercial operation, but proper writing is a sign of progress rather than a cause of progress. In this sense it can be equated with a medical practice as an early marker of progress. Once matured, the usefulness of the tool is remarkable to the point that it becomes, unexpectedly, an intellectual end in itself. In contrast to writing, it is the formation of small autonomous groups promoting self-interest by providing a useful commodity or service that, although developing in parallel with writing, are the true initiators of progress. The optimal small autonomous group is the koinon and its features are, for a second time, presented. It is proposed that independent self-interest groups are more likely in a heterarchical society because a commerce-guided society permits individuals to forego their allegiances to egalitarian kinships and thereby free to pursue specialized self-interests that prove useful as part of a settlement hierarchy.

A. Writing Systems and Societal Progress

Writing is commonly ascribed a pivotal role in human progress, but is that accurate? One reason for such an opinion is that it is through ancient writings that we know of ancient happenings. This is quite different from attributing to those writings a causal role in the happenings themselves. Furthermore, writing systems develop from simple markings, but, simple or complex, their modern translations display considerable imagination and literary license. The gifted prose and poetry of translators of ancient texts, especially myths and religious experiences, are wonderful to read because literal translations are rudimentary, leaving great scope for the imagination and personality of the creative translator. The *Iliad* in Homeric Greek may be an exception, but even it went through the redacting hands of experts of the Library of Alexandria.

It takes time for complex language to evolve from its simple roots, but writing evolves more slowly still. For example, spoken language is quickly affected by interaction with other languages, but a writing system is inherently conservative, in part because its value lies in providing historical records that remain accessible for a long time. It may have taken but two or three hundred years for Vulgar Latin to replace Classical Latin, then another two or three hundred years for Romance Languages to replace Vulgar Latin, but the same Greek script, Chinese logograms, and Sumerian cuneiform are identifiable over a span of 3,000 years. Yet society moves ahead regardless. The rapid evolution of Hippocratic medicine occurred despite the absence of a medical vocabulary.[1] The converse occurred: the written medical vocabulary that developed was the consequence of the clinical prowess of Hippocratic physicians.

A change in a writing system, meaning an increase in its vocabulary or complexity, is prompted by need, whether in commerce, managing a dominion, or advances in crafts and trades. It is as society changes that a writing system evolves, for writing is the consequence, not the cause, of change. The great advance of written characters representing solely syllabic sounds that would evolve into classical Greek not

---

[1] Hippocratic medicine nevertheless deserved a dictionary. See: Adams, W. H., *The Natural State of Medical Practice: Hippocratic Evidence*, Maitland (FL), 2019, the Appendix.

surprisingly occurred in the 12th C BC with the master traders of the Mediterranean and beyond, the Phoenicians. It is for such practical reasons that writing should be relegated to a secondary place in initiating mankind's march to progress.

It should be expected that writing and a true medical practice would develop concurrently, especially when the volume of information in a particular area increases beyond an individual's capability to remember and to master, regardless of whether that information is commercial or medical. It should also not be unexpected that the absence of one parallels absence of the other. And if both are absent, as they appear to be in eleven, and probably all, of the twelve lesser primary civilizations studied herein, there is likely a common explanation. It is argued here that the lack of a writing system in the twelve civilizations is an indication that in none had there been any societal progress, regardless of their civilizations' duration or size. Things may have gotten bigger, but not better. It is no surprise that egalitarian status was not associated with writing.

Where commercial activity existed, identification seals, numbers, and other marks were needed and were invented. These were tactical items relating to commerce, but the sphere of influence of the persons involved was often spanned by personal contact or a messenger. Simple inscribed forms were sufficient for tallying. Writing is a symbolization of language, and it was unnecessary if there was nothing about which to write, if direct communication was convenient and sufficient, or if the number of camels required for a number of bags of grain or the number of bricks needed for a wall was the level of complexity needed. It was only when specialization of goods and services occurred in a community and the knowledge and vocabulary so acquired expanded to the point that those providing special services could function better with access to permanent records that proper writing appeared. Statistical analysis earlier in this volume (p. 621*f*) indicated a strong association between writing and "progress" using a nascent medical profession as a marker. But whether medicine preceded writing is not analyzable with information at hand. Restated, it is likely that prosperity and specialization resulting from commercial success, rather than activities related to the commerce itself, that led to the invention of true writing.

The persistence of ancient writing in three of the four great riverine civilizations of chapters 3-6 might suggest a true written language was necessary for their prolonged survival as their populations grew and commerce expanded. But an alternative explanation is that it was only their initial primary civilizations (*i.e.*, predynastic Sumer and Protodynastic Egypt, and [probably] predynastic China and the Indus River civilization) that promoted true writing, for it was developed to assist in their provision of complex goods and services during the settlement hierarchy of early urbanization. It was only because of the military successes by subsequent regimes in Mesopotamia, Egypt and China that the succeeding secondary authoritarian civilizations found writing useful for secret knowledge and for commanding their dominions. We view writing differently now, but for the building of early empires writing was a tool for domination as well as for commerce, but not progress.

It can be proposed, therefore, that had any of the twelve lesser civilizations expanded in population and commerce, neither a writing system nor a medical profession would have ensued there was a point during the phase of commercial development that supported free enterprise. That point was not reached, and probably never would have been reached in any of the long-lived lesser civilization, for all retained prominent kinship elements. Complexity of commercial activity was insufficient to require anything more than seals or enumeration mnemonics such as the Norte Chico civilization "quipu," a device of strings that served for numeric memory. This does not in any way imply that the lesser civilizations could not have devised true writing systems. It merely indicates that their civilizations never approached, even in a thousand years, the complexity that prosperity and ingenuity of the common man and woman could provide. Ingenuity is not a characteristic of egalitarianism.

Seven thousand languages are known today, of which approximately 4,000 have writing systems, many being writing systems of primitive or recently extinct cultures/civilizations. It is thought, however, that most are neither used nor useful, and of the 7,000 languages fully half of them are spoken by no more than a few thousand persons. If a writing system is a requirement for societal progress, it is surely not apparent in those primitive or recently extinct cultures/civilizations that had, or have, one.

Finally, a number of written languages are recognized from the Bronze Age, but most, including the Cypro-Minoan syllabary, Linear A of the Minoan civilization, and the Harappan "script" of the Indus River Valley civilization, disappeared when their parent cultures disappeared. It is not being argued that written languages are of little use to their cultures, but it is obvious that a writing system is not essential to initiation of progress and that the presence of a writing system is no guarantor of survival.

The question is whether the lack of a written language prevents progress at an early stage, and the answer is "no." It is the lack of progress that prevents emergence of a writing system. In the realization of progress the decisive factor is the autonomous group with a common self-interest that has something to write about.

B. The Individualist vs. the Autonomous Group

Did early humans promptly see benefit in organizing into groups? It would seem the presence of children and the importance of family and kinship as a sympathetic force for ensuring security and survival would have prompted such behavior, although that may be judging the past by present standards. One might have expected to see a large settlement not too far from Eden's gate, with colonies gradually extending the inhabited region town by town as local subsistence became insufficient for the concentrated population. Instead, what seems to have been a purposeful flight from others of the same species occurred, and this would help explain the relentless early global spread of *Homo sapiens* in the absence of crowding. How/why did humans reach such disparate geographical regions rather than developing a flourishing large egalitarian society in one locale, and yet retain a pattern of thinking that produced similar results so far afield? Why did not Africa become fully inhabited first, with subsequent human colonization elsewhere a planned event? Why was the Tower of Babel considered necessary to bring together our species?[2] Was there something inherent in humans that, like cats, preferred a more solitary existence?

One aspect of the issue is group size, based on the observation by some that humans have little aggressiveness in small hunter-gatherer groups and that it is the appearance of larger communities that is associated with the tendency of some humans to exert control over others, a trait primarily observed in males.[3] A perspective of the small

---

[2] The *Book of Genesis* states that the Tower of Babel, Babel being the incipient Babylon, was a sign to God that humankind was opposing the command to disperse about the earth. The metaphorical application of different languages to halt this process was to ensure the desired dispersion.

[3] Prof. T. W. Luke, in his book, *Social Theory and Modernity* (Newbury Park (CA), 1990), comments on p. 107 that "natural man", who was once free by being a part of Nature, becomes

group preference is that all humans desire to control their own destinies and that it is not part of their nature to subject themselves to other humans. Thus, there is a tendency to disperse in small groups, as discussed earlier (see p. 637*f*).

The original group of two humans, which science has nicely placed in Africa but inconveniently well apart in distance and in time, has since been followed by ever larger groups.[4] This volume has focused much on groups of socially or genetically related individuals, from bands, tribes, and chiefdoms to states. But it was noted within these various expressions of egalitarian kinship that, in concept, an individual of superior competence reaped no personal benefit and an individual with an ingenious idea was prevented from implementing it. In this early egalitarian world individualism had no place, and the idea of freedom for the individual would have been considered nonsense.

Now, however, focus on a subgroup with a common interest operating within a large group. In Part I (p. 129) an excursus was dedicated to a description of a particular group, the *koinon*, considered an ancient Greek invention as applied to a communal polity or to a federation of city-states. The open and equal expression of opinions and ideas permitted in these freely-entered-into groups is proposed to have been applied to a variety of other organizations by the Greeks, one being a group of professional medical practitioners organized by Hippocrates. Because each physician member was autonomous this grouping of physicians was not an example of "groupism," which is a desire to belong to a group and thereby share in that group's particular value system and goals. In groupism members relinquish some of their individuality because the group becomes more important than any one individual and, in setting its course for members, the group achieves authority over them that either forces a member to act in a way that may not be in his best interest or, for the indecisive, uses the power of rhetoric or intrigue to make certain that what leadership considers the proper decision is taken. The Hippocratic physicians, in contrast, functioned as a network of individuals who shared a common goal in that each wished to improve the medical service he offered but the group had no purpose other than to provide open exchange of ideas and experience which each member might or might not elect to incorporate into his medical practice; there was no other purpose of the koinon than to serve as a reservoir of ever-increasing knowledge into which any member could dip. And that is the uniqueness of the koinon: it had no goal that was not consonant with the goal of every member and it had no role that could be commandeered for any one or a few members' personal benefit. The koinon was a network of autonomous individuals rather than an alliance or a consortium.

The point made here is that, in the temporal order of things, it was the relative freedom of early urbanization that prompted entrepreneurial independent action by individuals, but their actions in exploiting their commodity or service for personal gain were manifested through a group. And the reason for this is the superiority of a group over an individual in solving a problem. In medicine, for example, the care provided by a single individual in a band or tribe, whether a family member or a neighbor, was old news and incapable of improvement. But to have several individuals combine their ingenuity and promote their improved service to the community was, based on prior experience in an egalitarian world, a vast improvement. Thus, the group preceded the

---

unfree in society as social artifice works to dominate Nature. By accepting new social needs and duties, social man becomes something he really is not and generates a false objectivity that robs him of his true essence.

[4] See: Poznik, G. D., *et al.*, *Sequencing Y Chromosomes Resolves Discrepancy in Time to Common Ancestors of Males Versus Females*, in *Science*: 341:562-565, 2013.

individualist because no individual had ever been permitted to progress beyond mere empiricism. It was only after the possibility of improvement was discovered and implemented by the koinon that an individual could consider independent exploitation of his or her own ingenuity.

C. The Essential Role of the "Group" in Progress of a Society; the Koinon

There is a recently published book, *The Age of the Network*, that refers to ancient networking of small groups as a time of major progress of early civilization, their face-to-face techniques that led to our present enviable state now finally being acknowledged.[5] While this may be true, two points should be considered. (1) Mankind has since its inception been desirous of and capable of personal interactions to improve its condition. This capability is not brilliant or unexpected; it is a normal response to motivating circumstances. "Two heads are better than one" is not a new idea, although leave it to modern scholarship to confirm it as true.[6] The issue is not its ingenuity; the issue is what prevents it from happening, a theme than runs throughout the present work. (2) There are many types of human networks that fulfill a common need for a subpopulation, for example, a common interest such as ethnicity or dogma. The function of these groups is usually not only social interaction within the confines of the group, but also the amplification of the group's presence and voice in the greater society.[7] But the networks relevant to present topic are but two: networks of individuals and networks of groups. The former is the koinon; the latter is the heterarchy.

A heterarchy does not speak for the individual; it speaks for the organization or a network of organizations. Its power is related to the size and number of the organizations, and it is discussed below. In contrast, a koinon represents a single group that is a network of individuals. There are some semantic difficulties with this definition, for Greek confederations of city-states were called koinons, and yet they functioned more as a heterarchy. Thus, it has been the process, rather than composition, of the koinon that is used to define the term's meaning in this volume.

As it is presently understood, the ancient Greeks first developed this novel type of network. It may have existed earlier, perhaps even in prehistory, although there is no way of knowing. But as a society initiated urbanization there could be personal contact between like-minded individuals. Prosperity promotes specialization, and, as population increased, networks of individuals could more easily form to further common goals of self-interest, a desideratum previously unavailable to the smaller societies that lived and planned from day to day and worked within the confines of an egalitarian kinship. The personal networks so formed would have benefited each member and at the same time

---

[5] Lipnack, J., and Stamps, J., *The Age of the Network*, Essex Jct., Vermont, 1994, p. 48.

[6] See: Wooley, A. W., et al., *Collective Intelligence and Group Performance*, in *Current Directions in Psychological Science*, 24:420-424, 2015. And there is the common sense interpretation of C. S. Lewis: "Two heads are better than one, not because either is infallible, but because they are unlikely to go wrong in the same direction."

[7] See: Katz, N., et al., *Network Theory and Small Groups*, in *Small Group Research*, 35:307-332, 2004.

would spread throughout society as the group's particular commodity or service became popular.[8]

What is necessary for a koinon to form and successfully function? As a koinon is not a populist group or political party, and as it represents a group of people who provide specialized services or products, the upper limit of a koinon's size is, as stated above, small relative to the size of its community. Its members are equals when it comes to the function of the koinon: equal voice, equal opportunity. For physicians, they might be dispersed throughout the community rather than living and working in proximity to each other. The koinon can function regardless of the type of community governance, *e.g.*, hierarchy, oligarchy, tyranny, democracy, unless it or its members are directly threatened by that governance, for its network is apolitical. But it could not exist in an egalitarian society because the mere presence of specialization leading to personal aggrandizement inserts an inequality into the community that would be leveled, either by thwarting its development or by requiring that koinon members distribute their commodity or service to all in the community as an egalitarian duty. The motive for individualism in koinon members would thereby be nullified.

Unity of action is no requirement for a koinon, for its most important tool is communication between members. Indeed, it is the only implement used. There is a chronological requirement, and, based on analysis of ancient Greece and the Modern West, a medical koinon might need two or three centuries to develop and function as a profession within an established community susceptible to progress. Modern English dictionaries have fifty or more synonyms for "group," but none satisfactorily encompass the composition and function of the koinon. For this reason the ancient Greek word has been retained in Romanized form and in restricted usage for the present work.

D. Heterarchy vs. Koinon

The concept of heterarchy has been applied to many scholarly areas, including mathematics and neural physiology.[9] The importance of global informational exchange and business management also has prompted great interest in networking and heterarchies. There are general attributes that have been ascribed to hierarchy and heterarchy, and the differences can be profound in archetypal models. A summary of real or inferred characteristics of hierarchic and heterarchic "dynamics" concludes the former tends to rigidity, gender stratification, centralized control, a rigid class system, a focus on violence, imposed solutions, a predisposition to imperialism, authoritarianism, and a steady state, whereas the latter tends to flexibility, equal gender access, multi-modal market economy, multiple avenues for advancement, a focus on peace, pluralism, consensus orientation, and temporal fluctuation.[10] But to avoid caricatures, both

---

[8] This does not hold today as there are egalitarian communities that avoid capitalistic ventures while residing within modern democracies, for those democracies provide the physical, legal, and economic security that enables small egalitarian communities to exist and thrive, something previously impossible.

[9] For an introduction to heterarchy as it applies to anthropology see the overview of the concept by its early advocate, Dr. Carole Crumley, *Heterarchy and the Analysis of Complex Societies*, in *Archeological Papers of the American Archeological Association*, 6:1-5, 1995.

[10] See: Gill, R. B., *The Great Maya Droughts*, Albuquerque, 2000. This listing is a summary of the Table found on p. 65 of that publication.

hierarchy and heterarchy inevitably coexist in social symbiosis. Thus, there is a degree of confusion in its definition. Present context, however, is the role of heterarchy in the organization and function of commercial units within larger human settlements such as the city-states as defined on p. 13. It is important, therefore, to restrictively define the term:

> Heterarchy: A nongovernmental form of provincial management by fluctuating commercial interests.

It is key that heterarchy is an informal network of groups, not individuals, whereby each commercial interest has its leader and the overweening goal is the security and prosperity of its members. The shifting social importance of independent commercial organizations that operate independently of government is heterarchical, and the well-being and availability of the regional total workforce, the coordination of transport, and other inter-organizational issues for this heterarchy of organizations is justification for the describing a heterarchy as a "network."[11]

Archeological evidence of a heterarchy is primarily based on lack of evidence for a political hierarchy and elite groups. Thus, heterarchy is considered a consequence of managerial mechanisms now thought to better explain prosperity and social order in large archeologically egalitarian societies.

The medical koinon, while profoundly different from a heterarchy, has some similarities. The koinon, like a heterarchy, has no permanent head. On the other hand, the role of a leader in a koinon, should there be one, is that of a panel moderator rather than leadership directed by policy. Like a heterarchy it is a network, but it is a network of individuals rather than groups, and those individuals are functionally independent and not dependent in the delivery of their service upon the interventions of other members of the koinon, whereas commercial interests in a heterarchy can be either at variance with or assist each other. A koinon also resembles a heterarchy in that competition can provide a stimulus, although its response to the stimulus is to improve its function rather than obliterate competition. Finally, there is a group purpose in a heterarchy which may or may not fit comfortably with the individual member, whereas in a koinon each member has the option of saying "take it or leave it" and suffers no consequence if the latter is chosen. In Part I the local Chamber of Commerce in an American town was likened to a koinon (p. 131).

Very different, therefore, is the koinon from the heterarchical group. The koinon of a craft, service, or trade might number just a few members and function very well, although its social influence in comparison to other organizations would be diminutive. The significance of a heterarchical group, however, increases with group size: more work

---

[11] There is an important theory in social management that applies to economics: spontaneous order. This refers, in the opinion of many experts, to the "invisible hand" of Adam Smith, the guiding force that results in free markets producing better results than those originating from centralized government. The "invisible hand" is not a mystical force, although the details of its effectiveness are not fully understood. At its core is the idea that a group of free individuals in a free market, on its own and without direction from either external or internal organizing forces and with no particular goal or planning, will, by the commercial activity of individuals left alone to make their own decisions, arrive at an optimally functioning market. It produces order out of chaos, and there is no leadership whatsoever. The good result is the consequence of the conglomerate action of individuals, each acting without compulsion.

is done, more things produced, a greater population is reached, a spin-off group to add to the existing heterarchical structure more likely. Accumulation of power is inevitable, although its setting is variable. The smaller koinon is the initiator of progress; heterarchy is its exploiter. And this leads to a profound and perhaps unexpected conclusion that bears on the role of the heterarchical network in the history of civilizations.

E. Conclusion – Cities, the City-State, and Heterarchy

As a prelude to this Section, Dr. Ingolf Thuesen has proposed a four-stage process in which a community can evolve over time that may encompass heterarchy.[12] In the earliest stage a settlement develops that can interact with proximal settlements in such a way as to become the regional "central city." This process requires no chief or bureaucratic structure, as it is, in effect, the result of networks that develop at the individual or small group level. The subsequent three stages are the city-state, the city-state empire and the provincial city. According to this scheme, the stage that provides the window of opportunity for individual and group enterprise is the first stage. The general thesis of the first stage by Dr. Thuesen is similar to the role and effect of heterarchy, with the notable exception that he has the nuclear settlement preceding the development of trade patterns, whereas it is here posited that no cluster of settlements developed into a larger nuclear center until one was purposely formed by commercial interests, probably arising in market towns. His subsequent three stages are the consequence of political and military force. As the history of politics and warfare attract the most attention, it is no surprise that the first and transient entrepreneurial phase usually goes unmentioned in history, the final three stages chronologically engulfing the flickering beginning of progress. But it is that first networking stage, or shortly thereafter, that is proposed as the likely time for the initial collection of data that would appear in the classics of medicine in the five successful civilizations.

The role of heterarchy as an important force on the path to progress has been implied in this and preceding chapters, sometimes in the context of city-states and at times in hierarchies and egalitarian societies. From this it may be suspected that heterarchy can be viewed as a tool, one that is useful in any society but one that, while a capable temporary substitute for decision-making in a society, cannot be considered a permanent mechanism of governance. One reason for this thinking is that a heterarchy of commercial interests refers not to management of an entire society but only to a slice of that society. This is reasonable, for it seems unrealistic to suppose that an entire society, or civilization, can have as its primary governance a managerial policy that shifts from place to place, from department to department, or even from city-state to city-state, depending on trade or a manufactured product or other external event that causes the locus of influence to shift from one place to another.

But consider the following. In contrast to Erich Fromm's pessimistic opinion of the common man in his book, *Escape from Freedom* (see p. 426, footnote), the American experience revealed a population that, once it escaped authoritarian European bondage, reveled in its freedom and flourished, rather than seeking but another master.[13] In doing

---

[12] See: Thuesen, I., *The City-State in Ancient Western Syria*, in *Comparative Study of thirty City-State Cultures*, Copenhagen, 2000, M. H. Hansen, editor, p. 64.

[13] In a sense, Dr. Fromm is not completely contradicted, because the 20th C European populations upon which he based his analysis had nowhere to go to find freedom, nowhere to escape *to*. But in

this the diverse social organizations in America that developed throughout much of its history, including religious, commercial, industrial, and ethnic, can be considered an amalgamation of heterarchies in that they provided a contractual structure for local prosperity and growth that averted chaos while little central bureaucratic authority existed. Even today it is the prospering of autonomous industries, trades, crafts, organizations, guilds, sects, and brotherhoods/sisterhoods that, free from controls of the State, provide a continuity of culture, freedom and personal choice despite the unending political avarice and turmoil that attends each generation.

Thus, a role of heterarchy and its implied authority within the structure of a civilization can be traced from mankind's earliest settlements to the modern day. As archeological studies in the last century have disclosed, the move from hunter-gatherer to sedentism was for centuries a cautious movement and the original settlements were small. Rather than acting like a stab-inoculated culture of a bacterium and promptly extending its circumference homogeneously, humans chose instead to stay in small units, or settlements. Compared to nomadic groups early human settlements were smaller still, and this happened around the world in many cultures. People did not say, "Ah, the weather is improving, crops are bountiful, so let's move closer together so we can enjoy the pleasure of human company." No, thousands of years went by before cities came into being, and even then they did not come into being because they were desired. They came into being, despite the inconveniences they presented, because they were opportunities forbidden in egalitarian kinships. As the small human settlements matured and prospered, networks were formed between settlements, some near, some distant. Then, because of some commercial needs and benefits, including access to a workforce, efficiency in trading, security, and access to a convenience of transportation, the interests of one commercial venture sought to coalesce with the interests of other commercial ventures. Mutual benefit was found when several commercial ventures were conveniently located near each other. It was this commercially useful pattern that prompted enlarging settlements. The development of irrigation on a large scale was not intended as a nucleus about which urbanization would crystallize. Large-scale irrigation was a secondary response to an enlarging population fueled by commercialism. Thus, the early large towns and then cities were confederations of commercial enterprises. The larger aggregations of a population were not sought because of social enjoyments. Who, in those ancient days and in the absence of external threats of violence, would have preferred to live in a crowded walled city rather than a small village in the countryside. No, the attraction was not city lights. It was what the commercial interests provided: security, the hope of prosperity, and freedom from the regulated status of the egalitarian kinship. Cities were commercial, not social, inventions.[14] Once the benefits of these commercial confederations vanished, so did their populations.

---

addition to his analytical error of misinterpreting the tragic position many found themselves after WW I and unable to see any credible prospects for "self-realization," he not only confused a fear of freedom with a fear of chaos, but he also missed presenting the American experience, which might have led him to refrain from positing that communism would be mankind's ideal governance if only mankind would adjust its behavior accordingly.

[14] This possibility was raised by Blanton, et al., (*A Dual Processual Theory for the Evolution of Mesoamerican Civilization*, in *Anthropology*, 37:1-14, 1996) who identified a "corporate political strategy" whereby the sum of power in a population center was shared over a network of commercial interests that predated the rise of a leadership hierarchy. Also see the definition of "city" on p. 13, which requires only a discrete population in a defined space brought together for commercial

Given the social pattern just described, all city-states and traditional cities find their origins in heterarchy provided by confederations of commercial ventures.[15] This includes cities that sprang from colonies and modern cities purposefully designed to exploit a particular raw material or convenient piece of valuable geography. It is the pattern of commerce that has always been the spark of progress and prosperity. The exciting idea of the city being a wonderful development, a fount of enjoyment, learning, great institutions, and opportunity is a relatively modern perspective. For most people most of the time cities have instead been merely necessary institutions, often unhealthful ones. But present discussion concerns primary civilizations and the initiation of a centralized population that would evolve into a city. For urbanization during subsequent phases of civilizations up to modern times Dr. Monica Smith (cited above, on p. 3) has stated that in cities "kinship ties are reaffirmed and augmented, rather than destroyed" as neighborhoods and social interactions develop over time. This is not contested, although kinship in the ghetto should not necessarily be considered a positive attribute of cities.

As a focus of influence, heterarchy is to be reckoned with in originating what would become cities. But, as a piton upon which to attach the fragile thread of human liberty and the progress of mankind, it will fail the test. Its transcendental value in this effort lies in the following: (1) it provided an attractive haven for members of egalitarian kinships desiring to leave the security of the band or clan, (2) it provided a finite window of opportunity for progress during the development of a settlement hierarchy, (3) it provided a level of protection against hierarchical overreach once the latter emerged, (4) it provided a degree of durability that might give sufficient time for specialization and nascent professions to appear, (5) it provided a degree of stability within a community in times of hierarchical disruption, and (6) it provided a safety net in the life of the common man and woman over thousands of years. Its source of power resided in those who organized the production of bronze implements or those who bartered for a local storable crop and then "sold" it to a distant population that in return asked for more. It resided in those who had to invite, rather than to command, the local population to join in their commercial enterprise. A great debt is owed to heterarchy because the commercial world it harbored permitted mankind's escape from egalitarianism.

---

purposes. With this functional definition even size is not a characteristic of a city. Obviously the distinction between "town" and "city" becomes blurred, but (1) it is blurred anyway, and (2) a small town built around a commercial product can grow to be a large city, in which case "small" and "big" as arbitrarily assigned is the only adjectival distinction needed. All this does not deny the importance of attendant social needs, associations, and designs that develop in and contribute to city life, but at its heart the city, large or small, is a concentrated population that has crystallized around a commercial product.

[15] Or, to abbreviate the statement of Dr. Monica Smith, "...cities in the premodern world did not require a state level of political organization, only an initial impetus for settlement, ..." See: Smith, M. L., *The Social Construction of Ancient Cities*, Washington DC, 2010, the Introduction, p. 15. The only difference here is the author's opinion that this statement can be extended to include all cities.

CHAPTER THIRTY-EIGHT

ESCAPE FROM EGALITARIANISM

Ἐλευθέρους ἔθηκα
"I set them free."

Solon (638-558 BC), 36.15
Translation of John Lewis, from
his book, *Solon the Thinker*, London, 2006
(repeated here for of its ancient elegance)

After a definition of historicism and a review of its criticisms, it is argued that historicism may justifiably identify some basic threats to human progress and as an aspect of social science should not be discarded. It is further argued that historicism has yet to be fairly tested, for history has never recorded a "satisfactory" civilization. The negative social consequences of egalitarianism and the importance of smaller groups to progress are again discussed, and the wide gap between democracy and individualism is noted. Progress which emerged from release of the plebeian class is not the consequence of democracy. It is the consequence of the voluntary autonomous group fed and led by self-interest. That group is the koinon. Democracy is nonetheless useful, for it is the only form of governance that can accommodate the existence of koinons, meaning that it is the only form of governance that up to a point can resist the temptation to interfere with self-interest group activity. It is the not-so-subtle threat of today that such support can be withdrawn.

A. Historicism, This Book Thus Far, and Predicting the Future

Historicism has been a focus of attention by sociologists over the last two centuries in that it has been proposed that the study of historical patterns of human behavior and societal change should make it possible to predict not only the consequences of those patterns but the subsequent course of events. Dr. Karl Popper defined historicism thus: "… an approach to the social sciences which assumes that *historical prediction* is their primary aim, and which assumes that this aim is attainable by discovering the "rhythms" of the "patterns," the "laws" or the "trends" that underlie the evolution of history (*sic*)."[1] There are prominent sociologists, Dr. Popper in particular, who disagree with this theory, arguing that the future of mankind cannot be known unless all the factors that produced its course to date are understood, and they are not.

Not to counter the arguments of experts, yet there does seem reason to consider some factors more important than others in determining the course of human events. If this is true, at least some factors that seem inordinately important, especially if malevolent, might be identified and perhaps controlled or avoided to the benefit of future generations. It would be tragic if a lesson from the past that can keep us from repeating what demonstrably is an error is ignored. The final product, in agreement with Popper,

---

[1] See: Popper, K., *The Poverty of Historicism*, London, 2004, p. 3. The book was first published in 1957.

will be unknown, but the path there may be made less painful. It is in accord with that end that this volume has been presented for deliberation.

It is proposed that there is a critical juncture in the evolution of a society that, if the right moment is seized and right action taken, members of that society can provide the spark for initiating an intrinsic mechanism that will improve society's chances not only of survival but improvement in the lives of all its members. That moment does not occur in the earliest societies because populations are too small and life expectancy too short to accumulate knowledge. But, once a predictable surplus of a crop or a product provides the opportunity for commerce, prosperity fosters an increase in local population that can in turn benefit from communal projects, perhaps focusing on needs such as irrigation, sanitation, and roads. Specialization then emerges as an individual can now become an expert and join with others having a similar interest to exploit a newfound competence that would, by benefiting others, benefit himself or herself. The critical juncture is at hand and the basic tool for progress has been obtained, for now several individuals can focus their collective minds on a single issue.[2] Thus, success is attributable to groups of individuals, and it is the ability of a society to conceive, permit, support, and exploit the good news of such dedicated groups that will lead to the flowering of a society. Progress is beginning in this theoretical community, and it seems so simple and obvious.

But, using medical practice as a marker, in Part I focus was on the perversion of a group's actions by political authoritarianism. In Part II the emphasis has been on its prevention by egalitarianism, authoritarianism in a different guise. In Part I, the destructiveness of authoritarianism was not purposeful; at times, as in pharaonic Egypt, it even integrated early medical practitioners into the mechanism of governance once there was evidence of their popularity. Instead, the misappropriation of the nascent profession was used to facilitate control of the commoner population by an elite class. In Part II, egalitarianism was not inherently antagonistic to a group of medical practitioners, as such a profession had yet to be encountered. It was, instead, coercion of a more general nature, a negation of the idea that an individual could have a personal goal that was not integrated into the goal of society.[3] The profound stagnation inherent in egalitarianism is in part based on the assumption that, as bad as things are, things are as good as they will ever get and we must not lose what we have, or, in modern times, should be allowed to have. In the egalitarian's view, time and change will merely allow more power and wealth to be

---

[2] The implied nascent medical profession does not require an office or signage for its founding and success. At its earliest stage it might be face-to-face deliberation on what to do about a particular problem, the initial response being something like "I think Joe tried to ...... once, and it turned out OK. Let's ask him." It takes little for a person to be identified as qualified in medicine (which has its good and bad points). See for example p. 53 of the present volume where the popularity of the quasi-medical expertise of Heinrich Schliemann (1822-1890) during his excavations at Troy attracted ailing individuals from a large surrounding area, so desperate are we to find relief and an explanation for our ills and our pains.

[3] To be clear, the source of the problem is not the provision of medical care to all members of society. No one would ever make that argument. The source of the problem is, instead, the provider. With a central government as the provider, all benefits of the interested group, the koinon, are lost. Clinical medicine becomes a job rather than a profession. The judge of any attempt at innovation will be a central committee of disinterested persons guided by personal financial considerations, national economic policy, limited knowledge, and friendships. But the arguments against socialism are so vast and have been apparent for so long it is clear that logic is not an issue for the forces that daily march us closer to the intellectual stagnation that kept ancient kinships picking berries for thousands of years.

concentrated in fewer and fewer people, and this is not tolerable. It is better to equitably distribute what we have. Such a philosophy becomes even more powerful if change or progress is viewed not only as possible but dangerous: political activism then adds to the destructive nature of egalitarianism.

And so the present work has reinforced the idea that there has yet to be a long-lived satisfactory civilization. Some of the civilizations discussed in this volume surely persisted, several for a thousand years, but they were not "satisfactory." Living to an average age of 35 years, not knowing one's grandparents (and frequently not even parents) nor having their wisdom imparted, helplessly bearing the pain and suffering of trauma, disease, infirmity, and childbirth with nothing but hope or the risk of toxic botanicals as treatment, and serving as living tools of the powerful and fodder for warriors is no way to pass one's life. As we have no history of a satisfactory civilization, how will we know when one has arrived? The question is moot. The best to be expected is some sort of gradual improvement over what previously existed. A more realistic question is how can we continue our present success and avoid losing what has already been gained, for that loss occurred in the five successful civilizations described in chapters 2-5 and 16-17. And which threat is the greater, egalitarian stagnation or authoritarian misappropriation.

It is proposed, therefore, that historicism has yet to be given a fair trial, that initially successful human civilizations have been conquered or consistently superseded by authoritarian secondary civilizations within two or three centuries. As a result, there is no predictability to the course of human societies because those initially successful civilizations, shortly after their birth, were perverted. The source of that unpredictability has been the enforced product of elite factions or external forces rather than the preference of a society's members based on self-interest. Should societies evolve that are imbued with the freedom to proceed with actions dependent instead on the natural inclination, canvassed response, and thoughtful opinion of the full membership rather than an elite few or class, the options for action will be more focused, more carefully considered, less destructive, and thereby more predictable.

In other words, historicism, having overlooked the common man and woman who quantitatively and qualitatively are the source of beneficence in every society in which they have been provided opportunity, has predictably been unable to predict history's course. Historicism, therefore, has yet to be put to the test for the purpose intended, that purpose being the promotion of the best way forward to a more satisfactory society. Put in the context of chapter 36, there has been no society that has yet permitted, over an extended period, the operation of natural law. There is the possibility, of course, that such a test is presently under way, characterized appropriately by Dr. William McNeill (unfortunately recanted to a certain extent in his 1991 retrospective preface) in his popular 1963 book, *The Rise of the West: A History of the Human Community*, and will turn out to be permanently "more satisfactory."[4]

---

[4] Dr. McNeill's excellent and thoughtful book is, nevertheless, quite different in its focus and its conclusions than the present three-volume work, for he assigns the mechanism for progress to the interactions of civilizations, interactions that tend to be clashes. Humankind's progress, therefore, based on his analysis of the histories of mature civilizations, is the result of contributions from them all. This, of course, is completely at odds with the present work. And even though Dr. McNeill discusses progress in terms of all mankind (the "human community"), by combining the knowledge acquired by "clashes" (including physical coercion and war) with the realization that all human governance up to recent times has been strictly authoritarian, knowledge becomes a tool that

B. *Isagorial Theory of Human Progress* as Historicism

Definition of *Isagorial Theory of Human Progress*: A theory ascribing all apolitical advances for the betterment of mankind to unimpeded self-interest groups in which each member has equal opportunity to speak freely and share ideas about the group's common interest without fear of retribution. Axiomatically it excludes "betterments" that have been stolen, copied, derived by exploitation, or used for subjugation of others.

In determining the relevance to historicism of the Isagorial Theory as a predictor of the course of societies, the requirements arbitrarily selected to support a civilization's capability for progress were derived by an analysis of the ancient Greek city-state, Miletos. Similar data were then sought in a variety of civilizations, large and small, ancient and recent. It is concluded that the concept of progress has never had a chance to persist unimpeded for more than two centuries. Even today's massive expansion of knowledge in medicine that began in the modern West is but the work of little more than two centuries, doubts about its survival into the next century being a subject of debate. Despite a mechanism for transmission, *i.e.,* writing, "progress" as manifested in the ancient medical treatises was lost even though the works themselves were transmitted. But it is commonly claimed that forceful assimilation must have been necessary for our modern age to reap the benefit of ancient reason, for modern progress is based on an ever-increasing knowledge base since ancient times that has been passed down to us. This, however, is not the case. Once forceful assimilation occurred the assimilating power was unable to build upon and benefit from the formulation of progress it had received. It welcomed the messenger but could not comprehend the message. This explains why the modern age of science, including medicine, was reinvented anew in the 18th C rather than being an improvement on Hippocratic medicine of 4th C BC. A functional transfer of advances from a primary civilization to its subsequent secondary civilization is apparently difficult, if not impossible. The ancients may have passed down to us the stuff of history books, but the progress that has been passed on to us is only two or three centuries old.

What, then, is the relevance of the *Isagorial Theory of Human Progress* if progress must be repeatedly born, phoenix-like, over the ages only to fade away or evolve into meaningless canon? What must present generations think about the changes their progeny will encounter if today's civilization follows the path of all preceding civilizations and dissipates or, more likely, is taken not so gently under authoritarian wings? The following deductions from isagorial theory might be considered: (1) In an authoritarian world the greater the size of a population, the smaller is the significance of the individual. It is important, therefore, to minimize authoritarian mechanisms and to limit centralization of power. An exception may be defensive protections against threatening external authoritarian forces. (2) Egalitarian societies were present in all of the lesser civilizations analyzed herein, including the most enduring (>1,000 years) and unchanging societies. If there is any feature identifiable with crippling human potential for improvement, it is egalitarianism. Social egalitarianism as government policy is to be strictly avoided. (3) It is the unique role of the individual to innovate and enter with like-minded people into groups to further the development of good ideas. There is only one civilization that can be cited as promoting individual liberty, and that is Western

benefits an elite class, not the total of the human community. The mass of humankind is still without benefits of that knowledge except for such access as the elite class permits. "Progress" thus acquired is not considered progress in this book.

civilization. It is this respect for the individual that has placed the West in such a commanding position in the history of mankind. The third point, therefore, is to approximate Western constitutional governance, especially as originally intended in the United States of America, to defend the inherent freedom of the individual.

If isagorial theory is not seriously considered and individual liberty cannot be maintained, another authoritarian relapse can be reliably predicted and the respectability of historicism will unfortunately be restored.

C. Democracy's Origins and Role in Western Progress; Conclusion of the Argument

Dr. Barbara Geddes discusses various explanations for shifts to democracy, but a satisfactory one she feels is not available because the contexts of the various theories are narrow and specific, being tailored around a particular mechanism. She thinks explanations will vary according to the type of preceding authoritarianism.[5] Some consider economic development not to be a cause of democracy, but once the switch occurs prosperity stabilizes it.[6] Generally the assumption seems to be that democracy flows from a prior political state rather than by *de novo* design.

But is democratization the issue? Democracy has its etymological origin in the Greek δεμοκρατία (demokratia), "demos" referring to the people and "kratia" to political power. One of the earliest uses of the term was by Herodotus in his hypothetical discussion between Greeks and Persians of the merits of several types of governance. The word "demos" refers to the people of a place, in particular the people "of a deme," the deme at that time being defined geographically rather than ethnically and the defined place being either rural or urban. Ancient Athens had more than one hundred demes. Thus, the power in managing the course of the city-state was spread throughout the length and breadth of society regardless of wealth or status, although the right to vote rested solely with male citizens. Important to present discussion, democracy gave each voting citizen a vested interest in the success of his city-state by investing a small slice of political power in him. But it did not grant him individual liberties. The laws of that city-state were a separate issue, and while they may have granted him equal rights before the law they were no Bill of Rights. In effect, democracy granted the power to eligible citizens to have active membership in a political group of their choosing. There were usually subgroups of varying political perspectives, but individual liberty was not the issue. True, citizens were considered freeborn and therefore "free." But the basic definition of being born free meant not to be born a slave rather than to be born with certain unalienable rights which all mankind should share. And it is true that freedom of political speech assembly was guaranteed to citizens, an important advance. But to citizens of classical Greece, democracy in a city-state was not an invitation to function as a free agent but as a member of a large koinon (see definition of koinon, p. 14). Pericles' funeral oration makes it clear that the great virtue of democracy was its usefulness in stimulating individual motivation because self-interest was involved. But that individual motivation

---

[5] See: Geddes, B., *What Causes Democratization?*, in *Oxford Handbook of Comparative Politics*, Oxford, 2009, C. Boix and S. C. Stokes, editors, p. 612.
[6] See: Przeworksi, A., et al., *Democracy and Development: Political Institutions and Well-Being in the World, 1950-1990*, Princeton, 2000.

was good because it contributed to the winning of battles and assisting the survival of the Athenian city-state. It was not intended to promote the significance of the individual for that individual's benefit; it was use of self-interest as a tool for winning battles. In battle the motivated side was the one where personal interest was involved, not the interests of a distant king. But, as in political assembly, an army composed of the more motivated troops still had group interests at heart, namely the winning of the battle, something that an individual acting alone could not do. In this sense Athens and Sparta were as one in their desire to impel their soldiers to victory. They merely differed in the means: Sparta by indoctrination, Athens by motivation.

The importance of individualism to the individual also was not carried beyond the lip service of ancient Greece when it became a minion of the Roman Empire, or by the Roman Empire itself. Cicero declared "We are servants of the law in order that we may be free." The idea of the individual as a morally free agent was there, but it was as defined and permitted by the State. The concept of individualism came from a separate source: the evolution of Judeo-Christian ethic and each person's relation to God. But the onset of the European Dark Ages saw no evidence of improvement in mankind's prospects as the decline of the Roman Empire in the West was replaced by another ultimately authoritarian pan-European institution, the Church, the consequences being discussed in chapter 18, p. 291*ff.*

There has been generous acknowledgement by Western scholars since the 17th C of ancient Greek democracies as models for modern Western democracies. It represents, however, a *post hoc, ergo propter hoc* form of reasoning. It is argued here that the significance of the individual within society as presently understood finds its initiation solely in the Reformation; that it was freedom to determine one's personal association with God, whether through a church of one's choice or even directly, that emphasized the significance of the individual and, inasmuch as this association was more important than any other human consideration and applied to every human, it could not be infringed by secular authority.[7]

The push for political democracy in the West, therefore, had its origins in this religious "right" as first effectively put forward in medieval times by Martin Luther, who taught that salvation from sin was not something granted by the Church but by God through faith of the individual. The argument was, initially, strictly theological. Martin Luther made no literary or intellectual appeal to the rise of classical Greek democracy. He was a scholar of classical Greek, but his emphasis was solely apropos translation of the Bible from the Greek. It was the Reformation that would initiate collective action to protect the individual against authoritarian forces that would have had this religious inspiration contained, with the course to political freedom for the individual unplanned. But it was popular, and so, despite the colossus of the Church, Lutheranism as a distinct religious entity was widespread within three years of Luther's *95 Theses* of 1517.

---

[7] This is not an issue of "free will" as commonly understood, a concept with many complexities in philosophical and theological discussion. For example, Martin Luther did not believe in free will, for Satan interfered in all human endeavors. And, using English law as an example, Magna Carta of 1215, the Petition of Rights of 1628, and the Bill of Rights of 1689, except for conferring freedom of speech in Parliament, provided specific protections for the people against authoritarian governance but did not confer freedoms. Regarding the Bill of Rights of 1689, there was a statement in Henry Care's Proem of his 1682 classic, *English Liberties*, on the superiority of English governance over all others, for England was "nor yet a democracy or popular state, much less an Anarchy, where all confusedly are 'hail fellow well met'."

With moral righteousness and an appeal to conscience as an additional motivation, parliamentary governments in Europe over the next two-three centuries bit by bit replaced monarchism with democratic process. There had been many attempts, mostly brief, to foster democratic reform in earlier societies. This time, however, the common man and woman, rather than an advantaged class with political ambitions, were complicit in this invention, and now, assisted by not only legal protections from monarchism but also fewer restrictions on freedoms, it is they who would be the source of modern progress.

This is a restatement, although on a grander scale, of the same course of history that accompanied the evolution of medical practice: Greek medicine of Hippocrates flowered in the 5th and 4th C BC then promptly declined, disappearing altogether, but in the 18th C in the West medical practice began anew and flourished. Again, common men and women, the source of local medical practitioners throughout Western nations, brought science and discovery in medicine to the benefit of all mankind and did so unrelated to the Greek experience.

It is incorrect, therefore, to give credit for our Western success to "standing on the shoulders" of the ancient Greeks. No, the origin of our modern civilization is distinct in every way from that of ancient Greece. We can appreciate what the ancient Greeks accomplished in the realm of democracy. They were the first to show what was possible. But it is proposed here that even without any knowledge of the Greek experience it was Western civilization and the Reformation that led to the invention, again, of democratic governance, with the ultimate realization that an individual's freedom was a gift of God and not a grant from the State.

But democracy, the placing of political power in the hands of the governed, was never devised to foster individualism. In ancient times it might even be said that democracy was used to harness the benefits of individualism for purposes of society. In contrast, the Reformation, as a revolt against a pan-European authoritarian institution, in effect a kinship (arguably with an egalitarian face), allowed people to ponder alternative methods of governance. The praise of this maturation of free society is appropriately unbounded in the West. But it must be remembered that "progress" was first expressed thousands of years earlier in small self-interest groups that developed in a commercial environment that permitted the common people to free themselves from egalitarian kinships. In an analogous fashion, the immediate result of Martin Luther's *Theses* can be viewed similarly: a splintering of the bonds of an institutional kinship that, active at all levels of society, contributed to containment, coercively when necessary, of the consciences and habits of an entire continent.[8] Just as transient human progress was the consequence of release from egalitarian bonds in ancient times, modern progress would be the consequence of release from medieval European kinships. And immediately there was formation of numerous and heterogeneous smaller groups by people with a variety of religious convictions. Other attempts in preceding centuries had been met with defeat or extinction, but with the expanding ability to speak out in public and debate issues, intellectuals and parliaments over two or three centuries would recognize individualism beyond one's relationship with God as a desirable political and intellectual object. The

[8] Other important contributors included the small size of Dark Ages towns and cities, with populations rarely reaching 10,000, warfare, monasticism, and evolution of paternal kinships to avert chaos and to consolidate hereditary holdings within the scope of the Church. See, for example, Wareham, A., *The Transformation of Kinship and the Family in Late Anglo-Saxon England*, in *Early Medieval Europe*, Oxford, 2001, pp. 375-399.

theological concept of natural law became a political issue. There is no prior human experience with such a thing.

And so today we can appropriately praise the genius of many individuals prominent in many fields, and we can benefit from their inventions and discoveries. But this is possible only because the Reformation initiated the process whereby freedom of self-interest groups has become, within legal limits, unrestricted and without the necessity of patronage. The small groups have now become, in the West, modern universities, professions, and corporations, institutions that rely, and indeed exist, on the open expression of opinion equally from all their members and constituents who can speak freely without fear of retribution. Of all the intellectual dangers facing modern society, the greatest is a restriction on the functioning of self-interest groups, large and small, whether imposed externally or, in defiance of tenets of the koinon, imposed internally by their members. Such a purposeful hobbling of the common person within the confines of the large group, a modern rebinding of the individual to what the Leader considers or states to be the greater good of society, a denunciation of natural law, will have dire consequences.

The association of political democracies and progress gives the impression that there is a direct cause and effect between the two, and that the former led to the latter. This is incorrect. (1) One of the problems of democratic governance is the well-known tyranny of a majority, surely inimical to the individual and to progress.[9] It is a relatively recent phenomenon that the Constitution of the United States and many other constitutions have acknowledged the importance of protection of minorities and individuals that might be assaulted by unfair majority opinion. (2) That democracy was unnecessary for group liberty and subsequent progress seems obvious in that for four of the five "successful" early civilizations (Sumer, dynastic Egypt, Indus Valley civilization, and Longshan culture) democracy had yet to be invented, *i.e.,* long before ancient Greece. It was, instead, the relative absence of authoritarian forces that permitted initiation of progress. (3) Pericles praised Athenian democracy for its tolerance of differences among people; clearly there was a range of freedom of action that was tolerated, and it is not likely that this was unique to Athens. There also was the famous Greek aphorism: γνῶθι σεαυτόν, "know thyself," an expression of the increasing realization of self-worth that was also popular in medieval times. But the tolerance of others was voluntary, not guaranteed, and surely was not intended to be unanimously applied. It was accommodated but not promoted. It was a by-product of democracy, not a purpose.

No, the event that fostered progress in Athens was not democracy. It was the breakup of the phratry kinship structure. Once kinship allegiances were not mandatory

---

[9] Remember: J. S. Mill noted that "Society can and does execute…. a social tyranny more formidable that many kinds of political oppression." See Mill's *On Liberty*, 1859, and as footnoted in volume 1 of *The Natural State of Medical Practice: An Isagorial Theory of Human Progress*, Maitland (FL), 2019, pp. 307, 308. In a functional sense, the social tyranny of the majority can be likened to coercive egalitarianism. In the ante-bellum South, enslavement of a racial minority by a (voting) racial majority not only represented physical coercion by political authoritarian governance. It also was the purposeful denial of the ability of the enslaved to improve their lot resulting in a diminished ability to accommodate opportunity when freedom was obtained. In other words, just as egalitarian social pressure kept ancient and primitive peoples in a social prison of their own making that lasted for centuries, the tyranny of the majority, by keeping a racial minority in a social prison (but *not* of their own making), produced an equivalent effect that contributed in many quarters to continued victimization for several more generations.

and citizens could view their new status within a polity rather than a tribe, each person became an individual rather than a cipher. The key to this monumental change was not the fusion with democracy and its inevitable demands on patriotic duty; it was escape from the egalitarian kinship. It became easier for group freedom to make its appearance, for individuals could form local groups of their own choosing. While it is true that the small group, the koinon as defined herein, was itself democratic, *it was "democratic" in ideas, not in power*, for it had no power. But it provided a platform for expressing individual preferences, experiences and ideas regardless of the opinions and ideas of others. It was in the apolitical koinon through which individualism was displayed and an innovative idea based on personal self-interest rather than group self-interest could be proposed from which all could benefit. The ancient Greeks almost figured it out, for they could see the inadvertent benefits of personal liberty of individuals and small groups being manifested in science, medicine, and the arts. But it remained for the post-Reformation West over several centuries to actively seek it out and to institutionalize personal liberty on a vast scale to the benefit of the global population.

And so the Argument has been completed. It was first discerned during study of Hippocratic texts from early Classical Greece that only a committed and unrestricted group of common people, in this case medical practitioners, could have produced the early Hippocratic works and initiated true medical progress, and that group was identified by the Greek word "koinon," an acephalous small and democratic group committed to improving and promoting a common self-interest. By generalizing the relevance of the autonomous self-interest group to all civilizations, by assuming humankind is no more intelligent or moral than it was ten thousand years ago, and by using medicine as a sentinel species, it is clear that the inability to tolerate freedom of groups acting in self-interest prevents progress and is a marker of aberrant social evolution. It is shown that egalitarianism has inhibited social development just as political authoritarianism has prevented its proper maturation. Authoritarianism, in either its egalitarian or political camouflage, is to blame for the unfathomable misery endured over the ages by the common man and woman who, had they been left alone to collaboratively pursue their personal interests and to freely contribute to the course of society, could have obtained the betterment of all mankind thousands of years ago. It is the common man and woman who, motivated by personal interest, subtly guided by natural law, informed by common sense, and protected from repression that have been, are, and always will be the source of humanity's good fortune. It was meant to be so.

EPILOGUE TO PART II

In recounting the history and prehistory of medical practice a pattern has fallen into place that was unintended at this work's inception, namely, insight into the social circumstances surrounding the evolution of medical practice. As demonstrated in this volume, medical progress, recognized here as a surrogate for both pragmatic and intellectual progress, has always been prepared to emerge from the shadow of existential threats to life and well-being that can be acute, poignant, and demanding. The window of opportunity for that emergence, however, has been small and vulnerable. Had it been otherwise, much advanced knowledge of a modern nature might have been available in what we now call prehistory. Indeed, prehistoric human existence might have been significantly shorter had the escape from egalitarianism by our ancient forbears been successful. Based on data from the Population Reference Bureau it can be estimated that nearly 100 billion humans died between 50,000 BC and the 18th C AD, at which time the natural state of medical practice was reinstituted in the West and modern medicine and its scientific ramifications proceeded to mollify or prevent many of the miseries of humankind, dramatically improving what is bureaucratically termed QALY (Quality-Adjusted Life-Year), and doing so on a global scale.[1] It is a fanciful but fair deduction, given the evidence in this volume, that most of those suffering and dying before the age of modern medicine would have appreciated the benefits of improved medical care had the escape from egalitarianism been successful thousands of years earlier.

Nevertheless, with the remarkable progress that has been made in the past three centuries, perhaps mankind has finally, and permanently, ridded itself of an imposed serfdom that has led to entrapment of the mass of humanity and has shuffled off all past civilizations to their demise. But in doing so it has left historians with only the history of authoritarian machinations and the monuments recording the tragedies of human folly, rather than a chronicle of the common man and woman, from which to untangle the story of mankind. The real question to be posed is not what happened in our past. It is, instead, what did not happen. Although what did not happen will never be known, why matters happened as they did is now known. The root problem, having heretofore been overlooked, is demonstrated in the present work: authoritarianism in its many nefarious forms, one being social egalitarianism.

It is proposed that the recent efforts of the West, successful so far, and in retrospect the few and temporary successes of ancient times, can be attributed solely to liberty, but not of just liberty of the individual. More relevant for human progress is liberty of the autonomous group with focused self-interest, although the recognized importance of individual freedom in modern times permits the singular individual with an idea and a dream to become a force for progress, historically a novel event. The desire for and appreciation of liberty is inherent in every human heart, a component of the individual conscience, or "moral sense," traceable to natural law, that subtle human attribute that is neither genetic nor learned but has been instilled and available to all mankind since the first man and woman. Always, in the past, have authoritarian policies or doctrines pushed the good genie of our conscience back into the bottle as the authoritarian conscience ascended. In our age, however, a marvelous expansion of progress and an appreciation of liberty in promoting the welfare of all mankind can be

---

[1] See: Weinstein, M. C., Torrance, G., McGuire, A., *QALYs: The Basics*, in *Value in Health*, 12:S5-S9, 2009.

dated to the commencement of the Reformation.[2] Indeed, it may be stated that a natural state of medical practice, as defined and historically interpreted herein, has contributed to unprecedented healthful longevity because of adherence to natural law.[3] Let us, then, reconsider our attribution of today's manifold successes to great empires and great cities, to ethnic forbears, and to central planning. It is nothing like that; they are but the headline-catching flotsam on the far more interesting sea of humanity. Rejoice in the accomplishments of genius, but forget not that genius has abounded in every age and in every people as a well-kept secret, and that every person, in the appropriate place and at the appropriate time, can be considered a genius at something. Indeed, the unique genius of *Homo sapiens* is expressed best in the ability of that species to recognize the benefits of peaceful deliberation by free individuals for their varied ideas with a goal of self-interest focusing on the problem at hand. Unfortunately, it has been the rule of the jungle or the mob, *i.e.*, to take from or to control others, that has consistently delayed the establishment or speeded the demise of that principle of genius.

Briefly put, the broad-based success we enjoy in the West today, especially in healthful longevity, has been acquired in little more than two or three centuries. The road map for that success has been identified in this volume: the course of the history and prehistory of the natural state of medical practice coincides with the course of freedom, and freedom of conscience allows natural law and its corollary, spontaneous order, to be expressed through various human agencies. But present success is sporadic and human history suggests it is not permanent, for the unceasing authoritarian quest for control over, and uniformity of, every human endeavor using all necessary means of coercion remains today an increasingly threatening presence at home and globally. As we look about us today and witness the massive influx of foreign populations into Western democracies, an influx variously attributed to seeking asylum, fleeing poverty, and evading humanitarian disasters, what we are seeing is nothing more than an escape from the consequences of social egalitarianism, the principal difference today being the magnitude of the problem and the frantic efforts of egalitarian's emigrant who now knows, by virtue of modern communication, that he or she need not chance survival alone upon escaping into the jungle or the savannah, but that in that country just across the border there is a better life, liberty, and the possibility of happiness. More than just medical practice is in the balance.

THE END

---

[2] One must wonder what the consequences of the early 19th C "invention" of socialism would have been had it been more successful in shaping social policies in the West prior to the work of Pasteur, Maxwell, Curie, Roentgen, Edison, and Einstein, among many others. It is possible that many of the great discoveries and inventions that have produced our brave new world would never have transpired if egalitarian policies had full play. The idea that somehow those discoveries and inventions would have been inevitable is a catastrophic misinterpretation of history. In their absence we might still have been living in pre-Dickensian times. But there is an even greater revelation here. The Reformation initiated two parallel but complementary events: (1) it set the West on the path toward technical progress as mankind was gradually able to display its collective genius, and (2) by freeing up mankind's ability to freely consult its collective conscience, it directed that path toward a secular Eden. Unfortunately, political features of modern times indicate that path to be less and less likely to be travelled for long.

[3] The cause of the "healthful longevity" is due, of course, not just to medical diagnosis and treatment, but also to biological knowledge and supporting sciences upon which rest disease prevention, sanitation, epidemiology, nutrition and food supply, and veterinary services, among many. The success of medicine is but a marker of progress on many fronts within a population.

INDEX

CPSIA information can be obtained
at www.ICGtesting.com
Printed in the USA
LVHW071804030820
662268LV00020B/2698